RADIOLOGY DEPARTMENT
NATIONAL NAVAL MEDICAL CENTER
BETHESDA, MARYLAND 20889-5600

Fundamentals of
DIAGNOSTIC
RADIOLOGY

Fundamentals of
DIAGNOSTIC
RADIOLOGY

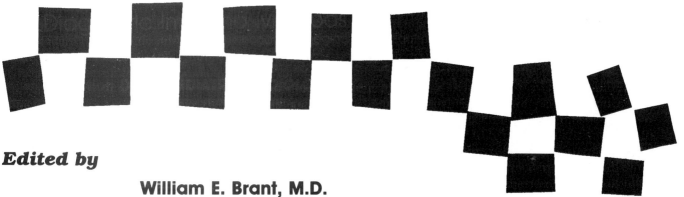

Edited by

William E. Brant, M.D.
Associate Professor of Radiology
Department of Radiology
University of California Davis
School of Medicine
Sacramento, California

Clyde A. Helms, M.D.
Professor of Radiology
Department of Radiology
University of California,
San Francisco
School of Medicine
San Francisco, California

Williams & Wilkins
BALTIMORE • PHILADELPHIA • HONG KONG
LONDON • MUNICH • SYDNEY • TOKYO

A WAVERLY COMPANY

Editors: William M. Passano III, Timothy H. Grayson
Project Manager: Victoria Rybicki Vaughn
Copy Editor: E. Ann Donaldson
Designer: Wilma E. Rosenberger
Illustration Planner: Wayne Hubbel
Cover Designer: Bob Och

Copyright © 1994
Williams & Wilkins
428 East Preston Street
Baltimore, Maryland 21202 USA

Portions of Section VIII are borrowed from Helms: Fundamentals of
Skeletal Radiology, 2nd ed.,courtesy of W.B. Saunders

Accurate indications, adverse reactions, and dosage schedules for
drugs are provided in this book, but it is possible that they may
change. The reader is urged to review the package information data of
the manufacturers of the medications mentioned.

Printed in the United States of America

Library of Congress Cataloging in Publication Data

Fundamentals of diagnostic radiology / edited by William E. Brant,
  Clyde A. Helms,
      p. cm.
    Includes bibliography references.
    ISBN 0-683-01011-5
    1. Diagnosis, Radioscopic.   2. Diagnostic imaging.   I. Brant,
  William E.   II. Helms, Clyde A.
    [DNLM: 1. Diagnostic Imaging.   WN 200 F981 1994]
  RC78.F86   1994
  616.07'57—dc20
  DNLM/DLC
  for LIbrary of Congress   93-34269
                                                                CIP

96 97 98
4 5 6 7 8 9 10

This book is dedicated to my children, Dan, Ryan, Jon, and Rachel, who add so much to the joy of life, and to all residents and medical students whose quest for knowledge adds so much to the joy of teaching.

WEB

To Nancy Marie Major, my beloved wife.

CAH

Foreword

Radiologists are avid readers; the plethora of radiologic texts is a testimony to this fact. Despite the recent push to subspecialization, most of us who teach diagnostic radiology are still approached by residents and students with the request for a recommendation for a good single-volume text. It is expected that such a text would also deal with the new advances in our field such as computed tomography, magnetic resonance imaging, and ultrasound. Until Drs. Brant and Helms undertook this difficult task, there was no easy response to the query for there was no publication that could fulfill these criteria.

The authors have garnered contributions from an outstanding group of radiologists who represent the broad areas of subspecialization and who have presented succinctly the basic elements of their disciplines.

This work fulfills a requirement for those who are contemplating a career in radiology or who are new to the field and desire a broad overview. Drs. Brant and Helms are to be congratulated on recognizing the need and carrying it out in exemplary fashion.

Theodore E. Keats, M.D.

Preface

Diagnostic radiology is a captivating specialty with an exploding body of knowledge that overwhelms the neophyte resident, yet must be learned to practice effectively. A wide variety of excellent, and usually, multivolume texts are available for study of each subspecialty area of radiology. What is lacking is a comprehensive, succinct, and modern text that beginning students of radiology can use to achieve that basic framework of knowledge needed to initiate their learning of diagnostic imaging. We wrote this text to provide a complete, yet concise, beginning in radiology. Each section of this book corresponds to a major subspecialty area on radiology, and deliberately, to categories for examination by the American Board of Radiology.

We visualize this monograph being used in two major fashions. We hope it will become the beginning resident's "first reader" and the graduating resident's "last reader." We provide an overview of the subject matter as residents begin their first rotations on chest or bone or gastrointestinal radiology. A few nights' study of the assigned section provides a working knowledge of the fundamentals of that topic. Practical clinical experience in their residency will provide the cookbook details of performing each imaging study. Our text provides the basic approach toward interpretation of each study. Once students have mastered the framework of the body of knowledge, they can fill in the details by study of the subspecialty texts and studious attendance at teaching conferences and film reading sessions. By the final year of residency, with radiology board examinations looming, residents want a comprehensive review source that covers everything they "need to know" to pass boards. While there is no way a text of any kind can cover "everything needed to pass boards," we hope this text will resurrect the accumulated knowledge of the residency experience and help the residents to organize it in a memorable and usable fashion that will give them confidence taking the board examinations, and, more importantly, practicing excellent radiology.

To accomplish these lofty goals we have selected as contributors individuals with a proven ability to teach practical, important, patient care-oriented radiology. They know what it takes to be an effective radiologist and they know how to teach it to others. The text emphasizes differential diagnosis and supplements these differential considerations with numerous tables. The tables from all chapters are grouped in a list for easy reference. Each subspecialty of radiology is covered, including nuclear radiology, a topic not contained in most radiology texts. Ultrasound, rather than being artifically sequestered as a separate section, is integrated into the sections identified by body system. This approach allows comparison of ultrasound to the other imaging modalities and more closely simulates the use of ultrasound in daily radiologic practice. Yet, all of the facets of ultrasound examination are covered including obstetrics, small parts, cardiac, and vascular sonography. Nuclear radiology is reviewed as a separate section as well as being integrated into body system discussions.

We have provided copious illustrations for each chapter. Each figure is comprehensively labeled with an abundance of arrows and letters so the beginning student can readily identify the important findings and orient to the anatomy displayed. We utilize all of the imaging modalities and stress current concepts of their importance in solving each diagnostic problem. Anatomy, as the basis for all diagnostic imaging, is extensively reviewed in the appropriate sections. While imaging modalities are developed and evolve with frightening speed, the basic principles of interpretation encompassing a firm understanding of anatomy and pathology change little. The latter is what is stressed in this book with examples of some of our best images. We emphasize the concept that a secure knowledge of anatomy and pathology can be applied to nuances of any existing or yet-to-be-developed imaging method to make a confident diagnosis. The student should avoid the concept of learning a checklist of findings for each disease on each imaging modality, but instead should stress understanding the disease process and the clinically applicable physics of each imaging method.

While obviously directed at the resident in diagnostic radiology, we hope that students and practitioners of other specialties will also find this book a useful reference and study guide as they use radiology in diagnosis.

We acknowledge the enthusiastic and professional assistance of personnel at Williams & Wilkins who provided us with constant encouragement and thoughtful suggestions. Tim Grayson, Will Passano, Editor-in-Chief, and Vicki Vaughn, Project Manager, were ardent driving forces promoting this book. Dr. Nancy Major, a resident in diagnostic radiology at the University of California, San Francisco, reviewed each chapter as it was written to provide us with invaluable resident perspective. Her insight resulted in numerous improvements and clarifications, and is deeply appreciated.

William E. Brant, M.D.
Clyde A. Helms, M.D.

Contributors

Jerome A. Barakos, M.D.
Neuroradiology
San Francisco, California

Robert M. Barr, M.D.
Clinical Instructor, Neuroradiology
University of California, San Francisco
Department of Radiology
San Francisco, California

John M. Bauman, M.D.
Chief, Nuclear Medicine Service
Madigan Army Medical Center
Tacoma, Washington

Peter W. Blue, M.D.
Chief, Nuclear Medicine Service and Department of Radiology
Moncrief Army Community Hospital
Fort Jackson, South Carolina
Professor of Radiology
University of South Carolina School of Medicine
Columbia, South Carolina

William E. Brant, M.D.
Associate Professor of Clinical Radiology
Department of Radiology
University of California Davis
School of Medicine
Sacramento, California

Jerrold T. Bushberg, Ph. D.
Technical Director, Nuclear Medicine
Associate Clinical Professor
Department of Radiology
University of California Davis Medical Center
Sacramento, California

Frederic A. Conte, M.D.
Chairman, Department of Radiology
David Grant United States Air Force Medical Center
Travis Air Force Base, California;
Assistant Clinical Professor
Department of Radiology
University of California Davis School of Medicine
Sacramento, California

Nancy J. Fischbein, M.D.
Diagnostic Radiology Resident
Department of Radiology
University of California, San Francisco School of Medicine
San Francisco, California

Erik H.L. Gaensler, M.D.
Medical Director, MRI Services
Alta Imaging Medical Group
Berkeley, California;
Assistant Clinical Professor of Radiology
University of California, San Francisco
San Francisco, California

Alisa D. Gean, M.D.
Assistant Professor of Radiology and Neurology
University of California, San Francisco
Chief of Neuroradiology
San Francisco General Hospital
San Francisco, California

Jeffrey L. Groffsky, M.D.
Diagnostic Radiology Resident
Department of Radiology
University of California, San Francisco Medical Center
San Francisco, California

Michael F. Hartshorne, M.D.
Professor of Radiology
Veterans Administration Medical Center
Associate Professor and Vice-Chairman
Department of Radiology
New Mexico School of Medicine
Albuquerque, New Mexico

Clyde A. Helms, M.D.
Professor of Radiology
Department of Radiology
University of California, San Francisco
School of Medicine
San Francisco, California

Arnold B. Honick, M.D.
Chief of Ultrasound
Department of Radiology
David Grant United States Air Force Medical Center
Travis Air Force Base, California;
Assistant Clinical Professor
Department of Radiology
University of California Davis Medical Center
Sacramento, California

Susan D. John, M.D.
Assistant Professor of Radiology and Pediatrics
Children's Hospital
University of Texas Medical Branch
Galveston, Texas

Jeffrey S. Klein, M.D.
Associate Clinical Professor
Radiology Department
San Francisco General Hospital
San Francisco, California

Kelly Koeller, M.D.
Lieutenant Commander, United States Navy
Neuroradiologist
Department of Radiology
Naval Hospital
San Diego, California

Todd E. Lempert, M.D.
Radiologist
Department of Radiology
Alta Bates Medical Center
Berkeley, California

Karen K. Lindfors, M.D.
Associate Professor of Radiology
Department of Radiology
University of California, Davis Medical Center
Sacramento, California

Cal L. Lutrin, M.D., Ch.B.
Medical Director, Nuclear Medicine Division
Sutter Memorial Hospital
Partner, Radiological Associates at Sacramento Medical Group,
   Inc.
Sacramento, California

Mike McBiles, M.D.
Lieutenant Colonel, United States Army
Chief, Nuclear Medicine Service
Fitzsimons Army Medical Center
Aurora, Colorado

Walter L. Olsen, M.D.
Staff Radiologist
Sharp Chula Vista Medical Center and Coronado Hospital
Chula Vista, California
Medical Director
Magnetic Resonance Institute of Chula Vista
Assistant Clinical Professor of Radiology
University of California, San Diego
La Jolla, California

Howard A. Rowley, M.D.
Assistant Professor of Radiology and Neurology
Department of Radiology
University of California, San Francisco
San Francisco, California

Scott R. Schultz, M.D.
Diagnostic Radiology Resident
Department of Radiology
University of California, San Francisco School of Medicine
San Francisco, California

David K. Shelton, Jr., M.D.
Assistant Professor of Radiology
Chief, Nuclear Medicine
Vice Chairman, Radiology
University of California, Davis Medical Center
Sacramento, California

David J. Seidenwurm, M.D.
Medical Director, Imaging Centers of Sacramento
Partner, Radiological Associates at Sacramento Medical Group,
   Inc.
Sacramento, California

Leonard E. Swischuk, M.D.
Deputy Chairman
Department of Radiology
Director, Division of Pediatric Radiology
The University of Texas Medical Branch
Children's Hospital
Galveston, Texas

Robert J. Telepak, M.D.
Associate Professor of Radiology
Department of Radiology
University of New Mexico School of Medicine
Albuquerque, New Mexico

James H. Timmons, M.D.
Chief, Diagnostic Imaging Service
Department of Radiology
Madigan Army Medical Center
Tacoma, Washington

Philip W. Wiest, M.D.
Assistant Professor of Radiology
University of New Mexico
Staff Radiologist
Veterans Administration Medical Center
Albuquerque, New Mexico

John E. Williams, M.D.
Chief, Angiography and Interventional Radiology
Department of Radiology
David Grant United States Air Force Medical Center
Travis Air Force Base, California;
Assistant Clinical Professor
Department of Radiology
University of California Davis Medical Center
Sacramento, California

Rhonda A. Wyatt, M.D.
Chief, Nuclear Medicine
David Grant United States Air Force Medical Center
Travis Air Force Base, California

Contents

List of Tables

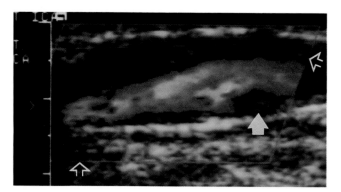

Figure 1.14

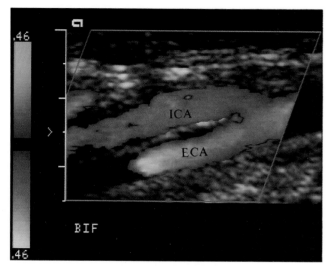

Color Plate Figure 21.1

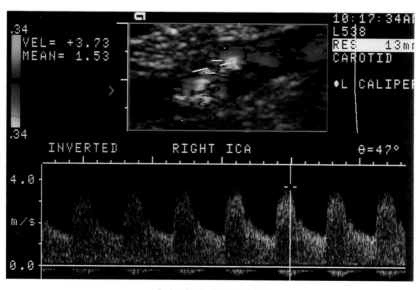

Color Plate Figure 21.2

Color Plate Figure 21.3

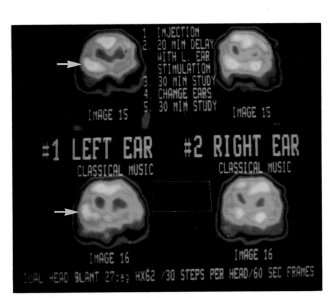

Figure 55.2

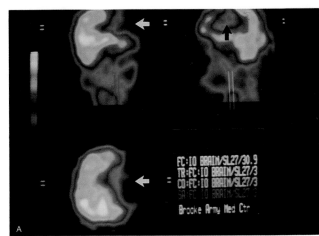

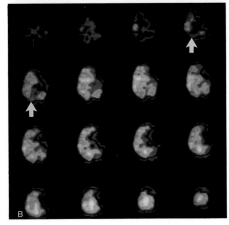

Figure 55.3 A, B

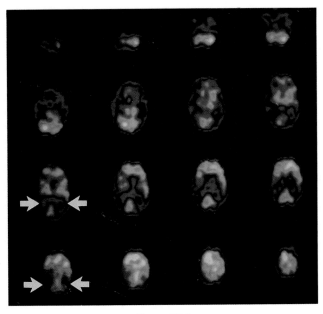

Figure 55.4

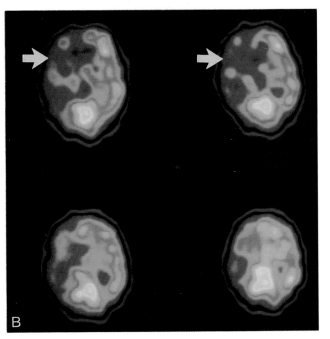

Figure 55.5 B

Section I   BASIC PRINCIPLES

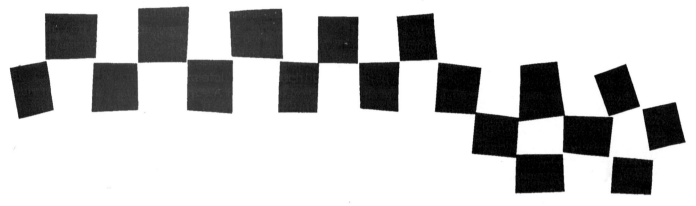

1 Diagnostic Imaging Methods

1

Diagnostic Imaging Methods

William E. Brant

Diagnostic radiology is a dynamic specialty that has undergone rapid change with continuing advancements in technology. Not only has the number of imaging methods increased but each one continues to undergo improvement and refinement of its use in medical diagnosis. This chapter will review the basics of the major diagnostic imaging methods and provide the basic principles of image interpretation for each method. Contrast agents commonly used in diagnostic radiology will also be discussed. The basics of nuclear radiology are discussed in Chapters 46 and 47.

PLAIN FILM RADIOLOGY

Plain film examination of the human body dates back to the genesis of diagnostic radiology in 1895, and remains fundamental to its practice.

Image Generation. X-rays are a form of radiant energy similar in many ways to visible light. However, x-rays differ from visible light in having a very short wavelength and in being able to penetrate many substances that are opaque to light (1). Plain film radiographs are produced by a photochemical interaction between x-rays and a screen coated with fluorescent particles inside a film cassette (Fig. 1.1). The fluorescent particles that are activated by x-rays emit light rays that expose photographic film within the cassette. As x-rays pass through the human body they are attenuated by interaction with body tissues (absorption and scatter), resulting in an image pattern recognizable as human anatomy (Fig. 1.2). The x-ray beam is produced by bombarding a tungsten target with an electron beam within an x-ray tube.

Naming Radiographic Views. Most radiographic views are named by the way that the x-ray beam passes through the patient. A posteroanterior (PA) chest radiograph is one in which the x-ray beam has passed through the back of the patient and exits through the front of the patient to expose an x-ray film placed against the patient s chest. An anteroposterior (AP) chest film is exposed by an x-ray beam passing through the patient from front to back. A craniocaudad (CC) mammograph is produced by passing a beam through the breast in a vertical cranial to caudad direction. Some views are named by identifying the position of the patient. Erect, supine, or prone views may be specified. A right lateral decubitus view of the chest is exposed with the patient lying on his or her right side with a horizontal x-ray beam passing through the chest. Films taken during fluoroscopy are named by the patient's position relative to the fluoroscopic table. A right posterior oblique view is taken with the patient lying with the right side of his or her back against the table and the left side elevated away from the table. The x-ray beam passes from the x-ray tube located beneath the table through the patient to the film located above the patient.

Principles of Interpretation. Plain film radiographs demonstrate five basic radiographic densities: air, fat, soft tissue, bone, and metal. Air attenuates very little of the x-ray beam allowing nearly the full force of the beam to blacken the film. Bone and metals attenuates a large proportion of the x-ray beam allowing very little radiation through to blacken the film. Thus, bone and metallic objects appear white on radiographs. Fat and soft tissues attenuate intermediate amounts of the x-ray beam, resulting in proportional degrees of film blackening. Thick structures attenuate more radiation than thin structures of the same composition. Anatomic structures are seen on radiographs when they are outlined in whole or in part by tissues of different x-ray density. Air in the lung outlines pulmonary vascular structures, producing a detailed pattern of the lung parenchyma (Fig. 1.3). Fat within the abdomen outlines the margins of the liver, spleen, and kidneys allowing them to be

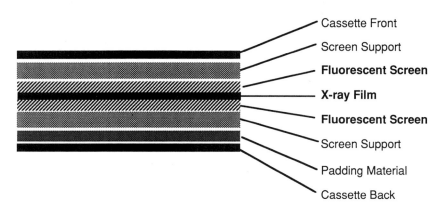

Figure 1.1.   X-ray Film Cassette. Diagram demonstrates a sheet of x-ray film between two fluorescent screens within a light-proof cassette.

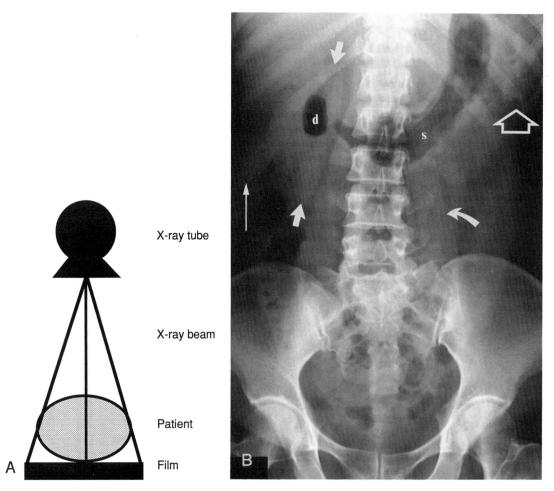

Figure 1.2.   Plain Film Radiographs. A. Diagram of an x-ray tube producing x-rays that pass through the patient and expose the radiographic film. **B.** Supine anteroposterior radiograph of the abdomen demonstrates normal anatomy. The stomach (s) and duodenum (d) are visualized because air in the lumen is of different radiographic density than the soft tissues that surround the gastrointestinal tract. The right kidney (between *short straight arrows*), edge of the liver (*long straight arrow*), edge of the spleen (*open arrow*), and the left psoas muscle (*curved arrow*) are visualized because fat outlines their soft-tissue density. The bones of the spine, pelvis, and hips are clearly seen through the soft tissues because of their high radiographic density.

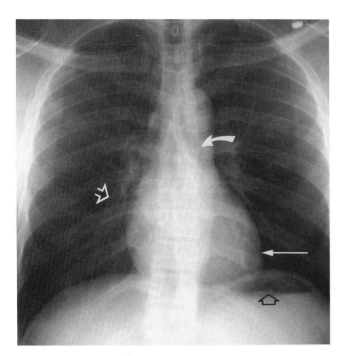

Figure 1.3. Erect PA Chest Radiograph. The pulmonary artery (*white open arrow*) is seen in the lung because the vessel is outlined by air in alveoli. The left cardiac border (*long arrow*) is crisply defined by adjacent air-filled lung. The left main bronchus (*curved arrow*) is seen because its air-filled lumen is surrounded by soft tissue of the mediastinum. An air-fluid level (*open black arrow*) in the stomach confirms the erect position of the patient during exposure of the radiograph.

visualized (Fig. 1.2**B**). The high density of bones allows their details to be visualized through overlying soft tissues. Metallic objects such as surgical clips are usually clearly seen because they highly attenuate the x-ray beam. Radiographic contrast agents are suspensions of iodine and barium compounds that highly attenuate the x-ray beam and are used to outline anatomic structures. Disease states may obscure normally visualized anatomic structures by silhouetting their outline. Pneumonia in the right middle lobe of the lung replaces air in the alveoli with fluid and silhouettes the right heart border (Fig. 1.4). Squire and Novelline (2) provide an excellent text on the fundamentals of radiographic interpretation.

Conventional Tomography provides radiographic slices of a living patient. This is done by simultaneously moving both the x-ray tube and the film about a pivot point centered in the patient in the plane of the anatomic structures to be studied (Fig. 1.5). Structures above and below the focal plane are blurred by the motion of the tube and film. Objects within the focal plane are visualized with improved detail due to the blurring of the overlying structures. Motion of the x-ray tube and film may be linear, circular, elliptical, spiral, or hypocycloidal. Tomography is a useful adjunct to conventional radiographs whenever improved detail is needed for diagnosis.

Fluoroscopy allows real-time radiographic visualization of moving anatomic structures. A continuous x-ray beam passes through the patient and falls onto a continuously fluorescing screen (Fig. 1.6). The faint light emitted by the fluorescing screen is amplified electronically by an image intensifier and the image is displayed on a television screen. Fluoroscopy is extremely useful to evaluate motion such as gastrointestinal peristalsis, movement of the diaphragm with respiration, and cardiac action. Fluoroscopy is also used to perform and continuously monitor radiographic procedures such as barium studies and catheter placements.

Angiography involves the opacification of blood vessels by intravascular injection of iodinated contrast agents. Conventional arteriography utilizes small flexible catheters that are placed in the arterial system usually via puncture of the femoral artery in the groin. Using fluoroscopy for guidance, catheters of various size and shape can be manipulated selectively into virtually every major artery. Contrast injection is performed by hand or by mechanical injector and is accompanied by timed rapid sequence filming or digital acquisition of the fluoroscopic image. The result is a timed series of images depicting blood flow through the artery injected and the tissues that it supplies. Conventional venography is performed by contrast injection of veins via distal puncture or selective catheterization.

CROSS-SECTIONAL IMAGING TECHNIQUES

Computed tomography (CT), magnetic resonance imaging (MR), and ultrasonography are techniques that produce cross-sectional images of the body. All three interrogate a three-dimensional volume or slice of patient tissue to produce a two-dimensional image. The resulting image is made up of a matrix of picture elements (pixels), each of which represents a volume element (voxel) of patient tissue. The tissue composition of the voxel is averaged (volume averaged) for display as a pixel. Computed tomography and MR assign a numerical value to each picture element in the matrix. The matrix of picture elements that make up each image is usually between 128 × 256 (32,768 pixels) and 560 × 560 (313,600 pixels), determined by the specified acquisition parameters (Fig. 1.7).

To produce an anatomic image, shades of gray are assigned to ranges of pixel values. For example, 16 shades of gray may be divided over a *window width* of 320 pixel values. Groups of 20 pixel values are each assigned one of the 16 gray shades. The middle gray shade is assigned to the pixel values centered on a selected *window level*. Pixels with values above the upper limit of the window width are displayed white, while pixels with values below the lower limit of the window width are displayed black. To optimally ana-

Figure 1.4. Right Middle Lobe Pneumonia. A PA erect chest radiograph demonstrates pneumonia (*P*) in the right middle lobe replacing air density in the lung with soft-tissue density and silhouetting the right heart border. The right hemidiaphragm (*black arrow*) is defined by air in the right lower lobe and remains visible through the right middle lobe infiltrate. The left heart border (*white arrow*) defined by air in the ligula remains well defined despite infiltrate in the left lower lobe.

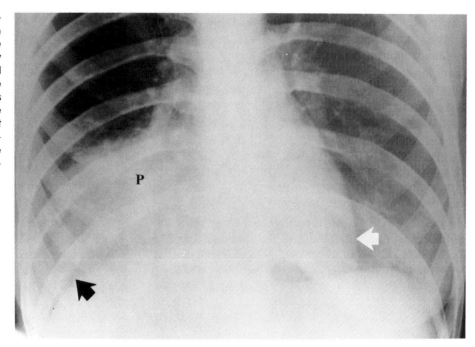

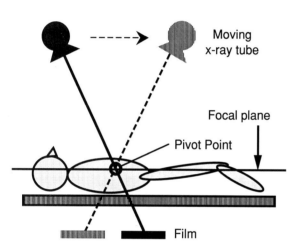

Figure 1.5. Conventional Tomography. In this technique the x-ray tube and film move about a pivot point at the level of the desired focal plane. Anatomic structures within the focal plane remain in sharp focus while the structures above and below the focal plane are blurred by the motion of the tube and film.

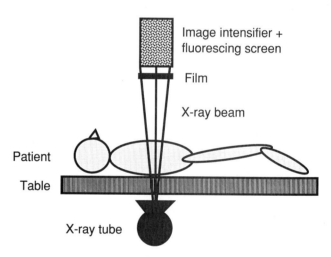

Figure 1.6. Fluoroscopy. Diagram of a fluoroscopic unit illustrates the x-ray tube located beneath the patient examination table and the fluorescing screen with the image intensifier positioned above the patient. Amplification of the faint fluorescing image by the image intensifier allows the radiation exposure to the patient to be kept at low levels during fluoroscopy. The real-time fluoroscopic images may be recorded on videotape. Radiographs are obtained by placing a film cassette between the patient and the image intensifier and exposing the film with a brief pulse of radiation.

lyze all of the anatomic information of any particular slice, the image is photographed at different window width and window level settings optimized for bone, air-filled lung, soft tissue, etc.

Computed Tomography

Computed tomography uses a computer to mathematically reconstruct a cross-sectional image of the body from measurements of x-ray transmission through thin slices of patient tissue (1). Computed tomography displays the imaged slice alone, without the superimposition of blurred structures seen with conventional tomography. A narrow, well-collimated

beam of x-rays is generated on one side of the patient (Fig. 1.8). The x-ray beam is attenuated by absorption and scatter as it passes through the patient. Sensitive detectors on the opposite side of the patient measure x-ray transmission through the slice. These measurements are systematically repeated many times from different directions as the x-ray tube rotates around the patient. Computed tomography numbers are assigned to each pixel in the image by a computer algorithm that uses as data these measurements of trans-

Matrix of CT Image

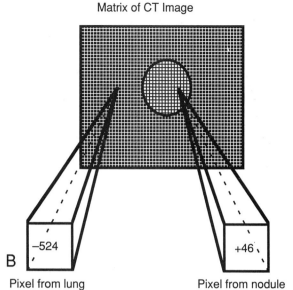

-524

+46

Pixel from lung   Pixel from nodule

Figure 1.7. Image Matrix. A. Magnified cone-down CT image of a pulmonary nodule (*N*). The pixels that make up the image are evident. The window width is set at 2000 with a window level of −600. **B.** Diagram of the matrix that constitutes the CT image. A pixel from

air-filled lung with a calculated CT number of −524 HU is dark gray, while a pixel from the soft tissue nodule with a calculated CT number of +46 is light gray.

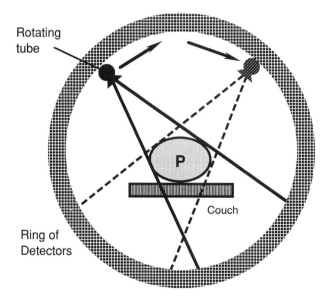

Rotating tube

P

Couch

Ring of Detectors

Figure 1.8. Computed Tomography. Diagram of a fourth-generation CT scanner. The patient is placed on an examination couch within the core of the CT unit. An x-ray tube rotates 360° around the patient (*P*) producing pulses of radiation that pass through the patient. Transmitted x-rays are detected by a circumferential bank of radiation detectors. X-ray transmission data is sent to a computer, which uses an assigned algorithm to calculate the matrix of CT numbers used to produce the anatomic cross-sectional image.

mitted x-rays. Computed tomography pixel numbers are proportional to the difference in average x-ray attenuation of the tissue within the voxel compared to that of water. A Hounsfield unit (HU) scale, named for the inventor of CT, is used. Water is assigned a value of 0 HU with the scale extending from − 1024 HU for

air to + 3000–4000 HU for very dense bone. Hounsfield units are not absolute values, but rather are relative values that vary from one CT system to another.

Voxel dimensions are determined by the computer algorithm chosen for reconstruction and the thickness of the scanned slice. Most CT units allow slice thickness specifications between 1 and 10 mm. Data for an individual slice are routinely acquired in 1–3 seconds. Advantages of CT compared to MR include rapid scan acquisition, superior bone detail, and demonstration of calcifications. Computed tomography imaging is generally limited to the axial plane.

Contrast Administration in CT

Intravenous contrast is administered in CT to enhance density differences between lesions and surrounding parenchyma, to demonstrate vascular anatomy and vessel patency, and to characterize lesions by their patterns of contrast enhancement. The normal blood-brain barrier of tight neural capillary endothelial junctions prevents access of contrast into the neural extravascular space. However, defects in the blood-brain barrier associated with tumors, stroke, infection, and other lesions allow contrast accumulation within abnormal tissue improving its visibility. In nonneural tissues the capillary endothelium has loose junctions allowing free access of contrast into the extravascular space. Contrast administration and timing of CT scanning must be carefully planned to optimize differences in enhancement patterns between lesions and normal tissues. For example, most liver tumors are predominantly supplied by the hepatic artery, while the liver parenchyma is predominantly supplied by the portal vein. Contrast given by bolus in a peripheral arm vein will arrive earliest in the hepatic artery and enhance (increase the CT density of) the tumor. Maximal enhancement of the liver parenchyma is delayed 1–2 minutes until the contrast has circulated through the intestinal tract and returns to the liver via the portal vein. Differentiation of tumor and parenchyma by contrast enhancement can thus be maximized by giving an intravenous bolus of contrast and performing rapid CT scanning of the liver in the first 2 minutes following contrast administration. Oral or rectal contrast is generally required to opacify the bowel for CT scans of the abdomen and pelvis. Bowel without intraluminal contrast may be difficult to differentiate from tumors, lymph nodes, and hematomas.

Computed Tomography Artifacts

Artifacts refer to components of the image that do not have anatomic correlates in tissue. Artifacts degrade the image and may cause errors in diagnosis (3).

Volume Averaging is present in every CT image and must always be considered in image interpretation. The displayed two-dimensional image is created from data obtained and *averaged* from a three-dimensional volume of patient tissue. Slices above and below the image being interpreted must be examined for sources of volume averaging that may be misinterpreted as pathology.

Beam Hardening Artifact results from greater attentuation of low-energy x-ray photons than high-energy x-ray photons as they pass through tissue. The mean energy of the x-ray beam is increased (beam hardening), resulting in less attenuation at the end of the beam than at its beginning. Beam hardening errors are seen as areas or streaks of low density extending from structures of high x-ray attenuation such as the petrous bones, shoulders, and hips.

Motion Artifact results when structures move to different positions during image acquisition. Motion is demonstrated in the image as prominent streaks from high- to low-density interfaces or as a blurred or duplicated image.

Streak Artifacts eminate from high-density sharp-edged objects such as vascular clips and dental fillings. Reconstruction algorithms cannot handle the extreme differences in x-ray attentuation between very dense objects and adjacent tissue.

Principles of CT Interpretation

Like all imaging analysis, CT interpretation is based upon an organized and comprehensive approach. Computed tomography images are viewed in sequential anatomic order examining each slice with reference to slices above and below. The radiologist must seek to develop a three-dimensional concept of the anatomy and pathology displayed. The study must be interpreted with reference to the scan parameters, slice thickness and spacing, administration of contrast, and artifacts. Optimal bone detail is viewed at bone windows, generally a window width of 2000 HU and a window level of 600 HU (Fig. 1.9). Lungs are viewed at lung windows with a window width of 1000–2000 HU and window levels of −500 to −600 HU. Soft tissues are examined at window width 400–500 HU and window level 20–40 HU. Narrow windows (width = 100–150 HU, level = 70–80 HU) increase the image contrast and are helpful for detection of subtle liver and spleen lesions.

Magnetic Resonance Imaging

Magnetic resonance imaging (MR) is a technique that produces tomographic images by means of magnetic fields and radiowaves (4). While CT evaluates only a single tissue parameter, x-ray attenuation, MR analyzes multiple tissue characteristics including hydrogen or proton density, T1 and T2 relaxation times of tissue, and blood flow within tissue. The soft tissue contrast provided by MR is substantially better than for any other imaging modality. Differences in the density of protons available to contribute to the MR signal discriminate one tissue from another. Most tissues are differentiated by significant differences in their characteristic T1 and T2 relaxation values. T1 and T2 are features of the three-dimensional molecular environment that surrounds each proton in the tissue imaged. T1 is a measure of a proton's ability to exchange energy with its surrounding chemical matrix. It describes how quickly a tissue can become magnetized. T2 conveys how quickly a given tissue loses its magnetization. Blood flow has a complex effect on the MR signal that may decrease or increase its intensity.

The complicated physics of MR is beyond the scope of this book. However, in simplest terms, MR is based upon the ability of a small number of protons within the body to absorb and emit radiowave energy when the body is placed within a strong magnetic field (4). Different tissues absorb and release radiowave energy at different, detectable, and characteristic rates. Two major components of MR machine settings selected by the operator are TR and TE. The time between administered radiofrequency (RF) pulses, or the time allowed for protons to align with the main magnetic field, is TR. The time allowed for absorbed radiowave energy to be released and detected is TE. T1-weighted images emphasize differences in the T1 relaxation times between tissues. T1-weighted images are ob-

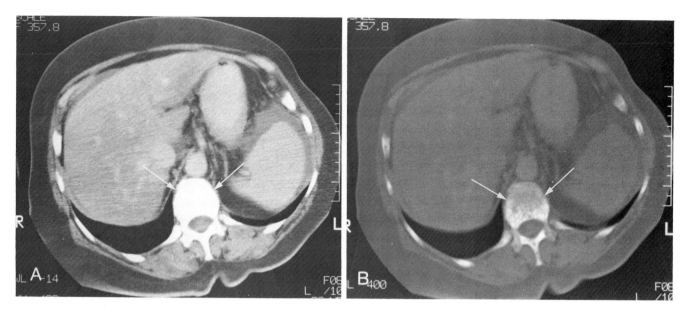

Figure 1.9. CT Windows. A. A CT image of the upper abdomen photographed with soft tissue windows (window width = 482, window level = 14) portrays the thoracic vertebra (*arrows*) entirely white with no bone detail. **B.** The same CT image rephotographed with bone windows (window width = 2000, window level = 400) demonstrates destructive changes in the vertebral body (*arrows*) which were due to metastatic lung carcinoma.

tained by selecting short TR (≤500 msec) and short TE (≤20 msec) settings. T1-weighted images usually provide the best anatomic detail and are good for identifying fat and subacute hemorrhage. T2-weighted images emphasize differences in the T2 relaxation times of tissues by selecting long TR (≥2000 msec) and long TE (≥80 msec) values. T2WI usually provide the most sensitive detection of pathologic lesions (Fig. 1.10). Proton density-weighted images utilize a long TR (2000-3000 msec) and a short TE (25-30 msec) to minimize T1 and T2 effect and accentuate proton density differences in tissues.

Magnetic resonance scans are obtained by placing the patient in a static magnetic field 0.02 to 4 tesla (T) in strength, depending upon the particular MR unit used. Low-field strength systems (<0.1 T), midfield systems (0.1–1.0 T), and high-field systems (>1.0 T) each have their own advantages and disadvantages. The choice of unit for imaging is based upon preference and local availability. A small number of tissue protons in the patient align with the main magnetic field and are subsequently displaced from their alignment by application of RF gradients. When the RF gradient is terminated, the displaced protons realign with the main magnetic field, releasing a small pulse of energy that is detected, localized, and then processed by a computer algorithm similar to that used in CT to produce an anatomic tomographic image. Images can be obtained in any anatomic plane. Standard spin-echo sequences produce a batch of images in about 10–20 minutes. Because the MR signal is very weak, prolonged imaging time is often required for optimal images. An entire series of images covering a specified body area is obtained during the imaging time as compared with CT, which produces images one slice at a time. Motion due to breathing and cardiac and vascular pulsation may degrade the image substantially. More recently available gradient-echo and fast spin-echo techniques have significantly decreased imaging times making breath-hold imaging practical (5, 6). Continued rapid-paced technological improvements are making MR image acquisition times comparable with CT. Magnetic resonance angiograms may be obtained by a variety of two- and three-dimensional gradient-echo, flow compensation, and RF presaturation techniques (7, 8).

The advantages of MR are its outstanding soft-tissue contrast resolution, ability to provide images in any anatomic plane, and absence of ionizing radiation. Magnetic resonance is limited by its inability to demonstrate dense bone detail or calcifications, long imaging times, limited spatial resolution compared with CT, limited availability in many geographic areas, and expense. Because of the physically confining space for the patient within the magnet, a number of patients experience symptoms of claustrophobia and require sedation, or are simply unable to tolerate MR scanning.

Safety Considerations. Magnetic resonance is contraindicated in patients who have electrically, magnetically, or mechanically activated implants including cardiac pacemakers, insulin pumps, cochlear implants, neurostimulators, bone-growth stimulators, and implantable drug infusion pumps (9). Patients with intracardiac pacing wires or Swan-Ganz catheters are at risk for RF current-induced cardiac

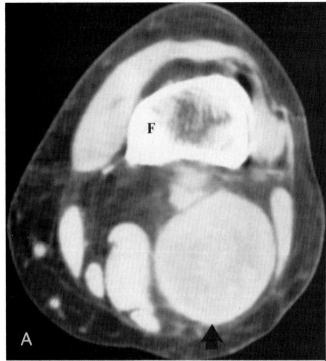

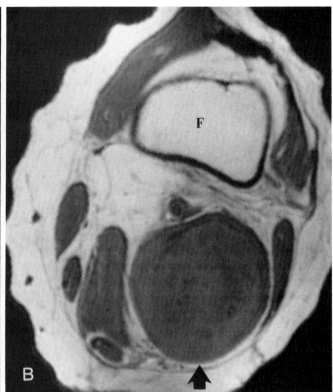

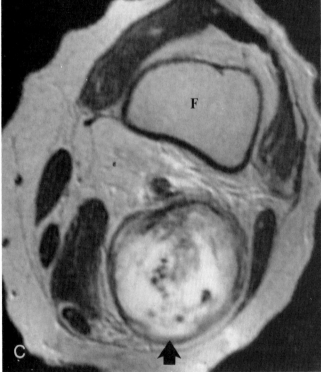

Figure 1.10.   Computed Tomography and MR of Soft-Tissue Tumor Left Thigh. A CT without intravenous contrast (**A**), T1-weighted spin echo MR (TR = 550, TE = 20) (**B**), and T2-weighted spin echo MR (TR = 2250, TE = 80) (**C**) of a granular cell myoblastoma (*arrow*) arising in the soft tissue of the posterior thigh. *F*, femur.

fibrillation and burns. Ferromagnetic implants such as cerebral vascular aneurysm clips, vascular clips, and skin staples are at risk for movement and dislodgment, burns, and induced electrical currents. Bullets, shrapnel, and metallic fragments may move and cause additional injury or become projectiles in the magnetic field. Metal workers and patients with a history of penetrating eye injuries should be screened with plain radiographs of the orbits to detect intraocular metallic foreign bodies that may dislodge and cause blindness. A number of implants have been confirmed to be safe for MR including nonferromagnetic vascular clips and staples, and orthopaedic devices composed of nonferromagnetic materials. Prosthetic heart valves with metal components and stainless steel Greenfield filters are considered safe because the in vivo forces affecting them are stronger than the deflecting forces of the electromagnetic field.

Magnetic Resonance Imaging Artifacts

Ferromagnetic Artifact is caused by focal distortions in the main magnetic field due to the presence of ferromagnetic objects such as orthopaedic devices, surgical clips and wire, dentures, and metallic foreign bodies in the patient (10). The artifact is seen as a signal void at the location of the metal implant, often with a rim of increased intensity and a distortion of the image in the vicinity.

Motion Artifact is common in MR because of prolonged image acquisition time. The image appears blurred or double-exposed.

Chemical Shift Misregistration occurs at interfaces between fat and water (10). Protons bound in lipid molecules experience a slightly lower magnetic influence than protons in water when exposed to an externally applied gradient magnetic field resulting in misregistration of signal location. The artifact is seen as a line of high-signal intensity on one side of the fat-water interface and a line of signal void at the opposite side of the fat-water interface.

Truncation Error occurs adjacent to sharp boundaries between tissues of markedly different contrast. The artifact is due to inherent errors in the Fourier transform technique of image reconstruction. It appears as regularly spaced alternating parallel bands of bright and dark signal.

Aliasing or image wraparound artifact occurs when anatomy outside the designated field of view but within the image plane is mismapped onto the opposite side of the image (10). For instance, on a midline sagittal brain MR image, the patient's nose may be artifactually displayed over the area of the posterior fossa.

Principles of MR Interpretation

Outstanding soft-tissue contrast is obtained in MR by designing imaging sequences that accentuate differences in T1 and T2 tissue relaxation times. Sequences that accentuate differences in proton density are fruitful in brain imaging but are generally less useful for extracranial soft-tissue imaging where proton density differences are small. Interpreting MR images depends upon a clear understanding of the biophysical basis of MR tissue contrast (11). Water is the major source of the MR signal in tissues other than fat. Mineral-rich structures such as bone and calculi, and collagenous tissues such as ligaments, tendons, fibrocartilage, and tissue fibrosis are low in water content and lack mobile protons to produce an MR signal. Therefore these tissues are low in signal intensity on all MR imaging sequences. Water in tis-

Table 1.1. Rules of MR Soft-Tissue Contrast

T1-weighted Images	T2-weighted Images
Short T1→High signal	Short T2→Low signal
Long T1→Low signal	Long T2→High signal

sue exists in at least two physical states: *free water* with unrestricted motion and *bound water* with restricted motion due to hydrogen bonding with proteins (11). Free water is found mainly in extracellular fluid, while bound water is found mainly in intracellular fluid. Intracellular water is both bound and free, and is in a condition of rapid exchange between the two states.

Free Water has long T1 and T2 relaxation times resulting in low signal intensity on T1-weighted images and high signal intensity on T2-weighted images (Table 1.1). Organs with abundant extracellular fluid and therefore large amounts of free water include the kidney (urine), ovaries and thyroid (follicles), spleen and penis (stagnant blood), prostate, testes, and seminal vesicles (fluid in tubules) (Table 1.2). Edema is an increase in extracellular fluid and therefore tends to have the effect of prolonging T1 and T2 relaxation times in affected tissues. Most neoplastic tissues have an increase in extracellular fluid as well as an increase in the proportion of intracellular free water resulting in their visualization with bright signal intensity on T2-weighted images (11). However, neoplasms in organs, such as the kidney, that are also rich in free or extracellular water may appear isointense or hypointense compared with the bright normal parenchyma on T2-weighted images. Neoplasms that are hypocellular or fibrotic appear dark on T2-weighted images because fibrotic tissue dominates their signal characteristics. Simple cysts, cerebrospinal fluid, urine in the bladder, and bile in the gallbladder all reflect the signal characteristics of free water.

Proteinaceous Fluids. The addition of protein to free water has the effect of shortening the T1 relaxation time and brightening the signal on T1-weighted images (11). T2 relaxation is also shortened but the T1 shortening effect is dominant even on T2-weighted images. Therefore, proteinaceous fluid collections remain bright on T2-weighted images. Proteinaceous fluids include synovial fluid, complicated cysts, abscesses, many pathologic fluid collections, and necrotic areas within tumors.

Soft Tissues with a predominance of intracellular bound water have shorter T1 and T2 times than tissues with large amounts of extracellular water. These tissues, including the liver, pancreas, adrenal glands, and muscle, have intermediate signal intensities on both T1- and T2-weighted images. Intracellular protein synthesis lowers T1 even more; therefore, muscle

Table 1.2.   MR of Tissues and Body Fluids[a]

Tissue/Body Fluid	Examples	T1-Weighted Image Signal	T2-Weighted Image Signal
Gas	Air in lung Gas in bowel	Absent	Absent
Mineral-rich tissue	Cortical bone Calculi	Absent	Absent
Collagenous tissue	Ligaments Tendons Fibrocartilage Fibrous tissue	Low	Low
Fat	Adipose tissue Fatty bone marrow	High	Intermediate to high
Cellular tissue High bound water	Liver Pancreas Adrenal glands Muscle Hyaline cartilage	Low	Low to intermediate
High free water tissue	Kidney Testes Prostate Seminal vesicles Ovary Thyroid Spleen Penis Simple cysts Bladder Gallbladder Edema Urine Bile Cerebrospinal fluid	Low	High
Proteinaceous fluid	Complicated cysts Abscess Synovial fluid Nucleus pulposus	Intermediate	High

[a]Modified from Mitchell DG, Burk DL Jr, Vinitski S, Rifkin MD. The biophysical basis of tissue contrast in extracranial MR imaging. AJR 1987;149:831–837.

that is less active in protein synthesis is lower in signal intensity on T1-weighted images than organs with more active protein synthesis. Benign tumors with a predominance of normal cells, such as focal nodular hyperplasia in the liver and nonhyperfunctioning adrenal adenomas, tend to remain isointense with their surrounding parenchyma on all imaging sequences. Hyaline cartilage has a predominance of extracellular water but the water is extensively bound to a mucopolysaccharide matrix. Therefore, its signal characteristics resemble cellular soft tissues and is intermediate in strength on most imaging sequences.

Fat. Protons in fat are bound to hydrophobic intermediate-sized molecules and exchange energy efficiently within their chemical environment. T1 relaxation time is short, resulting in a bright signal on T1-weighted images. T2 of fat is shorter than T2 of water, resulting in lower signal intensity for fat relative to water on strongly T2-weighted images. On images with lesser degrees of T2-weighting, T1 effect predominates and fat appears isointense or slightly hyperintense compared with water (11). Specialized fat-saturation imaging sequences may be employed to reduce the signal intensity of fat and enhance the visibility of pathologic processes within fat (Fig. 22.19) (12,13).

Flowing Blood. The MR signal of slow-moving blood, such as in the spleen, venous plexuses, and cavernous hemangiomas, is dominanted by the large amount of extracellular water resulting in low signal on T1-weighted images and high signal on T2-weighted images. Higher velocity blood flow, however, alters the MR signal in complex ways depending upon multiple factors (14). Protons may move out of the imaging plane between RF absorption and RF release, resulting in high velocity signal loss. Alternatively, blood may be replaced by fully magnetized blood from outside of the image volume, resulting in flow-related enhancement. Flow-related enhancement predominates in gradient-echo imaging, resulting in bright signal intensity (white blood) for flowing blood while high-velocity signal loss predominates in spin-echo imaging, resulting in signal void (black blood) in areas of flowing blood.

Hemorrhage. Magnetic resonance images of hemorrhage depend upon the age of the hemorrhage, the physical and oxidative state of hemoglobin, and the location of the hemorrhage (Table 1.3). Hemorrhage in the first few hours (hyperacute) is high in free water and thus has low signal on T1-weighted images and high signal on T2-weighted images. Immediately following intraparenchymal hemorrhage, red blood cells are saturated with oxygen, and contain oxyhemoglobin, which is not paramagnetic. Within a few hours red blood cells become desaturated and contain deoxyhemoglobin which is paramagnetic. Intracellular paramagnetic deoxyhemoglobin selectively shortens T2, reducing signal intensity on T2-weighted images. The most hypoxic and desaturated

Table 1.3.   MR of Hemorrhage[a]

Age	Dominant Component	T1-Weighted Image Signal	T2-Weighted Image Signal
Hyperacute (<1 day)	Free water Oxyhemoglobin	Low	High
Acute (1–6 days)	Deoxyhemoglobin	Low	Low
Chronic (>7 days)	Methemoglobin		
	Intracellular	High	Low
	Extracellular	High	High
Scar	Hemosiderin	Low	Low

[a]Modified from Mitchell DG, Burk DL Jr, Vinitski S, Rifkin MD. The biophysical basis of tissue contrast in extracranial MR imaging. AJR 1987;149:831–837.

portions of the hematoma have the lowest signal. The dark hematoma at this stage is often surrounded by high intensity due to encircling serum and edema. By approximately 1 week, intracellular deoxyhemoglobin is converted to intracellular methemoglobin beginning at the periphery of the clot. Intracellular methemoglobin is paramagnetic but has restricted motion and is heterogeneous in distribution, shortening T1 and selectively shortening T2, resulting in high signal on T1-weighted images and low signal on T2-weighted images. Lysis of red blood cells at 1 week to 1 month increases access of methemoglobin to water molecules, enhancing T1 shortening effect. T1 shortening predominates over T2 shortening even on T2-weighted images resulting in high signal on both T1- and T2-weighted images. The more dilute the concentration of extracellular methemoglobin (the more water is present), the higher the signal intensity on T2-weighted images.

At about the same time, as lysis of red blood cells is occurring centrally within the clot, releasing free methemoglobin, hemosiderin is being ingested by macrophages at the periphery of the clot. Hemosiderin is highly paramagnetic but water insolubility precludes close interaction with water and T1 shortening. Restricted motion of hemosiderin in its intracellular location causes local inhomogeneous magnetic susceptibility and T2 shortening. The result is low signal on both T1- and T2-weighted images. Edema surrounding the hypointense band of hemosiderin produces a concentric outer rim of hyperintensity as long as edema is present. Hemosiderin-laden macrophages quickly enter the blood stream removing hemosiderin from the hematoma in nonneural tissues and in areas of the brain where the blood-brain barrier is destroyed, such as in areas of hemorrhage into tumor. Where the blood-brain barrier is quickly repaired, the hemosiderin may remain in brain tissue for long periods of time and be seen as persisting low intensity. Differentiation of hematoma from other tissues generally requires at least two pulse sequences. Different areas of the hematoma may show signal intensity effects dominated by components in differing stages of evolution.

Ultrasonography

Ultrasound imaging is performed by using the pulse-echo technique (Fig. 1.11). The ultrasound transducer converts electrical energy to a brief pulse of high-frequency sound energy that is transmitted into patient tissues (1). The ultrasound transducer then becomes a receiver, detecting echoes of sound energy reflected from tissue. The depth of any particular echo is determined by the round-trip time of flight for the transmitted pulse and the returning echo, assuming an average speed of sound in tissue of 1540

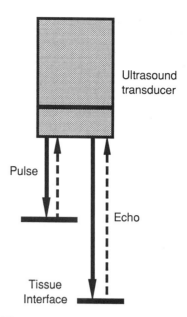

Figure 1.11. Ultrasound Pulse-echo Technique. The ultrasound transducer transmits a brief pulse of ultrasound energy into tissue. The transmitted ultrasound pulse encounters tissue interfaces that reflect a portion of the ultrasound beam back to the transducer. The depth of the tissue interface is determined by the round-trip time of flight for the transmitted pulse and the returning echo, assuming an average speed of 1540 m/sec for sound transmission in human tissue.

m/sec. The ultrasound instrument assumes that all returning echoes originate from along the line of site of the transmitted pulse. The composite image is produced by interrogating tissue in the field of view with multiple closely spaced ultrasound pulses. The shape and appearance of the resulting image depends upon the design of the particular transducer used (Fig. 1.12). Modern ultrasound units operate sufficiently quickly to produce near real-time images of moving patient tissue allowing assessment of respiratory and cardiac movement, vascular pulsations, peristalsis, and the moving fetus. Most medical imaging is performed using ultrasound transducers that produce sound pulses in the frequency range of 1–10 MHz. Higher frequency transducers (5–10 MHz) yield the greatest spatial resolution but are restricted by limited penetration. Lower frequency transducers (1–3.5 MHz) allow better penetration of tissues but at the cost of poorer resolution. High-frequency transducers are routinely used for endoluminal applications, examination of superficial structures such as thyroid, breast, and testes, and examination of infants, children, and small adults. Lower frequency transducers are used for most abdominal, pelvic, and obstetric applications.

Ultrasound examinations are performed by applying the ultrasound transducer directly onto the patient's skin using a water-soluble gel as a coupling

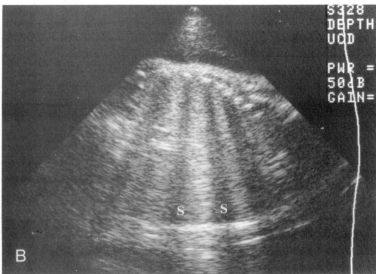

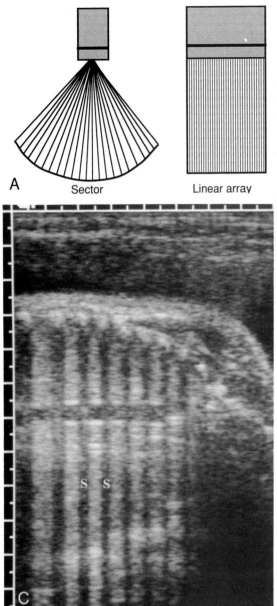

Figure 1.12.   Sector vs. Linear Array Ultrasound Transducers. A. Diagram of the diverging ultrasound beams transmitted by a sector transducer (*left*) and the parallel ultrasound beams transmitted by linear array transducer (*right*). Sector transducers have the advantage of wider field of view in the far field, while linear array transducers have a wider field of view in the near field. **B.** Sector transducer image of a fetus shows prominent shadowing (*S*) from the fetal ribs. Note how the width of the shadows expands with increasing depth because of the diverging ultrasound beams. **C.** Linear array transducer image of the same fetus shows parallel nonwidening shadows (*S*) from the fetal ribs. Note the improved visualization of structures in the near field.

agent to ensure good contact. Images may be produced in any anatomic plane by adjusting the orientation and angulation of the transducer and the position of the patient. The standard orthogonal planes—axial, sagittal, and coronal—allow for the easiest recognition of anatomy but may not be optimal for demonstration of all anatomic structures. The quality of all ultrasound examinations depends heavily upon the skill and diligence of the sonographer. Ultrasound examinations generally provide the most diagnostic information when they are directed at solving a particular clinical problem.

Visualization of anatomic structures by ultrasound is severely limited by bone and by gas-containing structures such as bowel and lung. Sound energy is nearly completely absorbed at interfaces between soft tissue and bone causing an acoustic shadow with limited visualization of structures deep to the bone surface. Soft tissue-gas interfaces cause near complete reflection of the sound beam eliminating visualization of deeper structures. Optimal visualization of many organs is performed through acoustic windows that allow adequate sound transmission. The liver is imaged through the windows of the intercostal spaces. The pancreas is visualized through the window of the left lobe of the liver. Pelvic organs are examined through the urine-filled bladder, which displaces the gas-filled bowel out of the pelvis. Ultrasound visualization of structures in the chest depends upon finding windows between bone and air-filled lung. Ultrasound examination may also be limited by surgical wounds, dressings, and skin lesions, which preclude firm

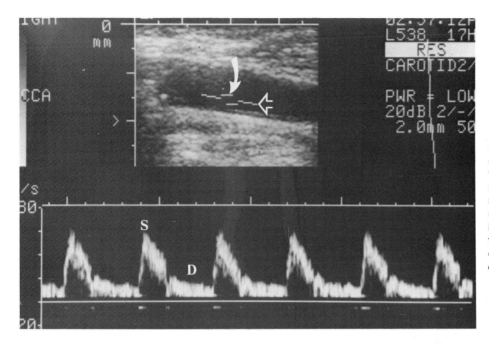

Figure 1.13. Duplex Doppler Ultrasound. Ultrasound image shows the Doppler spectrum of the right common carotid artery. The vertical scale shows blood flow velocity in meters per second. The horizontal scale shows time in seconds. The Doppler trace demonstrates peak velocities in systole (*S*) and low flow velocities in diastole (*D*). A 2-mm Doppler sample volume (*curved arrow*) is placed by the sonographer in the midportion of the artery visualized by real-time ultrasound. Only Doppler shifts originating from this sample volume are analyzed for display. The Doppler angle of 50° is communicated to the ultrasound unit computer by aligning the angle indicator (*open arrow*) parallel to the vessel walls.

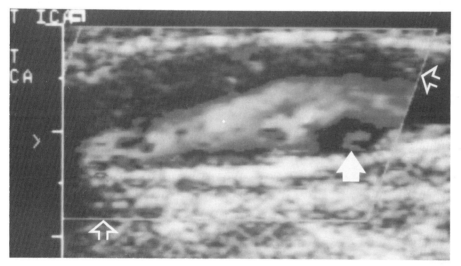

Figure 1.14 (Color Plates). Color Doppler Ultrasound. Flow in the left internal carotid artery is shown in color, while static portions of the ultrasound image are shown in shades of gray. The color Doppler field of view is indicated by the box outlined in white (*open arrows*). With the color map setting indicated by the bar on the left side of the image, blood flow relatively away from the transducer face is portrayed in shades of red, while blood flow relatively toward the transducer face is portrayed in shades of blue. The red-blue orientation of blood flow is easily changed by the sonographer by the flip of a switch on the ultrasound unit. A normal area of blood flow reversal in the carotid bulb is evident on this image (*closed arrow*).

transducer contact with the skin. Endoluminal techniques obviate many of the problems of surface scanning. Endovaginal transducers allow close and highly detailed visualization of the uterus and ovaries without intervening tissues. Endorectal tranducers allow intimate examination of the prostate gland.

Doppler Ultrasound is an important adjunct to real-time gray scale imaging. The Doppler effect is a shift in the frequency of returning echoes, as compared to the transmitted pulse, caused by reflection of the sound wave from a moving object. In medical imaging the moving objects of interest are red blood cells in flowing blood. If blood flow is relatively away from the face of the transducer the echo frequency is shifted lower. If blood flow is relatively toward the face of the transducer the echo frequency is shifted higher. The amount of frequency shift is proportional to the relative velocity of the red blood cells.

Thus, Doppler ultrasound can detect not only the presence of blood flow but can also determine its direction and velocity. The Doppler frequency shift is in the audible range producing a sound of blood flow that has additional diagnostic value. *Pulsed Doppler* utilizes a Doppler sample volume that is time-gated to interrogate only a select volume of patient tissue for the Doppler shift. *Duplex Doppler ultrasound* combines real-time gray scale imaging with pulsed Doppler to allow accurate placement of the Doppler sample volume in visualized blood vessels or specific areas of interest (Fig. 1.13). *Color Doppler ultrasound* combines gray scale and Doppler information in a single image (Fig. 1.14 Color Plates). Stationary tissue with echoes having no Doppler shift are displayed in shades of gray, while blood flow and moving tissue producing echoes having a detectable Doppler shift are displayed in color. Blood flow relatively toward the

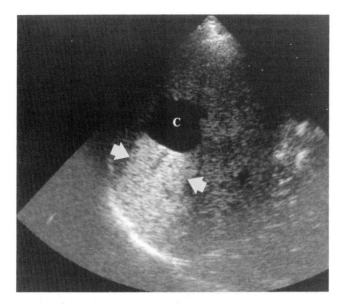

Figure 1.15.   Acoustic Enhancement. Ultrasound image of a simple cyst (C) in the liver demonstrates acoustic enhancement (arrows) as a band of bright echoes deep to the cyst.

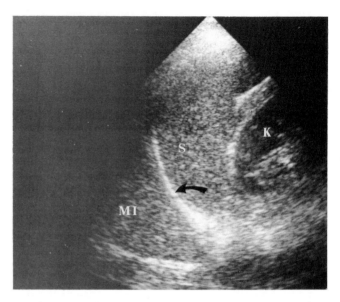

Figure 1.16.   Mirror-image Artifact. Longitudinal image of the left upper quadrant of the abdomen demonstrates the spleen (S), diaphragm (arrow), and artifactual mirror image (MI) of the spleen above the diaphragm. K, left kidney.

transducer face is usually displayed in shades of red while blood flow relatively away from the transducer face is displayed in shades of blue. Lighter color shades imply higher flow velocities.

Ultrasound Artifacts

Artifacts are extremely common in ultrasound imaging and must be recognized to avoid diagnostic errors (15). However, some artifacts, such as acoustic shadowing, are diagnostically useful.

Acoustic Shadowing is produced by near complete absorption or reflection of the ultrasound beam obscuring deeper tissue structures. Acoustic shadows are produced by bone, metallic objects, gas bubbles, gallstones and urinary tract stones. The presence of acoustic shadowing aids in the identification of all types of calculi (Fig. 23.21).

Acoustic Enhancement refers to the increased intensity of echoes deep to structures that transmit sound exceptionally well such as cysts, fluid-filled bladder, and gallbladder, and some solid masses such as lymphoma-replaced lymph nodes. The presence of acoustic enhancement aids in the identification of cystic masses (Fig. 1.15).

Reverberation artifact is caused by repeated reflections between strong acoustic reflectors. Returning echoes are re-reflected into tissues, producing multiple echoes of the same structures that are portrayed on the image progressively deeper in tissue because of prolonged time of flight of echoes eventually returning to the transducer. Reverberation artifact is seen as repeating bands of echoes of progressively decreasing intensity at regularly spaced intervals.

Mirror Image artifact is commonly evident when examining the upper abdomen and diaphragm. Multipath reflection from the strong sound reflection produced by the air-filled lung surface above the curving diaphragm results in depiction of liver or spleen tissue both below and above the diaphragm (Fig. 1.16).

Ring Down or comet tail artifact is seen as a pattern of tapering bright echoes trailing from small bright reflectors such as air bubbles and cholesterol crystals. The artifact may result from vibrations of the reflector or multiple short-path reverberations.

Principles of Ultrasound Interpretation

Interpretation of ultrasound examinations is best performed by the radiologist who has studied the images produced by the sonographer and who, with transducer in hand, has personally examined the patient. Ultrasound in the hands of a skilled physician is a dynamic extension of physical examination. The examining physician has the opportunity to query the patient regarding current and past symptoms, previous surgery, and pertinent medical history. Suspected masses can be palpated as well as examined by ultrasound. Artifacts are more easily differentiated from true components of the image by real-time examination. Active examination allows rapid assessment of three-dimensional anatomic relationships. The real-time ultrasound examination yields thousands of images within a few minutes. The hard copy recorded images serve only to document the dynamic real-time examination. All questions in interpretation should be answered by active sonographic examination.

Fluid-containing structures such as cysts, bile ducts, dilated calyces and ureters, and the distended bladder and gallbladder characteristically demonstrate well-defined walls, absence of internal echoes, and distal acoustic enhancement. Solid tissue demonstrates a speckled pattern of tissue texture with definable blood vessels. Fat is highly echogenic while solid organs such as liver, pancreas, and kidney demonstrate lower degrees of echogenicity. Lesions within or arising from organs demonstrate mass effect, with alteration of organ contour and displacement of blood vessels and alteration in tissue texture. Lesions of lower echogenicity (lower intensity echoes) than surrounding parenchyma are termed *hypoechoic*, while lesions of greater echogenicity (higher intensity echoes) than surrounding parenchyma are called *hyperechoic*. The term *anechoic* refers to the complete absence of echoes such as those within simple cysts. Cystic structures containing echogenic fluid such as blood, pus, or mucin may cause confusion in the sonographic differentiation of cystic and solid lesions. Echogenic cystic structures demonstrate the absence of internal blood vessels, fluid-fluid layering, shifting contents with transducer compression or change in patient position, and well-defined walls. Acoustic enhancement may or may not be present.

RADIOGRAPHIC CONTRAST AGENTS

Iodinated Contrast Agents

Iodinated water-soluble contrast agents are used extensively for intravascular applications in CT, urography, and angiography, and for arthrography, cystography, fistulography, and gastrointestinal opacification. Older, cheaper high-osmolar ionic agents are being replaced in many applications by newer, expensive low-osmolar agents because of safety considerations.

Ionic Contrast Agents (higher osmolality contrast agents) have been considered safe and effective for more than 40 years (16). All iodinated contrast agents have a chemical structure based upon a benzene ring containing three iodine atoms. Ionic media are acid salts (diatrizoate, iothalamate) that dissociate in water into a iodine-containing anion (−) and a cation (+), usually sodium or meglumine. To achieve a sufficient concentration of iodine for radiographic visualization, ionic agents are markedly hypertonic (up to 7 times the osmolality of body fluids). High osmolality and viscosity cause significant hemodynamic, cardiac, and subjective effects including vasodilation, heat, pain, osmotic diuresis, and decreased myocardial contractility. Following intravenous injection, contrast media are distributed quickly into the extracellular space. Excretion is by glomerular filtration, with slower vicarious excretion through the liver, biliary system, and intestinal tract when renal function is impaired.

Adverse reactions to intravenous contrast injection occur in about 5% of patients (16, 17). Most (95%) of the reactions are mild or moderate, while about 5% are severe. Death occurs as a result of contrast injection in about 1 in 40,000 patients. A feeling of warmth at the time of rapid ionic contrast injection is almost universal. Common reactions include nausea, vomiting, hives, and bronchospasm. Additional adverse effects include hypotension, bradycardia, vagal reactions, shock, seizures, and anaphylactoid reaction. Acute renal failure may also be precipitated by contrast injection. The patients at highest risk for contrast reactions include those with a history of previous contrast reaction, a history of allergies, the young (<1 year), the old (>60 years), and patients with heart disease, diabetes, or impaired renal function. An extended discussion of contrast media, adverse effects, and treatment is found in *The Contrast Media Manual* (16) and in the review by Bush and Swanson (17).

Lower Osmolality Contrast Agents (LOCA) have an osmolality reduced to about twice that of blood, resulting in a significant decrease in the already low incidence of adverse reactions. Reduction in osmolality is achieved by making compounds that are nonionic monomers (iopamidol, iohexol, ioversol), nonionic dimers (iotrol, iodixanol), or monoacidic dimers (ioxaglate). Reduced osmolality results in less hemodynamic alterations on contrast injection. A number of studies, none ideal in design, indicate at least a 50% reduction in the incidence of both minor and major adverse reactions (16). Because death is so uncommon, no study to date has included a sufficient number of patients to document a reduced incidence of fatal reactions. The cost ratio between LOCA and ionic media is as much as 13:1 in the United States. The decision to use LOCA or ionic media is heavily debated because of the huge cost implications. The decision to use LOCA in an individual patient must be based upon analysis of cost versus medical benefit versus legal implications (18, 19).

Magnetic Resonance Imaging Intravascular Contrast Agent

Gadopentetate Dimeglumine, gadolinium-labeled diethylenetriamine pentaacetic acid (Gd-DTPA), is a U.S. Food and Drug Administration (FDA) approved contrast agent for MR. Gadopentetate is used, similar to the use of iodinated contrast agents in CT, to identify regions of disruption of the blood-brain barrier, to enhance organs to accentuate pathology, and to document patterns of lesion enhancement.

Gadolinium is a rare-earth heavy metal ion paramagnetic substance that shortens the T1 and T2 relaxation times of hydrogen nuclei within its local magnetic field. At recommended doses Gd-DTPA shortens T1 to a much greater extent than it shortens T2. Signal intensity increases, as a result of T1 shortening, are best seen on T1-weighted images. However, when high tissue concentration is reached, such as in the renal collecting system, T2 shortening causes a significant loss of signal intensity which is best seen on T2-weighted images. The Gd-DTPA is injected intravenously, diffuses rapidly into the extracellular fluid and blood pool spaces, and is excreted by glomerular filtration. About 80% of the injected dose is excreted in 3 hours. Imaging is usually performed immediately after injection. Adverse reactions are uncommon and usually minor. They include headache, nausea, local pain, and coldness at the injection site. At the present time FDA approval is only for intravenous Gd-DTPA at a dose of 0.1 mmol/kg body weight for head and spine applications in patients 2 years and older. Pregnancy, lactation, and renal failure are considered contraindications.

Gastrointestinal Contrast Agents

Barium Sulfate is the standard contrast agent for routine fluoroscopic contrast studies of the upper and lower gastrointestinal tract. Modern formulations provide excellent coating of the gastrointestinal mucosa. "Thin," more fluid, suspensions are used for single-contrast studies, while "thick," more viscous, suspensions coat the mucosa for double-contrast examinations. Barium preparations are remarkably well tolerated. Aspiration of barium rarely causes a clinical problem. Small amounts are cleared from the lungs within hours; however, huge amounts may result in pneumonia. Suspected allergic reactions including hives, respiratory arrest, and anaphylaxis have been occasionally reported. Allergic reactions to latex used in enema balloons and rectal examination gloves have also been suggested. The major risk from the use of barium products is barium peritonitis resulting from the spill of barium into the peritoneal cavity. Barium deposits act as foreign bodies, inducing fibrin deposition and massive ascites. Bacterial contamination from intestinal perforation can lead to sepsis, shock, and death in up to 50% of patients (16).

Gas Agents. Air and carbon dioxide gas are effective and inexpensive contrast agents for both CT and fluoroscopic studies. A number of effervescent powders, granules, and tablets are available that release carbon dioxide on contact with water. These preparations are excellent for distending the stomach for CT or barium studies. Air injected directly into the gastrointestinal tract via a nasogastric or enema tube may be used to distend the stomach or colon.

Water-soluble Iodinated Contrast Media opacify the bowel lumen by passive filling rather than mucosal coating and are considered by most radiologists to be inferior to barium agents for routine fluoroscopic gastrointestinal studies. However, because of the high mortality associated with barium peritonitis, water-soluble agents are indicated whenever gastrointestinal tract perforation is suspected. Water-soluble agents are quickly reabsorbed through the peritoneal surface. Dilute solutions (2–5%) of ionic agents (Gastrografin or oral Hypaque) are routinely used in CT to opacify the gastrointestinal tract. Ionic contrast agents stimulate intestinal peristalsis, which promotes faster opacification of the distal bowel on CT and may be useful in the postoperative patient with ileus. The major risk of oral water-soluble agents is aspiration, resulting in chemical pneumonitis. Low-osmolar agents may be safer whenever aspiration is deemed a risk. Large volumes of hypertonic water-soluble agents in the gastrointestinal tract may result in hypovolemia, shock, and even death, especially in infants and debilitated adults.

References

1. Curry TS III, Dowdey JE, Murry RC Jr. Christensen's introduction to the physics of diagnostic radiology. 4th ed. Philadelphia: Lea & Febiger, 1990.
2. Squire LF, Novelline RA. Fundamentals of radiology. 4th ed. Cambridge: Harvard University Press, 1988.
3. Brant WE. Computed tomography artifacts. In Vogler JB, Helms CA, Callen PW, eds. Normal variants and pitfalls in imaging. Philadelphia: WB Saunders, 1986:3–12.
4. Balter S. An introduction to the physics of magnetic resonance imaging. Radiographics 1987;7:371–383.
5. Haacke EM, Tkach JA. Fast MR imaging: techniques and clinical applications. AJR 1990; 155:951–964.
6. Elster AD. Gradient-echo MR imaging: techniques and acronyms. Radiology 1993;186:1–8.
7. Edelman RR, Mattle HP, Atkinson DJ, Hoogewoud HM. MR angiography. AJR 1990;154:937–946.
8. Chien D, Edelman RR. Basic principles and clinical applications of magnetic resonance angiography. Semin Roentgenol 1992;27:53–62.
9. Shellock FG. MRI biologic effects and safety considerations. In Higgins CB, Hricak H, Helms CA, eds. Magnetic resonance imaging of the body. 2nd ed. New York: Raven Press, 1992:233–265.
10. Clark JA II, Kelly WM. Common artifacts encountered in magnetic resonance imaging. Radiol Clin North Am 1988;26:893–920.
11. Mitchell DG, Burk DL Jr, Vinitski S, Rifkin MD. The biophysical basis of tissue contrast in extracranial MR imaging. AJR 1987;149:831–837.
12. Semelka RC, Chew W, Hricak H, et al. Fat-saturation MR imaging of the upper abdomen. AJR 1990;155:1111–1116.
13. Simon JH, Szumonski J. Proton (fat/water) chemical shift imaging in medical magnetic resonance imaging—current status. Invest Radiol 1992;27:865–874.
14. von Schulthess GK. Blood flow. In Higgins CB, Hricak H, Helms CA, eds. Magnetic resonance imaging of the body. 2nd ed. New York: Raven Press, 1992:313–337.

15. Scanlan KA. Sonographic artifacts and their origins. AJR 1991;156:1267–1272.

16. Katzberg RW, ed. The contrast media manual. Baltimore: Williams & Wilkins, 1992.

17. Bush WH, Swanson DP. Acute reactions to intravascular contrast media: types, risk factors, recognition, and specific treatment. AJR 1991;157:1153–1161.

18. American College of Radiology. Current criteria for the use of water soluble contrast agents for intravenous injections. Reston, VA, 1990.

19. Caro JJ, Trindade E, McGregor M. The cost-effectiveness of replacing high-osmolality with low-osmolality contrast media. AJR 1992;159:869–874.

Section II   NEURORADIOLOGY

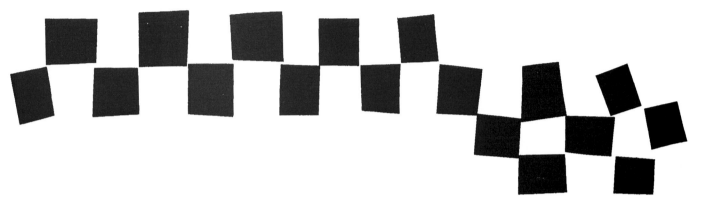

2

Introduction To Brain Imaging and Neuroanatomy Atlas

David J. Seidenwurm

IMAGING METHODS

CHOOSING THE CORRECT STUDY

With the bewildering array of examinations available for imaging the brain, it seems a hopeless task to decide which of them is best for a given clinical situation. To make matters easier, two imaging methods can be eliminated. Plain radiography is useless in emergency patient management and is only of value in the evaluation of bony lesions or the documentation of fracture for medical/legal reasons. Nuclear medicine brain scans are useful only in certain very limited settings and are discussed in Chapter 55. Even without these two, we still have to decide between CT, magnetic resonance imaging (MR), ultrasound, and angiography in the evaluation of the acute neurologic patient. We also need to decide whether to give intravenous contrast material. Angiography and ultrasound are used in the acute setting based upon the appropriate combination of CT, MR, and clinical findings; therefore, the only serious contenders for the "first test" for the brain are MR and CT.

As a general rule in brain imaging, one does CT early in the neurologic illness and MR in the more chronic and subacute cases. That is, if the onset of neurologic symptoms referable to the brain is within 48 hours, start with a CT. If the problem is older than 3 days, start with an MR. If the CT or MR suggests a primary vascular lesion such as an arteriovenous malformation or aneurysm, catheter angiography is indicated, but in the future, MR angiography will play an increasing role. If the CT or MR suggests tumor, give intravenous contrast. If the CT or MR fails to demonstrate an acute infarct and the symptoms suggest a transient ischemic attack or stroke, do a carotid Doppler ultrasound study. Do not give intravenous iodinated contrast for CT in the acute setting unless brain abscess or tumor is a strong consideration. Give gadolinium for MR whenever there is a clinical finding that suggests a specific neurologic localization, a seizure in an adult, or a strong history of cancer or infectious disease. There are exceptions to these guidelines, but very few. Follow the rules and you will be doing the right thing in most cases. Remember that these rules are general guidelines. Sometimes an MR will be required to clarify a questionable finding on CT. Also, remember that some patients are simply too sick to study easily with MR. These include multisystem trauma patients or those who require assisted ventilation. While there is an almost infinite variety of clinical syndromes related to the central nervous system, most patient referrals for diagnostic imaging of the brain can be divided into a limited number of categories (Table 2.1).

Acute Trauma patients have perhaps the most dramatic presentation. A noncontrast-enhanced CT scan is preferred because CT can be obtained quickly, and it is possible to perform this study on virtually any patient, no matter how sick. Furthermore, CT scanners are almost universally available in hospitals with emergency departments. In this setting the most important abnormalities to be detected are extracerebral hematomas. These lesions produce devastating neurologic symptoms that can be completely reversible if they are treated early. Intracerebral contusions are of secondary interest because they are more difficult to treat surgically, and the results of such treatment are less encouraging.

Stroke is an acute neurologic syndrome attributable to brain insult. In the stroke patient, a noncontrast CT scan is the preferred initial imaging study. Most strokes are bland infarcts, and in the acute phase the CT scan is normal or nearly normal. In stroke patients search for evidence of hemorrhage. A cerebral hematoma in the stroke patient suggests hypertensive hemorrhage or amyloid angiopathy, depending upon the distribution of the lesion and the age of the patient. Subarachnoid hemorrhage re-

Table 2.1. Preferred Neuroimaging Studies by Clinical Setting[a]

Clinical Presentation	CT Without Contrast	CT Contrast Enhanced	MR Without Contrast	MR Gadolinium Enhanced
Trauma	XX			
Stroke	XX			
Seizure		X		XX
Infection		X		XX
Cancer		X		XX
Acute Headache	XX			
Chronic Headache	X		XX	
Coma	XX			
Dementia	X		XX	

[a]XX, optimal study; X, acceptable substitute.

quires further evaluation by MR and/or angiography to search for an aneurysm or arteriovenous malformation. If no hemorrhage is seen, a bland infarct occult to CT scanning is presumed to be present. The absence of visible hemorrhage on CT allows the clinician to initiate anticoagulation or thrombolytic therapy in order to prevent progression of, or even reverse, the neurologic deficit.

Seizure patients present an interesting problem for the radiologist. If it is the patient's first seizure an intracranial tumor must be excluded. Contrast-enhanced MR or contrast-enhanced CT is the preferred approach. If the patient is in the immediate postictal state, or if residual neurologic deficit is present at the time of imaging, then a noncontrast CT scan should be obtained as the first study. If the seizure disorder is chronic, and particularly if it is refractory to medical therapy, a detailed MR examination including high-resolution coronal images of the medial temporal lobes is performed. In pediatric patients contrast enhancement is generally not required because congenital anomalies, rather than tumor, are the most common structural cause of seizures.

Infection and Cancer. In any patient in whom infectious disease or cancer is a strong consideration, contrast-enhanced MR is the preferred study. Parenchymal tumors and metastatic disease will be demonstrated with this study, and contrast-enhanced MR has the advantage of depicting meningeal disease much better than any other imaging modality. In some centers, contrast-enhanced CT is performed rather than contrast-enhanced MR. It is difficult to quantify the clinical impact of this choice of imaging strategy. It can be justified on grounds of economic cost and extensive clinical experience.

Headache is a frequent indication for imaging of the brain. Patients with severe acute headaches should be imaged with noncontrast head CT because of suspicion of subarachnoid hemorrhage, acute hy-

drocephalus, or an enlarging intracranial mass. The chronic headache patient is generally evaluated by MR. If the headache is not accompanied by local neurologic symptoms, a noncontrast MR scan is usually sufficient. However, if the headache is associated with focal neurologic complaints or clinical findings, then gadolinium-enhanced MR scanning is generally performed.

Coma. It is crucial to distinguish between a patient with acute confusional state or coma and a patient who is chronically demented. The patient may be comatose or acutely confused due to an intracranial hemorrhage and is studied urgently with noncontrast CT. However, many patients will be comatose because of functional or physiologic abnormalities of the brain rather than structural lesions demonstrable on neuroimaging studies. An acute infarct may be present, but may be invisible on CT.

Dementia. The chronic dementia patient is generally studied by noncontrast-enhanced MR. This is a screening examination for large frontal masses, hydrocephalus, and other treatable abnormalities that may result in a clinical picture indistinguishable from Alzheimer's disease. Furthermore, MR is employed to search for small vessel ischemic changes in the cerebral white matter, and small infarcts that may produce a clinical dementia picture similar to Alzheimer's disease. If these findings are not present, and the clinical picture is compatible, the clinician may offer a diagnosis of Alzheimer's disease.

ANATOMY

The basis of interpretation of the cross-sectional neuroimaging studies is a firm grounding in neuroanatomy and pathophysiology. The accompanying atlas (Figs. 2.1–2.36) depicts the topographic features of the brain that are relevant to clinical neuroradiology.

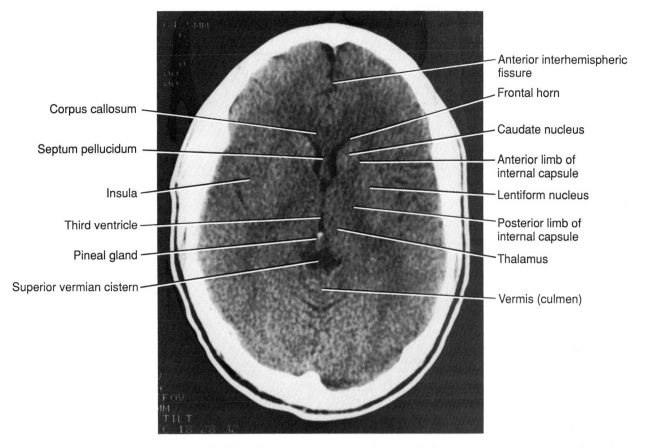

Corpus callosum

Septum pellucidum

Insula

Third ventricle

Pineal gland

Superior vermian cistern

Anterior interhemispheric fissure

Frontal horn

Caudate nucleus

Anterior limb of internal capsule

Lentiform nucleus

Posterior limb of internal capsule

Thalamus

Vermis (culmen)

Figure 2.1. Brain CT. Without intravenous contrast, axial plane through pineal gland.

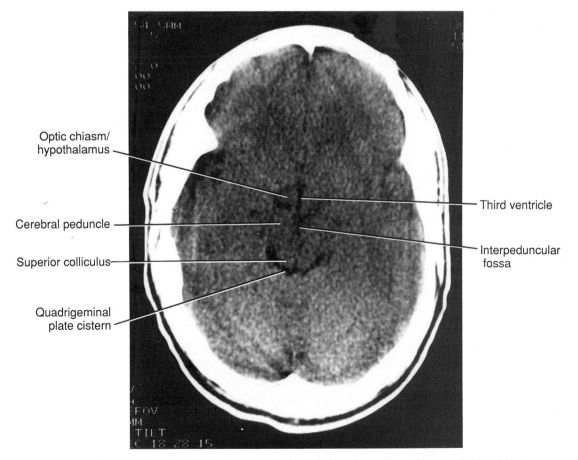

Optic chiasm/ hypothalamus

Cerebral peduncle

Superior colliculus

Quadrigeminal plate cistern

Third ventricle

Interpeduncular fossa

Figure 2.2. Brain CT. Without intravenous contrast, axial plane through quadrigeminal plate cistern.

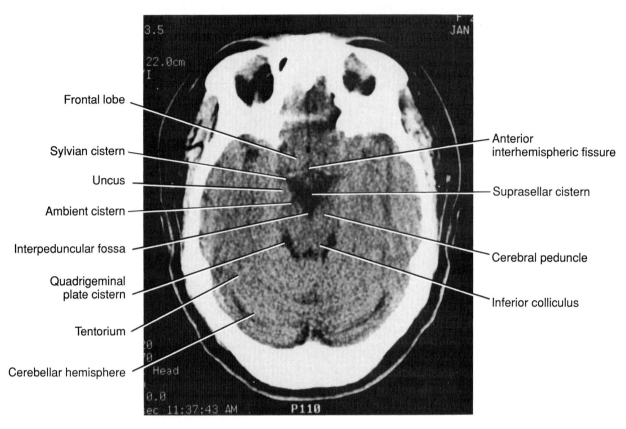

Figure 2.3. **Brain CT.** Without intravenous contrast, axial plane through cerebral peduncles and suprasellar cistern.

Frontal lobe

Sylvian cistern

Uncus

Ambient cistern

Interpeduncular fossa

Quadrigeminal plate cistern

Tentorium

Cerebellar hemisphere

Anterior interhemispheric fissure

Suprasellar cistern

Cerebral peduncle

Inferior colliculus

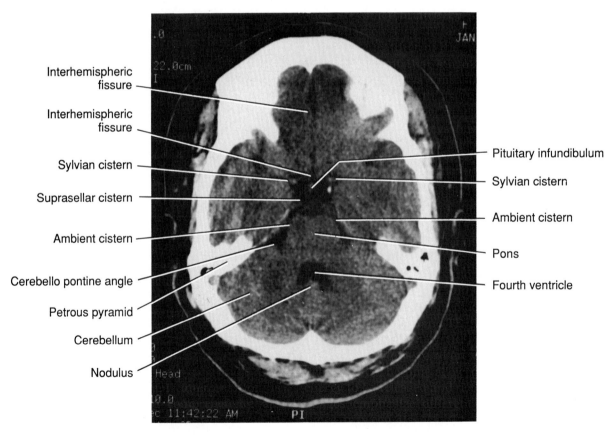

Figure 2.4. **Brain CT.** Without intravenous contrast, axial plane through the pons and fourth ventricle.

Interhemispheric fissure

Interhemispheric fissure

Sylvian cistern

Suprasellar cistern

Ambient cistern

Cerebello pontine angle

Petrous pyramid

Cerebellum

Nodulus

Pituitary infundibulum

Sylvian cistern

Ambient cistern

Pons

Fourth ventricle

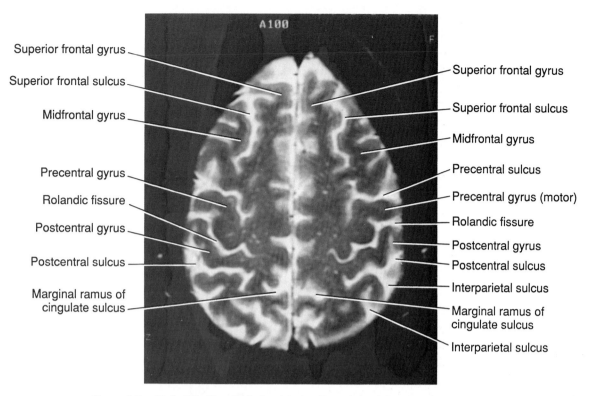

Superior frontal gyrus

Superior frontal sulcus

Midfrontal gyrus

Precentral gyrus

Rolandic fissure

Postcentral gyrus

Postcentral sulcus

Marginal ramus of cingulate sulcus

Superior frontal gyrus

Superior frontal sulcus

Midfrontal gyrus

Precentral sulcus

Precentral gyrus (motor)

Rolandic fissure

Postcentral gyrus

Postcentral sulcus

Interparietal sulcus

Marginal ramus of cingulate sulcus

Interparietal sulcus

Figure 2.5. **Brain MR.** T2-weighted, axial plan through frontal and parietal convexity.

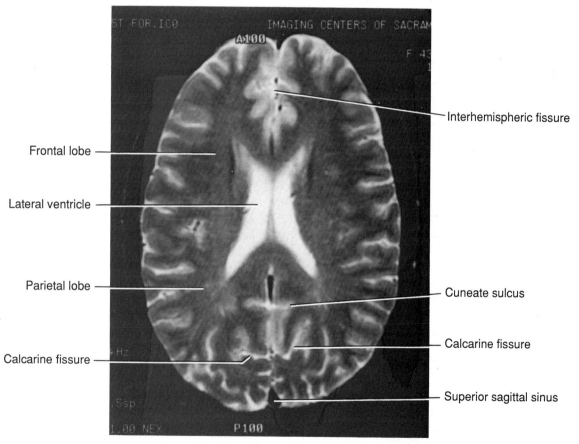

Frontal lobe

Lateral ventricle

Parietal lobe

Calcarine fissure

Interhemispheric fissure

Cuneate sulcus

Calcarine fissure

Superior sagittal sinus

Figure 2.6. **Brain MR.** T2-weighted, axial plane through body of the lateral ventricles.

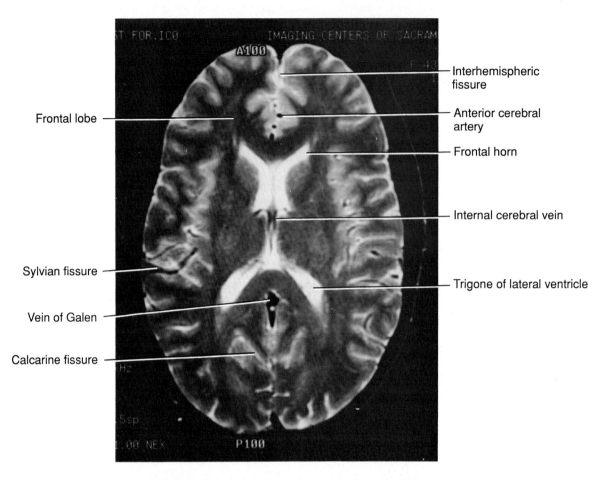

Figure 2.7. Brain MR. T2-weighted, axial plane through frontal horns and trigone of the lateral ventricles.

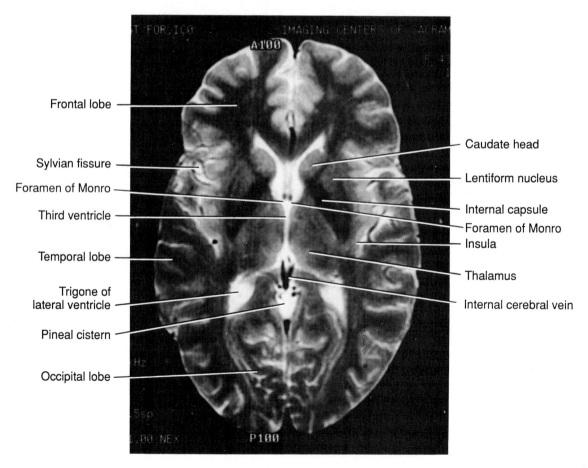

Figure 2.8. Brain MR. T2-weighted, axial plane through foramina of Monro and third ventricle.

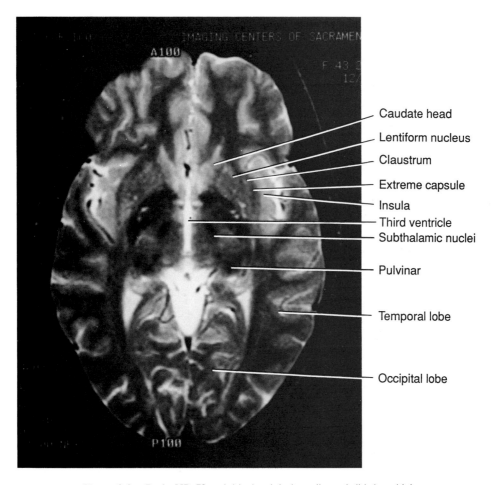

Figure 2.9. Brain MR. T2-weighted, axial plane through third ventricle.

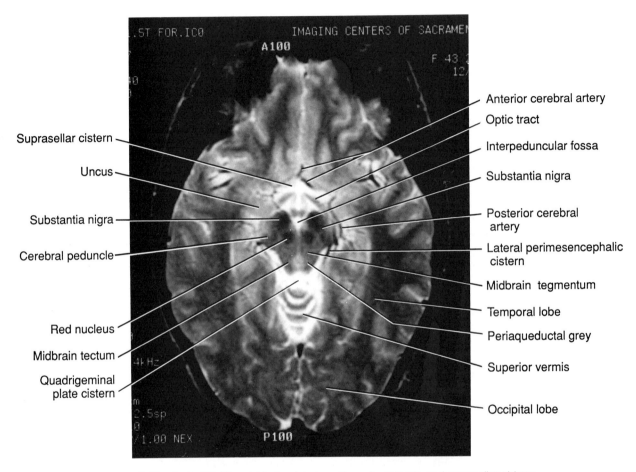

Figure 2.10.   Brain MR. T2-weighted, axial plane through midbrain and suprasellar cisterns.

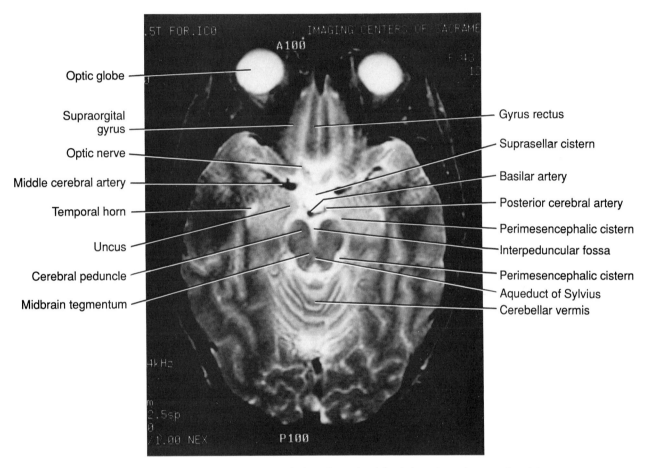

Optic globe

Supraorgital gyrus

Optic nerve

Middle cerebral artery

Temporal horn

Uncus

Cerebral peduncle

Midbrain tegmentum

Gyrus rectus

Suprasellar cistern

Basilar artery

Posterior cerebral artery

Perimesencephalic cistern

Interpeduncular fossa

Perimesencephalic cistern

Aqueduct of Sylvius

Cerebellar vermis

Figure 2.11. Brain MR. T2-weighted, axial plane through midbrain, vermis, and suprasellar cisterns.

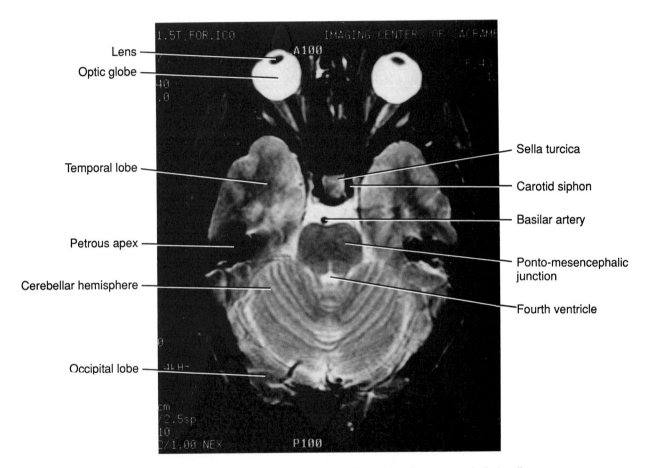

Lens
Optic globe

Temporal lobe

Petrous apex

Cerebellar hemisphere

Occipital lobe

Sella turcica

Carotid siphon

Basilar artery

Ponto-mesencephalic junction

Fourth ventricle

Figure 2.12.   Brain MR. T2-weighted, axial plane through pontomesencephalic junction.

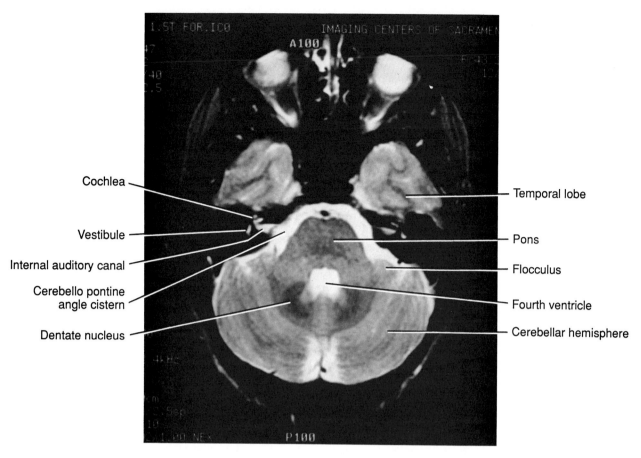

Cochlea

Vestibule

Internal auditory canal

Cerebello pontine
angle cistern

Dentate nucleus

Temporal lobe

Pons

Flocculus

Fourth ventricle

Cerebellar hemisphere

Figure 2.13.   Brain MR. T2-weighted, axial plane through pons.

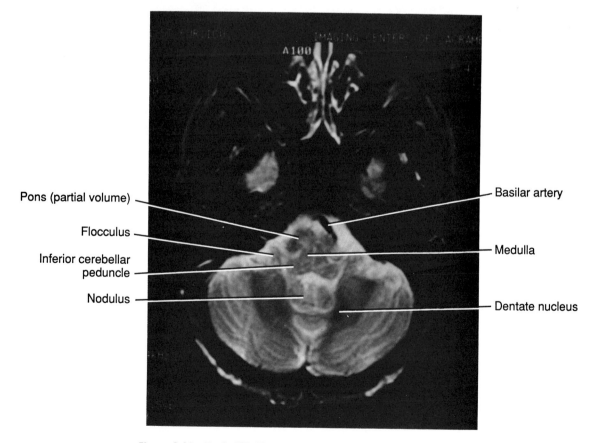

Pons (partial volume)

Flocculus

Inferior cerebellar
peduncle

Nodulus

Basilar artery

Medulla

Dentate nucleus

Figure 2.14.   Brain MR. T2-weighted, axial plane through medulla.

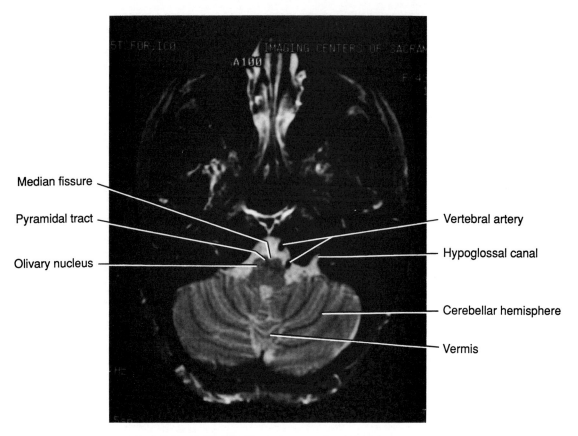

Median fissure

Pyramidal tract

Olivary nucleus

Vertebral artery

Hypoglossal canal

Cerebellar hemisphere

Vermis

Figure 2.15.   Brain MR. T2-weighted, axial plane through medulla.

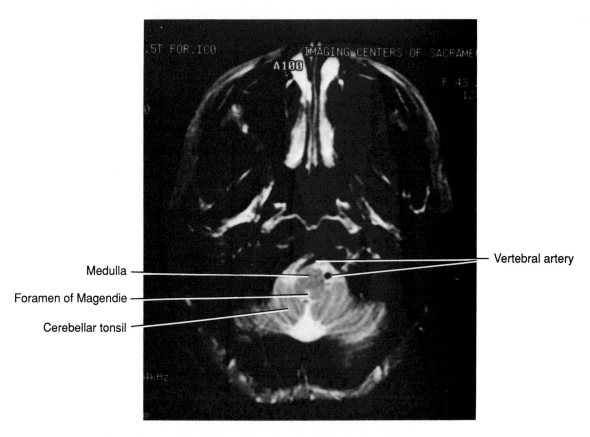

Vertebral artery

Medulla

Foramen of Magendie

Cerebellar tonsil

Figure 2.16.   Brain MR. T2-weighted, axial plane through foramen of Magendie.

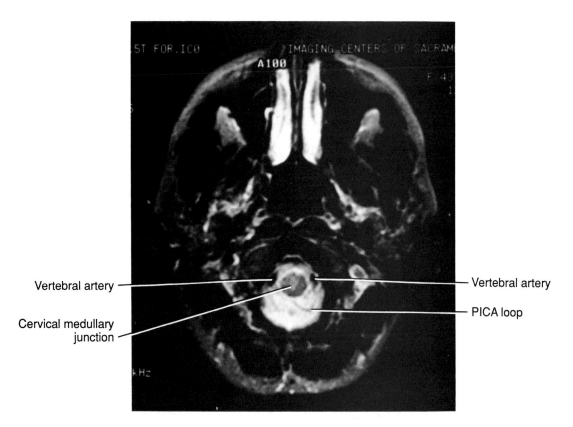

Vertebral artery

Cervical medullary
junction

Vertebral artery

PICA loop

Figure 2.17. **Brain MR.** T2-weighted, axial plane through cervical medullary junction.

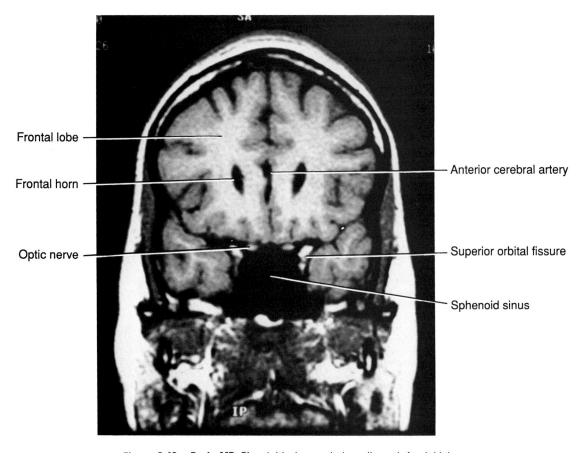

Frontal lobe

Frontal horn

Optic nerve

Anterior cerebral artery

Superior orbital fissure

Sphenoid sinus

Figure 2.18. **Brain MR.** T1-weighted, cornal plane through frontal lobes.

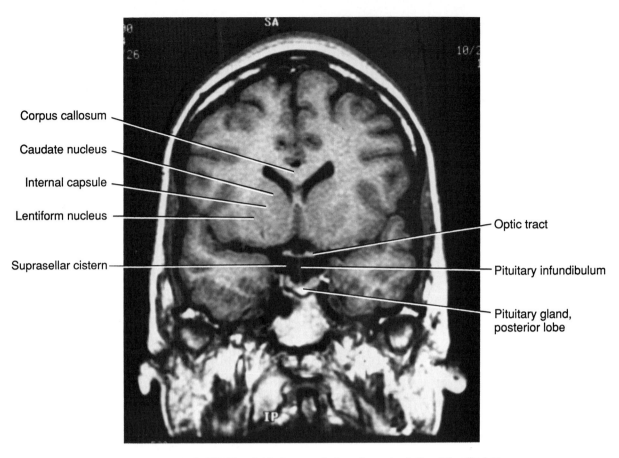

Corpus callosum

Caudate nucleus

Internal capsule

Lentiform nucleus

Suprasellar cistern

Optic tract

Pituitary infundibulum

Pituitary gland, posterior lobe

Figure 2.19. Brain MR. T1-weighted, coronal plane through pituitary infundibulum.

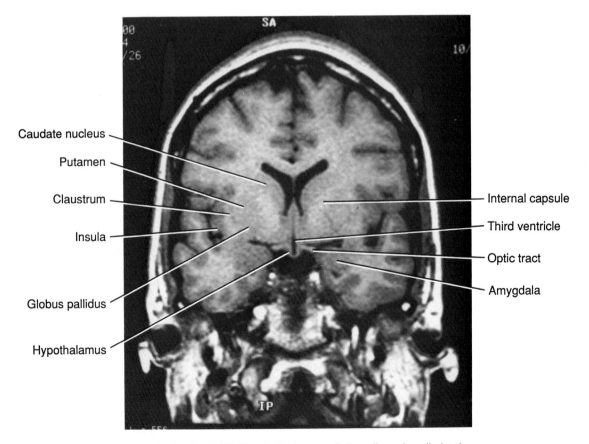

Caudate nucleus

Putamen

Claustrum

Insula

Globus pallidus

Hypothalamus

Internal capsule

Third ventricle

Optic tract

Amygdala

Figure 2.20. Brain MR. T1-weighted, coronal plane through optic tracts.

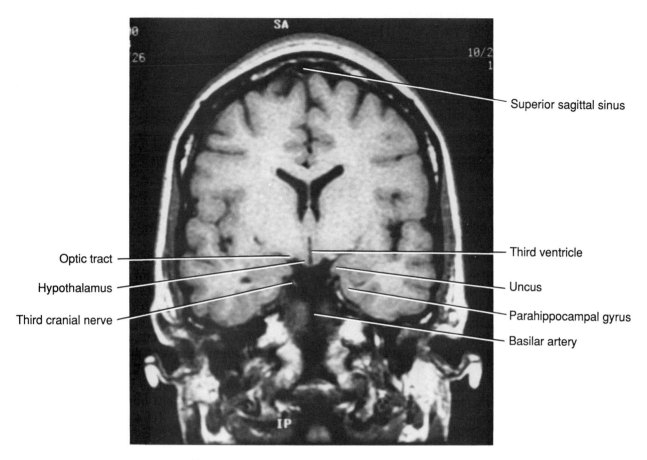

Figure 2.21. **Brain MR.** T1-weighted, coronal plane through hypothalamus.

Optic tract

Hypothalamus

Third cranial nerve

Third ventricle

Uncus

Parahippocampal gyrus

Basilar artery

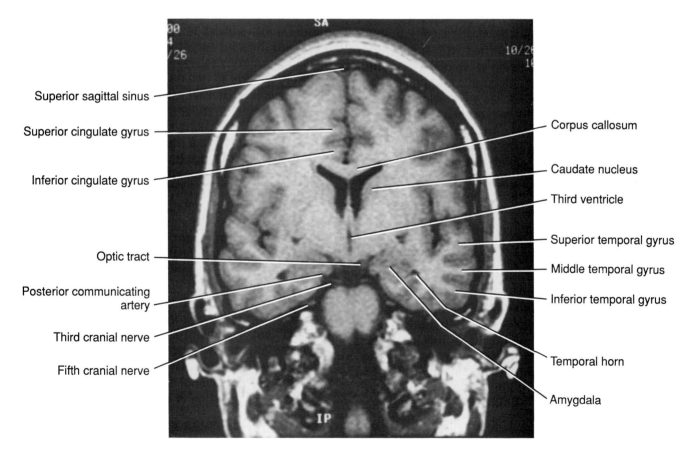

Figure 2.22. **Brain MR.** T1-weighted, coronal plane through anterior third ventricle.

Superior sagittal sinus

Superior cingulate gyrus

Inferior cingulate gyrus

Optic tract

Posterior communicating artery

Third cranial nerve

Fifth cranial nerve

Corpus callosum

Caudate nucleus

Third ventricle

Superior temporal gyrus

Middle temporal gyrus

Inferior temporal gyrus

Temporal horn

Amygdala

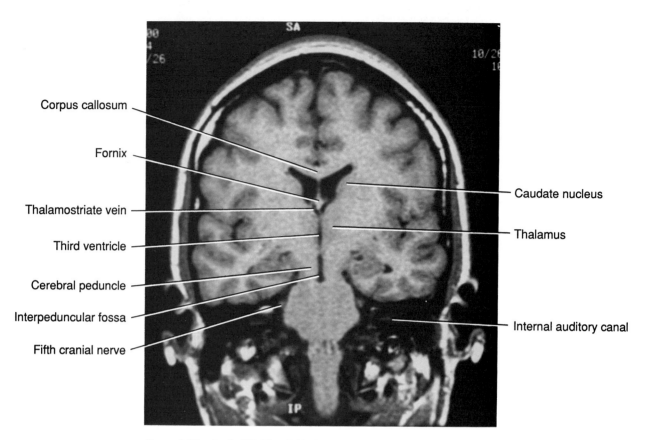

Figure 2.23.   Brain MR. T1-weighted, cornal plane through third ventricle.

Corpus callosum

Fornix

Thalamostriate vein

Third ventricle

Cerebral peduncle

Interpeduncular fossa

Fifth cranial nerve

Caudate nucleus

Thalamus

Internal auditory canal

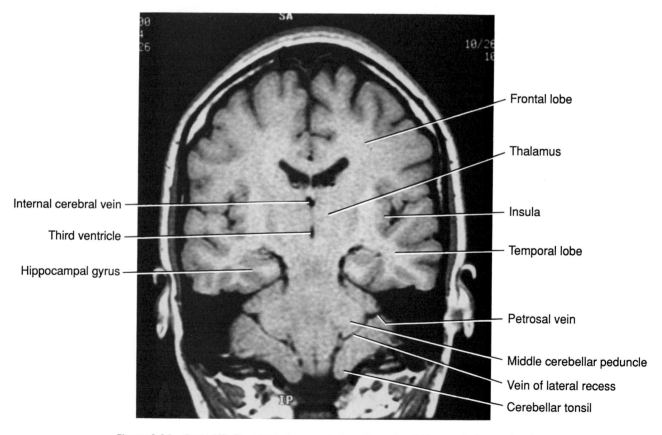

Figure 2.24.   Brain MR. T1-weighted, coronal plane through middle cerebellar peduncle.

Internal cerebral vein

Third ventricle

Hippocampal gyrus

Frontal lobe

Thalamus

Insula

Temporal lobe

Petrosal vein

Middle cerebellar peduncle

Vein of lateral recess

Cerebellar tonsil

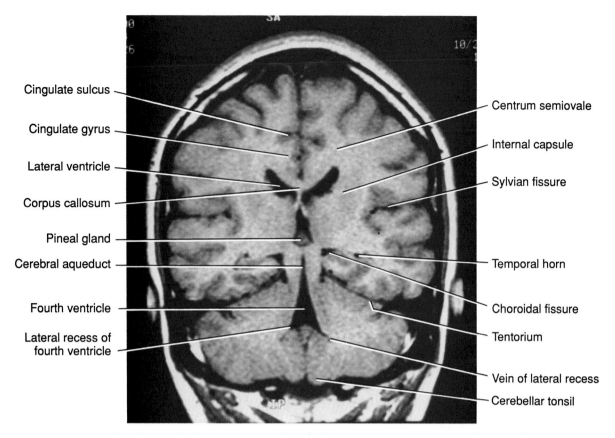

Cingulate sulcus

Cingulate gyrus

Lateral ventricle

Corpus callosum

Pineal gland

Cerebral aqueduct

Fourth ventricle

Lateral recess of
fourth ventricle

Centrum semiovale

Internal capsule

Sylvian fissure

Temporal horn

Choroidal fissure

Tentorium

Vein of lateral recess

Cerebellar tonsil

Figure 2.25. **Brain MR.** T1-weighted, coronal plane through cerebral aqueduct and fourth ventricle.

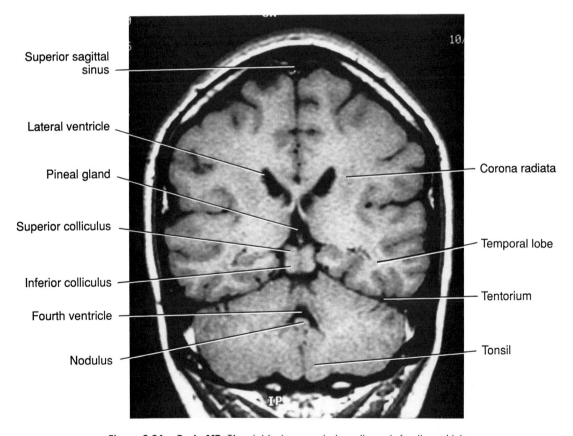

Superior sagittal
sinus

Lateral ventricle

Pineal gland

Superior colliculus

Inferior colliculus

Fourth ventricle

Nodulus

Corona radiata

Temporal lobe

Tentorium

Tonsil

Figure 2.26. **Brain MR.** T1-weighted, coronal plane through fourth ventricle.

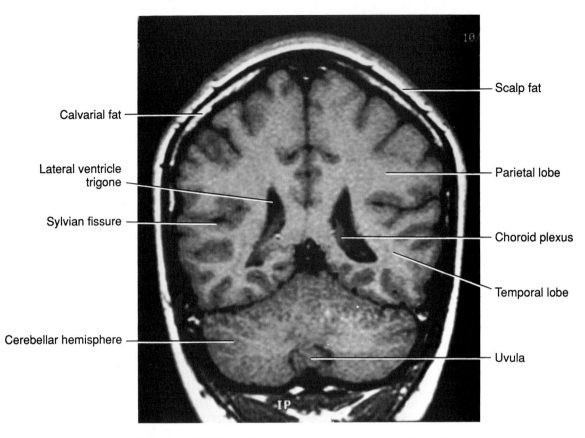

Calvarial fat

Lateral ventricle trigone

Sylvian fissure

Cerebellar hemisphere

Scalp fat

Parietal lobe

Choroid plexus

Temporal lobe

Uvula

Figure 2.27. Brain MR. T1-weighted, coronal plane through ventricular trigones.

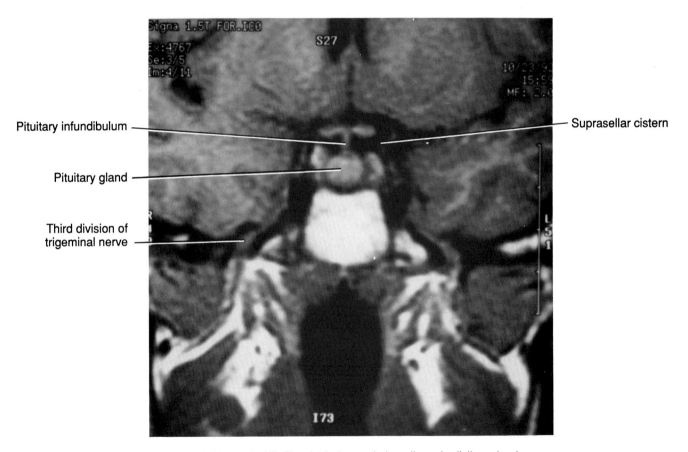

Pituitary infundibulum

Pituitary gland

Third division of trigeminal nerve

Suprasellar cistern

Figure 2.28. Brain MR. T1-weighted, cornal plane through pituitary gland.

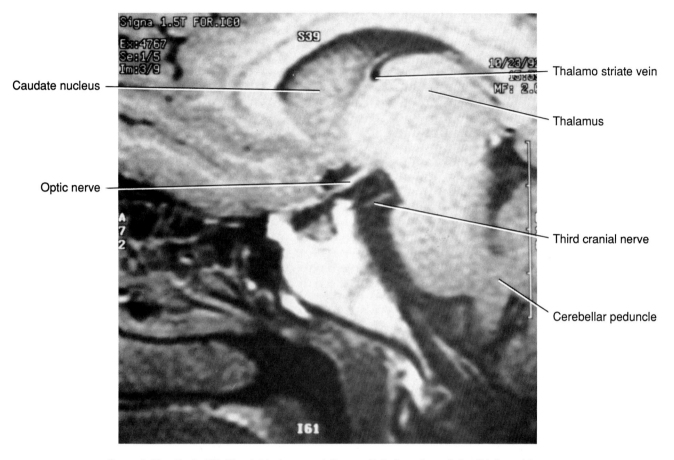

Caudate nucleus

Optic nerve

Thalamo striate vein

Thalamus

Third cranial nerve

Cerebellar peduncle

Figure 2.29.   Brain MR. T1-weighted, para-midline sagittal plane through the third cranial nerve.

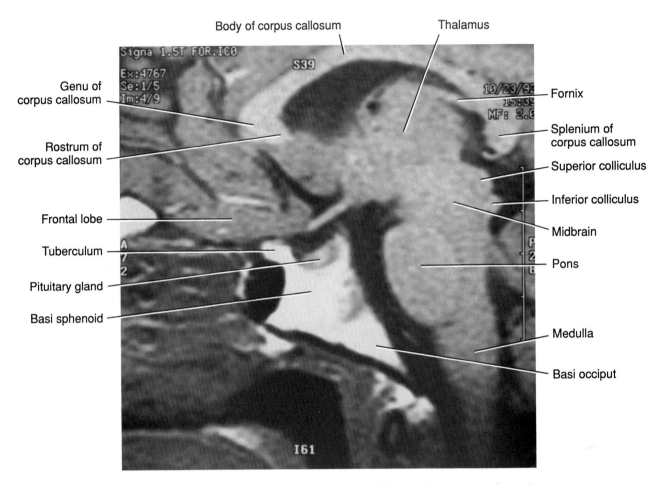

Figure 2.30.   Brain MR. T1-weighted, para-midline sagittal plane through parasellar region.

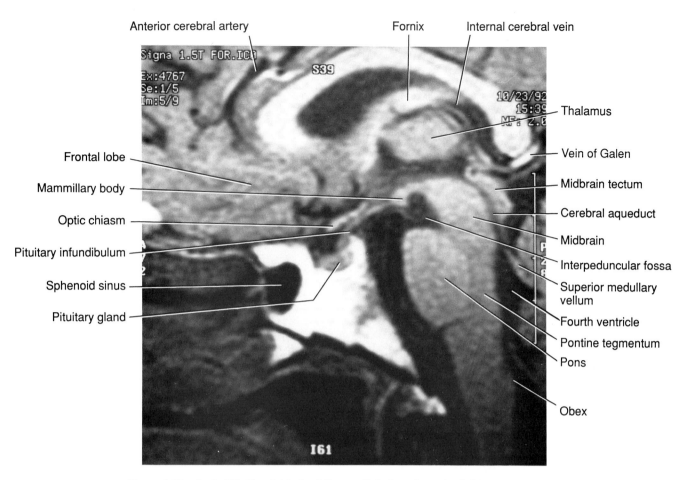

Anterior cerebral artery

Fornix

Internal cerebral vein

Frontal lobe

Mammillary body

Optic chiasm

Pituitary infundibulum

Sphenoid sinus

Pituitary gland

Thalamus

Vein of Galen

Midbrain tectum

Cerebral aqueduct

Midbrain

Interpeduncular fossa

Superior medullary vellum

Fourth ventricle

Pontine tegmentum

Pons

Obex

Figure 2.31. Brain MR. T1-weighted, midline sagittal plane through pituitary infundibulum.

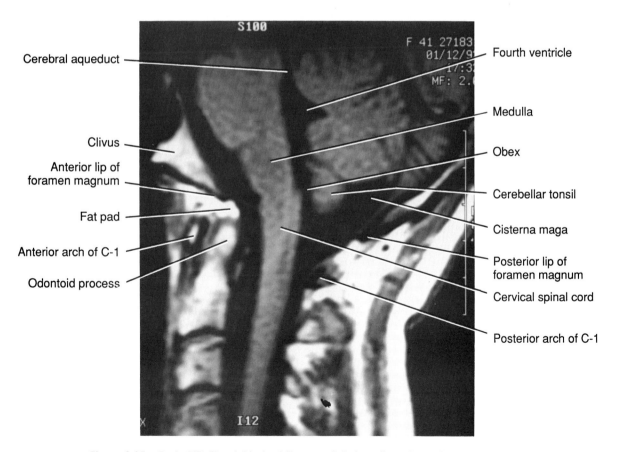

Cerebral aqueduct

Clivus

Anterior lip of foramen magnum

Fat pad

Anterior arch of C-1

Odontoid process

Fourth ventricle

Medulla

Obex

Cerebellar tonsil

Cisterna maga

Posterior lip of foramen magnum

Cervical spinal cord

Posterior arch of C-1

Figure 2.32. Brain MR. T1-weighted, midline saggital plane through craniocervical junction.

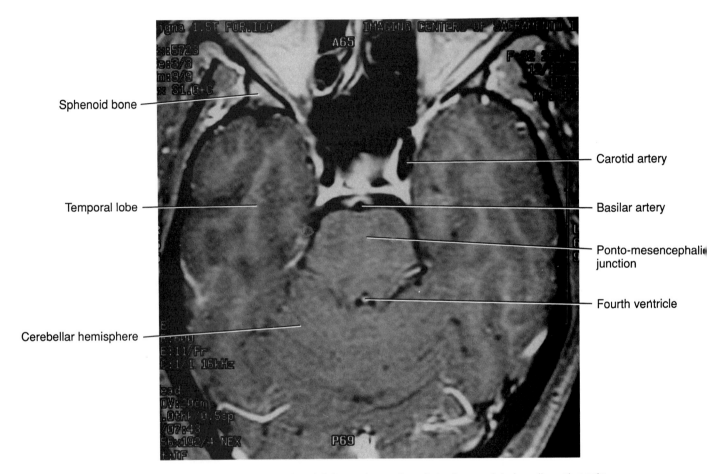

Sphenoid bone

Temporal lobe

Cerebellar hemisphere

Carotid artery

Basilar artery

Ponto-mesencephalic junction

Fourth ventricle

Figure 2.33.   Brain MR. T1-weighted, gadolinium-enhanced, posterior fossa, axial plane through ponto-mesencephalic junction.

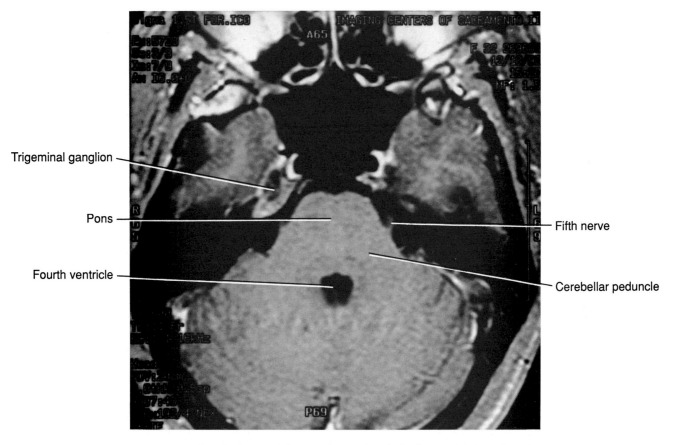

Figure 2.34. **Brain MR.** T1-weighted, gadolinium-enhanced, posterior fossa, axial plane through fifth cranial nerve.

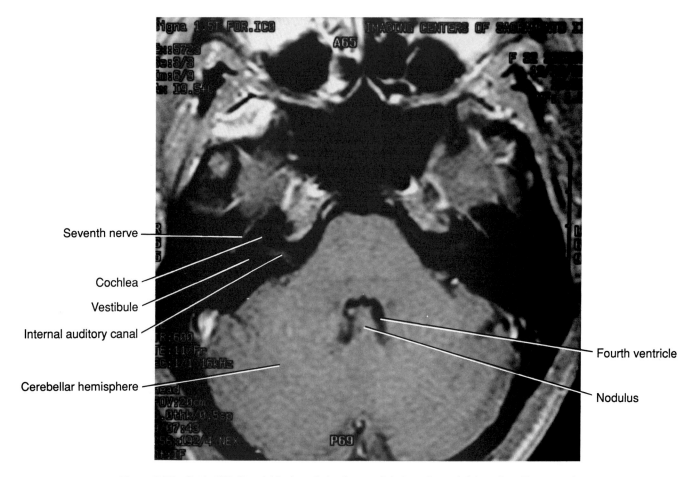

Seventh nerve

Cochlea

Vestibule

Internal auditory canal

Cerebellar hemisphere

Fourth ventricle

Nodulus

Figure 2.35. Brain MR. T1-weighted, posterior fossa, axial plane through internal auditory canal.

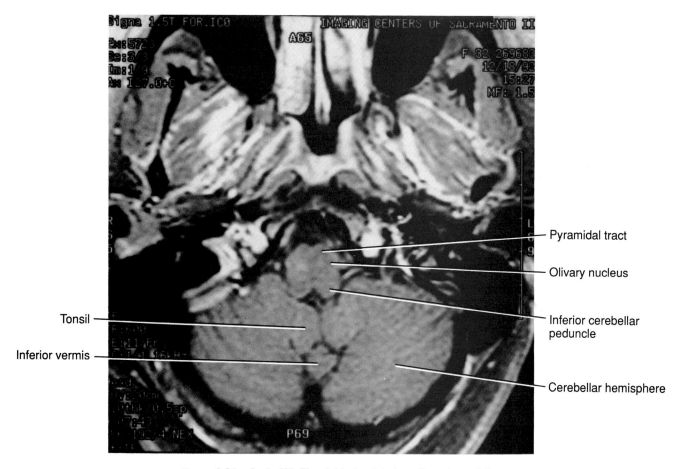

Tonsil

Inferior vermis

Pyramidal tract

Olivary nucleus

Inferior cerebellar peduncle

Cerebellar hemisphere

Figure 2.36. **Brain MR.** T1-weighted, axial plane through medulla.

Looking at the Brain. A few simple principles can be employed to ensure that no neurosurgical emergency is missed, even on a first cursory look at an emergency brain CT at midnight. The middle of the patient's brain should be in the middle of the patient's head and the two sides of the brain should look alike (Figs. 2.1–2.4). While there are important functional asymmetries between the right and left hemispheres, the anatomic underpinnings are subtle and play no role in clinical neuroradiology. Any shift of midline structures is presumed to represent a mass lesion on the side from which the midline is displaced. There are no "sucking" brain wounds that draw the midline toward them. If the interventricular septum (septum pellucidum) and third ventricle are located in the midline, no subfalcine herniation is present (Fig. 2.1).

Symmetry of the brain is the key to evaluation of the nervous system with radiologic studies. Only experience teaches how much asymmetry is within the range of normal variation. Generally, the sulcal pattern should be symmetric. The sulci on one side should be the same size as the corresponding sulci on the other side. The anterior interhemispheric fissure should be visualized (Figs. 2.1 and 2.5). Loss of sulci may represent compression due to mass, or opacification of cerebrospinal fluid (CSF) due to subarachnoid hemorrhage. The sulci should extend to the inner table of the skull. In older patients, however, mild atrophy is normal. Significant medial displacement of the sulci may represent compressed brain due to an extracerebral fluid collection such as a subdural or an epidural hematoma. Because these may be bilateral and similar in density to the brain, care needs to be taken in evaluating the periphery of the brain.

More subtle, but more important, signs of intracranial mass include distortion of the CSF spaces of the posterior fossa and around the base of the brain. The key structures are the quadrigeminal plate cistern and the suprasellar cistern (Figs. 2.2–2.4, 2.10, 2.11, 2.19). Because these CSF spaces are traversed by important neural structures, careful attention to these regions is essential. The quadrigeminal plate cistern in the axial plane has the appearance of a smile and should be symmetric (Figs. 2.2, 2.3). Any asymmetry must be suspect, and abnormality of this cistern may represent rotation of the brainstem due to transtentorial herniation, effacement of the cistern due to cerebellar or brainstem mass, or opacification of the cistern as in subarachnoid hemorrhage.

The suprasellar cistern should look like a pentagon or like the Jewish star, depending upon the angulation of the scan through it (Figs. 2.3, 2.4, 2.10, 2.11). The five corners of the pentagon are the interhemispheric fissure anteriorly, the sylvian cisterns anterolaterally, and the ambient cisterns posterolaterally. The sixth point of the Jewish star is in the interpeduncular fossa posteriorly. The cistern should have the appearance of CSF and structure should be symmetric. The anatomic continuations of this structure should be the same density as CSF. Significant asymmetry may be due to uncal herniation; central mass may be due to sellar or suprasellar tumor; opacification of the cistern may be due to subarachnoid hemorrhage or meningitis.

The final structure that must be evaluated is the ventricular system. it is best to start with the fourth ventricle in the posterior fossa because it is the most difficult to see on CT scanning (Fig. 2.4). Subtle asymmetries of the fourth ventricle may be the only sign of significant intracranial masses. The overall size of the ventricular system is assessed (Figs. 2.1, 2.2, 2.4, 2.6–2.16). Enlarged lateral ventricles and third ventricle in the setting of headache or with signs of intracranial mass may represent hydrocephalus, a potentially fatal yet easily treatable condition. Hydrocephalus is distinguished from enlargement of the ventricular system in atrophy by a discrepancy in the degree of ventricular and sulcal enlargement, and by a characteristic pattern of frontal horn and temporal horn enlargement and a round appearance of the anterior portion of the third ventricle.

When confronted with a CT scan under emergency conditions, ask yourself these five questions.
Is the middle of the brain in the middle of the head?
Do the two sides of the brain look alike?
Are the smile (quadrigeminal plate cistern) and the pentagon (suprasellar cistern) readily apparent?
Is the fourth ventricle in the midline and symmetrical in contour?
Are the lateral ventricles enlarged on the sulci effaced?

If these five questions are answered correctly, there is no neurosurgical emergency requiring immediate intervention. This approach leaves many important diagnoses unmade, but the diseases are either untreatable or the treatment can safely be delayed several hours.

The anatomy of the midline of the brain is extremely complex. Because the structures are not duplicated, principles of symmetry cannot be applied, and midline anatomy must be learned in detail. There are three prime locations to study. The first of these is the suprasellar and sellar region (Figs. 2.10–2.12, 2.18–2.22, 2.28–231). On virtually every MR examination, it is possible to localize the sella turcica, the pituitary gland, pituitary infundibulum, optic chasm, anterior third ventricle, mammillary bodies, and anterior interhemispheric fissure. Important vascular structures are also seen in this region. The tip of the basilar artery and the posterior cerebral arteries are seen posteriorly (Figs. 2.12, 2.22), and the anterior cerebral arteries are visualized anterior and superior to the sella (Fig. 2.10). We can see the anterior cerebral arteries traveling in the interhemispheric fissure (Figs. 2.7, 2.18). Slightly off the midline we see the S-shaped carotid siphons (Fig. 2.10), and the posterior communicating arteries. Parallel to the course of the posterior communicating artery we frequently see the third cranial nerve (Fig. 2.29). In the parasagittal location, associated with the optic chiasm, we also see the optic nerve anteriorly and the optic tract posteriorly (Figs. 2.10, 2.11, 2.29–2.31).

The next important region to study in the midline is the pineal region (Figs. 2.1, 2.8–2.11, 2.30, 2.31). In this area it is crucial to identify the midbrain, the midbrain tegmentum (frequently with a small lucency representing the decussation of the superior cerebellar peduncle), the aqueduct of sylvius, the midbrain tectum with superior and inferior colliculi, the pineal gland, and the superior cerebellar vermian lobules. If the precentral cerebellar vein can be seen in the superior vermian cistern, a mass here is unlikely.

Another region of paramount importance in the midline or immediately parasagittal image is the craniocervical junction (Figs. 2.17, 2.32). Historically, this has been a relative blind spot to the neuroradiologist, so it is particularly important to study this region. The anterior arch of C-1, the odontoid process, and the cervical occipital ligaments are present anteriorly. The sharp inferior edge of the clivus marks the anterior lip of the foramen magnum. The posterior lip is marked by the dark cortical margin of the occipital bone. An imaginary line drawn between these two points should cross no more than 3 mm above the inferior tip of the cerebellar tonsil. Furthermore, the obex, the most posterior projection of the dorsal medulla, should lie above this imaginary line. The only structures visible at this level within the calvarium and spinal canal are the cervical medullary junction and a tiny bit of cerebellar tonsilar tissue. Any other soft tissue in this location is pathologic.

ANALYSIS OF THE ABNORMALITY

Once an abnormality is detected, the goal of the radiologist is to categorize the finding and, if possible, make a specific diagnosis. Given the rather large number, and relatively infrequency, of specific findings of neurologic diseases it is essential to adopt a systematic analytic method in order to narrow the range of differential diagnostic possibilities. Armed with an amalgam of basic clinical, anatomic, and pathologic knowledge, we can create such a system.

The central question in neuroradiology for purposes of lesion analysis is the presence of mass or atrophy. Once the brain has completed its development, any injury resulting in tissue loss is permanent. While functional recovery can occur, tissue loss is virtually never restored. Whenever focal or tissue loss is identified, a strong inference is drawn that the lesion is permanent and untreatable. On the other hand, if the brain is expanded with normal structures displaced away from lesion, the lesion is probably active and potentially treatable. Therefore, the urgency for specific diagnosis is greater.

Mass. The concept of mass effect is an essential starting point. A mass in radiology is recognized by displacement of normal structures away from the abnormality. The term "mass" is used in a sense that differs somewhat from our understanding of mass in physics, where the central feature of mass is its gravitational affect. The term mass in neuroradiology is employed in the sense of an object occupying space. Since two solid objects cannot coexist in the same space, the mass displaces normal cerebral structures away from it. The normal midline structures may be shifted contralateral to the mass. The sulci adjacent to the mass may be effaced since the CSF occupying the sulci is displaced by the mass. Similarly, ipsilateral ventricular structures may be compressed by a mass, rendering the ipsilateral ventricle smaller than the contralateral ventricle. These specific points are summarized by the question: Is there too much tissue within the skull?

Atrophy. Conversely, an atrophic lesion is recognized by the widening of the ipsilateral sulci or enlargement of the ventricle adjacent to the lesion. We may ask the question: Is there too little brain? It is important to note that we have not listed shift of the midline toward the side of the lesion as sign of atrophy. A shift ipsilateral to an atrophic lesion is very unusual. It is only seen commonly in congenital hemiatrophy. Even if a complete hemispherectomy is performed, shift of the midline toward the side of the hemispherectomy defect is almost always a sign of mass in the remaining cerebral hemisphere, or an extraaxial mass compressing it.

When a pattern of diffuse cerebral atrophy is encountered, the first question we must ask is: What is the patient's age? If the patient is over 65 and has normal cognitive function, a diagnosis of age-appropriate cerebral atrophy can be made. Experience teaches us the range of normal to be expected for each age group. If the patient is demented, a diagnosis of Alzheimer's disease may be made on clinical grounds. It has been recently suggested that specific neuroradiologic features of Alzheimer's disease exist, such as focal atrophy of the hippocampal regions of the medial temporal lobe, but this has yet to be confirmed prospectively.

If the patient is under 65 years of age, a large number of relatively rare conditions discussed in Chapter 7 must be considered. It is most important for the radiologist to consider the reversible causes of cerebral atrophy. There are three common causes of reversible cerebral atrophy related to dehydration and starvation. Patients with Addison's disease or other causes of dehydration or abnormal fluid balance may occasionally present with a CT or MR picture of atrophy. With treatment, a more normal appearance of the brain can be restored. Anorexia nervosa and bulimia cause reversible nutritional cerebral atrophy. The relative contribution of dehydration and starvation in these conditions is difficult to determine. Alcoholism may also occasionally result in reversible "cerebral atrophy." Although the neurotoxic effect of the effects of alcohol are not reversible, it has been hypothesized that the accompanying nutritional deficiencies may be corrected, restoring a more normal appearance to the brain on imaging studies.

Should a mass be identified, the first question we must ask is: Is the mass intraaxial, within the brain expanding it, or extraaxial, outside the brain compressing it? This distinction is usually obvious. However, in some cases it is very difficult to distinguish between these two possibilities at a casual glance. This distinction is extremely important because intraaxial masses are more dangerous to the patient and less easily treated than extraaxial masses. Therefore, we concentrate on the diagnosis of extraaxial masses and orient our approach in a manner that maximizes the reliable detection of treatable disease. Intraaxial masses most commonly represent metastases, intracranial hemorrhages, primary intracranial tumors such as glioblastoma, and brain abscesses. Extraaxial masses most commonly represent subdural or epidural hematomas, meningiomas, neuromas, and dermoid or epidermoid cysts, and arachnoid cysts.

In order to distinguish an intraaxial from an extraaxial mass, it is crucial to concentrate on the margins of the mass. Just as the beach is more interesting than the open sea, the interface between the mass and the surrounding brain is more interesting than the center of the mass. Extraaxial masses generally possess a broad dural surface. In contrast, intraaxial masses are surrounded completely by the brain. In the posterior fossa the most reliable sign of an extraaxial mass is widening of the ipsilateral subarachnoid space. That is, the cerebellum and brain stem are displaced away from the bony margins of the calvarium by the mass. If we look at the margins of the mass we can see that the subarachnoid space is widened. In contrast, intraaxial masses demonstrate a narrow ipsilateral subarachnoid space. In the supratentorial compartment we evaluate a mass somewhat differently. With an intraaxial mass, the gyri become larger and larger and the sulci become smaller and farther apart as we approach the center of the mass. The sulci adjacent to an extraaxial mass, on the other hand, become smaller and smaller as we approach the mass.

With the multiplanar capability of MR we are frequently able to visualize the direct displacement of the brain away from the dura by an extraaxial mass. Occasionally, even this observation is difficult to make. When gadolinium is administered, extraaxial masses frequently demonstrate dural enhancement, whereas this is less common with intraaxial masses. Extraaxial masses tend to enhance homogeneously, e.g., meningioma or neuroma, or not at all, e.g., extracerebral hematomas and cysts. Intraaxial lesions tend to enhance in a ring-like or in an irregular fashion. In general, intraaxial masses tend to have more surrounding edema than extraaxial masses of the same size.

Once a mass is identified and its location within or outside the brain is established, the next question we ask is: Is this a solitary lesion or are these multiple lesions? In general, the implication is that a single lesion is more likely to be the result of isolated primary cerebral disease, and that multiple lesions are more likely to be manifestations of widespread or systemic diseases. A single ring-enhancing lesion within the brain may be considered a glioblastoma, although of course, a solitary metastasis cannot be excluded. Multiple ring-enhancing lesions within the brain more likely represent metastases or abscesses. If a single infarct is identified, it is likely to be caused by a lesion within the carotid artery ipsilateral to the lesion. If multiple infarcts are seen, they may represent border zone infarcts due to cardiac arrest or may be due to a cardiac source of emboli.

If a lesion is within the brain and primarily manifest by lucency on a CT scan, or increased signal on the T2-weighted MRI scan, the most important question is whether or not the lesion involves gray matter, white matter, or both. Diseases primarily involving white matter without mass effect are the subject of Chapter 7 and are the result of a wide array of causes. Lesions involving gray matter are usually due to infarct, trauma, or encephalitis. If the lesion has mass effect, these conditions may be said to be acute. If the lesion is atrophic, or there is tissue loss with this distribution, then the lesion may be said to be chronic.

If the white matter is exclusively involved and the lesion is expansile, a pattern of edema is present. Usually this will represent vasogenic edema caused by an intracerebral mass. The frond-like pattern of white matter extension and mass effect is typical. This form of edema results from disturbances in tight capillary junctions that occur in association with cerebral tumors, abscesses, or hematomas. This type of edema tends to progress relatively slowly and persist, over time. If there is relatively more edema compared to the size of the lesion, a tumor or abscess is considered to be more likely than a hematoma.

If there is white matter expansion and increased T2 signal or lucency on CT with gray matter involvement, cytotoxic edema is present. Cytotoxic edema is caused by increased tissue water content due to the neuropathologic response to cell death. In these cases, infarct, trauma, or encephalitis should be considered. This is called the gray matter pattern.

When a gray matter pattern is identified, the distribution of the gray matter abnormality within the brain allows us to distinguish infarct, trauma, and encephalitis. Infarcts are distributed according to vascular patterns described in Chapter 4. For example, if a wedge-shaped lesion involves the opercula of the sylvian fissure, and the underlying white matter and basal ganglia, a diagnosis of middle cerebral artery territory infarct is made. Similarly, if the medial aspect of the cerebral hemisphere anteriorly and over the convexity is involved, an anterior cerebral infarct is diagnosed. If the area of involvement falls immediately between two major vascular territories, a border zone or "watershed" infarct is likely. With multiple border zone infarcts, global hypoperfusion, due to cardiac arrest, must be suspected. If the deep gray matter structures bilaterally are involved, pure anoxia due to carbon monoxide poisoning or respiratory arrest should be considered.

Traumatic lesions occur in a characteristic fashion. They are detailed in Chapter 3. Because of the transmission of forces through the brain and the relationship of the brain to the surrounding skull, traumatic lesions tend to occur at the orbital frontal and frontal polar regions, the temporal poles, and the occipital poles in acceleration/deceleration injuries. A direct blow produces injury beneath the site of the blow and opposite the site of the blow. The lesion opposite the blow is called the contra coup injury. Clearly, this applies to closed-head trauma. Penetrating brain wounds are distributed according to the path of the missile or the location of the trauma.

The most common encephalitic disease, herpes simplex encephalitis, is also distributed in a characteristic fashion. This disease spreads from the oral and nasal mucosa to the trigeminal and olfactory ganglion cells and then transdurally to the brain. The most common locations for involvement in herpes simplex encephalitis are the medial temporal lobes adjacent to the trigeminal ganglia, and the orbital frontal regions adjacent to the olfactory bulbs. Other forms of encephalitis are less common and are diagnosed by typical clinical presentation, characteristic CSF findings, cultures, and mixed gray and white matter patterns of involvement at other sites within the brain (see Chapter 6).

The next question we must ask about a cerebral abnormality is whether it is associated with abnormal contrast enhancement. Enhancement of the brain parenchyma means that the blood brain barrier has broken down, and that the process is biologically active. In fact, in the astrocytoma tumor line an increase in enhancement correlates with higher tumor grade. However, enhancement does not imply malignancy. Infarcts, hemorrhages, abscesses, and encephalitis can all demonstrate contrast enhancement. However, in these nonneoplastic processes, enhancement only occurs in the acute phase and resolves with time.

You will note that we have saved patterns of signal intensity for the last area of discussion. These patterns are specific to the imaging modality or MR pulse sequence employed and are, therefore, the least generally applicable and, to a great extent, the least reliable radiologic findings. Knowledge of the physical basis for imaging with CT and MR is necessary in order to understand the pattern of signal intensities within the brain. However, as a starting point, one needs only to know that if an abnormality is white on CT or white on T1-weighted MR or black on T2-weighted MR, hemorrhage must be considered. This topic is discussed in Chapter 4.

See individual chapters for specific references.

Suggested Readings

Bannister R. Brain's clinical neurology, 5th ed. New York: Oxford, 1978.

Brodal A. Neurological anatomy in relation to clinical medicine, 3rd ed. New York: Oxford, 1981.

Carpenter MB. Text of neuroanatomy, 2nd ed. Baltimore: Williams & Wilkins, 1978.

DeGroot J. Correlative neuroanatomy, 21st ed. Norwalk: Appleton & Lange, 1991.

Escourolle R, Poirier J. Manual of basic neuropathology, 2nd ed. Philadelphia: WB Saunders, 1978.

Gluhbegovic N, Williams TH. The human brain. Philadelphia: Harper and Row, 1980.

Osborn AG. Handbook of neuroradiology. St. Louis: Mosby Yearbook, 1991.

Plum F, Posner JB. The diagnosis of stupor and coma, 3rd ed. Philadelphia: FA Davis, 1980.

Ramsey RG. Neuroradiology, 2nd ed. Philadelphia: WB Saunders, 1980.

Schochet SS, McCormick WF. Essentials of neuropathology. Appleton: New York, 1979.

Sox HC, Blatt MA, Higgins MC, Marton KI. Medical decision making. Stoneham: Butterworth, 1988.

3

Craniofacial Trauma

Robert Barr
Alisa D. Gean

HEAD TRAUMA

Imaging Strategy

COMPUTED TOMOGRAPHY

Imaging of head trauma in the emergency setting is performed to detect potentially treatable lesions before secondary neurologic damage occurs. Currently, this is best performed by computed tomography (CT) for several reasons: it is quick, widely available, accommodates monitoring equipment easily, and is highly accurate in the detection of acute intra- and extraaxial hemorrhage, as well as skull, temporal bone, facial, and orbital fractures.

Computed tomography images must be reviewed using multiple windows. A narrow window width is used to evaluate the brain, a slightly wider window width is used to exaggerate contrast between extraaxial collections and the adjacent skull, and a very wide window is used to evaluate the skull itself (see Figs. 3.1 and 3.6). Contiguous 5-mm sections through the brain provide sufficient detail, and can be obtained with modern scanners in well under 15 minutes. Thinner sections are used to evaluate the orbits, facial skeleton, and skull base. Intravenous contrast media is not used in the acute setting because it may mimic or mask underlying hemorrhage.

MAGNETIC RESONANCE IMAGING

Magnetic resonance imaging (MR) is less desirable than CT in the acute setting because of the longer examination times, difficulty in managing life-support and other monitoring equipment, inferior demonstration of bone detail, and lower sensitivity to acute hemorrhage. Magnetic resonance is superior to CT in the detection of nonhemorrhagic lesions, however, and is more sensitive to subacute and chronic hemorrhage. Further, lesions in the posterior fossa are often obscured on CT by beam-hardening artifact from the surrounding bone but are well seen on MR. In the majority of cases, MR is the modality of choice for patients with subacute and chronic head injury, and is recommended for patients with acute head trauma when neurologic findings are unexplained by CT. Magnetic resonance imaging is also more accurate in predicting long-term prognosis. With the development of faster imaging sequences, improved monitoring equipment, and greater scanner availability, MR is likely to play an increasing role in the evaluation of acute head trauma.

SKULL FILMS

Unfortunately, plain films continue to be used in evaluating patients with acute head trauma, despite abundant evidence that they are not helpful. Patients who are judged to be at low risk for intracranial injury based on a careful history and physical examination should be observed, and patients at high risk should be imaged by CT. Plain films virtually never demonstrate significant findings in the low-risk group, and are inadequate to characterize or exclude intracranial injury in the high-risk group. Further, the absence of skull fractures on plain films clearly does not exclude significant intracranial injury. In fact, in one large series of patients with fatal head injuries, 25% had normal skull films. The decision to obtain a head CT in the setting of trauma must be based on clinical grounds. Skull films are poor predictors of significant

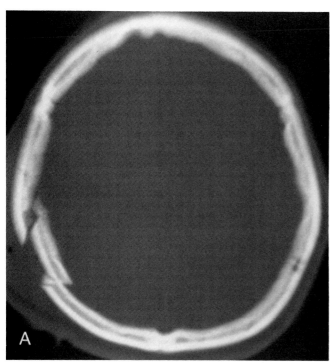
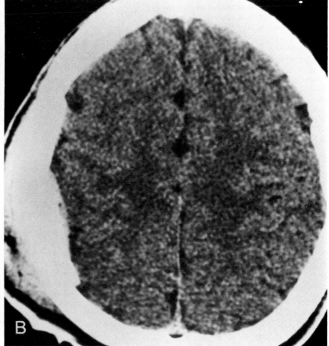

Figure 3.1. Depressed Skull Fracture. A. Axial CT scan demonstrates a right parietal depressed skull fracture with overlying soft-tissue selling. The fracture is well seen using a wide window in order to enhance contrast between bone and soft tissue. **B.** The narrower window demonstrates excellent contrast between gray and white matter but fails to show the fracture. A small extraaxial hematoma is seen in the right parietal area.

intracranial pathology and should not be used either to prevent or encourage further diagnostic evaluation.

Classification of Head Injury

The manifestations of head trauma can be divided into primary and secondary lesions. Primary lesions are those that occur at the time of trauma as a direct result of the traumatic force. Secondary lesions occur as a consequence of primary lesions, usually as a result of mass effect or vascular compromise. This division is clinically important because secondary lesions are often preventable, whereas primary injuries, by definition, have already occurred by the time the patient arrives in the emergency department.

Primary lesions include scalp injury, skull fractures, and extraaxial hemorrhage (epidural, subdural, subarachnoid, and intraventricular) as well as the different forms of neuronal injury. The four major types of primary neuronal injury are diffuse axonal injury (DAI), cortical contusions, intracerebral hematomas, and subcortical gray matter injury. Direct injury to the cerebral vasculature is another type of primary lesion.

The types of secondary lesions that will be discussed include cerebral swelling, brain herniation, hydrocephalus, ischemia/infarction, cerebrospinal fluid (CSF) leak, leptomeningeal cyst, and encephalomalacia. Brainstem injury, which is also divided into primary and secondary forms, will be discussed separately, as will injury from penetrating trauma and head injury from child abuse. Lastly, facial trauma will be discussed.

Primary Head Injury

SCALP INJURY

When interpreting CT scans for head trauma, it is helpful to begin by examining the extracranial structures for evidence of scalp injury or radiopaque foreign bodies. Scalp soft-tissue swelling is often the only reliable evidence of the site of impact. The subgaleal hematoma is the most common manifestation of scalp injury and can be recognized on CT or MR as a relatively well-defined soft-tissue swelling of the scalp located beneath the subcutaneous fibrofatty tissue and above the temporalis muscle and calvarium.

CALVARIAL FRACTURES

Nondisplaced linear fractures of the calvarium are the most common type of skull fracture. They may be difficult to detect on CT scans, especially when the fracture plane is parallel to the plane of section. Fortunately, isolated linear skull fractures do not require treatment. Surgical management is usually indicated for depressed and compound skull fractures, both of which are seen better on CT scans than plain films

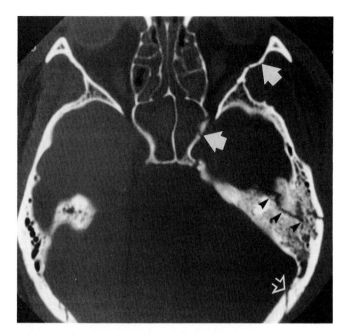

Figure 3.2. Longitudinal Temporal Bone Fracture. Axial CT scan shows a longitudinal left temporal bone fracture (*arrowheads*) with opacification of the mastoid air cells. Diastasis of the left lambdoid suture (*open arrow*) and fractures of the sphenoid sinus (*black arrow*) and left lateral orbital wall (*white arrow*) are also present.

(Fig. 3.1). Depressed fractures are frequently associated with an underlying contusion. Intracranial air ("pneumocephalus") may be seen with compound skull fractures or fractures involving the paranasal sinuses. Thin-section CT using a bone algorithm is the best method to evaluate fractures in critical areas, such as the skull base, orbit, or facial bones. Thin sections can also be helpful to evaluate the degree of comminution and depression of bone fragments.

TEMPORAL BONE FRACTURES

Thin-section, high-resolution CT scanning has led to a dramatic improvement in the ability to detect and characterize temporal bone fractures. Patients with fractures of the temporal bone may present with deafness, facial nerve palsies, vertigo, dizziness, or nystagmus. Clinical symptoms are often masked in the presence of other serious injuries, however. Physical signs of temporal bone fracture include hemotympanum, CSF otorrhea, and ecchymosis over the mastoid process ("Battle's sign"). Temporal bone fractures may be first suspected on standard head CT scans performed to exclude intracranial injury. Findings such as opacification of the mastoid air cells, fluid in the middle ear cavity, pneumocephalus, or occasionally, pneumolabyrinth, should raise the suspicion of a temporal bone fracture. Optimal evaluation of a suspected temporal bone fracture requires thin-section (1.5 mm) axial and direct coronal CT imaging using a bone algorithm.

Fractures of the temporal bone can be classified as longitudinal or transverse depending on their orientation relative to the long axis of the petrous bone. If the fracture parallels the long axis of the petrous pyramid it is termed a "longitudinal" fracture; fractures perpendicular to the long axis of the petrous bone are termed "transverse" fractures. "Mixed" fracture types also occur.

The longitudinal temporal bone fracture represents 70–90% of temporal bone fractures. It results from a blow to the side of the head. Complications include conductive hearing loss, dislocation or fracture of the ossicles, and CSF otorhinorrhea. Facial nerve palsy may occur, but is often delayed and incomplete. Sensorineural hearing loss is uncommon (Fig. 3.2).

The transverse temporal bone fracture usually results from a blow to the occiput or frontal region. Complications are usually more severe and include sensorineural hearing loss, severe vertigo, nystagmus, and perilymphatic fistula. Facial palsy is seen in 30–50% of these cases and is often complete. Transverse fractures may also involve the carotid canal or jugular foramen, causing injury to the carotid artery or jugular vein.

Mixed or complex temporal bone fractures represent about 10% of temporal bone fractures. They involve a combination of fracture planes and generally follow severe crushing blows to the skull. Patients with mixed temporal bone fractures have a high incidence of associated intracranial injury.

EXTRAAXIAL HEMORRHAGE

Epidural Hematoma. Epidural hematomas are usually arterial in origin and often result from a skull fracture that disrupts the middle meningeal artery. The developing hematoma strips the dura from the inner table of the skull, forming an ovoid mass that displaces the adjacent brain. They may occur from stretching or tearing of meningeal arteries without an associated fracture, especially in children. Overall, skull fractures are seen in 85–95% of cases. In about a third of patients with an epidural hematoma, neurologic deterioration occurs after a lucid interval.

Most epidural hematomas are temporal or temporoparietal in location, though frontal and occipital epidural hematomas can also occur. Venous epidural hematomas are less common than arterial epidurals and tend to occur at the vertex, posterior fossa, or anterior aspect of the middle cranial fossa. Venous epidural hematomas usually occur as a result of disrupted dural venous sinuses.

On CT, acute epidural hematomas appear as well-defined, high attenuation lenticular or biconvex extraaxial collections (Fig. 3.3). Associated mass effect with sulcal effacement and midline shift is frequently seen. Bone windows usually demonstrate an overlying

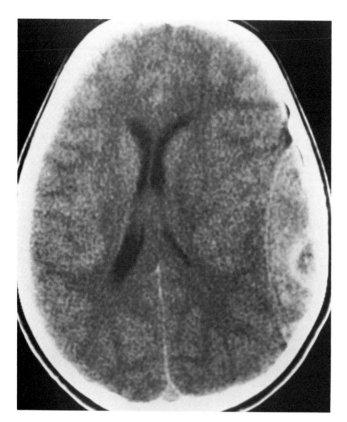

Figure 3.3. Epidural Hematoma. Axial CT scan demonstrates a biconvex high attenuation extraaxial collection causing mass effect on the left temporal lobe and mild midline shift (subfalcial herniation).

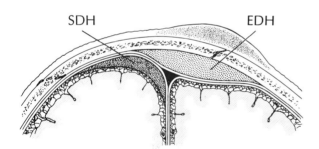

Figure 3.4. Epidural Versus Subdural Hematoma. Coronal diagram of the brain surface near the vertex demonstrates the characteristic locations of the epidural hematoma (*EDH*) compared with the subdural hematoma (*SDH*). Note how the EDH is located above the outer dural layer and the SDH is located beneath the inner dural layer. Only the EDH can cross the falx cerebri.

linear skull fracture. Because epidural hematomas exist in the potential space between the dura and inner table of the skull, they can cross the midline but will not cross the cranial sutures, where the dura is more firmly attached (Fig. 3.4). Occasionally an acute epidural hematoma will appear heterogeneous, containing irregular areas of lower attenuation. This finding indicates active extravasation of fresh unclotted blood into the collection and warrants immediate surgical attention.

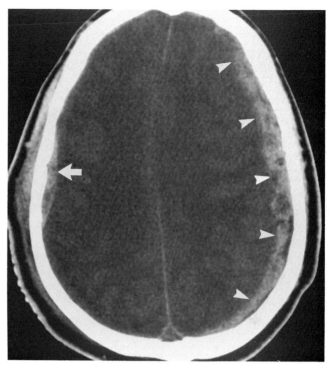

Figure 3.5. Left Subdural and Right Epidural Hematomas. Axial CT scan demonstrates a crescent-shaped high attenuation collection extending along the entire left hemisphere consistent with a subdural hematoma (*arrowheads*). Compare the appearance with that of a small epidural hematoma seen on the right (*arrow*) where overlying scalp soft-tissue swelling is also present.

Subdural Hematomas are usually venous in origin, resulting from stretching or tearing of cortical veins that traverse the subdural space en route to the dural sinuses. They may, however, also result from disruption of penetrating branches of superficial cerebral arteries. Because the inner dural layer and arachnoid are not as firmly attached as the structures that make up the epidural space, the subdural hematoma typically extends over a much larger area than the epidural hematoma. Patients with a subdural hematoma commonly present after acute deceleration injury from a motor vehicle accident or fall. The same mechanism can cause cortical contusions and DAI, which are frequently seen in association with acute subdural hematomas.

On axial CT, acute subdural hematomas appear as crescent-shaped extraaxial collections of high attenuation (Fig. 3.5). Small subdural hematomas may be masked by adjacent cortical bone when viewed on a narrow window width but will be seen with an intermediate window width (Fig. 3.6). Most subdural hematomas are supratentorial, located along the convexity. They are also frequently seen along the falx and tentorium. Because dural reflections form the falx cerebri and tentorium, subdural collections will not cross these structures (Fig. 3.4). However, unlike epidural hematomas, subdural hematomas

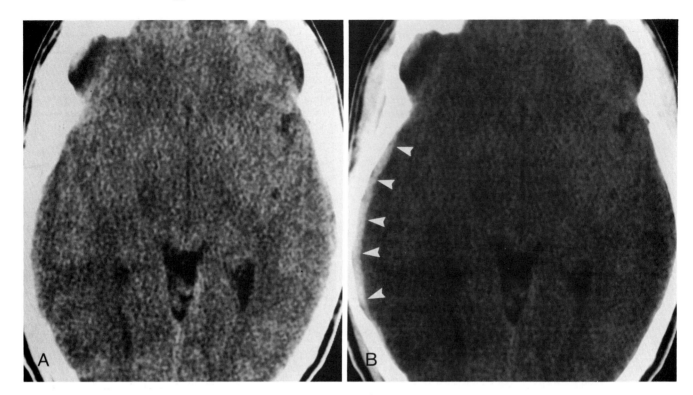

Figure 3.6. Subdural Hematoma Seen on Intermediate Window Only. On this axial CT scan, a small right temporal subdural hematoma is masked using a narrow window (**A**), but is clearly seen (*arrowheads*) with an intermediate (or subdural) window (**B**).

can cross sutural margins, and, in fact, are frequently seen layering along the entire hemispheric convexity from the anterior falx to the posterior falx. Diffuse swelling of the underlying hemisphere is common with subdural hematomas. Because of this, there may be more mass effect than would be expected by the size of the collection, and little or no reduction in midline shift after evacuation of a hemispheric subdural hematoma.

The CT appearance of subdural hematomas changes with time. Initially, extravasated blood is hyperdense, measuring 50–60 Hounsfield units (HU), relative to normal brain, which measures 18–30 HU. The density of an acute subdural hematoma initially increases slightly because of clot retraction. The density will then progressively decrease as protein degradation occurs within the hematoma. Occasionally, rebleeding occurs during evolution of a subdural hematoma causing a heterogeneous appearance from the mixture of fresh blood and partially liquefied hematoma (Fig. 3.7). A sediment level or "hematocrit effect" may be seen either from rebleeding or in patients with clotting disorders (Fig. 3.8). Chronic subdural hematomas have low attenuation values similar to CSF (Fig. 3.9). On noncontrast CT scans, it can be difficult to distinguish them from prominent subarachnoid space secondary to cerebral atrophy.

During the transition in appearance from acute to chronic subdural hematomas, an isodense phase occurs, usually between several days and 3 weeks after the acute event. Although the subdural hematoma itself is less conspicuous during this isodense phase, there are indirect signs on a noncontrast CT scan that should lead to the correct diagnosis. These include effacement of sulci, displacement of cortex with white matter "buckling," and midline shift (Fig. 3.10). Contrast enhancement can help identify nonacute subdural hematomas by demonstrating an enhancing capsule or displaced cortical veins. This is especially helpful in distinguishing chronic subdural hematomas from prominent subarachnoid spaces. Acute subdural hematomas may be isodense relative to the brain in patients with severe anemia.

The MR appearance of subdural hematomas depends on the biochemical state of hemoglobin, which varies with the age of the hematoma (see Chapter 4). Acute subdural hematomas are isointense to brain on T1-weighted images and hypointense on T2-weighted images. Magnetic resonance imaging is particularly helpful during the subacute phase, when the subdural hematoma may be isodense or hypodense on CT scans. T1-weighted images will demonstrate high signal intensity caused by the presence of methemoglobin in the subdural collection. This high signal clearly distinguishes subdural hematomas from most nonhemorrhagic fluid collections. Magnetic resonance imaging also reveals that subacute subdural hematomas frequently have a lentiform or biconvex appearance when seen in the coronal plane, rather than the crescent-shaped appearance that is characteristic on

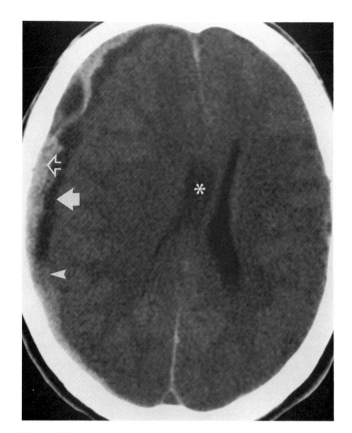

Figure 3.7. Acute and Chronic Subdural Hematoma. Axial CT scan demonstrates the heterogeneous appearance of superimposed acute and chronic subdural hematomas. The higher attenuation material (*open arrow*) represents fresh bleeding into a chronic, low attenuation subdural hematoma (**closed arrow**). Layering of acute blood products is seen in the posterior aspect of the collection (*arrowhead*). Midline shift or "subfalcial herniation" is also present, evidenced by displacement of the right lateral ventricle (*asterisk*) across midline.

axial CT scans (Fig. 3.11). The multiplanar capability of MR scanning is helpful in identifying small convexity and vertex hematomas that might not be detected on axial CT scans because of the similar attenuation of the adjacent bone.

Subarachnoid Hemorrhage is common in head injury but is rarely large enough to cause a significant mass effect. It results from the disruption of small subarachnoid vessels or direct extension into the subarachnoid space by a contusion or hematoma. On CT, subarachnoid hemorrhage appears as linear areas of high attenuation within the cisterns and sulci (Fig. 3.12). Subarachnoid collections along the convexity or tentorium can be differentiated from subdural hematomas by their extension into adjacent sulci. Occasionally the only finding is apparent effacement of sulci when the sulci are filled with small amounts of blood. In patients who are found unconscious after an unwitnessed event, it is important to remember that the detection of subarachnoid hemorrhage may indicate a ruptured aneurysm, rather than trauma, as the

primary etiology. In such cases, angiography needs to be considered.

Acute subarachnoid hemorrhage is more difficult to detect on MR than it is on CT scans because it is isointense to brain parenchyma. Subacute subarachnoid hemorrhage may be better appreciated on MR because of its high signal intensity at a time when the blood is isointense to CSF on CT. Chronic hemorrhage on MR scans may show hemosiderin staining in the subarachnoid space, which appears as areas of markedly decreased signal intensity on T1- and T2-weighted sequences ("superficial hemosiderosis"). Subarachnoid hemorrhage may lead to subsequent hydrocephalus by impaired CSF resorption at the level of arachnoid villi.

Intraventricular Hemorrhage is commonly seen in patients with head injuries and can occur by several mechanisms. First, it can result from rotationally induced tearing of subependymal veins on the surface of the ventricles. Another mechanism is by direct extension of a parenchymal hematoma into the ventricular system. Third, intraventricular blood can result from retrograde flow of subarachnoid hemorrhage into the ventricular system through the fourth ventricular outflow foramina. Patients with intraventricular hemorrhage are at risk for subsequent hydrocephalus by obstruction either at the level of the aqueduct or arachnoid villi.

On CT, interventricular hemorrhage appears as hyperdense material layering dependently within the ventricular system. Tiny collections of increased density layering in the occipital horns may be the only clue to intraventricular hemorrhage.

INTRAAXIAL INJURY

Diffuse Axonal Injury is one of the most common types of primary neuronal injury in patients with severe head trauma. As the name implies, DAI is characterized by widespread disruption of axons that occurs at the time of an acceleration or deceleration injury. The affected areas of the brain may be distant from the site of direct impact; in fact, direct impact is not necessary to cause this type of injury.

The incidence of DAI was likely underestimated until recently because of the difficulty in visualizing these lesions on existing imaging studies as well as on histologic specimens. Diffuse axonal injury is much better seen by MR than CT. This factor accounts to a large degree for the increased success of MR at explaining neurologic deficits after trauma and in predicting long-term outcome. Though MR has improved the detection of DAI in head trauma patients, the overall incidence of this form of injury is probably still underestimated, even with MR.

Patients with DAI are most commonly injured in high-speed motor vehicle accidents. These lesions

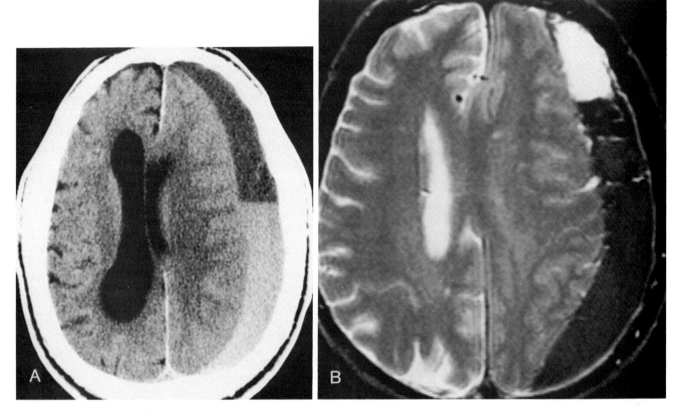

Figure 3.8. Subdural Hematomas with Hematocrit Effect. A CT scan (**A**) and T2-weighted MR scan (**B**) in two different patients show large left hemispheric subdural hematomas with fluid-fluid levels, known as the hematocrit effect. This appearance can be seen in patients with clotting disorders or in patients with rebleeding into an older subdural collection.

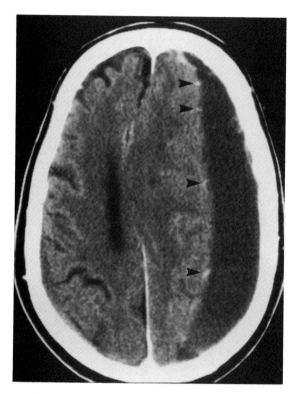

Figure 3.9. Chronic Subdural Hematoma. Contrast-enhanced CT scans shows a large water-density left subdural collection consistent with a chronic subdural hematoma. There is considerable mass effect with midline shift. Displaced cortical veins can be seen along the brain surface (*arrows*).

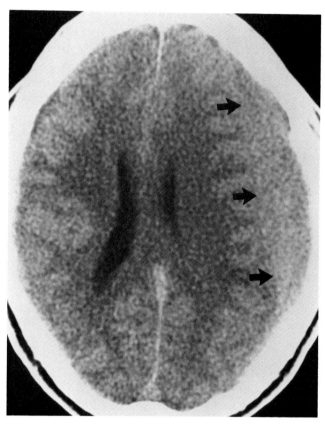

Figure 3.10. Subacute Subdural Hematoma on CT. Noncontrast CT scan shows an isodense left subdural hematoma with displacement of the underlying cortex (*arrows*), compression of the lateral ventricle, and mild midline shift.

have not been seen as a consequence of simple falls, such as when a patient falls from the standing position. Loss of consciousness typically starts immediately after the injury and is more severe than in patients with cortical contusions or hematomas.

On MR, nonhemorrhagic DAI lesions appear as small foci of increased signal on T2-weighted images (T2 prolongation) within the white matter (Fig. 3.13). The lesions tend to be multiple, with up to 15–20 lesions seen in patients with severe head injury. If seen on T1-weighted images, they appear as subtle areas of decreased intensity. Petechial hemorrhage causes a central hypointensity on T2-weighted images and hyperintensity on T1-weighted images within a few days as a result of intracellular methemoglobin. The conspicuity of DAI on MR diminishes over weeks to months as the damaged axons degenerate and the edema resolves. Residual findings might include nonspecific atrophy or hemosiderin staining, which can persist for years and is especially obvious on gradient-echo sequences (Fig. 3.14).

Diffuse axonal injury is seen in characteristic locations that correlate with the severity of the trauma. Patients with the mildest forms of injury have lesions confined to the frontal and temporal white matter,

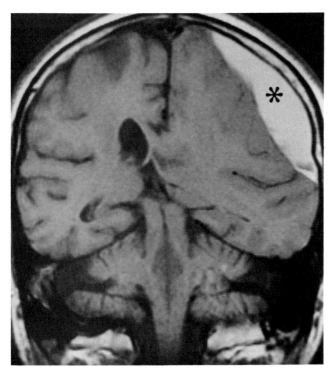

Figure 3.11. Subacute Subdural Hematoma on MR. Noncontrast coronal T1-weighted MR scan shows a well-defined, uniform, hyperintense extraaxial collection (*asterisk*) with associated mass effect on the left cerebral hemisphere. This represents a subacute subdural hematoma. The increased signal intensity on a T1-weighted sequence is attributable to methemoglobin. Subdural hematomas can appear crescent-shaped in the axial plane and biconvex in the coronal plane.

near the gray-white junction. The lesions typically involve the parasagittal regions of the frontal lobes and periventricular regions of the temporal lobes. Patients with more severe trauma have DAI involving lobar white matter as well as the corpus callosum, especially the posterior body and splenium. The corpus callosum accounts for about 20% of all DAI lesions. Initially thought to be caused by direct impact from the falx, experimental work shows that injury to the corpus callosum is most commonly caused by rotational shear forces, like all forms of DAI. The corpus callosum may be particularly susceptible to DAI because the falx prevents displacement of the cerebral hemispheres. Diffuse axonal injury of the corpus callosum is almost always seen in association with lesions in the lobar white matter. Diffuse axonal injury in the most severe cases involves the dorsolateral aspect of the midbrain and upper pons in addition to the lobar white matter and corpus callosum (see the section on "Brainstem Injury").

Computed tomography findings in DAI can be subtle or absent. Only about 20% of lesions contain sufficient hemorrhage to be visible on CT scans, accounting for the low sensitivity of this modality. Most common is the finding of small, petechial hemorrhages at the gray-white junction of the cerebral hemispheres or corpus callosum (Fig. 3.15). Ill-defined areas of decreased attenuation on CT may occasionally be seen with nonhemorrhagic lesions.

Cortical Contusions are areas of focal brain injury primarily involving superficial gray matter. Patients with cortical contusions are much less likely to have loss of consciousness at the time of injury than patients with DAI. Contusions are also associated with a better prognosis than DAI. They are very common in patients with severe head trauma and are usually well seen on CT scans. Contusions characteristically occur near bony protuberances of the skull and skull base. They tend to be multiple and bilateral and are more commonly hemorrhagic than DAI. Common sites are the temporal lobes above the petrous bone or posterior to the greater sphenoid wing, and the frontal lobes above the cribriform plate, planum sphenoidale, and lesser sphenoid wing (Fig. 3.16). Less than 10% of lesions involve the cerebellum. Contusions can also occur at the margins of depressed skull fractures.

The CT appearance of cortical contusions characteristically varies with the age of the lesion. Many nonhemorrhagic lesions are initially poorly seen but become more obvious during the 1st week because of associated edema. Hemorrhagic lesions are seen as foci of high attenuation within superficial gray matter (Fig. 3.17). These may be surrounded by larger areas of low attenuation secondary to surrounding edema. During the 1st week, the characteristic CT pattern of mixed areas of hypo- and hyperdensity ("salt and pep-

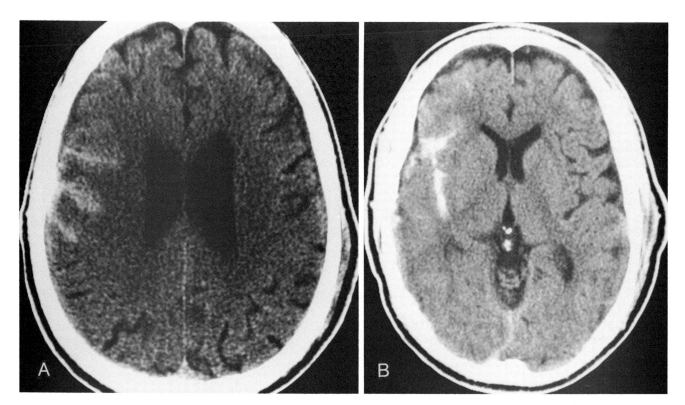

Figure 3.12. Subarachnoid Hemorrhage. Noncontrast axial CT scans in two different patients demonstrate high attenuation mate- rial within the sulci (**A**) and right sylvian fissure (**B**) consistent with sub- arachnoid hemorrhage.

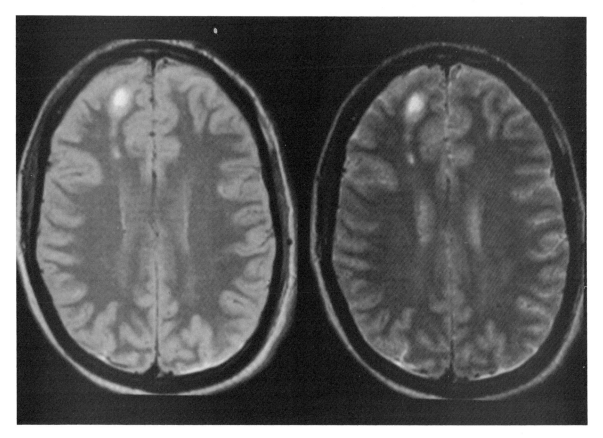

Figure 3.13. The MR Appearance of Acute DAI. Proton-density (*left*) and T2-weighted (*right*) MR images show several adjacent foci of high signal representing DAI in the right frontal parasagittal white matter.

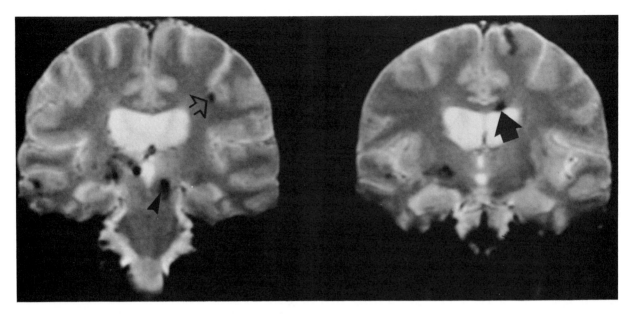

Figure 3.14.   The MR Appearance of Chronic DAI. Coronal gradient-echo images in a patient with a history of prior severe head trauma demonstrate numerous hypointense foci in a distribution characteristic of DAI, including the gray-white junction (*open arrow*), corpus callosum (*closed arrow*), and cerebral peduncle (*arrowhead*). Evidence of remote hemorrhage is especially conspicuous on gradient-echo sequences.

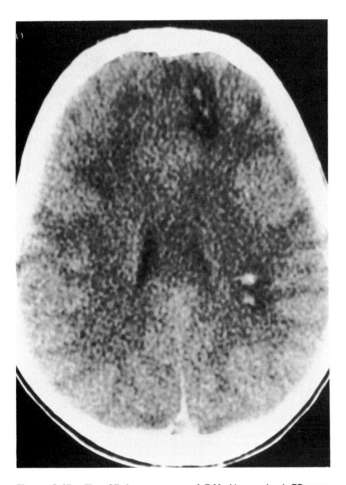

Figure 3.15.   The CT Appearance of DAI. Noncontrast CT scan shows punctate high attenuation foci with surrounding edema in the left frontal and parietal white matter consistent with hemorrhagic DAI. Additional lesions could be seen at other levels.

per" pattern) becomes more apparent. Occasionally, surgical decompression of the contused brain is required to alleviate severe mass effect. Areas of prior contusion can often be recognized as foci of encephalomalacia within the same characteristic locations described above.

On MR imaging, contusions appear as poorly marginated areas of increased signal on proton-density and T2-weighted sequences. They are recognized because of their characteristic distribution in the frontal and temporal lobes, and often have a "gyral" morphology. Hemorrhage causes a markedly heterogeneous pattern of signal intensity on all sequences which varies depending on the age of the lesion (Fig. 3.18). Hemosiderin staining from hemorrhage of any cause leads to markedly decreased signal intensity on T2-weighted images, especially at higher field strengths. This signal loss can persist indefinitely as a marker of prior hemorrhage.

Intracerebral Hematoma. Occasionally, intraparenchymal hemorrhage is seen that is not necessarily associated with cortical contusion but rather represents shear-induced hemorrhage from the rupture of small intraparenchymal blood vessels. This lesion is known simply as an intracerebral hematoma. Intracerebral hematomas tend to have less surrounding edema than cortical contusions because they represent bleeding into areas of relatively normal brain. Most intracerebral hematomas are located in the frontotemporal white matter, though they have also been described in the basal ganglia. They are often associated with skull fractures and other primary neu-

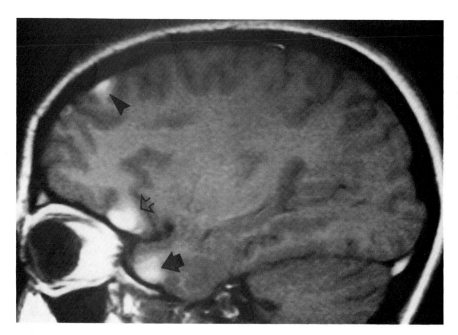

Figure 3.16. The MR Appearance of Cortical Contusion. Sagittal T1-weighted MR scan demonstrates multiple peripheral areas of increased signal intensity involving the inferior frontal (*open arrow*), anterior temporal (*closed arrow*), and superior frontal lobes (*arrowhead*) consistent with subacute hemorrhage from cortical contusion.

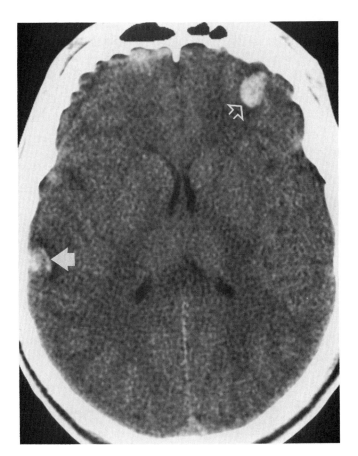

Figure 3.17. The CT Appearance of Cortical Contusion. Noncontrast CT scan reveals high attenuation lesions involving the left frontal (*open arrow*) and right temporal (*closed arrow*) gray matter consistent with hemorrhagic cortical contusions.

ronal lesions, including contusions and DAI. In the absence of other significant lesions, patients with in-

tracerebral hematomas can remain lucid after their injury. When symptoms develop, they commonly result from the mass effect associated with an expanding hematoma. Intracerebral hematomas can also present late secondary to delayed hemorrhage, which is another cause of clinical deterioration during the first several days after head trauma (Fig. 3.19).

Subcortical Gray Matter Injury is an uncommon manifestation of primary intraaxial injury and is seen as multiple, petechial hemorrhages primarily affecting the basal ganglia and thalamus. These represent microscopic perivascular collections of blood that may result from disruption of multiple small perforating vessels. These lesions are typically seen following severe head trauma.

Vascular Injuries as causes of intra- and extraaxial hematomas were discussed previously. Other types of traumatic vascular injury include arterial dissection or occlusion, pseudoaneurysm formation, and the acquired arteriovenous fistula. Arterial injury commonly accompanies fractures of the base of the skull. The internal carotid is the most often injured artery, especially at sites of fixation. These include its entrance to the carotid canal at the base of the petrous bone and at its exit from the cavernous sinus below the anterior clinoid process.

Magnetic resonance imaging findings of vascular injury include the presence of an intramural hematoma or intimal flap with dissection, or the absence of normal vascular flow void with occlusion. An associated parenchymal infarction might also be seen. There is a potential role for MR angiography in evaluating patients at risk for traumatic vascular injury. Conventional angiograms are usually needed to con-

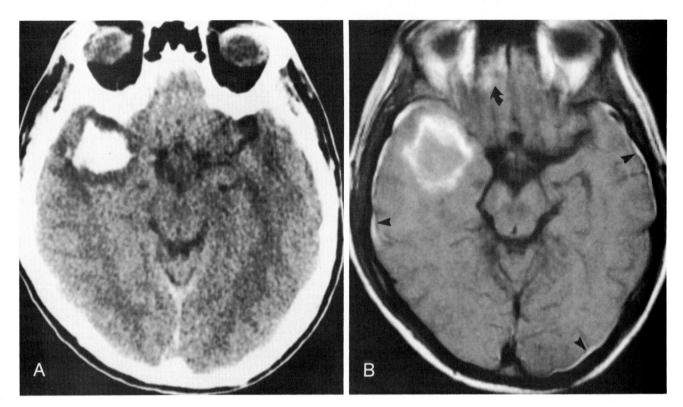

Figure 3.18.   Intracerebral Hematoma. A. Axial CT scan demonstrates a high attenuation mass within the right temporal lobe. **B.** The corresponding T1-weighted MR scan demonstrates a central region of isointensity consistent with acute hemorrhage (deoxyhemoglobin). The surrounding high signal intensity rim represents the conversion to methemoglobin, which begins to form at the periphery of a hematoma. High signal in the inferior right frontal lobe represents an associated frontal contusion (*curved arrow*). A small amount of subdural blood is also present bilaterally and is hyperintense (*arrowheads*).

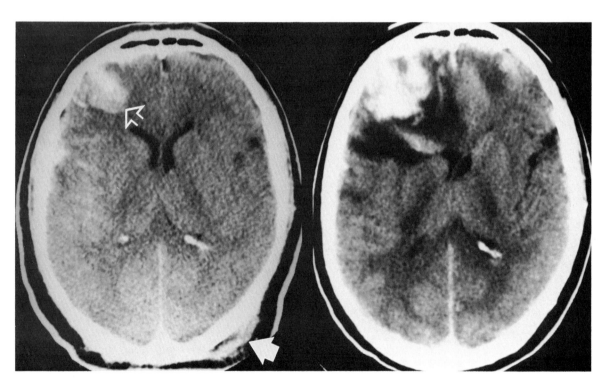

Figure 3.19.   Delayed Hemorrhage. Admission CT scan (*left*) shows a small right frontal hematoma without significant mass effect (*open arrow*). Left parietal soft-tissue swelling indicates the site of impact (*closed arrow*). A follow-up CT scan (*right*) was performed when the patient's clinical condition deteriorated and demonstrates marked increase in the size of the hematoma with increased edema, mass effect, and compression of the ipsilateral frontal horn.

firm and delineate dissections and may also show spasm or pseudoaneurysm formation in injuries to the vessel wall.

The carotid cavernous fistula (CCF) is a communication between the cavernous portion of the internal carotid artery and the surrounding venous plexus. The lesion typically follows a full-thickness arterial injury, resulting in venous engorgement of the cavernous sinus and its draining tributaries (e.g., the ipsilateral superior ophthalmic vein and inferior petrosal sinus). Findings may be bilateral because venous channels connect the cavernous sinuses. The CCF most often results from severe head injury. Skull base fractures, especially those involving the sphenoid bone, indicate patients at increased risk for associated cavernous carotid injury. The CCF may also result from ruptured cavernous carotid aneurysms. On MR, the CCF may manifest as enlarged superior ophthalmic vein, cavernous sinus, and petrosal sinus flow voids. There may be evidence of proptosis, swelling of the preseptal soft tissues, and enlargement of the extraocular musculature. Diagnosis usually requires selective carotid angiography with rapid filming to demonstrate the site of communication (Fig. 3.20). On occasion, patients present with findings weeks or months after the initial trauma.

Dural fistulas are also associated with trauma. For example, they may be caused by laceration of the middle meningeal artery with resultant meningeal artery to meningeal vein fistula formation. Drainage via meningeal veins prevents formation of an epidural hematoma. Patients may be asymptomatic or present with nonspecific complaints, including tinnitus.

MECHANISMS OF PRIMARY HEAD INJURY

Early research suggested that head injuries could be explained by areas of parenchymal compression and rarefaction caused by direct impact. Many authors still use the terms "coup" and "contrecoup" to describe intracranial lesions that characteristically occur both on and opposite the side of a blow to the head. More recently, however, Gentry and others have questioned the use of these terms, which they feel incorrectly imply that neuronal injury is caused by compression and rarefaction strains subsequent to direct impact.

Gennarelli et al. have shown in a primate model that all major types of intraaxial lesions, as well as subdural hematomas, can be produced purely by rotational acceleration of the head without direct impact. Only skull fractures and epidural hematomas require a physical blow to the head. Rotational acceleration causes damage by shear forces, rather than by compression-rarefaction strain. Compression-rarefaction strain is not felt to play a significant role in most head injuries.

The character of the accelerational force influences the type of injury produced. Cortical contusions and intracranial hematomas are more severe when the period of acceleration or deceleration is very short, whereas DAI and gliding contusions are associated with a longer acceleration or deceleration injury. Thus, DAI is more common in motor vehicle accidents while contusions and hematomas are more frequent in falls.

Secondary Head Injury

CEREBRAL SWELLING

Diffuse cerebral swelling is a common manifestation of head trauma. It may occur either because of an increase in cerebral blood volume or an increase in tissue fluid content. Hyperemia refers to an increase in blood volume, whereas cerebral edema refers to an increase in tissue fluid. Both lead to generalized mass effect with effacement of sulci, suprasellar and quadrigeminal plate cisterns, and compression of the ventricular system. Effacement of the brainstem cisterns indicates severe mass effect and may herald impending transtentorial herniation.

Cerebral swelling from hyperemia is most commonly seen in children and adolescents. The pathogenesis is poorly understood but appears to be due to loss of normal cerebral autoregulation. Hyperemia is recognized on CT as ill-defined mass effect, effacement of sulci, and *normal* attenuation of brain. Acute subdural hematomas are often associated with unilateral swelling of the ipsilateral hemisphere.

Diffuse cerebral edema occurs secondary to tissue hypoxia. Because of the increase in tissue fluid, edema causes *decreased* attenuation on CT images with loss of gray-white differentiation. The cerebellum and brainstem are usually spared and may appear hyperdense relative to the cerebral hemispheres (Fig. 3.21). Often the falx and cerebral vessels appear dense, mimicking acute subarachnoid hemorrhage. Focal areas of edema are frequently seen in association with cortical contusions and may contribute significantly to mass effect.

BRAIN HERNIATION

Several forms of herniation are seen secondary to mass effect produced by primary intracranial injury. These are not specific for head trauma and can be seen secondary to mass effect produced by other causes as well, including intracranial hemorrhage, infarction, or neoplasm (Fig. 3.22).

Subfalcial Herniation, in which the cingulate gyrus is displaced across the midline under the falx cerebri, is the most common form of brain hernia-

Figure 3.20. Carotid Cavernous Fistula.
A. A CT scan shows fullness in the right cavernous sinus (*open arrow*) and right proptosis, with swelling of the extraocular muscles (*closed arrows*) and preseptal soft tissues (*arrowheads*). **B.** Internal carotid angiogram in a different patient shows opacification of the cavernous sinus (*open arrow*) and jugular vein (*closed arrow*) during the arterial phase.

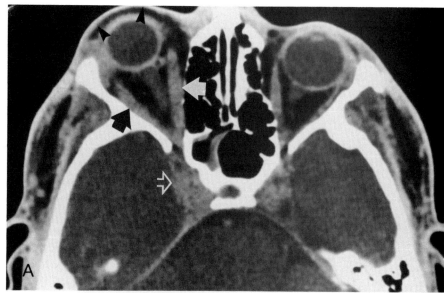

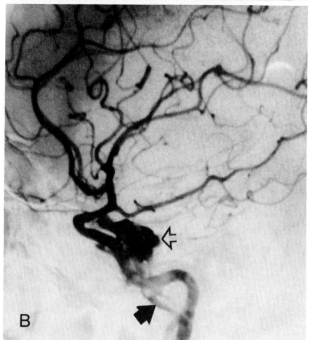

tion (Fig. 3.7). Compression of the adjacent lateral ventricle may be seen on CT scans, as well as enlargement of the contralateral ventricle from obstruction at the level of the foramen of Monro. Both anterior cerebral arteries (ACAs) may be displaced to the contralateral side. These patients are at risk of ACA infarction in the distribution of the callosomarginal branch of the ACA where it becomes trapped against the falx.

Uncal Herniation, in which the medial aspect of the temporal lobe is displaced medially over the free margin of the tentorium, is also common (Fig. 3.23). Uncal herniation causes focal effacement of the ambient cistern and the lateral aspect of the suprasellar cistern. Rarely, displacement of the brainstem causes compression of the *contralateral* cerebral peduncle against the tentorial margin, resulting in peduncular hemorrhage or infarction. The focal impression on the cerebral peduncle is known as "Kernohan's notch." Mass effect on the third cranial nerve and compression of the contralateral cerebral peduncle causes a recognizable clinical syndrome characterized by a blown pupil with ipsilateral hemiparesis.

TRANSTENTORIAL HERNIATION

The brain can herniate either downward or upward across the tentorium. Descending transtentorial herniation is recognized by effacement of the suprasellar and perimesencephalic cisterns. Pineal calcification, usually seen at about the same level as calcified choroid plexus in the trigones of the lateral ventricles, is displaced inferiorly. Large posterior fossa hematomas can cause ascending transtentorial herniation, in which the vermis and portions of the cerebellar hemispheres can herniate through the tentorial incisura. This is much less common than descending transtentorial herniation. Posterior fossa hematomas can also cause herniation of the cerebellar tonsils downward through the foramen magnum.

Finally, external herniation can occur in which swelling or mass effect causes the brain to herniate through a calvarial defect. This can be posttraumatic or occur at the time of craniotomy and prevent closure of the skull flap.

Hydrocephalus can occur after subarachnoid or intraventricular hemorrhage as a result of either impaired CSF reabsorption at the level of the arachnoid granulation or obstruction at the level of the aqueduct or fourth ventricular outflow foramina. Mass effect from cerebral swelling or an adjacent hematoma can also cause hydrocephalus by compression of the aqueduct or outflow foramina of the fourth ventricle.

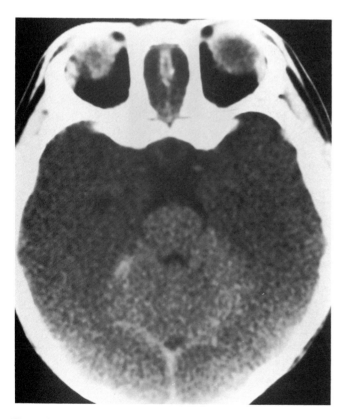

Figure 3.21. Diffuse Cerebral Edema. Noncontrast CT scan in an infant with diffuse cerebral edema following strangulation. There is a diffuse decrease in attenuation of the cerebral hemispheres with loss of gray-white differentiation. Sparing of the brainstem and cerebellum causes these structures to appear dense relative to the rest of the brain.

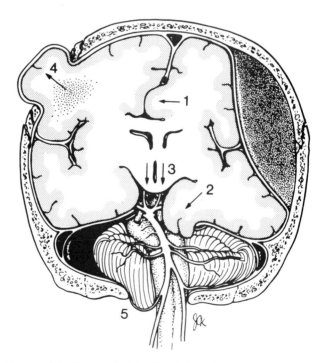

Figure 3.22. Types of Brain Herniation. Diagram of the major types of brain herniation. (*1*) Subfalcial herniation. (*2*) Uncal herniation. (*3*) Descending transtentorial herniation. (*4*) External herniation. (*5*) Tonsillar herniation.

Figure 3.23. Uncal Herniation. Contrast-enhanced CT scan shows compression of the left aspect of the brainstem, displacement of the left posterior cerebral artery (PCA) (*arrowheads*), and effacement of the ambient and crural cisterns. The temporal horns of the lateral ventricles are dilated, indicating obstructive hydrocephalus. Compression of the PCA during uncal herniation can lead to a PCA infarct.

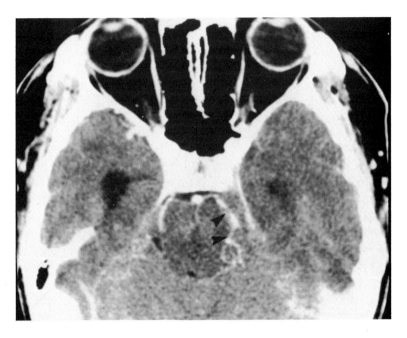

Asymmetric lateral ventricular dilation can be produced by compression of the foramen of Monro.

ISCHEMIA/INFARCTION

Posttraumatic ischemia or infarction can result from raised intracranial pressure, embolization from a vascular dissection, or direct mass effect on cerebral vasculature from brain herniation or an overlying extraaxial collection. In addition, patients may suffer diffuse ischemic damage from acute reduction in cerebral blood flow or from hypoxemia secondary to respiratory arrest or status epilepticus. Patterns of infarction from focal mass effect include anterior cerebral artery infarction from subfalcial herniation, posterior cerebral artery infarction from uncal herniation, and posterior inferior communicating artery infarction from tonsillar herniation. Ischemia or infarction secondary to globally reduced cerebral perfusion tends to occur in characteristic "watershed zones" and is not specific for trauma (see Chapter 4).

CEREBROSPINAL FLUID LEAK

The CSF leak requires a dural tear and can occur after calvarial or skull base fractures. Cerebrospinal fluid rhinorrhea occurs subsequent to fractures in which communication develops between the subarachnoid space and the paranasal sinuses or middle ear cavity. Cerebrospinal fluid otorrhea occurs when communication between the subarachnoid space and middle ear occurs in association with disruption of the tympanic membrane. Cerebrospinal fluid leaks can be difficult to localize, and can lead to recurrent meningeal infection. Radionuclide cisternography is highly sensitive for the presence of CSF extravasation; however, CT scanning with intrathecal contrast is required for detailed anatomic localization of the defect.

LEPTOMENINGEAL CYST

Leptomeningeal cyst or "growing fracture" is caused by a traumatic tear in the dura, which allows an outpouching of arachnoid to occur at the site of a suture or skull fracture. This leads to progressive, slow widening of the skull defect or suture presumably as a result of CSF pulsations. The leptomeningeal cyst appears as a lytic skull defect on CT or plain skull film, which can enlarge over time.

ENCEPHALOMALACIA

Focal encephalomalacia consists of tissue loss with surrounding gliosis and is a frequent manifestation of remote head injury. It may be asymptomatic or serve as a potential seizure focus. Computed tomography demonstrates fairly well-defined areas of low attenuation with volume loss. There may be dilation of adjacent portions of the ventricular system (Figs. 3.24 and 3.25). Encephalomalacia will follow CSF signal on MR sequences, except for gliosis, which appears as increased signal intensity on both proton-density and T2-weighted images. The appearance of encephalomalacia is not specific for posttraumatic injury, but the locations are characteristic: anteroinferior frontal and temporal lobes. Focal volume loss along the white matter tracts associated with cell death is known as wallerian degeneration and may be seen on CT and especially MR studies.

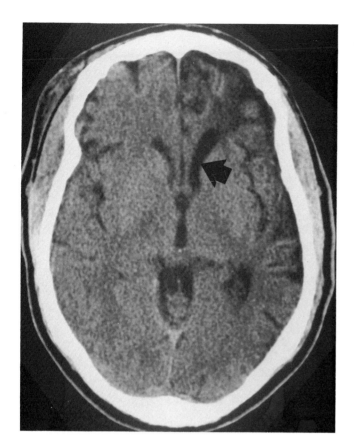

Figure 3.24. Posttraumatic Encephalomalacia. Axial CT shows a well-defined area of decreased attenuation involving gray and white matter of the left frontal lobe consistent with encephalomalacia. Dilation of the ipsilateral frontal horn (*arrow*) confirms the presence of tissue loss rather than a space-occupying lesion.

Brainstem Injury

Primary. The most common form of primary brainstem injury is DAI, which affects the dorsolateral aspect of the midbrain and upper pons (Fig. 3.26). The superior cerebellar peduncles and the medial lemnisci are particularly vulnerable. Both the location and lack of sufficient amounts of hemorrhage make this lesion difficult to diagnose on CT scans. Brainstem DAI is nearly always seen in association with lesions of the frontal or temporal white matter and corpus callosum. This distinguishes brainstem DAI from a rare form of primary injury caused by direct impact of the free margin of the tentorium on the brainstem. Primary brainstem injury may also occur in the form of multiple petechial hemorrhages in the periaqueductal regions of the rostral brainstem (see "Subcortical Gray Matter Injury"). They are not associated with DAI, although they occur in a similar distribution. This form of injury represents disruption of penetrating brainstem blood vessels by shear strain and carries a grim prognosis.

An extremely rare form of indirect primary brainstem injury is the pontomedullary separation or rent.

As the name implies, this represents a tear in the ventral surface of the brainstem at the junction of the pons and medulla. There is a spectrum of severity ranging from a small tear to complete avulsion of the brainstem. Pontomedullary separation can occur without associated diffuse cerebral injury. This lesion is usually fatal.

Secondary brainstem injury includes infarction, hemorrhage, or compression of the brainstem as a result of adjacent or systemic pathology. Brainstem infarction from hypotension-induced cerebral hypoperfusion is usually seen in conjunction with supratentorial ischemic injury. The brainstem may be relatively spared in hypoxic injury. Mechanical compression of the brainstem usually occurs in the setting of uncal herniation. There may be visible displacement or a change in the overall shape of the brainstem as a result of the mass effect. Neurologic injury caused by brainstem compression may be reversible in the absence of intrinsic brainstem lesions.

Brainstem lesions that occur as a result of downward herniation or hypoxia/ischemia usually involve the ventral or ventrolateral aspect of the brainstem, in contrast to primary brainstem lesions, which are most common in the dorsolateral aspect of the brainstem. A characteristic secondary brainstem lesion is the Duret hemorrhage. This is a midline hematoma in the tegmentum of the rostral pons and midbrain seen in association with descending transtentorial herniation. It is believed to result from stretching or tearing of penetrating arteries as the brainstem is caudally displaced (Fig. 3.27). The brainstem infarct is another type of secondary brainstem injury which typically occurs in the central tegmentum of the pons and midbrain.

Penetrating Trauma

Unlike blunt head trauma where diffuse injury often occurs secondary to acceleration-induced shear strain, in penetrating injury the damage is defined by the trajectory of the object. Penetrating sharp objects such as knives or glass cause tissue laceration along their course with resultant bleeding or infarction from vascular injury. Plain films or CT can be used to confirm and localize radiopaque intracranial foreign bodies. Leaded glass and metal are hyperdense on CT scans whereas wood is hypodense.

Gunshot wounds are among the most common causes of penetrating head trauma. They can cause the type of injuries seen in nonpenetrating trauma as well, because significant blunt force occurs from the bullet's impact on the skull. Metallic foreign bodies such as bullet fragments often cause significant streak artifact, which can obscure underlying injury. Tilting the CT gantry to change the plane of section helps minimize this artifact. The entry and exit sites

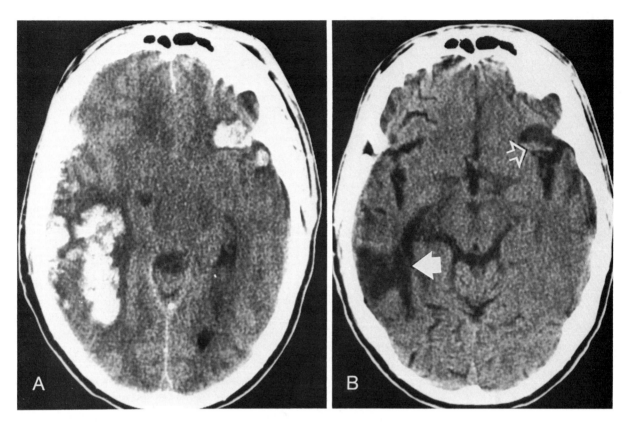

Figure 3.25.   Posttraumatic Encephalomalacia. Admission (**A**) and follow-up (**B**) scans in a patient with severe head trauma show the interval development of left frontal (*open arrow*) and right posterior temporal (*closed arrow*) encephalomalacia in the same locations as the initial intracerebral hematomas.

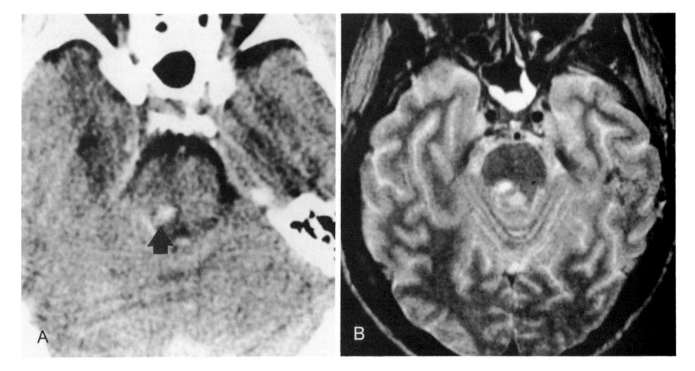

Figure 3.26.   Brainstem DAI. A. Noncontrast CT scan shows a punctate focus of increased attenuation representing focal hemorrhage from DAI of the brainstem (*arrow*). Note the characteristic lo-cation in the dorsolateral aspect of the brainstem. **B.** T2-weighted MR scan in a different patient shows a hyperintense lesion in a similar location.

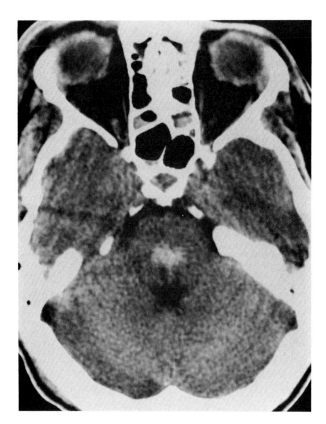

Figure 3.27. Duret Hemorrhage. Noncontrast CT scan performed 24 hours after severe head trauma shows a midline pontine hemorrhage. This type of secondary brainstem injury, known as the Duret hemorrhage, occurs in association with downward transtentorial herniation and can be distinguished from most primary brainstem injuries by its midline location (compare with Fig. 3.26).

can often be distinguished by the direction of beveling of the calvarial defect, or from the pattern of calvarial fracture. The bullet path can often be recognized on CT as a linear hemorrhagic strip (Fig. 3.28). Gunshot wounds in which the bullet crosses the midline or in which small fragments are seen displaced from the main bullet are associated with a poorer prognosis.

Additional complications of penetrating injury are caused by associated skull fractures and dural lacerations with resultant pneumocephalus, CSF leaks, and infection. Fragments of bone, skin, or hair that may be driven intracranially also increase the risk of subsequent abscess formation.

Predicting Outcome After Acute Head Trauma

The Glasgow coma scale, which stratifies patients with acute head trauma based on clinical findings including level of consciousness, brainstem reflexes, and response to pain, is not reliable at predicting long-term outcome. Likewise, CT findings, while extremely valuable in identifying patients with injuries requiring acute intervention, do not correlate well with prognosis. With the increasing use of MR in the setting of head trauma, however, there is growing evi-

dence that imaging studies will be helpful in determining a patient's prognosis after severe head injury. This is in large part because of the ability of MR to detect nonhemorrhagic injury, including DAI, and brainstem injury. Magnetic resonance imaging studies have shown good correlation between initial Glasgow coma scales and the number and distribution of DAI lesions. Numerous DAI lesions and the presence of DAI in the corpus callosum or brainstem are associated with more severe clinical findings and low initial scores on the Glasgow coma scale. Perhaps more important, however, is the finding that the number of DAI lesions and the presence of brainstem injury or corpus callosum DAI are associated with poor long-term outcome. The mean number of cortical contusions is not related to the final outcome except in cases with evidence of significant mass effect. There is also a poor correlation between the presence of an isolated epidural or subdural hematoma and long-term outcome, unless transtentorial herniation was also present.

Head Trauma in Child Abuse

It is important to consider the possibility of child abuse when pediatric patients present with intracranial injury; it is also important to recognize characteristic features in these suspected cases. Intracranial injuries can result either from a direct blow or from nonimpact acceleration forces, usually caused by vigorous shaking.

Skull fractures are caused by direct blows and represent the second most common skeletal injury after long bone fracture. As in adults, however, the decision to image the brain should not rest on the finding of bony injury, or significant lesions will be missed. Skull fractures are seen in approximately 50% of children with intracranial injuries from abuse. The subdural hematoma is the most commonly recognized intracranial complication from child abuse and is usually caused by nonimpact forces. One of the most characteristic patterns in child abuse is the presence of a posterior interhemispheric subdural hematoma, though it is not pathognomonic. In the perinatal period, this could result from birth trauma itself. Posterior interhemispheric subdural hematomas are seen on CT as hyperdense collections with a flat medial border along the falx and an irregular convex lateral border. Subdural hematomas may also be found along the convexity, over the tentorial surface, at the skull base, or in the posterior fossa. Occasionally low attenuation subdural fluid collections are seen in infants without any clear precipitating trauma or infection. These are known as benign subdural effusions of infancy. They are most common in infants 3–6 months old and appear similar to chronic subdural hemato-

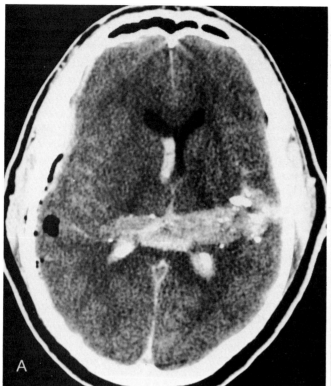

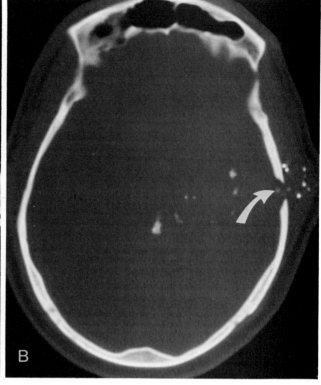

Figure 3.28. Gunshot Wound. A. Noncontrast CT scan shows hemorrhage delineating the bullet's path in this despondent southpaw. There is associated intraventricular and subarachnoid hemorrhage as well as pneumocephalus and a right subdural hematoma. **B.** Bone window shows the typical bevelled entry site (*arrow*) and scattered bullet fragments along the trajectory.

mas. Epidural hematomas are not frequently seen in child abuse.

The most common intraaxial manifestation of head injury related to child abuse is diffuse brain swelling. The initial swelling is believed to be caused by vasodilation associated with loss of autoregulation. At this stage, the injury may be reversible despite dramatic findings on imaging studies. Computed tomography scans show global effacement of the subarachnoid space and compressed ventricles. As the brain becomes edematous, the normal attenuation of gray and white matter may appear indistinguishable or even reversed. The cerebral hemispheres will demonstrate diffusely decreased attenuation. The brainstem, cerebellum, and possibly deep gray matter structures may be spared (Fig. 3.21). The other manifestations of intraaxial injury described above may also be seen in child abuse, including diffuse axonal injury and brainstem injury. Cortical contusions occur but are considered less common, possibly because the inner surface of the skull is relatively smooth in children. In infants, head trauma may lead to tears at the gray-white junction, especially in the frontal and temporal lobes.

Multiple injuries of various ages are also strongly suggestive of child abuse. Chronic sequelae of head injury in children includes chronic subdural collec-

tions (which may occasionally calcify), global cerebral atrophy, and encephalomalacia. While CT is the modality of choice for the evaluation of acute head injury in children, MR can help identify subdural collections of various ages or hemosiderin deposits from prior hemorrhages (Fig. 3.29). The ability of MR to identify these remote intracranial hemorrhages makes it an important tool in the evaluation of suspected child abuse. In some centers, it has been proposed as a necessary complement to the skeletal series. MR is also recommended when patients are clinically stable after head injury to help determine the full extent of injury and prognosis.

FACIAL TRAUMA
Imaging Strategy

Plain Films. Unlike head injury, facial trauma is initially evaluated by plain films. Indeed, many facial fractures can often be diagnosed by plain films alone and need no further imaging. Four views are usually adequate in the plain film evaluation of acute facial trauma. These are the Caldwell view, a shallow Water's view, a cross-table lateral view, and a submental vertex view. When patients are acutely injured and unable to cooperate with upright imaging, the Caldwell and Water's views can be obtained supine in the anteroposterior projection. Films obtained in the poster-

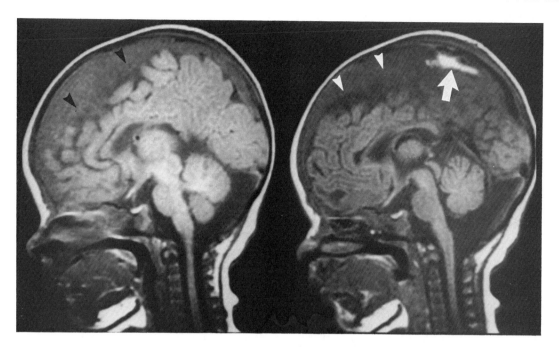

Figure 3.29.   Subacute and Chronic Interhemispheric Subdural Hematomas. Midline sagittal and parasagittal T1-weighted MR scans in a child demonstrate a low signal intensity chronic subdural hematoma (*arrowheads*) and superimposed high signal intensity subacute hematoma (*arrow*). The presence of intracranial injury of different ages is strong presumptive evidence of child abuse. The appearance is not pathognomonic for child abuse, however, since subdural hematomas do have a propensity to rebleed.

oanterior projection provide better bone detail and less magnification, and may be helpful if the initial films are difficult to interpret. The lateral and submental vertex views are both obtained with a horizontal beam, thus allowing the detection of air-fluid levels.

Computed Tomography is indicated when the clinical or plain film findings suggest complex facial fractures or complications such as extraocular muscle entrapment or optic nerve impingement. Further, it is important to remember that patients with facial fractures frequently have concurrent intracranial injury, especially victims of motor vehicle accidents. Imaging of the potential intracranial injury takes precedence in the acute management of these patients. If CT of the facial bones is required in patients suspected of having concurrent intracranial injury, it is usually performed after CT imaging of the brain or delayed several days until the patient is clinically stable.

Three- to five-millimeter sections (1.5 mm for the orbits) are usually obtained through the facial bones in the axial plane using a bone algorithm. The field of view should extend from the orbital roof to the superior alveolar ridge. The frontal sinus or maxillary dentition can be included if fractures are suspected in these areas. The mandible should be included when maxillary alveolar or palatal fractures are seen because of the high incidence of associated mandibular fractures in this setting. A standard algorithm with soft-tissue windows can be used to evaluate potential nonosseous injury, especially in the orbits. If there is no concern for a cervical spine injury, patients are also scanned in the direct coronal plane for better visualization of the orbital floors, palate, and floor of the anterior cranial fossa. Coronal reformations of axial images may be used when patients are unable to tolerate direct coronal scanning. Contrast is unnecessary except in the rare circumstance where vascular injury is being considered. Occasionally, three-dimensional reconstruction is used and may help plan operative repair of displaced or comminuted facial fractures.

Magnetic Resonance Imaging. The facial bones are difficult to visualize on MR scanning because they and the adjacent aerated sinuses are relatively void of signal. Computed tomography is the preferred modality for cross-sectional evaluation of facial injuries primarily because it provides excellent bone detail. Magnetic resonance imaging may be useful for injuries to orbital contents including the optic nerve, globe, and extraocular muscles. It is also useful for assessing potential vascular complications such as arterial dissections, pseudoaneurysms, and arteriovenous fistulas, and is the best way to evaluate trauma to the temporomandibular joint.

Angiography may be indicated when clinical or radiographic evidence suggests a vascular injury. Vascular injuries are more frequent with penetrating trauma, such as that occurring from gunshot or stab wounds. Fractures that extend through the carotid canal also predispose to vascular injury and may require angiographic evaluation.

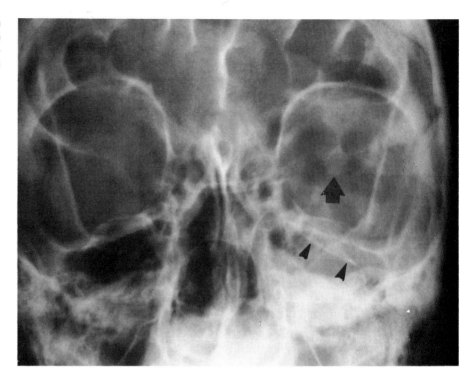

Figure 3.30. Orbital Emphysema on Plain Film. Air in the left orbit can be seen outlining the optic nerve (*arrow*) in this shallow Waters' view. An orbital floor fracture is also evident (*arrowheads*).

Indirect Signs of Injury

It is important to recognize the indirect signs of facial injury on plain films that provide objective evidence of trauma, help localize the site of impact, and direct attention to areas of potential bony injury. Soft-tissue swelling is the most commonly seen plain film finding in patients who sustain facial trauma. It may help localize the site of impact but does not necessarily indicate associated facial fractures or other more severe injury.

Paranasal sinus opacification suggests the presence of an associated fracture, particularly when air-fluid levels are seen. Just as the presence of a fluid level is relatively specific for acute sinusitis in the proper clinical setting, in the setting of acute trauma, it is highly suggestive of an associated fracture with resultant hemorrhage into an adjacent sinus. Fluid levels are most commonly seen in the maxillary, but may also be seen in the frontal or sphenoid sinuses. The ethmoids may become opacified with acute hemorrhage but are less likely to demonstrate fluid levels on plain films, probably because they contain internal septations.

Soft-tissue emphysema is also suggestive of associated fractures, depending on location. Orbital emphysema is most commonly caused by fracture of the thin medial orbital wall. Orbital floor blow-out fractures are less likely to cause orbital emphysema (Fig. 3.30).

Occasionally, facial films reveal important findings unrelated to fracture of the facial bones. For example, the films should be scrutinized for the presence of for-eign bodies that may not be clinically apparent. The craniocervical junction and upper cervical spine should be examined when included on the film. Nasopharyngeal and prevertebral soft-tissue swelling can indicate hemorrhage from cervical or skull base fractures. Pneumocephalus or depressed skull fractures are also occasionally seen. Rarely, shift of pineal calcification can be detected, indicating the presence of intracranial mass effect. Though plain films are usually no longer indicated for evaluation of head trauma, it still pays to remain alert to indirect manifestations of head trauma when reviewing facial films.

Nasal Fractures

Nasal bone fractures are the most common fractures of the facial skeleton. They can occur as an isolated injury or in association with other facial fractures. Nasal trauma frequently results in a depressed fracture of one of the paired nasal bones without associated ethmoidal injury. An anterior blow can fracture both nasal bones as well as the nasal septum. Associated fractures of the frontal process of the maxilla can be seen. Cartilaginous nasal injury cannot be diagnosed radiographically.

Nasal fractures are usually clinically evident and do not require radiologic diagnosis. Films of the nasal bone may document injury but are generally not useful for patient management and are often unnecessary. Fractures of the nasal bone may be transverse or longitudinal. Longitudinal fractures can be confused with the nasomaxillary suture and nasociliary grooves, which have the same orientation. Transverse

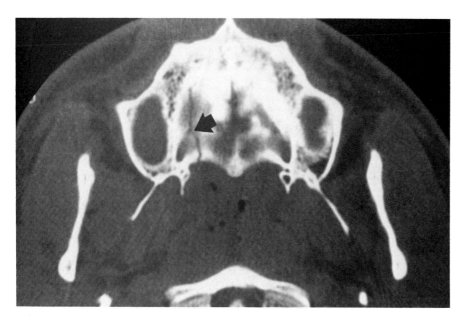

Figure 3.31. Palatine Fracture. Axial CT scan demonstrates a nondisplaced right palatine fracture in the characteristic parasagittal location (*arrow*).

fractures of the nasal bone are more common and are easily detected because they are oriented perpendicular to the normal suture line.

When films are obtained, remember to look for fractures of the anterior nasal spine of the maxilla, which may be associated with nasal fractures. One potentially serious injury that can be suggested on plain films or CT is a septal hematoma. Trauma to the septal cartilage may lead to hematoma formation between the perichondrium and cartilage, which can cause cartilage necrosis by disrupting the vascular supply. An organized hematoma can also cause breathing difficulty and may predispose to septal abscess formation.

Maxillary and Paranasal Sinus Fractures

Fracture of the maxillary alveolus is the most common isolated maxillary fracture. It frequently results from a blow to the chin that drives the teeth of the mandible into the maxillary dental arch. These fractures are usually demonstrated by dental films or panorex (panoramic radiographs), but can be seen on CT if the scan is extended inferior to the level of the palate. Associated fractures of the mandible are common with this form of injury, as predicted by the mechanism.

Fractures of the palatine process of the maxilla and horizontal plate of the palatine bone commonly occur in the sagittal plane near the midline (Fig. 3.31). Palatine fractures may also be seen in association with complex fractures of the midface.

The most common isolated sinus fracture involves the anterolateral wall of the maxillary antrum. The fracture may be seen directly or may be suspected by the finding of a maxillary sinus fluid level in the setting of acute trauma.

Isolated frontal sinus fractures can also occur and may be more serious if they extend intracranially. Frontal sinus fractures may be linear, or comminuted and depressed. Open (compound) frontal sinus fractures involve the posterior sinus wall (Fig. 3.32). These can lead to CSF rhinorrhea and recurrent meningitis or intracerebral abscess formation. Pneumocephalus may be seen in association with these fractures. Fractures of the medial wall and superior rim of the orbit frequently involve the frontal sinus.

Fractures of the sphenoid sinus are often seen in association with fractures of the orbital roof, nasoethmoid complex, midface, or temporal bone. Nondisplaced sphenoid sinus fractures may be subtle on CT. Angiography should be considered if there is a suspicion of associated vascular injury involving the cavernous portion of the internal carotid artery.

Orbital Trauma

FRACTURES

The orbit is involved in a number of facial fractures including the tripod, Le Fort, and nasoethmoidal complex fractures. Isolated orbital wall fractures usually involve either the medial wall or orbital floor. Medial wall fractures are detected on plain films by the presence of orbital emphysema and opacification of the adjacent ethmoid air cells. Medial wall fractures can be directly visualized well with axial or coronal CT scans. Bone displacement is usually minimal and muscle entrapment is unusual.

Orbital floor fractures are usually linear when seen in association with other facial fractures. These are

Figure 3.32. **"Open" Frontal Sinus Fracture.** Noncontrast CT scan demonstrates a severely comminuted fracture involving both walls of the frontal sinus (open fracture). The frontal sinus is opacified and subcutaneous air is present (*arrow*). Open fractures are prone to CSF leakage and meningitis or intracerebral abscess formation.

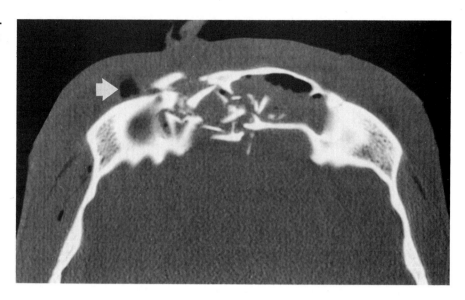

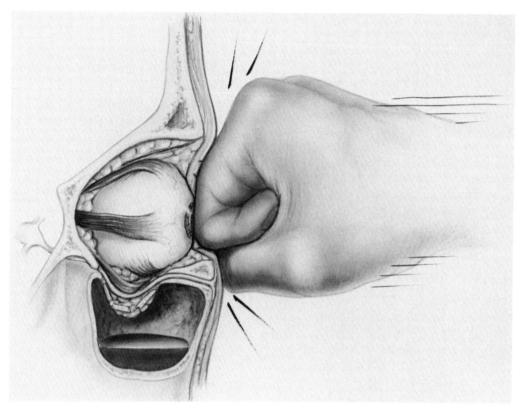

Figure 3.33.   Diagram of Orbital Floor Blow-out Fracture. Sudden increase in intraocular pressure from a direct blow to the eye can lead to a comminuted fracture of the orbital floor with herniation of orbital contents into the maxillary sinus. A fluid level in the sinus is often seen acutely secondary to bleeding.

rarely associated with entrapment. Comminuted orbital floor fractures, or blow-out fractures, may be seen as an isolated injury and result from a direct blow to the eye. Intraorbital pressure is acutely increased and relieved by fracture through the orbital floor (Fig. 3.33). The orbital rim remains intact in pure blow-out fractures. Blow-out fractures are often associated with herniation of orbital contents through the fracture. When the inferior rectus mus-

cle is compromised, patients will experience persistent vertical diplopia. Mild or transient diplopia can occur simply as a result of periorbital edema or hemorrhage. Rarely, fragments from an orbital floor fracture buckle upward into the orbit, an injury referred to as a "blow-in" fracture.

Plain film findings suggestive of orbital floor blow-out fractures include orbital emphysema, a fluid level in the ipsilateral maxillary sinus, indistinct orbital

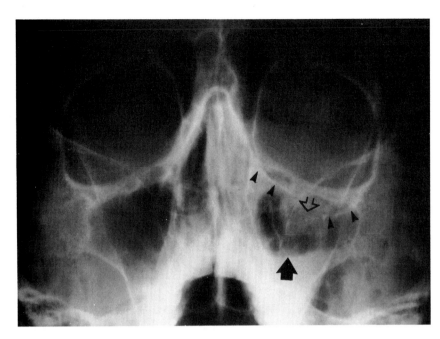

Figure 3.34. Orbital Floor Blow-out Fracture on Plain Film. Waters' view shows the major findings associated with an orbital floor blow-out injury: disruption of the orbital floor (*arrowheads*), soft-tissue mass in the superior aspect of the maxillary sinus (*open arrow*), and a maxillary sinus fluid level (*closed arrow*).

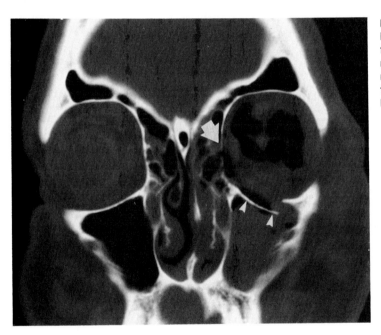

Figure 3.35. Orbital Floor Blow-out Fracture on CT Scan. Direct coronal CT scan shows a depressed left orbital floor fracture (*arrowheads*) with opacification of the ipsilateral maxillary sinus. Orbital air can be seen outlining the optic nerve (same patient as Fig. 3.30). A subtle medial wall fracture is also present (*arrow*), which likely accounts for the large amount of orbital emphysema in this case.

floor on Water's view, and soft tissue representing prolapsed orbital contents in the superior aspect of the maxillary sinus (Fig. 3.34). A bony spicule may be seen in the antrum representing the inferiorly displaced fracture fragment. Blow-out fractures are best seen on direct coronal CT images (Fig. 3.35). These should be obtained with the patient lying prone. In the supine position, fluid and debris in the maxillary antrum will layer against the orbital floor and could obscure soft tissue herniating through the fracture.

SOFT-TISSUE INJURY

Penetrating foreign bodies such as bullets, metal fragments, glass, or other sharp objects account for a significant amount of traumatic injury to the orbit. Thin-section CT is the method of choice for confirming the presence of foreign bodies and for this localization (Fig. 3.36). Computed tomography can usually clearly define the relationship of bone fragments or foreign bodies to critical structures such as the optic nerve, globe, or extraocular muscles (Fig. 3.37). Magnetic resonance imaging carries a potential risk of further injury by causing motion of intraocular ferromagnetic metal.

Traumatic optic neuropathy is seen in a significant number of patients with severe head trauma, and occasionally occurs in patients with relatively minor deceleration injury. Damage may be maximal

Figure 3.36. Intraocular Metallic Foreign Body. Axial (**A**) and coronal (**B**) CT scans confirm the presence of a metallic foreign body in the left globe.

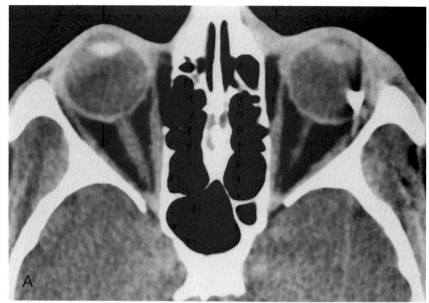

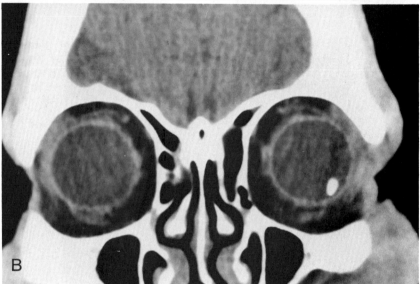

initially with unilateral blindness or decreased acuity, or may worsen in the first few days after the injury. When delayed worsening occurs, secondary optic nerve compression from edema or hemorrhage in the optic nerve sheath should be considered. Imaging studies, particularly CT scans, are indicated to detect fractures through the optic canal or orbital apex. Rarely, displaced fractures are responsible for direct injury to the optic nerve sheath. More commonly, these fractures are nondisplaced, but serve as evidence of severe stress transmitted to the orbital apex. Primary optic nerve injury may occur as a result of deceleration strain causing damage to the delicate meningeal vessels or direct neural disruption. Secondary optic nerve injury may occur as a result of swelling of the optic nerve within the rigid bony canal with subsequent mechanical compression and vascular compromise.

Fractures of the Zygoma

The zygoma, or "cheekbone," is one of the most common sites of injury in fractures that involve multiple facial bones. Zygomatic arch fractures may occur as an isolated finding, or as part of a zygomaticomaxillary complex ("tripod," "quadripod," or "trimalar") fracture. Comminution and depression are frequently seen with zygomatic arch fractures. On plain films, the zygomatic arch is best evaluated on the submental vertex view (Fig. 3.38). Deformity of the arch is a frequent finding in populations with a high incidence of facial trauma and clinical examination may be required to differentiate acute from chronic injury.

Zygomaticomaxillary complex fractures usually result from a blow to the face. The zygoma articulates with the frontal, maxillary, sphenoid, and temporal bones. Fractures are somewhat variable, but typically

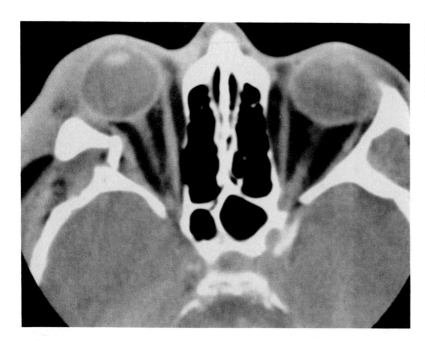

Figure 3.37. Lateral Orbital Wall Fracture with Impingement of Lateral Rectus Muscle. Noncontrast CT scan precisely localizes the site and degree of impingement on the right lateral rectus muscle in this patient with a comminuted fracture involving the zygomaticofrontal suture.

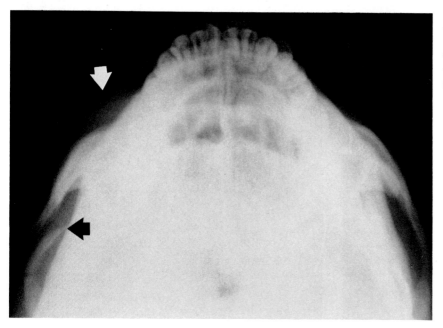

Figure 3.38. Right Zygomatic Arch Fracture. Submental vertex view shows a comminuted, depressed right zygomatic arch fracture (*black arrow*). Soft-tissue swelling anterior to the body of the zygoma is also seen (*white arrow*).

involve the zygomatic arch, zygomaticofrontal suture, infraorbital rim, orbital floor, lateral wall of the maxillary sinus, and lateral wall of the orbit. Injury to the infraorbital nerve is common secondary to fracture of the infraorbital rim at the infraorbital foramen. Diastasis of the zygomaticofrontal suture may injure the lateral canthal ligament or suspensory ligaments of the globe. Many of the fractures associated with this injury can be seen on both plain films and CT scans (Fig. 3.39). Associated findings on plain films include opacification of the ipsilateral maxillary antrum and posterior displacement of the body of the zygoma on the submental vertex view with overlying soft-tissue swelling.

Fractures of the Midface (Le Fort Fractures)

Complex fractures of the facial bones are frequently classified according to the method of Le Fort, who developed his theory by inflicting facial trauma on cadavers and analyzing the results. He described three general patterns of fractures that differ in location of the fracture plane across the face (Fig. 3.40). The three Le Fort fractures initially described are bilateral processes. All involve the pterygoid plates, which help anchor the facial bones to the skull. Though there is great variability in complex facial fractures, and the classic Le Fort injuries are rarely seen in their pure form, they remain a convenient way to categorize and describe basic patterns of injury. Frequently, similar

Figure 3.39. Zygomaticomaxillary Complex Fracture. A. Plain film shows diastasis of the left zygomaticofrontal suture (*open arrow*) and disruption of the orbital floor (*closed arrow*). An associated zygomatic arch fracture was seen on submental vertex view (not shown). **B.** A CT scan in a different patient shows comminuted left zygomatic arch fracture (*curved arrows*), with fractures of the anterior and posterolateral walls of the maxillary sinus (*arrowheads*). Associated signs of acute injury include soft-tissue swelling and partial opacification of the maxillary sinus.

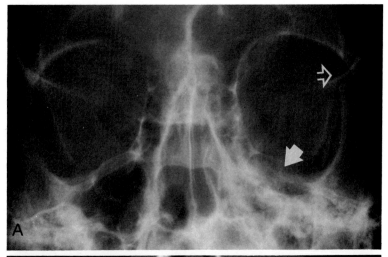
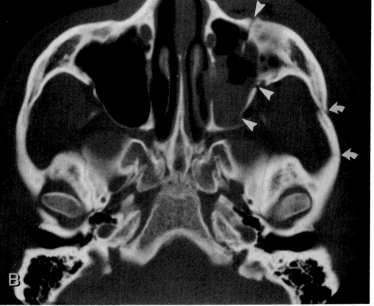

patterns of injury are seen on one side only and are known as "hemi-Le Forts." Combinations also occur, such as a Le Fort I pattern on one side and a Le Fort II pattern on the other.

The Le Fort I or "floating palate" fracture is a horizontal fracture through the maxillary sinuses. It extends through the nasal septum and walls of the maxillary sinuses into the inferior aspect of the pterygoid plates. The fracture plane is parallel to the plane of axial CT images but is recognized by the fracture of all walls of both maxillary sinuses (Fig. 3.41). It is well seen in the coronal plane. There may be an associated midpalatal or maxillary split fracture. The Le Fort I fracture is more often seen in the pure form than either the Le Fort II or Le Fort III fractures. It occasionally may be accompanied by a unilateral zygomaticomaxillary complex fracture.

The Le Fort II or "pyramidal" fracture describes a fracture through the medial orbital and lateral maxillary walls. It begins at the bridge of the nose and ex-

tends in a pyramidal fashion through the nasal septum, frontal process of the maxilla, medial wall of the orbit, inferior orbital rim, superior, lateral and posterior walls of the maxillary antrum, and midportion of the pterygoid plates. The zygomatic arch and lateral orbital walls are left intact. The Le Fort II is usually associated with posterior displacement of the facial bones, resulting in a "dish-face" deformity and malocclusion. The infraorbital nerve is frequently injured. Le Fort II fractures are rarely seen in the pure form.

The Le Fort III fracture, or "craniofacial dysjunction," is a horizontally oriented fracture through the orbits. It begins near the nasofrontal suture and extends posteriorly to involve the nasal septum, medial and lateral orbital walls, zygomatic arch, and base (superior aspect) of the pterygoid plates. Patients with a Le Fort III fracture also have dish-face deformity and malocclusion. Injury to the infraorbital nerve is less commonly seen than with Le Fort II fractures.

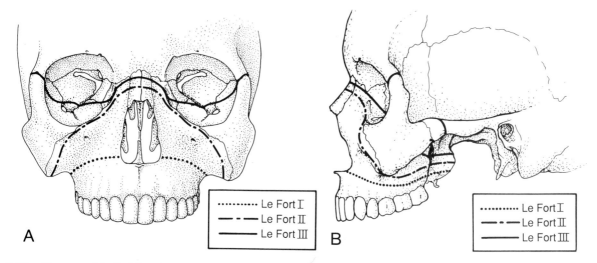

Figure 3.40. Diagram of Le Fort Fractures. Frontal (**A**) and lateral (**B**) projections demonstrate the patterns of facial fractures as originally described by Le Fort.

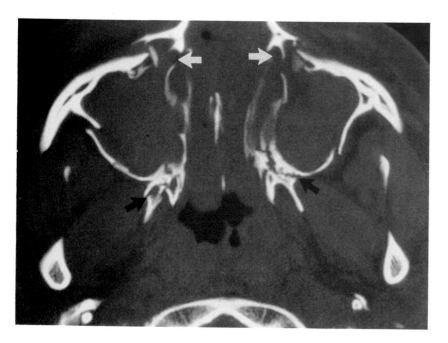

Figure 3.41. Le Fort I Fracture. Axial CT scan demonstrates comminuted fractures involving all walls of both maxillary sinuses with associated fractures through the pterygoid plates (*black arrows*). Both nasolacrimal ducts are also disrupted (*white arrows*). There is complete opacification of both maxillary antra.

A recognizable feature on plain films is the elongated appearance of the orbits on Water's and Caldwell views.

When interpreting CT scans obtained for facial trauma, it is probably best to describe the specific bones that are fractured on either side of the face. When appropriate, the Le Fort injury that best describes the distribution of fractures may also be used to categorize complex fractures.

Nasoethmoidal Fractures

Nasoethmoidal complex injuries describe the constellation of findings seen as a result of a blow to the midface between the eyes. This term encompasses a wide variety of different fracture complexes that are best described by listing the specific fractures seen on CT scans. These injuries may include fractures of the lamina papyracea, inferior, medial, and supraorbital rims, frontal or ethmoid sinuses, orbital roofs, nasal bone and frontal process of the maxilla, and sphenoid bone (Fig. 3.42). These fractures have also been called orbitoethmoid or nasoethmoid-orbital fractures because of the importance of the often associated orbital injuries. There may be associated fractures of the skull base and clivus. Other findings include orbital and intracranial air, opacification of the ethmoid and frontal sinuses, and depression of the midface. Nasoethmoidal fractures can be suspected on plain films when the lateral view shows posterior displacement of the nasion. Thin-section CT helps evaluate the extent of the injury and helps localize bony frag-

Figure 3.42. Nasoethmoidal Complex Fracture. Axial CT scan demonstrates a depressed fracture involving the root of the nose (*curved arrow*) and anterior ethmoids. Bilateral fractures of the medial orbital walls are also present (*large arrows*) with bilateral orbital emphysema.

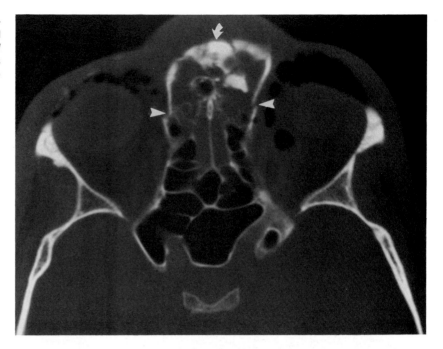

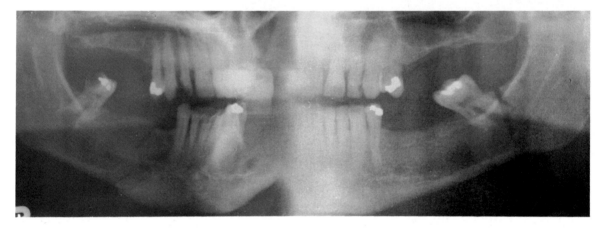

Figure 3.43. Panorex Film with Bilateral Mandibular Fractures. Fractures of the left mandibular angle (extending into the root of a molar tooth) and right horizontal ramus are both clearly seen on single panorex film.

ments that might encroach on the optic nerve or canal.

Complications of nasoethmoidal complex fractures depend on the location and extent of injury. Patients with fractures involving the floor of the anterior cranial fossa are prone to develop CSF leaks because of the high frequency of associated dural lacerations. The olfactory nerves are frequently injured when fractures extend to the cribriform plate. As mentioned earlier, orbital injuries are often seen as a component of nasoethmoid fractures. The globes or optic nerves may be damaged by displaced medial orbital wall fracture fragments.

Mandibular Fractures

Mandibular fractures are extremely common in patients with maxillofacial injury. Plain films are used in the initial evaluation of patients with suspected mandibular injury. The mandibular series includes posteroanterior, lateral, Towne, and bilateral oblique projections. Computed tomography or panoramic radiographs (panorex films) can also be used to evaluate mandibular injury (Fig. 3.43).

Mandibular fractures can be considered either simple or compound. Simple fractures are most common in the ramus and condyle and do not communicate externally or with the mouth. Compound fractures are those that communicate internally through a tooth socket or externally through a laceration (Fig. 3.44). Fractures of the body of the mandible are almost always compound fractures. Pathologic mandibular fractures can occur at sites of infection or neoplasm.

Mandibular fractures are frequently multiple or bilateral, and such fractures often involve the condyle (Fig. 3.45). Subcondylar fractures may be recognized

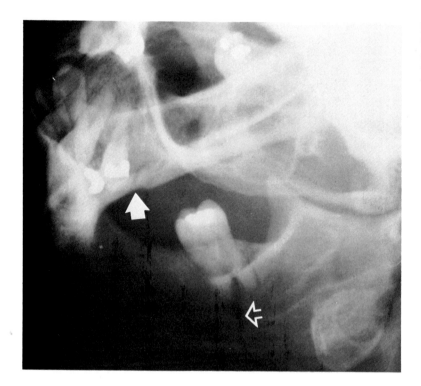

Figure 3.44. Compound Fracture of the Mandible. Oblique view of the mandible demonstrates a posterior ramus fracture extending through the adjacent tooth socket (*open arrow*). A contralateral fracture of the horizontal ramus is also present (*closed arrow*).

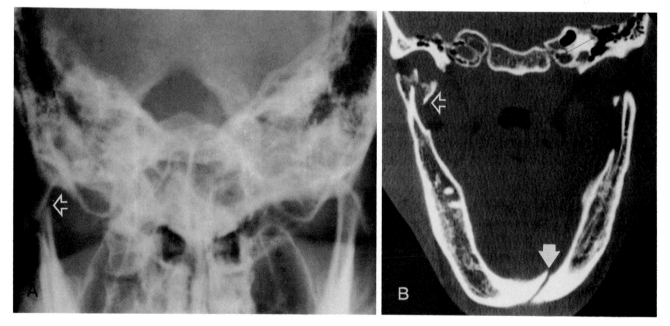

Figure 3.45. Plain Film and CT of Mandibular Condylar Fracture.
A. Plain film (Towne projection) shows a displaced right subcondylar fracture (*open arrow*). **B.** Axial CT in a different patient shows a right condylar fracture (*open arrow*) and an associated parasymphyseal fracture (*closed arrow*). The latter fracture is easily missed on plain films because of the oblique fracture plane.

on plain films by the "cortical ring" sign, a well-corticated density seen above the condylar neck on lateral views because of the horizontal axis of the fragment. A common pattern of injury is a unilateral condylar fracture with a contralateral fracture of the mandibular angle. The mandibular angle is also the most common site of isolated injury. Fractures of the ramus and coronoid processes are rare. Fractures through the symphysis or parasymphyseal region are common but difficult to diagnose on plain films because of the obliquity of the fracture plane. Fractures involving the dentoalveolar complex are also often missed on mandibular series and require intraoral dental films or CT for evaluation. Bilateral fractures through the mandibular body or comminuted fractures can lead to airway obstruction from posterior displacement of the tongue and free mandibular fragment.

Suggested Readings

Intracranial Injury

Adams JH. Pathology of nonmissile head injury. Neuroimaging Clin North Am 1991;1:397–410.

Eelkema EA, Hecht ST, Horton JA. Head trauma. In: Latchaw RE, ed. MR and CT imaging of the head, neck, and spine. 2nd ed. St. Louis: CV Mosby, 1991:203–265.

Gean AD. Imaging head trauma. New York: Raven Press, 1993.

Gennarelli TA, Thibault LE, Adams JH, et al. Diffuse axonal injury and traumatic coma in the primate. In: Dacey RG Jr, Winn HR, Rimel RW, Jane JA eds. Trauma of the central nervous system. New York: Raven Press, 1985:169–193.

Gentry LR, Godersky JC, Thompson B, Dunn VD. Prospective comparative study of intermediate-field MR and CT in the evaluation of closed head trauma. AJNR 1988;9:91–100.

Gentry LR, Godersky JC, Thompson B. MR imaging of head trauma: Review of the distribution and radiopathologic features of traumatic lesions. AJNR 1988;9:101–110.

Gentry LR. Head trauma. In: Atlas SW, ed. Magnetic resonance imaging of the brain and spine. 2nd ed. New York: Raven Press, 1991:439–466.

Hollerman JJ, Fackler ML, Coldwell DM, Ben-Menachem Y. Gunshot wounds. AJR 1990;155:685–702.

Cranial and Skull Base Injury

Bell RS, Loop JW. The utility and futility of radiographic skull examination for trauma. N Eng J Med 1971;284:236–239.

Gentry LR. Temporal bone trauma. Neuroimaging Clin North Am 1991;1:319–339.

Hackney DB. Skull radiography in the evaluation of acute head trauma: A survey of current practice. Radiology 1991;181:711–714.

Holland BA, Brant-Zawadzki M. High-resolution CT of temporal bone trauma. AJNR 1984;5:291–295.

Head Trauma in Child Abuse

Merten DF, Radkowski MA, Leonidas JC. The abused child: A radiological reappraisal. Radiology 1983;146:377–381.

Sato Y, Smith WL. Head injury in child abuse. Neuroimaging Clin North Am 1991;1:475–492.

Facial Trauma

DelBalso AM, Hall RE. Mandibular and dentoalveolar fractures. Neuroimaging Clin North Am 1991;1:285–303.

Kassel EE, Gruss JS. Imaging of midfacial fractures. Neuroimaging Clin North Am 1991;1:259–283.

Som PM. Sinonasal Cavity. In: Som PM, Bergeron RT, eds. Head and neck imaging, 2nd ed. St. Louis: CV Mosby, 1991:227–249.

4

Cerebrovascular Disease

Howard A. Rowley

Stroke is a clinical term applied to any abrupt non-traumatic brain insult—literally "a blow from an unseen hand." Strokes are caused by either brain infarction (75%) or hemorrhage (25%), and must be distinguished from other conditions causing abrupt neurologic deficits. *Infarction* is a permanent injury that occurs when tissue perfusion is decreased long enough to cause necrosis, typically due to occlusion of the feeding artery. *Transient ischemic attacks* (TIAs) are defined as transient neurologic symptoms or signs lasting less than 24 hours, which may serve as a "warning sign" of an infarction occurring in the next few weeks or months. Transient ischemic attacks are often due to temporary occlusion of a feeding artery. *Hemorrhage* is seen when blood ruptures through the arterial wall, spilling into the surrounding parenchyma, subarachnoid space, or ventricles.

Stroke is the third leading cause of death in the United States and major source of long-term disability among survivors. Treatment of ischemic stroke has been largely preventative or supportive in the past, but recent developments in neuroprotective drugs hold promise for more effective treatment in the near future. The patient with hemorrhage may harbor an aneurysm, vascular malformation, or other condition, each having important differences in treatment options. The radiologist plays a critical role in the triage and evaluation of all stroke patients. Selection of the proper imaging technique, recognition of early ischemic changes, differentiation of stroke from other brain disorders, and recognition of important stroke subtypes can have a significant impact on therapy and outcome.

This chapter reviews the pathophysiology of stroke, the time course of findings on computed tomography (CT) and magnetic resonance imaging (MR), patterns of arterial and venous occlusions, and overall radiologic approach to evaluation of the stroke patient.

ISCHEMIC STROKE

Etiologies

Despite our best clinical efforts, no clear source is ever identified in up to a quarter of patients with brain infarction. Among those with an established mechanism, about two thirds of infarcts are caused by thrombi and one third by emboli. Thrombi are formed at sites of abnormal vascular endothelium, typically over an area of atherosclerotic plaque or ulcer. Large-artery thrombosis in the neck may or may not cause distal infarction, depending on the time course of occlusion and available collateral supply. Small-vessel thrombi frequently occur in "end arteries" of the brain, accounting for about one fifth of infarcts ("lacunes"). Emboli may arise from the heart, aortic arch, carotid arteries, or vertebral arteries, causing infarction by distal migration and occlusion. There is obviously overlap between the thrombotic and embolic groups, since the vast majority of emboli begin as thrombi somewhere more proximal in the cardiovascular tree (hence the practical term, "thromboembolic disease"). Vasculitis, vasospasm, coagulopathies, global hypoperfusion, and venous thrombosis each account for 5% or fewer of acute strokes, but are important to recognize due to differing treatment and prognosis. A given patient's age, medical history, and type of stroke seen will help establish the major etiologic considerations (Table 4.1).

Pathophysiologic Basis for Imaging Changes

Neurons lead a precarious life. The brain consumes 20% of the total cardiac output to maintain its minute-to-minute delivery of glucose and oxygen. Since

Table 4.1. Differential Diagnosis of Ischemic Stroke by Age

Pediatric	Young Adult	Elderly
Congenital heart disease	Cardiac emboli	Atherosclerosis
Blood dyscrasias	Atherosclerosis	Cardiac emboli
Meningitis	Drug abuse	Coagulopathy
Arterial dissection	Arterial dissection	Amyloid
Trauma	Coagulopathy	Vasculitis
ECMO[a]	Vasculitis	Venous thrombosis
Venous thrombosis	Venous thrombosis	

[a]Extracorporeal membrane oxygenation.

there are no significant long-term energy stores (e.g., glycogen, fat), disruption of blood flow for even a few minutes will lead to neuronal death. The extent of injury depends upon both the duration and degree of vascular occlusion. Minor reduction in perfusion is initially compensated for by increased extraction of substrate, but injury becomes inevitable below a critical flow threshold (10–20 ml/100 g tissue/min versus normal 55 ml/100 g/min).

Certain cell types and neuroanatomic regions show selective vulnerability to ischemic injury. Gray matter normally receives 3–4 times more blood flow than white matter, and is therefore more likely to suffer under conditions of oligemia. Some subsets of neurons (e.g., cerebellar Purkinje cells, hippocampal CA-1 neurons) are injured more readily than others, possibly because of greater concentrations of receptors for excitatory amino acids. The slower metabolizing capillary endothelial cells and white matter oligodendrocytes are more resistant to ischemia than gray matter, but will also die when deprived of nutrients. Cells served by penetrating end arteries or those residing in the watershed zone between major territories have no alternate route for perfusion, and are therefore more prone to infarction. Damage will likely be more severe in a patient with an incomplete circle of Willis than in one with a complete arterial collateral pathway.

Ischemia causes a cascade of cellular level events leading to the gross pathologic changes detected in clinical imaging. Failure of membrane pumps permits efflux of K^+ and simultaneous influx of Ca^{2+}, Na^+, and water. This leads to cellular ("cytotoxic") edema, observed clinically as increased water content in the affected region. *Increased brain water is the fundamental change that allows us to detect areas of infarction by CT and MR.* Even a small increase in water content causes characteristic decreased attenuation on CT, low signal on T1-weighted MR, and high signal on T2-weighted MR. This edema peaks 3 to 7 days after infarction and is maximum in the gray matter. A smaller component of vasogenic edema also develops as the more resistant capillary endothelial cells lose integrity. (In contrast, tumor-associated edema is

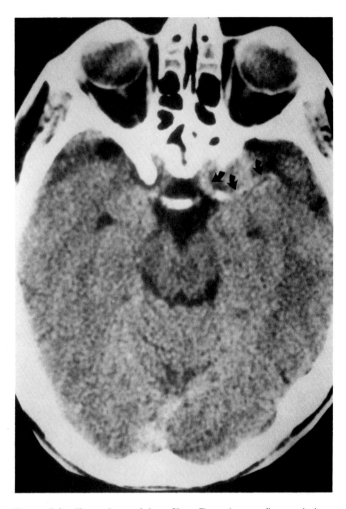

Figure 4.1. Hyperdense Artery Sign. Three hours after occlusion, high density is seen in the proximal left MCA (*arrows*). Acute thrombus fills the lumen.

primarily vasogenic and preferentially affects the white matter; see Chapter 5.)

Careful inspection of CT and MR images done within minutes to a few hours after vessel occlusion can give clues to ischemic injury, even before gross tissue edema or mass effect are seen. These "hyperacute" signs primarily relate to morphologic changes in the vessels rather than density or signal changes in the parenchyma. On CT, the actual thrombus may occasionally be seen in larger intracranial branches, resulting in the "hyperdense artery sign" (Fig. 4.1). On MR, the normal black signal of flowing blood within the lumen ("flow void") is immediately lost and may be replaced by an abnormal signal representing clot (Fig. 4.2). Loss of the flow void is best seen acutely in the large vessels (carotid siphon, vertebrobasilar vessels, middle cerebral branches). Dissolution of clot and improved collateral flow may occur within the first few days, leading to reestablishment of flow void on follow-up MR examination.

Computed tomography scans done within 6 hours of middle cerebral artery occlusion will commonly ex-

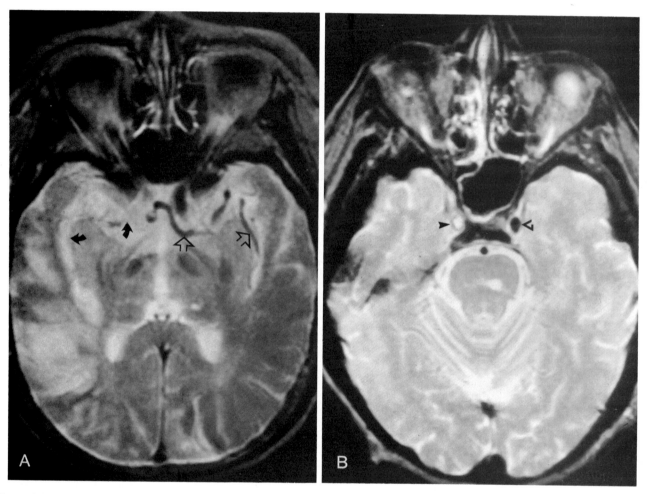

Figure 4.2.   Loss of Flow Void. Six hours after right internal carotid occlusion (**A**), there is a loss of vascular flow voids in the internal carotid artery and MCA branches (*arrows*) compared with the patent left side (*open arrows*). Hyperintensity is developing in the right posterior sylvian region, indicative of early edema on this T2-weighted image. A section below (**B**) shows complete occlusion of the right internal carotid artery in its cavernous segment (*arrowhead*), with normal flow void preserved on the left (*open arrowhead*). A lacune in the pons is evident.

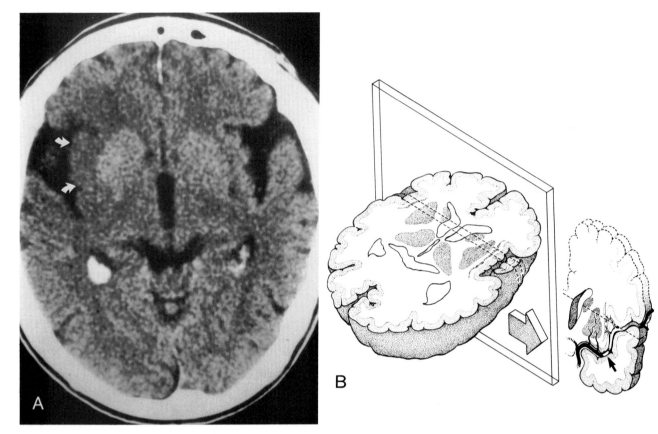

Figure 4.3.   Insular Ribbon Sign. A. A noncontrast CT done 4 hours after right MCA occlusion shows decreased attenuation and loss of gray-white borders in the right insular region (*arrows*). **B.** Diagram of the insula in transverse and coronal planes. The insular cortex, claustrum, and extreme capsule are infarcted because of occlusion of the MCA (*arrow*) beyond the lateral lenticulostriate vessels. (From Truwit CL, Barkovich AJ, Gean-Martin A, Hibri N, Norman D. Loss of the insular ribbon: another early CT sign of acute middle cerebral artery infarction. Radiology 1990;176:801–806.)

hibit the "insular ribbon sign," a subtle but important blurring of the gray-white layers of the insula due to early edema (Fig. 4.3). Magnetic resonance exams in the first few hours may show a similar loss of gray-white borders and slight crowding of sulci in areas destined to undergo infarction. Swelling noted on T1-weighted images may precede T2 hyperintensity, which typically develops at 6–12 hours after ictus. Beyond the first several hours, increased water in the infarcted tissue is most easily (and sometimes only) detected on T2-weighted sequences (Fig. 4.4).

In the subacute phase, edema leads to mass effect, ranging from slight sulcal effacement to marked midline shift with brain herniation, depending on the size and location of infarct. These changes peak at 3–7 days, with progressive brain softening (encephalomalacia) ensuing thereafter. One potential imaging pitfall, the "fogging effect," may be encountered on CTs done during the 2nd week after infarction as edema and mass effect are subsiding. At this stage, decrease in edema and accumulation of proteins from cell lysis balance one another such that brain morphology and density in the injured region can be nearly normal by CT. Fog-

ging effects are much less of a problem on MR because of its greater tissue sensitivity, particularly when contrast is used (Fig. 4.5). Edema or mass effect that persists beyond 1 month effectively rules out simple ischemia, and should raise the possibility of recurrent infarction or an underlying tumor.

In the weeks and months following infarction, macrophages remove dead tissue, leaving a small amount of gliotic scar and encephalomalacia behind. Cerebrospinal fluid takes up the space previously occupied by brain. The affected corticospinal tract atrophies (wallerian degeneration), leading to a shrunken appearance of the ipsilateral cerebral peduncle. If hemorrhage accompanied the infarct, hemosiderin may be seen grossly or detected as signal hypointensity by T2-weighted images. Widening of adjacent sulci and "ex vacuo" dilation of the ventricle occurs adjacent to the infarcted area (Fig. 4.6).

Hemorrhagic Transformation of Infarction

Reperfusion into infarcted capillary beds may secondarily lead to gross or microscopic hemorrhage, seen in up to half of infarcts. In most cases this takes

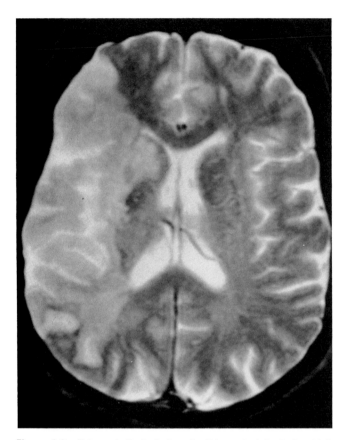

Figure 4.4. Edema in Early Ischemia. Edema is detected as high signal intensity and mild mass effect in the entire right MCA territory on this T2-weighted transverse image obtained 2 days after occlusion. Partial effacement of the right lateral ventricle is evident.

the form of microscopic leakage (diapedesis) of red blood cells, but on rare occasions a frank hematoma will form. Physical disruption of the capillary endothelial cells, loss of vascular autoregulation, and anticoagulation may all contribute to the development of these hemorrhages. Patients may develop headaches at the time of bleeding, but commonly have no new symptoms, presumably because the hemorrhage occurs within brain areas that are already dead or dysfunctional. Hemorrhagic infarction is confined to the territory of the infarcted vessel, whereas primary hemorrhage does not necessarily respect vascular boundaries. Intraventricular extension is uncommonly seen with hemorrhagic transformation and should raise the possibility of another process (such as hypertensive bleed or a ruptured arteriovenous malformation).

The peak time for hemorrhagic transformation is at about 1–2 weeks after infarction. It is usually manifest as a serpiginous line of petechial blood following the gyral contours of the infarcted cortex. These dots of hemorrhage are often patchy and discontinuous. On CT a faint line of high attenuation is observed, and on MR a bright signal is seen along the affected gyrus on the unenhanced T1-weighted images be-

cause of methemoglobin (Fig. 4.7**A**). (Alternate explanations for this bright signal have been offered, including laminar necrosis or calcification related to infarction; the practical point is to recognize this appearance as a feature of ischemia.) The petechial gyral pattern is not seen in primary brain hemorrhage and can be helpful in confirming the underlying ischemic etiology of a suspicious lesion. This is considered a normal part of the evolution of an infarct. Management in the presence of petechial hemorrhage is controversial, but most neurologists continue anticoagulation if there is a well-documented embolic source.

More extensive hemorrhagic transformation of the infarcted tissue may lead to the formation of a gross parenchymal hematoma. Here the blood does not conform to a gyrus and may form a clot indistinguishable from a primary hematoma. Large cortical infarcts are at somewhat higher risk for this type of change, compared with limited cortical or subcortical lesions. In contrast to the petechial gyral transformation just described, gross parenchymal hematomas tend to occur earlier and are more commonly associated with clinical deterioration. Anecdotal evidence suggests that reperfusion of a large cortical infarct during the first 24 hours may pose an especially high risk of hematoma formation. Frank hematomas seen on infarct follow-up studies should be reported promptly since anticoagulation therapy is contraindicated, even when the finding is incidental.

Use of Contrast in Ischemic Stroke

COMPUTED TOMOGRAPHY CONTRAST

A noncontrast CT remains the radiologic examination of choice for assessment of suspected acute stroke. The unenhanced study is necessary to help in triage of the patient. It serves to rule out hemorrhage, may define patterns of ischemic injury, shows areas of abnormal vascular calcification (e.g., giant aneurysms), and excludes mass lesions. This is important first-line information needed by the clinician faced with determining the need for lumbar puncture, vascular surgery, anticoagulation, cardiac evaluation, or other therapies. All acute stroke CTs should, however, be reviewed on the monitor since the unenhanced study may rarely show the need for intravenous contrast. A nonstroke lesion such as a tumor, abscess, or an isodense subdural hematoma might be suspected on the noncontrast examination and then be shown to better advantage with contrast.

The use of intravenous contrast for CT beyond the acute phase is slightly more controversial. Some radiologists feel contrast is contraindicated in brain infarction. They cite a slightly increased risk of seizures and other untoward central nervous system effects,

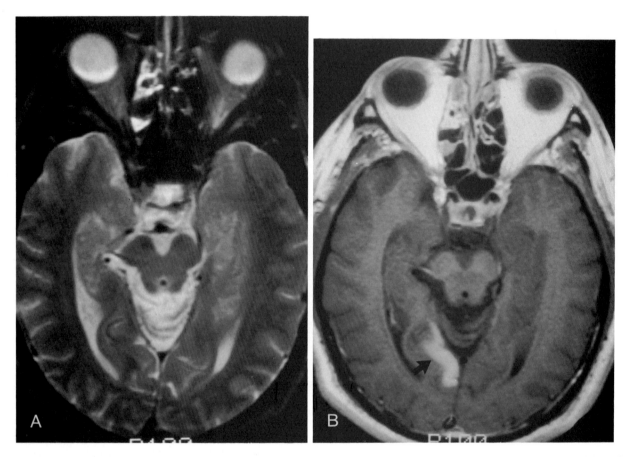

Figure 4.5.   Fogging Effect in Subacute Infarction. As edema and mass effect subside, but before development of atrophy, infarcts may be inconspicuous on unenhanced CT or MR images. **A.** Thirteen days after right PCA infarction, T2-weighted images are essentially normal in the occipital regions. **B.** T1-weighted images after gadolinium show enhancement of the infarcted deep right occipital cortex (*arrow*).

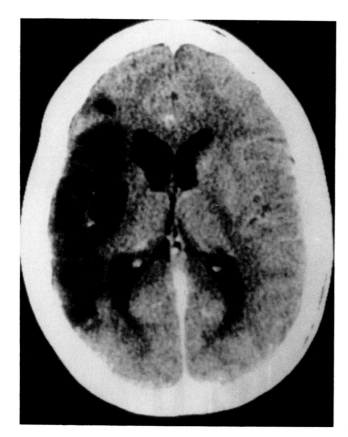

Figure 4.6. Chronic Infarction. Cystic encephalomalacia is present in the right MCA territory on CT 1 year after infarction. Note widening of the ipsilateral ventricle (ex vacuo dilation).

presumably because of a toxic effect of the contrast as it leaks through the abnormal blood-brain barrier. Most of these data, however, are based on studies using ionic contrast media. Others counter that this risk is exceedingly small and should not preclude its use. On the balance, use of nonionic contrast for CT seems reasonable when MR is not available and there is significant ambiguity about the diagnosis based on the noncontrast CT and clinical findings.

An intact blood-brain barrier normally excludes contrast from the brain. Leakage of macromolecular contrast agents through damaged vessels leads to local accumulation of iodine, seen as high attenuation (enhancement) of infarcted parenchyma. Blood-brain barrier breakdown underlies both hemorrhagic transformation and contrast enhancement of infarctions. Not surprisingly, then, these processes are seen at roughly the same time and often in combination. As with petechial gyral hemorrhage, a gyral pattern of enhancement (by CT or MR) is highly specific evidence of an underlying infarction. Computed tomography-detected enhancement of infarcted brain parenchyma typically begins at about 1 week, peaks at 7–14 days, often assumes a gyral pattern, and is less commonly observed in subcortical regions (Fig. 4.7B). Enhancement is seen in about half of the patients during the

1st week and in about two-thirds between weeks 1 and 4. As gliosis ensues and the blood-brain barrier is repaired, enhancement fades and then resolves by 3 months.

MAGNETIC RESONANCE CONTRAST

Most of the comments regarding the strategy, pathophysiology and enhancement patterns for CT also generally hold true for contrast in MR. Intravenous gadolinium diethylenetriamine pentaacetic acid and similar recently released gadolinium agents are very well tolerated by stroke patients and may give valuable information not readily available from the noncontrast MR. Stasis of gadolinium within vessels or leakage of contrast through an abnormal blood-brain barrier will shorten T1 relaxation of adjacent protons, leading to hyperintensity (enhancement) on T1-weighted images. As with CT, a noncontrast MR sequence is mandatory before contrast is given since both enhancement and subacute blood appear hyperintense on T1-weighted images. (This will be discussed in the "Hemorrhage" section.)

Intravascular enhancement on MR is commonly seen in the infarcted territory during the 1st week. This may be because of slow flow or vasodilation leading to stasis of gadolinium. The intravascular enhancement pattern may be detected within minutes of vessel occlusion, is seen in a majority of cortical infarcts at 1–3 days, and resolves by 10 days. The proximal trunks of more distally occluded arteries and leptomeningeal cortical channels are most prominently involved (Fig. 4.8). The area of vascular enhancement may extend beyond the T2 hyperintensity, possibly indicating recruitment of collateral supply at the ischemic border. Meningeal enhancement seen with meningitis, and dural enhancement seen postoperatively, can superficially resemble intravascular enhancement, but the distinction should be obvious on clinical grounds. Magnetic resonance imaging intravascular enhancement helps identify early strokes, dates them to less than 11 days old, and has no obvious CT counterpart.

Magnetic resonance imaging parenchymal enhancement occurs in a similar pattern to that seen on CT (and with the same time course seen by nuclear medicine infarct scans of the past). It may occur as early as day 1, but more typically begins after the 1st week, a time when intravascular enhancement is waning (Fig. 4.9). Virtually all cortical infarcts enhance on MR at 2 weeks. Elster has summarized this in his Rule of 3s: MR parenchymal enhancement peaks at 3 days to 3 weeks and resolves by 3 months.

The imaging time courses for CT and MR examinations in brain infarction are summarized in Table 4.2.

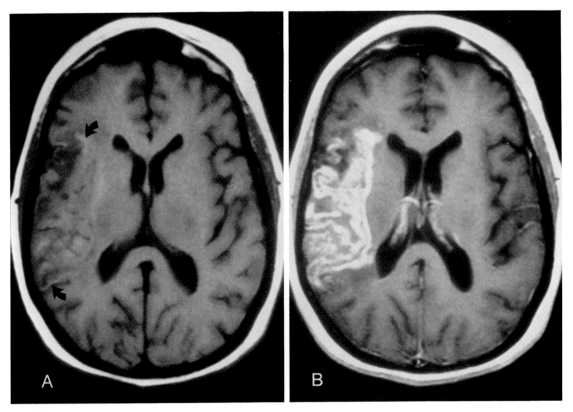

Figure 4.7. Petechial Hemorrhage and Gyral Enhancement in Subacute Infarction. A. Precontrast T1-weighted MR shows mild effacement of sulci in the right MCA territory. A few subtle areas of bright signal intensity scattered along the cortex indicate areas of petechial hemorrhage or laminar necrosis (*arrows*). **B.** Postcontrast T1-weighted image demonstrates marked gyral enhancement, a hallmark of subacute infarction.

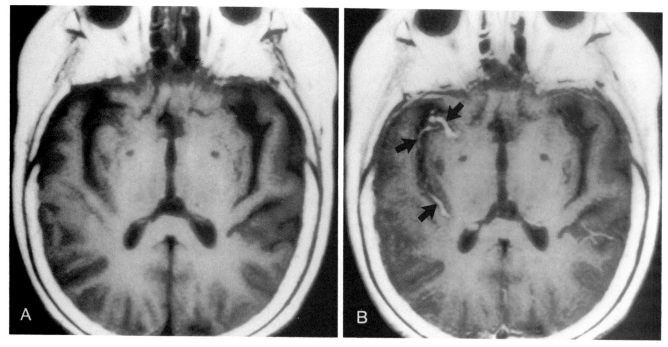

Figure 4.8. Intravascular Enhancement in Acute Infarction. Before (**A**) and after (**B**) contrast T1-weighted transverse images in acute right MCA infarction. There is mild sulcal effacement and prominent enhancement of sylvian branches of the MCA (*arrows*). Intravascular enhancement is seen only during the first 10 days after stroke.

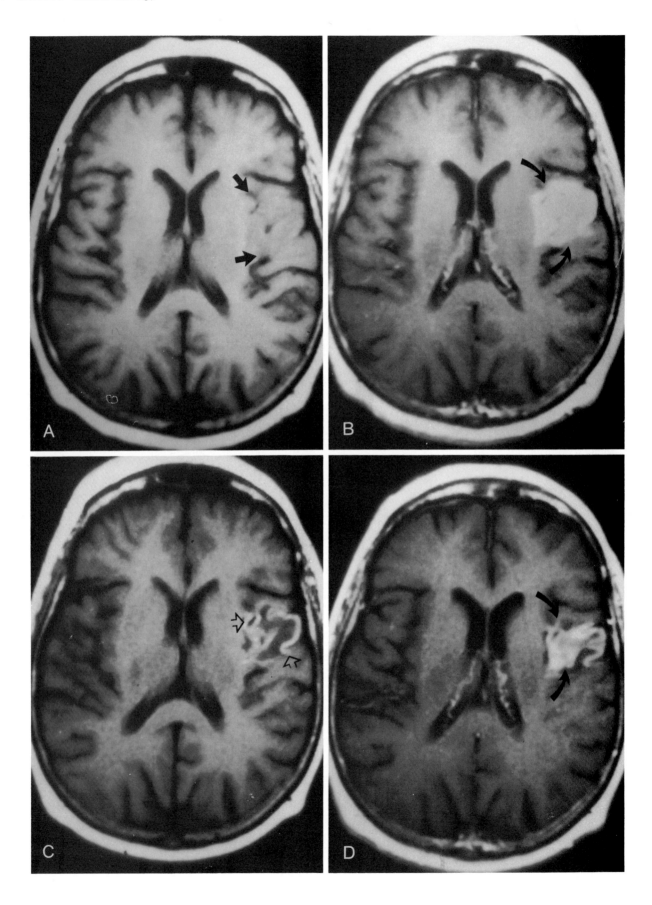

Pattern Recognition in Ischemic Stroke

Familiarity with the major vascular territories can help distinguish between infarction and other pathologic processes. The clinical time course and localization should be consistent with the imaging findings, and all should correspond to a known vascular distribution. Stroke localization is not necessarily synonymous with "focal." An ischemic event may cause a pattern of damage that is diffuse (hypoxic-ischemic injury), multifocal (vasculitis, emboli), or focal (single embolism or thrombus). The vessels causing stroke may be large or small, and may be on either the arterial or venous side. There is no such thing as a "funny" stroke; if it does not fit a vascular territory, the differential diagnosis changes (Fig. 4.10).

The relation of vascular anatomy to functional neuroanatomy is at the heart of clinicoradiologic correlation in stroke. Classically strokes and TIAs are divided into anterior (carotid territory) or posterior (vertebrobasilar territory) events. Patients with anterior circulation ischemia have been shown to benefit from carotid endarterectomy when the carotid artery is narrowed by at least 70% compared with its normal diameter. Surgery has not been proven beneficial for patients with lesser degrees of carotid stenosis or those with posterior territory TIAs, who therefore usually receive medical therapy (e.g., anticoagulation). Ischemia in the carotid territory may cause visual changes, aphasia, or sensorimotor deficits because of retinal, cortical, or subcortical damage. Vertebrobasilar strokes are more likely to cause syncope, ataxia, cranial nerve findings, homonymous visual field deficits, and facial symptoms opposite those of the body. A given deficit can be predicted from the known func-tional topography of the cortex and its connections through the internal capsule (Fig. 4.11).

The patterns of injury observed after occlusion of large arteries in the anterior and posterior circulations, small arteries in any region, and of the dural venous channels are reviewed in turn.

Anterior (Carotid) Circulation

INTERNAL CAROTID ARTERY

Thromboembolic disease in the internal carotid artery may cause TIAs or infarction in its middle cerebral artery (MCA) or anterior cerebral artery (ACA) branches or in the watershed zone between them. Embolic occlusion of the ophthalmic branch of the internal carotid artery may cause transient monocular blindness (amaurosis fugax). Observation of any of these patterns should prompt a careful look at the carotid arteries. The extent and distribution of ischemia observed depends upon the time course of occlusion, the degree of oligemia, and the available collateral supply. Complete carotid occlusions are occasionally found in asymptomatic patients with a well-developed collateral supply.

Atherosclerotic disease near the carotid bifurcation is responsible for the majority of ischemic events in the internal carotid artery territory. Arterial dissection, trauma, fibromuscular dysplasia, tumor encasement, prior neck radiotherapy, and connective tissue diseases may also cause significant carotid narrowing (Fig. 4.12). Hemodynamic effects begin to be seen when there is >80% reduction in area or >60% decrease in diameter. Lesions causing less severe narrowing may nonetheless become symptomatic when they serve as a nidus for thrombus formation or are

Table 4.2. Imaging Time Course after Brain Infarction

Time		CT	MR
Minutes		No changes	Absent flow void
			Arterial enhancement (days 1–10)
Hours	2–6	Hyperdense artery sign	Brain swelling (T1)
		Insular ribbon sign	(No signal Δ yet)
	6–12	Sulcal effacement	T2 hyperintensity
		± Decreased attenuation	
	12–24	Decreased attenuation	T1 hypointensity
Days	3–7	Maximum swelling	Maximum swelling
	3–21	Gyral enhancement (peak: 7–14 days)	Gyral enhancement (peak: 3–21 days)
			Petechial methemoglobin
	30–90	Encephalomalacia	Encephalomalacia
		Loss of enhancement	Loss of enhancement
		Resolution of petechial blood	Resolution of petechial blood

Figure 4.9. Evolution of Petechial Hemorrhage and Parenchymal Enhancement. Before and after contrast T1-weighted images in left sylvian cortical infarction. The acute study (**A** and **B**) shows non-hemorrhagic swelling (**A,** arrows) with prominent cortical enhance-ment (**B,** curved arrows). At 2-month follow-up (**C** and **D**) there is petechial hemorrhage (**C,** open arrows) and decreasing parenchymal enhancement (**D,** curved arrows). Parenchymal enhancement should resolve by 3 months.

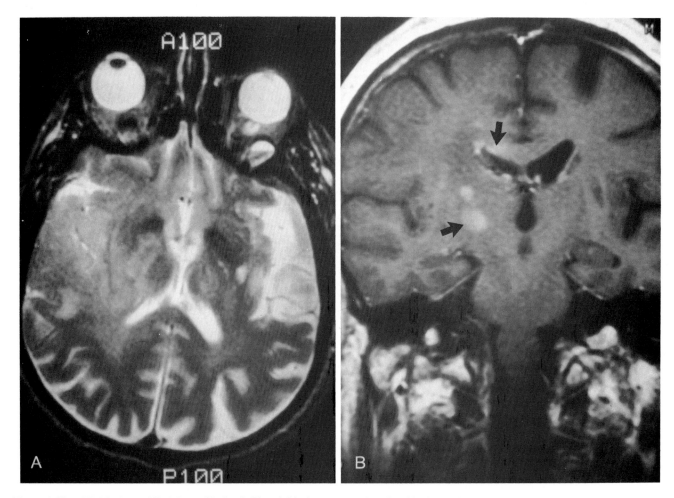

Figure 4.10.   Glioblastoma Mimicking a Stroke. A. T2-weighted axial section shows edema primarily in the right MCA territory, but with additional involvement of the medial temporal lobe, thalamus, and periatrial regions. **B.** Postcontrast coronal T1-weighted image shows patchy, nodular areas of enhancement in the basal ganglia and periventricular regions (*arrows*). Even with a strong clinical history for stroke-like onset, the nonvascular distribution and atypical enhancement pattern effectively exclude underlying infarction. When in doubt, follow-up imaging studies will usually clarify the diagnosis.

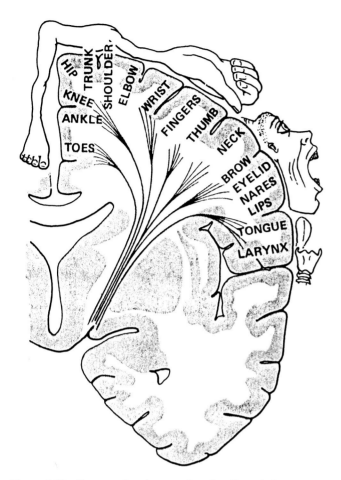

Figure 4.11. Homunculus. A coronal section through the precentral (motor) cortex depicts the topographic representation of the opposite side of the body. The face and hand areas are served by the MCA territory, the leg by the ACA. (From Gilman S., Winans SS. Essentials of clinical neuroanatomy & neurophysiology. Philadelphia: F.A. Davis Company, 1982.)

unmasked by hypotension. Studies have shown a clear benefit of endarterectomy in symptomatic patients with >70% stenosis but not for those with <30% narrowing. Ongoing studies should clarify the guidelines for the 30–70% group within the next 5 years.

Noninvasive screening of the carotid arteries may be achieved with either ultrasound or magnetic resonance angiography (MRA). The choice of ultrasound versus MRA depends upon the abilities of the available personnel and equipment. Sensitivity and specificity are as high as 85–90% for either technique. Both methods are used to noninvasively identify patients with hemodynamically significant disease who might then be referred for conventional angiography. Ultrasound is the most commonly employed screening examination in most centers. It has the advantage of portability, generally lower costs, and can be performed in patients with contraindications to MR/MRA. Ultrasound is more operator-dependent than MRA and is unable to reliably assess portions of the distal internal carotid artery near the skull base.

Transcranial Doppler sonography may extend the ability of ultrasound to examine the carotid siphon and intracranial branches. Magnetic resonance angiography can evaluate the entire course of the carotid and may be quickly performed in conjunction with the patient's brain MR study. It is a particularly good method for screening pediatric or elderly patients in whom conventional angiography may be technically more difficult.

Selective common carotid angiography remains the gold standard for carotid artery evaluation and is generally the method of choice for surgical planning. The study should cover the entire internal carotid artery, including cervical and cranial portions.Evaluation of the surgically inaccessible cranial segments (petrous, cavernous, and supraclinoid) is necessary to exclude high-grade intracranial stenoses or "tandem" lesions that might contraindicate endarterectomy.

ANTERIOR CEREBRAL ARTERY

The terminal bifurcation of the ICA is into the anterior and middle cerebral arteries (Fig. 4.13). The ACA is divided into three subgroups: the *medial lenticulostriate branches* serve the rostral portions of the basal ganglia; the *pericallosal* branches supply the corpus callosum; and the *hemispheric* branches serve the medial aspects of the frontal and parietal lobes (Fig. 4.14). About 5% of infarcts involve the ACA.

The medial lenticulostriates penetrate the anterior perforating substance to give variable supply to the anterior-inferior aspect of the internal capsule, putamen, globus pallidus, caudate head, and portions of the hypothalamus and optic chiasm. The largest of these vessels supplies the caudate head/anterior internal capsule region and is recognized as our friend, the recurrent artery of Heubner. Infarction in the medial lenticulostriate territory may cause problems with speech production (motor aphasia), facial weakness, and disturbances in mood and judgment.

Above the take-off of the lenticulostriates, the ACAs are interconnected by the anterior communicating artery. Each ACA ascends further, giving off branches to the frontal pole (orbitofrontal and frontopolar arteries). The ACAs terminate as a bifurcation into the (lower) pericallosal and (upper) callosomarginal branches. These arteries run parallel to the corpus callosum from front to back, giving supply to the medial cortex of the frontal and parietal lobes. As its name would imply, the pericallosal artery courses around and feeds the corpus callosum. The ACA branching patterns are quite variable from one patient to the next, with about 10% having only one pericallosal branch, which supplies both hemispheres, an "azygous" ACA (Fig. 4.15).

Unilateral damage in the ACA hemispheric branches will cause preferential leg weakness on the

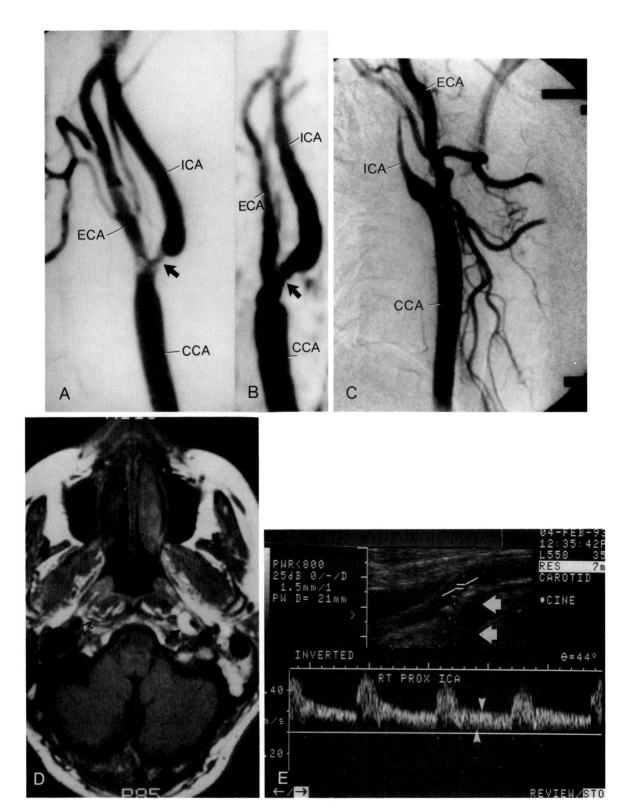

Figure 4.12. Carotid Disease. A. Atherosclerosis. Lateral view of the carotid bifurcation by conventional digital subtraction angiography. There is approximately 60% reduction in the diameter of the proximal internal carotid artery (*arrow*) compared with its normal caliber above. *CCA*, common carotid artery; *ICA*, internal carotid artery; *ECA*, external carotid artery and its branches. **B.** Atherosclerosis. Lateral maximum intensity projection from a two-dimensional time-of-flight MR angiogram in the same patient shows a very similar pattern of flow-related enhancement. **C.** Carotid dissection with a tapering occlusion in the internal carotid artery just above the bifurcation. **D.** Dissection in another patient with the mural crescent sign indicative of intramural thrombus in the petrous portion of the left internal carotid artery (*arrow*). T1-weighted transverse image. Note normal caliber flow void and scant amounts of fat surrounding the normal right internal carotid artery (*open arrow*). **E.** Carotid ultrasound showing evidence of calcified plaque with acoustic shadowing (*arrows*), vessel narrowing, and spectral broadening (between *arrowheads*) in a case of atherosclerosis.

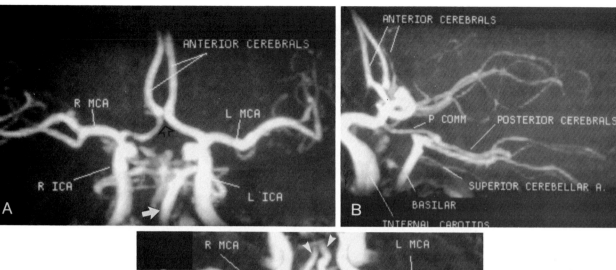

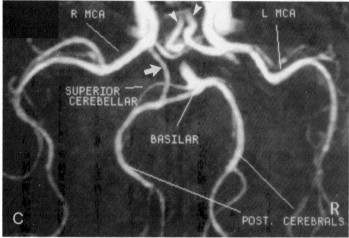

Figure 4.13. MR Angiography of the Normal Circle of Willis and Its Branches. A. The anterior (coronal) projection depicts the normal internal carotid arteries (*ICA*) with bifurcation into the ACA and MCA intracranial branches. The basilar artery and cerebellar branches project below (*arrow*). The ACA is very short in this patient but would be found at the *open arrow*. **B.** Lateral projection shows a single large posterior communicating artery (*P COMM*) connecting the anterior to posterior circulations. The superior cerebellar and poste-rior cerebral branches of the basilar artery are clearly shown. **C.** Submentovertex projection outlines the relationship of the major vessels to the circle of Willis. We are looking down the barrel of the internal carotid arteries and basilar artery. A single posterior communicating artery is again seen (*arrow*); the opposite side is likely hypoplastic. The ACAs project between the internal carotid arteries (*arrowheads*).

opposite side of the body (Table 4.3). Bilateral ACA infarctions lead to incontinence and an awake but apathetic state known as akinetic mutism. Infarction of the corpus callosum can cause a variety of interhemispheric disconnection syndromes including ideomotor apraxia (the inability to perform right hemisphere tasks when given cues from the dominant left hemisphere).

MIDDLE CEREBRAL ARTERY

The MCA supplies more brain tissue than any other intracranial vessel and is host to almost two-thirds of infarcts. Its offspring are the *lateral lenticulostriates*, which supply most of the basal ganglia region, and the *hemispheric branches*, which serve the lateral cerebral surface (Figs. 4.3 and 4.16).

The lateral lenticulostriates arise from the proximal MCA as numerous small perforating end arteries dis-tributed to the putamen, lateral globus pallidus, superior half of the internal capsule, and adjacent corona radiata, and the majority of the caudate. Isolated vascular lesions of the globus pallidus or putamen are commonly asymptomatic or may affect contralateral muscle tone and motor control. Lesions of the internal capsule or corona radiata may cause pure or mixed sensory and motor deficits on the opposite side of the body. Interruption of visual connections to the lateral geniculate nucleus results in a subtle type of contralateral homonymous hemianopsia. Rarely, the arcuate fasciculus pathway from Wernicke's to Broca's speech areas may be selectively infarcted, leading to a conduction aphasia (the inability to repeat or read aloud, despite preserved comprehension and fluency).

The MCA loops laterally through the insula where it bifurcates or trifurcates into its major cortical branches (Fig. 4.13**A**). The insula itself is supplied by

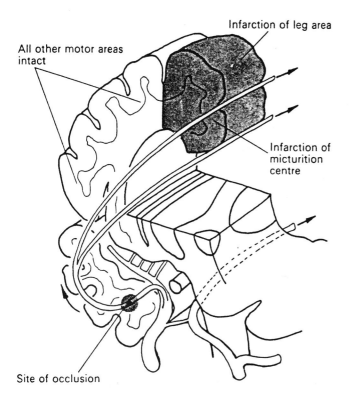

Figure 4.14.   An ACA Occlusion. An ACA occlusion causes infarction of the paramedian frontal cortex responsible for motor and sensory function of the Opposite Leg (*stippled area*). If bilateral, incontinence and akinetic mutism may also be seen. (From Patten J. Neurological differential diagnosis. New York: Springer Verlag, 1977.)

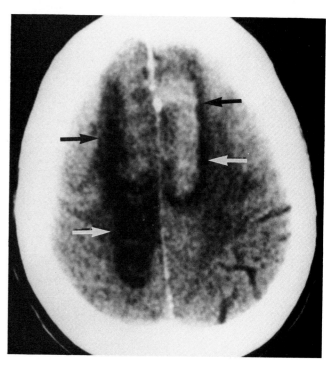

Figure 4.15.   Hemorrhagic Infarction. Hemorrhagic infarction in a bilateral ACA distribution (*arrows*) shown by noncontrast CT. This was an embolic stroke, presumably occluding an azygous ACA.

Table 4.3.   Functional Vascular Anatomy[a]

Vessel	Branch	Side	Deficit/Syndrome
ACA	Hemispheric	Either	Leg weakness
		Both	Incontinence, akinetic mutism
	Medial lenticulostriates	Either	Facial weakness
		Left	Dysarthria; ± motor aphasia
MCA	Hemispheric	Either	Face and arm > leg weakness
		Left	Motor aphasia (anterior lesion)
			Receptive aphasia (posterior lesion)
			Global aphasia (total MCA)
		Right	Neglect syndromes
			Visuospatial dysfunction
	Lateral lenticulostriates	Either	Variable lacunar syndromes
PCA	Hemispheric	Either	Hemianopsia
		Both	Cortical blindness
			Memory deficits
	Thalamoperforators	Either	Somnolence
			Sensory disturbances
Cerebellar	PICA, AICA[b], or SCA[c]	Either	Ataxia, vertigo, vomiting
			Coma if mass effect
			± Brain stem deficits
Watershed	ACA/MCA/PCA	Either	Man in a barrel syndrome
		Bilateral	Severe memory problems

[a]Assumes left hemisphere language dominance.
[b]Anterior inferior cerebellar artery.
[c]Superior cerebellar artery.

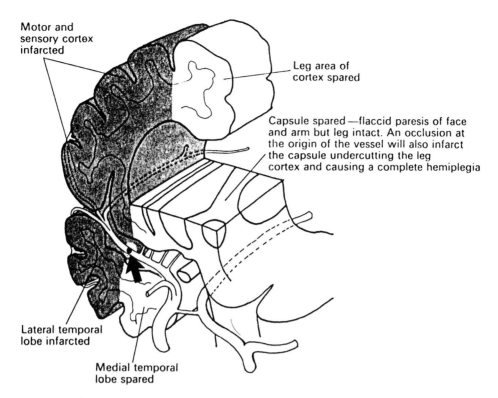

Motor and
sensory cortex
infarcted

Leg area of
cortex spared

Capsule spared —flaccid paresis of face
and arm but leg intact. An occlusion at
the origin of the vessel will also infarct
the capsule undercutting the leg
cortex and causing a complete hemiplegia

Lateral temporal
lobe infarcted

Medial temporal
lobe spared

Figure 4.16. An MCA Occlusion. An MCA occlusion distal to the lateral lenticulostriates (*large arrow*) causes infarction of the motor and sensory cortex of the arm and face (*stippled area*). More proximal occlusion will also affect the internal capsule, potentially adding leg deficits. (From Patten J. Neurological differential diagnosis. New York: Springer Verlag, 1977.)

hemispheric branches, not by the lateral lenticulostriates. When the proximal MCA is occluded, this insular region is furthest from any potential collateral supply, probably explaining the early appearance of edema, which gives rise to the "insular ribbon sign" (Fig. 4.3). The anterior hemispheric branches of the MCA supply the anterolateral tip of the temporal lobe (anterior temporal artery), the frontal lobe (operculofrontal arteries), and the motor and sensory strips (central sulcus arteries). Posterior hemispheric branches of the MCA supply the parietal lobe behind the sensory strip (posterior parietal artery), the posterolateral parietal and lateral occipital lobes (angular artery), and the majority of the temporal lobe (posterior temporal artery).

Occlusion of the rostral MCA branches of the dominant hemisphere will cause a motor (Broca) aphasia in which comprehension remains intact. Posterior branches in the dominant hemisphere supply Wernicke's area, causing a receptive aphasia when occluded. Posterior temporal branch occlusion may interrupt visual radiations, causing contralateral homonymous field defects. Involvement of either hemisphere's precentral gyrus (motor strip) will produce contralateral weakness that affects the face and arm more than the leg (Fig. 4.11). Contralateral cortical sensory loss occurs when the primary or association sensory cortex behind the central sulcus is affected. In the nondominant right hemisphere,

posterior MCA infarcts commonly cause bizarre impairment in visualospatial abilities and sometimes neglect (or nonrecognition) of the left body. Complete occlusion of the MCA beyond the lenticulostriates causes a combination of these deficits: contralateral face and arm hemiparesis, field defect, and either neglect or global aphasia, depending on which hemisphere is affected. Leg weakness may also be seen when the MCA stem is occluded, because of internal capsule involvement. These relationships are summarized in Table 4.3.

Posterior (Vertebrobasilar) Circulation

VERTEBRAL ARTERIES

The vertebral arteries usually originate from the subclavian arteries, ascend straight upward in the transverse foramina of vertebra C6 through C3, turn sharply through the C2-C1-foramen magnum levels, and unite anterior to the low medulla to form the basilar artery (Fig. 4.17). Atherosclerotic narrowing commonly affects the vertebral arteries at their origins and may affect the basilar artery over variable lengths. Narrowing of the cervical portion of the vertebral arteries may be because of compressive uncovertebral osteophytes. Rapid head turning (e.g., motor vehicle accidents) may stretch the vertebrals at the C1-2 level, leading to arterial dissection. Any of these conditions may cause vertebrobasilar ischemia via thrombotic or

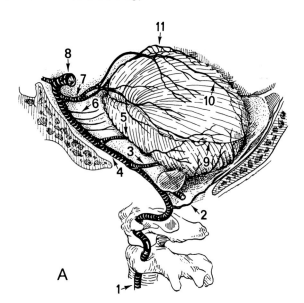

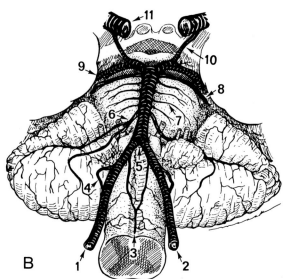

Figure 4.17. Vertebrobasilar arteries. A. Lateral view. *1*, left vertebral; *2*, posterior meningeal; *3*, PICA; *4*, basilar; *5*, anterior inferior cerebellar artery (AICA); *6*, pontine perforators; *7*, superior cerebellar artery (SCA); *8*, PCA; *9*, branches of the SCA and AICA in the horizontal fissure of the cerebellum; *10*, SCA hemispheric branches; *11*, superior vermian branches. **B.** Anterior view. *1*, Right vertebral; *2*, left vertebral; *3*, anterior spinal; *4*, PICA; *5*, basilar; *6*, AICA; *7*, pontine; *8*, SCA; *9*, PCA; *10*, posterior communicating; *11*, internal carotid artery. (From Osborn AG. Introduction to cerebral angiography. Philadelphia: Harper & Row, 1980.)

embolic mechanisms. Endarterectomy or angioplasty are sometimes feasible for correction of atherosclerotic lesions but have not gained wide acceptance. Anticoagulation and antiplatelet agents remain the mainstay of treatment for vertebrobasilar ischemia.

BASILAR ARTERY

The basilar artery is formed by the union of the two vertebral arteries. As it ascends between the clivus and brainstem, it sends large branches to the cerebellum and smaller perforating vessels to the brainstem. The basilar artery ends at its bifurcation into the posterior cerebral arteries just above the tentorium cerebelli. Occlusion of the basilar artery itself is usually rapidly fatal, because of infarction of respiratory and cardiac centers in the medulla. Occlusion of the perforating end arteries from the basilar artery causes focal brainstem infarction, usually manifest as cranial nerve dysfunction, ataxia, somnolence, and crossed motor or sensory deficits. These lesions characteristically respect the midline of the brainstem and often extend to the ventral surface (Fig. 4.18). Metabolic disturbances (e.g., central pontine myelinolysis) and hypertensive hemorrhages (most commonly in the pons) tend to be more centrally or diffusely located. Large or multiple lesions in the pons can cause a nightmarish syndrome of quadriparesis with intact cognition, the "locked in" state.

POSTERIOR CEREBRAL ARTERY (PCA)

The basilar artery ends at its bifurcation into the PCAs at the midbrain level, just above the tentorial hi-atus. The major branches of the PCA include the midbrain and thalamic *perforating vessels*, *posterior choroidal arteries*, and *cortical branches* to the medial temporal and occipital lobes (Fig. 4.19). Ten to 15% of infarcts occur in the PCA territory.

The proximal segments of the PCAs sweep posterolaterally around the midbrain, giving off small perforating branches to the mesencephalon and thalamus along the way. Midbrain infarction causes loss of the pupillary light responses, impaired upgaze, and somnolence because of damage of the quadrigeminal plate, third cranial nerve nucleii, and reticular activating formation, respectively. Proximal PCA perforators also supply the majority of the thalamus and sometimes portions of the posterior limb of the internal capsule. Thalamic infarction may cause a variety of disturbances, but contralateral sensory loss is the most common problem.

The posterior choroidal arteries arise from the proximal PCA to supply the choroid plexus of the third and lateral ventricles, pineal gland, and regions contiguous with the third ventricle. Isolated posterior choroid infarctions are rare because of the rich collateral supply through the choroid plexus.

Posterior cerebral artery cortical branches supply the inferomedial temporal lobe (inferior temporal arteries), superior occipital gyrus (parieto-occipital artery), and visual cortex of the occipital lobes (calcarine artery) (Fig. 4.20). Hemispheric PCA occlusions are usually from an embolic source. Inferomedial temporal infarction may cause memory deficits, which are severe when bilateral. Loss of the primary visual cor-

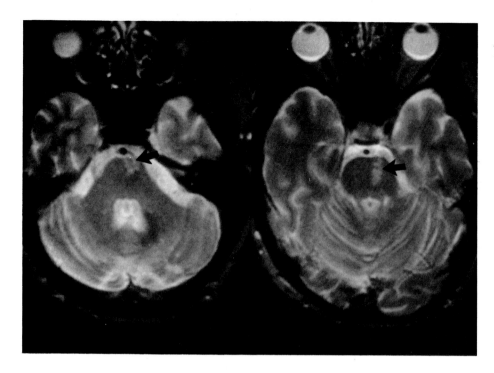

Figure 4.18. Brainstem Infarction. Adjacent transverse T2-weighted images show a left paramedian pontine infarct (*arrows*), which respects the midline.

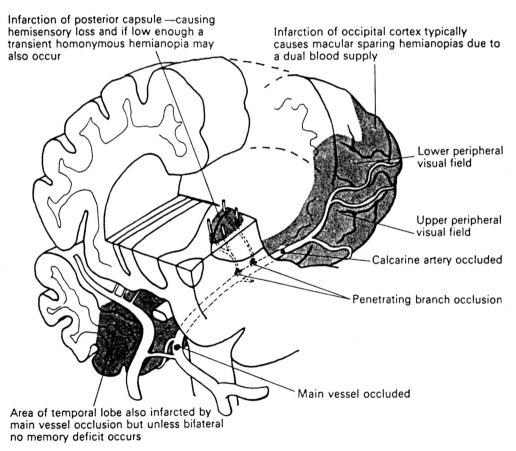

Infarction of posterior capsule —causing hemisensory loss and if low enough a transient homonymous hemianopia may also occur

Infarction of occipital cortex typically causes macular sparing hemianopias due to a dual blood supply

Lower peripheral visual field

Upper peripheral visual field

Calcarine artery occluded

Penetrating branch occlusion

Main vessel occluded

Area of temporal lobe also infarcted by main vessel occlusion but unless bilateral no memory deficit occurs

Figure 4.19. A PCA Occlusion. A PCA occlusion results in syndromes of memory impairment, opposite visual field loss, and sometimes hemisensory deficits. (From Patten J. Neurological differential diagnosis. New York: Springer Verlag, 1977.)

Figure 4.20. A PCA Infarction. Adjacent T2-weighted transverse images show involvement of the left occipital lobe and medial temporal lobe. The patient presented with a dense right homonymous visual field defect.

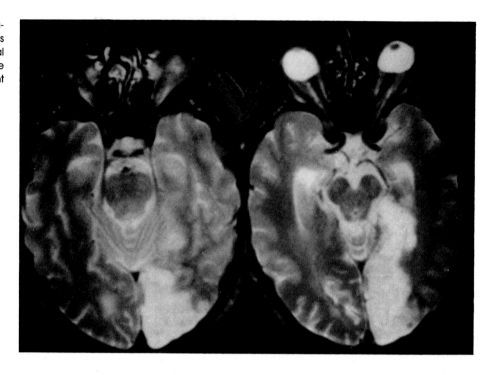

tex causes complete loss of vision in the opposite visual field (homonymous hemianopsia).

In about 20% of patients, one or both of the proximal PCA segments may be hypoplastic or absent. In these cases flow is derived from the internal carotid artery system via a prominent posterior communicating artery. This is commonly referred to as "fetal origin" of the PCA, since embryologically the PCA develops with the internal carotid artery. Since this is a fairly common variation, both vertebral and carotid disease should be considered when evaluating PCA infarctions.

CEREBELLAR ARTERIES

Headache, vertigo, nausea, vomiting, and ipsilateral ataxia are the hallmarks of cerebellar stroke; 85% are ischemic and 15% are primary hemorrhages. Clinically it is difficult to distinguish which cerebellar subterritory is involved and whether it derives from infarction or hemorrhage. *Because of clinical urgency, acute evaluation of suspected cerebellar strokes should be performed by CT.* Cerebellar hemorrhages and any infarctions with significant mass effect are neurosurgical emergencies requiring posterior fossa decompression. Multiplanar MR is preferred for evaluation beyond the acute phase, since beam-harding artifacts degrade posterior fossa images on CT.

Even though deficits related to the cerebellar territories are hard to distinguish clinically, it is important to recognize characteristic distributions in order to elucidate stroke mechanisms. Luckily, only a *SAP* would forget the correct order of cerebellar branches

going from top to bottom: the *s*uperior, *a*nterior inferior, and *p*osterior inferior cerebellar arteries (Fig. 4.17).

Superior Cerebellar Arteries. The upper parts of the cerebellum are supplied by the superior cerebellar arteries. These arise from the distal basilar as the last large branches beneath the tentorium cerebelli. The superior cerebellar arteries territory includes the superior vermis, middle and superior cerebellar peduncles, and superolateral aspects of the cerebellar hemispheres (i.e., the "roof" of the cerebellum). Most superior cerebellar arteries infarcts are embolic.

Anterior Inferior Cerebellar Arteries (AICA). These arteries arise from the proximal basilar artery to supply the anteromedial cerebellum and sometimes part of the middle cerebellar peduncle. The AICA is usually the smallest of the three major cerebellar hemisphere branches. Occlusion commonly causes ipsilateral limb ataxia, nausea, vomiting, dizziness, and headache.

Posterior Inferior Cerebellar Arteries (PICA). The bottom of the cerebellum is supplied by the posterior inferior cerebellar artery (PICA). The PICA is the first major intracranial branch of the vertebrobasilar system, usually arising from the distal vertebral artery 1–2 cm below the basilar origin. Its territory is variable but often includes the dorsolateral medulla, inferior vermis, and posterolateral cerebellar hemisphere. The PICA maintains a reciprocal relation with the AICA above it. If the PICA is large, then the ipsilateral AICA is usually small, and vice versa. This arrangement is sometimes referred to as the AICA-PICA loop.

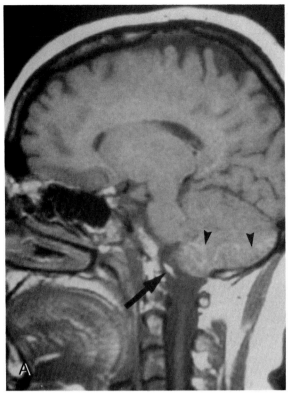

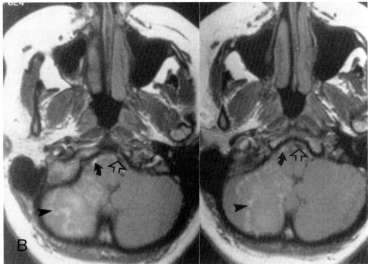

Figure 4.21. Vertebral Dissection with PICA Infarction. This patient developed neck pain and ataxia following a skiing accident. T1-weighted images without contrast. Sagittal (*A*) and transverse (*B*) images show high signal in the occluded right vertebral artery (*closed arrows*) with preserved flow void in the left vertebral (*open arrows*). There is hemorrhagic infarction in the right PICA territory (*arrowheads*).

The PICA is usually the largest cerebellar hemisheric branch and is the most commonly occluded. Occlusions may occur from extension of a vertebral dissection that began at the C1-2 level (Fig. 4.21). If only the cerebellar hemisphere is affected, ipsilateral limb ataxia, nausea, vomiting, dizziness, and headache are seen, just as for AICA infarcts. Involvement of the medulla in PICA infarction adds elements of Wallenberg's syndrome, ipsilateral ataxia, facial numbness, Horner's syndrome, contralateral body numbness, dysphagia, and dysarthria.

Watershed (Border Zone) Infarction

An episode of transient global hypoperfusion may result in bilateral infarctions in the watershed regions between arterial territories (also referred to as the border zones). Typical triggering events include cardiac arrest, massive bleeding, anaphylaxis, and surgery under general anesthesia. The border zones are regions perfused by terminal branches of two adjacent arterial territories (Fig. 4.22). When flow in one or both of the parent vessels falls below a critical level, the brain living in the watershed zone is the first to go. Unilateral watershed damage may be seen when carotid occlusion or stenosis is unmasked by global hypotension; in this case, the nonstenotic side recovers because of relative preservation of flow. Images show damage extending out from the "corners" of the lateral ventricles on higher sections (Fig. 4.23). Characteristic clinical findings include weakness isolated to the upper arms ("man in a barrel syndrome"), cortical blindness, and memory loss.

Small-Vessel Ischemia

LACUNES

There are small subcortical infarcts that may occur in any territory. They account for about 15–20% of all strokes. Lacunes are the 2–15 mm^3 cavities (literally, "little lakes") left in the brain as the result of occlusion of a penetrating artery causing infarction and ensuing encephalomalacia. Patients usually have a history of long-standing hypertension, leading to lipohyalinosis of the vessels and eventual thrombosis. Transient ischemic attacks precede the stroke in 60% of cases, and a stuttering course is common in the first 2 days. Pure motor or sensory syndromes may occur with these small lesions. Characteristic locations include the lenticular nucleus (37%), pons (16%), thalamus (14%), caudate (10%), and internal capsule (10%) (Fig. 4.24).

Internal Capsule Lacunes. These are an especially important subset of lacunes because they are quite common and cause characteristic syndromes. Axonal projections to and from the cortex must funnel through the internal capsule and brainstem where even tiny lacunes may cause major deficits. The internal capsule receives supply from multiple small perforating arteries at the base of the brain, all of which are common sites for lacunar infarction and hypertensive hemorrhages. Its contrib-

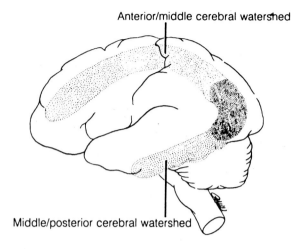

Anterior/middle cerebral watershed

Middle/posterior cerebral watershed

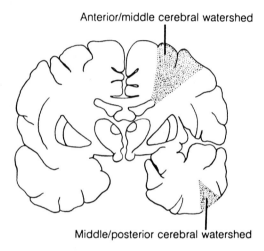

Anterior/middle cerebral watershed

Middle/posterior cerebral watershed

Figure 4.22. Watershed Ischemia. Stippled brain areas are served by terminal branches of adjacent parent arteries. The watershed zones are at highest risk of infarction when flow is reduced in one or both carotids. (From Simon RP, Aminoff MJ, Greenberg DA, eds. Clinical neurology. Norwalk, CT: Appleton & Lange, 1989.

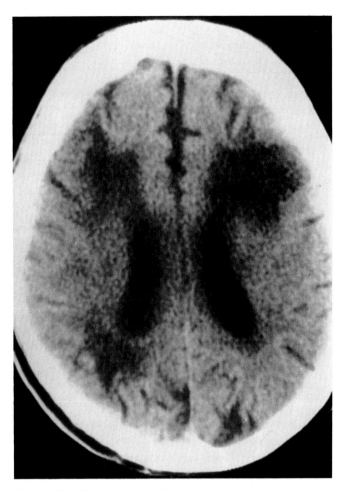

Figure 4.23. Watershed Infarctions. This patient developed upper arm weakness and memory deficits after resuscitation from cardiac arrest. The ACA/MCA border zones show infarction bilaterally near the vertex.

utors include the ACA and MCA lenticulostriates, the anterior choroidal branch of the internal carotid artery, and PCA thalamogeniculates. Isolated lesions of the anterior limb interrupt connections of the anterior frontal lobe, but are usually clinically silent. Beginning at the genu and working back, the capsule carries corticobulbar, *head*, *arm*, and then *leg* fibers in a somatotopically organized fashion (Fig. 4.25). (Our little homunculus man, *HAL*, stands in the posterior limb with his head at the genu, reclining with his head directed medially as he enters the cerebral peduncle.) Lesions in the posterior limb are clinically most important since they may cause severe sensory, motor, or mixed deficits. Lesions at the genu may disrupt speech production or swallowing, but generally become apparent only when bilateral.

Lacunes versus Perivascular Spaces. "État lacunaire" refers to a state of multiple lacunar infarctions. The term is still used in the literature and should be distinguished from the term "état criblé," which refers to enlarged perivascular spaces (Virchow-Robin spaces) that may develop around perforating vessels (Fig. 4.26). These normal spaces may simulate lacunes but have no associated neurologic deficit or other clinical relevance. By definition, Virchow-Robin spaces should follow cerebrospinal fluid intensity on all MR sequences, have no associated mass effect, and occur along the path of a penetrating vessel. Common locations include the medial temporal lobes and inferior one-third of the putamen and thalamus. Occasionally, they may be seen along the course of small medullary veins near the vertex (Fig. 4.27). Most perivascular spaces seen on MR are between 1 and 3 mm in diameter, but some may be 5 mm or larger. Enlarged perivascular spaces are observed as a normal variant in all age groups. Both increasing size and frequency are noted with increasing age.

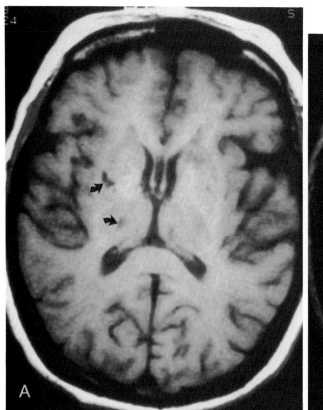
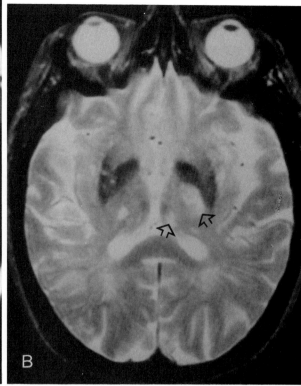

Figure 4.24. Lacunes. T1- (**A**) and T2- (**B**) weighted transverse images show small holes of cerebrospinal fluid intensity in the right thalamus and posterior putamen, likely representing old lacunes (*arrows*). New areas of edema and mass effect are seen in the left thalamus and inferior aspect of the internal capsule on the T2-weighted images (*open arrows*). The latter correspond to an acute right hemiparesis and sensory deficit, indicating recent lacunar infarction. (Bilateral hypointensity in the putamen and globus pallidus on the T2-weighted sequence represents normal iron deposition associated with aging.)

Small-Vessel Ischemic Changes. Small foci of T2 hyperintensity are commonly seen scattered throughout the brains of older patients, with or without clinical symptoms. These "UBOs" (unidentified bright objects) can cause considerable consternation. They are commonly associated with patchy or diffuse T2 hyperintensity in the centrum semiovale (Fig. 4.26). Pages could be filled with different authors' terms for related processes: small vessel ischemic disease, senescent change, Binswanger's disease, multiinfarct dementia, and leukoariosis, to name a few. There is no consensus on when these imaging changes should be considered abnormal, and when they simply represent a normal part of the aging process. At one end of the spectrum are patients who have collected enough tiny infarcts over the years to impair brain function. Individually or in small numbers these infarcts were presumably asymptomatic, but in aggregate lead to a multiinfarct dementia picture. At the other end of the spectrum are perfectly healthy patients who have presumably developed a speck of gliosis or occlusion of an inconsequential tiny vessel as a normal part of aging. The clinical findings must determine which of

these patients with unidentified bright objects needs further workup.

VASCULITIS

Patchy inflammatory changes in arterial walls may lead to either large or small vessel stroke. Vasculitis may be triggered by autoimmune disorders, drug exposure (heroin, amphetamines), polyarteritis nodosa, and idiopathic processes (e.g., giant cell arteritis). Vasculitic infarcts are often scattered across multiple vascular territories and therefore may produce atypical patterns of damage. Varying stages of inflammation, necrosis, fibrosis, and aneurysms may be seen simultaneously.

Cases of suspected vasculitis are evaluated by conventional cut-film angiography, which provides the highest possible resolution. Views of the intracranial circulation and the external carotid artery are reviewed in search of irregular focal narrowing. Positive sites may then be selected for biopsy confirmation. Sometimes the vessels affected are so small the angiogram is normal. In these cases, skin, nerve, muscle, or random temporal artery biopsy may be required to make the diagnosis. Diagnostic confirmation is im-

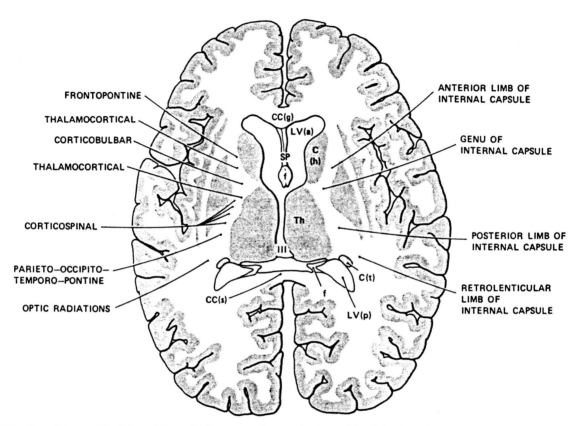

FRONTOPONTINE

THALAMOCORTICAL

CORTICOBULBAR

THALAMOCORTICAL

CORTICOSPINAL

PARIETO—OCCIPITO—
TEMPORO—PONTINE

OPTIC RADIATIONS

ANTERIOR LIMB OF
INTERNAL CAPSULE

GENU OF
INTERNAL CAPSULE

POSTERIOR LIMB OF
INTERNAL CAPSULE

RETROLENTICULAR
LIMB OF
INTERNAL CAPSULE

CC(g)
LV(a)
C
(h)
SP
f
Th
III
CC(s)
f
C(t)
LV(p)

Figure 4.25. Somatotopy of the Internal Capsule. Transverse diagram showing the main parts of the internal capsule (labeled on the right) and major fiber tracts passing through it (labeled on the left). *CC(g)*, genu of the corpus callosum; *CC(s)*, splenium of the corpus callosum; *C(h)*, caudate head; *C(t)*, caudate tail; *f*, fornix; *LV(a)*, anterior horn of the lateral ventricle; *LV(p)*, posterior horn of the lateral ventricle; *SP*, septum pellucidum; *TH*, thalamus; *III*, third ventricle. (From Gilman S, Winans SS. Essentials of clinical neuroanatomy & neurophysiology. Philadelphia: F.A. Davis Company, 1982.)

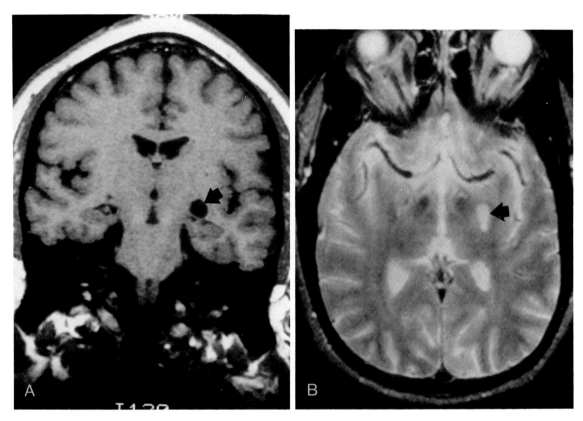

Figure 4.26.   Virchow-Robin Spaces. Coronal T1 (**A**) and transverse T2 (**B**) images show an enlarged but normal perivascular space (*arrows*) which exactly follows cerebrospinal fluid intensity. There is no mass effect, and the patient had no symptoms referable to this region.

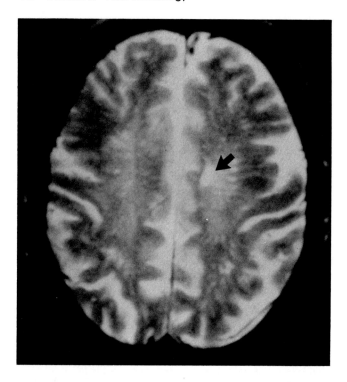

Figure 4.27. Small-Vessel Ischemic Changes and Perivascular Spaces. Transverse T2-weighted image at the level of the centrum semiovale shows numerous areas of hyperintensity. The radial, linear areas likely represent prominent cerebrospinal fluid spaces around small medullary veins. A rounded lesion (*arrow*) indicates a site of probable small infarction.

portant, since many of the vasculitides respond to steroids or cytotoxic drugs.

Venous Infarction

Venous occlusion is an uncommon but important cause of stroke. Characteristically venous infarcts occur in younger patients who present with headache, sudden focal deficits, and often seizures. Predisposing factors include hypercoaguable states, pregnancy, infection (spread from contiguous scalp, face, middle ear, or sinus), dehydration, meningitis, and direct invasion by tumor. Even though arterial supply is intact, blockage of outflow leads to stasis, deoxygenation of blood, and neuronal death. Continued perfusion into damaged, occluded vessels frequently leads to hemorrhage. Any dural sinus or cortical vein may be affected, but the most common are lateral, superior sagittal, and cavernous sinus occlusions.

A pattern of hemorrhagic infarction in the deep cortical or subcortical regions is usually present. These lesions tend to be rounded and may spare some overlying cortex, as opposed to the classic wedge-shaped arterial occlusions that grow larger toward the surface (Fig. 4.28). Venous infarctions may also be suspected when there is an apparent infarct not conforming to a known arterial territory.

The venous clot responsible may be seen indirectly as a filling defect in the superior sagittal sinus on contrast-enhanced CT, the "empty delta" sign (Fig. 4.29). The empty delta sign is usually present 1–4 weeks after sinus occlusion, but may be false-negative in the acute and chronic phases of the disease. Small venous occlusions are not reliably detected by CT. An appearance that mimics the empty delta sign has also been described in up to 10% of normal patients when CT scanning is delayed for more than 30 minutes after contrast infusion. This is probably because of differential blood pool clearance and dural absorption of contrast, effectively highlighting the dural margins of a normal venous sinus.

On MR, venous sinus thrombosis is suspected when venous flow voids are lost and confirmed when an actual clot is observed (Fig. 4.28). Normal but slowly flowing blood can sometimes cause high signal within veins, a potential MR pitfall in the diagnosis of venous occlusion. Magnetic resonance venography can be very helpful in equivocal cases. A combination of spin-echo MR and MR venography probably provides the best imaging evaluation for dural sinus occlusion. Intravenous digital subtraction angiography in the venous phase remains a suitable alternative in areas where MR is unavailable. This is one of the few uses of this technique, in which a large contrast bolus into the central venous system is followed digitally.

HEMORRHAGE

Hemorrhage occurs when an artery or vein ruptures, allowing blood to burst forth into the brain parenchyma or subarachnoid spaces. Although mixed patterns occur, hemorrhages are most conveniently divided into subarachnoid and parenchymal categories. Imaging studies are critical in determining the source of bleeding and in showing any associated complications. The location and pattern of hemorrhage help predict what the underlying lesion is and direct further workup.

Imaging of Hemorrhage

Hemorrhages are detected because of increased attenuation by CT and complex signal patterns related to iron oxidation by MR. In both cases, the formation of "clot," which has far less serum and therefore water than whole blood, also plays a role in the imaging findings. *A noncontrast CT should be performed when there is a question of acute hemorrhage, but MR is much more sensitive for evaluation of subacute or chronic hemorrhage* (Fig. 4.30).

The MR signal generated by blood depends upon a complex interplay of hematocrit, oxygen content, type

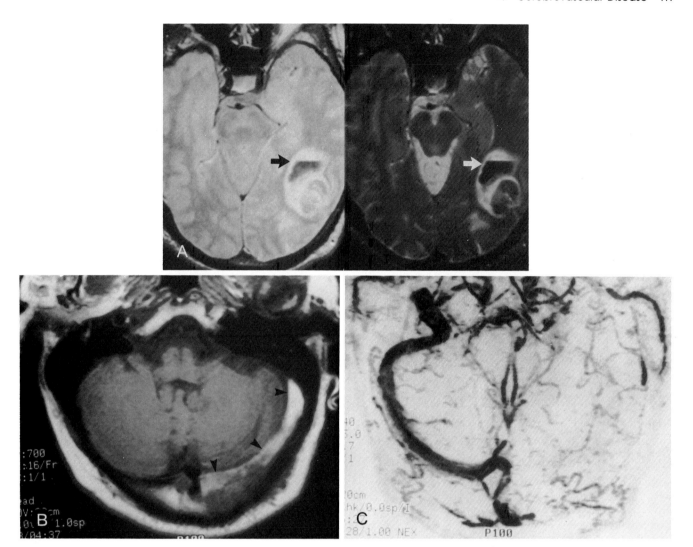

Figure 4.28. Transverse Sinus Occlusion with Venous Infarction.
A. This patient presented with headache and new focal seizures. First and second echo T2-weighted images show hemorrhage deep in the left posterior temporal region with with layering of blood clot (the hematocrit effect; *arrow*). Signal intensities suggest a dependent layer with intracellular methemoglobin or deoxyhemoglobin with a supernatant of extracellular methemoglobin. A small amount of edema surrounds the hematoma. **B.** Transverse noncontrast T1-weighted image through the posterior fossa shows hyperintensity in the left transverse sinus (*arrowheads*), consistent with thrombus-containing methemoglobin. **C.** Submentovertex projection from a two-dimensional time-of-flight MR angiogram confirms normal flow on the right, but lack of flow in the left transverse sinus.

of hemoglobin and chemical state of its iron-containing moieties, tissue pH, protein content of any clot formed, and the integrity of red blood cell membranes. Dominant among these mechanisms is the oxidation state and location of iron species related to hemoglobin. Oxygenated hemoglobin is sequentially converted to deoxyhemoglobin, methemoglobin, and then hemosiderin over time. The magnetic properties of the resultant degradation products change the MR relaxation rates of adjacent protons, allowing the hemorrhage to be detected. A small halo of surrounding edema is common in the subacute phase of parenchymal hemorrhage, sometimes making interpretation of signal changes quite complex. High-field scanners and gradient-echo sequences tend to improve conspicuity of subacute and chronic blood products. The general pattern of MR signal changes seen over time on a 1.5 tesla magnet is summarized in Table 4.4 and in Figure 4.31. Individual cases may of course vary somewhat from these simplified guidelines because of the multiple factors involved.

A brief stroll down physical chemistry lane will help us understand the complicated signal changes seen during the evolution of a hemorrhage. In order to change the signal characteristics of a tissue, hemorrhage must affect T1 or T2 relaxation. The sequential oxidation products of hemoglobin accomplish this because of changes in both magnetic properties and in molecular conformation. Iron within hemorrhage breakdown products changes the effective local magnetic field, a process known as magnetic susceptibility. This change in field is translated into an altera-

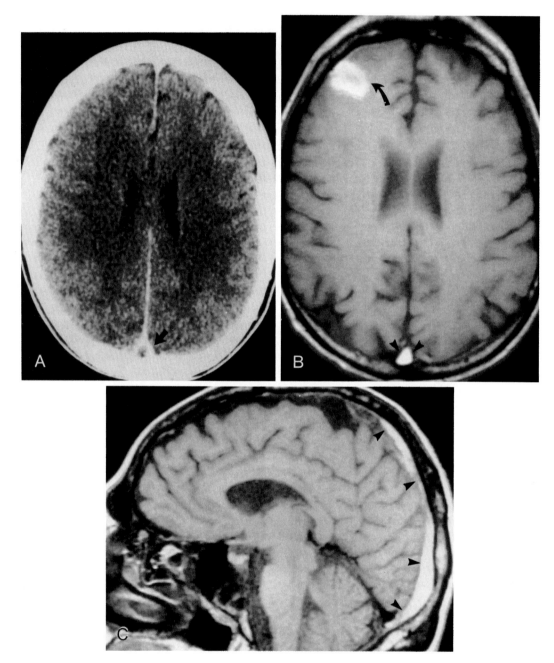

Figure 4.29. Superior Sagittal Sinus Thrombosis with Hemorrhagic Infarction. This patient was on chemotherapy for lymphoma when he developed headache and was found to have papilledema. Venous occlusion was probably because of dehydration. **A.** The initial contrast-enhanced CT shows a filling defect in the sagittal sinus—the empty delta sign (*arrow*). No hemorrhage was detected. He was treated with anticoagulants but presented 1 week later with worsening headaches. **B.** Follow-up axial noncontrast T1 MR shows high signal with mass effect in the right frontal lobe indicative of hemorrhagic infarction (*curved arrow*). The normal flow void of the superior sagittal sinus has been replaced by high signal clot (*arrowheads*). Hyperintense blood on T1 indicates presence of methemoglobin. **C.** Sagittal T1 image confirms clot in the superior sagittal sinus (*arrowheads*).

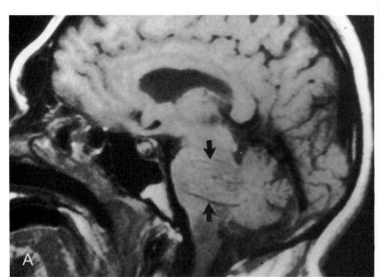
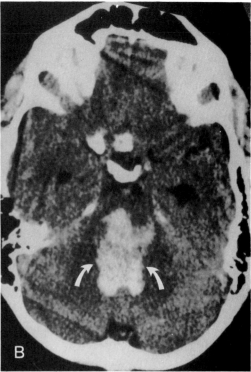

Figure 4.30. Insensitivity of MR to Hyperacute Blood. A patient anticoagulated because of posterior fossa TIAs suddenly lost consciousness while hospitalized. **A.** Sagittal T1 MR done within an hour shows a suggestion of mass effect in the posterior pons and region of the fourth ventricle (*arrows*). Little if any signal change is seen, probably because the blood is still in the oxy- and deoxyhemoglobin state. **B.** Noncontrast CT done immediately after MR confirms a very large hemorrhage (*curved arrows*).

Table 4.4. Evolution of Hemorrhage by MRI

Time	RBC[a]	Hemoglobin State	T1 Signal	T2 Signal
<1 Day	Intact	Oxyhemoglobin	Iso/dark	Bright
0–2 Days	Intact	Deoxyhemoglobin	Iso/dark	Dark
2–14 Days	Intact	Methemoglobin (intracellular)	Bright	Dark
10≥21 Days	Lysed	Methemoglobin (extracellular)	Bright	Bright
≥21 Days	Lysed	Hemosiderin/ferritin	Iso/dark	Dark

[a]Red blood cells.

tion in signal intensity because of acceleration or slowing of T1 and T2 relaxation rates. Changes in T1 relaxation occurs only within short-range (measured in angstroms) while T2 effects can be seen millimeters away.

Under normal conditions, circulating red blood cells contain a mixture of both oxy- and deoxyhemoglobin forms. During transit through the capillary bed, tissues extract oxygen according to metabolic needs, converting oxyhemoglobin to deoxyhemoglobin in the process. Neither of these forms have much detectable effect on T1 signal intensity in clinical images, but they may be distinguished because of their opposite effects on T2-weighted images. *Oxyhemoglobin* is a diamagnetic compound containing ferrous (Fe^{2+}) ions, *detected as high signal intensity on T2-weighted images* (particularly first echo). Deoxyhemoglobin also contains Fe^{2+} ions but is a para-

magnetic substance. The magnetic susceptibility of deoxyhemoglobin causes accelerated dephasing of spins on T2 or T2*-weighted images (e.g., gradient-recalled echo sequences), which results in signal loss. *Deoxyhemoglobin* is therefore *hypointense* on heavily T2-weighted images. These patterns of altered T2 signal are occasionally encountered on clinical images of acute hemorrhage. Perhaps more importantly, magnetic susceptibility effects of deoxyhemoglobin form the basis for a number of emerging functional MR methods.

When hemorrhage occurs, oxyhemoglobin is converted to deoxyhemoglobin at a rate dependent on local pH and oxygen tension. This takes place over hours for parenchymal hematomas but can be considerably delayed when oxygen-containing cerebrospinal fluid surrounds subarachnoid blood. This may explain why acute subarachnoid blood is relatively diffi-

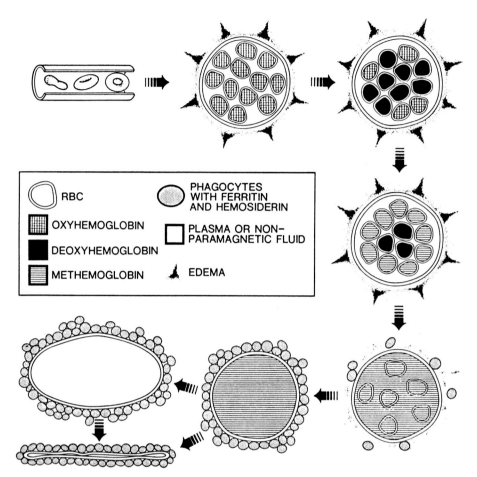

Figure 4.31. Biochemical Evolution of Hemorrhage. Within minutes of hemorrhage, a hematoma consists of intact red blood cells containing oxyhemoglobin. Over several hours, the clot begins to retract and the hemoglobin is oxidized from oxy- to deoxy- to methemoglobin. Methemoglobin tends to form in a ring that converges from the periphery to the center over time. Red cells lyse, releasing methemoglobin into the surrounding fluid. Macrophages break down the iron products into hemosiderin and ferritin, leaving a stain at the periphery of older hematomas. (From Atlas SW. Magnetic resonance imaging of the brain and spine. New York: Raven Press, 1991.)

cult to detect by MR. In parenchymal or extraaxial hematomas, further oxidation of deoxyhemoglobin leads to formation of methemoglobin, a ferric (Fe^{3+}) paramagnetic substance. This occurs over several days or longer, parallel in time course to lysis of red blood cells.

Methemoglobin causes a marked acceleration of T1 relaxation, leading to bright signal on T1-weighted images (Fig. 4.7**A**). This T1 shortening occurs with both intracellular and extracellular methemoglobin. The influence of methemoglobin on T2 relaxation is more complicated and depends on whether it is intra- or extracellular. Thus, methemoglobin contained within intact red cells is able to set up local field gradients between the cell and the protons outside; this magnetic susceptibility leads to signal loss on T2-weighted images. After cell lysis methemoglobin is dispersed throughout the tissue water, the gradient is lost, and T2 relaxation similar to cerebrospinal fluid is seen. T2-weighted images of subacute hematomas therefore show a "hematocrit effect": a dependent layer of intact cells exhibiting dark signal and a plasma supernatant showing bright signal (Fig. 4.28**A**).

Further oxidation of hemoglobin and breakdown of the globin molecule leads to accumulation of hemosiderin in the lysosomes of macrophages. Hemosiderin causes the gross rust-colored stain at the edges of an old hematoma seen at surgery or autopsy, even years after the index event. It is a paramagnetic ferric (Fe^{3+}) containing substance that is insoluble in water. As a result, hemosiderin shows no appreciable T1 effects but very prominent T2 shortening (dark signal) because of magnetic susceptibility effects. An area of remote hemorrhage will commonly be seen as atrophy alone on CT or T1-weighted MR, but a dark rim along the cleft on T2-weighted images implicates a prior bleed. Occasionally, large or recurrent subarachnoid hemorrhages will lead to diffuse hemosiderin deposition on the brain surface, a condition known as superficial hemosiderosis (or superficial siderosis).

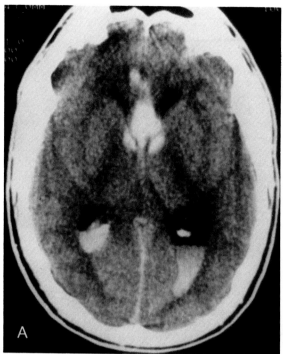

Figure 4.32. Ruptured Anterior Communicating Artery Aneurysm. This 21-year-old man collapsed immediately after snorting a line of cocaine. **A.** Noncontrast CT shows blood in the interhemispheric fissure and in the dependent portions of the lateral ventricles. Blood in the ventricles, cisterns, or layed in the sulci is subarachnoid by definition. **B.** Lateral view from a digital subtraction angiogram demonstrates a large anterior communicating artery aneurysm (*arrow*). Over half of drug abusers with intracranial hemorrhage will be found to have an underlying aneurysm or AVM.

SUBARACHNOID HEMORRHAGE (SAH)

The subarachnoid space is the cerebrospinal fluid-filled compartment that surrounds the blood vessels and communicates with the ventricular system. Subarachnoid hemorrhage is most commonly caused by anuerysm rupture. Arteriovenous malformations of the brain or spinal cord and vascular malformations involving the dura may also cause SAH, but usually in combination with parenchymal or subdural bleeding, respectively. Previously normal vessels may rupture into the subarachnoid space when damaged by drugs, trauma, or dissection. Subarachnoid hemorrhage may also occasionally be seen in patients with marked thrombocytopenia or other severe coagulopathies.

Patients with aneurysms may develop symptoms attributable to either bleeding or local mass effect. Sudden, severe headache is the most common symptom of aneurysm rupture, sometimes described by patients as the worst headache of their lives. Unruptured aneusyms or those with limited surrounding hemorrhage may also develop significant mass effect with or without headache. Classic presentations in this regard are the unilateral third nerve palsy because of a posterior communicating artery aneurysm, cavernous sinus syndrome because of an internal carotid artery/parasellar aneurysm, and optic chiasmal syndrome (bitemporal field defect) due to an anterior communicating artery aneurysm.

A patient who presents with subarachnoid hemorrhage is very likely to harbor a ruptured congenital (berry) aneurysm (Fig. 4.32). One to two percent of the population have aneurysms, thought to occur because of a congenital absence of the arterial media. Many of these aneurysms remain asymptomatic, but those greater than 3–5 mm are at increased risk for rupture. Berry aneurysms often occur near branch points of the circle of Willis. Eighty-five percent sprout from the anterior part of the circle of Willis, while 15% arise in the vertebrobasilar territory. Common locations include the anterior communicating (33%), MCA (30%), posterior communicating (25%), and basilar arteries (10%) (Fig. 4.31). Less commonly the ophthalmic artery, cavernous, or PICA are to blame. When distal branch aneurysms are seen, an episode of prior trauma or systemic infection should be considered (e.g., bacterial endocarditis with "mycotic" aneurysm). Other conditions associated with anuerysms include atherosclerosis, fibromuscular disease, and polycystic kidney diesase.

Even large acute SAHs easily seen by CT may be entirely missed on MR. Computed tomography is over 90% sensitive for the detection of acute SAH, probably because of the increased density of clotted blood.

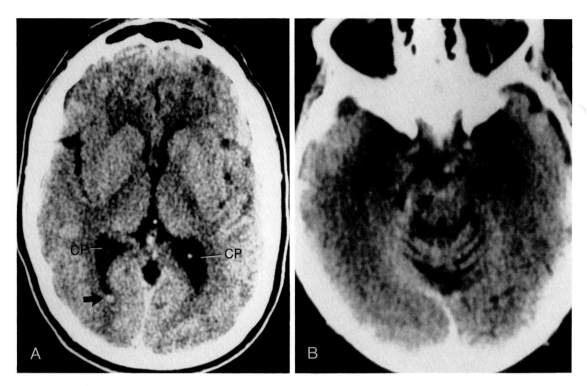

Figure 4.33. Subtle SAH by CT. The most sensitive areas for detecting SAH are the dependent parts of the occipital horns (**A**, *arrow*) and the interpeduncular fossa (**B**, *arrow*). The choroid plexus at the atrium of the lateral ventricle (**A**, *CP*) normally appears dense because of calcification or enhancement. The nondependent location of the choroid differentiates it from hemorrhage.

Subarachnoid hemorrhages may be quite difficult to detect even by CT when the patient's hematocrit is low, the amount of hemorrhage small, or there is a delay in scanning. In these cases, detection of red blood cells or xanthochromia by lumbar puncture may be the only way to confirm a suspected SAH. The most sensitive places to look for SAH on CT are the dependent portions of the subarachnoid space where gravity causes the blood to settle—the interpeduncular fossa and the far posterior aspects of the occipital horns (Fig. 4.33). Prompt scanning is important, since dissolution of subarachnoid blood reduces CT sensitivity to 66% by day 3.

About 15–20% of patients with subarachnoid bleeding will have multiple aneurysms. Because of this multiplicity, a "four-vessel" angiogram is needed on the initial evaluation. Sometimes special views or manuevers are needed to make the offending aneurysm rear its ugly head (e.g., opposite common carotid compression to fill the anterior communicating artery). When multiple aneurysms are present, the one that is largest or more irregular has focal mass effect, intraaneurysmal clot, or shows a change on serial examinations is likely to be the culprit. While MRA shows great promise for aneurysm evaluation in the future, it is not yet of proven reliability for the primary work-up of a patient presenting with SAH. The combination of MR and MRA probably detects the vast majority of aneurysms greater than 3 mm, making it a reasonable screening tool for some at-risk patients (strong family histories, polycystic kidney disease, etc.).

The location of blood in the subarachnoid spaces is imperfectly correlated with the location of a ruptured aneurysm, as subarachnoid blood can layer dependently. Sometimes a parenchymal clot will surround the site of hemorrhage, or thrombus may be seen in the aneurysm itself. When the routine screening CT shows SAH, sometimes fine sections through suspicious areas will demonstrate the aneurysm. Within a few days a focus of methemoglobin may sometimes pinpoint the bleeding site on MR. Unless there has been rebleeding, subarachnoid blood is generally inconspicuous on CT at 1 week.

Intravenous contrast will also potentially improve aneurysm localization and characterization (e.g., is there clot?). The condition of the patient and the philosophy of the surgeon determine which patients get contrast. Some surgeons operate within the first few days after hemorrhage, citing an early risk of rebleeding (20%) and the ability to aggressively manage hemodynamics once clipping is achieved. In this situation, contrast is not routinely administered because (a) the aneurysm needs to be characterized by angiography, not CT, for any surgical planning and (b) the contrast used for CT could limit the amount used in the subsequent angiogram or add to nephrotoxicity. Other centers routinely do the angiogram and operate

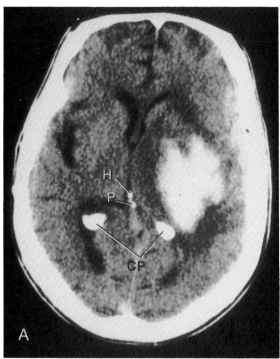
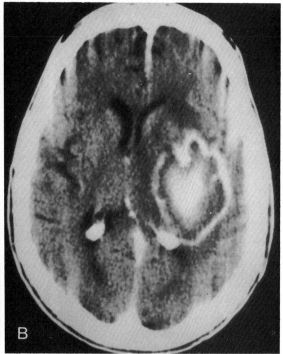

Figure 4.34. Hypertensive Putamenal Hemorrhage with Enhancement at 10 Days. The precontrast study (**A**) shows a large hematoma centered in the left putamen. Dense calcification of the choroid plexus (*CP*), pineal (*P*), and habenula (*H*) should not be mistaken for intraventricular extension. There is moderate mass effect and a small amount of surrounding edema. A ring of enhancement surrounds this benign hematoma (**B**), likely because of a vascular capsule. Resolving infarcts and hemorrhages normally show enhancement at the subacute phase.

after 10 days in order to avoid the period of maximal vasospasm (3–10 days). In this instance contrast may be administered on a more routine basis.

Follow-up studies are an integral part of SAH evaluation. The initial or subsequent CT may show communicating hydrocephalus, requiring a ventriculostomy or shunt. Episodes of possible rebleeding are evaluated with noncontrast CT. Postoperative angiography is used to assess adequacy of clip placement and to rule out vasospasm. Infarcts may also be seen in patients with elevated intracranial pressure or vasospasm, and are the main pathologic finding in patients whose condition continues to deteriorate after the initial SAH.

PARENCHYMAL HEMORRHAGE

Primary intraparenchymal hemorrhage occurs as a result of bleeding directly into the brain substance. Traumatic hemorrhages are not included in this section; they are discussed in Chapter 3. Parenchymal bleeds generally have a higher initial mortality than infarcts, but on recovery show fewer deficits than a similar-sized infarct. This is because hemorrhage tends to tear through and displace brain tissue, but can be resorbed. A similar-sized infarct is made up of dead rather than just displaced neurons. The main differential considerations are hypertensive hemor-

rhage, vascular malformations, drug effects, congophilic angiopathy, and bloody tumors.

Hypertensive Hemorrhages. Hypertensive bleeds are seen in the putamen (35–50%), the subcortical white matter (30%), the cerebellum (15%), thalamus (10–15%), and pons (5–10%) (Fig. 4.34). As with lacunes, lipohyalinosis of vessels is believed to be the primary predisposing pathologic feature, although miliary aneurysms in the vessel wall may also play a role. Small hypertensive hemorrhages may resolve with few deficits. Bleeds in the posterior fossa, those with a large amount of mass effect, or hemorrhages extending into the ventricular system have a relatively poor prognosis.

Vascular Malformations. These are far less frequently encountered than hypertension, but are a cause of hemorrhage which must be ruled out, especially in young patients. Vascular malformations develop because of a congenitally abnormal vascular connection that may enlarge over time. The relative frequency of vascular malformations as a cause of intracranial hemorrhage is about 5%. There are four main subtypes: arteriovenous malformations, cavernous malformations, telanagiectasias, and venous malformations.

Arteriovenous Malformations (AVMs). These are the most common type of brain vascular malformation. Arteriovenous malformations are an abnor-

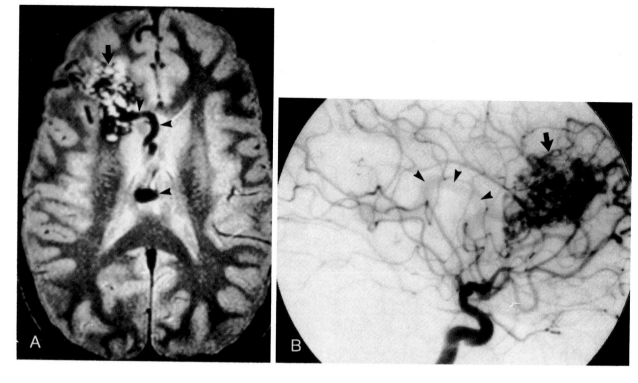

Figure 4.35.   Right Frontal AVM. An MR was performed because of headaches. **A.** Transverse T2-weighted image shows a large right frontal lesion (*arrow*) with a complex mixture of hyperintensity and hypointensity because of turbulent flow. A tortuous flow void headed toward the midline indicates a large draining vein (*arrowheads*). **B.** Digital subtraction angiography in the lateral projection (internal carotid artery injection) depicts the large frontal nidus (*arrow*) and tortuous draining vein (*arrowheads*).

mal tangle of arteries directly connected to veins without an intervening capillary network. About 80–90% are supratentorial, but any area may be affected. Most patients present with hemorrhage or seizures. Arteriovenous malformations have a 2–3% annual risk of bleeding, but the risk may double or triple in the 1st year after an initial bleed. Treatment depends on the age of the patient, symptoms, and philosophy of the attending physicians. Embolization, surgery, and radiotherapy all may play a role.

Unruptured AVMs typically appear as a jumble of enlarged vessels without mass effect (Fig. 4.35). Noncontrast CT will show a mixed attenuation lesion, sometimes with evidence of calcification. Magnetic resonance imaging demonstrates flow voids or complex flow patterns, sometimes leading to artifacts in the phase-encoding direction. T2 or T2*-weighted images may show dark signal intensity related to the AVM, a sign of prior hemorrhage with hemosiderin deposition. Intravenous contrast usually results in marked enhancement and therefore increased conspicuity of the AVM on both CT and MR studies. Feeding arteries and draining veins may show impressive enlargement well beyond the center (nidus) of the AVM. About 10% of AVMs will develop an associated aneurysm, generally on a feeding artery. Angiography remains the definitive method for evaluation of the AVMs anatomy.

Arteriovenous malformations can be difficult to detect soon after hemorrhage. Occasionally the AVM will obliterate itself at the time of rupture, but more commonly the resultant hematoma compresses and obscures many of the remaining vessels. Contrast studies may identify an enhancing portion of a vascular malformation adjacent to a hemorrhage. Normally, acute hemorrhage will not take up contrast unless there is an associated vascular malformation. A subacute hematoma of any cause may enhance because of a surrounding vascular capsule, and should not be mistaken for an AVM (Fig. 4.34).

Cavernous Malformations are thin-walled sinusoidal vessels (neither arteries nor veins) that may present with seizures or small parenchymal hemorrhages. These lesions may be asymptomatic and occur on a familial basis. Computed tomography scans and angiography are usually normal. Magnetic resonance will show a reticulated, often enhancing lesion with dark rim (hemosiderin) on T2.

Venous Malformations (or venous angiomas) are developmentally anomalous veins that drain normal brain. They are seen in 1–2% of patients studied by contrast MR but may easily be missed on CT or noncontrast MR. The classic appearance is of an enlarged, enhancing, stellate venous complex extending to the ventricular or cortical surface. The MR appearance is usually diagnostic, but venous phase angiography

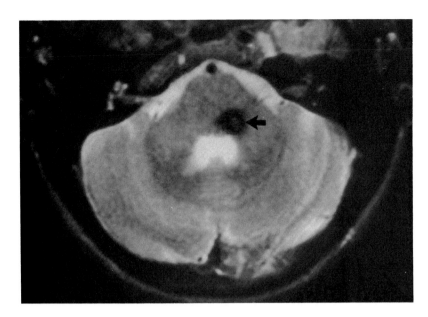

Figure 4.36. Pontine Occult Cerebrovascular Malformation. T2 transverse image showing a focal rim of marked hypointensity with slight central hyperintensity (arrow). The rim indicates ferritin or hemosiderin deposition, and the core represents subacute blood products or abnormal parenchyma related to the anomalous vessels.

may be needed in equivocal cases. Although these may bleed, treatment is somewhat controversial since they are commonly seen in asymptomatic patients and are often the only venous drainage for a brain region.

Telangiectasias are dilated capillary-sized vessels usually diagnosed at autopsy. These are generally small, solitary lesions found incidentally by MR. No treatment is necessary.

Occult Cerebrovascular Malformations. Computed tomography and MR cannot always reliably distinguish among these subtypes of small, angiographically occult ("cryptic") vascular malformations. The generic term occult cerebrovascular malformation is used to describe telangiectasias, cavernous malformations, and small, thrombosed AVMs. Occult cerebrovascular malformations are usually inconspicuous on CT but may be detected as a small area of calcification. On MR, an occult cerebrovascular malformation should be suspected when focal heterogeneous signal (acute/subacute blood) is seen with a surrounding ring of hypointensity (hemosiderin) (Fig. 4.36). Venous malformations may provide drainage for occult cerebrovascular malformations, but no feeding vessels should be seen. Unless recently ruptured, an occult cerebrovascular malformation should show no mass effect or edema. If all these criteria are met, conventional angiography may be unnecessary.

HEMORRHAGE DUE TO COAGULOPATHIES

Intracranial hemorrhage may also be because of blood dyscrasias. Chronic oral anticoagulation increases by eightfold the risk of intracranial hemorrhage. The association is particularly true when the coagulation parameters are extended beyond the recommended therapeutic range.

DRUG-ASSOCIATED HEMORRHAGE

Sympathomimetic drugs seem to provide an effective (if unintended) stress test for the presence of brain vascular anomalies (Fig. 4.32). Drugs such as amphetamines and cocaine have been commonly associated with intracranial hemorrhage. Symptoms develop within minutes to hours following the use of the drug. The genesis may be related to transient hypertension or arteritis-like vascular change similar to periarteritis nodosa. Up to 50% of drug abusers who suffer an intracranial hemorrhage have a demonstrable underlying structural cause such as an aneurysm or AVM.

AMYLOID ANGIOPATHY

Cerebral amyloid angiopathy or "congophilic" angiopathy is an increasingly recognized cause of intracranial hemorrhage, frequently lobar in nature. It is characterized by amyloid deposits in the media and adventitia of medium size and small cortical leptomeningeal arteries. It is not associated with systemic vascular amyloidosis. This angiopathy characteristically affects elderly individuals. Autopsy incidence rises steeply, ranging from 8% in the 7th decade to 22–35% in the 8th decade, 40% in the 9th decade, and 58% in persons older than 90. It is rarely seen in patients younger than 55. Cerebral amyloid angiopathy is associated with progressive senile dementia in about 30% of cases. Systemic hypertension is common in this age group but is not directly related to cerebral amyloid angiopathy. Amyloid is unique in that the associated cerebral infarcts and hemorrhages occur in superficial locations rather than in the deep white matter and basal ganglionic areas. These affect the occipital and parietal lobes, where the angiopathy

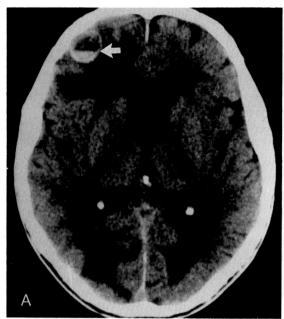 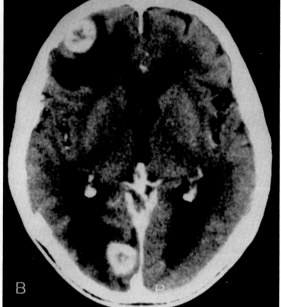

Figure 4.37. Hemorrhagic Metastases. This patient with known oat cell carcinoma of the lung presented with new onset seizures. The precontrast CT (**A**) shows a rounded bloody mass in the right frontal lobe with a hematocrit layer (*arrow*). Marked white matter edema surrounds this lesion and is also seen in the right occipital lobe. Postcontrast (**B**) there is irregular ring enhancement of the bloody lesion and a second discrete focus is identified in the occipital lobe. The degree of surrounding edema, focal and irregular enhancement, and nonvascular distribution implicate metastases and not stroke.

tends to predominate. Cerebral amyloid angiopathy should come to mind when an elderly, frequently demented patient presents with new or recurrent superficial hemorrhages.

PRIMARY HEMORRHAGE VERSUS HEMORRHAGIC NEOPLASM

Intracranial tumors are an uncommon but well-recognized cause of intracranial hemorrhage. They account for 1–2% of bleeds in autopsy series and as high as 6–10% in clinical radiologic series. Tumor necrosis, vascular invasion, and neovascularity may contribute to the pathogenesis of hemorrhagic neoplasms. Glioblastomas are the most common primary brain tumors to hemorrhage, while in the metastatic category bronchogenic carcinoma, thyroid, melanoma, choriocarcinoma, and renal cell carcinoma often bleed (Fig. 4.37). It may be possible to distinguish between a hemorrhagic neoplasm and a primary (benign) intracranial hemorrhage based on the MR findings. Intratumoral bleeds tend to be more complex and heterogeneous than benign hematomas. The expected evolution of blood products is commonly delayed with tumors, possibly because of profound intratumoral hypoxia. If a patient is scanned in the acute phase, lack of enhancement beyond the hematoma strongly supports a primary intracranial hemorrhage. If there is an enhancing component, then lesions such as tumor or AVM must be considered. In the subacute phase, however, a resolving hematoma

may develop a thin area of ring enhancement of its own (Fig. 4.34). Both acute hemorrhage and hemorrhagic neoplasms may cause an edematous reaction, although in the tumors edema is more predominant. In a benign intracranial hypertensive bleed, the edema should begin to substantially resolve within a week, while in the presence of a neoplasm it should persist. With a resolving benign hematoma, a fully circumferential hemosiderin ring begins to develop at about 2–3 week's time on MR. In the hematoma associated with tumor, this hemosiderin ring may be absent or incomplete. These useful differential features are summarized in Table 4.5. Sometimes when the findings are ambiguous, a follow-up examination in 3–6 weeks will clarify the diagnosis, avoiding a biopsy.

PRIMARY HEMORRHAGE VERSUS HEMORRHAGIC TRANSFORMATION OF INFARCTION

As discussed in the ischemic stroke section, it may also be difficult to distinguish between primary intracranial hemorrhage and hemorrhagic infarction. In hemorrhagic infarction, arterial occlusion causes infarction of the parent vessel itself along with its brain territory. If clot dissolution occurs or if collateral flow ensues, blood may then be extruded from the damaged vessel wall. Hemorrhagic infarctions therefore tend to be in classic vascular distributions and infrequently show much mass effect. They usually ex-

Table 4.5. Features of Benign vs. Malignant Intracranial Hemorrhage

Sign	Benign	Malignant
Evolution of blood products	Peripheral to central	Irregular, complex
Hemosiderin rim	Complete	Delayed, incomplete
Surrounding edema	Minimal/mild	Moderate/severe
Acute enhancement patterns	Minimal (unless AVM)	Moderate/severe

hibit some degree of contrast enhancement, since blood-brain barrier breakdown is present by definition. They are not associated with intraventricular blood, which may accompany a primary hemorrhage. Primary hemorrhage is characterized by disruption of the blood vessel wall, leading to extravasation of blood into the surrounding tissues, sometimes at a distance from the damaged vessel. Unlike hemorrhagic infarcts, primary hemorrhages may therefore cross vascular boundaries.

References

Atlas SW. Intracranial vascular malformations and aneurysms. Radiol Clin North Am 1988;26:821–837.

Atlas SW, ed. Magnetic resonance imaging of the brain and spine. New York: Raven Press. 1991.

Barkovich AJ, Atlas SW. Magnetic resonance imaging of intracranial hemorrhage. Radiol Clin North Am 1988;26:801–820.

Berman SA, Hayman LA, Hinck VC. Correlation of CT cerebral vascular territories with function: I. Anterior cerebral artery. AJR 1980;135:253–257.

Berman SA, Hayman LA, Hinck VC. Correlation of CT cerebral vascular territories with function: III. Middle cerebral artery. AJNR 1984;5:161–166.

Bousser M-G, Barnett HJM. Cerebral venous thrombosis. In: Barnett HJM, Mohr JP, Stein BM, Yatsu FM, eds. Stroke: pathophysiology, diagnosis and management. New York: Churchill Livingstone, 1992:517–538.

Braffman BH, Zimmerman RA, Trojanowski JQ, Gonatas NK, Hickey WF, Schlaepfer WW. Brain MR: Pathologic correlation with gross and histopathology. 1. Lacunar infarction and Virchow-Robin spaces. AJNR 1988;9:621–628.

Brown JJ, Hesselink JR, Rothrock JF. MR and CT of lacunar infarcts. AJNR 1988;9:477–482.

Elster AD, Moody DM. Early cerebral infarction: Gadopentetate dimeglumine enhancement. Radiology 1990;177:627–632.

Gomori JM, Grossman RI. Mechanisms responsible for the MR appearance and evolution of intracranial hemorrhage. Radiographics 1988;8:427–440.

Hayman LA, Berman SA, Hinck VC. Correlation of CT cerebral vascular territories with function: II. Posterior cerebral artery. AJR 1981;137:13–19.

Hayman LA, Taber KH, Ford JJ, Bryan RN. Mechanisms of MR signal alteration by acute intracerebral blood: Old concepts and new theories. AJNR 1991;12:899–907.

Osborn AG. Introduction to cerebral angiography. Philadelphia: Harper & Row, 1980.

Savoiardo M, Bracchi M, Passerini A, Visciani A. The vascular territories in the cerebellum and brainstem: CT and MR study. AJNR 1987;8:199–209.

Truwit CL, Barkovich AJ, Gean-Marton A, Hibri N, Norman D. Loss of the insular ribbon: Another early sign of acute middle cerebral artery infarction. Radiology 1990;176:801–806.

Ulmer JL, Elster AD. Physiologic mechanisms underlying the delayed delta sign. AJNR 1991;12:647–650.

Vintners HV. Cerebral amyloid angiopathy, a critical review. Stroke 1987;18:311–324.

Yuh WTC, Crain MR, Loes DJ, Greene GM, Ryals TJ, Sato Y. MR imaging of cerebral ischemia: Findings in the first 24 hours. AJNR 1991;12:621–629.

5

Central Nervous System Neoplasms

Kelly Koeller

BASICS OF IMAGING

Fortunately, neoplasms of the central nervous system (CNS) are rare, with an incidence of approximately 20,000 new cases in the United States each year. For a disease entity that is comparatively uncommon, these lesions garner exceptional interest because of the dramatic and often catastrophic alteration these tumors produce in patients' lives. About 15–20% of all intracranial neoplasms will occur in patients less than 15 years of age. Within this age range, 70% of tumors will be located within the posterior fossa and metastatic lesions are rare. CNS tumors follow leukemia as the most common types of cancer in this age group. In patients older than 15 years, about 70% of CNS neoplasms will be supratentorial, and metastatic lesions are more common, making up about 30% (according to the Armed Forces Institute of Pathology) of all CNS neoplasms.

While CNS neoplasms have been categorized classically (and often with considerable controversy) by neuropathologists according to their cell of origin, it is most helpful for the radiologist to also think of these lesions by their anatomic location within the CNS. This chapter will consider CNS masses not only by their histologic composition but also by their differential diagnoses based on their specific locations.

Classification

With some modifications, the classification scheme proposed by Bailey and Cushing in the 1920s remains the most widely used for classifying tumors by cells of origin. Basically, this scheme recognizes 7 cell types that give rise to CNS neoplasms (Table 5.1). These include glial cells (composed of astrocytes, oligodendrocytes, and ependymal cells), nerve sheath cells (composed of Schwann cells and fibroblasts), mesenchymal tissue (composed of meninges, blood vessels, and bone), lymphocytes and leukocytes, germ cells, neuroepithelial cells, and finally endo-, meso-, and ectodermal elements. Mature neurons do not divide and thus cannot produce neoplastic growth. Each of the cell types listed in Table 5.1 give rise to a particular type of neoplasm. For instance, glial cells give rise to gliomas, of which astrocytomas are, by far, the most common. In addition, oligodendrogliomas and ependymomas are part of the glioma family. If the cell of tumor origin is not a glial cell, then it is considered a nonglial tumor. These tumors include tumors of primitive bipotential precursors and nerve cells, nerve sheath tumors, mesenchymal tumors, lymphoreticular tumors and leukemia, tumors of maldevelopmental origin, and finally the phakomatoses. The histologic composition of these tumors is important to the radiologist because it directly impacts on the location of the tumor. Since glial tumors originate from glial cells, it stands to reason that these tumors must be of the brain parenchyma itself. Conversely, barring an invasive nonglial tumor, we will usually not see a nonglial primary tumor within the brain itself.

Clinical Presentation

The clinical presentation of a CNS neoplasm is almost always related to increased intracranial pressure, seizures, or a focal neurologic deficit secondary to the tumor mass (1). When the mass is in certain key locations or when the mass is of sufficient size,

Table 5.1. Intracranial Neoplasms and Their Cells of Origins

Type of Cell	Neoplasm
Glial Cells	
Astrocyte	Astrocytoma
Oligodendrocyte	Oligodendroglioma
Ependyma	Ependymoma
Nonglial Cells	
Nerve sheath cells	
Schwann cells	Schwannoma
Fibroblasts/Schwann cells	Neurofibroma
Mesenchymal cells	
Meninges	Meningioma
Blood vessels	Hemangioblastoma
Bone	Osteocartilaginous tumors, sarcoma
Lymphocytes, leukocytes	Primary
	Non-Hodgkin's lymphoma
	Histiocytosis X
	Rare: leukemia, myeloma
	Secondary
	Lymphoma
	Myeloma
	Leukemia
Germ cells	Germinoma
	Teratomatous types (embryonal carcinoma, yolk sac, teratoma, choriocarcinoma)
Neuroepithelial cells	Craniopharyngioma
	Rathke's cleft cyst
Endo-, meso-, ectoderm elements	Epidermoid/dermoid tumors
	Lipoma
	Hamartoma

portions of the brain may be pushed across the midline (subfalcine herniation) or through the tentorial incisura (uncal herniation and central descending transtentorial herniation). Subfalcine (or cingulate) herniation is the most common type of herniation. A midline shift of 3 mm or greater is significant. The falx is a very tough fibrous structure that is very resistant to any sort of displacement.

The uncus is the hooked extremity of the parahippocampal formation of the medial temporal lobe. Uncal herniation often compromises the many tracts running through the brainstem as well as nearby cranial nerves, particularly the oculomotor (III) nerves, which will result in ipsilateral pupillary dilation (or "blown pupil"). On imaging studies, effacement of the ambient cistern, downward displacement of the pineal gland, and contralateral hydrocephalus are the hallmarks of uncal herniation (2). Central herniation (or central descending transtentorial herniation) is the downward displacement of the lower brainstem and cerebellum without horizontal displacement. It is most commonly seen in bilateral or midline masses, and results in complete obliteration of the cisternal spaces (3).

The mass effect of an intracranial neoplasm may produce increased intracranial pressure or hydrocephalus secondary to obstruction of the flow of cerebrospinal fluid (CSF) as it circulates through the ventricles and into the subarachnoid space. In either case, the increased pressure may produce a classic triad of headaches, nausea and vomiting, and papilledema (caused by partial obstruction of the venous outflow from the optic nerve). This classic triad has a variable presentation, occurring early in the course, late in the course, or never (4). In addition, altered mental status (particularly with bilateral frontal lobe tumors), or alterations in equilibrium (commonly seen in cerebellar or eighth cranial nerve tumors) may be present. Intracranial neoplasms usually present with an indolent course marked by progressive headache and focal neurologic deficit, but may also present abruptly.

Approach to a Radiographic Abnormality

The detection of an intracranial abnormality on any imaging study should immediately cause the radiologist to ask three questions. By far the most important question to ask is, "Is it a mass?" It is important to consider that abnormal signal intensity on either a magnetic resonance imaging (MR) or computed tomography (CT) scan does not necessarily equate to a "mass." To call a lesion a mass, it must have mass effect; that is, it must displace normal structures of the brain. Differentiation of a small neoplasm from a small infarct however may be very difficult. The clinical presentation may allow differentiation. When it does not, a follow-up imaging study (preferably an MR) in 3 weeks time is often helpful. Virtually all (about 96%) of the infarcts will be smaller in size by 3 weeks. If the lesion is the same size or larger at 3 weeks, a neoplasm should be favored. Also, as detailed in Chapter 4, a subacute infarct will often show signs of subtle hemorrhage. In some circumstances, it may be necessary to perform a second follow-up scan in 3 weeks after the first follow-up. Obviously, as the treatment of tumor and infarct are dramatically incongruous, the differentiation of a tumor and an infarct is critical to appropriate clinical management of the patient.

The second most important question to ask is, "Is the mass intraaxial or extraaxial?" An intraaxial mass is a mass that is of the brain itself (i.e., arises from brain parenchyma). An extraaxial mass refers to everything outside the brain (i.e., arachnoid, meninges, dural sinuses, skull, etc.). The ventricular system is also considered extraaxial. Determining the (intra or extraaxial) origin of a mass allows the radiologist to formulate an appropriate differential diagnosis. Extraaxial lesions are characterized by "white matter buckling" or inward compression of the white matter

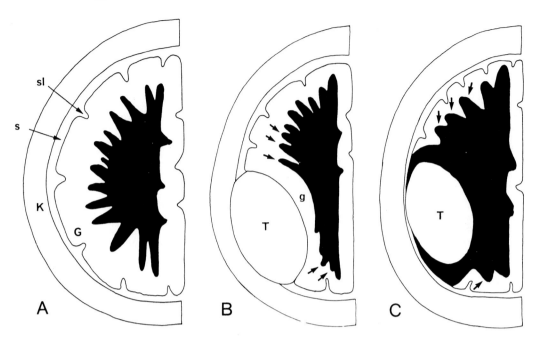

Figure 5.1. Extra- vs. Intraaxial Location for Intracranial Lesions. The presence of "white matter buckling" may provide a valuable clue in determining whether an intracranial mass is intra- or extraaxial in location. **A.** Diagrammatic representation of normal axial plane image at the level of centrum semiovale. Fronds of white matter (*black area*) insinuate themselves into cortical gray matter (G). *s*, subarachnoid space; *sl*, sulcus. **B.** Extraaxial tumor (*T*) crowds fronds of white matter producing white matter buckling. *g*, gray matter. **C.** Intraaxial tumor (*T*) expands white matter, thickening white matter fronds. Tumor is bathed by white matter edema. (From George AE, Russell EJ, Kricheff II. White matter buckling: CT sign of extraaxial intracranial mass. AJNR 1:425–430, 1980.)

(often with thinning of the fronds of the white matter), and maintenance of the gray-white matter interface (Fig. 5.1). An intraaxial mass, in contradistinction, expands the white matter, thickens its fronds, and blurs the gray-white matter interface. However, white matter buckling is not foolproof in differentiating extra- from intraaxial lesions. Where extensive white matter edema is present, no buckling of the white matter may occur. Therefore, while the white matter buckling sign is helpful when present, its absence does not necessarily indicate that a lesion is intraaxial (5).

The third question often posed is, "Where is the tumor margin?" The answer is that it is not possible by any imaging technique currently available to positively identify the margin of an intacranial neoplasm. By their very nature, virtually all glial malignancies will have, despite a grossly well-circumscribed appearance, some microscopic invasion into the surrounding brain parenchyma. The current wisdom is to treat the entire region of abnormal hyperintensity on T2-weighted images, and not just the region of enhancement on the T1-weighted postcontrast sequence (6).

Trying to make a histologic diagnosis from an MR or CT scan is fraught with hazard. However, it is possible to render an intelligent analysis of the mass, including assessment of signal intensities and enhancement characteristics, and to present an accurate differential diagnosis.

Imaging Protocol

In the 1990s, the imaging evaluation of intracranial neoplasms is best conducted by MR, which is far superior to CT because of its multiplanar capability, increased contrast resolution, and lack of ionizing radiation. In limited circumstances, CT is advantageous. Computed tomography is still superior to MR in the assessment of calcification, although the use of gradient-recalled echo sequences increases the sensitivity of MR to calcification. Computed tomography is invaluable for the evaluation of bony abnormalities such as erosion of the skull base.

A basic MR evaluation of a patient suspected of having an intracranial neoplasm includes a sagittal T1-weighted image sequence followed by an axial T2-weighted image sequence. An unenhanced T1-weighted image sequence is performed to allow distinction between inherent T1 shortening, such as in hemorrhage, and contrast enhancement. Depending on the location of the tumor, either the axial or coronal plane is selected for this sequence. For temporal lobe and midline lesions, the coronal plane often provides the best delineation of the tumor. Whatever plane is chosen for the precontrast sequence, it is imperative that a postcontrast sequence be done in the same plane to accurately assess tumor enhancement. To assist neurosurgical planning, at least two imaging planes (usually axial and coronal) should be used

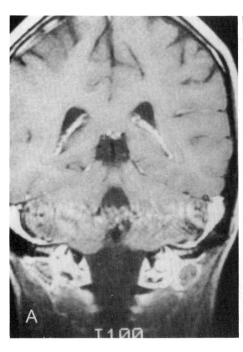
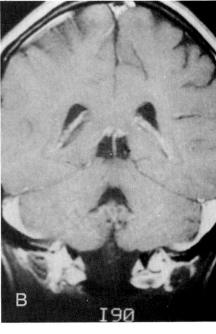

Figure 5.2. Flow Compensation in Posterior Fossa Imaging. Postcontrast images show the improvement in visualization of posterior fossa structures by employing flow compensation technique. **A.** Without flow compensation: significant phase artifact generated from the enhancing dural sinuses degrades the image. **B.** With flow compensation: the image is markedly improved.

for the postcontrast T1-weighted sequences. A sagittal postcontrast T1-weighted sequence will facilitate the placement of radiation ports, if radiation therapy is warranted. The performance of all of these sequences can be completed within 1 hour on current high-field (1.5 T) units.

In the evaluation of posterior fossa lesions imaging in all three orthogonal planes postcontrast is ideal. The postcontrast images should be performed with gradient-moment nulling (flow-compensating) technique, to decrease phase artifact generated by the dural sinuses (Fig. 5.2).

Appearance of Tumors

The radiologic appearance of CNS tumors varies with cellular composition and the presence or absence of hemorrhage and calcification. On CT, intraaxial neoplasms will typically appear as hypointense masses with a variable amount of surrounding white matter edema, the area of which roughly correlates with the aggressiveness of the tumor. On MR the mass is usually dark on T1 (T1 prolongation) and bright on T2 (T2 prolongation) with variable surrounding white matter edema. The presence of calcification within the tumor usually produces marked hypointensity on T1-weighted and T2-weighted images. However, occasionally, calcification, because of the surface area of the crystals producing T1 shortening, may appear bright on T1-weighted images (7).

The appearance of intracranial parenchymal hemorrhage usually depends on the age of the blood. In hyperacute (less than 6 hours) hemorrhage, the predominant oxyhemoglobin will produce T1 and T2 prolongation (dark on T1, bright on T2). When the hem-

orrhage has been present for 6 to 24 hours, the effect of deoxyhemoglobin predominates and the lesion has mild T1 prolongation (dark on T1-weighted images) and moderate T2 shortening (darker on T2-weighted images). Some time around 3–4 days, methemoglobin begins to predominate, first being intracellular, producing T1 and T2 shortening (bright on T1-weighted images, dark on T2-weighted images) and then, as the red blood cells begin to lyse, becoming extracellular where the lesion has T1 shortening and T2 prolongation (bright on T1- and T2-weighted images). In chronic hemorrhages (those older than 10–14 days), hemosiderin appears, producing a rim of extreme T2 shortening. This peripheral black rim occurs because of migrating macrophages, which carry the hemosiderin to the periphery of the hemorrhage. On CT, acute hemorrhage (less than 1 week old) has increased attenuation (appearing bright) compared with brain tissue. By 1 to 3 weeks after the hemorrhage, the signal becomes isodense with brain parenchyma. After 3 weeks, the focus of hemorrhage will be hypodense to brain parenchyma, simulating the attenuation of CSF. This evolution of blood breakdown products is illustrated in detail in Chapter 4.

The appearance of intratumoral hemorrhage reflects the heterogeneous nature of the tumor and is quite different than benign parenchymal hemorrhage. Intratumoral hemorrhage is often intermittent, producing a heterogeneous mixture of the various blood breakdown products just described. In addition, hemorrhage may occur in cystic or necrotic portions of the tumor, creating blood-blood or blood fluid levels. Debris from the necrotic mass will also contribute to this heterogeneous mixture. Normal deoxyhemoglobin evolution is delayed such that it will persist for longer than the usual 3–4 days after hemorrhage. The typical hemosiderin ring does not occur with intratumoral hemorrhage, probably due to interference with the migration of the macrophages by viable tumor at the margins. In cases where there is confusion as to the nature of an intracranial hemorrhage, the presence of a nonhemorrhagic mass adjacent to the hemorrhage, the persistence of T2 prolongation (most likely representing edema or tumor itself), and mass effect all suggest intratumoral hemorrhage instead of a simple parenchymal hematoma (8). Gadolinium administration is often helpful in these cases, as benign hematomas should not have as significant an enhancing rim as hematomas in tumors.

Because of their high vascularity, certain neoplasms are noted for their propensity to hemorrhage. Choriocarcinoma among primary tumors and metastasis from melanoma, thyroid carcinoma, and renal carcinoma have this characteristic. In the setting of multiple hemorrhagic lesions within the brain, these tumors should be considered. Multiple cryptic arteriovenous malformations, either occurring de novo or secondary to radiation therapy, can have a similar appearance.

Besides hemorrhage, two other entities may produce focal T1 shortening on MR scans. Lipomas or other neoplasms that contain fat (e.g., dermoid) will have marked T1 shortening and intermediate signal on T2-weighted images following the signal intensity of subcutaneous fat. The presence of chemical shift artifact on T2-weighted images associated with such a lesion helps to confirm the presence of fat. Melanin, as seen in melanotic melanoma, also follows the same signal intensities as fat on T1- and T2-weighted images, distinguishing melanin from hemorrhage.

Tumors of high cellular density, usually those with small cells such as lymphoma, pineoblastoma, neuroblastoma, or medulloblastoma, are usually hyperdense compared with brain tissue on CT. In addition, metastasis from melanoma, lung carcinoma, colon carcinoma, and breast carcinoma may be hyperdense. On MR, these same tumors typically are hypointense on T2-weighted images, with the appearance presumably being related to a high nucleus:cytoplasm ratio of the tumor cells, which produces less free water and thus less T2 prolongation. However, on occasion, isoor hyperintensity may be seen because of heterogeneity of the tumor matrix.

Contrast enhancement, whether from the iodinated contrast agents used in CT or the paramagnetic gadolinium agents used in MR, works on the same principle: the breakdown of the blood-brain barrier. Unlike nonneural endothelium, the endothelium of the cerebral capillaries allows the passage of only small molecules through their tight junctions and narrow intercellular gaps. The macromolecules of contrast agents are too large to pass this barrier under normal circumstances (9). The blood-brain barrier breaks down in many pathologic states, including intra- and extraaxial tumors (either primary or metastatic), inflammatory diseases, subacute infarcts, postoperative gliosis, and radiation necrosis. However, some tumors, particularly low-grade neoplasms, will not show enhancement, presumably because they form new capillaries that are quite similar to the native cerebral capillaries, and the blood-brain barrier is left intact. More aggressive neoplasms have fenestrated capillaries, allowing the passage of contrast media, and image enhancement. However, the fact that a lesion enhances only means that there is breakdown of the blood-brain barrier, and the presence or absence of enhancement cannot be used to categorically state that a lesion is malignant or benign (Fig. 5.3). In addition, some specialized areas of the brain, such as the choroid plexus, pituitary and pineal glands, tuber cinereum, and area postrema, have no blood-brain barrier and will normally enhance after administration of a contrast agent (9).

The Postoperative Patient

In the evaluation of the postoperative brain tumor patient, timing is of the essence. Ideally, these patients should have an MR scan performed within 72 hours after surgery to serve as a baseline scan for future follow-up. Scar tissue, which occurs in all patients who have had neurosurgical transgression of the blood-brain barrier, takes about 72 hours to fully develop and enhances after administration of contrast. Once formed, the scar tissue in the operative site and dura, may persist for weeks to months. Since most malignant brain tumors have some enhancement, if the patient can be scanned within this 72-hour "window," enhancement can be interpreted as being secondary to residual tumor and not to granulation tissue. After 72 hours, it becomes difficult to distinguish between enhancing tumor and enhancing scar tissue.

Postoperative neurosurgical patients are often not ideal candidates for scanning in an MR unit, and usually require monitoring of vital signs to assure their safety. If proper monitoring and life-support equipment (e.g., shielded pulse oximeter and oxygen) and personnel for MR are not available, a contrast-enhanced CT can be substituted.

Postradiation Changes

Many malignant tumors will be treated by a combination of chemotherapy and radiation therapy following surgical debulking. Typical radiation doses are in the range to 5000–5400 rads (50 to 54 Gy), most often

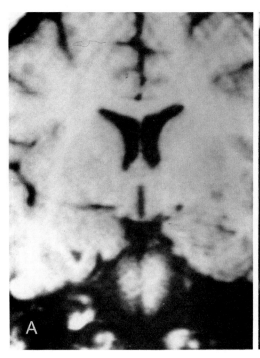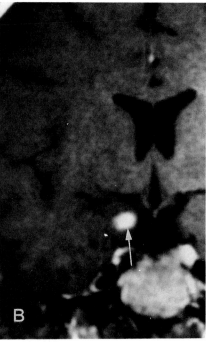

Figure 5.3.   Enhancement: Benign or Malignant? Patient with long history of medically refractory seizures. Intense enhancement (*arrow*) of temporal lobe lesion pathologically proven to be a ganglioglioma, a low-grade neoplasm.

delivered in fractionated doses (about 180 rads each visit) over several weeks. As a consequence of these hefty doses, radiation injury may occur. This occurs in two forms: focal radiation necrosis and diffuse white matter injury. Radiation necrosis is seen on imaging studies as having mass effect and enhancement, whereas diffuse radiation injury presents as T2 hyperintensity, without mass effect or enhancement, and is more commonly seen following whole-brain or large-volume radiation. Clinically, radiation necrosis occurs with focal neurologic deficits, while diffuse white matter injury is often asymptomatic. When radiation necrosis occurs in the vicinity of the operative site (and this is where it is most likely to occur), it is not possible, by any imaging method currently available, to reliably distinguish it from tumor recurrence (10). White matter hyperintensity on T2-weighted images, due to diffuse radiation injury will conform to the selected radiation ports, and should not be misinterpreted as vasogenic edema from the tumor.

SPECIFIC NEOPLASMS

It is hazardous, in many circumstances, to suggest a specific *histologic* diagnosis based on the imaging characteristics alone. However, taking into account other factors such as the location of the tumors (intraaxial, extraaxial, intraventricular, sellar, pineal region) and clinical information (age, sex, endocrinologic data, etc.), the differential diagnosis can be limited to just a few possibilities and sometimes a single most likely entity. Some intracranial tumors have a definite predilection for one gender and are listed in Table 5.2.

Table 5.2.   Tumor Predominance by Gender

Females	Males
Meningioma (4:1)	Pineal germinoma (10:1)
Neurofibroma	Pineal parenchymal tumor (4-7:1)
Pineocytoma	Medulloblastoma (3:1)
Pituitary tumor	GBM (3:2)
	Choroid plexus papilloma (2:1)
	CNS lymphoma
	Hamartoma of the tuber cinereum

Glial Tumors

Gliomas, derived from glial cells (astrocytes, oligodendrocytes, ependymal cells), account for 40–50% of all primary CNS neoplasms.

ASTROCYTOMAS

Astrocytomas account for 70% of all gliomas. These neoplasms have been graded according to degree of histologic malignancy. Originally, astrocytomas were divided into four grades: grades 1 and 2 for low-grade tumors, and grades 3 and 4 for high-grade tumors. Glioblastoma multiforme, the most malignant form of astrocytomas, was considered a grade 4 lesion. Today, there has been greater use of a three-tiered system with well-differentiated (fibrillary) astrocytoma at one end, anaplastic astrocytoma occupying an intermediate grade, and the highly malignant glioblastoma multiforme (GBM)/highly anaplastic astrocytoma (HAA) at the other end. Glial tumors do not have a capsule, and therefore are all malignant. However, the low-grade fibrillary astrocytomas are usually so slow-growing, and

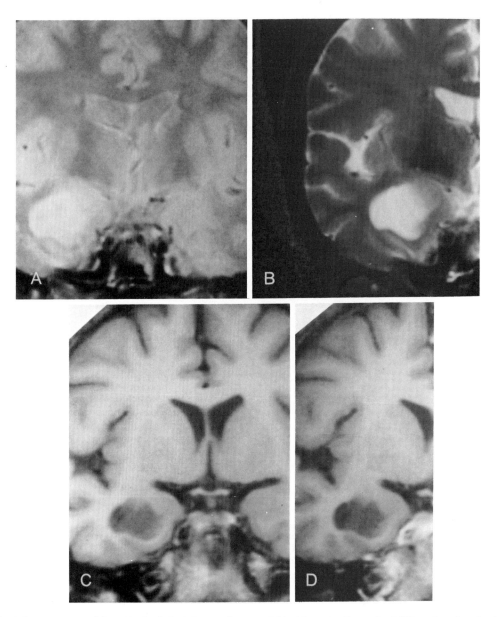

Figure 5.4.   Typical Appearance of Low-grade Astrocytoma. A and B. Hyperintense well-defined temporal lobe mass on T2- weighted images. Precontrast (**C**) and postcontrast (**D**) T1-weighted images show hypointense mass without enhancement.

exhibit such nonaggressive behavior, that patients with these tumors often do well with surgical resection alone.

The low-grade or "benign" astrocytoma and the high-grade or "malignant" astrocytoma have clinical and pathologic features that aid in distinguishing the two. Benign astrocytomas occur in young patients, usually children and adults aged 20–40 years old. They are well-demarcated tumors without necrosis or neovascularity, are rarely hemorrhagic, and are often cystic. They show calcification in 20% of cases and rarely have surrounding edema. On CT, they are hypodense with little or no enhancement. On MR, compared with gray matter, they are hypointense on T1-weighted images, hyperintense on T2-weighted images, and show minimal enhancement (Fig. 5.4).

Table 5.3.   Intraaxial Lesions with Marked Surrounding Edema

Metastasis
Abscess
Glioma
Radiation necrosis

In contrast, the malignant astrocytoma tends to occur in patients older than 40 years of age. These tumors are poorly delineated microscopically although they may appear well-circumscribed grossly. Necrosis, hemorrhage, and neovascularity are common. Surrounding white matter edema is very common (Table 5.3). On CT, they are typically heterogeneous with intense enhancement, often in a ring-like pattern. On MR they are iso- to hypointense compared with gray

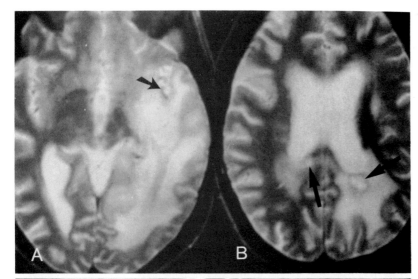

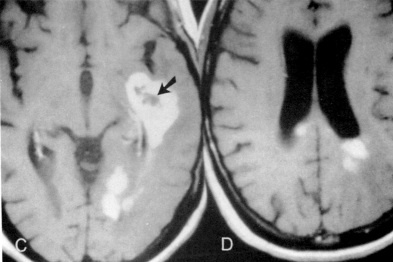

Figure 5.5.   Glioblastoma Multiforme. A and B. Axial T2-weighted images show large areas of hyperintensity predominantly in the left cerebral hemisphere. Note the dark rim lesions (*small arrows*) of anterior left temporal lobe and of left posterior periventricular area. Also note the abnormal hyperintensity (*large arrow*) extending across the splenium of corpus callosum. **C and D.** Postcontrast T1-weighted images through the same levels as in **A** and **B** show multiple enhancing lesions corresponding to areas of T2 hyperintensity. Central area of hypointensity (*arrow*) within left temporal lesion was proven pathologically to be necrosis, characteristic of GBMs.

matter on T1-weighted images and hyperintense on T2-weighted images. A ring-like pattern following contrast may be seen (Fig. 5.5).

Astrocytomas demonstrate a paradox in their gross appearances. The well-differentiated low-grade astrocytomas insinuate themselves through the neurons and other supporting cells that make up the "scaffold" of the brain parenchyma, whereas the highly-malignant GBM is macroscopically better circumscribed. All astrocytomas are poorly circumscribed upon microscopic examination. All will show extension into normal brain tissue beyond the expected margin of the tumor noted on gross inspection. If necrosis is present, the lesion is considered to be a GBM/HAA; if no necrosis is present, the lesion is considered an anaplastic astrocytoma. As GBM and HAA have essentially the same biologic behavior, they can be considered synonymous.

Gliomas spread from their native site in four ways. They may spread by way of natural passages or along subpial or subependymal surfaces. They may spread via the white matter tracts, such as the corona radiata, corticospinal tracts, corpus callosum, and commissures. Finally, tumors may spread across the meninges.

Glioblastoma Multiforme (GBM)

Glioblastoma multiforme (GBM) is the most malignant and most common form of glioma. The peak age of incidence is 45–55 years old, with males slightly more commonly affected. The deep white matter of the frontal lobe, the largest lobe in the brain, is the most common location, followed by the temporal lobe and basal ganglia.

The radiologic appearance reflects the pattern of necrosis, hemorrhage, and neovascularity seen pathologically. The classic appearance of a GBM on either CT or MR is an expansile mass with central necrosis, ring-enhancement, and a large surrounding region of white matter edema (11). On noncontrast CT, GBMs are heterogeneous and lobulated with marked surrounding white matter edema. Calcification occurs

Table 5.4.   Ring-enhancing Lesions ("MAGIC DR")

Metastasis
Abscess
Glioma
Infarct
Contusion
Demyelinating disease
Resolving hematoma

occasionally. Necrosis and hemorrhage are common. The most common hemorrhagic neoplasms in the brain are GBM, metastasis, and oligodendroglioma. On contrast-enhanced CT, more than 90% of GBMs will show at least some enhancement, usually in an irregular, occasionally nodular, ring-like pattern. On MR the tumor nidus commonly shows T1 and T2 prolongation (dark on T1-weighted images, bright on T2-weighted images) compared with gray matter (Fig. 5.5). Because of cellular debris from the necrosis, the signal intensity of these "cystic areas" is usually different than normal CSF.

Besides GBMs, many other lesions can present as ring-enhancing masses. A convenient method to remember these is by the mnemonic "magic doctor" (MAGIC DR) (Table 5.4). The first three entities (metastasis, abscess, and glioma) are in order of frequency. The irregular ring of a neoplasm is often distinct from the smooth ring usually seen in cerebral abscesses (compare Fig. 5.5 with Fig. 6.3**A**). Furthermore, an abscess rim typically is hyperintense on T1-weighted images and hypointense on T2-weighted images, features not commonly noted in tumors (12).

Gliobastoma multiforme tends to be a highly vascular tumor with multiple dark holes representing flow voids within vessels seen on T2-weighted images. Gliobastoma multiforme is one of two entities (CNS lymphoma is the other) that may have bihemispheric spread through the corpus callosum. Because of the imaging appearance of these GBMs, they are known as "butterfly gliomas." White matter edema does not occur in the corpus callosum because its commissural fibers do not conduct edema fluid. White matter or vasogenic edema also cannot travel through projection fibers of the internal capsule that run from the cerebral cortex to the lower centers. In the presence of an intraaxial neoplasm, any T2 hyperintensity seen in the corpus callosum or internal capsule must be considered secondary to neoplastic spread.

For the highly malignant anaplastic astrocytoma and GBM, chemotherapy and radiation therapy are standard treatment protocols at present. Following treatment, GBMs typically decrease in size in association with some symptomatic improvement. Treated lesions are often extensively necrotic and calcified. However, usually within 1 year after surgery, radioresistant cells proliferate and the lesion recurs. Therefore, the prognosis for these patients is much worse than intermediate-grade moderately anaplastic astrocytomas. Gliobastoma multiforme has an 8–12% 2-year survival while moderately anaplastic astrocytomas have 38–50% 2-year survival. New treatment modalities, such as gamma-knife surgery and more advanced chemotherapy protocols, may alter these dismal statistics.

Low-grade Astrocytoma

Low-grade astrocytoma is characterized by slow growth and a longer clinical course. Patients often have productive lives for many years after diagnosis. Intermediate-grade anaplastic and low-grade astrocytomas account for 20–30% of all gliomas. Males are slightly more frequently affected, and the peak incidence is between 30 and 40 years old. In children, they tend to occur in optic pathways, hypothalamus, and the third ventricle. In adults, the lesions are supratentorial within the hemispheres.

Low-grade astrocytomas are pathologically divided into the low-grade fibrillary astrocytoma, the pilocytic (cerebellar cystic) astrocytoma, and the subependymal giant cell astrocytoma seen in tuberous sclerosis. Gemistocytic astrocytomas and pleomorphic xanthoastrocytomas are extremely rare. Approximately 10% of low-grade astrocytomas will degenerate into a more aggressive form (13).

On CT and MR, these lesions generally have variable amounts of surrounding white matter edema and have variable mild and heterogeneous enhancement. Less than 50% will show enhancement. They may not have any abnormal T2 hyperintensity and may not even be apparent on either noncontrast or contrast-enhanced CT.

Calcification (in 25% of cases) and hemorrhage may be present. Necrosis does not occur. Tumors are usually poorly marginated with mild mass effect (Fig. 5.4). The variable appearance occasionally makes distinction from an acute infarct difficult. In these cases a follow-up scan can be crucial in separating the two.

Subependymal giant cell astrocytoma has a strong association with tuberous sclerosis, occurring in up to 10% of patients. It is very rare in patients who do not have this syndrome. Any mass discovered in the region of the foramen of Monro in a young patient should provoke investigation for other manifestations of tuberous sclerosis, such as subependymal and cortical hamartomas. Subependymal giant cell astrocytomas are benign and slow-growing, with calcification a common feature. Because of their location within the foramen of Monro, these tumors almost always produce some degree of hydrocephalus. On MR, they are typically iso- to slightly hyperintense to gray matter on T1-weighted images, and hyperintense to gray matter on T2-weighted images, with some heterogeneity noted because of the calcification. With contrast, they usually enhance. Tuberous sclerosis is discussed in greater detail in Chapter 8.

Juvenile pilocytic astrocytomas will be discussed in the section on posterior fossa tumors.

GLIOMATOSIS CEREBRI

Gliomatosis cerebri is a rare disease that is the result of widespread infiltration of neoplastic astrocytes with varying degrees of differentiation. Despite the diffuse involvement of the brain seen pathologically and on imaging studies, the clinical symptoms are often mild. Peak incidence is between 20 and 40 years of age. Frequently, the lesion appears to smolder for weeks to years before erupting into a full-blown GBM or HAA. Radiotherapy may temporarily improve the radiologic appearance and improve clinical symptoms. Because these are uncommon lesions, the long-term prognosis is not well defined but is probably poor. Invariably, the CT in patients with gliomatosis cerebri is normal, as the lesions are isodense to normal brain parenchyma and do not enhance. However, on MR, the lesion is characterized by diffuse T1 and T2 prolongation throughout the white and gray matter, particularly the hypothalamus, basal ganglia, and thalami. Mass effect and enhancement are minimal (14). Distinction between the gray and white matter is often lost. This appearance can be quite similar to that seen in progressive multifocal leukoencephalopathy seen in immunocompromised patients.

OLIGODENDROGLIOMAS

Oligodendrogliomas account for about 5% of all gliomas (about 2–3% of all intracranial neoplasms). They are more common in adults with a peak age of 35–40 years old. Slow growth with prolonged survival is characteristic. However, the postoperative survival rates are relatively poor, with 50% 5-year survival and 10–30% 10-year survival. The tumor is supratentorial in 85% of cases. Calcification is present pathologically in 100% of oligodendrogliomas, and is seen in about 70% of CT studies. However, it is important to remember that, because astrocytomas, which calcify in about 25% of cases are far more common than oligodendrogliomas, a calcified tumor in the brain is more likely to be an astrocytoma than an oligodendroglioma. Hemorrhage and cysts occur about 20% of the time. Hematogenous or subarachnoid spread is uncommon. About half of the time, these tumors present as a heterogeneous mixed glioma (e.g., oligoastrocytoma). On MR, they are usually hypointense to gray matter on T1-weighted images and hyperintense on T2-weighted images. Surrounding edema is seen in only about one-third of cases. With contrast, about two-thirds show some enhancement, although the degree of enhancement is variable. They are most com-

Table 5.5. Posterior Fossa Masses in Children

Tumor	Location in Relation to Fourth Ventricle	Appearance
Medulloblastoma	Posterior (vermis)	Hyperdense on CT Hypointense on T1-weighted images Variable on T2-weighted images
Juvenile pilocytic astrocytoma	Lateral/posterior	Cystic, with solid mural nodule that enhances intensely
Ependymoma	Within	Foraminal extension Heterogeneous (CT and MR) Inhomogeneous enhancement
Brainstem glioma	Anterior	Expansile brainstem Iso- to hypodense on CT Hypointense on T1-weighted images Hyperintense on T2-weighted images

monly located in the frontal lobes and often extend to the cortex, where they may erode the calvarium. The appearance, in an adult, of a heterogeneous calcified mass within the periphery of a frontal lobe with calvarial erosion and relative absence of edema should suggest the diagnosis of an oligodendroglioma (15).

Posterior Fossa Neoplasms in Children

The posterior fossa is the most common site for intracranial neoplasms in the pediatric population. Medulloblastomas and cerebellar astrocytomas account for about two-thirds of all posterior fossa neoplasms in children, with ependymoma and brainstem glioma comprising the remaining one-third (Table 5.5). Symptoms related to cerebellar dysfunction (ataxia, nausea and vomiting, etc.) dominate the clinical picture in all of these lesions.

MEDULLOBLASTOMA

The first problem with medulloblastomas is what to call them. There is a controversy among neuropathologists as to the exact nature of these neoplasms because of histologic similarities between several neoplasms predominantly seen in children. Medulloblastomas, called by some primitive neuroectodermal tumors, are the second most common pediatric brain tumor (second only to astrocytomas) and the most common pediatric posterior fossa tumor. Peak occurences are at 4–8 years and at 15–35 years. They

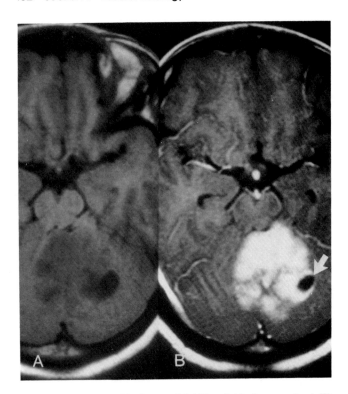

Figure 5.6. Medulloblastoma. Axial T1-weighted precontrast (**A**) and postcontrast (**B**) images demonstrate fairly well-circumscribed and intensely enhancing posterior fossa mass that lies in the region of the vermis and extends slightly into left cerebellar hemisphere. Well-defined area of hypointensity (*arrow*) along the left lateral margin of enhancing mass represents a cyst, a not uncommon feature of these tumors.

may occur at any age, but 75% of patients are less than 15 years of age. Males are more commonly affected. Clinical presentation is usually nausea, vomiting, and headaches. Medulloblastomas are found only in the posterior fossa, originating most commonly from the vermis, and extending into the fourth ventricle. Most adults with these tumors will have them located within the cerebellar hemispheres. They are highly malignant, exhibiting rapid growth that almost always leads to hydrocephalus.

Medulloblastomas are believed to arise from residual bipotential precursor cells of the germinal matrix. They are usually solid, hyperdense masses on CT. Cystic change or necrosis occurs in up to 50% of cases and calcification occurs in up to 20%. Hemorrhage is rare. According to Barkovich (16), the most reliable way to differentiate these tumors from astrocytomas is on a noncontrast CT scan, where the astrocytoma will usually be hypodense and the medulloblastoma will almost never be hypodense. On MR, they are usually hypointense to gray matter on T1-weighted images and have an extremely variable appearance on T2-weighted images, probably reflecting the varying nucleus to cytoplasm ratio. Cerebellopontine angle involvement is rare. Surrounding edema is almost always seen. With contrast, there is intense and fairly

homogeneous enhancement of the tumor (Fig. 5.6). Blurring of cerebellar folia on the midline sagittal MR image can be a helpful differentiating feature and reflects the infiltrative nature of these neoplasms (16).

Therapeutically, these tumors are challenging because of their tendency to spread via the subarachnoid spaces, which has occurred in up to 50% cases at the time of diagnosis. CSF metastases are found in the ventricular system, at the operative site, and in the thecal sac of the spinal canal. Postcontrast MR scans demonstrate lesions as brightly enhancing foci, "studding" the meninges. It is particularly important that MR evaluation of the spinal canal with gadolinium be performed preoperatively. Postoperative granulation tissue and hemorrhagic debris can create either the illusion of "drop" metastasis or mask true lesions during the first 6–8 weeks after surgery. Systemic metastasis occur in about 5% of cases, with the skeleton being the most common site (17).

CEREBELLAR ASTROCYTOMAS

Cerebellar astrocytomas occur with virtually identical incidence as medulloblastomas. Most are of a distinct subset, the juvenile pilocytic astrocytoma (JPA). Early morning headache and vomiting are typical early symptoms, and there is eventual development of ataxia if no intervention is sought. There is an increased frequency of these tumors with neurofibromatosis (8). While 60% are located within the posterior fossa, these tumors may also occur supratentorially, where common locations include the optic pathways and cerebral hemispheres. Most (85%) of the posterior fossa tumors originate within the vermis, but 30% extend into the cerebellar hemispheres.

There are two basic forms of these tumors. Half are cystic with a mural nodule, and have a benign character with a 94% 25-year survival rate. The other half are solid masses with or without a necrotic center, and are more aggressive, with a 40% 5-year survival rate. Calcification occurs in 20% of cases, usually in the solid tumor types. Hemorrhage is very unusual.

On CT, they present as a well-delineated vermian or hemispheric mass with the solid portion being iso- or hypodense to brain tissue. On MR, they are iso- or hypointense to gray matter on T1-weighted images and hyperintense to gray matter on T2-weighted images. The cystic portion usually contains proteinaceous fluid and therefore will not exactly follow the signal intensity of CSF. Surounding edema is rare. The solid component of the tumor enhances to some degree, but is of variable intensity. The mural nodule of the cystic forms will enhance intensely (Fig. 5.7). On noncontrast MR, one should exercise caution in ascribing hypointensity on T1-weighted images and hyperintensity on T2-weighted images within a mass to be "cystic." Truly cystic lesions can only be confidently iden-

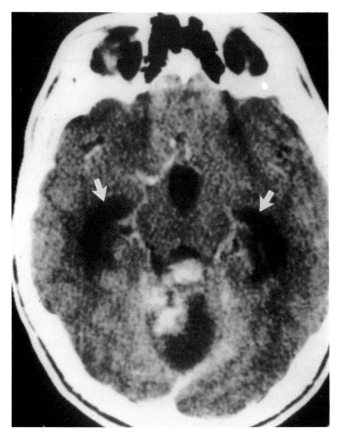

Figure 5.7. Juvenile Pilocytic Astrocytoma. Axial postcontrast CT scan shows heterogeneous posterior fossa mass with both cystic and solid enhancing components. Hydrocephalus is evidenced by the dilated temporal horns (arrows). Hemangioblastomas may also appear as cystic posterior fossa masses with mural nodules. The age of the patient is a useful discriminator between JPAs (peak age, 9 years) and hemangioblastomas (peak age, 35 years).

tified by the presence of fluid-fluid levels or wave pulsation.

The appearance of a cystic mass with an enhancing mural nodule should suggest two possible diagnoses, JPA and hemangioblastomas. Juvenile pilocytic astrocytomas much more commonly occur in children, with a peak age of birth to 9 years. Hemangioblastomas have a peak age of 35 years and are the most common primary intraaxial neoplasm of the posterior fossa in an adult. Other possible posterior fossa lesions include infection (especially toxoplasmosis), other cystic gliomas, and metastasis.

EPENDYMOMA

Ependymoma accounts for about 5–6% of all intracranial neoplasms and are primarily tumors of children and adolescents. A benign subtype of ependymoma known as subependymoma occurs in the middle-aged and elderly population, and characteristically is intraventricular in location. Ependymomas are the most common spinal cord tumor. In children, 60–70% of ependymomas occur within the posterior

fossa, with 70% of those centered within the fourth ventricle. The 30% that occur supratentorially are usually parenchymal in location. Symptoms are insidious in onset, and are related to increased cerebellar pressure from obstruction of the fourth ventricle or cerebellar ataxia. Most tumors are benign. Most are solid but 20% of cases are composed of myxopapillary elements, making them soft and conforming to the shape of whatever structure they are within. Calcification occurs in 50%. Subarachnoid seeding is rare, and its presence should suggest the possibility of a malignant ependymoma. A characteristic feature of these tumors is extension through the foramen of Luschka into the cerebellopontine angle or through the foramen of Magendie into the cisterna magna and through the foramen magnum. This feature of extension helps differentiate ependymomas from the other pediatric posterior fossa masses. They are difficult to cure and have a high recurrence rate with 25–50% 5-year survival.

On CT, these tumors are isodense masses with a mixture of calcification, cystic change, and even hemorrhage, producing an overall heterogeneous appearance. This pattern is also seen on MR where they are slightly hypointense to gray matter on T1-weighted images and hyperintense to gray matter on T2-weighted images. With contrast, there is inhomogeneous enhancement of the solid component. A posterior fossa mass extending through the foramen magnum strongly favors the diagnosis (Fig. 5.8) (16).

BRAINSTEM GLIOMA

These astrocytomas account for about 15% of all pediatric CNS neoplasms. There is no sex predilection and the peak incidence is between 3 and 10 years of age. Like other astrocytomas, they infiltrate through the normal tracts and produce expansile enlargement of the brainstem, creating cranial nerve palsies, pyramidal tract signs, and ataxia as a consequence. Because of the nature of the tumor and the delicate structures (e.g., cranial nerve nuclei) located within this region, chemotherapy and radiation therapy, rather than surgery, are the treatment options. However, brainstem gliomas nearly always recur within 2 years after completion of the therapy, and the overall prognosis is poor (10–30% 5-year survival).

Detection of brainstem gliomas may be difficult. Identification of three imaging features will prove helpful in suggesting the diagnosis. First, exophytic growth into the adjacent cisternal spaces occurs in about 60% of cases. Second, if the ventral portion of the pons extends anteriorly to the margin of the basilar artery (which normally lies within the midline indentation of the ventral pons), then abnormal enlargement of the pons is present and a cause should be identified. The differential diagnosis of pontine en-

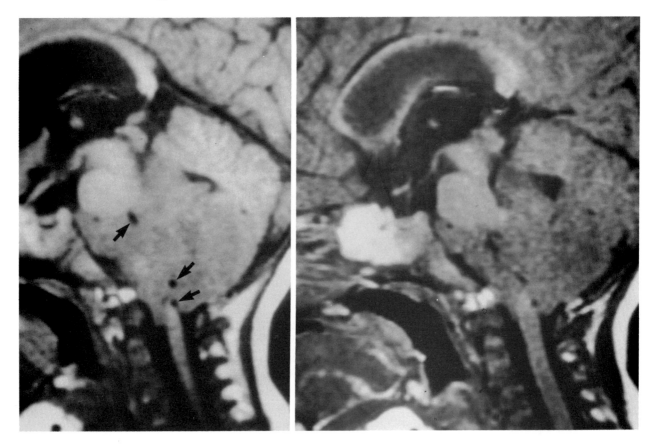

Figure 5.8. Ependymoma. Sagittal noncontrast T1-weighted images in a 4-year-old patient with ataxia. A lobulated mass extends inferiorly through the foramen magnum. The mass also extended through the foramen of Luschka (not shown). The tumor is centered within the fourth ventricle with only a small portion of the fourth ventricle still visible at the superior margin of mass. The dark holes (*arrows*) contained within the mass represent vessels surrounded by this soft tumor.

largement also includes encephalitis, tuberculoma, acute disseminated encephalomyelitis, infarction, resolving hematoma, and vascular malformation. The presence of blood breakdown products makes detection of one of the vascular causes straightforward on MR. However, encephalitis and tuberculoma cannot be distinguished from a brainstem glioma based on imaging characteristics alone. Third, alteration of the normal fourth ventricle contour provides a useful clue. The floor of the fourth ventricle may be flattened, the ventricle itself may be displaced posteriorly, and if there is involvement of the lateral recesses, the ventricle will be rotated. In cases where the tumor grows exophytically into the cerebellar hemispheres, it may mimic a cerebellar astrocytoma. Occasionally a brainstem glioma may involve not only the pons but also the medulla and the cervical cord. When a brainstem glioma extends through the foramen magnum, it may resemble an ependymoma. However, ependymomas are separate from the brainstem, and typically enhance more vigorously than brainstem gliomas.

On CT, brainstem gliomas present as focal hypo- to isodense expansion of the brainstem with extremely variable enhancement that may change with time. The degree of enhancement does not correlate reliably with the grade of the tumor. The adjacent cisterns may be compressed. On MR, typical prolongation of T1 and T2 is seen (Fig. 5.9). The T2-weighted images are of most value in assessing the true extent of the tumor as the signal hyperintensity of the tumor contrasts sharply with the relative low signal of normal white matter. Because of the slow growth of these tumors, hydrocephalus is not usually seen. Hemorrhage or cysts occur in about 25% of cases (16).

Nonglial Tumors

PRIMITIVE NEUROECTODERMAL TUMORS

Classification of this tumor and differentiation from medulloblastoma is controversial. Because of the diverse heterogeneity of the cells that compose these neoplasms, neuropathologists have disagreed as to their exact nature. It is believed that they arise from bipotential precursor cells of the germinal matrix with the ability to differentiate along either glial or neuronal cell lines. Similar histology is also seen in other "-blastoma" lesions—ependymoblastoma, pineoblastoma, spongioblastoma, and neuroblastoma.

Primitive neuroectodermal tumors occur supratentorially in two-thirds of cases and are much more

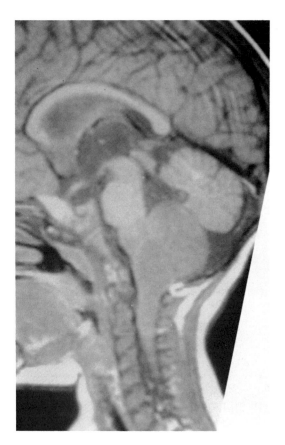

Figure 5.9. Brainstem Glioma. Midline sagittal T1-weighted images in a young child with progressive ataxia. The large mass, slightly hypointense to normal surrounding brainstem, has a large exophytic component and also involves the upper cervical cord.

Table 5.6. Congenital Brain Tumors in Infants Less Than 60 Days Old[a]

Teratoma—most common, ⅓ to ½ of all tumors, ⅔ supratentorial
PNET—curvilinear, sparse calcification
Astrocytoma
Choroid plexus papilloma
Ependymoma
Medulloepithelioma
Germinoma
Angioblastic meningioma
Ganglioglioma

[a]Adapted from Buetow PC, Smirniotopoulos JG, Done S. Congenital brain tumors: a review of 45 cases. AJNR 1990;11:793–799.

common in children than adults. However, the age distribution in some types of PNETs, such as neuroblastoma, are more equally weighted between adult and pediatric populations (18). Along with teratomas, they are one of the most common congenital intracranial neoplasms (Table 5.6) (19). Primitive neuroectodermal tumors typically present with symptoms of increased intracranial pressure or seizures. Overall, they carry a very poor prognosis, with a mean survival of only 5 months (19). The most common appearance is a large well-demarcated heterogeneous mass within the deep cerebral white matter. Heterogeneity is sec-

ondary to necrosis, hemorrhage, and calcification. Hydrocephalus is very common. A periventricular or intraventricular location is common with neuroblastomas (18). The solid portions of the tumor are usually hyperdense on CT and iso- to hypointense to gray matter on T2-weighted images, probably reflecting decreased amounts of intracellular water, and show at least some enhancement.

CENTRAL NERVOUS SYSTEM LYMPHOMA

The incidence and demographics of CNS lymphoma are changing rapidly as a consequence of acquired immunodeficiency syndrome (AIDS). Once considered extremely rare as a primary neoplasm, this tumor (almost always a B-cell non-Hodgkin's lymphoma) now accounts for more than the previously reported 1% of all brain tumors. Also at increased risk are other immunocompromised patients, such as those who have had organ transplantation or who have congenital immunodeficiencies. Confusion, lethargy, and memory loss are common. Most patients will have elevated protein and decreased glucose within the CSF, but positive cytology is rare. An impressive response to corticosteroids is quite common, even as soon as 8 hours after administration (20). In spite of lymphomas being highly radiosensitive, the overall prognosis is very dismal even with treatment because of the associated systemic diseases present, especially in the case of AIDS (21).

The classic apearance of CNS lymphoma, particularly in those with AIDS, is multifocal well-demarcated enhancing lesions scattered within the cerebral white matter tracts, often in a periventricular distribution (Fig. 5.10). Most (85%) are supratentorial. Calcification and hemorrhage are rare. The lesions generate relatively little edema for their size. Subependymal spread is common and bihemispheric involvement via the corpus callosum (similar to butterfly glioma) may be seen. Usually the enhancement is focal rather than the ring-like pattern commonly seen with toxoplasmosis. Toxoplasmosis lesions do not exhibit subependymal spread and are more likely to be located within the corticomedullary junction or within the basal ganglia. Both lymphoma and toxoplasmosis lesions are hypointense to white matter on T1-weighted images. However, hypointensity to white matter on T2-weighted images or hyperdensity on CT (again reflecting the high density of small cells) strongly suggests lymphoma. While the only certain method available to differentiate between these two etiologies is biopsy, an empiric trial of anti-*Toxoplasma* therapy for 3 weeks is frequently employed, and the lesions are reassessed by imaging. If the lesions are not regressing in size, then a stereotactic biopsy may be performed to secure the diagnosis (22). Other considerations in the differ-

Figure 5.10. CNS Lymphoma. A 69-year-old immunocompromised patient with altered mental status of progressive nature. **A and B.** Postcontrast axial CT scans show multiple areas of enhancement in a predominantly periventricular distribution. Involvement of the genu of the corpus callosum and subependymal spread (within the frontal horns) is also seen.

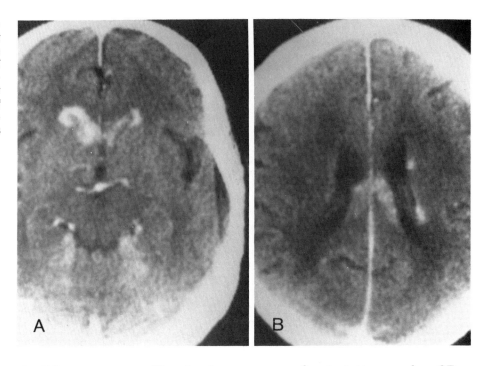

Table 5.7. Most Common Metastases to the CNS

Intraaxial	Extraaxial	Hemorrhagic
Lung carcinoma	Breast carcinoma	Melanoma
Breast carcinoma	Lymphoma	Renal carcinoma
Melanoma	Prostate carcinoma	Thyroid carcinoma
Colon carcinoma	Neuroblastoma	Choriocarcinoma

ential diagnosis include metastasis and focal cerebritis.

Secondary involvement of the brain by systemic lymphoma more commonly involves the leptomeninges instead of the brain parenchyma itself. Differential diagnosis in these cases would include meningioma and leptomeningeal carcinomatosis.

METASTASIS

Metastasis to the CNS from extracranial sites account for about 32% of all intracranial neoplasms. Metastases may be intraaxial (most commonly from lung, breast, melanoma, and colon carcinomas), extraaxial, dural (most commonly breast carcinoma, lymphoma, prostate carcinoma, and neuroblastoma), or within the subarachnoid spaces or skull (Table 5.7). They may occur at any age but most frequently present in older age groups, often with seizures or focal deficits. Clinically silent metastases are most common in patients with oat cell carcinoma, lung carcinoma (especially adenocarcinoma), and melanoma (8).

While most metastases are multiple, up to 30% are solitary (with melanoma, lung, and breast carcinoma the most likely primaries). About 10% of metastases, especially those from melanoma, thyroid carcinoma, and renal cell carcinoma are hemorrhagic (Fig. 5.11).

The classic appearance of metastatic spread on CT or MR is one of multiple foci, located at the cortical-white matter junction, hypodense on CT, hypointense on T1-weighted images, and variable signal intensity on T2-weighted images, with marked edema surrounding each lesion. As with vasogenic edema seen in other neoplastic processes, there is sparing of the cortical gray matter. With contrast administration, there is intense enhancement, which is variable in its form (ring or nodular) (Fig. 5.12). Studies have documented the advantage of contrast, particularly gadolinium on MR, in the detection of more lesions compared with plain spin-echo images, contrast-enhanced CT (23), or even double-dose delayed CT (24). As recently shown, it has been suggested that the sensitivity of metastatic detection may be increased even further by high-dose gadolinium MR (25). These are important considerations as single metastasis may be treated by surgical resection, whereas multiple lesions are more commonly treated by radiotherapy. Most (80–85%) metastatic lesions occur supratentorially, with the exception of renal cell carcinoma, which has a predilection for the posterior fossa. Postcontrast MR is especially helpful in the detection of cortically based lesions that do not demonstrate much edema in the surrounding parenchyma.

Dural (either epidural or subdural) metastasis is the most common form of extraaxial metastasis, seen in 18% of autopsy series. When symptoms occur, they are often secondary to compression of brain parenchyma or dural venous sinus thrombosis. Skull lesions, usually secondary to breast, lung, prostate, or renal carcinoma, give rise to epidural metastases. Subdural lesions are believed to result from hematog-

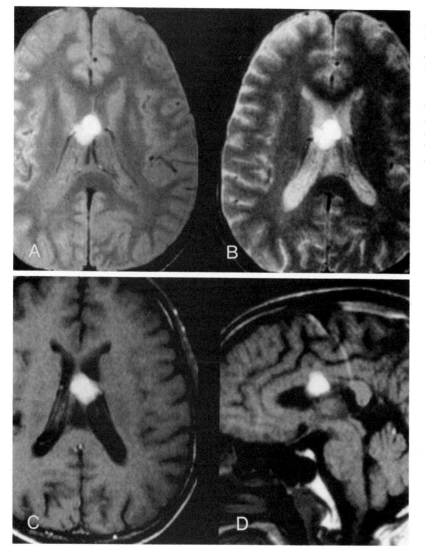

Figure 5.11. Thyroid Metastasis. An adult patient with florid pulmonary metastases (not shown) from thyroid carcinoma and recent onset of headaches. Axial T2-weighted images (**A,** first echo; **B,** second echo) show hyperintense mass of corpus callosum body. Hyperintensity persists on axial (**C**) and sagittal (**D**) T1-weighted images (without contrast), confirming the hemorrhagic nature of the lesion. Melanoma and metastases from renal cell carcinoma and choriocarcinoma are the most common metastases to hemorrhage. Among primary tumors, GBM and oligodendroglioma are the most common to do so.

Figure 5.12. Cerebral Metastasis. Axial T2-weighted images (**A**) show prominent T2 prolongation consistent with vasogenic edema surrounding lesion within the left posterior frontal lobe. Note the mildly hypointense ring representing the margin of the mass. Postcontrast axial T1-weighted images (**B**) show intense ring enhancement with central hypointense area. The irregular shape of the rim (compared with the usual smooth wall of an abscess) is a clue to the true nature of this lung metastasis. Compare to Fig. 6.3**A**.

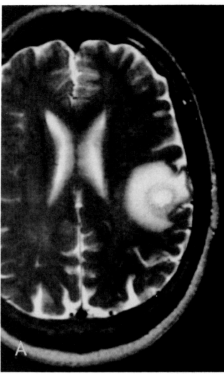 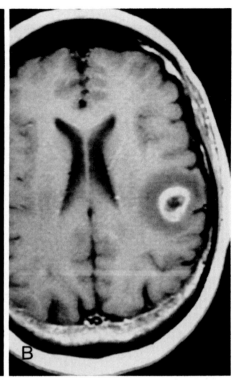

enous spread and, in the case of spine lesions, spread from pelvic tumors by way of Batson's plexus, the epidural collection of spinal veins (26). Epidural and subdural metastases both have a biconvex shape, but can be distinguished by the presence of adjacent skull involvement in epidural metastasis.

Leptomeningeal carcinomatosis deserves special mention because its appearance may exactly mimic meningitis. Characterized by cranial nerve palsies because of its involvement of the basilar cisterns, it is the result of leptomeningeal spread by primary CNS malignancies, extracranial adenocarcinomas (especially of lung or breast origin), leukemia, or lymphoma. Postcontrast MR is far more sensitive than contrast-enhanced CT in the detection of leptomeningeal enhancement. However, even with this technique, not all cases will be detected, and the presence of hydrocephalus in a patient with a known malignancy should suggest this diagnosis as a possibility (26).

Skull metastasis may present a special problem on MR imaging. As with metastases to the spinal vertebral bodies, the administration of contrast will often obscure lesions of the bone marrow that are easily visible on noncontrast T1-weighted image sequences. For this reason, noncontrast T1-weighted images should always be obtained in cases of suspected skull metastasis. While CT with bone windows is superior in detecting subtle bone erosion, MR, with its increased contrast resolution and multiplanar capabil-

ity, easily outperforms CT in the evaluation of epidural and intracranial extension of skull metastasis.

GANGLIOGLIOMA AND GANGLIOCYTOMA

Gangliogliomas are composed of both glial cells and differentiated neurons. Gangliocytomas or ganglioneuromas are pure neuronal tumors without glial components. Both of these tumors are part of spectrum of ganglion neoplasms that includes, ganglioneuroblastoma, anaplastic ganglioglioma, and neuroblastoma, in increasing order of malignancy. Gangliogliomas and gangliocytomas, which account for about 1% of all intracranial neoplasms, are relatively low-grade neoplasms with good prognoses, with a peak age of incidence between 10 and 20 years, but occurring at any age. No sexual predilection is noted. Clinical presentation, often with long-standing symptoms (belying their slow growth), is in the form of focal seizures or hypothalamic dysfunction, depending on their location (16).

While the temporal lobe is the most common location, these lesions may occur anywhere, even within the spinal cord. On CT, these tumors are most often hypo- or isodense well-circumscribed lesions with little associated mass effect or surrounding edema. Calcification is a frequent (35%) feature. They are often peripheral in location. Enhancement varies between absent to completely homogeneous. On MR, they are usually hypo- to isointense relative to gray matter on T1-weighted images and almost always hyperintense to gray matter on T2-weighted images. There is noth-

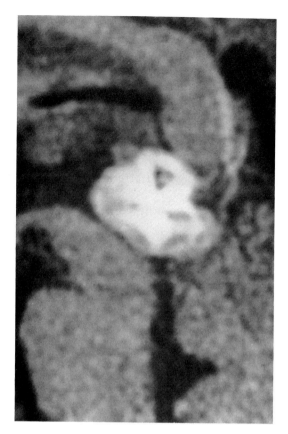

Figure 5.13. Pineal Germinoma. A postcontrast sagittal T1-weighted image in a young adult patient with onset of Parinaud's syndrome. There is heterogeneous enhancement of lobulated pineal mass. It is not possible to distinguish pineal germinomas from pineal parenchymal tumors on the basis of an imaging study alone.

ing specific about this appearance. When these tumors occur in the region of the hypothalamus, another consideration is hypothalamic glioma. When they occur peripherally, the differential diagnosis includes low-grade astrocytoma, oligodendroglioma, and dysembryoplastic neuroepithelial tumor, a benign tumor of neuroepithelial origin seen in patients with medically refractory partial seizures (27). When they occur in the cerebellum, gangliogliomas are indistinguishable from Lhermitte-Duclos disease (28).

Pineal Region Masses

Germ cell tumors constitute the most common type of neoplasms of the pineal region, accounting for 60% of all pineal masses (Fig. 5.13). Pineal parenchymal tumors such as pineoblastoma (malignant) and pineocytoma (benign) compose 14% of pineal masses. The remaining 26% is divided among glioma (from adjacent brain parenchyma), meningioma (from the tentorium) (Fig. 5.14), and miscellaneous lesions such as arachnoid cyst, vein of Galen aneurysm, lipoma, and pineal cyst (Table 5.8). No distinction can be made on imaging studies between germinomas and pineal parenchymal tumors. However, a calcified

pineal mass in a female is more likely to be secondary to a pineocytoma, whereas in a male this same appearance is more likely to be a germinoma. Anytime calcification in the pineal region exceeds 1 cm in size, a pathologic pineal process should be suspected (29).

The size and location of pineal region masses are important imaging characteristics to be conveyed to the neurosurgeon. If a lesion does not contain a large supratentorial component, the preferred infratentorial approach can be performed (31).

Germ Cell Tumors are well-defined, usually midline masses occurring most commonly (65%) in the region of the pineal gland, where they account for about 60% of all pineal region masses. Germinomas are by far the most common intracranial germ cell tumors. They also occur in the suprasellar region (35%), and are most commonly seen in children and young adults, with peak incidence around puberty. Cerebrospinal fluid dissemination is common. Histologically, germinomas are similar to testicular seminomas and ovarian dysgerminomas. In the pineal region, males are much more commonly affected than females (10:1). Typical clinical presentation is related to compression of the sylvian aqueduct, producing hydrocephalus or compression of the superior colliculus, producing Parinaud's syndrome. Curiously, in the case of suprasellar germinomas, there is no sex predilection. Tumors arise in the floor of the third ventricle and rarely extend into the basal ganglia. Because of compression of the optic chiasm and infundibulum, visual changes and symptoms related to hypothalamic dysfunction (emotional disturbance, diabetes insipidus, precocious puberty, etc.) are common.

In either the pineal or suprasellar regions, germinomas have the same appearance on CT: iso- to hyperdense well-circumscribed mass. "Engulfment" of the normal physiologic pineal calcification is a distinguishing feature of germinomas from pineal parenchymal tumors, which more commonly produce an "exploded" appearance of this calcification (32). On MR, hypointensity on T1-weighted images and hyperintensity on T2-weighted images is most common. Hypointensity on T2-weighted images is occasionally present and favors germinoma over pineal tumor. As with pineal parenchymal tumors, intense enhancement on either CT or MR is the rule (Fig. 5.13). In the final analysis, there are no discriminating factors on imaging studies between pineal parenchymal tumors and germinomas that allow accurate differentiation.

Teratomas, embryonal carcinoma, choriocarcinoma, and endodermal sinus tumor are much less common than germinomas. Teratomas usually occur at an earlier age than germinomas and have a variable radiographic appearance and biologic behavior. Besides the pineal region (their most common location), teratomas also occur in the third ventricle and poste-

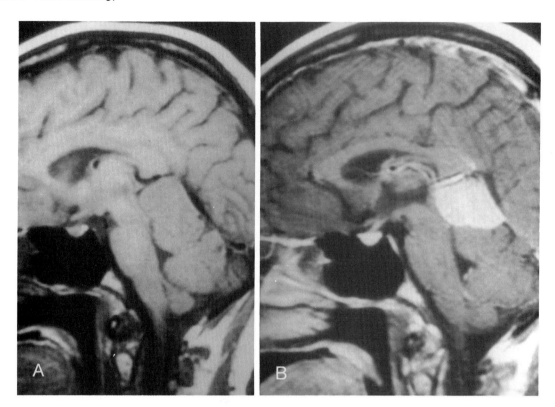

Figure 5.14.   Tentorial Meningioma. Midline sagittal precontrast **(A)** and postcontrast **(B)** T1-weighted images of dural-based, intensely enhancing mass compressing the superior portion of the cerebel- lum and the tectum. The pineal gland itself is not evident, as it is being severely flattened by the expanding meningioma.

Table 5.8.   Pineal Region Masses

Germ cell tumors (60%)
   Germinoma
   Teratoma
   Embryonal carcinoma
   Endodermal sinus tumor
   Choriocarcinoma
Pineal parenchymal tumors (14%)
   Pineocytoma
   Pineoblastoma
Others
   Pineal cyst
   Glioma
   Meningioma (tentorial)
   Vein of Galen aneurysm
   Arachnoid cyst
   Lipoma

rior fossa. Because they contain all three germ cell lines, they will usually be extremely heterogeneous on CT and MR with a mixture of fat, calcification, and cysts. Hydrocephalus is frequent, and enhancement is variable. A midline heterogeneous mass in a child should suggest this diagnosis.

Embryonal carcinoma, choriocarcinoma, and endo- dermal sinus tumor are highly malignant types of germ cell tumors. All are frequently hemorrhagic but have no specific radiographic features. α-Fetoprotein may be elevated in the blood and CSF with embryonal cell carcinoma, teratoma, or choriocarcinoma. Human chorionic gonadotropin may be elevated in choriocarcinoma or teratoma. Germinomas are not associated with elevated human chorionic gonadotro- pin or α-fetoprotein levels. Microneurosurgical tech- niques allow relatively safe open biopsy of suspicious pineal masses for much more accurate pathologic confirmation of the diagnosis (31).

Pineocytoma and Pineoblastoma are true pin- eal tumors that account for 14% of all pineal masses. Pineoblastomas are histologically and radiographi- cally similar to medulloblastoma and have been cate- gorized as part of the PNET group by some neuropa- thologists. These are highly malignant neoplasms, occurring primarily in young children, although they may be seen in patients up to 30 years of age. They are rarely well-circumscribed, demonstrating a lobular contour, local invasion, and frequent calcification. In- tratumoral hemorrhage is rare. Similar to other PNETs, CSF spread is common. There is a rare vari- ant in the form of "trilateral retinoblastoma" seen in patients who have bilateral retinoblastomas and a pineoblastoma.

Pineocytomas, on the other hand, are most com- monly seen in adults although they too may occur at any age. In contrast with pineoblastomas, most are well-demarcated, noninvasive, and slow growing. They are often calcified. Much less commonly than pineoblastomas, they may metastasize with CSF spread. On either CT or MR, they cannot be reliably differentiated from either pineal germinomas or from pineoblastoma.

Both pineal parenchymal tumors are iso- to hyperdense on CT. On MR, they are usually iso- to hypointense on T1-weighted images. There is much variability in signal intensity of these tumors on T2-weighted images, with most being iso- to hyperintense to gray matter. Both the native tumor and their metastases enhance intensely with contrast.

Pineal Cysts are common (~40% in autopsy series) and have internal signal intensity similar to that of CSF (30). The lack of CSF pulsation may cause slightly higher signal on T1- and on T2-weighted images. No enhancement of the cyst itself is seen and no internal architecture is noted. If the cyst is eccentric to the pineal gland itself, it may be difficult to differentiate this lesion from a small pineal neoplasm. They may produce slight flattening of the superior colliculus but do not cause Parinaud's syndrome (paralysis of upward gaze) or hydrocephalus. Very rarely, they may hemorrhage.

Sellar Masses

PITUITARY ADENOMAS

Pituitary adenomas account for about 10–15% of all intracranial tumors and constitute the most common sellar masses, being five times more common than craniopharyngiomas and Rathke's cleft cysts. Based on their size, they are considered either microadenomas (10 mm size or less) or macroadenomas (>10 mm size). In general, about 75% of adenomas are hormonally active, and most of these will be microadenomas. The other 25% are nonsecreting adenomas, and most of these will be macroadenomas. There is a topographical relationship of the secretory cells within the pituitary gland and, in a general sense, depending on the clinical signs and symptoms, this can be used to focus attention on particular sections of the gland. Prolactinomas and growth hormone-secreting adenomas are more commonly located within the lateral aspects of the gland. Adenomas with secretion of ACTH, TSH, or follicle-stimulating hormone/luteinizing hormone are more common in the central region of the gland. Clinical symptoms are related to the type of hormone secreted. For instance, ACTH-producing tumors produce Cushing's disease, and growth hormone-producing tumors produce acromegaly in adults and gigantism in children. Prolactinomas are the most common (40–50%) of the secreting adenomas and are marked clinically by amenorrhea, galactorrhea, or impotence. A serum prolactin level of >150 ng/ml almost always indicates a prolactinoma, and levels >1000 ng/ml herald invasion into the cavernous sinus. Normal prolactin levels are <20 ng/ml.

Magnetic resonance imaging has supplanted CT as the best imaging modality to detect pituitary tumors. Microadenomas are usually detected best on coronal T1-weighted images as focal areas of hypointensity (on noncontrast studies) compared with the rest of the pituitary gland (Fig. 5.15). Occasionally they may be isointense or even hyperintense on noncontrast studies. Other clues to the presence of a microadenoma include deviation of the infundibulum, asymmetric convexity of the pituitary gland, and mild down-sloping of the roof of the sphenoid sinus. In general, gadolinium contrast increases the conspicuity of these often small neoplasms. Gadolinium contrast reveals these small tumors as hypointense foci within the gland on immediate postcontrast scans or as hyperintense foci on delayed (about 30 minutes) scans. In addition, the use of narrow windows is essential to optimize visualization of these small lesions.

Macroadenomas are never a problem to visualize on MR. When they are heterogeneous because of cyst formation or hemorrhage (Fig. 5.16), and differentiation from a craniopharyngioma or parasellar meningioma is difficult, the use of contrast may be helpful (Fig. 5.17). Macroadenomas most commonly present because of optic chiasm or nerve compression, hydrocephalus, cranial nerve palsies, or occasionally anterior pituitary dysfunction. These lesions are isointense to gray matter on T1-weighted images and characteristically produce "draping" of the optic chiasm over the top of the tumor. Invasion of the cavernous sinus can be accurately diagnosed when there is tumor tissue between the internal carotid artery flow void and the *lateral* wall of the cavernous sinus (26).

CRANIOPHARYNGIOMA AND RATHKE'S CLEFT CYST

Both of these entities arise from squamous epithelial remnants of the anterior lobe of the pituitary gland. Craniopharyngiomas are derived from the pars tuberalis and Rathke's cleft cyst arise from the pars intermedia. However, whereas Rathke's cleft cysts are usually asymptomatic, craniopharyngiomas are frequently symptomatic because of their larger size. Symptoms related to increased intracranial pressure, optic nerve or chiasm compression, or hypothalamic symptoms are common. There are two age peaks seen in craniopharyngiomas, between 5 and 10 years old, and between 50 and 60 years old. It is the most common suprasellar mass in the pediatric population. Most craniopharyngiomas involve both intrasellar and suprasellar compartments (70%), whereas 20% are intrasellar only and 10% are purely extrasellar. Solid

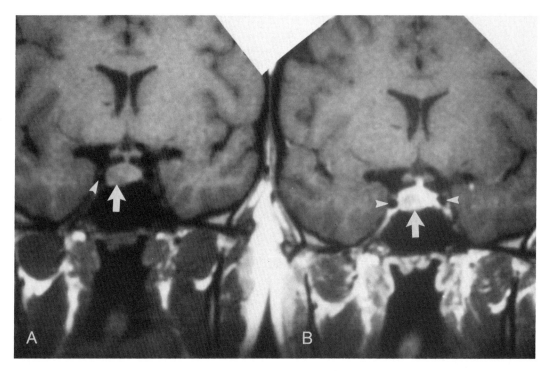

Figure 5.15. Pituitary Microadenoma. A. Precontrast, thin-section coronal T1-weighted images through the sella in patient with elevated prolactin levels show prominent right aspect of the gland with slight hypointensity (*arrow*), compared with the normal pituitary gland to the left. Down-sloping of the sphenoid roof is also seen. **B.** With contrast, the lesion is slightly more conspicuous, measuring 8 mm in transverse diameter. Note the normal flow voids (*arrowheads*) of the internal carotid arteries and the normal enhancement of the cavernous sinuses.

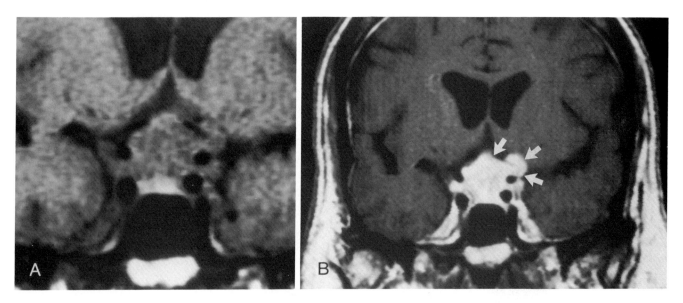

Figure 5.16. Pituitary Macroadenoma. Coronal T1-weighted images without (**A**) and with (**B**) contrast show enhancing mass (*arrows*) extending beyond the lateral margin of cavernous sinus and flow voids of the left internal carotid artery.

and cystic components are typical, with the fluid of the cyst often containing cholesterol crystals and grossly having the appearance of "crank-case oil." On CT, the classic appearance of a craniopharyngioma is a large cystic-appearing sellar/suprasellar mass with an enhancing rim and evidence of some calcification. In children calcification is seen in up to 80% of cases (compared with 40% for adult cases). On MR, because of the presence of the liquid cholesterol, the classic finding of hyperintensity on T1- and T2-weighted images, corresponding to the cystic portion, is most common (Fig. 5.18). However, some craniopharyngiomas will not contain fluid, but instead will be a solid nodule that may be completely calcified. Enhance-

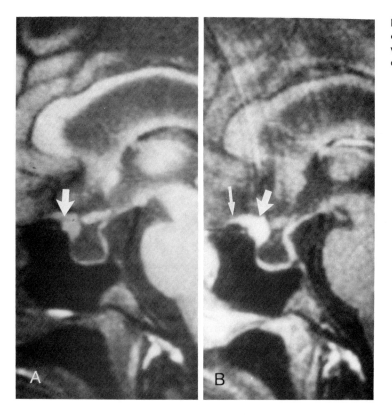

Figure 5.17. Tuberculum Sella Meningioma. Suprasellar enhancing mass (*arrows*) in the region of tuberculum sella with extension along the planum sphenoidale (*small arrow*), a highly characteristic feature of parasellar meningiomas.

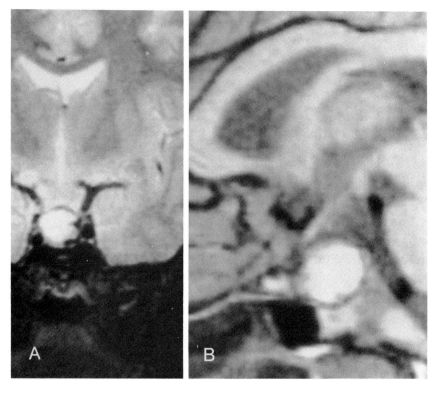

Figure 5.18. Craniopharyngioma. A. Coronal T2-weighted images through the sella in a patient with mild visual symptoms. A hyperintense intrasellar mass with suprasellar component is seen. **B.** Sagittal T1-weighted images show that the hyperintense signal is maintained, consistent with the presence of liquid cholesterol within these tumors.

Table 5.9. Suprasellar Masses ("SATCHMO")

Sella tumor, Sarcoid
Aneurysm, Arachnoid cyst
Teratoma
Craniopharyngioma
Hypothalamic glioma, Hamartoma of tuber cinereum, Histiocytosis
Meningioma
Optic glioma

ment of the rim and any soft-tissue component is noted.

Rathke's cleft cyst are either purely intrasellar (66%) or intra- and suprasellar (33%). The cyst contents are variable. Most commonly, a mucoid fluid fills the cyst. Less commonly, serous fluid or desquamated cellular debris occupies the cyst. Because of this variability, they may be hyperintense on T1- and T2-weighted images, appearing identical to craniopharyngiomas, or they may be iso- to hypointense on either sequence because of cellular debris mimicking the appearance of a solid nodule. A key to differentiating Rathke's cleft cyst from craniopharyngiomas is their lack of enhancement.

A complete differential diagnosis (and time-tested mnemonic) for suprasellar masses is contained in Table 5.9.

Nerve Sheath Tumors

SCHWANNOMA/NEUROFIBROMA

There are three types of nerve sheath tumors: schwannomas (also known as neurilemomas or neurinomas), neurofibromas, and malignant nerve sheath tumors, which are very rare and will not be discussed further. Schwannomas arise from Schwann cells, which form the myelin sheaths of axons. They are focal, encapsulated, and affect the cranial nerves, most often the vestibulocochlear (VIII) nerve and trigeminal (V) nerve. They are often cystic, with hemorrhage and necrosis common. Comprising about 8% of all intracranial neoplasms, they are most common in adults. Virtually 100% of patients with bilateral acoustic schwannomas will have neurofibromatosis type II. Symptoms depend on the cranial nerve involved. For instance, sensorineural hearing loss is very common in acoustic schwannomas. Depending on their size and location, hydrocephalus, brainstem compression, or neuropathy may be present.

On CT, these are iso- to hypodense masses that homogeneously enhance with contrast. On MR, it is advantageous to perform thin-section (3 mm) axial and coronal T1-weighted images through the internal auditory canal to demonstrate these neoplasms that are hypointense to gray matter on T1-weighted images and hyperintense to gray matter on T2-weighted images. As with CT contrast, they enhance intensely

with gadolinium. The larger a schwannoma is, the more likely it is to show heterogeneity because of cysts, hemorrhage, or necrosis.

Acoustic schwannomas are located within the internal auditory canal, being either completely intracanalicular or extending from the canal into the cerebellopontine angle. The internal auditory canal is frequently enlarged. Differentiation from a cerebellopontine meningioma may be difficult. The single most helpful imaging feature to distinguish an acoustic schwannoma from a meningioma is extension of the enhancement along the course of the seventh and eighth nerves, seen in about 80% of acoustic schwannoma cases (Fig. 5.19). Sometimes a meningioma will be obvious because of its broad dural tail (Fig. 5.20). A precontrast or fat-suppressed sequence will detect the unlikely intracanalicular lipoma, which will appear identical to an acoustic schwannoma tumor on postcontrast images. Other cerebellopontine angle lesions include epidermoid tumors (Fig. 5.21) and nonacoustic (cranial nerves V, IX-XI) schwannomas. A mnemonic for cerebellopontine angle lesions is given in Table 5.10.

Trigeminal schwannomas can be identified by their location within the pontine cistern at the midpons level between the trigeminal ganglion located in Meckel's cave (just posterolateral to the cavernous sinus) and the brainstem (Fig. 5.22). Extension through the ganglion and into the foramen ovale, foramen rotundum, or superior orbital fissure may be seen. Less commonly, schwannomas may also involve cranial nerves IX-XI.

Neurofibromas arise from fibroblasts and Schwann cells, are fusiform, and involve the cutaneous exiting spinal nerves. They are rarely cystic, hemorrhagic, or necrotic. Neurofibromas, which are rarely solitary, are more commonly seen in the spine as part of neurofibromatosis types I and II. The most common clinical presentation is that of multiple radiculopathies or cord compression. These tumors are discussed in greater detail in Chapter 8.

Tumors of Mesenchymal Origin

MENINGIOMA

Meningioma is the most common extraaxial neoplasm of adults and accounts for 15% of all primary intracranial neoplasms, second only to gliomas. The peak age of incidence is 50–60 years old. For both intracranial (2:1) and intraspinal (4:1) meningiomas, females are more commonly affected. Because the tumors are hormonally sensitive, they may increase in size during pregnancy. Up to 9% are multiple and are associated with neurofibromatosis. They are rare in children unless associated with neurofibromatosis. Pediatric meningiomas are more likely to be malig-

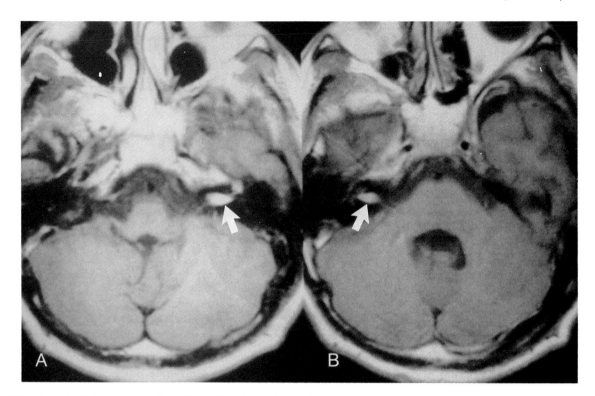

Figure 5.19. Acoustic Schwannoma. A and **B.** Postcontrast axial T1-weighted images show bilateral intracanalicular acoustic schwannoma (*arrows*) in a patient with neurofibromatosis type 2. Ex- tension into the internal acoustic canal and lack of a broad dural base differentiate this entity from meningioma.

nant. Most meningiomas are benign and slow grow- ing tumors that are most frequently found in parasagittal or convexity locations (50%). Other loca- tions include sphenoid wing (20%), olfactory groove/ planum sphenoidale (10%), parasellar region (10%), and miscellaneous locations (10%) including the ven- tricles (the most common site in children), tentorium, and optic nerve sheath. About 2–3% occur within the spine, with the thoracic spine the most common loca- tion.

Meningiomas arise from meningothelial arachnoid cells (villi), probably with some contribution from du- ral fibroblasts and pial cells. Intraventricular mening- iomas arise from arachnoidal cell rests within the cho- roid plexus. There are five basic types: meningothelial (syncytial), transitional, fibroblastic, hemangioperi- cytoma/angioblastic, and malignant meningioma. Two basic shapes (globular and en plaque) are seen.

Meningiomas present some of the most classic roentgenologic findings of any disease process. Even on plain skull films, these tumors can be suspected by focal sclerosis, prominent dural grooves from enlarged middle meningeal arteries, and calcification. On CT, they are well-defined, hyperdense (85%) masses with variable surrounding edema with intense and homo- geneous enhancement (Fig. 5.23). Hyperostosis of the adjacent inner table is noted about 40% of the time. Calcification is seen in 10–20%. The key to diagnosis is the broad dural base of these extraaxial masses. Ad-

jacent dural thickening (the "dural tail") (Figs. 5.17 and 5.20) is seen in about 60% of cases, but is not specific for meningiomas and does not necessarily in- dicate involvement by meningioma tumor cells (33, 34). Hemorrhage is rare but cysts are not uncommon.

On MR, meningiomas are characterized by iso- to hypointensity to gray matter on T1-weighted images and iso- to hyperintense to gray matter on T2- weighted images. Hyperintensity on T2-weighted images almost always correlates with a syncytial or angioblastic type of meningioma. Heterogeneity is the rule because of the presence of cysts, vessels, or calci- fication. Often, there may be a hypointense rim around the tumor. Prominent pial blood vessel flow voids are frequently (80%) noted on MR and provide evidence of the extraaxial nature of the tumor. Cere- brospinal fluid clefts around the margins of the tumor also confirm the extraaxial location in 80% of cases. Invasion of the dural margin interface is highly spe- cific for a dural process (26). Special attention should be given to possible involvement of the dural sinuses as this finding carries important significance in neu- rosurgical planning. Because of this feature, MR is su- perior to CT in overall evaluation of these tumors. Any diminution in the caliber of a dural sinus adjacent to a meningioma is highly suspicious for involvement. Further evaluation with MR angiography or conven- tional angiography may confirm this finding and pro- vide evidence for or against complete occlusion.

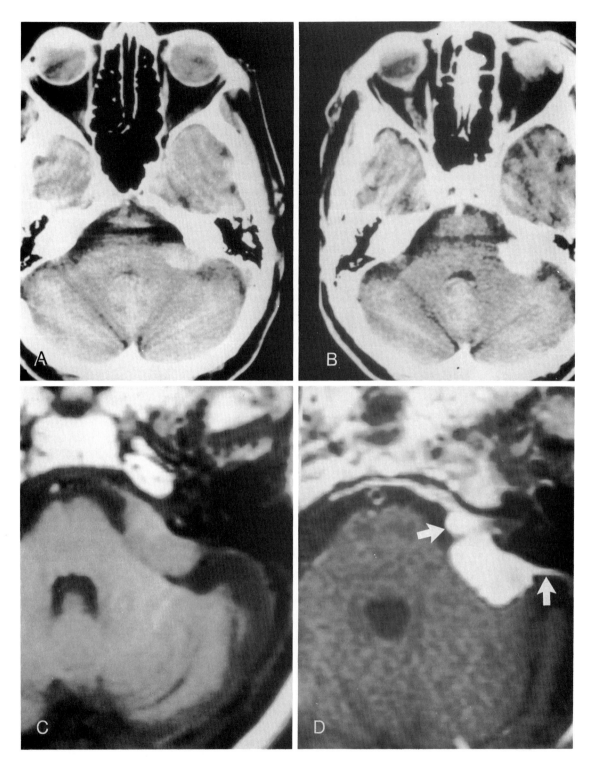

Figure 5.20. Cerebellopontine Angle Meningioma. Noncontrast (**A**) and contrast (**B**) CT scans show a left cerebellopontine mass that intensely enhances. Noncontrast (**C**) and contrast (**D**) T1-weighted images show an extraaxial lesion with broad dural base and intense enhancement. There is no extension along the neurovascular bundle of internal acoustic canal. Note the dural tails (*arrows*) extending anteriorly and posteriorly within the cerebellopontine angle.

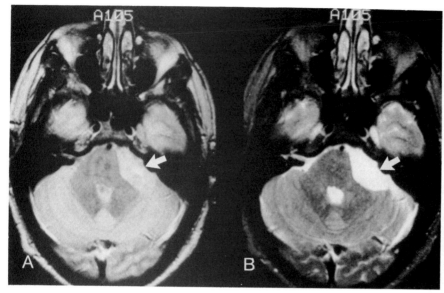
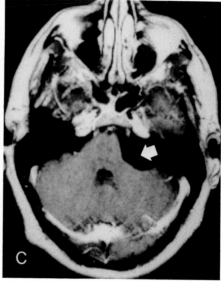

Figure 5.21.   Epidermoid Tumor. Axial T2-weighted images (**A,** first echo; **B,** second echo) show left cerebellopontine angle mass (*arrows*) that closely follows signal intensity of CSF. Postcontrast T1-weighted images (**C**) show no enhancement of the extraaxial mass (*arrow*), which again has signal intensity similar to that of CSF.

Table 5.10.   Cerebellopontine Masses ("AMEN")[a]

	T1WI	T2WI	Gd
Acoustic schwannoma (80%)	Hypo	Hyper	Yes
Meningioma (11%)	Iso to hypo	Iso to hyper	Yes
Ependymoma (4%)	Hypo	Hyper	Yes
Neuroepithelial cyst (arachnoid, epidermoid) (5%)	CSF	CSF	No

[a]T1WI, T1-weighted images signal compared with gray matter; T2WI, T2-weighted images signal compared with gray matter; Gd, gadolinium enhancement; Iso, isointense; Hypo, hypointense; Hyper, hyperintense; CSF, follows signal of cerebrospinal fluid.

Angiographically, meningiomas present a classic appearance. During the arterial phase, there is an early dense tumor blush with a radial arrangement of the vessels. This blush persists well into the venous phase. Because the blush "comes early and stays late," some (not necessarily this author) have called this "the in-law sign" (Fig. 5.24). In addition, enlarged dural vessels and arteriovenous shunting may be noted. The most common blood supply to meningiomas is from branches of the external carotid artery, primarily the middle meningeal artery. The anterior meningeal arteries (arising from the ophthalmic arteries) and the posterior meningeal arteries (arising from the vertebral arteries) may also provide blood supply to these tumors. Preoperative embolization of these vessels often facilitates neurosurgical resection.

Malignant variants of meningiomas are rare, occurring in about 1% of cases. It is not possible to reliably distinguish malignant from nonmalignant meningiomas based on imaging characteristics alone.

HEMANGIOBLASTOMA

Capillary hemangioblastomas are benign neoplasms of endothelial origin. They are most common in young and middle-aged adults, and are the most common primary intraaxial neoplasm of the posterior fossa in adults. Approximately 4–20% occur as part of the von Hippel-Lindau syndrome (discussed in the chapter 8) in which case they are often multiple. They most often occur in the cerebellar hemispheres, but other sites of involvement include the spinal cord (especially the cervical portion), medulla, and even the cerebral hemispheres (very rare). As they contain no capsule, recurrence is common if only partial resection is performed. Because the tumor nidus receives its blood supply from the pia mater, the nodule (which represents the tumor itself) is always superficial in location (35). Calcification is very rare. The classic appearance is a well-defined cystic mass with an intensely enhancing mural nodule (60% of cases). Up to 40% are entirely solid. On MR, they appear as cystic masses with hypointensity to gray matter on T1-weighted images and hyperintensity to gray matter on T2-weighted images. Surrounding edema may be present. Serpiginous flow voids within the nodule may be seen. In the less common presentation of a solid mass, the margins are usually ill-defined and occasionally hemorrhage is present. Because of the highly vascular nature of the nodule, intense enhancement is the rule (Fig. 5.25). If CT or MR is negative in highly clinically suspicious cases, angiography may be helpful in revealing small (less than 1 cm) lesions.

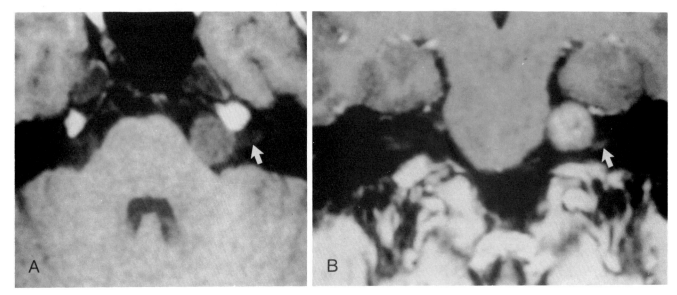

Figure 5.22. Trigeminal Schwannoma. A. Axial T1-weighted images in a patient with dizziness show isointense mass in the cisternal space near the vicinity of the internal auditory canal. Note the portion of the seventh and eighth nerve complex (*arrow*) displaced by mass. **B.** Postcontrast coronal T1-weighted images show homogeneous enhancement. Again note the seventh and eighth nerve complex (*arrow*) displaced by this schwannoma from the trigeminal nerve.

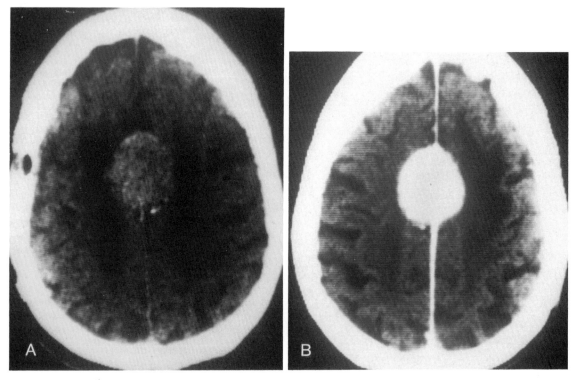

Figure 5.23. Meningioma. Precontrast (**A**) and postcontrast (**B**) CT images of falcine meningioma. On the precontrast study, the mass is hyperdense to normal brain parenchyma. With contrast, there is intense enhancement. One-half of all meningiomas occur parasagittally or along the convexity.

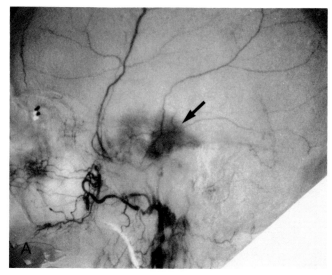

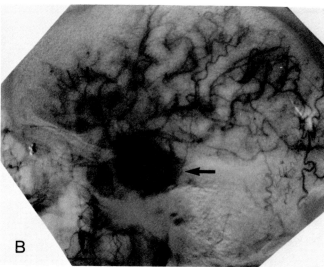

Figure 5.24. Meningioma on Angiogram. Selective external carotid injection (**A**) demonstrates early blush (*arrow*) on arterial phase, while **B** shows persistent staining on venous phase. This coming early and staying late has been referred to as the "in-law sign."

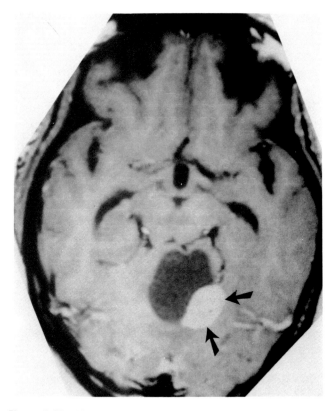

Figure 5.25. Hemangioblastoma. The classic appearance on a postcontrast axial T1-weighted image of cystic posterior fossa mass, with intensely enhancing mural nodule (*arrows*), which represents the tumor itself.

Tumors of Maldevelopmental Origin

EPIDERMOID AND DERMOID

Epidermoid and dermoid are congenital neoplasms that result from enclosure of ectodermal elements when the neural tube closes. Epidermoid tu-

mors account for about 1% of all intracranial neoplasms, whereas dermoid tumors, as intracranial masses, are much less common. Both are benign and characterized by slow growth. The peak age of incidence is 40 to 50 years old for epidermoids and 20 to 30 years old for dermoids. While epidermoid tumors are composed of squamous epithelium alone, dermoid tumors contain mesodermal elements as well. They both contain keratin but dermoid tumors are also composed of fat and calcification. Epidermoids are most often located off the midline at the skull base (i.e., cerebellopontine angle, parasellar, or the posterior fossa) while dermoids are characteristically midline masses, most common in the inferior vermis or at the vallecula. Symptoms from epidermoids are produced by compression of adjacent structures, most commonly the cranial nerves. Symptoms from dermoid tumors are secondary to obstruction of CSF pathways, chemical meningitis (secondary to rupture of the dermoid), or infection if associated with a sinus tract. A comparison of epidermoid and dermoid tumors is given in Table 5.11.

On imaging studies, the differing compositions produce different signal intensities. Epidermoid tumors are well-circumscribed lobulated masses that, because of CSF within the interstices of the tumor, most commonly have signal intensities on both CT and MR that follow that of CSF (hypodense on CT, hypointense on T1-weighted images, and hyperintense on T2-weighted images) (Fig. 5.21). Rim enhancement following contrast may be seen. On occasion, epidermoids contain enough liquid cholesterol (similar to craniopharyngioma) to produce T1 shortening (hyperintensity) of the mass (36). The primary differential diagnosis is an arachnoid cyst. If the diagnosis is in doubt, the definitive study is a cisternogram that demonstrates contrast filling the interstices of the epidermoid (producing a "cauliflower-like" appearance), whereas an arachnoid cyst will have a smooth margin. Sometimes this cauliflower appearance can be appreciated on thin-section T1-weighted images.

Dermoid tumors, on the other hand, typically have signal characteristics that follow that of fat (low density on CT, hyperintense on T1-weighted images, and intermediate to hypointense on T2-weighted images, with signal suppression on fat saturation images) (Fig. 5.26). They do not enhance unless infected. Heterogeneity of the mass may be seen because of calcification and other soft-tissue components. The presence of a fat-fluid level is al-

Table 5.11. Epidermoid vs. Dermoid Tumors

Characteristic	Epidermoid	Dermoid
Frequency	Common	Uncommon
Peak age	40–50	20–30
Germ cells	Ectoderm	Ectoderm and mesoderm
Location	Off midline (CPA,^{a} parasellar, posterior fossa)	Midline (pericerebellar, suprasellar)
Imaging	Follows CSF most commonly, lobulated with interstices	Some portion will follow fat

^{a}cerebellar-pontine angle.

most pathognomonic. If no heterogeneity is present, it is impossible to distinguish dermoid tumors from lipomas. Occasionally, dermoids rupture into the subarachnoid space, producing a chemical meningitis. In this situation, multiple foci of T1 shortening will be seen extraaxially and the patient is almost always quite ill, with some fatalities reported. In the presence of an intracranial dermoid, the nasofrontal and occipital regions of the scalp should be evaluated to detect a sinus tract.

LIPOMA

Intracranial lipomas are usually asymptomatic and incidental findings on imaging studies. They occur in all ages and are most common in the midline, in the corpus callosum, quadrigeminal plate, and suprasellar regions. Lipomas are thought to arise from incomplete resorption of the primitive meningeal tissue in the development of the subarachnoid cisterns (8). Lipomas in the pericollosal region are commonly associated with agenesis of the corpus callosum (Fig. 5.27). As expected for a fatty mass, they are low density on CT, occasionally containing calcification. On MR, they exhibit T1 and mild T2 shortening, following the signal intensity of subcutaneous fat. They do not enhance. The presence of either a chemical shift artifact or signal suppression on a fat saturation T1-weighted image establishes the diagnosis.

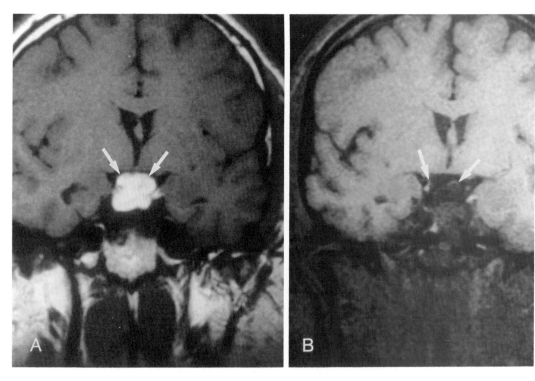

Figure 5.26. Dermoid Tumor. Coronal T1-weighted images (**A**) show a hyperintense suprasellar mass (*arrows*). With fat-suppression technique (**B**), the signal of the dermoid tumor becomes iso- intense following the signal of subcutaneous fat, confirming the nature of the lesion.

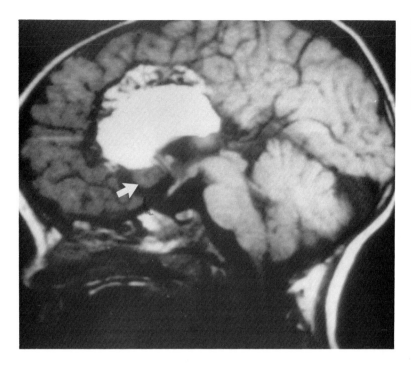

Figure 5.27. Lipoma with Agenesis of Corpus Callosum. Sagittal T1-weighted images shows a large hyperintense midline mass. The development of a lipoma in this location prevents normal development of the corpus callosum. Note that only a portion of the genu (*arrow*) is present in this case, with the remaining structures of the corpus callosum absent.

ARACHNOID CYSTS

Arachnoid cysts account for about 1% of all intracranial masses and are congenital in nature. "Secondary" or "acquired arachnoid cysts" are in reality leptomeningeal cysts resulting from prior inflammatory process (meningitis, hemorrhage, etc.). True arachnoid cysts are created by secretion of CSF from the cells lining the cyst and are therefore intraarachnoidal. They are most common (50%) in the middle cranial fossa where they may be quite large. Other sites include the frontal convexity, the suprasellar and quadrigeminal cisterns, and the posterior fossa. If they attain sufficient size to obstruct CSF flow or compress the brain, they become symptomatic.

They follow the attenuation/signal intensity pattern of CSF on CT and MR. Remodeling of the adjacent bone may be seen. Hemorrhage may occur after trauma or spontaneously. Unless infection is present, no enhancement is noted.

The differential diagnosis for the posterior fossa arachnoid cyst includes enlarged cisterna magna, epidermoid, and Dandy-Walker malformation. Enlarged cisterna magna and epidermoid may be difficult to distinguish from an arachnoid cyst based on CT or MR. Intrathecal injection of iodinated contrast will fill the cisterna magna but not the arachnoid cyst, demonstrate the fronds of the epidermoid, or the arachnoid cyst's smooth margins. Dandy-Walker cysts are extensions of the fourth ventricle, whereas an arachnoid cyst will be separate from the fourth ventricle (16).

Neuroepithelial Tumors

COLLOID CYST

This tumor of the anterior-superior third ventricle is the most common intraventricular neuroepithelial cyst. They account for less than 1% of all intracranial tumors yet they are important because of their propensity to cause acute hydrocephalus by obstructing the foramina of Monro. The classic presentation is acute onset of a severe headache that can be reproduced by the patient tilting the head forward. Occasional fatalities have been reported. Some colloid cysts are entirely cystic and others have a heterogeneous composition of old hemorrhage, cholesterol crystals, and various ions producing a variable appearance on CT and MR. On CT, most are hyperdense to brain tissue. On MR hyperintensity on T1-weighted images is most common (Fig. 5.28). Rim enhancement is seen in 40%. Other lesions that occur in the anterior-superior third ventricle are listed in Table 5.12. Dense enhancement suggests a lesion other than colloid cyst (37).

CHOROID PLEXUS PAPILLOMA

Choroid plexus papilloma is a rare neuroepithelial tumor that is most common in the first decade but can also be seen in adults. They account for only about 0.5% of all intracranial neoplasms. The atrium of the lateral ventricle is the most common site in children, while the fourth ventricle is the most common site in adults. The clinical presentation of choroid plexus papilloma is often related to increased intracranial pressure and hydrocephalus, which occur because of marked increase in production of CSF by these tumors. CSF resorption is also reduced because

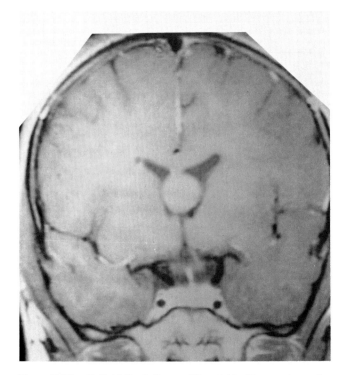

Figure 5.28. Colloid Cyst. Coronal T1-weighted image shows the typical appearance, with the characteristic location in the third ventricle.

Table 5.12. Masses of the Anterosuperior Third Ventricle

Colloid cyst
Meningioma
Choroid plexus papilloma
Hamartoma
Glioma
Vascular lesion
Granulomatous lesion

Table 5.13. Most Common Lateral Ventricle Masses by Location and Age[a, b]

Age (years)	Foramen of Monro	Body	Trigone
0–5		PNET Teratoma CPP	CPP
6–30	Subependymal GCA JPA	Epend JPA	Epend Oligodendrog
>30	Metastasis	Subepend GBM	Meningioma

[a]Adapted from Jelinek J, Smirniotopoulos JG, Parisi JE, Kanzer M. Lateral ventricular neoplasms of the brain: differential diagnosis based on clinical, CT, and MR findings. AJNR 1990;11:567–574.
[b]CPP, choroid plexus papilloma; GCA, giant cell astrocytoma; Epend, ependymoma; Oligodendrog, oligodendroglioma; Subepend, subependymoma.

of hemorrhage and increased protein content within the CSF. Malignant degeneration in the form of choroid plexus carcinoma occurs in 10–20% of cases (38).

Table 5.14. Intraventricular Masses[a]

The major players
  Astrocytoma—most common frontal horn lesion, least enhancement
  Colloid cyst—foramen of Monro, most common third ventricle mass
  Meningioma—most common atrial lesion
  Ependymoma—most common body of lateral ventricle lesion
  Medulloblastoma—fourth ventricle (by direct extension), third and lateral ventricles by seeding
  Craniopharyngioma—second most common third ventricle mass
  Choroid plexus papilloma/carcinoma—lateral ventricle >third ventricle, enhance intensely
Others
  Cysticercosis—fourth > anterior third ventricle, change position with head tilting
  Epidermoid—fourth ventricle
  Ependymal/arachnoid cyst—third ventricle most common
  Dermoid—fourth ventricle and frontal horn
  Subependymoma—fourth ventricle, frontal horn
  Arteriovenous malformations—lateral and fourth ventricles
  Teratoma

[a]Adapted from Morrison G, Sobel DF, Kelly WM, Norman D. Intraventricular mass lesions. Radiology 1984;153:435–442.

On CT, these are well-defined masses that are iso- to hyperdense and typically have the shape of a cauliflower (Fig. 5.29). Engulfment of the glomus of the choroid plexus is a distinguishing feature. Choroid plexus calcification in the first decade of life is atypical and suggests the possibility of a choroid plexus papilloma. On MR, they are isointense to gray matter on T1-weighted images. These highly vascular tumors enhance markedly. Carcinomatous degeneration is suggested by heterogeneity or parenchymal invasion with white matter edema. Differential diagnoses for intraventricular masses based on age and location are provided in Tables 5.13 and 5.14.

Subarachnoid spread of either choroid plexus papilloma or choroid plexus carcinoma is possible. The prognosis of choroid plexus papillomas is quite favorable if resected before irreversible damage secondary to hydrocephalus or repeated hemorrhage has occurred. The prognosis for choroid plexus carcinoma is more guarded.

HAMARTOMA OF THE TUBER CINEREUM

An "Aunt Minnie" in neuroradiology, these rare congenital malformations of normal neuronal tissue are more common in boys who usually have precocious puberty, seizures, developmental delay, and hyperactivity. They are well-circumscribed, round or oval masses centered in the region of the tuber cinereum (at the base of the infundibulum). They do not calcify or hemorrhage. On CT and MR, they have the same signal intensity as brain tissue (possibly slightly hyperintense on T2-weighted images) and do not enhance (Fig. 5.30) (16). Along with the characteristic

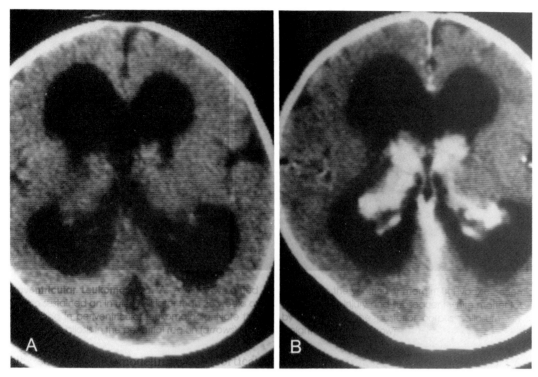

Figure 5.29.   Choroid Plexus Papilloma. Precontrast (**A**) and post-contrast (**B**) CT scans. Note the enlarged ventricles and the extremely prominent choroid plexus formation bilaterally. Hydroceph-alus results from increased production of CSF and decreased resorption secondary to proteinaceous debris and hemorrhage.

Figure 5.30.   Hamartoma of Tuber Cinereum. This lesion was found in a young adult with diabetes insipidus. Hamartomas may vary in size from 1 to 2 mm to larger lesions such as this one (arrows). Sagittal midline MR.

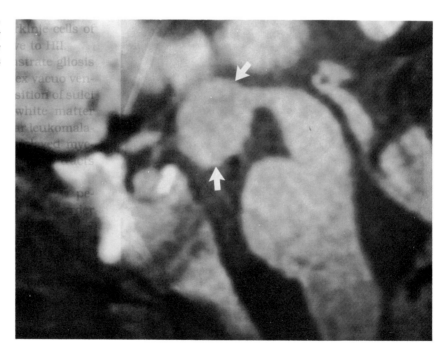

location, a stalk connecting the mass with the tuber cinereum or mamillary bodies cinches the diagnosis.

References

1. Netter FH. The CIBA collection of medical illustrations, nervous system. Summit, NJ: CIBA-Geigy Corporation, 1986: 115.
2. Mattle HP, O'Reilly GV, Edelman RR, Johnson KA. Brain: spontaneous hemorrhage. In: Edelman RR, Hesselink JR, eds. Clinical magnetic resonance imaging. Philadelphia: WB Saunders, 1990:512.
3. Hahn F, Gurney J. CT signs of central descending transtentorial herniation. AJNR 1985;6:844–845.
4. Fetell MR, Stein BM. Tumors: general considerations. In: Rowland LP, ed. Merritt's textbook of neurology. Philadelphia: Lea & Febiger, 1989:275–367.
5. George AE, Russell EJ, Kricheff II. White matter buckling: CT sign of extraaxial intracranial mass. AJNR 1980;1:425–430.
6. Kelly PJ, Daumas-Duport C, Scheithauer BW, Kall BA, Kispert DB. Stereotactic histologic correlation of CT- and MR-defined abnormalities in patients with glial neoplasms. Mayo Clin Proc 1987;62:450–459.
7. Henkelman RM, Watts JF, Kucharczyk W. High signal intensity in MR images of calcified brain tissue. Radiology 1991;179:199–206.
8. Atlas SA. Intraaxial neoplasms. In: Atlas SA, ed. Magnetic resonance imaging of the brain and spine. New York: Raven Press, 1991:223–326.
9. Sage MR. Blood-brain barrier: phenomenon of increasing importance to the imaging clinician. AJR 1982;138:887–898.
10. Valk PE, Dillon WP. Radiation injury of the brain. AJNR 1991;12:45–62.
11. Burger PC. Malignant astrocytic neoplasms: classification, pathologic anatomy, and response to therapy. Semin Oncol 1986;13:16–26.
12. Haimes AB, Zimmerman RD, Morgello S. MR imaging of brain abscess. AJNR 1989;10:279–291.
13. Russell DS, Rubenstein LJ. Pathology of tumors of the central nervous system. 5th ed. Baltimore: Williams & Wilkins, 1989.
14. Spagnoli MV, Grossman RI, Packer RJ, et al. Magnetic resonance imaging determination of gliomatosis cerebri. Neuroradiology 1987;29:15–18.
15. Lee Y-Y, Tassel PV. Intracranial oligodendrogliomas: imaging findings in 35 untreated cases. AJNR 1989;10:119–127.
16. Barkovich AJ. Pediatric neuroimaging. 1st ed. New York: Raven Press, 1990:149–203.
17. Olson EM, Tien RD, Chamberlain MC. Osseous metastasis in medulloblastoma: MRI findings in an unusual case. Clin Imaging 1991;15:286–289.
18. Davis PC, Wichman RD, Takei Y, Hoffman JCJ. Primary cerebral neuroblastoma: CT and MR findings in 12 cases. AJNR 1990;11:115–120.
19. Buetow PC, Smirniotopoulos JG, Done S. Congenital brain tumors: a review of 45 cases. AJNR 1990;11:793–799.
20. Hochberg FH, Miller DC. Primary central nervous system lymphoma. J Neurosurg 1988;68:835–853.
21. So YT, Beckstead JH, Davis RL. Primary central nervous system lymphoma in acquired immune deficiency syndrome: a clinical and pathological study. Ann Neurol 1986;20:566–572.
22. Dina TS. Primary central nervous lymphoma versus toxoplasmosis in AIDS. Radiology 1991;179:823–828.
23. Sze G, Milano E, Johnson C, Heier L. Detection of brain metastasis: comparison of contrast-enhanced MR with unenhanced MR and enhanced CT. AJNR 1990;11:785–791.
24. Davis PC, Hudgins PA, Peterman SB, Hoffman JC Jr. Diagnosis of cerebral metastasis: double-dose delayed CT vs contrast-enhanced MR imaging. AJNR 1991;12:293–300.
25. Yuh WTC, Engelken JD, Muhonen MG, Mayr NA, Fisher DJ, Ehrhardt JC. Experience with high-dose MR imaging in the evaluation of brain metastasis. AJNR 1992;13:335–345.
26. Goldberg HI. Extraaxial brain tumors. In: Atlas SA, ed. Magnetic resonance imaging of the brain and spine. New York: Raven Press, 1991:327–378.
27. Koeller KK, Dillon WP. Dysembryoplastic neuroepithelial tumors: MR appearance. AJNR 1992:13:1319–1325.
28. Castillo M, Davis PC, Takei Y, Hoffman JCJ. Intracranial ganglioglioma: MR, CT, and clinical findings in 18 patients. AJNR 1990;11:109–114.
29. Juhl JH. Paul and Juhl's essentials of Roentgen interpretation. 4th ed. Philadelphia: Harper & Row, 1981:359.
30. Lee DH, Norman D, Newton TH. MR imaging of pineal cysts. J Comput Assist Tomogr 1987;11:586–590.
31. Edwards MSB, Hudgins RJ, Wilson CB, Levin VA, Wara WM. Pineal region tumors in children. J Neurosurg 1988;68:689–697.
32. Ganti SR, Hilal SK, Stein BM, Silver AJ, Mawad M, Sane P. CT of pineal region tumors. AJR 1986;146:451–458.
33. Goldsher D, Litt AW, Pinto RS, Bannon KR, Kricheff II. Dural "tail" associated with meningiomas on Gd-DTPA-enhanced MR images: characteristics, differential diagnostic value, and possible implications for treatment. Radiology 1990;176:447–450.
34. Tokumaru A, O'uchi T, Eguchi T, et al. Prominent meningeal enhancement adjacent to meningioma on Gd-DTPA-enhanced MR images: histopathologic correlation. Radiology 1990;175:431–433.
35. Lee SR, Sanches J, Mark AS, Dillon WP, Norman D, Newton TH. Posterior fossa hemangioblastomas: MR imaging. Radiology 1989;171:463–468.
36. Gao P-Y, Osborn AG, Smirniotopoulos JG, Harris CP. Epidermoid tumor of the cerebellopontine angle. AJNR 1992;13:863–872.
37. Waggenspack GA, Guinto FCJ. MR and CT of masses of the anterosuperior third ventricle. AJNR 1989;10:105–110.
38. Coates TL, Hinshaw DB, Peckman N, et al. Pediatric choroid plexus neoplasms: MR, CT, and pathologic correlation. Radiology 1989;173:81–88.

6

Central Nervous System Infection

Walter L. Olson

Central nervous system (CNS) infections commonly require evaluation by radiologists. Because these infections often have dire neurologic consequences, early diagnosis and management is crucial. Computed tomography (CT) and magnetic resonance imaging (MR) have significantly aided this effort. For example, prior to CT, pyogenic abscesses of the brain carried a 30–70% mortality rate. The mortality rate has dropped to less than 5% in recent years, largely because of the ability of CT to accurately diagnose the abscess and monitor the efficacy of treatment. Magnetic resonance imaging is playing an increasing role in the evaluation of CNS infection, because of improved sensitivity for detecting early infections. However, since CT and MR are highly accurate, the choice of modality often depends on the clinical situation. Gravely ill patients are usually better evaluated by CT, which is faster, less susceptible to patient motion artifact, and permits closer patient monitoring. Magnetic resonance imaging is generally preferable in the clinically stable patient.

PARENCHYMAL INFECTIONS

Pyogenic Cerebritis and Abscess

Pyogenic infections of the brain may develop by direct extension following trauma, surgery, sinusitis, dental infections, or otomastoiditis. Hematogenous infections may also occur, especially in patients with lung infections, endocarditis, or congenital heart dis-ease. Anaerobic bacteria are the most common organisms overall. *Staphylococcus aureus* infection is common after surgery or trauma. Gram-negative rod, pneumococcal, streptococcal, nocardial, and actinomycetic infections also occur with some frequency. The frontal and parietal lobes are most affected, especially in patients with sinus infections and hematogenous spread. The temporal lobe or cerebellum are involved in patients with spread from otomastoiditis.

Clinical symptoms in patients with pyogenic brain infections may be mild or severe. Usually there is headache. There may be varying degrees of lethargy, nausea, vomiting, and fever. Fever is absent in more than 50% of the cases. Meningeal signs are present in only 30% of patients. Focal neurologic deficits, papilledema, nuchal rigidity, and seizures often develop rapidly, over the course of a few days, in distinction to tumors. There is often, but not invariably, an elevated white blood count. Cerebrospinal fluid (CSF) findings are often nonspecific and are usually not obtained because of the risk of lumbar puncture in the setting of a brain mass.

Pathologically, there are four stages of evolution of a brain abscess, which correlate with the imaging findings.

Early cerebritis. Within the first few days of infection, the infected portion of brain is swollen and edematous. Areas of necrosis are filled with polymorphonuclear leukocytes, lymphocytes, and plasma cells. Organisms are present in both the center and periphery of the lesion, which has ill-defined margins. Computed tomography scans may be normal, or show an area of low density. There may be mild mass effect and patchy areas of enhancement within the lesion. On MR the lesion shows increased signal on proton density and T2-weighted images, with low or isointensity on T1-weighted images. Published experience with contrast enhancement on MR scans in the early cerebritis stage is limited, but patchy enhancement similar to that seen with CT is to be expected. A ring of enhancement is not present at this stage, distinguishing it from the later three stages. Unfortunately, these imaging features are nonspecific and can be seen with tumors or infarcts. The clinical features are therefore most important in

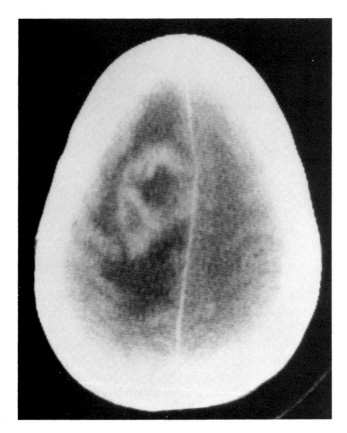

Figure 6.1. Cerebritis. This contrast-enhanced CT scan demonstrates irregular enhancement peripherally and low density centrally. There is surrounding low-density vasogenic edema. This is typical of the late cerebritis stage of pyogenic infection.

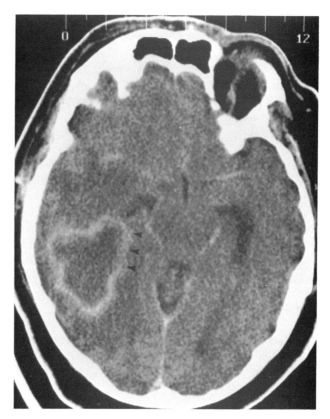

Figure 6.2. Pyogenic Cerebral Abscess. There is thin, smooth, well-defined contrast enhancement in the capsule of this right temporal lobe abscess imaged with CT. The enhancement is thinnest medially, (*arrowheads*) which is typical of pyogenic abscesses. This patient had a dental infection and developed a headache that progressed to lethargy, weakness, and coma within a few days. Surgery revealed an actinomycotic abscess.

making the correct diagnosis. If the diagnosis can be made at this stage, nonsurgical treatment with antibiotics is often effective.

Late Cerebritis stage occurs within 1 or 2 weeks of infection. Central necrosis is increased with fewer organisms detected pathologically. There is vascular proliferation at the periphery of the lesion with more inflammatory cells, which represents the brain's effort to contain the infection. Not surprisingly, this results in thick, irregular contrast enhancement at the edges of the lesion on imaging studies (Fig. 6.1). Vasogenic edema is seen outside the enhancing rim at this stage as well. Delayed scans may show central filling in with contrast. No discrete low-signal capsule is evident on T2-weighted MR imaging, in distinction to some mature abscesses. This stage can also be treated effectively with antibiotic therapy, but distinguishing late cerebritis from an early abscess or tumor can be difficult, and surgery is often performed.

Early Capsule. With time, the infection is walled off as a capsule of collagen and reticulin forms in the inflammatory, vascular margin of the infection. Macrophages, phagocytes, and neutrophils are also present in the capsule. The necrotic center contains very few organisms. This is the early capsule stage of

brain abscess formation. Contrast-enhanced CT and MR scans show a well-defined rim of enhancement (Fig. 6.2). The rim tends to be low in signal on T2-weighted MR. Centrally there is necrosis (low density on CT, low signal on T1-weighted MR, high signal on intermediate and T2-weighted MR). There is prominent surrounding vasogenic edema.

Late Capsule. In the late capsule stage, the rim of enhancement becomes even more well defined and thin, reflecting more complete collagen in the abscess wall (Fig. 6.3). Multiloculation is common. The capsule often exhibits characteristic MR features that are helpful diagnostically at this stage. On T1-weighted images, the capsule is usually iso- or hyperintense to white matter, and on T2-weighted images it is usually hypointense to white matter (Fig. 6.4). These signal characteristics suggest paramagnetic T1 and T2 shortening, similar to that seen in hematoma evolution (see Chapter 4). However, hemorrhage is not often found pathologically, and the paramagnetic effects may be secondary to the presence of free radicals produced by macrophages in the capsule. In any case, the MR appearance of the capsule is fairly specific for ab-

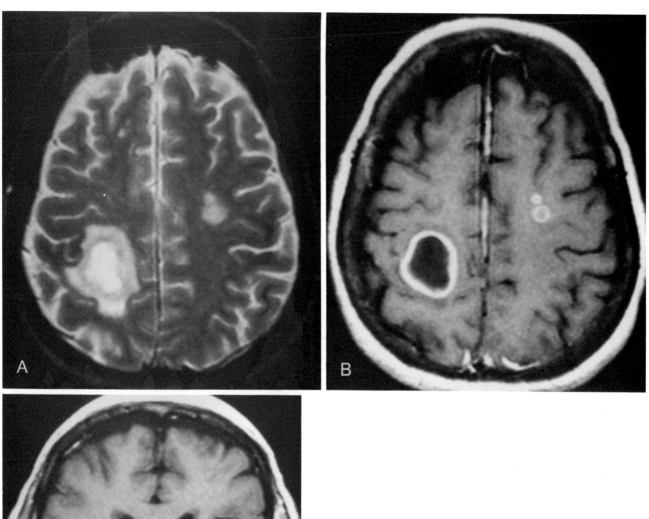

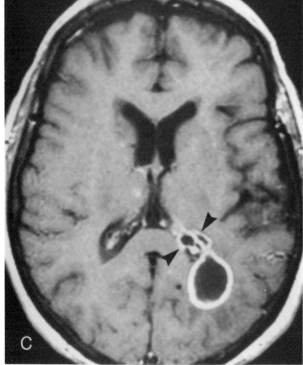

Figure 6.3. Multiple Pyogenic Abscesses. A. A T2-weighted MR scan reveals a right parietal mass lesion with high-signal intensity centrally and low-signal intensity peripherally within the capsule. There is surrounding high-signal intensity edema. Two smaller high-signal lesions are present on the left. **B.** A gadolinium-enhanced T1-weighted MR scan shows thin, smooth enhancement of all three lesions. **C.** More inferiorly the contrast-enhanced T1-weighted scan reveals a fourth abscess that has extended into the atrium of the left lateral ventricle (*arrowheads*). The enhancement pattern and intraventricular extension favor the diagnosis of abscess over tumor. These lesions proved to be abscesses that cultured anaerobic streptococcus. (Case courtesy of Dr. Vincent Burke, Atherton, California.)

scesses, as capsules are unusual in tumors. The medial aspect of the enhancing capsule is often (about 50% of the time) thinner than the lateral aspect (Figs. 6.2 and 6.3). This reflects decreased blood supply and fibroblast migration centrally compared with cortically; recall that the blood supply at the gray-white junction runs superficial to deep. This thin medial rim predisposes to intraventricular rupture with resulting ventriculitis (Figs. 6.3 and 6.4). Rupture leads to ependymitis, seen as enhancement of the lining of the ventricle, and sometimes abnormal density/signal intensity of the CSF.

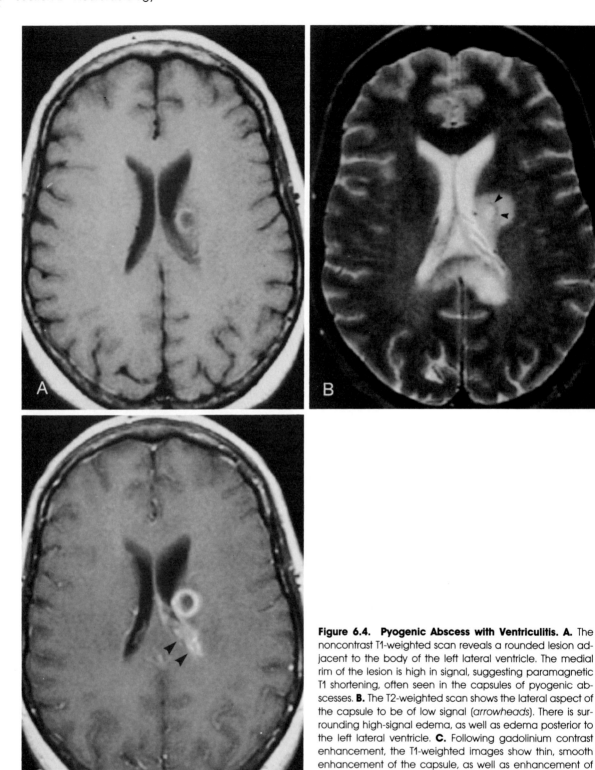

Figure 6.4. Pyogenic Abscess with Ventriculitis. A. The noncontrast T1-weighted scan reveals a rounded lesion adjacent to the body of the left lateral ventricle. The medial rim of the lesion is high in signal, suggesting paramagnetic T1 shortening, often seen in the capsules of pyogenic abscesses. **B.** The T2-weighted scan shows the lateral aspect of the capsule to be of low signal (*arrowheads*). There is surrounding high-signal edema, as well as edema posterior to the left lateral ventricle. **C.** Following gadolinium contrast enhancement, the T1-weighted images show thin, smooth enhancement of the capsule, as well as enhancement of the ependyma of the left lateral ventricle (*arrowheads*), indicating intraventricular extension and ventriculitis.

The principal differential diagnosis of pyogenic abscess includes tumor-resolving hematoma and atypical infarcts. The clinical features, combined with the appearance of a thin enhancing rim, thinnest medially, much edema, and paramagnetic effects in the capsule (with no blood products centrally) should strongly suggest a brain abscess. Multiple loculations and/or enhancement of the ependyma, if present, should clinch the diagnosis.

Septic Embolus. Infections that begin with a septic embolus may not have the typical appearance of an abscess. The embolus frequently causes an infarct that dominates the imaging findings. Depending on the size of the embolus, there may be a small, rounded area of enhancement or a larger wedge-shaped cortical infarct. As with other embolic infarcts, hemorrhage may occur. Because of the nonviable, infarcted tissue with a poor blood supply, a typical capsule may not form. A thicker, more irregular ring of enhancement that persists within an area of infarction should suggest the diagnosis.

A solitary abscess is usually treated surgically. If the abscess is in a critical area of the brain, a sterotactic needle aspiration is performed to provide culture material to determine antibiotic therapy. If there is significant mass effect, or if the lesion is in a relatively "safe" area, a formal drainage or resection is performed. If there are multiple abscesses, or if the patient is at high surgical risk, antibiotic therapy alone is used. Imaging studies should be performed frequently (about once a week) to monitor the efficacy of treatment and to assess for complications such as ventriculitis, infarction, or hydrocephalus.

Mycobacterial Infections

The most common form of CNS mycobacterial infection is tuberculous meningitis, which will be discussed later in this chapter. Focal mycobacterial infection of the brain occurs in two forms: tuberculoma and abscess.

Tuberculoma. In the early 1900s one-third of all brain mass lesions in England were tuberculomas. Because of improved prevention and treatment, these lesions are now unusual in developed countries. In developing areas of the world, however, tuberculomas account for up to 15–30% of brain masses. There is a predilection for the extremes of age—children and the elderly. The infection spreads to the brain hematogenously from the lungs. In developed countries tuberculomas usually result from reactivation of quiescent disease, although only 50% of patients have a known history of previous tuberculosis. Most lesions in adults are supratentorial, involving the frontal or parietal lobes. Sixty percent of tuberculomas in children are in the posterior fossa, usually the cerebellum. Multiple lesions are common. Most tuberculomas are not associated with tuberculous meningitis. Clinical features include headache, seizures, papilledema, and focal neurologic signs. Fever is seen only rarely. The CSF is almost always abnormal, showing elevated protein and reduced glucose. An abnormal chest x-ray is present in up to 50% of patients. These lesions can be treated medically if there are characteristic clinical and imaging features. Surgery is often performed when the diagnosis is in doubt, for medical treatment failures, and for large lesions.

Noncontrast CT scans show one or more iso- or slightly hyperdense mass lesions. Multiple lesions are present about 50% of the time. Thick rim enhancement is common postcontrast (Fig. 6.5**A**). The center of the tuberculoma is usually more dense than the fluid-like center of a pyogenic abscess, because of caseous necrosis. Smaller lesions may show a solid enhancement pattern. A "target" appearance with a central zone of enhancement or central calcification surrounded by rim enhancement is an uncommon but helpful finding, strongly suggesting the diagnosis. Calcification is present in less than 5% of cases at the initial diagnosis, but is commonly seen with treatment as the lesions resolve. Surrounding edema is usually present. On MR, tuberculomas usually have a low signal rim, reflecting the fibrous wall, which enhances markedly. Centrally there is a proteinaceous fluid-type signal. Smaller lesions, or those containing calcifications, may be entirely low in signal, especially on T2-weighted images (Fig. 6.5**B**). Surrounding edema is usually better seen with MR than with CT scans. Paramagnetic effects (increased signal on T1-weighting and marked decrease in signal on T2-weighting) in the tuberculoma wall, similar to that seen in pyogenic abscesses, have not yet been described. The differential diagnosis includes tumor, pyogenic abscess, fungal and parasitic infections, and sarcoidosis.

Tuberculous Abscess is a rare complication, seen primarily in immunocompromised patients. Abnormal T-cell function prevents the normal host response of tuberculoma formation with caseous necrosis. Symptoms develop more rapidly than with tuberculomas. The imaging features are similar to that seen with pyogenic abscesses. Atypical mycobacterial infections are also more common in immunocompromised patients.

Fungal Infections

Fungal infections of the CNS can be grouped into endemic and cosmopolitan categories. Endemic fungal infections are geographically restricted. They can occur in immunocompetent and immunosuppressed patients. Cosmopolitan fungal infections occur worldwide, usually in immunosuppressed patients, infants, the elderly, or chronically ill, with the exception of cryptococcosis, which also occurs in patients with normal immunity.

The most common endemic fungal infections in the United States are coccidioidomycosis, North American blastomycosis, and histoplasmosis. These infections usually manifest as granulomatous meningitis, as will be discussed. Focal parenchymal lesions are unusual. Central nervous system involvement is a manifestation of disseminated infection, with hematogenous spread, usually from pulmonary disease.

Coccidioidomycosis occurs in the southwestern United States. Most infected patients are asympto-

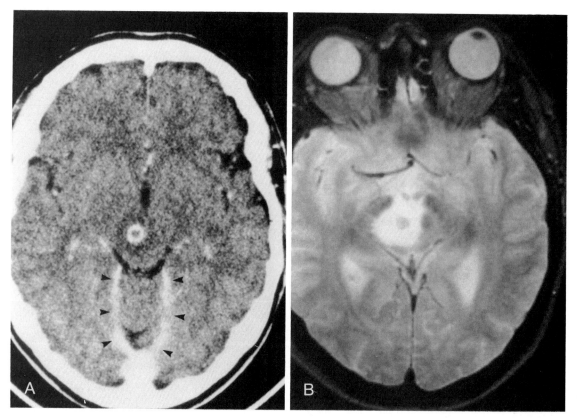

Figure 6.5.   Midbrain Tuberculoma. A. The contrast-enhanced CT scan shows a ring-enhancing lesion in the right side of the midbrain with surrounding low-density edema. Most tuberculomas this size are solid or show thick rim enhancement. Thick enhancement of the tentorial edges is due to tuberculous meningitis (*arrowheads*), helping to distinguish this lesion from a pyogenic abscess. However, meningitis is often absent in patients with tuberculoma. **B.** The T2-weighted MR scan shows that the lesion is in the right red nucleus. The high-signal edema is more apparent than on the CT scan, reflecting the increased sensitivity of MR in detecting alterations in brain water content.

matic or have mild respiratory symptoms. Less than 1% of patients develop disseminated infection and meningitis. Focal parenchymal granulomas are rare.

Blastomycosis occurs in the Ohio and Mississippi River valleys. Central nervous system involvement occurs in 6–33% of disseminated cases. Meningitis is the most frequent presentation, but parenchymal abscesses and granulomas occur more frequently than with coccidioidomycosis. Epidural granulomas and abscesses also occur in the head and spine, usually from direct extension from bone infection. Up to 40% of focal brain lesions are multiple.

Histoplasmosis is usually a benign, asymptomatic infection, occurring in the midwest and southern United States. Dissemination is unusual and only a small percent of disseminated cases involve the CNS. Meningitis is most common, but multiple or solitary granulomas may occur. Abscesses are unusual. As seen on CT or MR, most fungal granulomas are small and show solid or thick rim enhancement (Fig. 6.6). Fungal abscesses, as seen with blastomycosis, have a similar appearance as pyogenic abscesses already described. Meningeal enhancement from men-

ingitis is a common accompanying feature. Hydrocephalus is also common, especially with coccidioidomycosis.

The most common cosmopolitan fungal infections are cryptococcosis, aspergillosis, mucormycosis and candidiasis. These infections also usually present as meningitis, but focal parenchymal lesions are fairly common.

Aspergillosis involves the CNS in 60–70% of patients with disseminated disease. The infection may arise from hematogenous spread or by direct extension from an infected paranasal sinus. Parenchymal disease usually takes the form of an abscess; granulomas are unusual. Infarcts or hemorrhage from blood vessel invasion may occur, but are less common than in mucormycosis, which is highly angioinvasive.

Mucormycosis.   *Mucor* invades the brain usually by direct extension from the sinuses, nose, or oral cavity, but hematogenous spread also occurs. Almost all patients are diabetic or otherwise immunocompromised. The mortality rate in treated diabetic patients is 65–75%, and worse in immunocompromised patients.

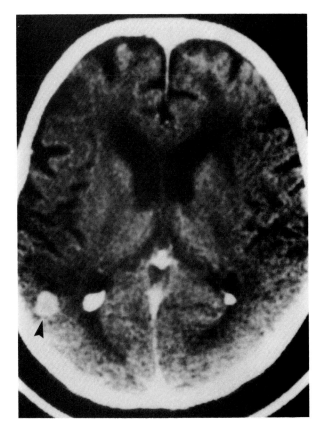

Figure 6.6. Histoplasmosis Granuloma. This patient had disseminated histoplasmosis with several lesions in the brain and spine. This contrast-enhanced CT scan shows a solidly enhancing lesion near the atrium of the right lateral ventricle (*arrowhead*). Most fungal granulomas are small and show either solid or thick rim enhancement. (Case courtesy of Dr. J.R. Jinkins, San Antonio, Texas.)

Candidiasis usually causes meningitis, but granulomas and small abscesses may occur. Spread to the CNS is usually hematogenous.

Imaging studies in patients with CNS aspergillosis or mucormycosis will reveal single or multiple mass lesions with varying degrees of peripheral enhancement. The amount of enhancement depends on the compromised host's ability to fight the infection. Surrounding edema is variable in amount. Smaller lesions will show a solid enhancement pattern. The lesions are often in the base of the brain adjacent to diseased sinuses. Infarcts, intra- or extraaxial hemorrhage, and meningeal enhancement can be seen with CT or MR if T2*-weighted gradient-echo techniques and T1-weighted sequences before and after gadolinium enhancement are used. A lesion with peripheral enhancement, cortical sparing, and a nonvascular distribution is more likely to be an abscess than an infarct, but it is often difficult to distinguish the two. In cases of CNS candidiasis, meningeal enhancement or multiple small enhancing microabscesses are seen.

Cryptococcosis is the most frequently reported CNS fungal infection. It occurs in patients with normal immune function in about 50% of cases. This is also an extremely common infection in patients with acquired immunodeficiency diseases (AIDS) as will be discussed later. Infection of the CNS occurs via hematogenous spread from the lungs. Serologies and CSF studies are valuable in making the diagnosis: about 90% of patients have antigen in the CSF and/or antibody in the serum. The usual manifestation is meningitis. Granulomas can occur and are usually multiple; abscesses are less common. A recently reported characteristic cryptococcal lesion is the gelatinous pseudocyst. This is a cystic lesion, usually in the basal ganglia, representing enlarged Virchow-Robin spaces filled with the organism. These lesions are usually found only in immunocompromised patients (see Fig. 6.27). Computed tomography scans in patients with cryptococcosis are usually normal, reflecting relatively mild meningeal involvement in most cases. Mass lesions are seen in about 10% of cases. Cryptococcomas are shown as small, usually multiple, solid enhancing, peripheral parenchymal nodules. Calcifications within a granuloma are occasionally seen. Gelatinous pseudocysts are smooth, round, low-density masses in the basal ganglia that show no contrast enhancement. With the improved sensitivity of MR, meningeal and parenchymal lesions are seen more frequently than with CT. Leptomeningeal nodules are often only seen on T1-weighted, contrast-enhanced MR as multiple tiny enhancing lesions near the basal cisterns and sulci. Diffuse meningeal enhancement is unusual. Granulomas may show either solid or ring enhancement. Gelatinous pseudocysts and dilated Virchow-Robin spaces are better seen with MR than with CT. These are nearly isointense with CSF on all sequences and do not enhance.

Parasitic Infections

Parasitic infections are common throughout much of the third world, but are relatively uncommon in the industrialized nations. The most common infections likely to be encountered in the United States are cysticercosis, echinococcosis, toxoplasmosis, and rarely amebiasis. Central nervous system involvement in malaria, trypanosomiasis, paragonimiasis, sparganosis and schistosomiasis are rarely encountered in the United States and will not be discussed.

Cysticercosis is caused by the larvae of the pork tapeworm, *Taenia solium*. Infestation occurs via the fecal-oral route. The eggs are shed by humans, the definitive host, and then ingested by the intermediate host, pigs or humans. The life cycle can be completed in the pig, but not in humans. The eggs form oncospheres (primary larvae) that hatch in the intestine and are hematogenously distributed throughout the body and form cysticerci (secondary larvae). The cysticerci cannot develop further in humans and eventu-

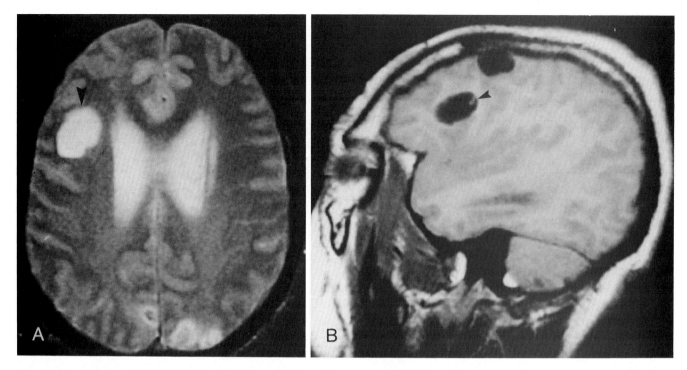

Figure 6.7.   Cysticercosis. A. T2-weighted MR shows a right frontal lesion isointense with CSF (*arrowhead*). There is no surrounding edema, indicating that this is early in the course of the disease. Three smaller lesions are present posteriorly. **B.** The T1-weighted parasagittal image in the same patient shows two cysticercal cysts that are isointense with CSF. A scolex is visible in one of the cysts (*arrowhead*).

ally die. The cysticerci that reach the CNS may infest the parenchyma, meninges, ventricles, or spine. This disease is fairly frequently encountered in the southwestern United States in Latin American immigrants. Seizures occur in over 90% of patients. Cysticercosis is the most common cause of seizures in Latin America. Encephalitic symptoms are also common. Treatment is with the drug praziquantel.

Parenchymal cysticercosis is the most common type. Early in the infestation the viable cysts appear as small (usually 1 cm or less), solitary or multiple rounded lesions that are low density on CT and isointense to CSF on MR (Fig. 6.7). The lesions are usually peripherally distributed near the gray-white junction or in the gray matter. A small marginal nodule representing the scolex is sometimes seen (Figs. 6.7**B** and 6.8). There is usually no enhancement or edema at this stage. When the cyst dies, the fluid within it leaks into the surrounding brain, causing inflammation. This produces clinical symptoms of an acute encephalitis, which may be severe, depending on the number of lesions. Imaging studies now reveal ring-enhancing lesions with surrounding edema (Fig. 6.8). The cyst fluid is of increased density on CT and increased signal compared with CSF on T1- and T2-weighted MR. As the dead cyst degenerates, it becomes smaller, showing nodular enhancement, and then calcifies. Computed tomography scans at this late stage show small, peripheral calcifications, with

no edema or enhancement (Fig. 6.9). With MR, the calcifications are best seen on T2-weighted or T2*-weighted gradient-echo images, but are better demonstrated by CT than MR.

Intraventricular cysticercosis is similar to the parenchymal variety in pathogenesis and appearance (Fig. 6.10). The cysts are usually isodense and isointense to CSF, making them difficult to visualize. Magnetic resonance imaging is superior to CT for imaging, as subtle signal changes and lack of CSF pulsations within the cyst makes them more visble. Enhancement may or may not be present, depending on the stage, similar to the parenchymal form. The cysts may obstruct the foramen of Monro, the third ventricle, or aqueduct, resulting in hydrocephalus. If acute hydrocephalus occurs, death may rapidly ensue. Ventriculitis occurs if the cyst ruptures.

Meningeal infestation is known as meningobasal (since the basal cisterns are most frequently involved) or racemose cysticercosis (Latin for "clusters"). The cysts lack a scolex but may grow by proliferation of the cyst wall. The cysts may grow in grape-like clusters (Fig. 6.11) or conform to the shape of the cistern. No mural nodules or calcifications are seen. Computed tomography scans show CSF density cysts in the basal cisterns. Magnetic resonance imaging reveals cysts that are isointense with CSF, often with mural enhancement or diffuse meningeal enhancement. Hydrocephalus is commonly observed.

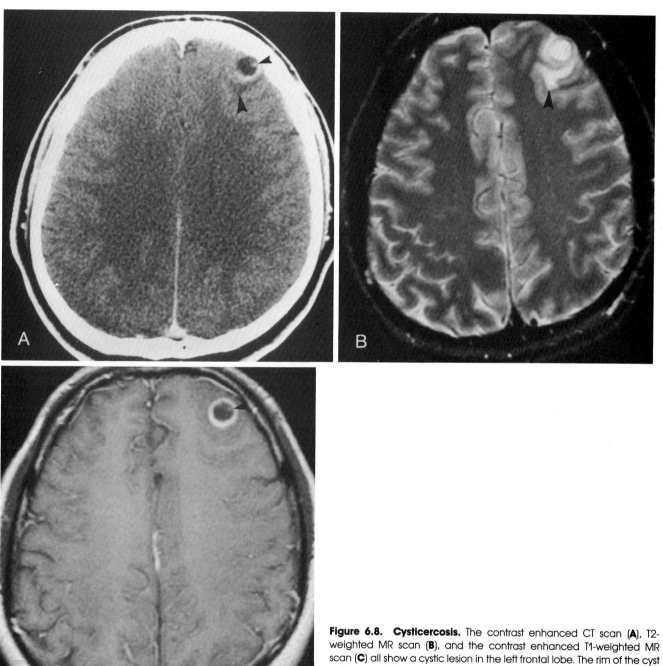

Figure 6.8.   Cysticercosis. The contrast enhanced CT scan (**A**), T2-weighted MR scan (**B**), and the contrast enhanced T1-weighted MR scan (**C**) all show a cystic lesion in the left frontal lobe. The rim of the cyst enhances with contrast and there is surrounding edema (*large arrowheads*) indicating that the cyst has died and that fluid has leaked out, inciting an inflammatory response. The scolex is visible (*small arrowheads*).

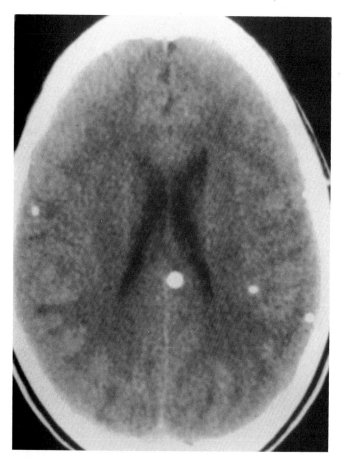

Figure 6.9. Late-stage Cysticercosis. This unenhanced CT scan shows multiple calcifications in the gray matter and gray-white junction, typical of late stage cysticercosis.

Spinal cysticercosis is usually intradural, but can be either intra-or extramedullary. Intramedullary lesions are best seen with MR as solid or ring-enhancing cord lesions similar to that seen in the brain parenchyma. Extramedullary cysts are analogous to the racemose form and are also best evaluated with MR.

Echinococcosis, also known as hydatid disease, occurs in South America, Africa, Central Europe, the Middle East, and rarely in the southwestern United States. The etiologic agent is the dog tapeworm and man is an intermediate host. Hydatid cysts are more frequently present in the lung and liver, but the brain is involved in 1–4% of cases. The cysts are usually solitary, unilocular, large, round, and smoothly marginated. They are most often supratentorial, in the middle cerebral artery territory. There may rarely be mural calcification. With CT the fluid within the cyst is usually isodense with CSF. There is usually no surrounding edema or abnormal contrast enhancement, unless the cyst has ruptured, leading to an inflammatory reaction. A report of a typical hydatid cyst imaged with MR showed a large, smooth spherical cyst with fluid isointense to CSF on T1-and T2-weighted images. There was no edema, but contrast was not administered. A recent case report of a pontine hyatid cyst showed fluid nearly isointense to CSF on the T1-weighted images but hyperintense to CSF on T2-weighted images. There was mild edema and contrast enhancement in the posterior aspect of the wall of the cyst.

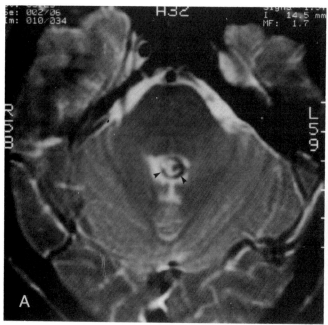

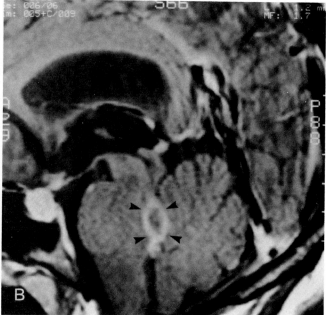

Figure 6.10. Intraventricular Cysticercosis. A. The T2-weighted MR scan shows a rounded lesion with a low-signal rim (*small arrowheads*) in the fourth ventricle. A low-signal scolex is seen in the left side of the cyst. **B.** The contrast-enhanced T1-weighted sagittal scan shows enhancement of the cyst and ependyma of the fourth ventricle, from rupture of the cyst (*large arrowheads*).

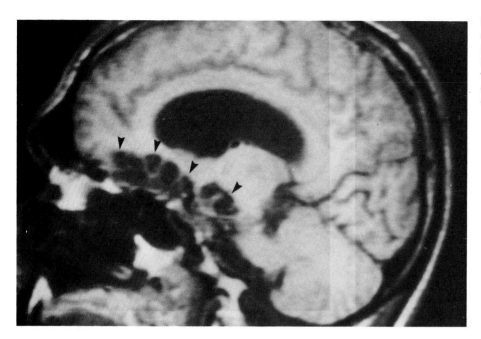

Figure 6.11. Subarachnoid (Racemose) Cysticercosis. There are multiple cysts in a grape-like cluster in the basal cisterns on this parasagittal T1-weighted scan (*arrowheads*). These cysts lack a scolex, but grow by proliferation of the cyst wall.

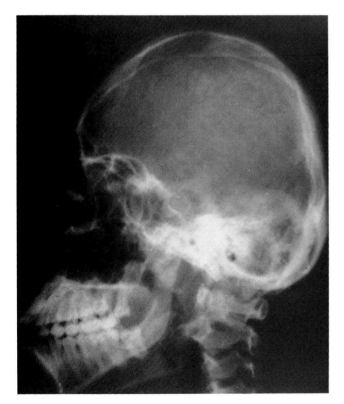

Figure 6.12. Microcephaly. A lateral skull film shows a small cranial vault, as can be seen in congenital toxoplasmosis or other TORCH (Toxoplasmosis; Other, which includes syphilis, Rubella, Cytomegalovirus, and Herpes) infections.

Toxoplasmosis is caused by the protozoa *Toxoplasma gondii*, which occurs worldwide. The disease may be either congenital or acquired. The acquired form is seen primarily in immunocompromised patients and is very common with AIDS. The congenital form results when the mother eats poorly cooked meat or is infected from a cat during pregnancy. A diffuse encephalitis of the fetal brain ensues, usually causing severe destruction. The infant is usually born with microcephaly (Fig. 6.12), chorioretinitis and mental retardation. Imaging studies reveal atrophy, dilated ventricles, and calcifications. The calcifications occur in the periventricular white matter, basal ganglia and cerebral hemispheres. This is in distinction to congenital cytomegalovirus (CMV) in which the calcifications are usually periventricular only.

Amebic Meningoencephalitis is sometimes seen in the southern United States. The amebae enter the nasal cavity of patients swimming in infested freshwater ponds or pools. There is direct extension through the cribiform plate to the brain. A severe meningoencephalitis results, which is usually fatal. Imaging studies often underestimate the severity of the disease. Early in the infection there may be meningeal and/or gray matter enhancement. Later there is diffuse white matter edema. There are a few reports of single or multiple, ring or solid enhancing lesions with surrounding edema in patients with amebic brain abscesses.

Spirochete Infections

Neurosyphilis develops in about 5% of patients with syphilis who are not treated for the primary infection. Involvement of the CNS occurs in the tertiary stage of the disease. Because of effective antibiotic therapy, neurosyphilis is rare. However, there has been a significant increase in incidence since the AIDS epidemic. Patients with neurosyphilis are usually asymptomatic. Symptomatic patients may have an aseptic meningitis, tabes dorsalis, general paresis, or meningovascular disease. Imaging studies are usu-

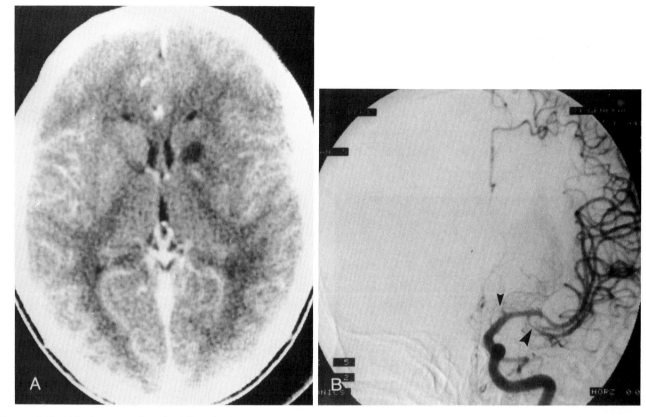

Figure 6.13. Meningovascular Syphilis. A. The contrast-enhanced CT scan reveals a small infarct in the left striate nucleus in this 21-year-old patient with meningovascular syphilis. **B.** A left internal carotid arteriogram in the frontal projection on another patient with meningovascular syphilis shows occlusion of the left anterior cerebral artery (*small arrowhead*) and narrowing of branches of the left middle cerebral artery (*large arrowhead*). Both patients improved with penicillin therapy.

ally normal in patients with tabes dorsalis, but rarely gummas are found. These usually appear as small enhancing nodules. Meningovascular syphilis presents as an acute stroke syndrome or a subacute illness with a variety of symptoms. Pathologically there is thickening of the meninges and an arteritis. Imaging studies reveal small infarcts of the basal ganglia, white matter, cerebral cortex, or cerebellum (Fig. 6.13**A**) The infarcts may exhibit patchy or gyriform enhancement, best seen with MR. Meningeal enhancement is unusual, but cranial nerve enhancement in patients with syphilitic cranial neuritis has been described. Angiography in patients with meningovascular neurosyphilis reveals multiple segmental constrictions and/or occlusions of large and medium-sized arteries, including the distal internal carotid, anterior cerebral, middle cerebral, posterior cerebral, and distal basilar arteries (Fig. 6.13**B**)

Lyme Disease is a multisystem spirochetal infection caused by *Borrelia burgdorferi*. It is found worldwide in deer, mice, raccoons, and birds. It is spread to humans via ticks, especially the deer tick. The disease occurs most frequently on the east coast, but midwestern and west coast cases also are reported. The disease begins as a flu-like illness, with a rash and an expanding skin lesion at the tick bite site. In a small

percentage of patients, cardiac, arthritic, or neurologic symptoms develop. Neurologic abnormalities are found in 10–15% of patients. A variety of symptoms, including peripheral neuropathies, radiculopathies, myelopathies, encephalitis, meningitis, pain syndromes, cognitive disorders, and movement disorders have been reported. Treatment with antibiotics and corticosteroids may have variable results. Magnetic resonance imaging is the modality of choice for imaging these patients. Magnetic resonance scans show multiple small white matter lesions similar to that seen with multiple sclerosis. The lesions can be found in the supra- and infratentorial white matter tracts. The lesions often enhance with contrast, in a nodular or ring pattern, depending on the size. There may be meningeal enhancement. The differential diagnosis includes multiple sclerosis and other demyelinating processes.

Viral Infections

The most common viral infections of the CNS include CMV, herpes simplex, varicella-zoster, and the human immunodeficiency virus. Rubella was once a devastating fetal viral infection, but is now uncommon because of widespread immunization.

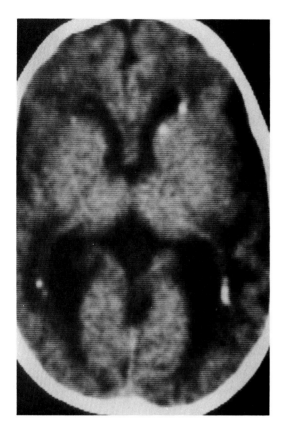

Figure 6.14. Congenital Cytomegalovirus Infection. A noncontrast CT scan shows multiple periventricular high-density calcifications and low-density areas of encephalomalacia. The calcifications in congenital CMV infection tend to be periventricular only, as in this case. With congenital toxoplasmosis, calcifications may be found throughout the brain.

Cytomegalovirus is a DNA virus in the herpesvirus family. It causes symptomatic CNS disease primarily through congenital transmission. A maternal CMV infection results in transplacental transmission to the fetus in 30–50% of cases and symptomatic disease in 5%. Symptomatic neonates may have hepatosplenomegaly, jaundice, cerebral involvement (psychomotor retardation), chorioretinitis and deafness. Mental retardation and deafness are present in 20% of cases. Infection in the first trimester results in necrosis in the germinal matrix, which may lead to migrational anomalies or calcification. The most common finding with CT scanning is periventricular calcification (Fig. 6.14). There are usually no basal ganglia or cortical calcifications as are seen in congenital toxoplasmosis. Parenchymal atrophy and ventriculomegaly are common. The disease has been diagnosed in utero with obstetrical sonography. Periventricular hyperechoic calcifications, preceded by hypoechoic periventricular ring-like zones, are characteristic findings. Hydranencephaly may also be seen. Magnetic resonance imaging is reported to show delayed or abnormal myelination in most cases. Paraventricular cystic lesions adjacent to the occipital horns of the lateral ventricles,

and oligo- or pachygyria, have also been reported on MR scans of patients with congenital CMV infection. Magnetic resonance imaging is less sensitive than CT in showing the periventricular calcifications.

Herpes simplex encephalitis occurs most frequently in neonates. The infant is usually infected during descent through the birth canal when the mother has genital (type II) herpes. Occasionally there is transplacental transmission before delivery, but this usually results in spontaneous abortion. The infection causes a severe encephalitis, which is either fatal or has severe neurologic consequences. The patient usually presents with seizures in the 2nd to 4th week. If the patient survives, varying degrees of microcephaly, mental retardation, microphthalmia, enlarged ventricles, intracranial calcifications, and multicystic encephalomalacia may occur. Early in the course of the encephalitis, CT scans may reveal bilateral patchy areas of decreased density in the cerebral white matter and cortex, with relative sparing of the basal ganglia, thalami, and posterior fossa structures (Fig. 6.15**A**). This progresses to areas of necrosis, which are sometimes hemorrhagic and may eventually calcify. Multicystic encephalomalacia is the end result. Increased density in the cortical gray matter is characteristic in this late stage (Fig. 6.15**B**).

Ventriculomegaly with periventricular calcifications are most pronounced in the congenital form of herpes simplex encephalitis acquired in utero. With MR there is decreased gray-white matter contrast early in the infection, reflecting gray matter edema. Later there is decreased signal on the T2-weighted images within the thinned cortical gray matter.

In adults, herpes simplex infection may cause encephalitis or cranial neuritis. The infection usually is secondary to reactivation of latent herpes simplex type I. Patients with herpes encephalitis present with the gradual onset of personality changes, dysphasia, and focal neurologic deficits. Seizures and coma may occur. An inconstant but characteristic electroencephalographic finding is a localized spiked and slow wave pattern. Early diagnosis is crucial since there is a greater than 70% mortality rate in untreated patients. Unfortunately, CSF studies are often negative. Treatment is with vidarabine, which significantly reduces mortality, but many survivors have permanent deficits. Computed tomography scans show a poorly defined area of decreased density in one or both temporal lobes (Fig. 6.16). The predilection for the temporal lobes is because the virus is usually latent within the trigeminal ganglion. The frontal lobes may also be involved. The insular cortex is often involved, but the adjacent putamen is usually spared. There is usually swelling with mass effect. Streaky enhancement is variable. The CT findings are not usually seen before the 5th day of symptoms. With MR, the findings may be

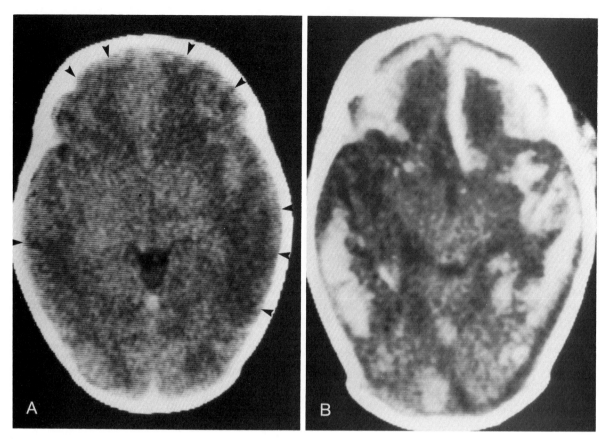

Figure 6.15. Neonatal Herpes. A. There is low density and swelling in the frontal and temporal lobes (*arrowheads*) on the noncontrast CT scan of this neonate with herpes type II infection in the acute stage. **B.** Several months later, the noncontrast CT scan on this same infant reveals widespread gray matter calcification, typical of late-stage neonatal herpes infection.

identified somewhat sooner. There is a nonspecific pattern of increased signal on the intermediate and T2-weighted images in the temporal and/or frontal lobe(s) with sparing of the putamen (Fig. 6.17**A**). Early on, meningeal enhancement may be seen (Fig. 6.17**B**). Later there may be parenchymal enhancement or evidence of hemorrhage. The differential diagnosis includes infarct, early bacterial cerebritis, and other types of viral encephalitis.

Varicella Zoster virus may rarely cause an encephalitis that is similar to that caused by herpes simplex. Another unusual manifestation is the syndrome of herpes zoster ophthalmicus and delayed contralateral hemiparesis caused by cerebral angiitis. In this syndrome, there are cerebral infarcts due to a large and medium vessel angiitis on the same side as ophthalmic zoster skin manifestations. Imaging studies show typical infarcts and angiography shows segmental areas of narrowing and/or beading of the arteries. Herpes zoster may also cause cranial neuritis, which may involve any of the cranial nerves. The most commonly involved is the facial nerve, resulting in the Ramsay Hunt syndrome. Clinically, there is ear pain and a facial paralysis accompanied by a vesicular eruption about the ear. Computed tomography scans

are usually normal, but MR may reveal increased contrast enhancement of the facial nerve.

Acute Disseminated Encephalomyelitis is an acute demyelinating disease that occurs after a viral infection, following a vaccination, or sometimes spontaneously. It probably has an autoimmune basis, since organisms are not isolated from brain tissue. Symptoms develop acutely with fever, headache, and meningeal signs. Seizures, focal neurologic deficits, stupor, and coma may develop. The mortality rate is 10–20%. T2-weighted MR is much more sensitive than CT in identifying lesions of increased signal intensity in the white matter. The lesions are usually multiple, but few in number. The appearance is similar to that seen in multiple sclerosis, but with a monophasic clinical course. Acute hemorrhagic leukoencephalitis is a severe variant of acute disseminated encephalomyelitis, which is often fatal. Pathologically there is perivascular hemorrhagic necrosis, primarily in the centrum semiovale. The hemorrhage is microscopic and is not seen with CT. The MR appearance is multiple foci of increased white matter intensity on T2-weighted images which look similar to severe multiple sclerosis, but are monophasic. The

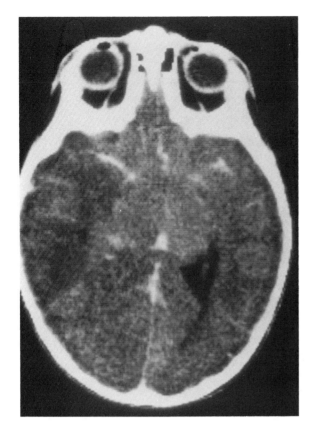

Figure 6.16. Adult Herpes Encephalitis. Both temporal lobes are of low density and appear swollen, especially on the right, on this contrast-enhanced CT scan. The appearance is similar to cerebral infarcts, but the clinical presentation is usually different.

major imaging feature is a rapid progression of low-density white matter areas over the course a few days.

Subacute Sclerosing Panencephalitis is caused by a variant of the measles virus. It typically occurs in children and young adults who had measles before age 2. The disease causes a progressive dementia, seizures, and paralysis leading to death. There is no treatment. Imaging studies may reveal extensive white matter lesions and atrophy. Enhancement of the white matter lesions can be seen with MR when there is active demyelination.

Progressive Multifocal Leukoencephalopathy is a demyelinating disease caused by a papovavirus (the Creutzfeldt-Jakob agent). It occurs only in immunosuppressed patients and has an increased incidence in patients with AIDS, as will be discussed.

Encephalitis can be caused by a variety of viruses not already discussed, including the togaviruses (arboviruses) that result in California, St. Louis, western equine and eastern equine encephalitis, Epstein-Barr virus, mumps, measles, rubella, and enteroviruses. *Rickettsia* and *Mycoplasma pneumoniae* may also produce encephalitis. Rasmussen's encephalitis is a devastating disease of childhood, most likely of viral etiology. There are intractable seizures and pro-

gressive neurologic deficits. The disease usually affects one cerebral hemisphere. Imaging studies show severe atrophy of the involved hemisphere. Positron-emission tomography scans show the hemisphere to be hypometabolic.

Creutzfeldt-Jakob Disease is caused by a slow virus infection of the brain. Clinically, there is a rapidly progressive dementia leading to death. Serial imaging studies rapidly progress from normal to marked cortical atrophy over the course of months. T2-weighted MR will also reveal progressive diffuse white matter high signal intensity. Abnormal signal intensity in the basal ganglia and thalamus has also been reported.

EXTRAAXIAL INFECTIONS
Meningitis

Meningitis can be caused by bacteria, mycobacteria, fungi, parasites, and viruses. Bacterial meningitis is caused by *Haemophilus influenzae*, *Neisseria meningitidis*, and *Streptococcus pneumoniae* in over 80% of cases. *Escherichia coli*, group B streptococcus, and *Listeria monocytogenes* occur commonly in neonates. The bacteria most commonly enter the meninges during a systemic bacteremia, but can spread directly from infected sinuses or after surgery or trauma. Patients present with a relatively acute onset of fever, a stiff neck, and headache followed by a decrease in mental status. Cerebrospinal fluid studies are usually diagnostic and imaging studies are generally not required. Computed tomography scans may be performed in the emergency setting in acutely comatose patients or in patients with a nonspecific headache, but are usually normal. The inflammatory exudate caused by the meningitis may occasionally produce high density within the subarachnoid spaces similar to that seen in subarachnoid hemorrhage.

The increased density is often more pronounced in the peripheral sulci than in the basal cisterns, unlike most cases of aneurysmal bleeding. If contrast is given there may or may not be meningeal enhancement. Computed tomography and MR are more often used later in the course of meningitis when there are suspected complications such as hydrocephalus, cerebritis/abscess, ventriculitis, and venous or arterial infarctions. The hydrocephalus that may develop is usually of the communicating type, reflecting decreased function of the arachnoid villi in absorbing CSF. Subdural effusions may be seen in infants, especially with *H. influenzae* meningitis. With CT and MR, subdural effusions appear as thin collections, along the surface of the brain, isodense/isointense with CSF (Fig. 6.18). These sterile effusions can be identified with sonography in infants. Echogenic sulci, ventriculomegaly, and abnormal parenchymal

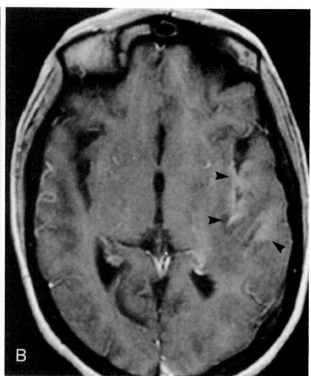

Figure 6.17.   Presumed Herpes Encephalitis. A. The intermediate-weighted MR scan reveals abnormal high signal in the insula and posterior temporal lobe with moderate mass effect. There is sparing of the putamen, which is typical of herpes. This was a patient with AIDS with multiple herpes skin lesions and herpes pharyngitis, who presented with an acute encephalitis that did not respond to anti-biotics. Toxoplasmosis titers in the CSF were negative and the patient was presumed to have herpes. Biopsy was refused and the patient died within 5 days. **B.** The T1-weighted postcontrast scan on this patient reveals meningeal and patchy gray matter enhancement (*arrowheads*), often present in cases of herpes encephalitis.

echogenicity have also been reported in infants with bacterial meningitis imaged with ultrasound.

Tuberculous Meningitis is the most common form of CNS tuberculosis. It is usually caused by *Mycobacterium tuberculosis*, but atypical mycobacteria, such as *M. avium-intracellulare* can cause meningitis in AIDS patients. Tuberculous meningitis has a predilection for infants and children, but is seen in all age groups. The disease spreads to the meninges hematogenously from the lungs, but the chest x-ray is normal in 40–75% of patients. The tuberculin skin test is also frequently negative. Clinically, there is usually a subacute or insidious onset of headache, malaise, weakness, apathy, or focal neurologic findings. Imaging studies will show enhancing, thickened meninges, especially near the base of the brain (Fig. 6.19), unlike bacterial meningitis where the peripheral meninges are more often involved. The often marked thickening of the meninges also distinguishes tuberculous and other granulomatous meningitides from pyogenic meningitis. The thick exudate in the basal cisterns may extend into the Virchow-Robin spaces, causing a vasculitis. This frequently leads to infarcts, better detected with MR than with CT. Communicating hydrocephalus is another relatively common complication.

The differential diagnosis of tuberculous meningitis includes fungal meningitis, racemose cysticercosis, sarcoidosis, and carcinomatous meningitis. Fungal meningitis usually causes thick meningeal enhancement in the basal cisterns, as with tuberculosis (Fig. 6.20). Enhancement is variable with cryptococcosis, depending on the immune status of the patient. Hydrocephalus is common, but infarcts and extension into the brain occur less frequently than with tuberculosis or pyogenic meningitis. Racemose cysticercosis may show thick meningeal enhancement, but cystic lesions in the cisterns are also frequently found (Fig. 6.11). Sarcoidosis involves the CNS in up to 14% of patients at autopsy, but only rarely causes neurologic symptoms. It primarily affects the leptomeninges, so that abnormal meningeal enhancement is seen with CT or MR. Focal parenchymal enhancing mass lesions or nonenhancing small white matter lesions may also be seen.

Viral Meningitis is caused most commonly by the enteroviruses, but can be caused by mumps, togaviruses, herpes simplex, lymphocytic choriomeningitis virus, and the human immunodeficiency virus (HIV). Most patients do not require treatment and neurologic deficits are uncommon. Imaging studies are typically normal.

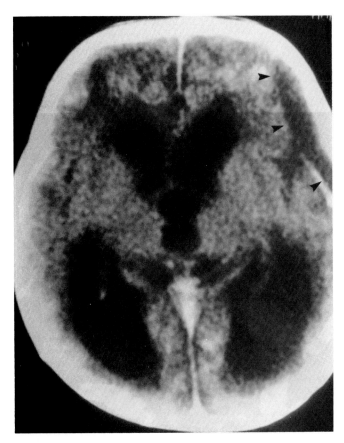

Figure 6.18. Subdural Effusion. A contrast-enhanced CT scan on this 6-year-old patient with *H. influenzae* meningitis reveals a subdural collection nearly isodense with CSF (*arrowheads*). Subdural effusions are common with *H. influenzae* meningitis. There is also enlargement of the lateral and third ventricles because of communicating hydrocephalus, which is a common complication of meningitis.

Subdural and Epidural Infections

Extraaxial pyogenic infections may also involve the epidural or subdural spaces. An epidural abscess may be caused by penetrating injuries, surgery, sinusitis, mastoiditis, orbital infection, or rarely by hematogenous spread. Computed tomography scans show an inwardly convex, extraaxial collection with increased density compared with CSF (Fig. 6.21). The inner margin usually enhances with contrast. There may be adjacent sinusitis or skull abnormalities. Magnetic resonance imaging is probably more sensitive in demonstrating these lesions, and can do so in multiple planes. The strong dural attachments prevent rapid expansion of epidural abscesses. However, a subdural empyema may spread rapidly throughout the subdural space, which is acutely life-threatening. Cortical venous thrombosis resulting in venous infarcts is a common result of these infections. Subdural empyemas are caused by the same conditions that produce epidural abscesses. Both CT and MR can demonstrate

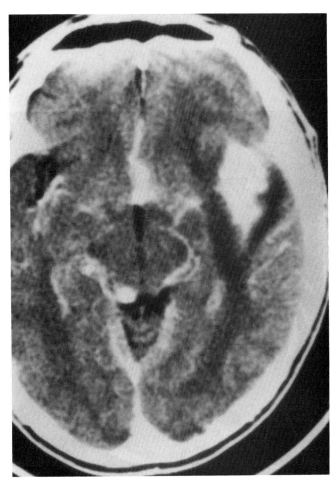

Figure 6.19. Tuberculous Meningitis. The contrast-enhanced CT scan shows marked abnormal contrast enhancement in the left sylvian fissure, interhemispheric fissure, ambient cistern, and along the tentorium. This thick, irregular enhancement in the basal cisterns is typical of a pachymeningitis such as tuberculosis or fungal meningitis. The CT scans in patients with bacterial meningitis are usually normal, or may reveal subtle increased density or enhancement in the peripheral sulci.

these subdural collections which usually have enhancing inner margins. Magnetic resonance imaging is more sensitive in showing smaller lesions because of the problem of partial volume averaging with the calvarium with CT. Magnetic resonance imaging is also better at detecting venous thrombosis and venous infarcts.

Mild, smooth dural, or meningeal enhancement may be seen after brain surgery, especially with MR (Fig. 6.22). The enhancement can persist for years and should be considered benign in this clinical setting. It most likely reflects a chemical meningitis due to perioperative hemorrhage.

ACQUIRED IMMUNODEFICIENCY SYNDROME

The CNS is a common site of involvement in patients with AIDS. Nearly 40% of AIDS patients will develop neurologic symptoms, and 10% present with

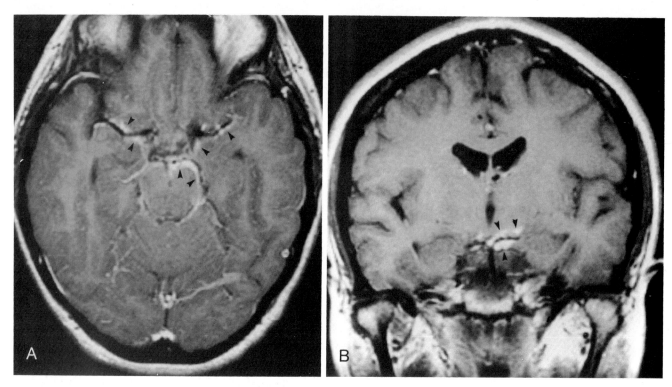

Figure 6.20. **Coccidioidomycosis Meningitis.** Contrast-enhanced, T1-weighted axial (**A**) and coronal (**B**) scans reveal abnormal enhancement of the meninges in the basal cisterns (*arrowheads*).

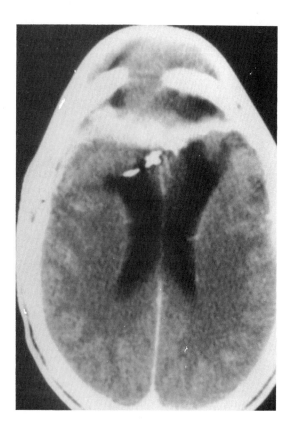

Figure 6.21. **Epidural Abscess.** This patient had a penetrating injury to the frontal bone several months prior to this contrast-enhanced CT scan. There is medium density pus extending through the calvarial defect into the epidural space. The inner margin enhances markedly. Surgical clips are present near the frontal horn of the right lateral ventricle.

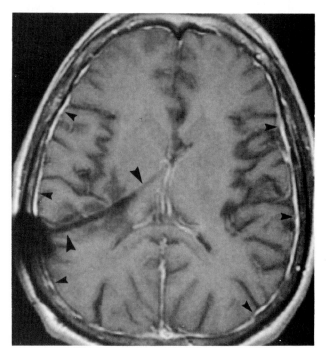

Figure 6.22. **Benign Postoperative Meningeal Enhancement.** Several years after brain surgery, this T1-weighted contrast-enhanced MR scan reveals smooth, but definitely abnormal enhancement of the dura (*small arrowheads*). There were no signs of infection or tumor recurrence. A ventricular shunt tube is seen on the right (*large arrowheads*).

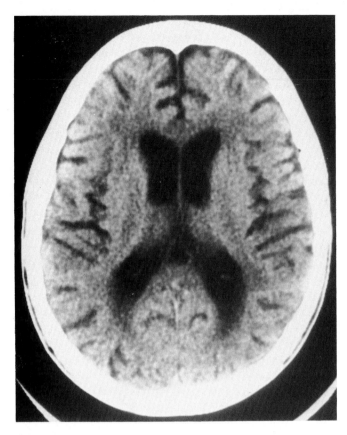

Figure 6.23.   AIDS-related Atrophy. A noncontrast CT scan reveals enlarged ventricles and sulci in this 24-year-old patient with AIDS. This is the most common abnormality found on brain imaging of patients with AIDS. It often correlates with the AIDS dementia complex.

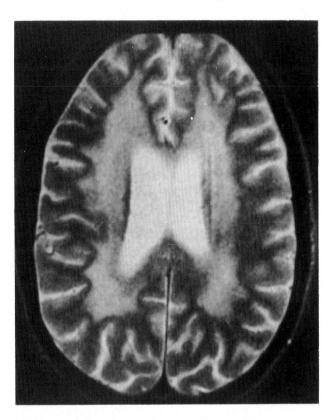

Figure 6.24.   AIDS White Matter Disease. This young patient clinically had the AIDS dementia complex. The T2-weighted MR scan shows widespread abnormal high signal in the periventricular white matter, as is frequently the case with this syndrome.

CNS disease as the earliest manifestation of the syndrome. A variety of infections and neoplasms may be diagnosed in these patients. The most common infections include HIV encephalitis, toxoplasmosis, cryptococcosis and other fungal infections, CMV and herpes meningoencephalitis, mycobacterial infection, progressive multifocal leukoencephalopathy (PML), and meningovascular syphilis. Primary CNS lymphoma is by far the most common tumor, but metastatic lymphoma, gliomas, and rarely, Kaposi's sarcoma may also occur.

HIV Encephalitis. The etiologic agent in AIDS, HIV, is neurotropic, infecting the brain in nearly 30% of patients at autopsy. Pathologically, HIV infection results in vacuolation of the white matter, with areas of demyelination and multinucleated giant cells. The centrum semiovale is involved most severely, but all white matter tracts, including the brainstem and cerebellum, may be affected. The cortical gray matter is usually spared. Clinically, patients with HIV encephalitis develop a subcortical dementia known as the AIDS dementia complex (ADC). Infants and children with HIV encephalitis exhibit loss of developmental milestones, apathy, failure of brain growth, and spastic paraparesis. This is the most common form of CNS

disease in pediatric patients with AIDS, as opportunistic infections and CNS tumors are unusual.

Diffuse Atrophy is the most common manifestation of HIV infection of the brain on neuroimaging studies, present in about 30% of all patients with AIDS (Fig. 6.23). This is largely central atrophy, reflecting the predominant white matter involvement. The degree of atrophy usually correlates with the severity of dementia. White matter lesions are also commonly seen in patients with the ADC. Magnetic resonance imaging is significantly more sensitive than CT for detecting these abnormalities. A diffuse pattern of increased signal in the deep white matter or multiple small punctate white matter lesions on T2-weighted images are the most common findings. The punctate lesions do not correlate well with symptoms and may be incidental findings of no clinical significance. The lesions do not exhibit mass effect or abnormal contrast enhancement.

The most severe cases of HIV brain infection show extensive bilateral areas of abnormal signal throughout the periventricular white matter, brainstem, and cerebellum (Fig. 6.24). In these severe cases, CT may also be abnormal, showing low density without enhancement in the white matter. Such severe involvement almost always correlates with severe encepha-

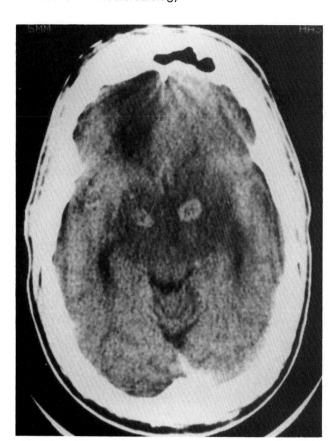

Figure 6.25. Toxoplasmosis. A contrast-enhanced CT scan reveals bilateral ring-enhancing lesions in the basal ganglia of this patient with AIDS. There is marked surrounding low-density edema. The basal ganglia are a common site for toxoplasmosis.

lopathy. The clinical and imaging abnormalities may respond to treatment with the antiviral agent azathioprine (AZT). Decreased metabolism has been demonstrated in the white matter of patients with ADC studied with localized phosphorus-31 nuclear magnetic resonance spectroscopy. In infants and children with HIV infection, atrophy is the most common observation, followed by calcifications in the basal ganglia. White matter calcifications and low-density lesions are also sometimes seen.

Toxoplasmosis is the next most common CNS infection in AIDS occurring in about 10% of patients. *Toxoplasma gondii* is an obligate intacellular protozoan that is ubiquitous throughout the world, causing subclinical or mild infection in a large percentage of the population. In the United States, between 20 and 70% of the population are seropositive for toxoplasmosis. In AIDS patients, CNS toxoplasmosis usually results from reactivation of the previously acquired infection. A necrotizing encephalitis usually results, with the formation of multiple thin-walled abscesses. Patients present clinically with headache, fever, lethargy, a decreased level of consciousness, and focal signs which initially can be confused with the

subacute encephalitis of HIV infection. Neuroimaging studies are therefore crucial in patient management.

The typical appearance of CNS toxoplasmosis is that of multiple enhancing mass lesions with surrounding vasogenic edema (Figs. 6.25 and 6.26). The lesions are usually relatively small, between 1 and 4 cm in diameter. The larger lesions usually exhibit ring enhancement, while the smaller lesions are usually solid. The lesions are usually of increased signal on precontrast T2-weighted images, but there may be central areas of decreased signal from calcification or hemorrhage, especially after antibiotic treatment. The basal ganglia is a favored site, but white matter and cortical lesions are also common. The main differential consideration is primary CNS lymphoma, which will be discussed later. A clinical and imaging response to antitoxoplasmosis antibiotics will usually distinguish between toxoplasmosis and lymphoma in most cases (Fig. 6.26). Biopsy is usually reserved for atypical cases or when there is no response to antibiotics. Other infections or tumors may occasionally mimic toxoplasmosis, but are unusual. Fungal and mycobacterial abscesses have been described. Bacterial abscesses are exceedingly rare in AIDS patients.

Fungal Meningitis. Although fungal abscesses and granulomas are unusual, fungal meningitis is a common complication of AIDS, occuring in 5–15% of patients. Cryptococcosis is the most common fungal infection, although histoplasmosis, candidiasis, aspergillosis, and coccidioidomycosis also occur. The meningitis caused by these agents is usually mild because of the diminished inflammatory response of the immunocompromised host. Therefore, there is usually little or no enhancement of the meninges, and imaging studies are usually normal. The diagnosis is made when there are elevated cryptococcal antigen titers in the serum and CSF.

As already mentioned, cryptococcosis may sometimes present as dilated Virchow-Robin spaces filled with cryptococcus organisms, known as gelatinous pseudocysts. These cysts appear as rounded, smoothly marginated lesions in the basal ganglia that are nearly isodense and isointense to CSF (Fig. 6.27). There is no enhancement following contrast administration, which distinguishes these lesions from toxoplamosis.

Progressive Multifocal Leukoencephalopathy is an infection of immunosuppressed patients caused by a papovavirus (the Creutzfeldt-Jakob agent). The incidence of PML in AIDS patients is between 2 and 7%. It can also occur in other immunosuppressed patients, such as transplant recipients and leukemics, but does not occur in immunocompetent patients. The infection causes demyelination and necrosis, primarily involving white matter. Clinical symptoms include mental status changes, blind-

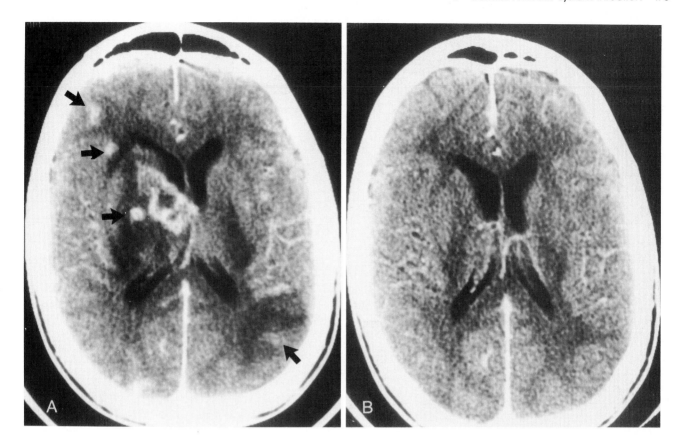

Figure 6.26. Toxoplasmosis. A. A contrast-enhanced CT scan shows a large right basal ganglia enhancing mass, and several other small enhancing lesions (*arrows*). The small size and multiplicity of the lesions favors toxoplasmosis over lymphoma. **B.** Following 2 weeks of antibiotic therapy, the contrast-enhanced CT scan reveals complete resolution of the lesions, typical for toxoplasmosis.

ness, aphasia, hemiparesis, ataxia, and other focal findings. There is a progressive course to death within months. In non-AIDS immunosuppressed patients, PML has a predilection for the occipital lobes, but in AIDS patients, any part of the brain may be involved. Because it is primarily a white matter process, MR is superior to CT in showing the lesions of PML. Magnetic resonance imaging reveals focal lesions of increased signal on T2-weighted images and decreased signal on T1-weighted images within the white matter (Fig. 6.28). Computed tomography shows white matter lesions of decreased density. The lesions may be solitary or multifocal. Mass effect and contrast enhancement are almost always absent, which are important distinguishing features. Rarely, both gray and white matter are involved, simulating an infarct.

Virus Infection. Cytomegalovirus infection is a common CNS infection in patients with AIDS pathologically, but does not usually result in frank tissue necrosis, and is usually subclinical. Cytomegalovirus meningoencephalitis is occasionally imaged as areas of demyelination or enhancement, especially near the ventricles. Herpes virus and varicella zoster virus infection are also only occasionally imaged. In patients with AIDS, these viral infections often have a more be-

nign clinical course and imaging appearance because of a diminished immune response.

Intracranial Mycobacterial Infections occur in a small percentage of patients with AIDS. Most of these patients are intravenous drug abusers. Most patients present with meningitis. Imaging studies in these patients reveal communicating hydrocephalus and/or meningeal enhancement. Tuberculomas and tuberculous abscesses are less common.

Primary CNS Lymphoma is by far the most common intracranial tumor associated with AIDS. Up to 6% of patients with AIDS will develop this tumor. It is the main differential diagnostic consideration along with toxoplasmosis when a mass lesion is found in patients with AIDS. Patients present with symptoms of a space-occupying lesion, as with toxoplasmosis. Solitary or multiple enhancing mass lesions are found with neuroimaging studies (Fig. 6.29). The lesions are usually centrally located within the deep white matter or basal ganglia, but cortical lesions also occur. The tumor may spread across the corpus callosum, which does not usually occur with toxoplasmosis. With MR imaging, there is variable signal intensity, with areas of low or high signal on T2-weighted images, and iso- or low signal on T1-weighted images. With CT, the lesions are often isodense with gray matter. The lesions

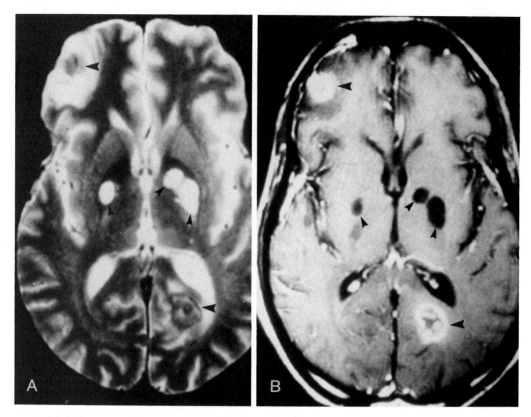

Figure 6.27. Cryptococcosis and Toxoplasmosis. A. The T2-weighted MR scan reveals multiple rounded lesions, isointense to CSF in the basal ganglia (*small arrowheads*). There is no surrounding edema. Darker lesions with surrounding edema are present in the right frontal and left occipital areas (*large arrowheads*). **B.** The contrast-enhanced T1-weighted MR scan again reveals the basal gan-

glia lesions to be isointense with CSF (*small arrowheads*). There is no contrast enhancement. The appearance of these lesions is typical of gelatinous pseudocysts of cryptococcosis. These lesions represent dilated Virchow-Robin spaces filled with cryptococcus organisms. The right frontal and left occipital lesions do enhance with contrast (*large arrowheads*), as is typical of toxoplasmosis.

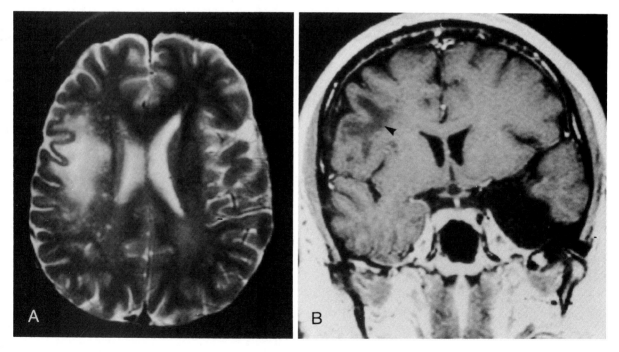

Figure 6.28. Progressive Multifocal Leukoencephalopathy. A. There is an area of abnormal high signal intensity in the right corona radiata on this T2-weighted image. There is no significant mass effect. **B.** On the contrast-enhanced T1-weighted image, the lesion is

of low signal intensity (*arrowhead*), and does not enhance. These are typical features of PML, which was proven with biopsy in this patient with AIDS. Incidentally, a left temporal arachnoid cyst can be noted.

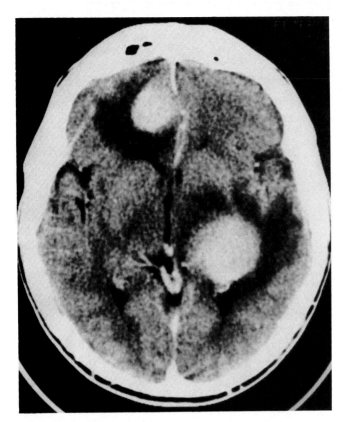

Figure 6.29.   Primary CNS Lymphoma. There are two solidly enhancing mass lesions with surrounding edema on this CT scan of a patient with AIDS. The relatively large size and solid enhancement pattern are more suggestive of lymphoma than toxoplasmosis, as was proven in this case.

almost always enhance with contrast, in either a ring or solid pattern. The imaging appearance is often indistinguishable from toxoplasmosis. The main distinguishing features are size and number. Toxoplasmosis is more frequently multiple and the lesions are usually smaller than with lymphoma. Isointensity with white matter on T2-weighted MR and diffuse, homogeneous contrast enhancement favors lymphoma.

A target-like double ring appearance has also been seen frequently with lymphoma. High signal on T2-weighted MR (often with a low-signal rim) and ring enhancement following contrast administration favors toxoplasmosis. Toxoplasmosis is also more common than lymphoma. Unfortunately, there is a great deal of overlap in the imaging appearance of these two mass lesions, which can coexist in the same patient. For this reason, some authors advocate biopsy when enhancing mass lesions are found in patients with AIDS. However, in most institutions, an empirical trial with antitoxoplasmosis antibiotics is usually attempted prior to biopsy. Clinical and radiologic improvement usually are seen within 2 weeks.

References

1. Enzmann DR, ed. Imaging of infections and inflammations of the central nervous system: Computed tomography, ultrasound, and nuclear magnetic resonance. New York: Raven Press, 1984.
2. Federle MP, Megibow A, eds. Radiology of AIDS. New York: Raven Press, 1988.
3. Fitz CR. Inflammatory diseases of the brain in childhood. AJNR 1992;13:551–567.
4. Haimes AB, Zimmerman RD, Morgello S, et al. MR imaging of brain abscesses. AJNR 1989;10:279–291.
5. Han BK, Babcock DS, McAdams L. Bacterial meningitis in infants: Sonographic findings. Radiology 1985;154:645–650.
6. Olsen WL. Neuroradiologic abnormalities in AIDS. Curr Probl Diagn Radiol 1988;17:89–100.
7. Rauch RA, Jinkins JR. Infections of the central nervous system. Curr Opinion Radiology 1991;3:16–24.
8. Sze G, Zimmerman RD. The magnetic resonance imaging of infections and inflammatory diseases. Radiol Clin North Am 1988;26:839–859.
9. Tien RD, Chu PK, Hesselink JR, Duberg A, Wiley C. Intracranial cryptococcosis in immunocompromised patients: CT and MR findings in 29 cases. AJNR 1991;12:283–289.
10. Weingarten K, Zimmerman RD, Becker RD, Heier LA, Haimes AB, Deck MDF. Subdural and epidural empyemas: MR imaging. AJNR 1989;10:81–87.

7 ■

White Matter and Neurodegenerative Diseases

Jerome A. Barakos

DEMYELINATING DISEASES
    Primary Demyelination
    Ischemic Demyelination
    Infection-Related Demyelination
    Toxic and Metabolic Demyelination
DYSMYELINATING DISEASES
CEREBROSPINAL FLUID DYNAMICS
NEURODEGENERATIVE DISORDERS

In contrast to gray matter, which contains neuronal cell bodies, white matter is composed of the long processes of the neurons. These axonal processes are wrapped by myelin sheaths and it is the lipid composition of these sheaths from which white matter is named. This chapter will examine a host of diseases that are characterized by their involvement of white matter. This will be followed by a discussion of hydrocephalus and neurodegenerative disorders.

With the marked sensitivity of T2-weighted magnetic resonance (MR) images, lesions of the white matter are readily detected. The difficulty that confronts the radiologist is that a wide spectrum of neurologic diseases may involve the white matter, and these lesions are often nonspecific in nature. Nevertheless an understanding of these white matter diseases, their clinical features, and parenchymal patterns of involvement is important in arriving at a useful differential diagnosis. Cerebral white matter diseases are classified into two broad categories, demyelinating and dysmyelinating. Demyelination is an acquired disorder that affects normal myelin. In contrast, dysmyelination is an inherited disorder affecting the formation or maintenance of myelin.

DEMYELINATINIG DISEASES

Demyelinating disease can be divided into four main etiologies: (1) primary, (2) ischemic, (3) infectious, and (4) toxic and metabolic (Table 7.1).

Primary Demyelination

MULTIPLE SCLEROSIS

Multiple sclerosis (MS) is the classic example of a primary demyelinating disease. Multiple sclerosis affects more than a quarter of a million people in the United States alone. The age of onset is between 20 to 40 years with only 10% of cases involving individuals older than 50. There is a slight female predominance of 1.5 to 1. Several environmental factors have been associated with MS, such as higher geographic latitudes and upper socioeconomic status. However, the etiology of MS remains unclear. The classic clinical definition of MS is multiple central nervous system lesions separated in both time and space. Patients may present with virtually any neurologic deficit, but most commonly present with muscle weakness, paresthesia, and visual or urinary disturbances. A key characteristic of MS symptoms is their multiplicity and tendency to vary over time. In fact, the clinical course of MS is characterized by unpredictable relapses and remissions of symptoms. The diagnosis can be confirmed with laboratory findings consisting of abnor-

Table 7.1. Classification of White Matter Diseases

Primary demyelination	Toxic and metabolic
Multiple sclerosis	demyelination
Vascular ischemic	Central pontine myelinolysis
demyelination	Marchiafava-Bignami
Deep white matter infarcts	syndrome
Lacunar infarcts	Wernicke-Korsakoff syndrome
Vasculitis	Radiation injury
Dissection	Necrotizing
Embolic	leukoencephalopathy
Migraine	Dysmyelination
Post anoxic	Metachromatic
Infection related demyelination	leukodystrophy
Progressive multifocal	Adrenal leukodystrophy
leukoencephalopathy	Leigh's disease
HIV encephalitis	Alexander's disease
Acute disseminated	
encephalomyelitis	
Subacute sclerosing	
panencephalitis	
Lyme disease	

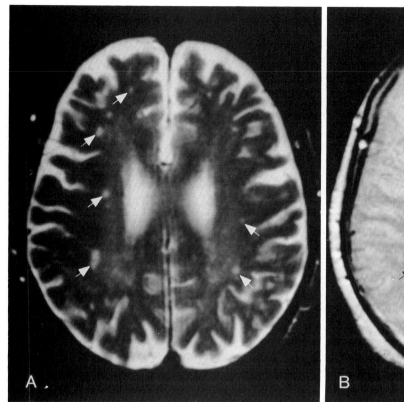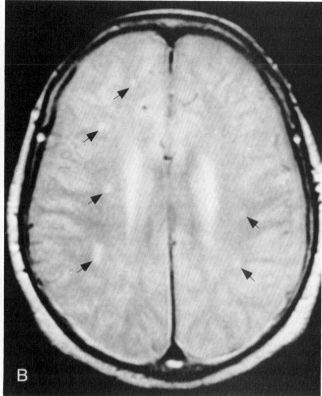

Figure 7.3. Ischemic Demyelination. Deep white matter ischemic lesions in a 67-year-old female presenting with unrelated symptoms (headaches). Axial first and second echo T2-weighted images demonstrate multiple punctate lesions involving the deep cerebral white matter (*arrows*). Note that these lesions can be distinguished from Virchow-Robin spaces since they are visible on the first echo sequence. In contrast, perivascular spaces are of CSF signal intensity and would be isointense on the first echo, and thus imperceptible.

spinal cord MS lesions (approximately 70–80%) will have associated plaques in the brain. Therefore, performing an MR scan of the head may confirm the diagnosis, thus avoiding a spinal cord biopsy.

Ischemic Demyelination

Although MR imaging is extremely sensitive in the detection of white matter lesions, the major difficulty in arriving at a diagnosis is that these lesions are often nonspecific. Thus, distinguishing MS lesions from other white matter lesions can be difficult. The most common white matter lesions are ischemic in origin.

AGE-RELATED DEMYELINATION

Small-vessel ischemic changes within the deep cerebral white matter are seen with such frequency in the older population (>60 years) that they can be considered a normal part of aging (Figure 7.3) (5). This represents an arteriosclerotic vasculopathy of the penetrating cerebral arteries (6). The deep white matter is more susceptible to ischemic injury as compared to the gray matter because it is supplied by long, small-caliber penetrating arteries. These vessels become narrowed by arteriosclerosis and lipohy-

aline deposits. The result is the formation of small ischemic lesions primarily involving the deep cerebral and periventricular white matter as well as the basal ganglia. The cortex, subcortical "U" fibers, central corpus callosum, medulla, midbrain, and cerebellar peduncles are usually spared because of their dual blood supply, which decreases their vulnerability to hypoperfusion.

Histologically, these areas of infarction demonstrate axonal atrophy with diminished myelin. Early neuropathologists noted the areas of paleness associated with these changes and coined the term "myelin pallor." These white matter changes have received many names over the years including leukoaraiosis, microangiopathic leukoencephalopathy, and subcortical arteriosclerotic encephalopathy. However, none of these terms are very satisfying as they do not accurately reflect all the changes observed histologically, and overstate the clinical significance of these lesions. A more appropriate term may simply be "age-related white matter ischemia." These small ischemic white matter lesions are often asymptomatic and clinical correlation is always required before a diagnosis of subcortical arteriosclerotic encephalopathy or multiinfarct dementia (Binswanger's disease) is made (7). Note that the white matter infarcts just described differ

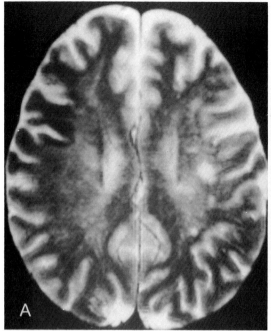

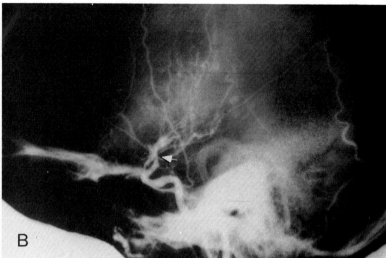

Figure 7.4. Vasculitis. T2-weighted sequence (**A**) demonstrates left hemispheric white matter lesions in a 42-year-old female. Although in a 60-year-old person these lesions may simply represent age-re-lated white matter ischemic changes, these findings are distinctly abnormal in a younger patient. Left internal carotid arteriogram (**B**) reveals severe supraclinoid stenosis (*arrow*), the result of vasculitis.

from lacunar infarcts. Lacunae refer to small infarcts (5–10 mm) occurring within the basal ganglia, typically the upper two thirds of the putamina. Nevertheless, both lacunar and deep white matter infarcts have similar etiologies and are the result of disease involving the deep penetrating arteries.

Small white matter lesions are more prominent in any patient with a vasculopathy, whether it is related to atherosclerosis (age, hypertension, diabetes) or to a vasculitis (lupus, polyarteritis nodosa, Behçet's syndrome). In younger individuals causes include vasculitis, embolic disease, hypoxia, dissection, and migraine (Figure 7.4). Differentiating these lesions related to ischemic changes from MS lesions can be difficult, especially in the older patient. This is important since 10% of patients who present with MS are over the age of 50. Of course, clinical testing and history are helpful. Additionally, deep white matter infarcts tend to spare the subcortical arcuate fibers and the corpus callosum, both of which are often involved with MS. Recent work has also shown that involvement of the callosal-septal interface is relatively specific for MS (Figure 7.5) (8, 9).

Several conditions can mimic white matter disease.

EPENDYMITIS GRANULARIS

This is a common normal anatomic finding that is seen on virtually every MR image of a normal head (10). This consists of an area of high signal on the T2-weighted images at the tips of the frontal horns.

These foci range in size from several millimeters up to a centimeter in width. Histologic studies of this subependymal area reveal a loose network of axons with low myelin count. This porous ependyma allows transependymal flow of CSF, resulting in a focal area of T2 prolongation. Unfortunately this entity has been given a name that sounds more like a disease entity, ependymitis granularis, rather than a histologic observation.

PROMINENT PERIVASCULAR SPACES

These can also mimic deep white matter or lacunar infarcts. As blood vessels penetrate into the brain parenchyma they are enveloped by CSF and a thin sheath of pia. These CSF-filled perivascular spaces are called Virchow-Robin spaces, and present as punctate foci of high signal on the T2-weighted sequence (11). They are typically located in the centrum semiovale (high cerebral hemispheric white matter) and the lower basal ganglia at the level of the anterior commissure, where lenticulostriate arteries enter the anterior perforated substance. These perivascular spaces are typically 1–2 mm in diameter but can be considerably larger (Figure 7.6). They can be seen as a normal variant at any age but become more prominent with increasing age as atrophy occurs.

An important means for differentiating a periventricular space from a parenchymal lesion is the use of the proton density-weighted image (first echo T2-weighted image) (5). On the proton density-weighted

Figure 7.5. Multiple Sclerosis. Sagittal first and second echo T2-weighted images of a 32-year-old female with MS demonstrate a multitude of lesions involving the callosal-septal interface (*arrows*). This location is a frequent site of MS involvement.

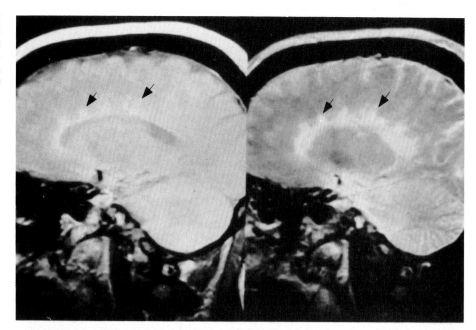

Figure 7.6. A large perivascular space in a 32-year-old male (*arrow*) shown in sagittal and coronal T1-weighted sequences (**A**), which demonstrate a well-rounded, right-sided lesion along the course of the lenticulostriate arteries as they enter the basal ganglia through the anterior perforated substance. Although perivascular spaces are typically 1 to 2 mm in diameter, they can be considerably larger. First and second echo T2-weighted coronal images (**B**) demonstrate that this lesion parallels the signal intensity of CSF on all imaging sequences, and is imperceptible on the proton density sequence (*arrow*). An old cavitated lacunar infarction may have a similar appearance and differentiation can be difficult, requiring clinical history.

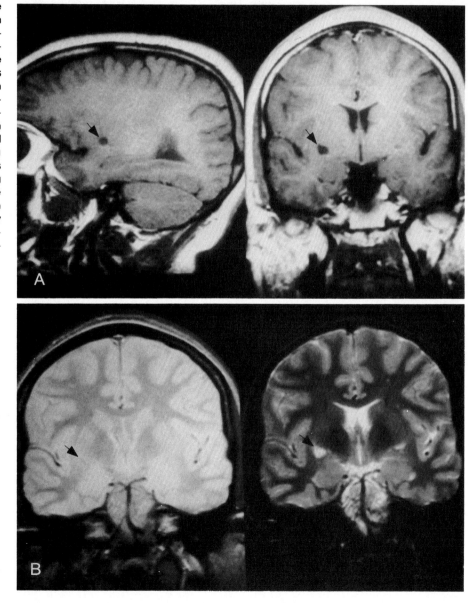

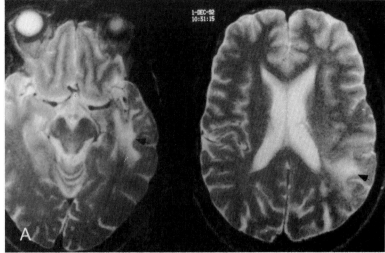
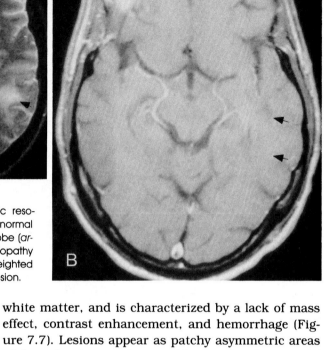

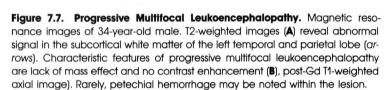

Figure 7.7. Progressive Multifocal Leukoencephalopathy. Magnetic resonance images of 34-year-old male. T2-weighted images (**A**) reveal abnormal signal in the subcortical white matter of the left temporal and parietal lobe (*arrows*). Characteristic features of progressive multifocal leukoencephalopathy are lack of mass effect and no contrast enhancement (**B**), post-Gd T1-weighted axial image). Rarely, petechial hemorrhage may be noted within the lesion.

sequence, CSF has similar signal intensity as white matter. A perivascular space is composed of CSF, and will parallel CSF signal intensity on all sequences, i.e., isointense on proton density sequence. In contrast, ischemic lesions, unless cavitated with cystic change, will be bright on the proton density sequence. Therefore, both a deep infarct and a perivascular space will be bright on the second echo T2-weighted image, but only the infarct will remain bright on the first echo image. An additional differentiating feature is that lacunar infarcts, as described above, tend to occur in the upper two-thirds of the putamina and are usually larger than 5 mm. In contrast, periventricular spaces are typically smaller, bilateral, and often symmetric within the inferior third of the putamina.

Infection-Related Demyelination

Infectious agents may result in white matter disease and most commonly are viral.

PROGRESSIVE MULTIFOCAL LEUKOENCEPHALOPATHY

Progressive multifocal leukoencephalopathy is being seen with increased frequency because of an expansion in the acquired immunodeficiency syndrome (AIDS) population (12). Progressive multifocal leukoencephalopathy represents a reactivation of a latent papovavirus. This is usually seen in immunocompromised patients, particularly individuals with AIDS, lymphoma, organ transplantation, and disseminated malignancies. Progressive multifocal leukoencephalopathy typically involves the deep cerebral

white matter, and is characterized by a lack of mass effect, contrast enhancement, and hemorrhage (Figure 7.7). Lesions appear as patchy asymmetric areas of demyelination with a predilection for the parietal region. These lesions rapidly progress and coalesce into larger confluent areas. Although most lesions involve supratentorial white matter, gray matter and infratentorial involvement are being identified more frequently. Progressive multifocal leukoencephalopathy is relentlessly progressive, with death ensuing within several months from the time of onset.

HUMAN IMMUNODEFICIENCY VIRUS (HIV) ENCEPHALITIS

In patients with AIDS, HIV encephalitis may result in diffuse white matter involvement, which can mimic progressive multifocal leukoencephalopathy (Figure 7.8) (13). The HIV encephalitis causes a progressive dementia and is believed to reflect a direct viral infection of the glial cells. Typical imaging features consist of a diffuse bilateral, relatively symmetric supratentorial white matter signal abnormality involving a large area. The HIV encephalitis can also present with more localized involvement with patchy ill-defined margins.

Demyelination may follow a viral illness, the result of a viral-induced autoimmune response to white matter (14).

ACUTE DISSEMINATED ENCEPHALOMYELITIS (ADEM)

ADEM typically occurs following a viral illness or vaccination, with measles, rubella, and mumps being the most common agents (15). Demyelinating lesions

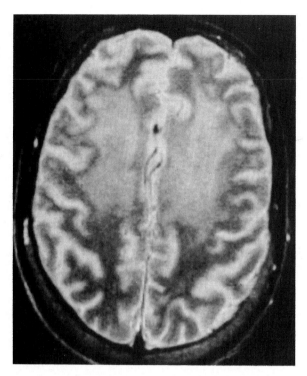

Figure 7.8. HIV Encephalitis. T2-weighted image of a 27-year-old male demonstrates diffuse hyperintensity of the deep cerebral white matter.

associated with ADEM typically begin approximately 2 weeks following viral infection, with the clinical onset of seizures and focal neurologic deficits. In the majority of cases there is spontaneous resolution of symptoms but permanent sequelae can be seen in up to 20% of patients with some even progressing to death. Lesions primarily involve white matter, but gray matter may also be affected. Magnetic resonance imaging demonstrates multifocal or confluent white matter lesions similar to multiple sclerosis (Figure 7.9). A differential feature is that ADEM is a monophasic illness, unlike MS, which has a remitting and relapsing course.

SUBACUTE SCLEROSING PANENCEPHALITIS (SSPE)

SSPE represents a reactivated, slowly progressive infection caused by measles virus. Children between the ages of 5 and 12, who had measles usually before the age of 3, are typically affected. Magnetic resonance imaging demonstrates patchy areas of periventricular demyelination as well as lesions of the basal ganglia. The disease course is variable and may be rapidly progressive or very protracted.

LYME DISEASE

Lyme disease is a spirochete infection (*Borrelia burgdorferi*) that results in white matter lesions that are indistinguishable from MS (Figure 7.10) (16). The

vector of transmission to humans is the ixodid tick (*Ixodes dammini*) which commonly infests deer and mice. The course of human infection has been divided into three stages, which starts with a migrating erythematous rash. The most prominent neurologic symptoms occur during the second stage, several weeks following the onset of the rash, and include cranial nerve palsies, irritability, and memory and sleep disorders. Since treatment with antibiotics is both simple and curative, one must have a high index of suspicion for this entity in endemic areas when encountering white matter lesions identical to multiple sclerosis.

Toxic and Metabolic Demyelination

CENTRAL PONTINE MYELINOLYSIS

Central pontine myelinolysis is a disorder that results in characteristic demyelination of the central pons. This is most commonly seen in patients with electrolyte abnormalities, particularly involving hyponatremia, that are rapidly corrected giving rise to the term "osmotic demyelination syndrome" (17). This condition occurs most commonly in children and alcoholics with malnutrition. Occasionally, cases have been associated with diabetes, leukemia, and infections. Typical clinical presentation is that of a rapidly evolving corticospinal syndrome with quadriplegia and a "locked-in" state where the patient is mute and unable to move but is not comatose. Patients tend to be extremely ill and often have a very poor prognosis. Magnetic resonance imaging characteristically demonstrates abnormal high signal on T2-weighted images corresponding to the regions of central pontine demyelination (Figure 7.11). Extrapontine sites of involvement such as the basal ganglia and thalamus are not unusual.

MARCHIAFAVA-BIGNAMI SYNDROME

This is a rare form of demyelination seen most frequently in alcoholics. This condition was first described in Italian red wine drinkers, but has since been reported with other types of alcohol as well as in nonalcoholics. The disease is characterized by demyelination involving the central fibers (medial zone) of the corpus callosum. Onset is usually insidious, with the most common being nonspecific dementia. No adequate therapy exists and the disease is usually slowly progressive, resulting in death.

WERNICKE-KORSAKOFF SYNDROME

Although pathologically indistinguishable, Wernicke and Korsakoff syndromes are clinically distinguishable and both are the result of thiamine defi-

Figure 7.9. Acute Disseminated Encephalomyelitis. T2-weighted (**A**) and post-Gd T1-weighted sequence (**B**) in a 7-year-old boy who presented with deteriorating mental status 1 week following viral gastroenteritis. Imaging findings reveal multiple subcortical white matter lesions. The patient improved following treatment with steroids.

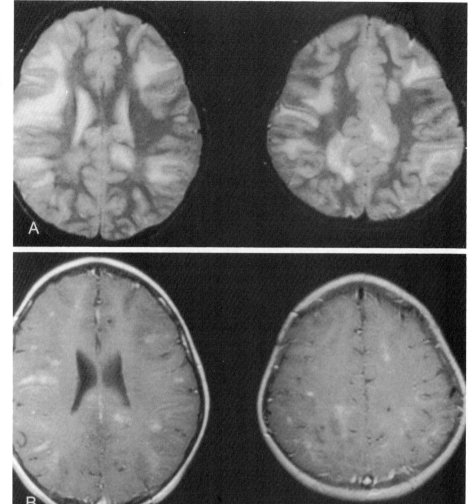

Figure 7.10. Lyme Disease. First and second echo T2-weighted axial images of a 30-year-old male demonstrate periventricular lesions mimicking MS. The patient presented several weeks following a migrating erythematous rash. Diagnosis was confirmed via serum spirochete-specific IgM immunofluorescence. Symptoms resolved following treatment with antibiotics.

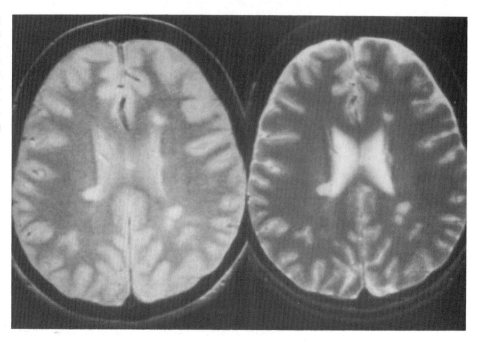

ciency. In both cases patients present with dementia. Magnetic resonance imaging demonstrates lesions of the basal ganglia, thalamus, and brainstem with periaqueductal involvement. Additionally, atrophy of the mammillary bodies may be seen. Except for the mammillary body involvement, these findings are very similar to Leigh's disease, discussed below.

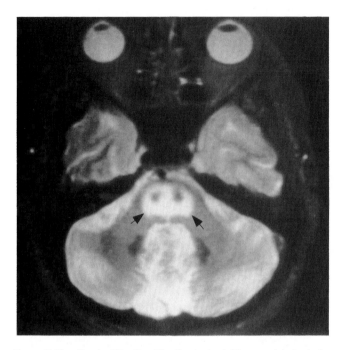

Figure 7.11. Central Pontine Myelinolysis. A 52-year-old alcoholic was admitted with a serum sodium of 110 mEq/ml. Following rapid normalization of sodium, the patient became comatose. This T2-weighted image demonstrates a well-defined high signal within the central pons (*arrows*).

RADIATION LEUKOENCEPHALITIS

Radiation may result in damage to the white matter secondary to arteritis and associated ischemic injuries. Radiation leukoencephalitis usually requires a cumulative dose in excess of 4000 rads delivered to the brain and occurs 6 to 9 months following treatment. Findings consist of areas of abnormal high signal on T2-weighted images, typically involving diffuse areas of confluent white matter extending to involve the subcortical U fibers in the distribution of the irradiated brain (Figure 7.12). Note that this represents an indirect effect of radiation on the brain, and results from an arteritis (endothelial hypertrophy, medial hyalinization, and fibrosis) involving small arteries and arterioles.

RADIATION NECROSIS

In contrast to the rather benign nature of radiation leukoencephalitis, radiation necrosis is the major hazard related to CNS radiation. Radiation necrosis is strongly dose-related, and is less commonly seen today, because of greater fractionation of CNS radiation doses. It may occur several weeks to years following irradiation, and can be progressive and fatal. Radiation necrosis typically presents as an enhancing lesion, with mass effect and ring enhancement, or as multiple foci of enhancement, mimicking recurrent neoplasm (Figure 7.13). It is found most commonly in or near the irradiated tumor bed, but sometimes is more remote from the tumor bed. It is theorized that the partially injured brain parenchyma within and adjacent to the tumor bed is more susceptible to radiation injury, thus accounting for the distribution of radiation necrosis. Following resection of a brain

Figure 7.12. Radiation Leukoencephalitis. Magnetic resonance image of a 57-year-old female 1 year following whole brain radiation for metastatic breast carcinoma to the brain. T2-weighted coronal and axial images reveal confluent areas of high signal involving the periventricular white matter. The patient was entirely asymptotic, returning for a routine follow-up examination.

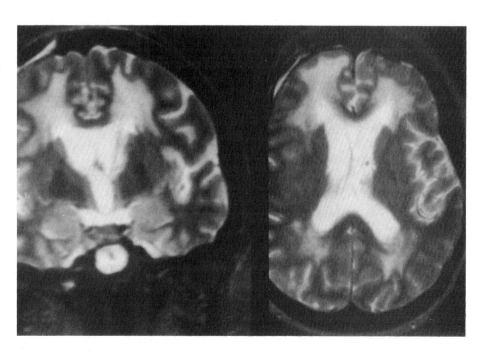

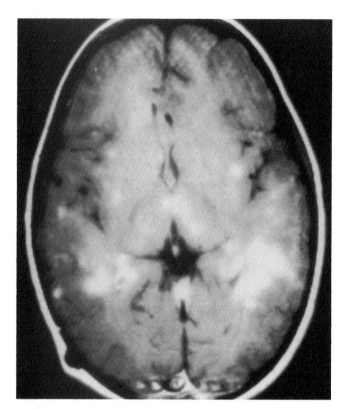

Figure 7.13. Radiation Necrosis. Radiation necrosis in a 7-year-old male presenting 16 months following irradiation of a posterior fossa glioma. Post-Gd T1-weighted image reveals multiple scattered foci of contrast enhancement. Review of radiation ports revealed that all lesions were confined to the port.

neoplasm with subsequent radiation therapy, it can be very difficult to differentiate tumor recurrence from radiation-associated necrosis. In such a case, serial MR scans are required to evaluate for tumor recurrence and progression. The use of positron emission tomography has also been reported to be useful in distinguishing tumor recurrence from radiation necrosis, since the former will be active metabolically and the latter will not (Figure 7.14).

It has been noted that when methotrexate chemotherapy (intrathecal or systemic) is administered in combiniation with CNS radiation, these agents may result in marked white matter changes. It is believed that low doses of radiation alter the blood-brain barrier, allowing increased penetration of methotrexate to neurotoxic levels. This has been noted most frequently in children being treated for leukemia where two specific conditions have been described. The first has been called *mineralizing microangiopathy*, which is seen in up to one-third of these children. The result is diffuse destructive changes to the brain characterized by symmetric corticomedullary junction and basal ganglia calcifications. There is also diffuse signal abnormality throughout the white matter. A more serious but less common complication of combined radiation and methotrexate therapy is called *necro-*

tizing leukoencephalopathy. This process results in widespread damage to the white matter consisting of demyelination, necrosis, and gliosis. Magnetic resonance imaging reveals large, diffuse, confluent areas of white matter signal abnormality with cortical sparing. Clinically these children may have symptoms ranging from slight reduction in cognitive function to progressive dementia, seizures, hemiplegia, and coma.

DYSMYELINATING DISEASES

The disease processes that have been described up until this point are demyelinating, since they represent the destruction of normal myelin. In contrast, the dysmyelinating conditions, also referred to as leukodystrophies, are disorders where myelin is abnormally formed or cannot be maintained in its normal state because of an inherited enzymatic or metabolic disorder. Although most of these conditions are not treatable, establishing a diagnosis is valuable to provide a prognosis, and allow for genetic counseling. These conditions are characterized by the progressive destruction of myelin due to the accumulation of various catabolites, depending on the specific enzyme deficiency. Children often present clinically with progressive mental and motor deterioration. Radiographically, these diseases present with diffuse white matter lesions that are very similar to one another; however, some distinguishing features do exist (Table 7.2). Factors that are helpful in differentiation include the age of onset as well as the pattern of white matter involvement. Ultimately, biochemical and enzymatic analysis allow a specific diagnosis to be made. Dysmyelinating diseases are rather uncommon, and we will focus on a few of the classic conditions.

METACHROMATIC LEUKODYSTROPHY

Metachromatic leukodystrophy is the most common of the leukodystrophies. It is transmitted by an autosomal recessive pattern and is due to a deficiency of the enzyme arylsulfatase A. The most common type is an infantile form, presenting at approximately 2 years of age with gait disorder and mental deterioration. There is steady disease progression with death occurring within 5 years from the time of onset. Magnetic resonance demonstrates progressive symmetrical areas of white matter involvement, which is nonspecific.

ADRENAL LEUKODYSTROPHY

Adrenal leukodystrophy is a sex-linked recessive condition and thus is found only in boys. Typical age of onset is between 5 and 10 years. As the name im-

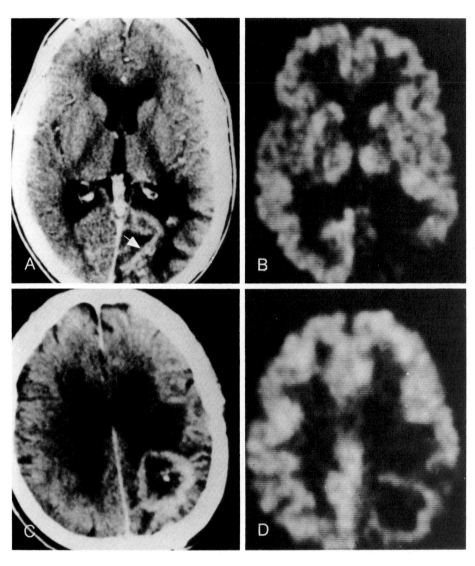

Figure 7.14. Tumor Recurrence. Contrast-enhanced computed tomogram (CT) and positive emission tomogram (PET) (^{18}F-2-fluoro-2-D-deoxyglucose). **A.** The CT reveals a new linear area of enhancement (*arrow*) within the tumor bed 10 months following surgery and focal irradiation for a high-grade glioma. The PET demonstrates no significant activity in this area, suggesting that the enhancement represents radiation necrosis. **B.** A CT of a different patient 6 months following surgery and focal irradiation for a high-grade glioma reveals a focus of ring enhancement. The PET reveals increased metabolic activity in this region, suggesting recurrent tumor.

Table 7.2. Dysmyelinating Diseases

	Head Size	Age of Onset (years)	White Matter Involvement	Gray Matter Involvement
Metachromatic leukodystrophy	Normal	Infantile form 1–2 years Juvenile form 5–7 years	Diffusely affected	None
Adrenoleukodystrophy	Normal	5–10	Symmetric occipital and splenium of corpus callosum	None
Leigh's disease	Normal	<5	Focal areas of subcortical white matter	Basal ganglia and periaqueductal gray
Alexander's disease	Normal to large	≤1	Frontal	None
Canavan's disease	Normal to large	≤1	Diffusely affected	Vacuolization of cortical gray matter

plies, these patients often have symptoms related to the adrenal gland such as adrenal insufficiency or abnormal skin pigmentation. Adrenal leukodystrophy has a striking predilection for the visual and auditory pathways, presenting with symmetric involvement of the periatrial white matter with extension into the splenium of the corpus callosum (Figure 7.15).

LEIGH'S DISEASE

This is also called necrotizing encephalomyelopathy, and commonly manifests in infancy or childhood (usually younger than 5 years). It has histopathologic findings similar to Wernicke's encephalopathy, hence the suspicion that it is related to an inborn defect in

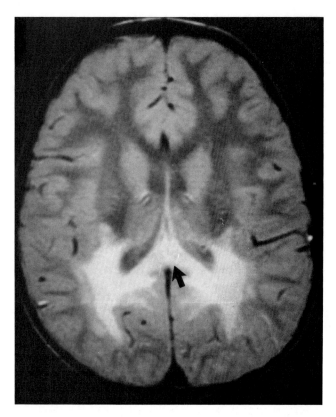

Figure 7.15. Adrenal Leukodystrophy. Adrenal leukodystrophy in a 6-year-old boy who presented with gradual gait disturbance and adrenal insufficiency. Axial T2-weighted image reveals high signal within the occipital white matter extending into the splenium of the corpus callosum (*arrow*).

thiamine metabolism. Clinical findings are extremely variable and often nonspecific. Symmetrical focal necrotic lesions are found in the basal ganglia and thalamus, as well as in the subcortical white matter (Fig. 7.16). Lesions may also extend into the midbrain, medulla, and posterior columns of the spinal cord. A characteristic finding is involvement of the periaqueductal gray matter. However, in contrast to Wernicke-Korsakoff syndrome there is sparing of the mammallary bodies.

ALEXANDER'S AND CANAVAN'S DISEASE

This is the rarest of the leukodystrophies and may appear as early as the first few weeks of life. Patients often have an enlarged brain, and thus have macrocephaly on examination. Typically, these patients present with delayed developmental milestones. In Alexander's disease, white matter lesions often begin in the frontal white matter and progress posteriorly (Figure 7.17).

CEREBROSPINAL FLUID DYNAMICS

In patients with acute hydrocephalus, transependymal flow of CSF may mimic periventricular white matter disease. Cerebrospinal fluid is produced predominately by the choroid plexus of the lateral, third, and fourth ventricles. Cerebrospinal fluid flows from the lateral ventricles into the third ventricle through the foramina of Monro, then by way of the cerebral aqueduct into the fourth ventricle. The CSF leaves the ventricular system via the lateral and medial fourth ventricular foramina, foramen of Luschka and Magendie, respectively. The CSF then travels

Figure 7.16. Leigh's Disease. Leigh's disease in a 2-year-old patient presenting with seizures. Axial T2-weighted sequence demonstrates high signal in the caudate nuclei, and putamina (*arrows*). The involvement of the periaqueductal gray matter (*arrowhead*) is suggestive of Leigh's disease.

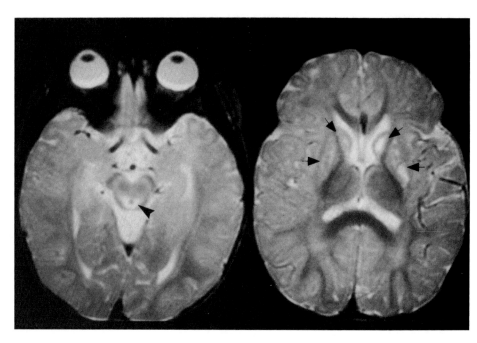

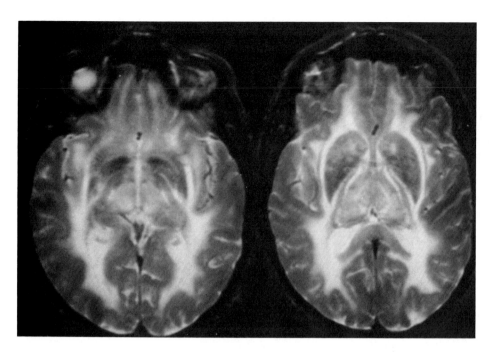

Figure 7.17. Alexander's Disease. Alexander's disease in a 16-month-old child who presented with progressive spastic quadriparesis and macrocephaly. T2-weighted axial images reveal diffuse high signal extending throughout the deep cerebral white matter as well as both the internal and external capsules.

through the basilar cisterns and over the surfaces of the cerebral hemispheres. The principal site of absorption is into the venous circulation through the arachnoid villi, which project into the dural sinuses, primarily the superior sagittal sinus. Although the principal routes of CSF production and absorption are as outlined above, a significant amount of CSF may be both produced and reabsorbed via the ependymal lining of the ventricles. This transependymal flow of CSF can become a very important means of CSF reabsorption during ventricular obstruction.

HYDROCEPHALUS

Hydrocephalus is caused by an obstruction of the CSF circulatory pathway and is classified into two principal types, noncommunicating and communicating. Noncommunicating hydrocephalus refers to an obstruction occurring within the ventricular system, which prevents CSF from exiting the ventricles. In contrast, with communicating hydrocephalus the level of obstruction is beyond the ventricular system, being located within the subarachnoid space. Thus, CSF is able to exit the ventricular system but fails to undergo normal resorption by the arachnoid villi. In communicating hydrocephalus most of the ventricular system is enlarged whereas with noncommunicating hydrocephalus dilation occurs up to the point of obstruction. It should be noted that the fourth ventricle often does not dilate because of the relatively confined nature of the posterior fossa. As a result, communicating hydrocephalus with a normal fourth ventricle may look like noncommunicating hydrocephalus with an obstruction occurring at the level of the aqueduct. Additionally, dilation of the

fourth ventricle is evidence for a communicating hydrocephalus, but not a reliable sign because obstruction at the outlet foramina of the fourth ventricle (Luschka and Magendie) may give a similar appearance.

EX-VACUO VENTRICULOMEGALY

Distinction must be made between hydrocephalus and ex-vacuo ventriculomegally, the result of parenchymal atrophy. With atrophy, the loss of brain matter results in prominence of all CSF spaces, cerebral sulci as well as ventricles. In contrast, with hydrocephalus the ventricles are enlarged but the sulci, especially the sylvian cistern, remain normal or mildly effaced. The third ventricle and temporal horns are particularly helpful in making this distinction. Both of these ventricular spaces are surrounded by tissue that is not typically subject to significant atrophy. The third ventricle is surrounded by the thalamus (gray matter) and there is a relative paucity of white matter in the temporal lobes. This is in contrast to the large amount of white matter surrounding the lateral ventricles, which may become atrophic. Thus, enlargement of the third ventricle with bowing of its lateral and inferior recesses, as well as temporal horn enlargement, suggests hydrocephalus (Fig. 7.18). Bowing and stretching of the corpus callosum, easily detected on the sagittal images, is an additional finding that is suggestive of hydrocephalus.

Subarachnoid hemorrhage and meningitis are the most frequent causes of hydrocephalus, and may result in either communicating or noncommunicating hydrocephalus, with obstruction at any level of the ventricular system, basilar cisterns, or at the arach-

Figure 7.18. Hydrocephalus. Axial first and second echo T2-weighted images in a 67-year-old male with tuberculous meningitis. The ventricles clearly are dilated out of proportion to the cerebral sulci. This finding, in addition to the bowing of the inferior third ventricle recesses (*arrows*), is characteristic for hydrocephalus.

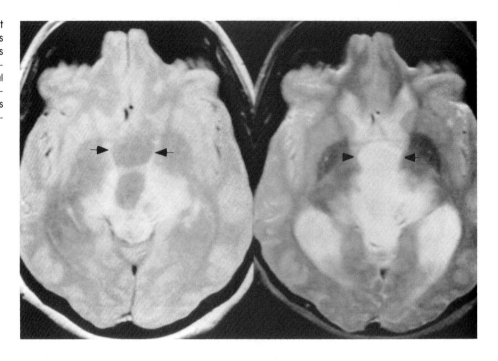

noid villi. The obstruction is because of adhesions and inflammation, and thus no obstructing mass is typically detected. Noncommunicating hydrocephalus can be the result of either an acquired or congenital obstructive process. Benign congenital webs may form across the cerebral aqueduct, resulting in aqueductal stenosis. Additionally, the Chiari and Dandy-Walker malformations are felt to represent adhesions occurring at the outlet foramina of the fourth ventricle and posterior fossa. A variety of neoplasms may result in obstructive hydrocephalus, often in very characteristic locations. Colloid cysts typically block the anterior third ventricle; pineal tumors and tectal gliomas obstruct the aqueduct; and ependymomas and medulloblastomas interrupt CSF flow at the level of the fourth ventricle. Whenever hydrocephalus is detected, it is important to inspect the ventricles for an obstructing mass. A location that should be specifically evaluated is the cerebral aqueduct. On routine axial and sagittal images, a normal pulsatile flow void should be detected, otherwise the diagnosis of aqueductal stenosis should be considered.

The duration of hydrocephalus affects the imaging findings. In acute hydrocephalus there is insufficient time for compensatory mechanisms, and as a result, a striking amount of transependymal CSF flow is noted. This results in a dramatic accumulation of high signal in the periventricular white matter on T2-weighted images. However, in chronic forms of hydrocephalus, compensatory mechanisms have occurred and the degree of transependymal flow is minimal (Figure 7.19).

NEURODEGENERATIVE DISORDERS

Neurodegenerative disorders frequently have no known cause, and result in progressive neurologic deterioration, faster than expected for the patient's given age.

ALZHEIMER'S DISEASE

Alzheimer's disease is the most common neurodegenerative disease and the commonest cause of dementia. Neuroimaging studies demonstrate diffuse atrophy, which is the result of neuronal loss. Although overlap does exist with normal degrees of age-related atrophy, certain regions tend to be more severely affected with Alzheimer's disease. Specifically, the hippocampal formation is consistently and heavily involved; therefore, marked enlargement of the temporal horns, suprasellar cisterns, and sylvian fissures may be useful in discriminating Alzheimer's disease from normal aging.

PARKINSONISM

Parkinsonism is the most common basal ganglia disorder, and one of the leading causes of neurologic disability in individuals over age 60. It is characterized clinically by tremor, muscular rigidity, and loss of postural reflexes. Parkinsonism is a result of a deficiency of the neurotransmitter dopamine caused by dysfunction of the dopaminergic neuronal system, specifically the pars compacta of the substantia nigra. A variety of parkinsonian syndromes exist including Parkinson's disease, progressive supranuclear palsy, and striatonigral degeneration. Idiopathic Parkin-

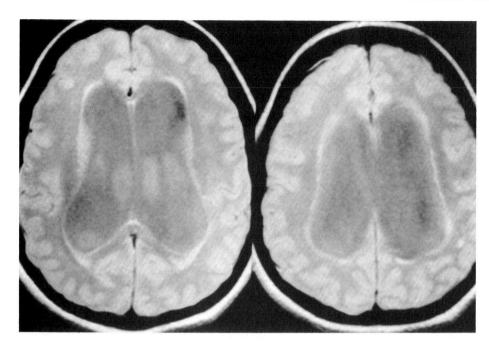

Figure 7.19. Chronic Hydrocephalus. Chronic hydrocephalus in a 40-year-old patient following traumatic subarachnoid hemorrhage. Note that only minimal periventricular transependymal CSF flow is identified on the axial proton density images reflecting the chronic nature of this process. As opposed to acute hydrocephalus where transependymal flow is common, sufficient time has elapsed for compensatory methods of CSF resorption to take place.

son's disease is known as paralysis agitans, and affects 2–3% of the population sometime during their life. Magnetic resonance imaging occasionally may reveal thinning of the pars compacta. The substantia nigra is made of the pars compacta (high-signal intensity band on T2-weighted images) posteriorly, which is sandwiched between the pars reticularis anteriorly and the red nuclei posteriorly. Thus with thinning of the pars compacta, the high-signal intensity band between the pars reticularis and the red nuclei is lost.

NORMAL PRESSURE HYDROCEPHALUS (NPH)

NPH is a chronic form of hydrocephalus. The classic clinical triad is that of dementia, gait disturbance, and urinary incontinence. In this condition, the CSF pressure is within normal limits, but a slight gradient exists between the ventricular system and the subarachnoid space because of an incomplete subarachnoid CSF block. This is most commonly from a previous subarachnoid hemorrhage or meningeal infection. The result is diffuse ventriculomegaly, which is out of proportion to the degree of sulcal prominence. However, differentiating mild hydrocephalus from atrophic ventriculomegaly can be very difficult. In addition to cross-sectional studies, radioisotope studies may be of value. The classic findings on radioisotope cisternogram are early entry of the radiopharmaceutical into the lateral ventricles, with persistence at 24 and 48 hours, and with considerable delay in the ascent to the parasagittal region. Differentiating normal pressure hydrocephalus from atrophic ventriculomegaly can be very difficult on imaging studies, and unfortunately no imaging study is very useful in making this diagnosis. It is important to realize that this is not a radiographic diagnosis, and

close correlation of clinical findings with radiographic results is required in making this diagnosis. The definitive diagnosis is made upon demonstrating clinical improvement following ventricular shunting.

The following are degenerative diseases of the extrapyramidal nuclei.

HUNTINGTON'S DISEASE

Huntington's disease is a progressive hereditary disorder that appears in the 4th and 5th decades. It is characterized by a movement disorder (typically choreathetosis), dementia, and emotional disturbance. Huntington's disease is inherited in an autosomal dominant pattern with complete penetrance. Although neuroimaging studies demonstrate diffuse cortical atrophy, the caudate nucleus and putamen are most severely affected. The caudate atrophy results in characteristic enlargement of the frontal horns, which take on a heart-shape configuration.

WILSON'S DISEASE

Also known as hepatolenticular degeneration, Wilson's disease is an inborn error of copper metabolism that is associated with hepatic cirrhosis and degenerative changes of the basal ganglia. A deficiency of ceruloplasmin (serum transport protein of copper) exists, which results in deposition of toxic levels of copper in various organs. Patients present with varied neurologic and psychiatric findings including dystonia, tremor, and rigidity. The Kayser-Fleischer ring, an intracorneal deposit of copper, is virtually diagnostic of the disease when present (75% of cases). Magnetic resonance findings include diffuse atrophy with signal abnormalities involving the deep gray matter nuclei and deep white matter.

Besides these neurodegenerative diseases, abnormalities of the basal ganglia can be caused by a wide range of etiologies. Toxins such as carbon monoxide or methanol poisoning may result in signal abnormalities of the basal ganglia, characteristically the globus pallidus. Magnetic resonance demonstrates low signal on T1- and high signal on the T2-weighted sequences. Recently, T1-shortening (high signal on T1-weighted image) has been described within the basal ganglia and brainstem associated with hepatic dysfunction, such as hepatic encephalopathy as well as hyperalimentation. The cause of these findings has not been fully determined. Occasionally, calcification of the basal ganglia may also appear as high signal on the T1-weighted sequence. This is the result of the hydration layer effect, where water molecules that are adjacent to the calcification have reduced relaxation times. This is the same effect that causes T1 shortening with proteinaceous fluids. As a result, any condition that results in basal ganglia calcifications may demonstrate T1 shortening within the basal ganglia.

References

1. Scott TF. Diseases that mimic multiple sclerosis. Postgrad Med 1991;89:187–191.
2. Reischies FM, Baum K, Brau H, Hedde JP, Schwindt G. Cerebral magnetic resonance imaging findings in multiple sclerosis. Relation to disturbance of affect, drive, and cognition. Arch Neurol 1988;45:1114–1146.
3. Gutling E; Landis T. CT ring sign imitating tumour, disclosed as multiple sclerosis by MRI: a case report. J Neurol Neurosurg Psychiatry 1989;52:903–906.
4. Honig LS, Sheremata WA. Magnetic resonance imaging of spinal cord lesions in multiple sclerosis. J Neurol Neurosurg Psychiatry 1989;52:459–466.
5. van Swieten JC, van den Hout JH, van Ketel BA, Hijdra A, Wokke JH, van Gijn J. Periventricular lesions in the white matter on magnetic resonance imaging in the elderly. A morphometric correlation with arteriolosclerosis and dilated perivascular spaces. Brain 1991;114:(Pt 2)761–774.
6. Lechner H, Schmidt R, Bertha G, Justich E, Offenbacher H, Schneider G. Nuclear magnetic resonance image white matter lesions and risk factors for stroke in normal individuals. Stroke 1988;19:263–265.
7. Morris JC, Gado M, Torack RM, McKeel DW Jr. Binswanger's disease or artifact: a clinical, neuroimaging, and pathological study of periventricular white matter changes in Alzheimer's disease. Adv Neurol 1990;51:47–52.
8. Gean-Marton AD, Vezina LG, Marton KI, et al. Abnormal corpus callosum: a sensitive and specific indicator of multiple sclerosis. Radiology 1991;180:215–219.
9. Gean AD, Weinstein MA. New MR imaging findings in multiple sclerosis. Radiology 1991;179:591–594.
10. Sze G, De Armond SJ, Brant–Zawadzki M, Davis RL, Norman D, Newton TH. Foci of MRI signal (pseudo lesions) anterior to the frontal horns: histologic correlations of a normal finding. AJR 1986;147:331–337.
11. Heier LA, Bauer CJ, Schwartz L, Zimmerman RD, Morgello S, Deck MD. Large Virchow-Robin spaces: MR-clinical correlation. Am J Neuroradiol 1989;10:929–936.
12. Trotot PM, Vazeux R, Yamashita HK, et al. MRI pattern of progressive multifocal leukoencephalopathy (PML) in AIDS. Pathological correlations. J Neuroradiol 1990;17:233–254.
13. Olsen WL, Longo FM, Mills CM, Norman D. White matter disease in AIDS: findings at MR imaging. Radiology 1988;169:445–448.
14. Boulloche J, Parain D, Mallet E, Tron P. Postinfectious encephalitis with multifocal white matter lesions. Neuropediatrics 1989;20:173–175.
15. Miller DH, Robb SA, Ormerod IE, et al. Magnetic resonance imaging of inflammatory and demyelinating white-matter diseases of childhood. Dev Med Child Neurol 1990;32:97–107.
16. Fernandez RE, Rothberg M, Ferencz G, Wujack D. Lyme disease of the CNS: MR imaging findings in 14 cases. Am J Neuroradiol 1990;11:479–481.
17. Miller GM, Baker HL Jr, Okazaki H, Whisnant JP. Central pontine myelinolysis and its imitators: MR findings. Radiology 1988;168:795–802.

8

Pediatric Neuroimaging

Todd E. Lempert

Specific areas of pediatric neuroimaging are sufficiently different from adult neuroimaging to warrant a separate discussion in this chapter. These areas are normal patterns of myelination, hypoxic ischemic brain injury, congenital lesions, migration anomalies, and phakomatoses (neurocutaneous syndromes).

IMAGING PARAMETERS/SEDATION

Magnetic resonance imaging (MR) has established itself as the procedure of choice for pediatric neuroimaging, although specific situations where ultrasound and computed tomography (CT) scanning remain advantageous will be described.

Sedation is usually required for children under 6 years old. Pediatric sedation protocols should be performed in conjunction with pulse oximetry monitoring at a minimum. A pediatric-equipped crash cart should be available along with personnel who are skilled at pediatric sedation techniques. Pediatric Advanced Life Support (PALS) training, a course offered through the American Heart Association, provides a useful review for radiologists.

NORMAL PATTERNS OF MYELINATION

Any discussion of pediatric neuroimaging has to begin with normal myelination as a frame of reference. T1- and T2-weighted sequences allow observation of the myelination process. T1-weighted images provide a detailed view of actively myelinating structures in the first 8 months of life. Areas that become myelinated stand out as high signal on T1-weighted images against a background of low signal intensity, unmyelinated white matter. This is because the myelin sheath (a lipid) is hydrophobic; therefore, myelinated white matter has a decreased amount of water, the source of mobile hydrogen protons, which form the basis of the MR signal. An oversimplified memory aid is to remember that myelinated white matter parallels the signal intensity of fat on T1- and T2-weighted sequences.

Heavily weighted T2-images (long TR/TE = 3000/120) are recommended in the age range of 0–12 months. The water content of the infant brain is high, and heavily T2-weighted images are needed to discriminate between many brain structures that have similar long T2 relaxation times. The myelination landmarks given in Table 8.1 are based on sequences performed at 1.5 tesla. Other field strength magnets may show differing patterns of myelination with the patients age.

At birth, normal myelination by MR imaging generally involves the dorsal lentiform nucleus, lateral geniculate nucleus, dorsal brainstem, cerebellar peduncles, ventrolateral thalamus, posterior limb of the internal capsule, and corticospinal tract extending into the perirolandic (pre- and postcentral) white matter Fig. 8.1).

T1-weighted images are useful for assessing myelination in the first 8 months, thereafter the T2-weighted images become more important. In general, myelination proceeds from dorsal to ventral, caudad to cephalad, and from central to peripheral.

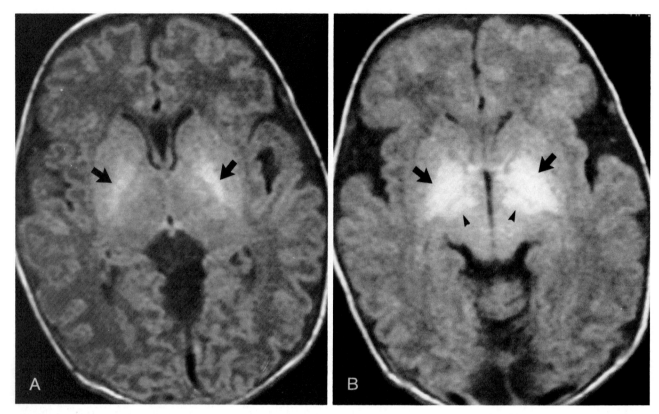

Figure 8.1.   Normal Myelination—Newborn. T1-weighted image of a newborn infant. **A.** The level of the internal capsule shows normal high signal intensity of the posterior limb of the internal capsule (*arrows*). Note the absence of high signal intensity in the anterior limb.

B. At a slightly lower level, the ventral lateral thalamus (*arrowheads*) and lentiform nuclei (*arrows*) are high signal intensity, consistent with myelination in these areas present at birth.

Table 8.1.   Myelination Landmarks By Age

Age (months)	Location/Appearance
Newborn	Dorsal brainstem, ventrolateral thalamus, lentiform nucleus, central corticospinal tracts: high signal, T1
	Posterior limb internal capsule posterior portion: low signal, T2
3	Anterior limb internal capsule: high signal, T1
	Cerebellar white matter: high signal, T1
4	Splenium of corpus callosum: high signal, T1
	Centrum semiovale: high signal, T1
6	Genu of corpus callosum: high signal, T1
	Splenium of corpus callosum: low signal, T2
8	Subcortical white matter: high signal, T1
	Genu: low signal, T2
11	Anterior limb internal capsule: low signal, T2
14	Occipital white matter: low signal, T2
16	Frontal white matter: low signal, T2
18	Adult appearance except for terminal myelination zones periatrial, adjacent to frontal horns

Evaluation of every pediatric brain image obtained by MR should begin with an assessment of myelin development. This important step will help determine the presence or absence of myelination delay and provide a framework for interpretation of suspected neuropathology.

The anterior limb of the internal capsule demonstrates high signal intensity on T1-weighted images by 3 months (Fig. 8.2). The corpus callosum provides the next set of landmarks, with the splenium becoming high signal on T1-weighted images by 4 months and the genu by 6 months. At 6 months the splenium becomes low signal intensity on T2-weighted images, but the unmyelinated peripheral white matter remains high signal (Fig. 8.3). With growth, the deep white matter gradually assumes the adult low signal intensity on T2-weighted images, with some high signal intensity persisting in the terminal myelination zones on T2-weighted images (Figs. 8.4 and 8.5).

Delayed Myelination. The differential diagnosis of delayed myelination includes a wide variety of disorders, including in utero insult (e.g., hypoxic ischemia or infection), metabolic/nutritional disorders, and leukodystrophy (Pelizaeus-Merzbacher disease). Delayed myelination also shows excellent correlation with clinical measures of developmental delay.

In utero insults have been shown to cause delayed myelination in both premature and term neonates. Look for other findings of hypoxic ischemic injury (HII) in conjunction with myelination delay. Nutritional deficiencies due to diet or malabsorption syndromes cause myelination delay because of an inade-

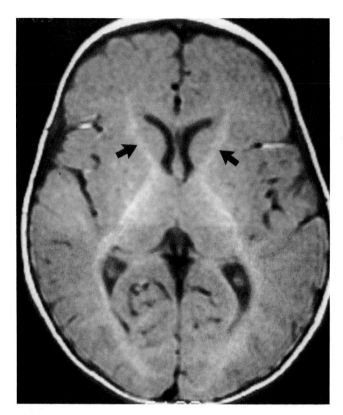

Figure 8.2. Normal Myelination—3 Months. Axial T1-weighted image of a 3-month-old infant. The level of the internal capsule shows extension of high signal into the anterior limb of the internal capsule, reflecting progressive myelination of this region (*arrows*).

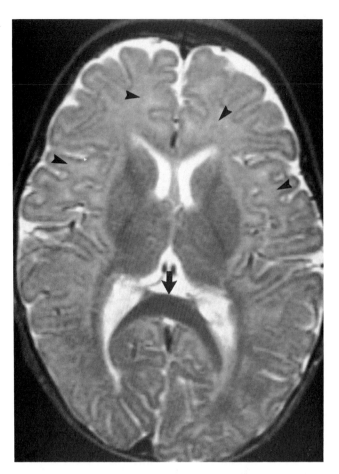

Figure 8.3. Normal Myelination—6 Months. Axial T2-weighted image of a 6-months-old infant at the level of the corpus callosum. The splenium of the corpus callosum is low signal intensity on T2-weighted images (*arrow*), but the unmyelinated deep and superficial cerebral white matter is high signal intensity (*arrowheads*).

quate supply of myelin precursors. Similarly, inborn errors of metabolism (amino and organic acidopathies) cause delayed myelination.

Pelizaeus-Merzbacher Disease is a rare X-linked leukodystrophy that demonstrates an arrest of myelin development, usually in the neonatal period. It can mimic other etiologies of delayed myelination because it shows lack of myelin formation only, not myelin formation followed by destruction (typical of many other leukodystrophies). A follow-up scan can be helpful in detecting a pattern of arrested myelination such as Pelizaeus-Merzbacher disease.

Developmental delay is a nonspecific term, used because of the large percentage of cases of myelination delay that have no known cause, but are related to a clinical diagnosis of developmental retardation (developmental function less than 80% of chronologic age).

In summary, if a particular MR scan shows myelination delay (corrected for any prematurity), a careful search for additional clues may yield a diagnosis.

HYPOXIC ISCHEMIC BRAIN INJURY

Unfortunately, HII is very common in the pediatric population. Knowledge of brain development and the reproducible patterns of brain damage can help answer questions about the severity of the insult and the timing of the injury. Patterns of brain injury can be divided into first and second trimester, late third trimester and perinatal, and postnatal. These patterns are summarized in Table 8.2.

The first and second trimesters of embryonic growth are characterized by rapid development of key brain structures. Hypoxic ischemic insults to the developing brain at this time are often severe and may arrest or alter further brain development. Hypoxic ischemic injury can be broadly divided into focal HII and diffuse HII. Focal HII causes an arrest/alteration in brain development manifested as focal cell migration disorders. Diffuse HII leads to generalized damage as seen in entities such as hydranencephaly and cortical dysplasias.

Hydranencephaly represents ischemic infarction of both cerebral hemispheres, and is believed to be due to early occlusion of both carotid arteries, or possibly a severe in utero infection. The pattern of destruction is characterized by little or no supratentorial brain tissue (Fig. 8.6). Another pattern that mimics this appearance is early severe hydrocephalus,

Table 8.2.   Imaging of Hypoxic Ischemic Brain Injury

Time	Deep Gray	Cortex	Other
1st Trimester	Spared	Cortical dysplasias Hydranencephaly	
<26 Weeks	Spared	Spared	Periatrial injury No gliosis Ex vacuo enlargement
>28 Weeks	Spared	Spared	Periatrial gliosis: high signal, T2
Term	Spared	Watershed infarcts Ulegyria	Variable deep, superficial white matter gliosis and atrophy Myelination delay Injury to hippocampi, pons

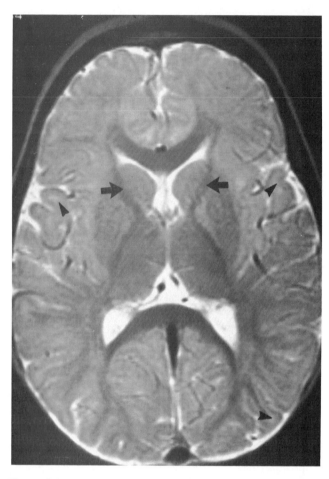

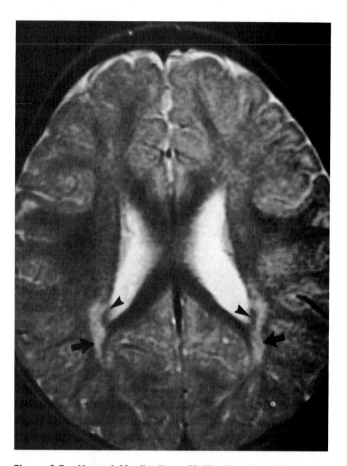

Figure 8.4.   Normal Myelination—11 Months. Axial T2-weighted image of an 11-month-old infant at the level of the atria of the lateral ventricles. Note that the anterior limb of the internal capsule is now low signal on T2-weighted images (*arrows*). There has been progressive myelination of central white matter (low signal), but the subcortical white matter (*arrowheads*) is still unmyelinated and high signal intensity.

Figure 8.5.   Normal Myelination—18 Months. Axial T2-weighted image of a normal 18-month-old infant. The process of normal myelination is essentially complete except for terminal myelination zones, which show persistent high signal (*arrows*) in the periatrial region. A thin hypointense band of white matter separates the terminal myelination zone from the atrial margin (*arrowheads*).

although in cases of hydrocephalus, a thin rind of cortical gray matter is usually evident, whereas in hydranencephaly there is usually nearly complete infarction of all supratentorial cerebral tissues in the vascular distribution of the carotid arteries with preservation of the thalami and cerebellum.

Hypoxic ischemic injury is a common type of insult (along with in utero infection) that causes disorders of neuronal migration and cortical dysplasias. This is because any severe insult to the developing brain can lead to an arrest of normal neuronal migration. Disorders of neuronal migration are described in "Migration Anomalies."

Injuries in the second and third trimester correlate with the location of arterial border zones, which are areas uniquely sensitive to watershed infarction. These border zones, in general, move centrifugally as the brain develops. The zones start in the immediate

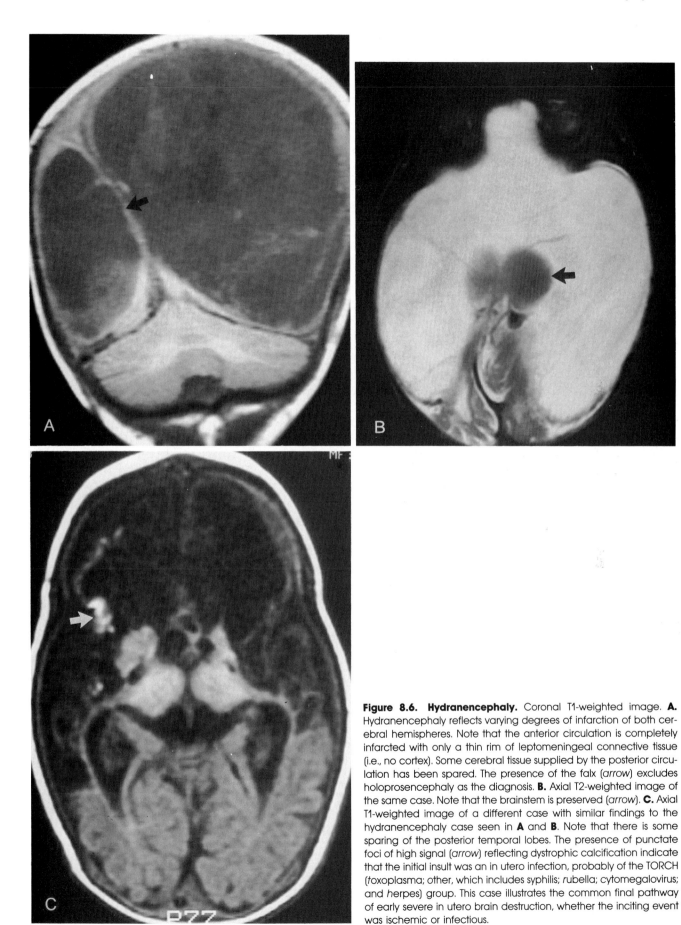

Figure 8.6. Hydranencephaly. Coronal T1-weighted image. **A.** Hydranencephaly reflects varying degrees of infarction of both cerebral hemispheres. Note that the anterior circulation is completely infarcted with only a thin rim of leptomeningeal connective tissue (i.e., no cortex). Some cerebral tissue supplied by the posterior circulation has been spared. The presence of the falx (*arrow*) excludes holoprosencephaly as the diagnosis. **B.** Axial T2-weighted image of the same case. Note that the brainstem is preserved (*arrow*). **C.** Axial T1-weighted image of a different case with similar findings to the hydranencephaly case seen in **A** and **B**. Note that there is some sparing of the posterior temporal lobes. The presence of punctate foci of high signal (*arrow*) reflecting dystrophic calcification indicate that the initial insult was an in utero infection, probably of the TORCH (*t*oxoplasma; *o*ther, which includes syphilis; *r*ubella; *c*ytomegalovirus; and *h*erpes) group. This case illustrates the common final pathway of early severe in utero brain destruction, whether the inciting event was ischemic or infectious.

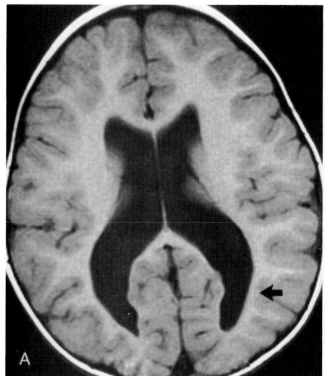

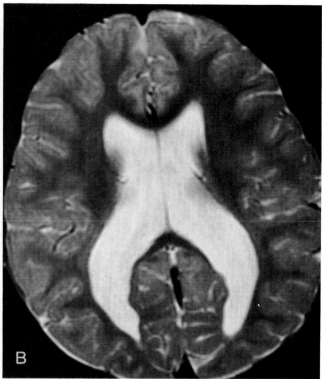

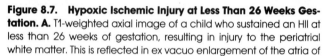

Figure 8.7. Hypoxic Ischemic Injury at Less Than 26 Weeks Gestation. A. T1-weighted axial image of a child who sustained an HII at less than 26 weeks of gestation, resulting in injury to the periatrial white matter. This is reflected in ex vacuo enlargement of the atria of the lateral ventricles. The severe periatrial white matter thinning has resulted in close apposition of a sulcus to the ventricular margin (*arrow*). **B.** The lack of periventricular gliosis is consistent with an insult occurring at 26 weeks of gestational age or less.

periventricular region and move outward into more peripheral white matter and cortical gray matter. Hence, injuries to second- and third-trimester fetuses are characterized by ischemic infarction in the periatrial and, less commonly, periventricular border zones. These areas of peritrigonal white matter undergo neuronal loss, leading to atrophy. The resulting atrial margin is often crenulated where necrotic periventricular white matter cysts have been incorporated. The loss of white matter leads to ex vacuo enlargement of the atria. Fetuses less than 26 weeks do not exhibit a significant response of gliosis. Therefore, HII to fetuses less than 26 weeks causes periventricular (periatrial) white matter thinning and atrial enlargement (Fig. 8.7).

Periventricular Leukomalacia. After 26 weeks, the brain responds to HII by gliosis in the periatrial region. Damage to the periventricular region is termed periventricular leukomalacia. This is best seen on proton-density weighted images. Periventricular leukomalacia can be differentiated from the normal peritrigonal terminal myelination zones by noting an extension of high signal on T2-weighted images to the ventricular margin. This is due to a loss of the normal thin myelinated white matter roof (tapetum) of the atrium of the lateral ventricle. Periatrial white matter

thinning and atrial enlargement are also evident (Fig. 8.8).

In the late third trimester and perinatal period there is continuing centrifugal extension of the arterial border zones sensitive to watershed infarction. Infants born at term who sustain insults during this period will demonstrate infarcts in the peripheral white matter and cortex (Fig. 8.9). Watershed infarctions occur at border zone regions between arterial distributions of major cerebral vessels.

The important border zones are (*a*) in the parasagittal cerebrum, between anterior and middle cerebral arteries. This leads to an apearance of bilateral infarcts in the paramedian cortex, and subsequent gliosis of subcortical white matter. (*b*) The posterior convexity, between the anterior, middle, and posterior cerebral arteries is another important border zone. Hypoxic ischemic injury shows bilateral parieto-occipital watershed infarcts. (*c*) Also inportant is the medial surface between the anterior and posterior cerebral arteries. Other brain areas affected by HII include the mesial temporal lobes (hippocampus). The temporal lobe infarcts may evolve to cause ex vacuo enlargement of the temporal horn of the lateral ventricle and/or mesial temporal sclerosis. Mesial temporal sclerosis is a condition characterized by neuronal loss and gliosis confined to the hippocampus, leading to

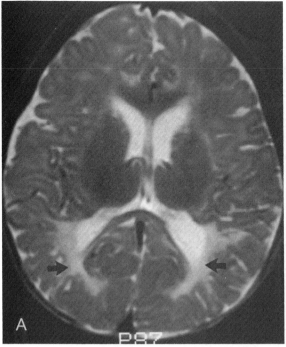
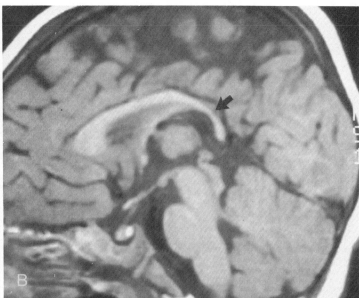

Figure 8.8.   Periventricular Leukomalacia. A. Axial T2-weighted image of a child who sustained an in utero HII later than 26 weeks of gestational age, resulting in periventricular leukomalacia. Note the high signal intensity due to gliosis in the periatrial region (*arrows*) that extends to the ventricular margin. **B.** Hypoxic ischemic injury causes white matter injury and subsequent white matter loss, as evidenced by thinning of the posterior corpus callosum, on this sagittal T1-weighted image (*arrow*).

partial complex seizures. A remodeling of subcortical infarcts occurring in the depths of sulci that spare the overlying gyri form a charactristic pattern of mushroom-shaped gyri called ulegyria.

The brainstem may be affected with selective neuronal loss of cranial nerve nuclei or neurons of the pons (pontosubicular necrosis). The Purkinje cells of the cerebellum also appear to be sensitive to HII.

Term infants with HII can also demonstrate gliosis of affected periventricular white matter, ex vacuo ventricular enlargement, and resulting apposition of sulci to the ventricular surface because of white matter loss, a pattern we saw with periventricular leukomalacia. Associated sequelae of HII include delayed myelination and thinning of large white matter tracts such as the corpus callosum.

Remember, term infants will primarily show peripheral damage corresponding to peripheral border zones. Periatrial damage, white matter loss, and delayed myelination are associated findings. Thus, the patterns of in utero HII can be correlated with gestational age (Table 8.2).

Hypoxic Ischemic Injury and the Premature Infant

Premature infants present special challenges because we often image the brain of infants that are developmentally immature. The first step is to under-

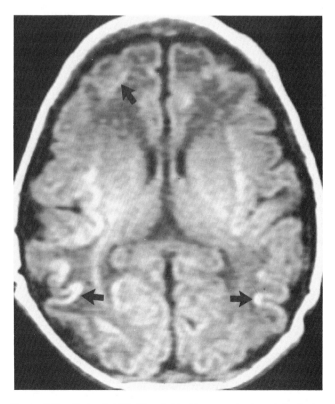

Figure 8.9.   Perinatal HII. T1-weighted image of a term infant who sustained partial HII injury in the perinatal period. Peripheral (cortical) hemorrhagic petechial infarcts (*arrows*) are seen in anterior and posterior watershed distributions.

Figure 8.10. Grade I Subependymal Hemorrhage. Neonatal neurosonogram. The coronal plane shows echogenic foci (*arrows*) anterior to the caudothalamic groove, consistent with grade I echogenic subependymal hemorrhage.

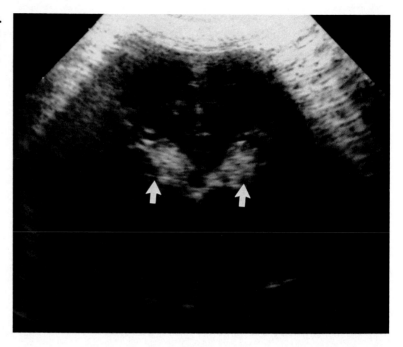

stand the degree of prematurity and subtract the intervening time interval. For example, if we image an infant that is 2 months old, but was delivered 2 months prematurely, we would expect to see the appearance of a newborn term infant. Premature infants are also special because extrauterine life places many severe stresses on the developmentally immature brain. Premature infants still have periventricular border zones of sensitivity to HII. Damage to the periventricular regions, leading to varying degrees of periventricular leukomalacia, is common in premature infants. In severe cases, white matter undergoes cystic necrosis and subsequently becomes incorporated into the margins of the ventricle.

Germinal Matrix Hemorrhage. The germinal matrix, a zone of proliferating, richly vascularized neuroectodermal cells, is also exquisitely sensitive to injury. The response of this region to disturbances in cardiorespiratory function, whether caused by apnea, hypoxia, acidosis, bradycardia, unstable blood pressure, or impaired cerebral blood flow autoregulation, lead to rupture and hemorrhage of fragile blood vessels within the germinal matrix. Premature infants at risk for germinal matrix hemorrhage are best evaluated by serial neonatal neurosonography. Isolated germinal matrix hemorrhage, termed grade I subependymal hemorrhage, has the typical sonographic acute appearance of an echogenic focus directly anterior to the caudothalamic notch (Fig. 8.10). The original hemorrhage eventually matures, either by disappearing entirely or evolving into a subependymal cyst. Bleeding may occur in the germinal matrix alone, or dissect into the parenchyma, or rupture into the ventricle (Fig. 8.11). Table 8.3 presents the classification system used for germinal matrix hemorrhage.

Term infants rarely have subependymal hemorrhage since developmentally, their germinal matrix has involuted and their arterial border zones have moved peripherally. This leads to a number of useful rules.

1. Isolated periventricular leukomalacia in the term infant is only rarely due to birth-related hypoxic ischemic events.
2. Gliosis in the periatrial region (seen best on proton-density scans) is due to injury to the developing brain at 28 weeks' gestational age or older.
3. Ex vacuo atrial enlargement without gliosis reflects injury prior to 26 weeks.

Profound versus Partial Hypoxic Ischemic Brain Injury

Differing injury patterns can be detected by MR, which distinguishes between term infants subjected to severe hypoxic ischemic insults, and those with milder or partial episodes of hypoxia/anoxia. Examples of profound hypoxic ischemic events include full cardiorespiratory arrest and complete placental abruption. The MR appearance will vary depending on the age of the patient and whether the injury is evaluated acutely, subacutely, or in the chronic phase.

Profound Perinatal HII tends to damage central brain areas with relative sparing of the cerebral cortex. Evaluated acutely (immediate to 3 days) by CT scanning, these infants may show injury to deep gray matter structures (basal ganglia and thalamus) with relative cortical sparing. In newborn infants this may lead to the peculiar appearance of deep gray matter

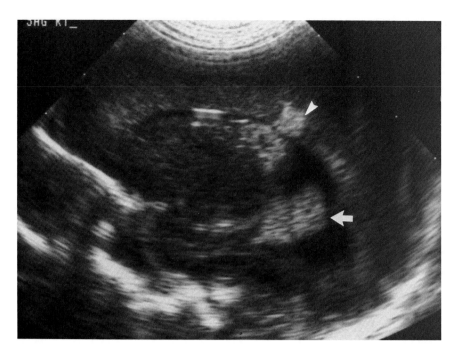

Figure 8.11. Grade IV Subependymal Hemorrhage. Parasagittal neonatal neurosonogram. This grade IV hemorrhage demonstrates an echogenic irregular choroid (*arrow*), reflecting adherent clot. Ventriculomegaly is also seen. The intraparenchymal extension of hemorrhage signifying a grade IV bleed is evident as an echogenic focus extending out from the ventricle (*arrowhead*).

Table 8.3. Classification of Subependymal Hemorrhage

Grade	Location/Appearance	Prognosis
I	Subependymal only, uni/bilateral	80% normal or mild neurodevelopmental impairment
	Echogenic focus seen anterior to caudothalamic groove	
II	Transependymal rupture into ventricle	75% normal or mild impairment
	Echogenic cast of clot in ventricle	
	Irregular contour of choroid suggests adherent clot	
	Echogenic clot dangles into occipital horn	
	Ventricle not expanded	
	Follow-up required to exclude hyrocephalus	
III	Similar to grade II but ventricle expanded	Increased morbidity
	Follow-up required to exclude hydrocephalus	Increased incidence of permanent hydrocephalus
IV	Intraparenchymal extension of hemorrhage	43% severe impairment
	Sequelae may be porencephalic cyst	Higher mortality, permanent hydrocephalus rate

structures becoming isodense to surrounding white matter, a very subtle abnormality.

Profound HII in the perinatal period evaluated acutely (up to 3 weeks) by MR will show mottled, globular high signal on T1-weighted images in the basal ganglia (posterolateral lentiform), and ventral/lateral thalamus (Fig. 8.12). These same areas show mottled low signal intensity on T2-weighted images. The signal intensity abnormalities may reflect hemorrhagic byproducts. Additionally, similar signal intensity abnormalities may be present in the tegmentum of the midbrain, lateral geniculate nuclei, and hippocampi (Fig. 8.13). The cortical damage is not often readily apparent in the acute phase.

In the subacute period (3 weeks to 3 months), the signal intensity of the basal ganglia damage may be variable on T2-weighted images. Damage to the cortex and white matter becomes more evident.

Profound HII in the perinatal period evaluated chronically (>3 months) predominantly shows evolv-

ing injury to central gray matter: the posterolateral lentiform nuclei, and ventral/lateral thalami. The small area of cortex involved is the perirolandic cortex (pre- and postcentral gyri). The affected areas evaluated chronically have evolved in their appearance because of atrophy and gliosis (high signal on T2-weighted images) (Fig. 8.14). Table 8.4 summarizes the imaging findings in profound perinatal hypoxic ischemic brain injury.

The basal ganglia regions are also extremely sensitive to toxic and metabolic processes and will exhibit a relatively nonspecific response to these nonhypoxic insults as well (Fig. 8.15).

Profound Postnatal HII tends to injure a much larger proportion of cerebral cortex, with relative sparing of the perirolandic cortex. Postnatal HII damages the corpus striatum (globus pallidas, putamen, caudate) and tends to spare the thalamus (Table 8.5).

Partial Perinatal HII. Partial or milder hypoxic ischemic events in the perinatal period tend to spare

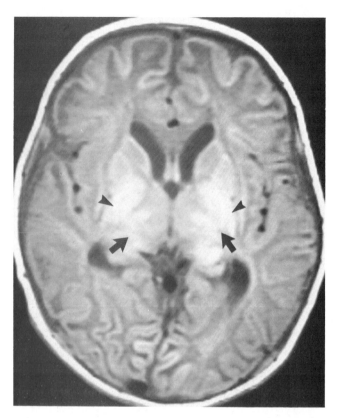

Figure 8.12. Profound Perinatal HII—Acute. Axial T1-weighted image of a term infant evaluated acutely by MR. Mottled high signal intensity is seen in the posterolateral lentiform nuclei, (*arrowheads*) and ventrolateral thalami (*arrows*). These high signal intensity areas most likely represent blood breakdown products.

central brain areas and will damage more peripheral gray matter. These peripheral infarcts are often located in watershed zones as previously described. The peripheral infarcts will often progress over time to petechial gyral hemorrhage and eventually to areas of cortical thinning. Marked diminution and high signal on T2-weighted images of the subcortical and deep white matter is also seen.

Acute hypoxic ischemic damage can be difficult to discern in newborn infants. Here are some helpful hints.

1. Unmyelinatined white matter is bright on T2-weighted images, making infarcts less apparent.
2. T1-weighted images can be a source of confusion. Do not confuse normal areas of T1 hyperintensity in areas of normal active myelination (basal ganglia, thalami, cerebral peduncles, perirolandic white matter) with the petechial hemorrhage due to profound HII. Petechial hemorrhage occurs in the putamina and thalami as punctate clumps on T1-weighted images and as blurred normal margins between the posterior limb of the internal capsule and the thalamus on T2-weighted images. Subtle punctate hyperintensity of a gyrus may in-

dicate petechial hemorrhage on T1-weighted images.
3. Cerebral edema is often not well seen on MR images. A CT scan may be more appropriate.
4. An extremely useful sign of infarction is the loss of normal gray matter hypointensity amidst a sea of hyperintense (unmyelinated) white matter on T2-weighted images.

Prolonged partial HII in the perinatal period evaluated acutely may show a global pattern of injury and severe low density of the cerebral hemispheres on CT scanning, due to diffuse edema. The cerebellum is relatively resistant to injury, leading to the "white cerebellum" sign. The CT sign shows a normal cerebellum appearing relatively white against a background of edematous supratentorial brain. Magnetic resonance imaging appears relatively insensitive to signs of edema in infants, and CT is still the preferred modality for assessing supratentorial brain edema. A correlate, however, to the CT white cerebellum sign has been described. This is the "'dark cerebellum sign" on MR. The normal cerebellum appears uniformly dark compared with the relatively hyperintense ischemic supratentorial brain.

Summary

The developing brain shows continually shifting areas of brain vulnerability to HII and changing brain response. A general knowledge of these regions and the evolving response of the damaged brain is necessary to sort out differing patterns of brain injury. Ultrasound is the best modality for demonstrating germinal matrix hemorrhage. Computed tomography is useful in demonstrating early signs of brain edema and hemorrhage. Magnetic resonance imaging is able to demonstrate many of the characteristic conditions associated with HII, including selective neuronal loss, watershed infarction, selective thalamic and basal ganglia necrosis, pontosubicular necrosis, hippocampal necrosis, periventricular leukomalacia, white matter thinning, and delayed myelination.

CONGENITAL LESIONS

Congenital lesions cannot be lumped into convenient categories by appearance. Most are "'Aunt Minnies," i.e., unique in their appearance. Some of the entities that share common features are clustered together.

Septo-Optic Dysplasia

Septo-optic dysplasia is defined as hypoplasia of the optic nerves and absence of the septum pellucidum. Complete or partial absence of the septum pellucidum can be seen. There is also variable hypo-

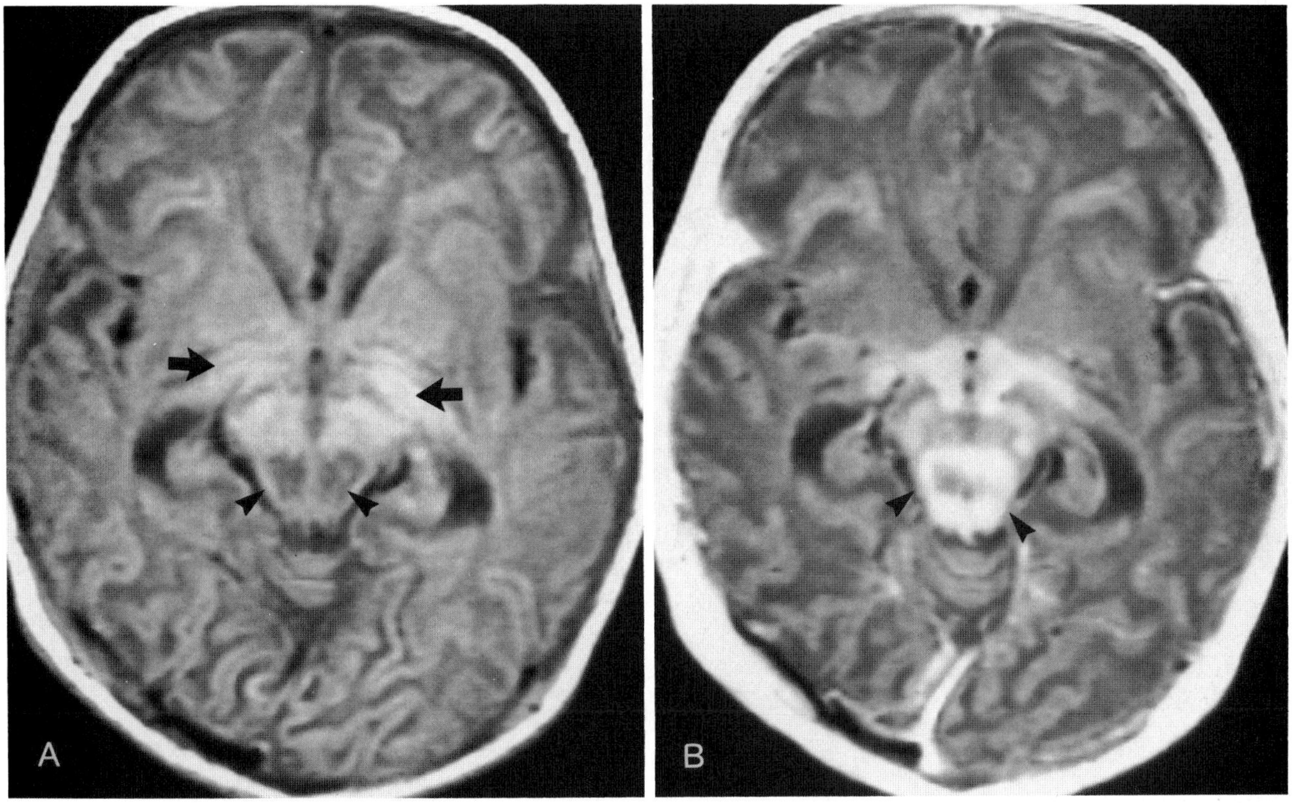

Figure 8.13. Profound Perinatal HII—Acute. A. T1-weighted image at the level of the midbrain (same case as in Fig. 8.12). Mottled high signal intensity is seen in the lateral geniculate nuclei (*arrows*) and abnormal low signal is seen in the midbrain tegmentum (*arrowheads*). The actively myelinating regions such as the midbrain teg- mentum are particularly susceptible to injury. **B.** T1 axial image following gadolinium administration shows blood-brain barrier breakdown caused by ischemia in the midbrain tegmentum (*arrowheads*).

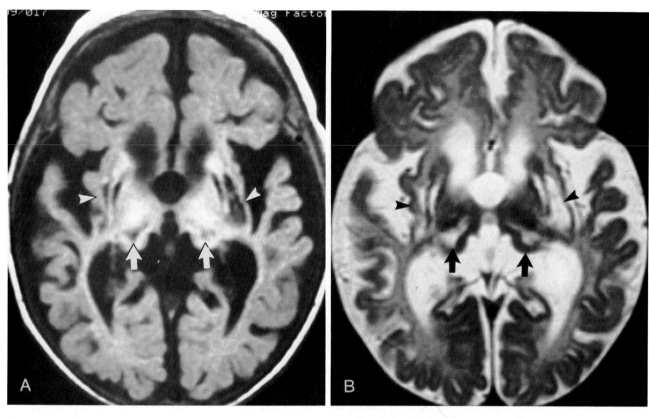

Figure 8.14.   Profound Perinatal HII—Chronic. Profound perinatal HII in a term infant evaluated chronically shows the evolving changes on MR. **A.** T1-weighted image shows neuronal loss in the posterolateral lentiform (*arrowheads*) and ventrolateral thalami (*ar-* *rows*). Marked periatrial white matter atrophy is also seen. **B.** T2-weighted image shows high signal intensity in the posterolateral lentiform (*arrowheads*) and ventrolateral thalami (*arrows*) caused by neuronal loss and gliosis.

Table 8.4.   Imaging of Profound Perinatal HII[a]

Time	Deep Gray (PLL, VLT[b])	Cortex	Other
Acute	Isodense to white matter on CT Mottled high signal, T1 Mottled low signal, T2	Normal	
Subacute	Variable signal, T1, T2	Perirolandic cortex: high signal, T2; Low signal, T2	Atrophy: hippocampi, lateral geniculate, midbrain tegmentum Deep, superficial perirolandic white matter gliosis and atrophy, high signal, T2 variable myelination delay
Chronic	High signal, T2	Perirolandic cortex: high signal, T2; Thinned gyri, atrophy	Atrophy: hippocampi, lateral geniculate, midbrain tegmentum Deep, superficial perirolandic white matter gliosis and atrophy, high signal, T2 variable myelination delay

[a]Adapted from Barkovich AJ. MR and CT evaluation of profound neonatal and infantile asphyxia. AJNR 1992;13:959–972.
[b]PLL, posterolateral lentiform; VLT, ventrolatral thalamus.

plasia of the optic nerves. A fundoscopic examination of the optic nerves is often a helpful correlate (Fig. 8.16). Endocrine abnormalities are common, as well as associated migration anomalies.

Holoprosencephaly

This spectrum of disorders classified as alobar, semilobar, and lobar holoprosencephaly all relate to failed cleavage of the developing brain. Holoprosencephaly also presents with orbital hypotelorism and varying degrees of facial dysmorphism.

Alobar Holoprosencephaly. The alobar form is a severe malformation with a dismal prognosis. This type of holoprosencephaly is distinctive, consisting an anterior rind of brain tissue and a posterior monoventricle which communicates with a dorsal cyst. The thalami are fused and the septum pellucidum, corpus callosum, and falx are absent (Fig. 8.17).

This form of holoprosencephaly only really needs to be discriminated from two other entities— hydranencephaly, which represents bilateral in utero cerebral hemisphere infarction, and severe hydrocephalus, with secondary pressure atrophy of the septum pellucidum. A reliable discriminating sign of alobar holoprosencephaly are the tips of the upside-down U-shaped mantle of brain tissue. These ends of the "'U" are known as the hippocampal ridges, and are best seen in the axial plane.

Semilobar Holoprosencephaly is less severe, and shows partial fusion of the hemispheres. The corpus callosum and the septum pellucidum are absent or dysgenic. There is a high association with migration anomalies (abnormalities of cortical development) (Fig. 8.18). The posterior portion of the interhemispheric fissure and falx are usually formed in cases of semilobar holoprosencephaly.

Lobar Holoprosencephaly is characterized by a more normal-appearing brain. Typically, there is partial absence of a frontal interhemispheric fissure. The absent septum pellucidum and the relatively normal brain gives this entity an overlap with septo-optic dysplasia. The body and splenium of the corpus callosum are usually present with the genu and rostrum absent (dysgenic corpus callosum).

The absence of the septum pellucidum is a constant helpful feature of the holoprosencephalies. Any portion of a visible septum pellucidum excludes holoprosencephaly, and should prompt consideration of severe hydrocephalus or agenesis of the corpus callosum. Remember, absence of the septum pellucidum is strongly associated with other malformations, including anomalies of the face and cerebral cortex (schizencephaly, polymicrogyria, and pachygyria). Coronal T1 images are extremely helpful in demonstrating a narrow portion of hemisphere fusion, confirming the diagnosis of holoprosencephaly.

Agenesis of the Corpus Callosum

The corpus callosum forms from front to back and myelinates from back to front. These facts help discriminate a number of callosal anomalies and mye-

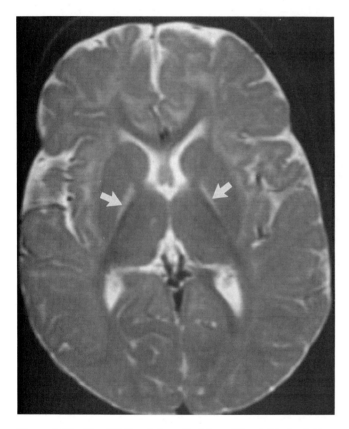

Figure 8.15. Non-HII Basal Ganglia Injury. T2-weighted axial image of a child at the level of the basal ganglia. A wide variety of metabolic and inflammatory insults can affect the basal ganglia. In this case, neonatal kernicterus has damaged the basal ganglia (globus pallidus) (*arrows*) and the subthalamic nuclei (not shown), a somewhat different pattern than HII. This case illustrates the relatively nonspecific response of the basal ganglia to *non*hypoxic ischemic injury. (Courtesy of Dr. Majeed Al-Mateen.)

Table 8.5. Imaging of Profound Postnatal HII[a]

Deep Gray Matter	Cortex	Other
Damage to corpus striatum: high signal, T2	Majority of cortex injured: high signal T2	Atrophy: hippocampi, lateral geniculate
Relative sparing of thalami	Relative sparing of perirolandic cortex Thinned gyri	

[a]Adapted from Barkovich AJ. MR and CT evaluation of profound neonatal and infantile asphyxia. AJNR 1992;13:959–972.

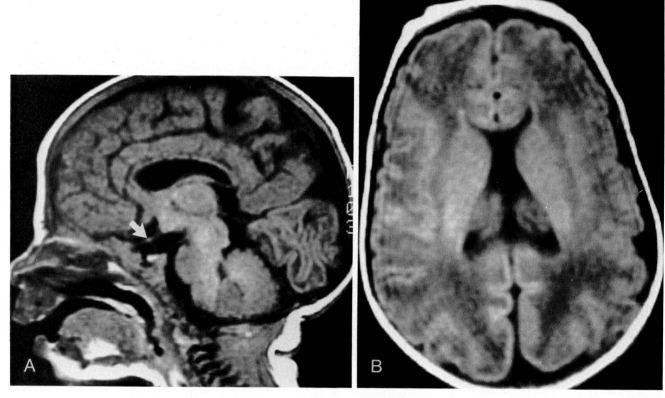

Figure 8.16.   Septo-optic Dysplasia. A. Sagittal T1-weighted image shows a hypoplastic optic nerve (*arrow*), an inconstant finding on MR imaging of septo-optic dysplasia. **B.** Axial T1-weighted image shows absence of the septum pellucidum, characteristic of septo-optic dysplasia.

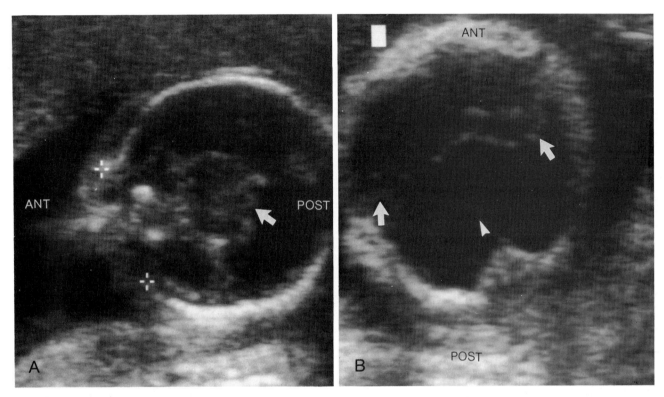

Figure 8.17.   Alobar Holoprosencephaly. A. An axial obstetrical ultrasound through the fetal brain demonstrates the in utero appearance of alobar holoprosencephaly. This severe disorder consists of a monoventricle, with absence of the septum pellucidum, corpus callosum, and falx. The thalami are fused (*arrow*). The white markers are placed over the orbits to measure the degree of hypotelorism. **B.** An axial image at a slightly higher level shows the posterior tips of the mantle of cerebral tissue, termed hippocampal ridges (*arrows*), characteristic of holoprosencephaly. This mantle is displaced forward within the calvarium by the posterior monoventricle. The monoventricle communicates with the cerebrospinal fluid space called the dorsal sac (*arrowhead*).

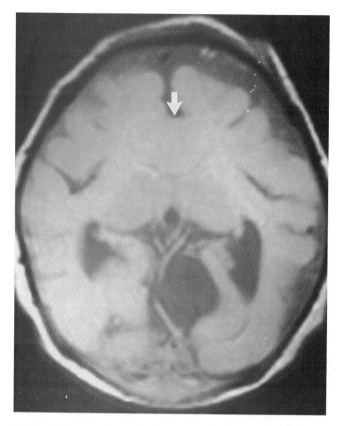

Figure 8.18. Semilobar Holoprosencephaly. An MR image of semilobar holoprosencephaly shows partial fusion of the anterior cerebral hemispheres (*arrow*).

lination questions. Following these principles, partial agenesis of the corpus callosum will result in formation of the genu, but absence of the dorsal body and splenium.

Two conditions deviate from the typical callosal agenesis appearance. Both secondary destruction of the corpus callosum and holoprosencephaly can result in nonsequential segments of absent callosum. The resultant dysgenic callosal pattern thus yields valuable clues regarding brain development and a correct diagnosis. For example, a callosum *only* missing a genu segment may indicate an insult to the brain after development of the corpus callosum, or lobar holoprosencephaly (if the septum is absent), which exhibits disorganized callosal development.

The imaging appearance is variable, ranging from complete to partial absence of callosal tissue. Concomitant with the absence of the corpus callosum is failure to form the cingulate sulcus. Without the supporting white matter fibers, there is alteration of the ventricles with "'steer-horn frontal ventricles" in the coronal plane or a "'racing car" ventricular appearance in the axial plane (Fig. 8.19). This is due to redirection of longitudinal callosal fibers (Probst bundles) along the medial ventricular walls. An interhemi-

spheric cyst may be seen, frequently in communication with the third ventricle.

It is important to describe a potential pitfall in interpretation. Occasionally, callosal hypogenesis will be accompanied by relative prominence of the hippocampal commissure. The hippocampal commissure should not be mistaken for the splenium, erroneously signaling "'atypical callosal hypogenesis" or callosal dysgenesis.

Callosal Lipoma

Lipomas of the corpus callosum have imaging criteria that are similar to other intracranial lipomas in other locations. Lipomas are high signal intensity on T1-weighted images, and cause chemical shift artifact along the frequency encoding direction of the scan. T2-weighted images show a diminution in signal intensity, although some fast-spin echo sequences will have high signal intensity from fat. Lipomas do not cause mass effect, and vessels course through these lesions unperturbed. Lipomas of the corpus callosum are associated with callosal anomalies (Fig. 8.20). Other common locations of intracranial lipomas include the pericallosal, quadrigeminal, and suprasellar cisterns. Less common locations include cerebellopontine angle, sylvian fissure, cerebellar vermis (Fig. 8.21), and the lamina terminalis.

Cephaloceles

Cephaloceles represent the failure of the skull and dura to close over the brain, leading to a herniation of intracranial contents through the defect. Meningoceles reflect herniation of the leptomeninges alone, while encephaloceles are associated with herniation of brain and leptomeninges. Occipital encephaloceles are the most common. Other locations include frontoethmoidal, parietal, and sphenoidal regions. The brain remaining inside the calvarium is typically stretched and distorted toward the defect. Frontoethmoidal encephaloceles are associated with craniofacial anomalies (including hypertelorism), and a higher incidence of callosal abnormalities (Figs. 8.22 and 8.23).

Sphenoid encephaloceles are often occult and present as a nasopharyngeal mass that contains variable amounts of herniated third ventricle, hypothalamus, and optic chiasm.

MIGRATION ANOMALIES

This group of disorders reflects varying patterns of arrested migration of neurons toward the brain surface. Many of the discrete layers of the cortex are formed by directed migration of specific neurons from the subependymal regions outward. Cells destined to

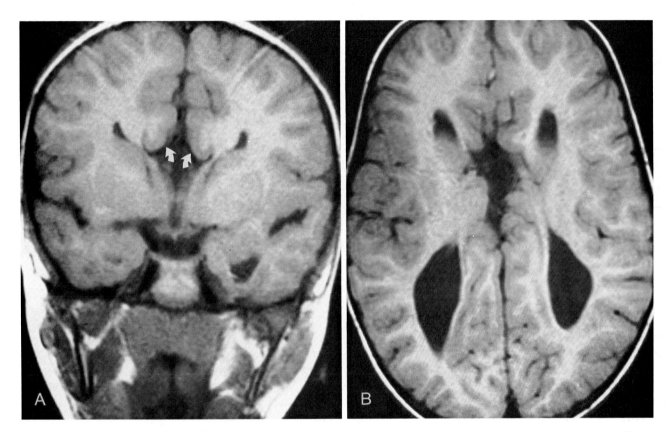

Figure 8.19. Agenesis of the Corpus Callosum. A. Coronal T1-weighted image shows steer-horn shape of the frontal horns of the lateral ventricle. There is absence of the midline corpus callosal tissue and cingulate sulcus (*arrows*). **B.** T1 axial image of the same case showing the racing car configuration of the ventricles. The frontal horns look like the front wheels and the atria of the lateral ventricles look like the larger rear tires on a racing car.

Figure 8.20.   Callosal Lipoma. A. Sagittal T1-weighted image shows a high signal intensity lipoma of the corpus callosum (*arrow*) with accompanying hypogenesis of the posterior body and splenium of the corpus callosum. (Courtesy of Dr. Robin Shanahan.)

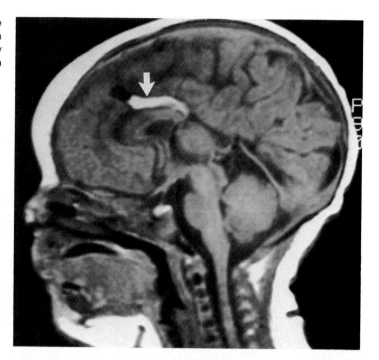

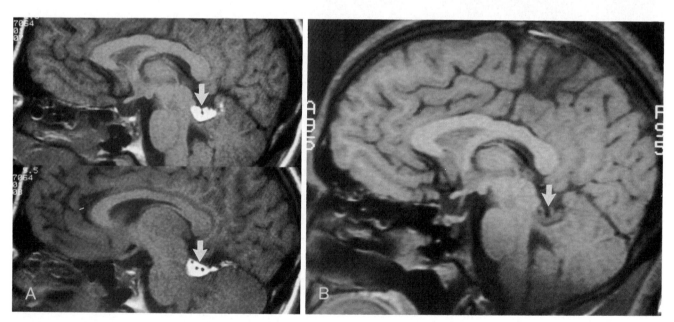

Figure 8.21.   Cerebellar Vermis Lipoma. A. T1-weighted sagittal image shows a lipoma of the superior vermis (*arrows*). Note that a vessel courses through the lipoma unperturbed. **B.** A fat saturation T1-weighted image shows the suppression of fat signal from the image, confirming the diagnosis of lipoma (*arrow*).

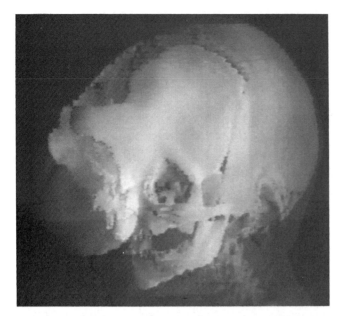

Figure 8.22. Frontal Encephalocele. A three-dimensional reformation CT image of a dramatic frontal encephalocele shows the calvarial defect and a soft-tissue sac herniating out through the defect.

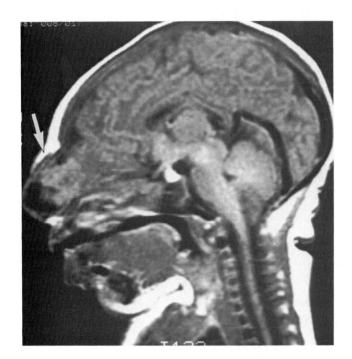

Figure 8.23. Frontal Encephalocele. T1-weighted MR image of a frontal encephalocele shows herniation of brain and meninges through the defect *arrow*). (Courtesy of Dr. Michael Taekman.)

become cortical gray matter end up in the wrong place following arrested migration.

Lissencephaly/Agryia

Lissencephaly and agryia are synonymous terms for the most severe disorder in this spectrum: absence of gyri. The lack of sulcation gives a smooth figure-of-

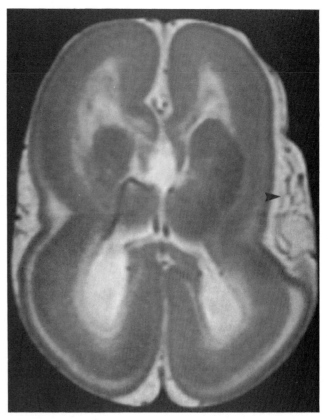

Figure 8.24. Lissencephaly. Axial T2-weighted image of lissencephaly. The brain has a smooth agyric appearance with an abnormally thickened multilayered cortex. The anomalous cortical venous drainage pattern is also seen (*arrowhead*).

eight appearance to the brain. The cortex is abnormally thick (Fig. 8.24), and multilayered. The premature infant's brain can mimic the appearance of lissencephaly. However, the history of prematurity and the normal-thickness cortex distinguish the premature infant.

Pachygyria/Polymicrogyria

Polymicrogyria and pachygyria are both milder disorders of neuronal migration than agyria. They are similar in appearance and prognosis. These entities are called cortical dysplasias. For simplicity's sake, lesions with these characteristics can be described as representing either polymicrogyria or pachygyria. Pachygyria, however, is seen as broad, thick gyri, with shallow sulci. Polymicrogyria is characterized by a thick mantle of gray matter with multiple small gyri. Underlying white matter gliosis in polymicrogyria can sometimes help differentiate it from pachygyria. In both poly- and pachygyria the normal interdigitating fingers of subcortical white matter are absent. These anomalies produce an abnormally thickened cortex with little or no sulcation, but in distinction to lissencephaly, they are more focal (Figs. 8.25 and 8.26).

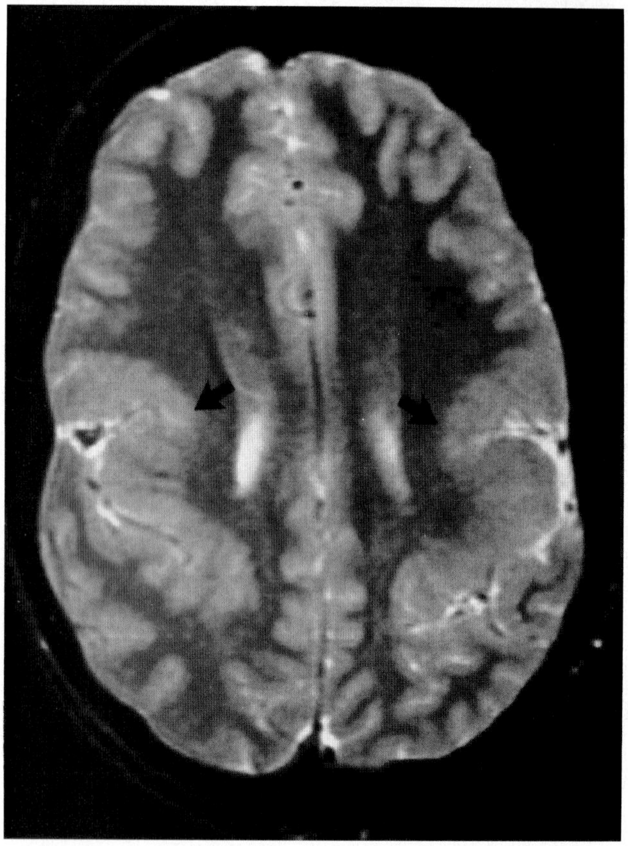

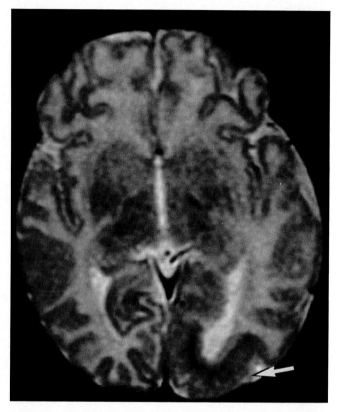

Figure 8.25.   Polymicrogyria. Bilateral areas of focal cortical thickening with deep clefting are seen in both hemispheres in this case of polymicrogyria (*arrows*).

Figure 8.26.   Pachygyria. A more focal area of smooth cortical thickening is seen in this more subtle case of focal pachygyria (*arrow*).

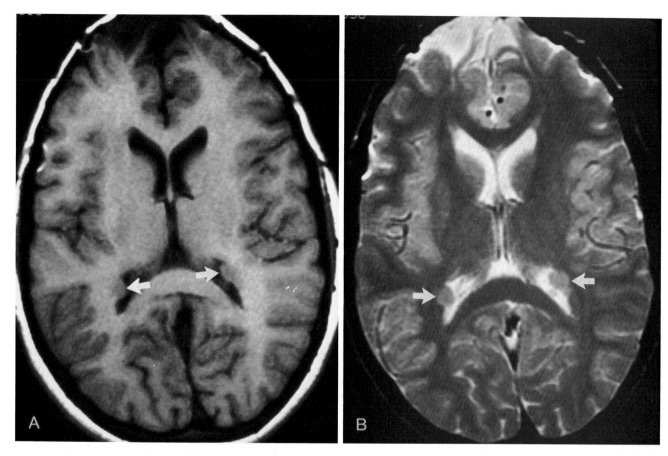

Figure 8.27. Heterotopic Gray Matter. A. A T1-weighted image demonstrates heterotopic gray matter (*arrows*) along the ependymal surface of the ventricle. Damage to the frontal lobes was sec- ondary to trauma. **B.** A T2-weighted image at the same level again shows the heterotopic nodules that parallel gray matter signal in all sequences (*arrows*).

Cortical dysplasias also show anomalous cortical venous drainage, which should not be confused with the abnormal vessels seen in arteriovenous malformations. Since polymicrogyria and pachygyria reflect an in utero insult resulting in arrested cell migration, other associated anomalies are common. These include heterotopic gray matter, schizencephaly, and callosal hypogenesis. Sometimes a whole hemisphere contains poly- and pachymicrogyric changes. This condition is called hemimegalencephaly.

Heterotopic Gray Matter

Disrupted migration of neurons can result in trapped nests of gray matter deep within the brain. These islands of gray matter can be seen anywhere between the ependymal surface and the subcortical white matter. These foci are called heterotopic gray matter. Heterotopic gray matter appears isointense to normal gray matter on all imaging sequences. These lesions do not enhance with gadolinium and do not calcify (Fig. 8.27). The only really important mimic of heterotopic gray matter are the lesions seen in tuberous sclerosis, which do calcify. Most heterotopic gray matter is nodular, although band heterotopias can be seen.

Schizencephaly

Schizencephaly represents abnormal gray matter-lined clefts that deeply invaginate the brain. A pial/ependymal seam communicates with the ventricle. All other clefts that do not extend to the ventricle are polymicrogyric clefts. Multiple imaging planes are often necessary to optimally visualize the clefts. The clefts can be either open lip or closed lip in appearance Fig. 8.28).

All of the migration anomalies can present with seizures as the clinical manifestation. When imaging a child for seizures, careful examination for mass lesions should be followed by scrutiny for anomalies of neuronal migration. If a gyrus looks suspiciously thickened, image it again in another plane. Schizencephaly is differentiated from porencephalic cysts by the presence of a gray matter-lined cleft. Porencephalic cysts are lined by a thin layer of white matter.

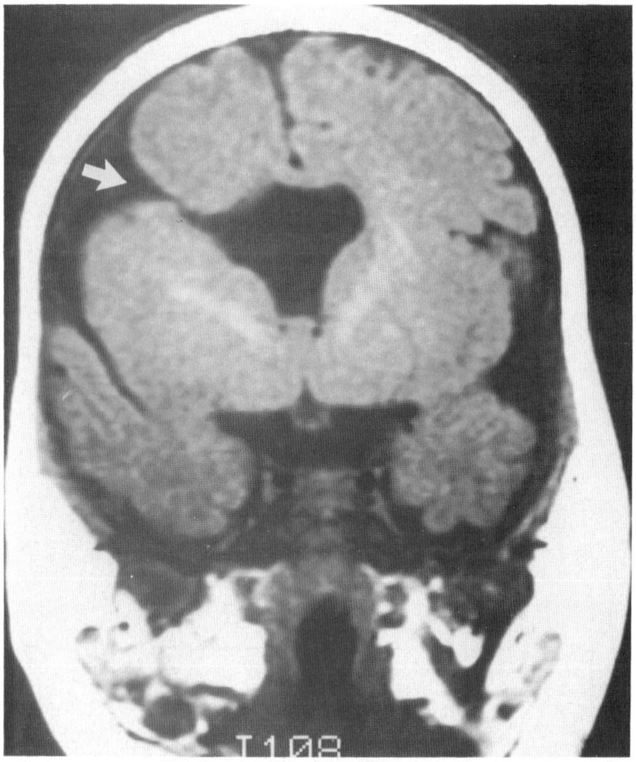

Figure 8.28.   Schizencephaly. An open-lip schizencephaly is seen on the coronal T1-weighted image. The cleft is lined by thickened polymicrogyric gray matter (*arrow*).

Chiari II Malformation

Chiari II malformations involve the brain and spine. Chiari II malformations are the serious neural tube disorders that are screened for in maternal prenatal ultrasound and α-fetoprotein programs. Starting from the head down, the key abnormalities are described.

SUPRATENTORIAL BRAIN

Nearly all patients will present with hydrocephalus. Most cases show partial or complete agenesis of the corpus callosum. The falx cerebri is often fenestrated, resulting in herniation of individual gyri across midline. The massa intermedia (midline rounded mass of gray matter connecting the thalami on sagittal images) is enlarged. The posterior cingulate gyrus is often dysplastic.

POSTERIOR FOSSA

Most of the hindbrain findings in Chiari II malformation derive from a diminutive posterior fossa with brain structures squeezed superiorly, inferiorly, and anteriorly. The cerebellum is squeezed up against the tentorium, down through the foramen magnum (tonsillar herniation), and forward around the brainstem.

The fourth ventricle is squeezed into a small vertical slit. The pons and medulla are also squeezed inferiorly, and with fixed attachments of the upper cervical spinal cord, a cervicomedullary kink often develops as the medulla buckles down past the tethered cord (Fig. 8.29).

SPINE

Most Chiari II malformations present with myelomeningocele. A myelomeningocele represents a failure to close the caudal end of the neural tube during development. This splayed open neural tube also fails to induce a dural or bony covering (Fig. 8.30).

Chiari I Malformations consist of cerebellar tonsillar ectopia (tonsils extend >5 mm below the foramen magnum). Although patients may be asymptomatic, alterations of cerebrospinal fluid dynamics at the level of the foramen magnum are believed to give rise to cervical spinal cord syrinx in some patients (Fig. 8.31). Similarly, Chiari II malformations are associated with cord syrinx (Fig. 8.32).

Cystic Lesions of the Posterior Fossa

A simple working classification of cystic posterior fossa malformations is to consider them within the spectrum of Dandy-Walker malformations. In distinction to Chiari malformations, Dandy-Walker malformations are characterized by a large posterior fossa (a high tentorial insertion). The posterior fossa is filled by a cystically dilated fourth ventricle that exerts mass effect (Fig. 8.33). Hypoplasia or absence of the cerebellar vermis and cerebellar hemispheres are associated findings. Hydrocephalus is also common in this disorder, as is callosal hypogenesis. From this definition follow the other entities within the spectrum: Dandy-Walker variant and megacisterna magna.

A Dandy-Walker variant shows a normal-sized posterior fossa, hypoplasia or absence of the vermis and cerebellar hemispheres, but no significant mass effect. Megacisterna magna shows a normal-sized posterior fossa and relatively normal cerebellar hemispheres and vermis. It is characterized by a prominent cisterna magna cerebrospinal fluid space without mass effect. Megacisterna magna exerts no mass effect, in distinction from retrocerebellar arachnoid cysts and epidermoid neoplasms. Mass lesions cause an inward convex bowing of brain tissue at their interface, and long-standing masses will cause smooth erosion of the inner table of the skull.

THE PHAKOMATOSES

The phakomatoses are a group of syndromes that are grouped together because they all share neurologic and cutaneous manifestations.

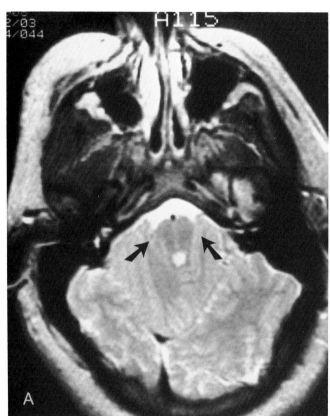

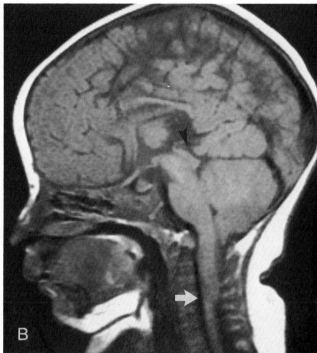

Figure 8.29.   Chiari II Malformation. A. Axial T1-weighted image of a Chiari II malformation demonstrates how the small posterior fossa squeezes the cerebellum around the brainstem (*arrows*). **B.** Saggital T1-weighted image shows beaking of the tectum (*arrowhead*) and downward displacement of the cerebellar tonsils. A cervicomedullary kink is identified (*arrow*). (Courtesy of Dr. John Zovickian.)

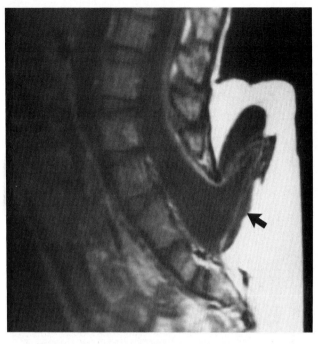

Figure 8.30.   Myelomeningocele. Sagittal T1-weighted image of a myelomeningocele in a case of Chiari II malformation. The myelomeningocele sac contains neural tissue and meninges and protrudes through the dysraphic posterior elements of the lumbar spine (*arrow*).

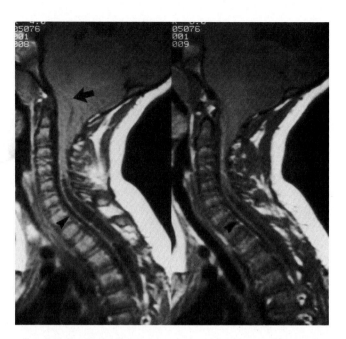

Figure 8.32.   Chiari II Malformation. Image also shows syrinx formation in the cervical cord (*arrowhead*). Note the more crowded appearance of the posterior fossa as compared with the Chiari I malformation shown in Figure 8.31 and the effaced fourth ventricle (*arrow*).

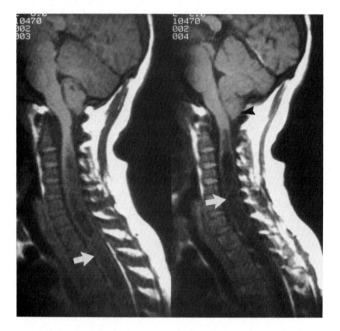

Figure 8.31.   Chiari I Malformation. An altered cerebrospinal fluid flow dynamics around the foramen magnum from tonsillar ectopia (*arrowhead*) in this Chiari I malformation has resulted in a cervical cord syrinx (*arrows*).

Neurofibromatosis

Neurofibromatosis is divided into type I (von Recklinghausen's disease), with distinct neurocutaneous manifestations, and neurofibromatosis II (NF-II).

NEUROFIBROMATOSIS I (NF-I)

Neurofibromatosis I (NF-I) is characterized by skin lesions (café au lait spots), neurofibromas, and ocular findings. The findings in the brain consist of tumors and non-neoplastic lesions in the white matter and globus pallidus.

Neurofibromatosis I is associated with a high incidence of gliomas. The most common gliomas involve the optic pathways. A typical tumor causes fusiform enlargement of the optic nerve (Fig. 8.34). However, the chiasm, optic tracts, and optic radiations can also become involved. Typically, the tumors show poor or no contrast enhancement, consistent with a low histologic grade. Parenchymal involvement along optic pathways is seen as hyperintense signal on T2-weighted images. Other parenchymal gliomas are also seen (Fig. 8.35).

Hyperintense foci in deep cerebral and cerebellar white matter are commonly seen on T2-weighted images. These lesions wax and wane when analyzed over serial scans, do not cause mass effect, and do not enhance (Figs. 8.36 and 8.37). In general, the lesions tend to regress with increasing age. Lesion progression in a child more than 10 years old warrants close follow-up to rule out neoplastic transformation. Significant enlargement, new mass effect, and gadolinium enhancement may herald degeneration into gliomas. The exact histology of these lesions is not known. The

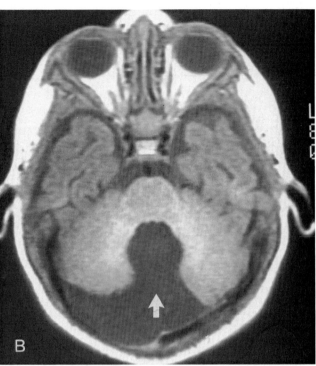

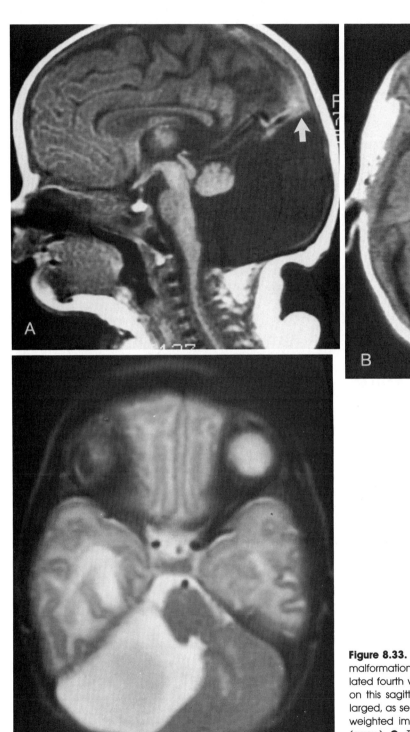

Figure 8.33.   Dandy-Walker Malformation. A. Dandy-Walker malformation characteristically will demonstrate a cystic dilated fourth ventricle and vermian agenesis, as demonstrated on this sagittal T1-weighted image. The posterior fossa is enlarged, as seen by a high torcular insertion (*arrow*). **B.** Axial T1-weighted image shows the cystically dilated fourth ventricle (*arrow*). **C.** This case demonstrates some of the features of Dandy-Walker malformation, but there is asymmetric hypoplasia of the right cerebellar hemisphere.

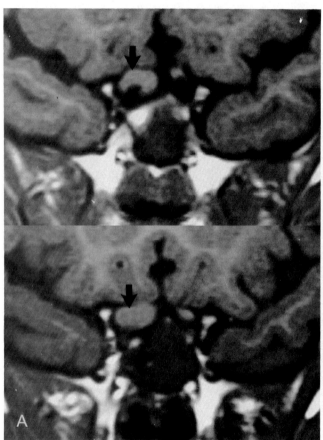

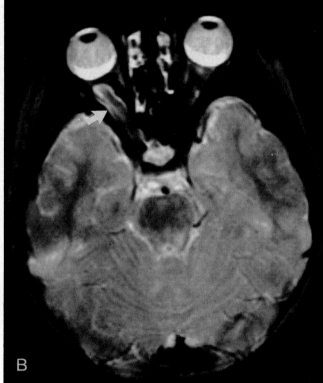

Figure 8.34.   Neurofibromatosis—Optic Glioma. A. Optic nerve gliomas in NFI are fusiform enlargements of the nerve on thin-section coronal T1-weighted images (*arrows*). **B.** Axial T2-weighted image at the midorbit level shows the fusiform enlargement of the right optic nerve (*arrow*). (Courtesy of Dr. Gamal Boutros.)

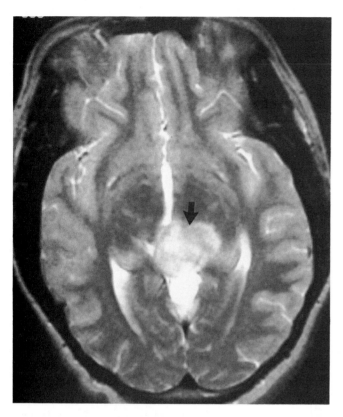

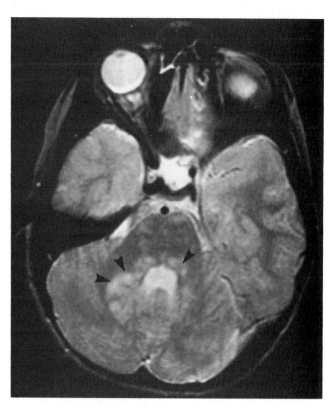

Figure 8.35. Neurofibromatosis—Glioma. T2-weighted axial image shows an exophitic tectal glioma (*arrow*), seen in this patient with NFI.

Figure 8.36. Neurofibromatosis Non-neoplastic Lesion. T2-weighted image of NFI shows multifocal areas of hyperintense signal in both middle cerebellar peduncles (*arrowheads*).

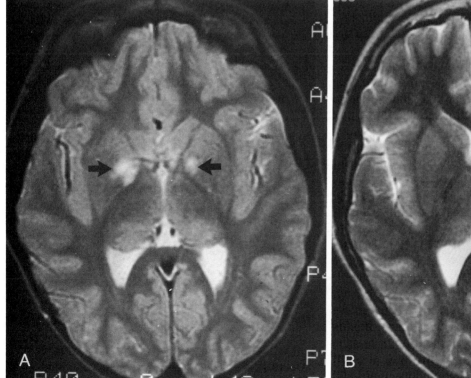

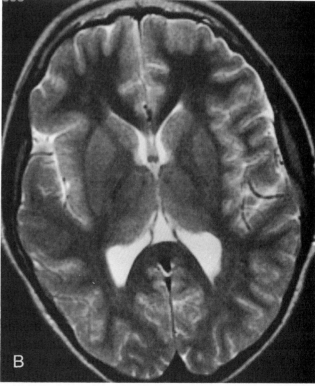

Figure 8.37. Neurofibromatosis—Non-neoplastic Lesions. A. Hyperintense foci on T2-weighted images are seen in the basal ganglia in this patient with NF-I (*arrows*). **B.** The lesions are seen to regress on a 4-year follow-up scan.

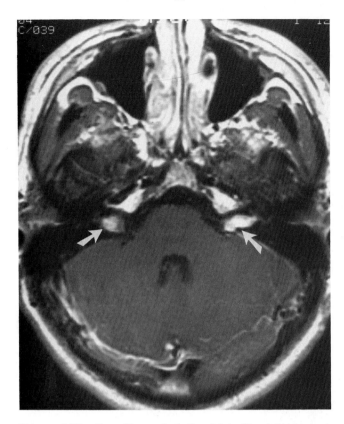

Figure 8.38. Neurofibromatosis-II. Axial T1-weighted post-gadolinium image in a patient with neurofibromatosis type II shows bilateral enhancing acoustic schwannomas of the eighth cranial nerves (*arrows*). (Courtesy of Dr. Ronald Shallat.)

globus pallidi also exhibit abnormal hyperintense signal on both T1- and T2-weighted images.

Neurofibromatosis I has other manifestations, which include plexiform neurofibromas (rope-like masses of neural tissue in subcutaneous soft tissues), vascular lesions, aneurysms, ectasias stenoses, moya-moya syndrome, spinal lesions (neurofibromas, meningoceles, scoliosis), and osseous lesions (sphenoid/lambdoid dysplasia, pseudoarthrosis, rib abnormalities).

Neurofibromatosis II (NF-II), also called central neurofibromatosis, differs considerably from NF I. The key features of NF II are bilateral acoustic schwannomas and meningiomas (Fig. 8.38). Neurofibromatosis II also has spinal manifestations, which include neurofibromas, meningiomas, ependymomas, and schwannomas of other cranial nerves.

Tuberous Sclerosis

Tuberous sclerosis is another distinctive neurocutaneous disorder. The skin lesions are adenoma sebaceum and ash-leaf spots. Brain lesions consist of subependymal harmartomas and cortical tubers (Fig. 8.39). Some of the subependymal nodules near the foramen of Monro can enlarge, cause mass effect, and invade brain tissue. Locally aggressive nodules are called subependymal "'giant cell astrocytomas" (Fig. 8.40).

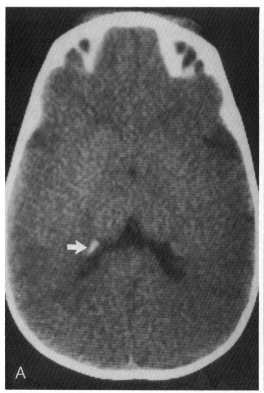

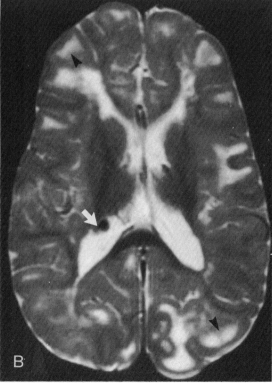

Figure 8.39. Tuberous Sclerosis. A. An axial slice from a CT scan in a patient with tuberous sclerosis shows a single calcified ependymal tuber (*arrow*). **B.** A T2-weighted image shows the same ependymal tuber seen on the CT scan. The tuber is seen as low signal intensity nodule (*arrow*). The subcortical tubers are also well demonstrated (*arrowheads*).

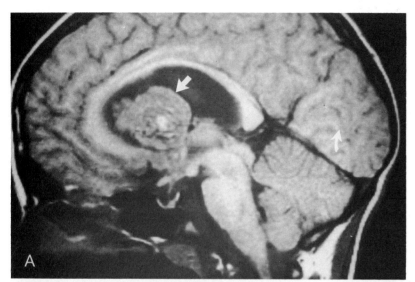

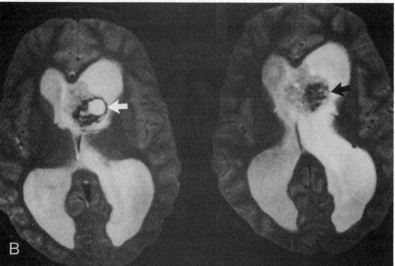

Figure 8.40.   Tuberous Sclerosis. A. In another case of tuberous sclerosis, the sagittal T1-weighted image demonstrates a giant cell astrocytoma arising in the region of the foramen of Monro (*arrow*). **B.** Axial T2-weighted image of a giant cell astrocytoma with concomitant hydrocephalus. The lesion is heterogeneous signal intensity (*arrows*).

Both cortical and subependymal lesions can undergo age-dependent calcification (Fig. 2.20). Subependymal nodules represent hamartomas, and before

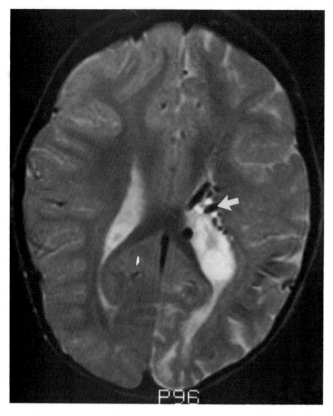

Figure 8.41.   Sturge-Weber Syndrome. Axial T2-weighted image illustrating the dilated ependymal veins seen in Sturge-Weber syndrome. The veins are serpentine flow voids bordering the ependymal surface of the ventricle (*arrow*).

calcification they tend to parallel white matter signal on MR images. Subependymal nodules are distinct from heterotopic gray matter in their signal characteristics and tendency to calcify. Calcified nodules may be isointense or hyperintense on T1-weighted images. Enhancement of nodules at the foramen of Monro does not determine malignant transformation to a giant cell astrocytoma, rather look for brain invasion to make this distinction. Cortical tubers are usually hypointense on T1-weighted images and hyperintense on T2-weighted images, and may calcify.

Sturge-Weber Syndrome

Sturge-Weber syndrome, or encephalotrigeminal angiomatosis, features angiomatous lesions of the skin and meninges. The facial lesion (a skin angioma called a port-wine nevus) appears in the ophthalmic division of the fifth cranial nerve. The pathologic entity seen in the brain is pial angiomatosis. These pial angiomas undergo age-dependent calcification and appear on CT scans as gyral cortical calcifications. The pial angiomatosis results in chronic ischemia of the gray matter, leading to gyral atrophy and underlying gliosis.

Another sequela of pial angiomatosis is alteration of normal superficial cortical venous drainage with concomitant enlargement of deep and subependymal veins (Fig. 8.41). These dilated subependymal veins can mimic arteriovenous malformations. Gadolinium enhancement can reveal the full extent of pial angiomatosis, and is helpful in cases where calcification atrophy has not yet occurred (Fig. 8.42). Young children may show subtle hypointensity of the underlying

Figure 8.42. Sturge-Weber Syndrome. A young patient with Sturge-Weber syndrome with before (*left*) and after (*right*) gadolinium T1-weighted images demonstrating the full extent of pial angiomatosis (*arrow*). Gadolinium may be particularly useful in younger patients who do not yet demonstrate cortical calcifications. (Courtesy of Dr. Jean Hayward.)

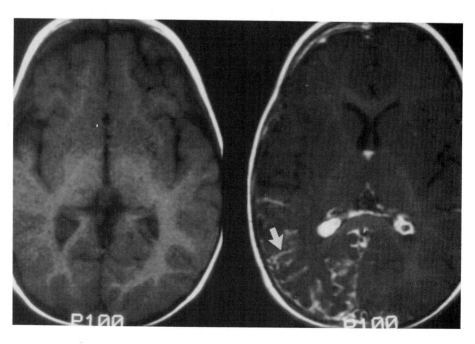

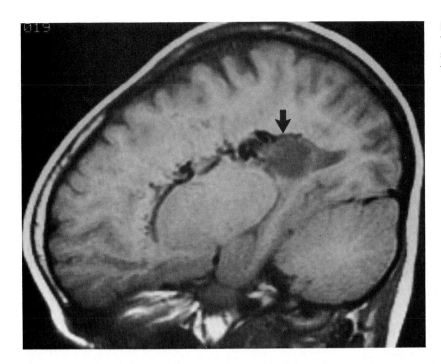

Figure 8.43. Sturge-Weber Syndrome. Saggital T1-weighted image in this case of Sturge-Weber syndrome shows ipsilateral choroid plexus hypertrophy (*arrow*).

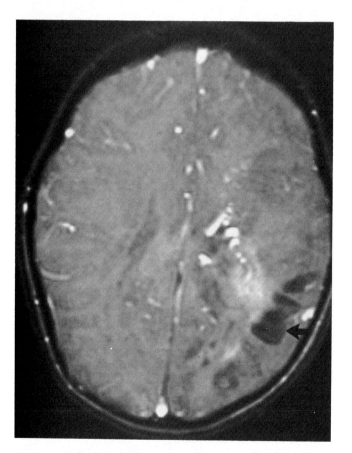

Figure 8.44. Sturge-Weber Syndrome. Gradient-recalled echo images accentuates the magnetic susceptibility artifact associated with the cortical calcifications (*arrow*) of Sturge-Weber syndrome.

white matter on T2-weighted images without calcification of the cortex. Ipsilateral choroid plexus hypertrophy is another feature of this entity (Fig. 8.43). Use gradient-recalled echo technique on MR images to accentuate the presence of calcium (Fig. 8.44).

von Hippel-Lindau Syndrome

von Hippel-Lindau syndrome is an inherited disorder consisting of retinal angiomas, and cerebellar and spinal hemangioblastomas. Hemangioblastomas are considered benign neoplasms and the presence of multifocal spinal cord nodules near the pia-arachnoid surface represents multicentric tumors, not drop metastasis.

Characteristic features of cerebellar hemangioblastomas include a well-circumscribed cystic lesion with an enhancing mural nodule. Other appearances include solid tumors, solid masses with central cysts, and a cyst alone (Figs. 8.45 and 8.46). Another helpful finding is a large blood vessel leading to the nodule. The small multifocal hemangioblastoma nodules are seen near the pial surface of the cerebellum or spinal cord (Fig. 8.47).

Although they are considered benign neoplasms, recurrance rates of up to 25% are reported. These vascular lesions are prone to sudden spontaneous hemorrhage. Gadolinium-enhanced MR imaging is the examination of choice for preoperative evaluation. Other associations with von Hippel-Lindau syndrome include renal cell carcinoma, and angiomas of the liver and kidney.

Figure 8.45. von Hippel-Lindau Syndrome. Axial T1-weighted images in a patient with von Hippel-Lindau syndrome. The left image is pregadolinium and the right image is postgadolinium injection. Some of the lesions are cystic, and one of the enhancing foci (*arrow*) was seen to represent a mural nodule on a lower image.

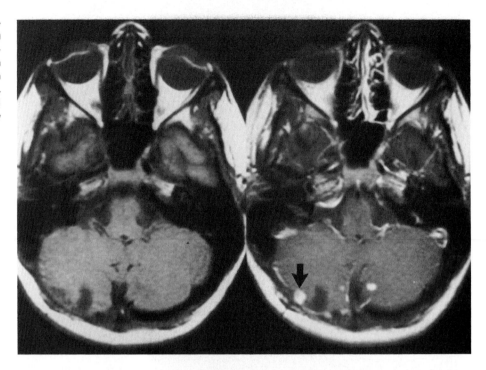

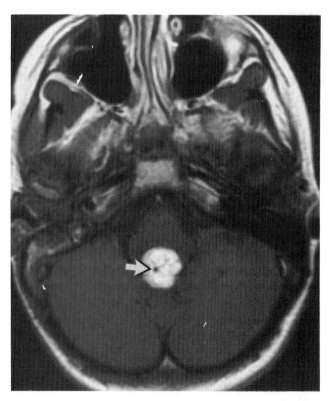

Figure 8.46. von Hippel-Lindau Syndrome. von Hippel-Lindau syndrome has a variable appearance, as demonstrated in this case of a solid enhancing mass in the fourth ventricle. A central speck of hypointensity represents a blood vessel (*arrow*). (Courtesy of Dr. Nora Wu.)

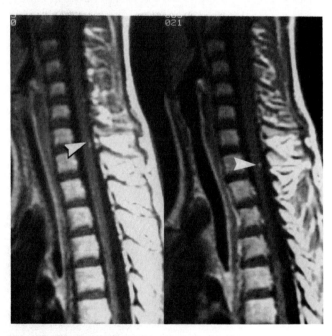

Figure 8.47. Spinal Cord Hemangioblastoma. Multicentric pial-based hemangioblastomas are seen on T1-weighted, gadolinium-enhanced thoracic spine images as punctate enhancing foci (*arrowheads*).

Suggested Readings

Barkovich AJ. *Pediatric neuroimaging.* New York: Raven Press, 1990.

Barkovich AJ. MR and CT evaluation of profound neonatal and infantile asphyxia. AJNR 1992;13:959–972.

Barkovich AJ, Truwit CL. Brain damage from perinatal asphyxia. AJNR 1990;11:1087–1096.

Rorke LB, Zimmerman RA. Prematurity, and destructive lesions in utero. AJNR 1992;13:517–536.

Smirniotopoulos JG, Murphy FM. The phakomatoses. AJNR 1992;13:725–746.

Truwit CL, Lempert TE. *Pediatric neuroimaging: a casebook approach.* DPS Press, distributed by Williams & Wilkins Baltimore, 1992.

9

Head and Neck Imaging

Jerome A. Barakos

"Head and neck" is a collective term used to describe the extracranial structures, and includes areas such as the skull base, orbits, temporal bone, paranasal sinuses, neck, and pharynx. The head and neck region encloses a tremendous spectrum of tissues in a compact space with almost every organ system being represented, including the digestive and respiratory tract, nervous, osseous, and vascular systems. Because of this anatomic complexity the head and neck region tends to be an area approached with considerable trepidation. However, accurate assessment of this area can be accomplished by understanding both the normal anatomy and the scope of pathologic entities that may occur. We will begin our discussion by considering lesions of the paranasal sinuses and nasal cavity. This will be followed by a review of the skull base, the deep spaces of the neck, lymph nodes, orbit and finally congenital head and neck lesions.

Imaging Methods

Both high-resolution computed tomography (CT) and magnetic resonance (MR) imaging can be used to exquisitely display the normal and pathologic anatomy of the head and neck. While each has advantages and disadvantages, the selection of CT versus MR is often based on which technique the patient is more likely to tolerate. If a patient has difficulty handling his or her oral secretions because of prior head and neck surgery, particularly following tracheotomy or partial glossectomy, he or she may have significant hardship lying still for the time required for MR scanning. In such cases the rapid imaging time of CT (1–3 seconds per image) is more likely to yield a study unmarred by motion artifact. Since calcification is better depicted with CT, this is the modality of choice when looking for obstructing salivary ductal calculi, or for the detection of osteomyelitis. In contrast, MR has outstanding sensitivity for the discrimination of soft tissues. As a result, MR will often better demonstrate the full extent of a primary lesion. Additionally, the direct multiplanar capability of MR often allows for better evaluation of pathologic entities. For example, because of the axial orientation of the palate, floor of the mouth, and skull base, pathology in these areas is best studied in the coronal plane.

PARANASAL SINUSES AND NASAL CAVITY
Sinusitis

Inflammatory disease is the most common pathology involving the paranasal sinuses and nasal cavity. Acute sinusitis is characterized by the presence of air-fluid levels and is typically caused by a viral upper respiratory tract infection. In chronic sinusitis, changes include mucoperiostal thickening as well as osseous thickening of the sinus wall. Soft-tissue findings suggestive of sinusitis are most readily detected on the T2-weighted images, as they are most often high in signal. An exception are chronic sinus secretions that have become so desiccated that they yield no signal and may mimic an aerated sinus. These sinus concretions and the bony wall thickening associated with chronic sinusitis will be most easily appreciated on CT.

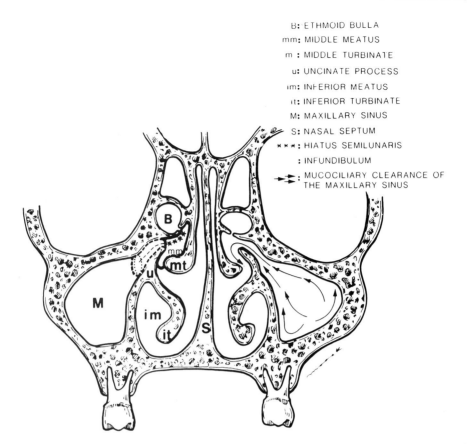

B: ETHMOID BULLA
mm: MIDDLE MEATUS
m : MIDDLE TURBINATE
u: UNCINATE PROCESS
im: INFERIOR MEATUS
it: INFERIOR TURBINATE
M: MAXILLARY SINUS
S: NASAL SEPTUM
✕ ✕ ✕: HIATUS SEMILUNARIS
: INFUNDIBULUM
➤➤: MUCOCILIARY CLEARANCE OF
THE MAXILLARY SINUS

Figure 9.1. Osteomeatal Unit (OMU). This coronal line drawing demonstrates the anatomy of the OMU. On the right side of the drawing lines with arrows show the normal route of mucocilliary clearance. Patterns of obstruction shown on the left side of the drawing include infundibular pattern (heavy *dashed line*) and the OMU pattern (*solid line*). Coronal CT far surpasses plain sinus films in evaluation problems of the OMU for potential relief through endoscopic surgery. (From Babbel RW, Harnsberger HR, Sonkens J, Hunt S. Recurring patterns of inflammatory sinonasal disease demonstrated on screening sinus CT. AJNR 1992;13:903–912.)

Endoscopic sinonasal surgery, for the evaluation and treatment of inflammatory sinonasal disease, is being performed with increasing frequency. Direct coronal sinus CT provides exquisite definition of sinonasal anatomy and provides for preendoscopic sinus assessment (Fig. 9.1). Knowledge of the anatomy of the lateral wall of the nasal cavity and routes of mucociliary drainage of the paranasal sinuses is critical to understanding patterns of inflammatory sinonasal disease. A major area of mucociliary drainage is the middle meatus, known as the osteomeatal unit. It is important to note that disease limited to the infundibulum of the maxillary ostium will result in isolated obstruction of the maxillary sinus. In contrast, a lesion located in the hiatus semilunaris (middle meatus) results in obstruction of some or all of the ipsilateral maxillary sinus, anterior and middle ethmoid air cells, as well as the frontal sinus. This last pattern of sinonasal disease has been described as the osteomeatal pattern of obstruction.

Several common complications are associated with sinusitis and include inflammatory polyps, mucous retention cysts, and mucoceles.

Inflammatory Polyps. Chronic inflammation leads to mucosal hyperplasia, which results in mucosal redundancy and polyp formation. Most often these polyps blend imperceptibly with the mucoperiosteal thickening and cannot be clearly differentiated. When an antral polyp expands to the point where it prolapses through the sinus ostium, it is referred to as an antrochoanal polyp. Although these polyps may not be associated with chronic sinusitis, they are similar to inflammatory polyps in that they represent areas of reactive mucosal thickening. Their characteristic appearance is that of a soft-tissue mass extending from the maxillary sinus to fill the ipsilateral nasal cavity and nasopharynx. Often the ostium of the maxillary sinus will be enlarged in relation to the mass effect of the polyp. The importance in recognizing such a lesion is that if it is surgically snared like a nasal polyp without regard for its antral stalk, it will recur.

Mucus Retention Cyst simply represents an obstructed mucous gland within the mucosal lining. These lesions have a characteristic rounded appearance, with the maxillary sinus being most commonly involved.

Mucocele is similar to a retention cyst, but instead of a single mucous gland becoming obstructed, the entire sinus is obstructed. This typically occurs because of a mass obstructing the draining sinus ostium. The characteristic feature of a mucocele is frank expansion of the sinus with associated bony thinning and remodeling. The frontal sinus is the sinus most commonly involved with a mucocele, followed by the ethmoid, maxillary, and sphenoid sinuses. If the mucocele becomes infected it demonstrates peripheral enhancement and is called a mucopyocele.

Tumors

Inverting Papilloma. A variety of papillomas occur within the nasal cavity but most attention has focused on the inverting papilloma. Inverting papillomas are named based on their histologic appearance. In this condition the neoplastic nasal epithelium inverts and grows into the underlying mucosa. These papillomas are not believed to be associated with allergy or chronic infection since they are almost invariably unilateral in location. Inverting papillomas occur exclusively on the lateral nasal wall centered on the hiatus semilunaris. Since there is an increased association with squamous cell carcinoma, it is recommended that these lesions be surgically resected with wide mucosal margins.

Juvenile Nasopharyngeal Angiofibroma are typically seen in adolescent males presenting with epistaxis. The tumor arises from fibrovascular stroma of the nasal wall adjacent to the sphenopalatine foramen. This is a benign tumor that can be very locally aggressive. In an adolescent male presenting with a nasal mass and epistaxis, it is important to have a high clinical suspicion for this lesion as life-threatening hemorrhage may result if a biopsy is performed. The tumor characteristically fills the nasopharynx and bows the posterior wall of the maxillary sinus forward. The tumor enhances markedly with contrast administration on CT, differentiating the lesion from the rarer lymphangioma. Preoperatively, interventional radiology may play a role in embolizing these lesions and making them less vascular, providing for easier surgical resection.

Malignancies. The tissues within the paranasal sinuses and nasal cavity that give rise to malignancies include squamous epithelium, lymphoid tissue, and minor salivary glands. Therefore the corresponding malignancies are squamous cell carcinoma, lymphoma, and minor salivary tumors. Since the entire upper aerodigestive tract is lined with squamous epithelium, it follows that squamous cell carcinoma is the most common malignancy (80–90%) of not only the paranasal sinuses and nasal cavity, but of the entire head and neck. Squamous cell carcinoma of the sinuses is often clinically silent until it is quite advanced. Early symptoms are usually related to obstructive sinusitis. Imaging findings consist of an opacified sinus with associated bony wall destruction. These findings are nonspecific and do not allow differentiation from non-Hodgkin's lymphoma or a minor salivary gland malignancy. The presence of marked head and neck or systemic adenopathy may suggest the diagnosis of lymphoma.

Minor salivary glands are dispersed throughout the upper aerodigestive tract but are most highly concentrated in the palate. Any of these minor salivary glands found throughout the head and neck may give rise to a salivary malignancy. The most common salivary malignancies include adenoid cystic carcinoma, adenocarcinoma, and mucoepidermoid carcinoma.

An esthesioneuroblastoma is an additional malignancy that should be mentioned when describing lesions of the nasal cavity. The esthesioneuroblastoma is a tumor that arises from the neurosensory receptor cells of the olfactory nerve and mucosa. Thus, this lesion may originate anywhere from the cribiform plate to the turbinates. This tumor is often quite destructive by the time of diagnosis and is found high within the nasal vault (Fig. 9.2). Involvement of the cribiform plate with extension into the anterior cranial fossa is not uncommon.

In assessing the size and extent of a sinus or nasal lesion it is often difficult to differentiate the lesion from associated obstructed sinus secretions. In such instances heavily T2-weighted sequences are of value since, in general, sinus secretions will be brighter than the malignancy, which is often isointense to muscle.

SKULL BASE

The skull base extends from the nose anteriorly to the occipital protuberance posteriorly and is composed of five bones: the ethmoid, sphenoid, occipital, temporal, and frontal bones. The skull base contains many foramina through which both vascular and neurologic structures pass. Because the skull base has an undulating surface with an axial orientation and a minimal craniocaudad dimension, coronal imaging is essential in its evaluation.

Tumors of the Skull Base

Tumors may arise intrinsic to the skull base or extend to involve the skull base either from above or below. Any lesion from the paranasal sinuses and nasal cavity as already described may extend to involve the skull base. Other lesions that may extend to involve the skull base are paragangliomas, neural sheath tumors (schwannoma and neurofibroma), and meningiomas. Most malignant lesions of the skull base are metastatic.

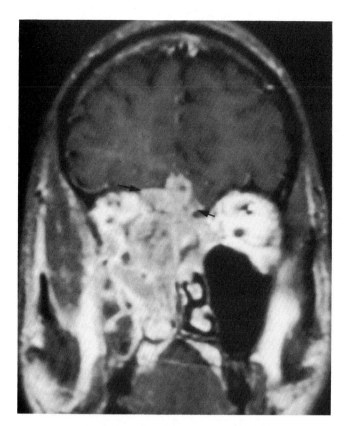

Figure 9.2. Esthesioneuroblastoma. Coronal fat-suppressed post-gadolinium T1-weighted sequence. A large destructive mass is identified in the nasal cavity and extending through the cribriform plate into the anterior cranial fossa (*arrows*). This degree of frank bony destruction is unusual for squamous cell carcinoma and lymphoma.

Primary Malignant Neoplasms are relatively uncommon comprising only about 2–3% of skull base tumors. The three most common primary malignant tumors are chondrosarcoma, osteogenic sarcoma, and chordoma. *Chondrosarcomas* are malignant tumors that develop from cartilage. Since the skull base is preformed in cartilage there is a predilection for chondrosarcoma to involve the skull base. A preferred site of origin is parasellar in location at the petroclival junction. *Osteogenic sarcoma* is typically the result of prior radiation therapy or malignant transformation of Paget's disease. *Chordoma* is a bone neoplasm that arises from remnants of the primitive notochord. These tumors may be found anywhere along the craniospinal axis with 35% of lesions involving the clivus, 50% the sacrum, and 15% the vertebral bodies. Radiographically, this lesion is characterized as a destructive bony lesion with predilection for the spheno-occipital synchondrosis. On a sagittal image, the spheno-occipital synchondrosis is occasionally seen as a horizontal line in the midclivus, midway between the sella and the basion (tip of clivus). The skull base, like any bone, may also be affected by metastases, myeloma, plasmacytoma, fibrous dysplasia, and Paget's disease.

Temporal Bone

Although a thorough discussion of the temporal bone is beyond the scope of this chapter, we will focus on some highlights. The most common diseases involving the temporal bone are inflammatory in nature and include cholesteatomas. Eustachian tube dysfunction with resultant decreased intratympanic pressure is believed to be the basic defect responsible for inflammatory disease of the middle ear and mastoid.

Cholesteatoma is an epidermoid cyst composed of desquamating stratified squamous epithelium. These cysts enlarge because of the progressive accumulation of epithelial debris within their lumen. They may be either congenital (2%) or acquired (98%). Congenital cholesteatomas originate from epithelial rests within or adjacent to the temporal bone. Acquired cholesteatomas originate from the stratified squamous epithelium of the tympanic membrane. These begin as localized tympanic membrane retraction pockets. The diagnosis of a cholesteatoma is based on the detection of a soft-tissue mass within the middle ear cavity, typically with associated bony erosion. The superior portion of the tympanic membrane (pars flaccida) retracts easily and is the most common sight for formation of an acquired cholesteatoma. Cholesteatomas arising in this area originate within Prussak's space (superior recess of the tympanic membrane), which is located medial to the pars flaccida between the scutum and the neck of the malleus. Thus, soft tissue in this region, with subtle erosion of the scutum and medial displacement of the ossicles, reflects a cholesteatoma. Note that when associated fluid or inflammatory tissue is present, these cannot be differentiated from cholesteatoma, since they have similar densities.

Although otoscopically most cholesteatomas can be easily diagnosed, the clinician cannot judge the size and full extent of the lesion. As a result, CT plays an important role in determining the size of the lesion, status of the ossicles, the labyrinth, the tegmen, and the facial nerve. Magnetic resonance imaging has a limited role in the evaluation of bony erosive lesions of the temporal bone since the lack of landmarks does not allow localization of the process, and gives no information concerning the status of the ossicles and other bony structures.

Cholesterol Granuloma, also know as giant cholesterol cyst, is a lesion of the temporal bone that has recently received considerable attention. Cholesterol granuloma is a type of granulation tissue that may involve the petrous apex. These lesions represent petrous apex air cells that have become partially obstructed and are filled with cholesterol debris and hemorrhagic fluid. Because of their hemorrhagic components, these lesions are characterized by high signal on both T1- and T2-weighted sequences.

SUPRAHYOID HEAD AND NECK

The suprahyoid head and neck is traditionally divided into compartments that include the nasopharynx, oropharynx, and oral cavity. Understanding the division between these spaces is essential to accurately determine and describe the full extension of mucosal lesions. The term "nasopharynx" is frequently misused. It is often utilized as a nonspecific term to describe any area in the upper aerodigestive tract. In fact, the nasopharynx refers to a very specific portion of the pharynx. The nasopharynx lies above the oropharynx, and is divided from the oropharynx by a horizontal line drawn along the hard and soft palates. Posteriorly the nasopharynx is bounded by the pharyngeal constrictor muscles and anteriorly by the nasal cavity at the nasal choana (paired funnel-shaped openings between the nasal cavity and the nasopharynx). Below the hard palate lie the oral cavity and oropharynx. These two areas are divided by a ring of structures that includes the circumvallate papillae along the posterior aspect of the tongue, tonsillar pillars, and the soft palate.

These traditional compartments are important for describing the spread of mucosal-based lesions, of which squamous cell carcinoma is the most common malignancy. In contrast to this division, multiple facial planes divide the deep head and neck into spaces that form true compartments. It is important to realize that these deep spaces are unrelated to the traditional division of the head and neck, since tumors within these spaces traverse the neck without regard to this traditional division. Therefore, when describing deep head and neck lesions the traditional pharyngeal subdivisions are of limited value, and most radiologists have adapted a spacial approach to the head and neck as described next, popularized by H. Ric Harnsberger.

The deep anatomy of the head and neck is subdivided by layers of the deep cervical fascia into the following spaces: (a) parapharyngeal, (b) superficial mucosal, (c) carotid, (d) parotid, (e) masticator, (f) retropharyngeal, and (g) prevertebral. When evaluating a patient with pathology in the deep head and neck, it is important to determine within which space the pathology lies. Since only a limited number of structures are located within each compartment, these are the structures from which pathology will arise. Therefore only specific pathology will be found within these separate fascial spaces, markedly limiting the differential diagnosis. For example, the principal structures within the parotid space are the parotid gland and the parotid lymph nodes. As a result, if a parotid space mass is identified, the diagnosis is primarily limited to either nodal disease or a parotid tumor. Each of these seven spaces will be reviewed in detail (Table 9.1). Note that while this spacial division is popular with radiologists, the surgeons and oto-

Table 9.1.   Deep Compartments of the Head and Neck

Compartment (Space)	Contents	Pathology
Mucosal	Squamous mucosa Lymphoid tissue (adenoids, lingual tonsil) Minor salivary glands	Carcinoma, lymphoma, minor salivary gland tumors, juvenile angiofibroma, rhabdomyosarcoma
Parapharyngeal	Fat Trigeminal nerve (V₃) Internal maxillary artery Ascending pharyngeal artery	Minor salivary gland tumors, lipoma, cellulitis/abscess, schwannoma
Parotid	Parotid gland Intraparotid lymph nodes Facial nerve (VII) External carotid artery and retromandibular vein	Salivary gland tumors, metastatic adenopathy, lymphoma, parotid cysts
Carotid	Cranial nerves IX–XII Sympathetic nerves Jugular chain lymph nodes Carotid artery Jugular vein	Schwannoma, neurofibroma, paraganglioma, metastatic adenopathy, lymphoma, cellulitis, abscess, meningioma
Masticator	Muscles of mastication Ramus and body of mandible Inferior alveolar nerve	Odontogenic abscess, osteomyelitis, direct spread of squamous cell carcinoma, lymphoma, minor salivary tumor, sarcoma of muscle or bone
Retropharyngeal	Lymph nodes (lateral and medial retropharyngeal) Fat	Metastatic adenopathy, lymphoma, abscess/cellulitis
Prevertebral	Cervical vertebrae Prevertebral muscles Paraspinal muscles Phrenic nerve	Osseous metastases, chordoma, osteomyelitis, cellulitis and abscess

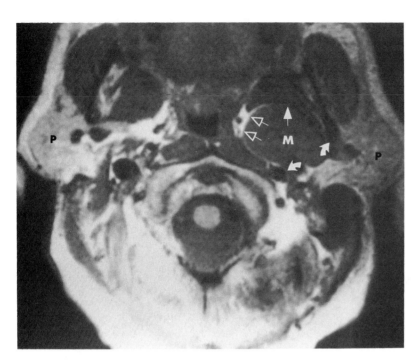

Figure 9.3. Parotid Benign Mixed Cell Adenoma (Plemorphic Adenoma). Axial T1-weighted sequence through the level of the oropharynx. A mass (*M*) is identified that displaces the parapharyngeal space medially (*open white arrows*) and the masticator space anteriorly (*white arrow*). There is widening of the stylomandibular notch (distance from the carotid space to the mandible (*curved arrows*)), which is characteristic of a deep lobe parotid lesion. Note that the lesion is sharply demarcated from the normal parotid tissue (*P*).

laryngologists occasionally use different terms, e.g., retrostyloid space instead of carotid space.

Parapharyngeal Space

The parapharyngeal space is a triangular fat-filled compartment that extends from the skull base to the submandibular gland region. It is located at the center of the surrounding spaces and is compressed or infiltrated in a characteristic fashion by masses originating from the various spaces (1). The importance of the parapharyngeal space is not that pathology may originate within it, but that it serves as an important landmark of mass effect in the deep face. When a lesion occurs in any of the four surrounding spaces, there will be characteristic impression on the parapharyngeal fat space, which will suggest the space of tumor origin.

The parapharyngeal space is surrounded by the carotid space posteriorly, parotid space laterally, masticator space anteriorly, and the superficial mucosal space medially. Therefore, the parapharyngeal space will be compressed on its medial surface by masses originating from the mucosal surface, anteriorly displaced by carotid sheath masses, medially displaced by parotid masses, and posteriorly and medially displaced by masses within the masticator space. Thus, by assessing the location and displacement pattern of the parapharyngeal space, one can assign a space of origin to a deep facial mass (Fig. 9.3).

Superficial Mucosal Space

The superficial mucosal space includes all structures on the airway side of the pharyngobasilar fascia.

The principle structure within this space is the mucosa of the upper aerodigestive tract, which consists of squamous epithelium, submucosal lymphatics, and hundreds of minor salivary glands. The pharyngobasilar fascia represents the superior aponeurosis of the superior pharyngeal constrictor muscle, which inserts into the skull base. This tough fascia separates the mucosal space from the surrounding parapharyngeal space. Lesions originating within the superficial mucosal space may invade deep to the mucosal surface, resulting first in lateral displacement and then obliteration of the parapharyngeal space. However, many early lesions that begin within the mucosal space present as only mild mucosal irregularities or asymmetries (Fig. 9.4). This space is easily evaluated by the clinician and thus the radiologist should have a low threshold for suggesting the presence of abnormalities within this space. In children there is frequently prominent adenoidal tissue that fills the nasopharynx. As long as there is no invasion of deep facial places and no systemic adenopathy, this is considered normal (Fig. 9.5).

Benign Lesions. The most common benign lesions arising in the mucosal space are Thornwald cysts and lesions related to minor salivary gland tissue. *Thornwald cysts* are found in the midline and have high intensity on T2-weighted images (Fig. 9.6). They are believed to be remnants of notochordal tissue aberrantly located in the nasopharynx, and have an incidence of approximately 4% in normal patients. Lesions arising from minor salivary glands include retention cysts and benign neoplasms. Retention cysts represent an obstructed gland similar to those found within the paranasal sinuses. The most com-

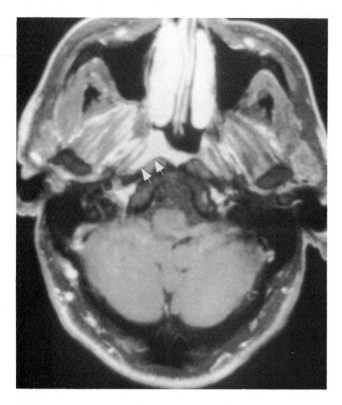

Figure 9.4. Squamous Cell Carcinoma. Axial postgadolinium fat-suppressed T1-weighted sequence through the level of the naso-pharynx. Contrast-enhancing soft tissue fills the right fossa of Rosenmüller (*white arrows*). Although this lesion does not grossly invade the underlying parapharyngeal tissues, there were submandibular nodal metastases.

mon benign neoplasm is the benign mixed cell tumor (pleomorphic adenoma). Both of these lesions present as well-circumscribed rounded lesions that have high signal intensity on T2-weighted images.

Tumors. The most common malignant neoplasms of the mucosa are squamous cell carcinoma, non-Hodgkin's lymphoma, and minor salivary gland malignancies. Of these, squamous cell carcinoma is by far the most common. Unfortunately, these malignancies all appear similar on CT and MR imaging. Initially there is mass effect, often associated with lateral compression or obliteration of the parapharyngeal space, followed by invasion of the skull base. An early triad of radiographic findings consists of (*a*) superficial naso-pharyngeal mucosal asymmetry, (*b*) ipsilateral retro-pharyngeal adenopathy, and (*c*) mastoid opacification. Mastoid opacification is an important early warning sign (Fig. 9.7). This finding is easily detected on the T2-weighted sequence and suggests potential dysfunction of the eustachian tube, frequently the result of tumor infiltration. This finding alerts the radiologist to carefully evaluate the mucosa of the naso-pharynx. Note that both the nasopharynx and the mastoid air cells are included on every head MR scan and these areas should not be overlooked in routine head studies. Contrast enhancement with gadolinium is useful in detecting subtle perineural spread of neoplasm, particularly along cranial nerves extending into the skull base. This is particularly true of adenoid cystic carcinoma, which has a marked propensity for perineural spread and is the most common minor salivary gland malignancy (Fig. 9.8).

Squamous Cell Carcinoma of the nasopharynx, despite being the most common malignancy of the pharynx is a relatively rare lesion in the Caucasian population, with an incidence of about 1 in 100,000 people

Figure 9.5. Adenoidal Hypertrophy. Axial first and second echo T2 in a 5-year-old child. Marked adenoidal tissue fills the nasopharynx, expanding the fossa of Rosenmüller bilaterally. Additionally, lateral pharyngeal nodes (*arrows*) are clearly visualized. These findings are typical for a child. The age of the patient and the lack of infiltration into the underlying soft tissues suggest that this is a normal finding.

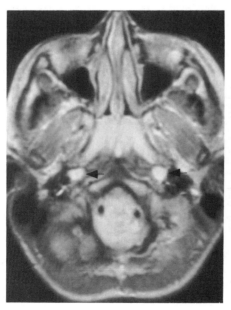
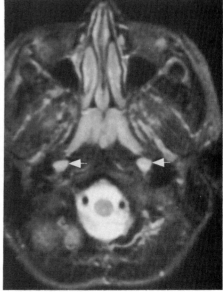

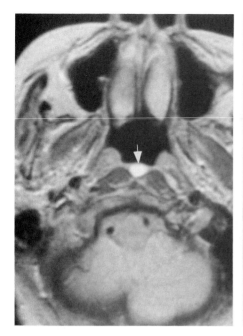

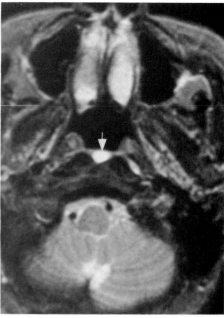

Figure 9.6. Thornwald's Cyst. Axial first and second echo T2-weighted sequence. A high signal intensity lesion is noted in the superficial mucosa (*arrows*). This midline location is characteristic of a Thornwald's cyst and is found in 1–2% of the normal population.

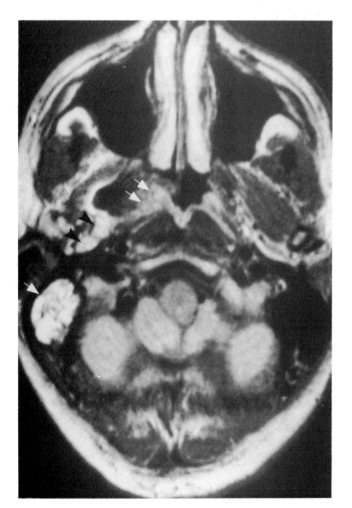

Figure 9.7. Nasopharyngeal Malignancy. Axial postgadolinium T1-weighted sequence. Triad of nasopharyngeal malignancy consists of (*a*) mucosal mass of the lateral nasopharynx (fossa of Rosenmüller) (*double white arrows*), (*b*) lateral retropharyngeal nodes (*arrowheads*), and (*c*) mastoid opacification (*white arrow*). Mastoid opacification is the result of dysfunction of the eustachian tube due to the nasopharyngeal mass.

per year. This is in contrast to rates 20 times higher in Asia, particularly southern regions of China. Although smoking and alcohol abuse are not a causal association, both environmental and genetic factors do play a role. Specifically immunoglobulin A antibodies to the Epstein-Barr virus have been associated with nasopharyngeal carcinoma.

Non-Hodgkin's Lymphoma involving the mucosa cannot be differentiated from squamous cell or minor salivary gland carcinoma. However, non-Hodgkin's lymphoma frequently has systemic manifestations with extranodal and extralymphatic sites of involvement, which are atypical for these other malignancies (2). Thus, the presence of these associated findings may suggest the diagnosis of lymphoma.

Carotid Space

Masses of the carotid space deviate the parapharyngeal space anteriorly and separate or anteriorly displace the carotid and jugular vein. They sometimes displace the styloid process anteriorly, which narrows the stylomandibular notch (space between the styloid process and the mandible). This is a characteristic feature that distinguishes these lesions from deep parotid space lesions which widen the stylomandibular notch.

Pseudomasses. When evaluating carotid space tumors there are several pseudomasses of the carotid space that must be taken into account. These pseudomasses are vascular variants that may be mistaken for a mass both clinically and radiographically. Asymmetry of the internal jugular veins is the most common variation in the vascular anatomy of the neck. Marked asymmetry between the jugular veins is common, with the right vein typically being larger. Additionally, the jugular veins may demonstrate con-

Figure 9.8.   Recurrent Adenoid Cystic Carcinoma. Coronal postgadolinium fat-suppression T1-weighted images. A 50-year-old patient status post resection of nasal septum and turbinates for adenoid cystic carcinoma. Follow-up examination reveals a recurrent mass (*M*) with extension into the right pterygopalatine fossa (*arrows*). Adenoid cystic carcinoma has a marked propensity for perineural spread, which allows the tumor to extend rapidly into noncontiguous spaces. Once the tumor enters the pterygopalatine fossa, it may extend into the orbit via inferior orbital foramen, cavernous sinus via foramen rotundum, and the infratemporal fossa via pterygomaxillary fissure. Once in the cavernous sinus tumor it can travel back along the cisternal portion of the trigeminal nerve into the brain stem.

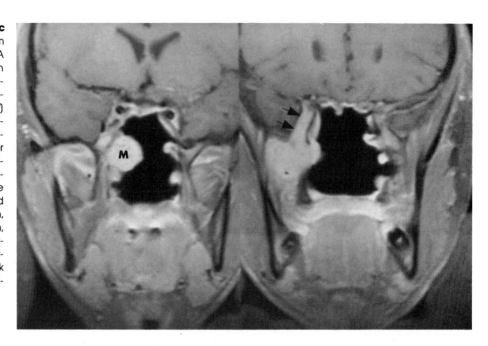

siderable variability in the degree of signal within their lumen. This venous intraluminal signal is frequently asymmetric, and should not be mistaken for thrombosis. It is important to follow these vessels on serial images to demonstrate their tubular nature, otherwise they may easily be confused for adenopathy. Tortuosity of the carotid artery may present as a submucosal pulsatile mass in the pharynx. This variation, which is frequently seen in the elderly, is easily detected on CT or MR imaging and obviates the need for further diagnostic work-up unless a posttraumatic aneurysm is suspected.

Tumors. Most carotid space masses are benign neoplasms and arise from the nerves located within the carotid sheath. The most common lesions are paragangliomas and nerve sheath tumors such as schwannomas and neurofibromas. *Paragangliomas* are vascular tumors that arise from neural crest cell derivatives. These lesions are named according to the nerves from which they arise and their location of origin. When arising from the carotid body, at the carotid bifurcation, they are called *carotid body tumors* (Fig. 9.9). These tumors may also arise from the ganglion of the vagus nerve (glomus vagale), along the jugular ganglion of the vagus nerve (glomus jugulare), and around Arnold's and Jacobson's nerves in the middle ear (glomus tympanicum) (3).

Clinically, patients present with a painless, slowly progressive neck mass that may be pulsatile with an associated bruit. Since these lesions are located within the carotid sheath there are often associated slowly progressive cranial neuropathies (cranial nerves IX-XII) (Fig. 9.10) (4). Paragangliomas are often multiple (5–10%) and in familial cases are multiple as

high as 25–33% of the time. Therefore, if a lesion is detected, it is essential to look for a second one.

Angiographically, paragangliomas are very vascular, with a strong blush in the capillary phase. Treatment often consists of surgical resection. Interventional radiology plays an important role in performing preoperative embolization, making these lesions much less vascular and easier to resect at the time of surgery. On CT scanning, paragangliomas and neuromas are both densely enhancing and are typically indistinguishable. In contrast, on MR imaging, paragangliomas are characterized by multiple flow voids and prominent enhancement (Figs. 9.11 and 9.12) (5). These features reflect the vascular nature of this lesion. Note that these findings, although suggestive of a paraganglioma, are not pathognomonic since, on occasion, a very vascular schwannoma may also have associated flow voids.

In addition to the neurogenic lesions of the carotid space, the other major source of pathology are lymph nodes. In fact, the principal malignancy of the carotid space are squamous cell nodal metastases. A major nodal chain is located within the carotid space, the deep cervical jugular chain. Any pathology that involves lymph nodes (metastases, lymphoma, infection, benign hyperplasia) may therefore be found within the carotid space.

Parotid Space

Masses arising from the deep lobe of the parotid gland will deviate the parapharyngeal space medially. Unlike carotid space masses, deep parotid masses push the styloid process and carotid vessels posteriorly. This results in characteristic widening of the stylomastoid foramen (Fig. 9.3). The structures

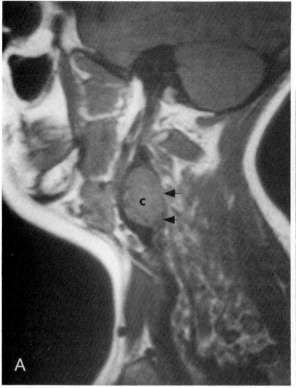

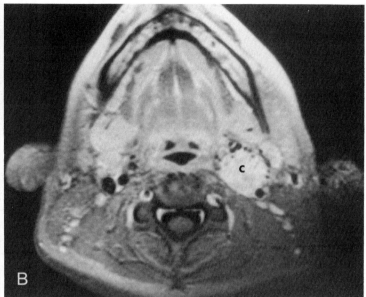

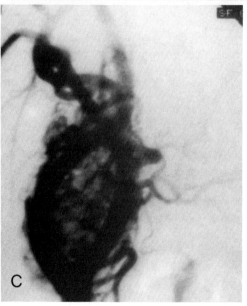

Figure 9.9. Carotid Body Tumor (C). Sagittal T1 **(A)**, axial postgadolinium fat-suppression T1 **(B)**, and angiogram **(C)**. A mass located between the carotid bifurcation, with splaying of the internal and external carotid artery, is characteristic of a carotid body tumor. The multiple flow voids in the axial image supports this diagnosis of a paraganglioma. The angiogram confirms the marked vascularity of this lesion. Angiography is helpful in providing preoperative embolization, making the lesion less vascular and easier to remove surgically.

within the parotid space that may give rise to pathology include the parotid gland and lymph nodes. The parotid gland is the only salivary gland to have lymph nodes contained within its capsule. This reflects the embryogenisis of the parotid gland, where its late encapsulation results in the presence of 10–20 nodes within the substance of parotid gland. Thus pathology of the parotid space includes salivary gland tumors and nodal disease.

Parotid Tumors. Most parotid tumors are benign (80%), and most of these are benign mixed cell tumors (pleomorphic adenomas) or Warthin's tumors (benign salivary gland tumor). Malignant tumors, which account for 20% of all parotid lesions, include adenocystic carcinoma, adenocarcinoma, squamous cell carcinoma, and mucoepidermoid carcinoma. Magnetic resonance and CT imaging cannot with certainty differentiate benign from malignant disease. Both benign and malignant disease may present as well-circumscribed lesions. Tumor homogeneity, unsharp margins, as well as signal intensity are poor predictors of histology. Nevertheless, both CT and MR imaging are useful in portraying the relationship of the tumor to surrounding normal anatomy, and to

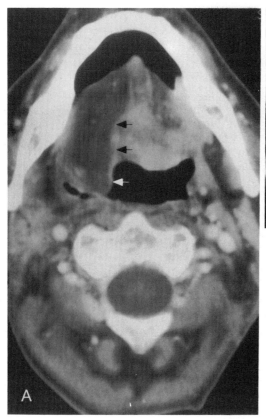

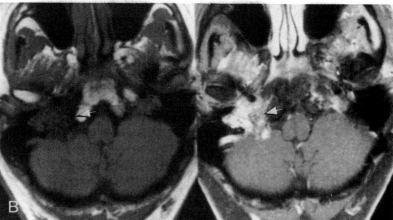

Figure 9.10. Glomus Jugulare Tumor. A. Axial contrast-enhanced CT. There is fatty atrophy of the right tongue (hypoglossal nerve palsy) (*black arrows*) and patulousness of the right oropharynx (vagus nerve palsy) (*white arrow*). In order for multiple cranial nerves to become affected, the most common site of involvement is where they are located together. For cranial nerves IX through XII, they arise in close proximity at the skull base. Therefore, when more than one of these cranial nerves is involved this suggests a skull base lesion. **B.** Axial T1, pre- and postgadolinium fat suppression. Glomus jugulare. Contrast-enhancing mass is identified extending through the right jugular foramen into the posterior fossa.

verify the location of a nonpalpable parotid mass before biopsy. A feature clearly suggestive of malignancy is infiltration into deep neck structures such as the masticator or parapharyngeal space (6). Clinical involvement of the facial nerve is another ominous finding suggestive of malignancy.

The presence of multiple lesions within the parotid space may be seen with several conditions including adenopathy, either inflammatory or malignant. Another possibility is the Warthin's tumor (benign salivary gland tumor), which is multiple 10% of the time. Parotid cysts have been seen in collagen vascular disease and more recently described in patients with acquired immunodeficiency syndrome (AIDS) (Fig. 9.13) (7). These parotid cysts, also known as lymphoepithelial cysts, are believed to be the result of partial obstruction of the terminal ducts by surrounding lymphocytic infiltration.

Masticator Space

The masticator space is formed by a superficial layer of the deep cervical fascia that surrounds the muscles of mastication and the mandible. It extends from the angle of the mandible superiorly to the skull base, and extends over the temporal muscle. The muscles of mastication include the temporalis, medial and lateral pterygoid, and the masseter. In addition, branches of the trigeminal nerve and the internal maxillary artery, surrounded by fat, are located within this space. Masses of the masticator space displace the parapharyngeal space medially and posteriorly.

Most masses of the masticator space are infectious in origin. They result from either dental caries or are secondary to dental extraction. A mass will surround the mandible and may extend along the temporalis muscle. Pseudotumors of the masticator space are common. Atrophy of the musculature can occur from compromise of the third division of the fifth cranial nerve. This is most commonly seen in patients with head and neck neoplasms with perineural extension along the trigeminal nerve. Occasionally, an accessory parotid gland is palpable in the masticator space along the anterior surface of the masseter muscle and can be mistaken for a mass.

Primary Malignancies of the masticator space are very uncommon. Malignancies of this space most often result from the extension of oropharyngeal or tongue base squamous cell carcinoma to involve the muscles of mastication (Fig. 9.14). In addition, tumor or infection from oropharyngeal or nasopharyngeal lesions may spread along the third division of the fifth cranial nerve, allowing the tumor to spread through the foramen ovale into the cavernous sinus (Fig. 9.15). From this location, tumor may extend posteriorly along the cisternal portion of the trigeminal nerve to the brainstem.

Primary malignancies of the masticator space include sarcomas arising from muscle, chondroid, or

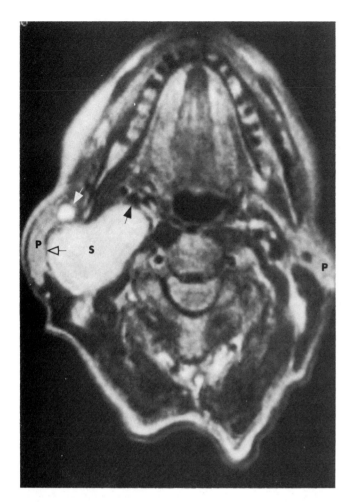

Figure 9.11. Schwannoma. Axial T2-weighted sequence through the floor of the mouth. A homogeneous mass (S) displaces the carotid space anteriorly (*black arrow*) and the parotid space (P) laterally (*open arrow*). Anterior displacement of the carotid artery is characteristic of a carotid space mass. The lack of associated flow voids suggests this lesion is a schwannoma as opposed to a paraganglioma. High signal within the right retromandibular vein (*white arrow*) is due to partial compression. Normal flow void is seen in the opposite retromandibular vein.

nerve elements. In addition, sarcomas of the bone such as osteosarcoma and Ewing's sarcoma may be seen. Non-Hodgkin's lymphoma will occasionally involve the mandible or extraosseous soft tissues of the masticator space.

Retropharyngeal Space

The retropharyngeal space is a potential space that lies posterior to the superficial mucosal space and pharyngeal constrictor muscles and anterior to the prevertebral space. A mass within this space results in characteristic posterior displacement of the prevertebral muscles. The facial planes in this area are complex, but can be simplified into a single compartment. This space is significant since it serves as a potential conduit for the spread of tumor or infection from the pharynx to the mediastinum (Fig. 9.16) (8). In con-

trast to the carotid and parotid spaces, in which inflammatory disease and metastases account for a minority of lesions, most retropharyngeal space lesions are due to infection or nodal malignancy (9). This space is most often involved by nodal malignancy because of lymphoma or metastatic head and neck squamous cell carcinoma. These tumors frequently affect the retropharyngeal nodes, which include medial and lateral nodes. The lateral retropharyngeal nodes, also known as nodes of Rouviere, are normal when seen in younger patients, but must be viewed with suspicion with increasing age (>30 years). In addition, head and neck infections may sometimes extend into the retropharyngeal space, gaining access to this space through lymphatics. Neck infections are most often the result of tonsillitis, dental disease, trauma, endocarditis, and systemic infections such as tuberculosis. With the advent of antibiotics, infections occur much less commonly but often are seen in immunosuppressed patients. On routine T1- and T2-weighted sequences it can be difficult to differentiate an abscess from cellulitis, as both can be isointense to muscle on T1 and hyperintense on T2. Gadolinium is of value in making this differentiation, as an abscess will demonstrate a rim of contrast enhancement.

Prevertebral Space

The prevertebral space is formed by the prevertebral fascia, which surrounds the prevertebral muscles. Masses of the prevertebral space displace the prevertebral muscles anteriorly. This allows prevertebral lesions to be easily differentiated from retropharyngeal processes, which will displace these muscles posteriorly. The structures that give rise to the preponderance of pathology in this space are the cervical vertebral bodies. Any process that involves the vertebral bodies, such as tumor (metastasis, chordoma, etc.) or osteomyelitis may extend anteriorly to involve this space (Fig. 9.11).

Transpacial Diseases

Occasionally, masses may not be localized to one of these described spaces. Such masses are often secondary to lesions involving anatomic structures that normally transgress spaces. These would include three categories: (a) lymphatic masses (lymphangioma); (b) neural masses (neurofibroma, schwannoma) and (c) vascular masses (hemangioma). Differentiation between these subtypes can occasionally be made by virtue of signal intensity characteristics. For instance, neurofibromatosis often involves several peripheral nerves and has a characteristic low intensity center on T1-weighted image sequences. This is distinctly different from both lymphatic and vascular masses. Lymphangiomas and hemangiomas are con-

Figure 9.12.   Glomus jugulare. Sagittal T1-weighted image through the carotid space. A large mass (*J*) extends from the carotid space through the jugulare foramen (*arrowheads*) into the posterior fossa. The presence of numerous flow voids is suggestive of a vascular lesion such as a paraganglioma.

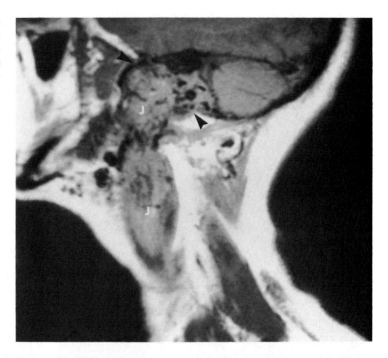

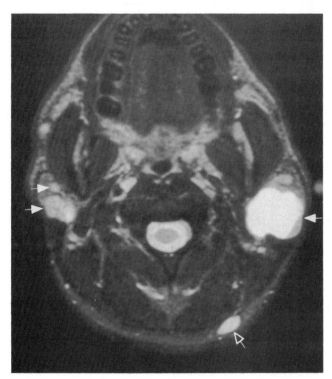

Figure 9.13.   AIDS-related Parotid Cysts. Axial T2-weighted sequence through the level of the oropharynx. Multiple cysts are seen within the parotid glands bilaterally (*arrows*). These are believed to be the result of lymphatic obstruction due to human immunodeficiency virus infection. Incidently, a sebaceous cyst is noted in the left posterior neck (*open arrow*).

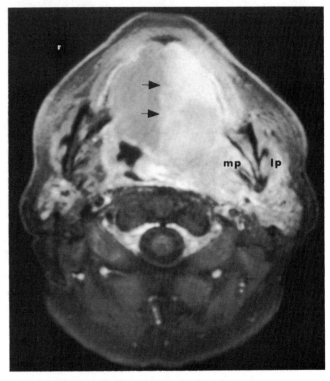

Figure 9.14.   Squamous Cell Carcinoma of the Tongue. Axial postgadolinium fat-suppression T1-weighted sequence through the level of the oropharynx. A left tongue base squamous cell carcinoma extends posteriorly along the oropharyngeal wall into the masticator space (medial and lateral pterygoid muscles (*mp* and *lp*). Malignancies of the masticator space are most frequently the result of the direct posterior extension of oropharyngeal squamous cell carcinoma. In this example, the left half of the tongue (*arrows*) is diffusely enhancing. Following denervation of the hypoglossal nerve, the muscles of the tongue first undergo a denervation myositis where they demonstrate diffuse enhancement. Later, the muscles will atrophy and become fatty replaced.

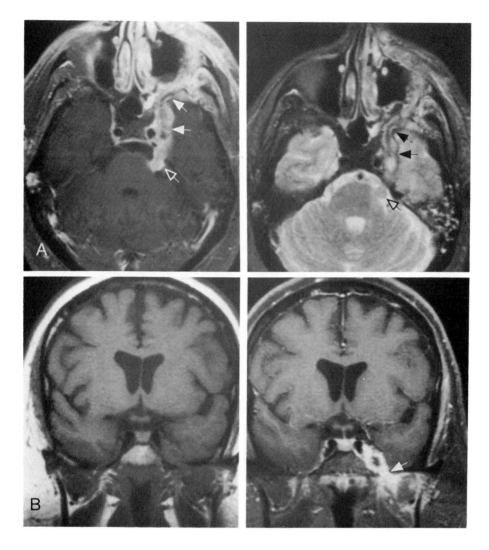

Figure 9.15. Masticator Space Infection. **A.** Axial postgadolinium fat-suppression T1- and T2-weighted images through the level of the nasopharynx. Mucormycosis infection in an immunocompromised host (diabetic ketoacidosis). Soft-tissue infiltration involves the left malleolar soft tissues and extends along the maxillary division of the trigeminal nerve (V₂) (*arrows*) into the cavernous sinus. From the cavernous sinus, contrast-enhancing tissue extends along the cisternal portion of the trigeminal nerve (*open arrows*) to the brain stem. **B.** Coronal T1, pre- and postgadonlinium fat-suppression. Contrast enhancement is seen filling the cavernous sinus and extending through the foramen ovale (*arrow*) into the masticator space along the mandibular division of the trigeminal nerve (V₃).

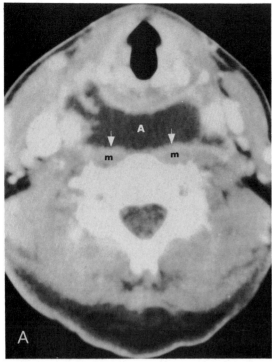

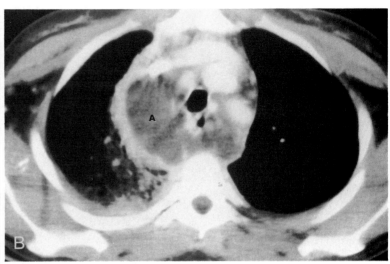

Figure 9.16.   Retropharyngeal Abscess. Axial postcontrast CT through the level of the larynx (*A*) and the upper mediastinum (*B*). A large fluid collection (*A*) is identified extending from the retropharyngeal space into the upper mediastinum. The posterior displacement of the prevertebral muscles (*m*) (*arrows*) identifies this collection as being retropharyngeal as opposed to prevertebral.

genital abnormalities that look quite similar on MR. Hemangiomas may have phleboliths, which may only be detected on CT. Both entities have increased signal intensity on T2-weighted images and infiltrate the various spaces. These two entities should be entertained in a patient with chronic history of facial swelling who has CT or MR evidence of an infiltrative process that bridges several spaces.

LYMPH NODES

Once a neoplasm of the head and neck is detected, the assessment of lymph nodes is a vital part of tumor staging. The presence of a single ipsilateral malignant node reduces the patient's expected survival by 50% (10). Thus, the detection of nodal disease is paramount for both prognostic reasons as well as for therapeutic planning (11). Computed tomography and MR imaging play a vital role in the staging of head and neck neoplasms, since clinical staging has many shortcomings. The full size and extent of the primary neoplasm can rarely be accurately determined clinically. At least 15% of malignant nodes are clinically occult because of their deep location, and thus are not palpable by the clinician (12). Additionally, the overall error rate in assessing the presence of adenopathy by palpation is between 25 and 33% (13). Thus, CT or MR imaging is vital in obtaining the most accurate pretreatment planning information.

There are at least 10 major lymph node groups in the head and neck, and knowledge of the location of these cervical lymph node chains and the usual modes of spread of head and neck disease is essential to be able to successfully analyze CT and MR scans (14, 15). However, a complete discussion of all the head and neck nodal chains is beyond the scope of this text. We will focus on the principal lymph node group of the neck which is the internal jugular chain (16). These lymph nodes serve as the final common afferent pathway for lymphatic drainage of the entire head and neck. This chain of nodes follows the oblique course of the jugular vein beneath and adjacent to the anterior border of the sternocleidomastoid muscle. The jugulodigastric node is the highest node of the internal jugular chain and is located where the posterior belly of the digastric muscle crosses this chain, near the level of the hyoid bone. This lymph node is immediately posterior to the submandibular gland and provides lymphatic drainage from the tonsil, oral cavity, pharynx, and submandibular nodes.

The jugulodigastric node and submandibular nodes may normally measure up to 1.5 cm in diameter. All other nodes of the head and neck are considered abnormal if greater than 1.0 cm in diameter (17). When an enlarged node is encountered, differentiating between a benign reactive node and a malignant one can be difficult. Several features that suggest malignancy are (*a*) peripheral nodal enhancement with central necrosis, (*b*) extracapsular spread with infiltration of adjacent tissues, and (*c*) matted conglomerate mass of nodes. Nodal size itself is a less reliable indicator of malignancy but is often used since the other differentiating features are frequently not available. If size criteria alone are used, approximately 70% of enlarged nodes are secondary to metastatic disease

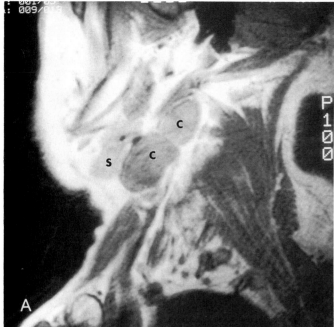

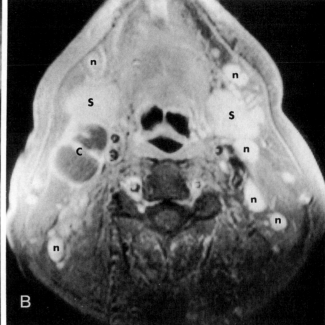

Figure 9.17. Squamous Cell Carcinoma - Cystic Node Metastasis. Sagittal T1-weighted image (**A**) and axial postgadonlinium fat-suppression T1-weighted image (**B**). A 43-year-old patient presented with a 6-month history of a right-sided neck mass that would swell during upper respiratory tract infections. images revealed a multiseptated cystic lesion (**c**) in the right jugular nodal chain. On biopsy this proved to be a squamous cell, cystic nodal metastasis. Although this lesion may appear similar to a branchial cleft cyst, the presence of multiple additional nodes (*n*) is unusual. A branchial cleft cyst may demonstrate a thickened wall with septations, depending on current or previous infections. *S*, submandibular gland.

and 30% are caused by benign reactive hyperplasia. Note that the features described as characteristic for malignancy are the same as for infection and the two cannot be differentiated (Fig. 9.17). Fortunately, the distinction is often easily made clinically.

ORBIT

Both CT and MR imaging are valuable in orbital imaging, each with distinct merits. When evaluating for calcification, such as in retinoblastoma in a child with leukocoria, or for bony fracture following trauma, CT is the modality of choice. On the other hand, MR with its multiplanar capability and superior soft-tissue discrimination has proven to be of tremendous value in orbital imaging. For most orbital abnormalities, including evaluation of the visual pathways, MR is the procedure of choice.

Understanding the spatial anatomy of the orbit is valuable since knowledge of the contents of the spaces provides insight into the naturally occurring lesions that develop within each space. The retrobulbar space contains both the extraconal and the intraconal spaces, which are separated by the muscle cone. This muscle cone, formed by the extraoccular muscles (superior, inferior, medial and lateral rectus; superior oblique; and levator palpebrae superior) and a fibrous septum, form a cone with its base at the posterior of the globe and apex at the superior orbital fissure.

When identifying an intraconal lesion, an essential issue is whether the lesion arises from the optic nerve sheath complex or is extrinsic to it. If the lesion arises from the optic nerve sheath complex the most common lesions are optic nerve glioma and optic sheath meningioma.

Optic Nerve Glioma is the most common tumor of the optic nerve, and typically occurs during the first decade of life (Fig. 9.18). There is a high association with neurofibromatosis type 1. The characteristic imaging finding is that of enlargement of the optic nerve sheath complex that may be tubular, fusiform, or eccentric with kinking. Some optic nerve gliomas have extensive associated thickening of the perioptic meningies. Histologically, this reflects peritumoral reactive meningeal change that has been termed "arachnoidal hyperplasia or gliomatosis." This finding is often seen in patients with neurofibromatosis.

Optic Sheath Meningiomas arise from meningoendothelial cells of the arachnoid layer of the optic nerve sheath. These lesions assume a circular configuration and grow in a linear fashion along the optic nerve. Optic sheath meningiomas demonstrate a characteristic "tram track" pattern of linear contrast enhancement, since the nerve sheath enhances and not the nerve itself. Magnetic resonance easily displays any extension along the optic nerve sheath through the orbital apex (Fig. 9.19). In contrast to optic nerve gliomas, meningiomas may invade and grow

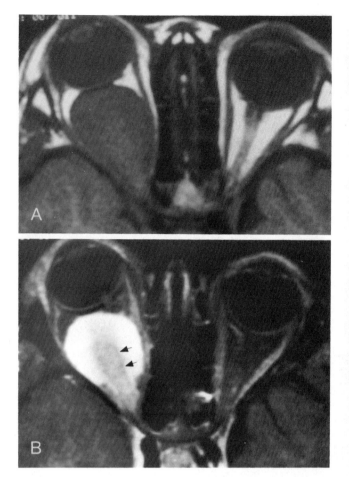

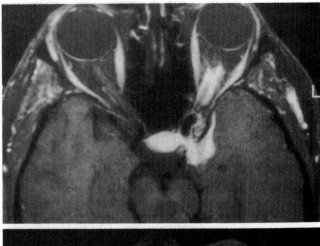

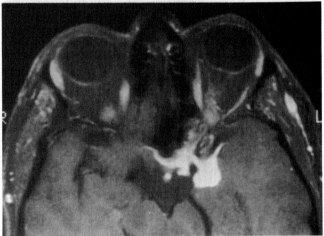

Figure 9.18.   Optic Nerve Glioma. Axial pregadolinium (**A**) and postgadolinium (**B**) fat-suppressed T1-weighted images through the orbits. A large mass is identified involving the right optic nerve. Following the administration of contrast, the enlarged optic nerve (*arrows*) is identified coursing through markedly thickened optic sheath soft tissue. This soft tissue represents arachnoidal hyperplasia, which is a finding associated with optic gliomas in patients with neurofibromatosis.

Figure 9.19.   Optic Sheath Meningioma. Axial postgadolinium fat-suppression T1-weighted image through the orbits. "Tram track" enhancement involves the left optic nerve sheath, and the tumor is seen extending into the middle cranial fossa.

through the dura, resulting in an irregular and asymmetrical appearance. Additionally, optic sheath meningiomas may be extensively calcified, whereas optic nerve gliomas rarely have any calcification.

Vascular Lesions. A variety of vascular lesions may develop intraconally. The four lesions we will consider include capillary hemangioma, lymphangioma, cavernous hemangioma, and varix. These are readily distinguished by a combination of imaging and clinical findings including the patient's age. *Capillary hemangiomas* develop in infants (younger than 1 year) and are diagnosed within the first weeks of life. Although these lesions may grow rapidly in size, they typically plateau during the first year or two then regress spontaneously. On imaging studies, a capillary hemangioma presents as an infiltrative soft-tissue complex, often with multiple vascular flow voids. *Lymphangioma* is one of the most common orbital tumors of childhood (3–15 years).

Lymphangiomas are characterized by their propensity to bleed and often contain blood degradation products. An acute hemorrhage may result in marked expansion of the lesion with sudden proptosis (Fig. 9.20). Magnetic resonance imaging reveals a multiloculated, lobular mass with characteristic signal heterogeneity caused by blood degradation products (Fig. 9.21). *Cavernous hemangiomas* are the most common orbital mass in adults. In contrast to the other vascular lesions of the orbit, hemangiomas are characterized as a sharply circumscribed, rounded mass (Fig. 9.22). These lesions demonstrate diffuse enhancement, sometimes with a mottled pattern. The *venous varix* is an enormously dilated vein that is characterized by its marked change in size with the Valsalva maneuver.

Superior Ophthalmic Vein is well visualized on MR imaging studies. Pathology includes thrombosis and enlargement. Thrombosis often occurs in conjunction with cavernous sinus thrombosis and presents as loss of the normal flow void, with signal intensity related to the age of the thrombus. Enlargement of the superior ophthalmic vein may also be seen with cavernous carotid fistulas (Figs. 9.23 and 9.24). These are either spontaneous or posttraumatic and may present with pulsating exophthalmos and bruit.

Lymphoma and Pseudotumor are two important lesions that may present with similar imaging findings. Lymphoma tends to present in middle-aged patients (mean age, 50 years) with painless proptosis. In contrast, pseudotumor presents with painful proptosis with chemosis and ophthalmoplegia. On imaging studies both lymphoma and pseudotumor are diffusely infiltrating lesions involving and extending into any retrobulbar structures (Fig. 9.25). Several reports have suggested that T2 shortening of the tumor (dark on T2) is suggestive of pseudotumor (Fig. 9.26). Nevertheless, the distinction between these two entities frequently remains very difficult clinically, radiographically and even histopathologically. When a diffusely infiltrative orbital mass is encountered in a young child, rhabdomyosarcoma should be a consideration.

Thyroid Ophthalmopathy is a common lesion and is the most frequent cause of unilateral or bilateral proptosis in the adult. Most patients will have clinical or laboratory evidence of hyperthyroidism, but 10% will not, and are referred to as "euthyroid ophthalmopathy." Imaging findings consist of enlargement of the extraocular muscles with sparing of the tendinous attachments to the globe (Fig. 9.27). This is in contrast to pseudotumor, which typically

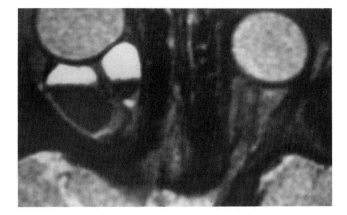

Figure 9.20. Lymphangioma. Axial T2-weighted image reveals a cystic retrobulbar lesion with a hematocrit effect. Hemorrhage into a lesion is a characteristic feature of lymphangiomas and may be responsible for the rapid development of proptosis.

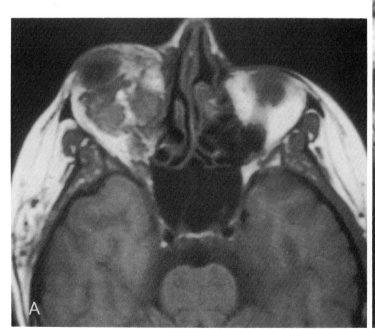
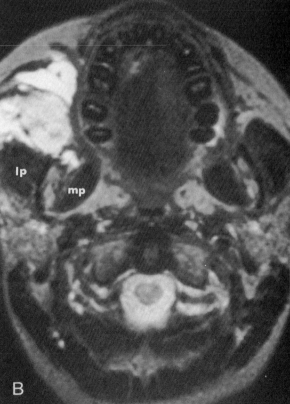

Figure 9.21. Lymphangioma. Axial T1- (**A**) and T2-weighted (**B**) images through the orbit and the midface, respectively. A heterogeneous lesion extends from the right orbit through the inferior orbital fissure into the masticator space. The heterogeneous signal of this lesion as well as its tendency to extend across facial spaces is characteristic for a lymphangioma. *lp*, lateral pterygoid muscle; *mp*, medial pterygoid muscle.

involves the muscle attachments to the globe. The muscles involved in decreasing order are the inferior, medial, lateral, and superior rectus. Eighty percent of patients have bilateral muscle involvement. In some cases the extraoccular muscles may be normal, and exophthalmos is the result of increased retrobulbar fat.

The extraconal space primarily contains fat and the lacrimal gland. However, many lesions involving the extraconal space are the result of tumor or inflammation extending from surrounding structures such as a sinus-related subperiosteal space abscess. Lesions arising from within the extraconal space are primarily lacrimal. A lesion of the lacrimal gland is very nonspecific since the lacrimal gland can be involved by a wide variety of lesions. These lesions can be divided into inflammatory (e.g., sarcoid, Sjögren's syndrome) and neoplastic. Neoplasms of the lacrimal gland include epithelial and lymphoid. Epithelial tumors are any of the lesions that may affect the salivary glands, such as benign mixed cell tumor or adenoid cystic carcinoma. Lymphoid tumors include lymphoma and pseudotumor. Although none of these lesions have specific imaging findings, a dermoid is one lesion that does have a characteristic finding consisting of a fat-fluid level (Fig. 9.28).

CONGENITAL LESIONS

As a general approach, neck masses in children tend to be benign and include congenital lesions (thyroglossal duct cysts, branchial cleft cysts, and lymphangiomas/cystic hygromas) as well as reactive lymphadenopathy secondary to infection (18). When malignancy is entertained, the two most common lesions in the pediatric age group are lymphoma, followed by rhabdomyosarcoma (19).

Thyroglossal Duct Cysts

Thyroglossal duct cysts account for about 90% of congenital neck lesions and usually are found in children, but may be seen in adults (20). The thyroglossal

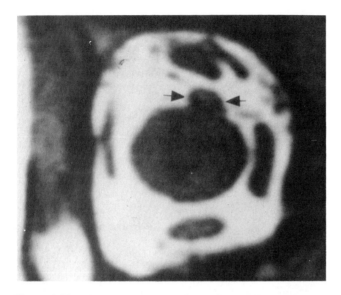

Figure 9.22.　Cavernous Hemangioma. Coronal T1-weighted image through the mid-orbit. A well-circumscribed retrobulbar mass is identified. The optic nerve is clearly visualized as separate from the mass (arrows). The well-circumscribed nature of this mass is characteristic of a cavernous hemangioma, and is the most common orbital mass in an adult.

Figure 9.23.　Carotid Cavernous Fistula. Axial T1-weighted image through the level of the upper orbit. A large flow void is identified in the right cavernous sinus (white arrows). The right superior ophthalmic vein is abnormally dilated (open arrows), while the left vein is normal (black arrows).

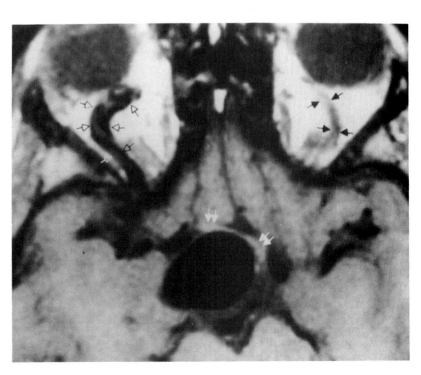

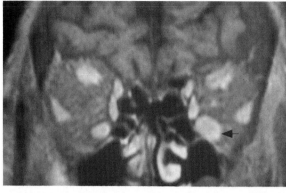

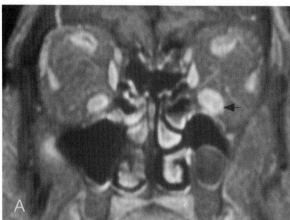

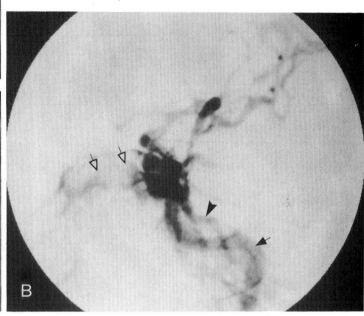

Figure 9.24. Cavernous Carotid Fistula. A. Coronal post-gadolinium fat-suppression T1-weighted image. A 35-year-old female presented with left proptosis. Coronal images reveal mild enlargement of the left inferior rectus muscle. Clinical symptoms were consistent with thyroid ophthalmopathy. At surgery, for apex decompression due to deteriorating vision, massive blood loss ensued. **B.** Coronal projection, left internal carotid artery injection (*arrow*).

Contrast is identified rapidly filling the cavernous sinus (*open arrows*) and inferior petrosal sinus (*arrowhead*). The cavernous sinuses and superior ophthalmic veins were entirely normal on MR in retrospective evaluation. This represents a case of spontaneous cavernous carotid fistula without significant drainage into the superior ophthalmic veins. Extraocular muscle enlargement has many causes, one of which is venous congestion due to a cavernous carotid fistula.

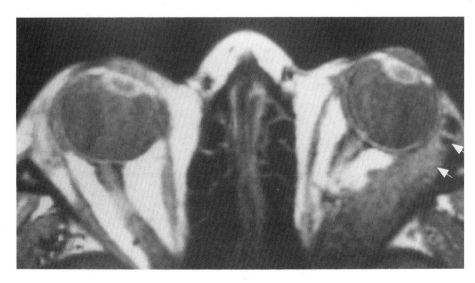

Figure 9.25. Pseudotumor. Axial T1-weighted image through the orbits. A diffusely infiltrating lesion is identified extending along the lateral rectus muscles. This lesion extends anteriorly to involve the tendinous insertion of the muscle to the globe (*arrows*). This is a feature that distinguishes pseudotumor from thyroid ophthalmopathy, in which the muscle insertion is spared.

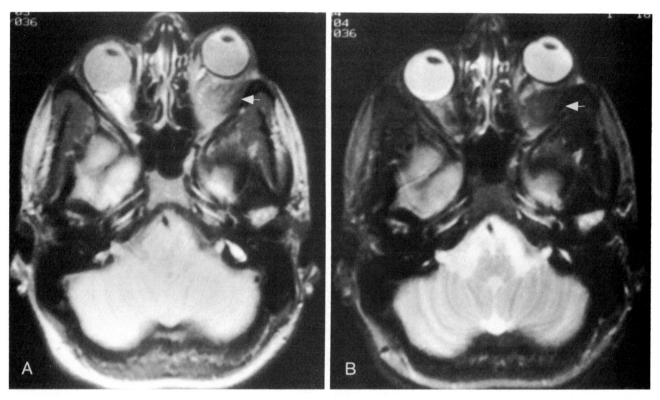

Figure 9.26. Pseudotumor. Axial first and second echo T2-weighted image. A soft-tissue mass (*arrow*) is located in the left orbit with associated proptosis. This lesion demonstrates T2 shortening (dark on T2) on the heavily T2-weighted sequence. This finding is useful in helping to differentiate lymphoma from pseudotumor, which otherwise present very similarly.

Figure 9.27. Thyroid Ophthalmopathy. Coronal T1-weighted image through the midorbits. Marked extraocular muscle enlargement is identified, involving primarily the medial and inferior rectus muscles. Thyroid ophthalmopathy is the most common cause of proptosis in the adult. Severe muscle hypertrophy may result in orbital apex compression and loss of vision.

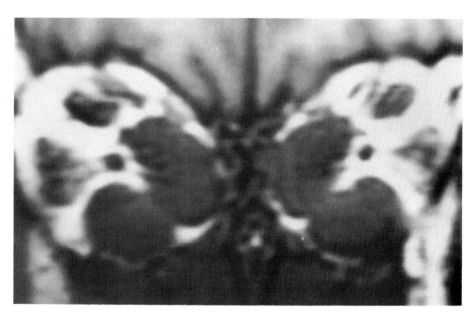

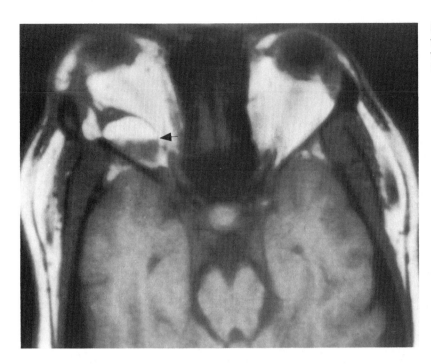

Figure 9.28. Dermoid. Axial T1-weighted image. A well-circumscribed mass is found in the lateral orbit, which demonstrates a fat-fluid level (*arrow*). This finding is characteristic for a dermoid.

duct represents an epithelial-lined tract along which the primordial thyroid gland migrates. This tubular structure originates from the foramen cecum (at the tongue base) and extends anterior to the thyrohyoid membrane and strap muscles before ending at the level of the thyroid isthmus. The duct normally involutes by 8 to 10 weeks of gestation. Because the duct is lined with secretory epithelium, a cyst may form along any portion of the thyroglossal duct that fails to involute, giving rise to a thyroglossal duct cyst. Additionally, thyroid glandular tissue can be arrested anywhere along the course of the thyroglossal duct, giving rise to ectopic thyroid tissue. Seventy-five percent of thyroglossal duct cysts are midline, and most are located at or below the level of the hyoid bone in the region of the thyrohyoid membrane (21). In fact, thyroglossal duct cysts are the most common midline neck mass. However, 25% are located in an off-midline location.

Surgery is the treatment of choice for these lesions since they may become infected. These lesions tend to recur if incompletely resected. As a result, sagittal MR imaging is ideal for determining the full extent of the lesion prior to surgery. On CT and MR scanning, these lesions appear as cystic masses with a uniformly thin peripheral rim of capsular enhancement, with occasional septations (Fig. 9.29). Differential diagnostic considerations include necrotic anterior cervical nodes, thrombosed anterior jugular vein, abscess, or obstructed laryngocele.

Branchial Cleft Cysts

Structures of the face and neck are derived from the branchial cleft apparatus, which consists of six branchial arches. A branchial cleft cyst, sinus, or fistula may develop if there is failure of the cervical sinus or pouch remnants to regress. Although branchial abnormalities can arise from any of the pouches, the majority (95%) arise from the second branchial cleft (22). The course of the second branchial cleft begins at the base of the tonsillar fossa and extends between the internal and external carotid arteries. Thus, second branchial cleft cysts are typically found along this pathway, anterior to the middle portion of the sternocleidomastoid muscle and lateral to the internal jugular vein at the level of the carotid bifurcation. The usual clinical presentation is that of a painless neck mass along the anterior border of the sternocleidomastoid muscle, presenting during the first to third decade. These lesions tend to vary in size over time, often enlarging with upper respiratory tract infections (23).

Branchial cleft cysts are readily identified on CT and MR as well-circumscribed cystic lesions. Wall thickness, irregularity, and enhancement are related to active or prior infections. With MR imaging, the T1-weighted signal characteristics of the cyst may be either hypo- or hyperintense (Fig. 9.30). This signal variability is related to proteinacious cyst contents. Differential diagnostic considerations include necrotic nodes, abscesses, cystic neural lesions, and thrombosed vessels.

Lymphangiomas and Cystic Hygromas

Lymphangiomas are congenital malformations of lymphatic channels. These lesions are benign and nonencapsulated. Histologically they are classified as

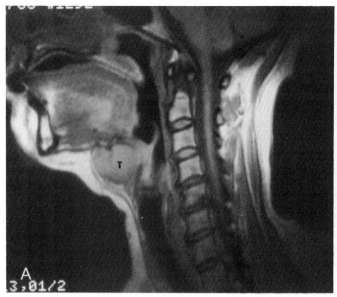

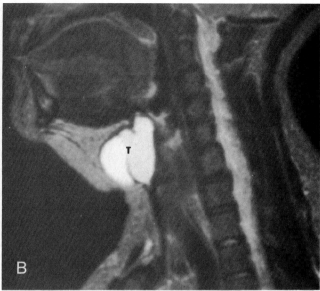

Figure 9.29. Thyroglossal Duct Cyst. Sagittal T1- (**A**) and T2-weighted (**B**) sequences. A well-defined cystic structure (*T*) is seen below the tongue base. A cystic lesion in this location is highly suggestive of a remnant of the thyroglossal duct.

capillary, cavernous, or cystic. Any of these histologic types can be found in a lesion, but the preponderance of a certain type dictates how the lesion is classified. The capillary lymphangiomas are composed of capillary-sized, thin-walled lymphatic channels. In contrast, cavernous lymphangiomas are composed of moderately dilated lymphatics with a fibrous adventitia. Cystic hygromas represent enormously dilated lymphatic channels.

The lymphatic system develops from primitive embryonic lymph sacs that are derived from the venous system. If these sacs fail to communicate with the venous system, they dilate with lymphatic fluid. Thus, lymphangiomas represent sequestrations of the primitive embryonic lymph sacs. If this defect is localized, the result is an isolated cystic hygroma. However, extensive defects in this communication are incompatible with life, and results in fetal hydrops. Various congenital malformation syndromes occur in association with fetal cystic hygromas including Turner's syndrome, fetal alcohol syndrome, Noonan's syndrome, and several chromosomal aneuploidies.

Most lymphangiomas present by 2 years of age (90%), with 50% presenting at the time of birth. This early presentation reflects that the time of greatest lymphatic development occurs in the first 2 years of life.

Cystic hygromas appear as painless compressible neck masses that, if large enough, will transilluminate. The lesions commonly occur in the posterior triangle of the neck, but may be found in the floor of the mouth. On imaging studies these lesions are multiloculated cystic masses with septations (Fig. 9.31).

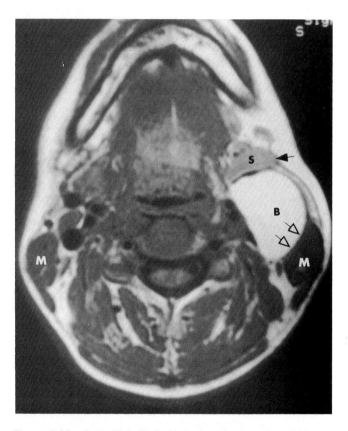

Figure 9.30. Branchial Cleft Cyst. Axial T1-weighted sequence through the floor of the mouth. A well-rounded, noninfiltrating lesion (*B*) is seen anterior to the left sternocleidomastoid muscle (*M*), which is displaced posteriorly (*open arrows*). The submandibular gland (*S*) is displaced anteriorly (*arrow*). Branchial cleft cysts may occasionally display high signal on the T1-weighted sequence, the result of T1 shortening effect of proteinacious fluid.

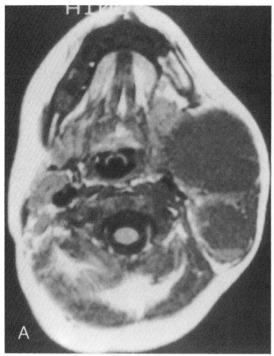

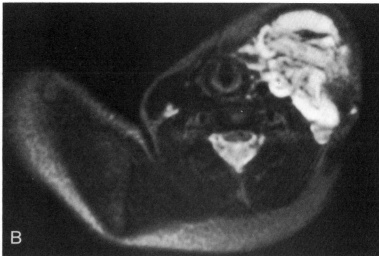

Figure 9.31. Cystic Hygroma. Axial T1- (**A**) and T2-weighted (**B**) images at the level of the floor of the mouth and the larynx, respectively. A 2-month-old infant presented with a left neck mass. This lesion is multiloculated and extends within the soft tissues of the anterior neck. The heterogeneous signal on the T2-weighted sequence is characteristic of a cystic hygroma or lymphangioma.

The thickness of the septations and walls is related to prior infections. Since the lesions are easily compressible, they do not displace adjacent soft-tissue structures, and this may prove a helpful differentiating feature from other cystic lesions, such as necrotic lymph nodes. These lesions also have a propensity to hemorrhage into themselves. This may result in a dramatic increase in the size of the lesion. On imaging studies one can expect a fluid-fluid level and sometimes signal characteristics associated with hemorrhage.

References

1. Carrau RL, Myers EN, Johnson JT. Management of tumors arising in the parapharyngeal space. Laryngoscope 1990;100:583–589.
2. Harnsberger HR, Bragg DG, Osborn AG. Non-hodgkin's lymphoma of the head and neck: CT evaluation of nodal and extranodal sites. AJNR 1987;8:673–677.
3. Biller HF, Som P, Lawson W, Rosenfeld R. Glomus vagale tumors. Ann Otol Rhinol Laryngol 1989;98:21–26.
4. Leonetti JP, Brackmann DE. Glomus vagale tumor: the significance of early vocal cord paralysis. Otolaryngol Head Neck Surg 1989;100:533–537.
5. Vogl T, Bruning R, Schedel H, et al. Paragangliomas of the jugular bulb and carotid body: MR imaging with short sequences and Gd-DTPA enhancement. AJR 1989;153:583–587.
6. Freling NJM, Molenaar WM, Vermey A, et al. Malignant parotid tumors: clinical use of MR imaging and histologic correlation. Radiology 1992;185:691–696.
7. Holliday RA, Cohen WA, Schinella RA, et al. Benign lymphoepithelial parotid cysts and hyperplastic cervical adenopathy in AIDS—risk patients: a new CT appearance. Radiology 1988;168:439–441.
8. Davis WL, Harnsberger HR, Smoker WRK, Watanabe AS. Retropharyngeal space: evaluation of normal anatomy and disease with CT and MR imaging. Radiology 1990;174:59–64.
9. Batsakis JG, Sneige N. Parapharyngeal and retropharyngeal space diseases. Ann Otol Rhinol Laryngol 1989;98:320–321.
10. Kalnins IK, et al. Correlation between prognosis and degree of lymph node involvement in cancer of the oral cavity. Am J Surg 1977;134:450.
11. Johnson JT. A surgeon looks at cervical lymph nodes. Radiology 1990;175:607–610.
12. Ali S, Tiwari RM, Snow GB. False positive and false negative neck nodes. Head Neck 1985;8:78–82.
13. Stern WBR, Silver CE, Zeifer BA, Persky MS, Heller KS. Computed tomography of the clinically negative neck. Head Neck Surg 1990;12:109–113.
14. Reede D, Bergeron RT. CT of cervical lymph nodes. J Otolaryngol 1982;11:411–418.
15. Mancuso AA, Harnberger HR, Muraki AS, Stevens MH. Computed tomography of cervical and retropharyngeal lymph nodes: normal anatomy, variants of normal, and applications in staging head and neck cancer. Part II: Pathology. Radiology 1983;148:715–723.
16. Mancuso AA, Harnberger HR, Muraki AS, Stevens MH. Computed tomography of cervical and retropharyngeal lymph nodes: normal anatomy, variants of normal, and applications in staging head and neck cancer. Part I: Normal anatomy. Radiology 1983;148:709–714.
17. Mancuso AA, Maceri D, Rice D, Hanafee W. CT of cervical lymph node cancer. AJR 1981;136:381–385.
18. Sonnino RE, Spigland N, Laberge JM, Desjardins J, Guttman FM. Unusual patterns of congenital neck masses in children. J Pediatr Surg 1989;24:966–969.

19. Putlley FJ. The diagnosis of head and neck masses in children. Otolaryngol Clin North Am 1970;3:277–289.

20. Allard RHB. The thyroglossal cyst. Head Neck Surg 1982;5:134–146.

21. Thomas JR. Thyroglossal duct cyst. Ear Nose Throat J 1979;58:512–517.

22. Pounds LA. Neck masses of congenital origin. Pediatr Clin North Am 1981;28:841–844.

23. Telander RI, Deane SA. Thyroglossal and branchial cleft cysts and sinuses. Surg Clin North Am 1977;57:779–791.

10

Nondegenerative Diseases of the Spine

ERIK H. L. GAENSLER

This chapter focuses on nondegenerative diseases of the spinal cord, meninges, and paraspinous soft tissues, and is divided into sections discussing inflammation, infection, neoplasms, vascular diseases, congenital malformations, and trauma (1–5). The spine is composed of vertebrae, which house the spinal cord, and thereby represents a "border zone" between the central nervous system (CNS) and musculoskeletal system (this is true politically as well as anatomically—with both neurosurgeons and orthopaedic surgeons claiming the spine as their province). Disc degeneration, spinal stenosis, and primary osseous tumors involving the vertebrae are covered in separate chapters.

Common Clinical Syndromes

Patients with spine disorders present with focal or diffuse "back pain," radiculopathy, or myelopathy, and the clinical syndromes produced by degenerative disease and nondegenerative disease can be difficult to distinguish. Focal back pain without neurologic compromise is not usually an emergency, although it is virtually an epidemic in our society, with tremendous implications in terms of lost productivity. Focal back pain can be due to a wide variety of both degenerative and nondegenerative processes. In the low back, the causes most commonly are orthopaedic, such as muscle and ligament strain, facet joint dis-

ease, or discogenic disease that does not compromise the nerve roots. However, vertebral metastases or infectious discitis may also cause focal back pain. Since degenerative disease of the spine is far more common than nondegenerative disease, nondegenerative processes may initially be overlooked, with disastrous consequences. Therefore, a good clinical history that specifically addresses any previous cancers, or ongoing fevers and chills, is crucial in raising the index of suspicion for a nondegenerative process. When history and physical findings are nonspecific, as often is the case, imaging procedures become central to the diagnosis.

In patients with spinal neurologic findings, an attempt should be made to distinguish between the clinical syndromes of myelopathy and radiculopathy, as they differ in significant respects, including degree of urgency. Important distinctions between radiculopathy and myelopathy are summarized in Table 10.1.

Myelopathy results from compromise of the spinal cord itself, due to mechanical compression, intrinsic lesions, or inflammatory processes loosely grouped under the term "myelitis." Classic symptoms include bladder and bowel incontinence, spasticity, weakness, and ataxia. With cord compression, a motor or sensory level may develop, and is helpful in focusing the imaging examination. However, the lesion may be several vertebral bodies higher than the apparent dermatomal sensory level, particularly in the thoracic region. Myelopathy often presents without a clear sensory level, and complete screening of the cord from the cervicomedullary junction to the conus is required.

The spinal cord is part of the CNS and, like the brain, has limited healing powers. In fact, the spinal cord in many respects is less tolerant of injury than the brain. A small benign mass, such as a 2-cm epidural hematoma or meningioma, may permanently damage the cord, because of the small diameter of the spinal canal. A similar-sized mass is often asymptomatic within the voluminous calvarium. The "plasticity" of the brain, whereby remaining cortex can assume the function of injured areas through a complex network of redundant axons, is well documented, particularly in younger patients. The spinal cord, which consists of long linear neuronal tracts, has far less plasticity.

Table 10.1. Myelopathy vs. Radiculopathy

	Myelopathy	Radiculopathy
Cause	Spinal cord compromise	Spinal nerve compromise
Typical disease processes	Extramedullary disease: cord compression due to epidural mass effect	Osteophytic spurring (especially C-spine)
		Disc herniations
	Intramedullary disease: tumor, inflammation AVMs, SDAVFs[a]	Extramedullary and paraspinous tumors and inflammatory processes compromising nerve roots
Neurologic findings	Ataxia	Weakness and diminished reflexes in specific muscle groups, dermatomal sensory deficits
	Bowel and bladder incontinence	
	Babinski's sign	
Accuracy of clinical localization	Often poor; lesion may be several levels higher than anticipated	Usually quite good
Urgency for imaging (of acute presentations)	High—little recovery expected with deficits untreated >24 hour	Low—short delay for conservative treatment usually entails little risk
Preferred imaging modality	MR has no substitute as the initial screening exam	CT, especially with intrathecal contrast is still excellent, particularly in C-spine

[a]Spinal dural arteriovenous fistula.

After 24 hours of acute cord compression, there is little hope for significant recovery of function. Therefore, an acute myelopathy is an emergency, where the radiologist should do everything to facilitate prompt imaging, preferably with magnetic resonance imaging (MR), for reasons that will be discussed below.

Radiculopathy results from impingement of the spinal nerves, either within the canal, lateral recesses, or neural foramina. This compromise, typically because of mass effect, results in specific dermatomal sensory deficits and muscle group weakness. These are outlined in any neurology or physical diagnosis text, and are worth knowing. The most common causes include disc herniations and, in the cervical spine, uncovertebral joint spurring, although malignant and infectious processes can equally compromise spinal nerves. The peripheral nervous system, unlike the CNS, has significant ability to withstand injury and to regenerate. Therefore, pure radicular symptoms, although at times excruciatingly painful, rarely represent a surgical emergency. Extensive epidural neoplasms and infections may present with mixed myelopathic and radicular signs. These patients must be imaged with the urgency of a pure cord syndrome.

Imaging Methods

Plain Radiographs of the spine used to be the initial test in every spine evaluation, but with newer techniques this is no longer logical or cost-effective. Radiographs continue to be the mainstay for ruling out trauma to the vertebral column (discussed Chapter 36), and other acute screening settings. Plain films are indispensable for correct localization in the operating room. Radiographs have a great deal of useful information to offer when evaluating degenerative processes, particularly with extensive osteophyte formation in the cervical spine. Flexion and extension plain films used to be the only dynamic imaging technique for assessment of spine stability. Magnetic resonance imaging now also can be done in flexion and extension, which can be useful in evaluating cord compression which is positional (see Fig. 10.8).

In nondegenerative disease, careful attention should be paid to the integrity of the vertebral bodies and pedicles, frequent sites of metastases. However, early infiltrative changes in the marrow space, easily seen on MR, cannot be detected by plain films. The classic radiographic findings of widened interpedicular distance with tumors, and midline bony spurs with diastematomyelia, are rarely seen except on board examinations.

Myelography. The definitive indications for plain film myelography are limited, and include survey for leptomeningeal drop metastases if the MR examination is equivocal, suspected spinal vascular malformations, complex postoperative cases, and patients in whom MR is contraindicated. Water-soluble nonionic contrast media have low toxicity, and have replaced metrizamide, an older agent, although the term "metrizamide myelogram" has stuck. Pantopaque (iophendylate), an even older oil-based iodinated medium, is almost never used. *Ionic contrast agents are absolutely contraindicated for myelography*, as they can result in severe inflammation, seizures, arachnoiditis, and death.

The recommended dosage of nonionic contrast in adults depends on the region to be studied, the size of the patient, and the size of thecal sac. A convenient and conservative rule of thumb in adults is not to exceed 3 g of intrathecal iodine, which works out to 17 ml of 180 mg/ml, 12.5 ml of 240 mg/ml, or 10 ml of 300 mg/ml, three of the standard concentrations. In general, lumbar myelography should be performed using contrast media with a concentration between 180 and 240 mg/ml, and cervical and/or thoracic myelography should be performed with 200–300 mg/ml. The smaller the area of the subarachnoid space, the denser the contrast must be for good plain films. With the high contrast sensitivity of computed tomography (CT), 180 mg/ml is more than adequate, and small doses (5 ml), or dilution of the full dose with time (3–4 hours delay if a full dose is given) is required for proper iodine concentration to avoid CT artifacts. Full-dose plain film myelography was already in decline before MR because of CT myelography, which can be done with lower doses of intrathecal contrast.

Myelography begins with a lumbar puncture, with the patient in prone position under fluoroscopy. The preferred puncture site depends on the clinical findings, and usually is the upper lumbar region, inferior to the posterior elements of L-2 or L-3. This injection level will avoid most disc herniations and spinal stenosis, which are usually worse at lower levels, and the conus, which in adults lies between T-12/L-1 and L-1/L-2 disc spaces. Care should be taken to place the needle near the midline in order to reduce the chances of an extra-arachnoid injection, or spearing of an exiting nerve root. Contrast should be injected only after spontaneous CSF backflow is established. The complications of poor needle placement include subdural and epidural injection. Examples of these complications are well illustrated in older neuroradiology textbooks, and have medicolegal implications, so if in doubt where the contrast is going, stop, take frontal and lateral plain films, and examine them carefully. Avoid any air bubbles in the tubing system, as they can cause filling defects easily confused with drop metastases. If tumor or infection is suspected, collect adequate CSF for chemistry, cultures, and cytology if this has not already been done. For routine degenerative cases, CSF examination has not proved worthwhile.

C1-2 punctures are rarely required, and are inherently more dangerous than lumbar injection, as direct injury to the cord or a low-lying posterior inferior cerebellar artery loop can occur. The puncture is best done under lateral fluoroscopy, placing the needle in the posterior third of the spinal canal between C-1 and C-2. Classic indications include known blocks caudally, or the need for dense opacification of the cervical and upper thoracic spinal canal for plain films. Today, one of the rare good reasons for a C1-2 puncture would be complete spine block in the midthoracic region identified by lumbar myelography, with the need to define the upper extent of the block—in a patient with a pacemaker precluding MR. If the pacemaker were not an issue, MR would have been the study of choice as the marrow space can be examined, and the MR is far quicker, more comfortable,

and, most importantly, safer for the patient. Even if there is no technical complication with a myelogram, patients with spine block can deteriorate from the subtle fluid and pressure shifts that inevitably accompany needle placement in the subarachnoid space, a syndrome known as "spinal coning." The multiple steps in the evaluation of spine block by plain film myelography followed by CT are shown in Figure 10.1. Contrast this with the simplicity and elegance of MR as shown in Figure 10.2.

Space-occupying lesions of the spinal canal are classified according to their location as intramedullary, intradural-extramedullary, and extradural. This distinction can be made on myelography, as well as on CT and MR, and is critical in formulating a differential diagnosis. Intramedullary lesions are usually confined to the spinal cord itself, but may be exophytic. Extramedullary lesions are by definition outside the cord, but may be either intra- or extradural. A summary of the radiologic appearance and differential diagnosis for each lesion location is outlined in Table 10.2. Remember that the lesion must be seen in at least two (and preferably three) 90° orthogonal planes, since large intradural lesions may simulate an extradural mass on any single view. Similarly, bilateral extradural disease can flatten the cord, increasing its apparent anteroposterior dimension in sagittal view, giving the false impression of an intramedullary mass (Fig. 10. 3). Correlation with axial imaging is invaluable in this regard. Also remember that lateral lesions, such as lateral disc herniations, may be completely missed by myelography. In most cases today, a CT is performed after myelography.

Computed Tomography. The decline of plain film myelography for degenerative disease was initially because of CT, especially CT with intrathecal contrast, which is superior to myelography in diagnostic accuracy. However, CT now steadily is being replaced by MR for most screening examinations of the spine. Low-dose CT myelography remains the gold standard in cases where the limits of the thecal sac or nerve root sleeves need to be precisely defined, such as in complex postoperative states. Small leptomeningeal (drop) metastases can be identified; however, MR with gadolinium has largely replaced CT myelography as the initial screening examination for drop metastases. In the cervical spine, CT remains the most reliable way to assess foraminal stenosis.

Computed tomography has been less effective in depicting intramedullary diseases of the spinal cord such as primary tumors, myelitis, and syringohydromyelia. These conditions are better evaluated with MR. For example, a nonexpansile multiple sclerosis (MS) plaque will escape detection on any imaging examination except MR.

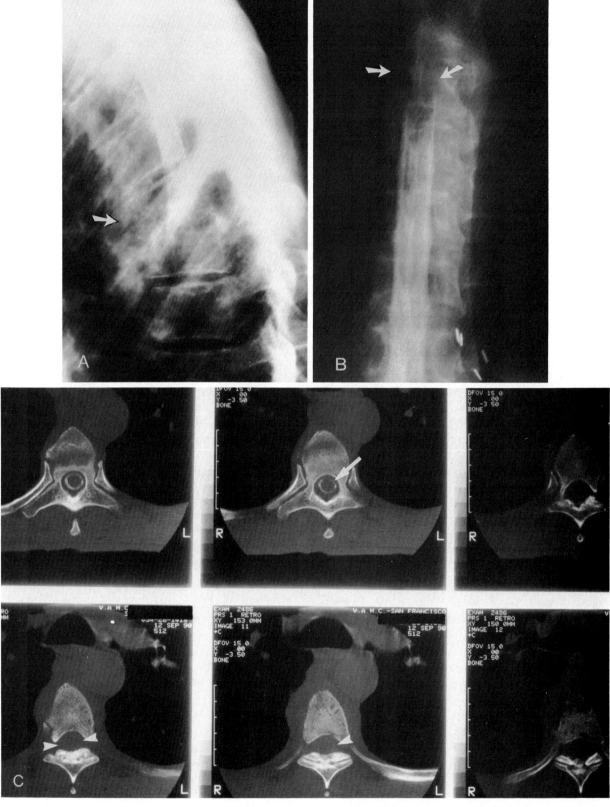

Figure 10.1. Acute Cord Compression. Middle-aged patient with acute myelopathy and midthoracic back pain, worked up the "old-fashioned" way. **A.** Plain film done in the emergency department shows compression fracture of a midthoracic vertebrae (*arrow*). **B.** Lumbar myelogram shows complete block to contrast in the midthoracic vertebrae (*arrows*). A portable C-arm fluoroscope then had to be obtained to do a C1-2 puncture, followed by a cervical and upper thoracic myelogram (not shown). **C.** Upper thoracic CT- myelogram images show gradual effacement of the subarachnoid space (*arrow*), which disappears at site of the block (*arrowheads*). **D.** Sagittal reconstruction enables assessment of the entire process in a single image, showing cord compression centered around an abnormal disc space (*arrow*), consistent with infection, which was proven at laminectomy. Note the gradual effacement of the subarachnoid space (*arrowheads*). Total elapsed time for procedures **A** to **D**: 3 hours—not bad for this technique!

Magnetic Resonance Imaging has done for the spinal canal what CT did for the calvarium, allowing for the first time a noninvasive "look inside." Therefore, it has become the examination of choice for any disorder of the spine resulting in myelopathy. The key to MR's success has been its superior soft-tissue contrast (including the ability to evaluate the marrow compartment), multiplanar capabilities, noninvasiveness, and high sensitivity to gadolinium enhancement, recently heightened further by fat saturation techniques.

Magnetic resonance scanning techniques for the spine continue to improve, and with the wide variety of imaging systems available, it makes little sense to recommend specific protocols in a general text. A few general guidelines follow. Surface coils are an absolute must in order to obtain adequate signal to noise in most systems. Motion "suppression" techniques, such as anterior radiofrequency saturation bands, gradient moment nulling, and cardiac/respiratory gating, are critical to reduce motion artifact. This is particularly important on T2 spin echo images of the cervical and thoracic spine, which remain the gold standard for evaluating intrinsic cord disease. Gradient-echo imaging has reduced imaging time and allowed for the rapid acquisition of myelographic "white CSF" images.

Gradient-echo images are less sensitive for marrow space evaluation, because of susceptibility effects from the bony trabeculae. Short TR inversion recovery (STIR) probably offers the highest sensitivity for marrow space edema, but until recently STIR has been time-consuming, with poor signal to noise. "Fast inversion recovery" techniques, however, have recently been developed, and will likely become standard in the near future. Ultrathin section imaging (<1 mm) without interslice gaps is now performed with three-dimensional Fourier transformation and now rivals CT for thin slice profiles, critical in the cervical spine for examination of the foramina.

There are, however, some pitfalls with spinal MR, which include motion sensitivity, imprecise detection of calcium, and occasional false-negatives with contrast examinations. Despite motion compensation techniques, both physiologic and patient motion remain problematic. Patient movement will tend to ex-

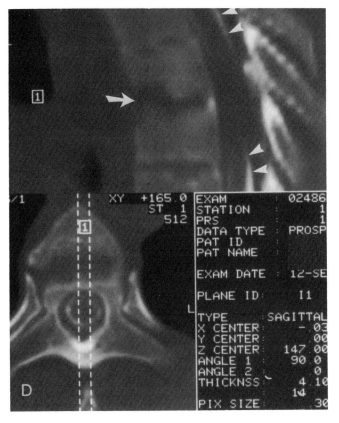

Figure 10.1D.

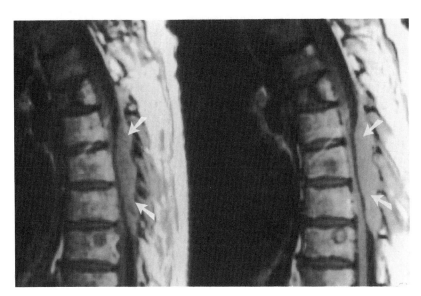

Figure 10.2. Acute Cord Compression—MR. Evaluation of a thoracic cord compression, the easy way—compare with Figure 10.1. A middle-aged patient presented to a physician's office with acute myelopathy. This emergency MR using T1 sagittal and axial sequences took 20 minutes, was completely noninvasive, and gives excellent detail of the marrow space, unavailable on CT. The epidural soft tissue mass (*arrows*) turned out to be lymphoma.

aggerate osseous encroachment of the spinal canal and neural foramina, as far more movement occurs during the 12 minutes it may take to do a three-dimensional Fourier transformation cervical spine axial image than a 2-second CT slice. Spin echo MR techniques are generally inferior to CT in the detection of subtle calcification. This may be important in defining small osteophytic spurring, ossification of the posterior longitudinal ligament, identifying retropulsed bone fragments following trauma, or characterizing calcification in tumors. Gradient recalled techniques may overestimate the size of calcific struc-

Table 10.2. Differential Diagnosis of Spinal Lesions by Location[a]

LOCATION AND IMAGING APPEARANCE

DIFFENTIAL DIAGNOSIS

A. INTRADURAL   INTRAMEDULLARY

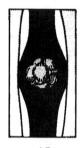 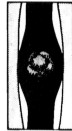 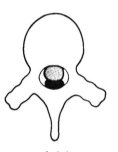

AP   Lateral   Axial

Cord appears widened in all views. The CSF space appears thinned on all sides in all views.

Ependymoma
Astrocytoma
Hemanigioblastoma
Lipoma/(Epi)Dermoid
Syringohydromyelia
Intramedullary AVM
Rare site: met/abscess

B. INTRADURAL   EXTRAMEDULLARY

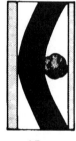 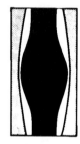

AP   Lateral   Axial

The contrast/CSF forms acute angles with the mass (which may have a dural attachment—"marble on the carpet"). This results in a "meniscus" around the mass, and a widened contrast column between the cord and the mass on one side, with effacement of the CSF on the other.

DIFFERENTIAL DIAGNOSIS

Meningioma
Schwannoma/neurinoma
Neurofibroma
Hemangiopericytoma
Lipoma/(Epi) Dermoid
Arachnoid cyst/adhesion
Drop/leptomeningeal met
Veins (extramed AVM)

C. EXTRADURAL

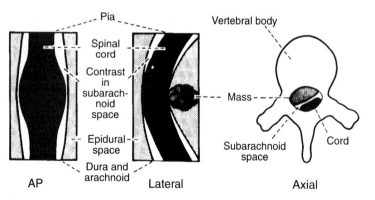

AP   Lateral   Axial

The dura and the sac will be displaced together, away from the mass. The CSF angles around the mass will be obtuse with a "marble under the carpet" appearance. The cord may be widened in one plane by pressure from the mass, with contrast material thinned on both sides of the cord.

DIFFERENTIAL DIAGNOSIS

Degenerative
　Herniated disc
　Synovial cyst
　Osteophyte
　Rheumatoid pannus
Non-Degenerative
　Metastasis
　Abscess
　Hematoma
　1° tumor expansion
　　or invasion
　Epidural lipomatosis

[a]Adapted from Latchaw RE, ed. MR and CT of the head, neck, and spine. 2nd ed. St. Louis: Mosby, 1991.

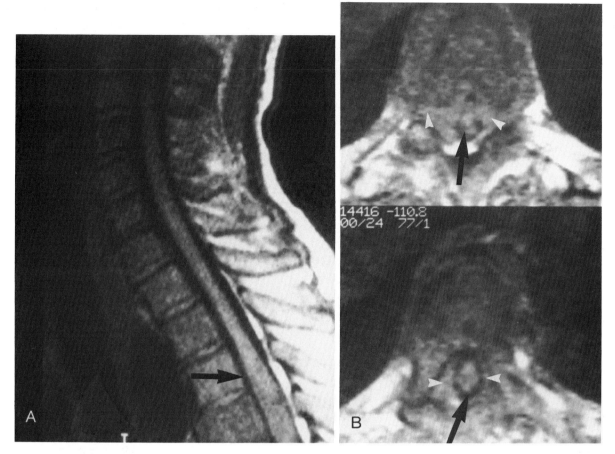

Figure 10.3. Extramedullary Tumor. This patient presented with myelopathy with an upper thoracic sensory level. **A.** On this midline sagittal image, the spinal cord appears widened (*arrow*), suggestive of an intramedullary lesion. The patient was unable to stay still for additional images. **B.** Subsequent reimaging in the axial plain shows that extramedullary tumor (*arrowheads*) has flattened the cord (*arrow*) from its sides, increasing its anteroposterior dimensions, giving the spurious impression of intramedullary expansile process on the midline sagittal images. The moral is the same as on plain films: always look at pathology in two (preferable 90° opposed) orthogonal planes.

tures, because of susceptibility effects. Gadolinium is essential in the evaluation of infection and intrathecal metastases, but may obscure vertebral metastases by making them isointense with surrounding marrow fat (Fig. 10.4). Also, it is difficult to evaluate hemorrhage on postcontrast images. Always obtain a pre-contrast T1 "scout" image to avoid these latter two pitfalls.

Spinal Angiography is technically demanding, dangerous in untrained hands, and difficult to interpret. There is no reliable spinal "circle of Willis" allowing collateral flow from multiple sources, although some variable interconnected vascular arcades exist. Therefore, an inadvertent catheter-induced complication can have tragic consequences. Excellent texts exist on spinal angiography, but this area has increasingly become the province of interventional neuroradiologists, who can both diagnose and often treat spinal arteriovenous malformations—the main indication for spinal angiography.

Nuclear Medicine Bone Scans give a comprehensive view of the skeleton when searching for me-

tastases. If a new focus of vertebral isotope uptake is noted, and plain films fail to show an abnormality, MR is increasingly used because of its excellent delineation of the marrow space and any associated spinal cord compression. Bone scans are highly sensitive but quite nonspecific, as both degenerative and nondegenerative processes will show increased uptake. When such patients are referred for MR, it is critical to be aware of the bone scan findings in order to protocol the examination appropriately.

Ultrasound has limited applications in the spine, as in adults the posterior elements obscure the potential acoustic window. However, in neonates the unossified posterior elements provide a window through which spinal anomalies can be evaluated, and excellent work has been done in this highly specialized area. Once the laminae have been removed surgically, intraoperative ultrasound has proven to be an excellent tool for the evaluation of the spinal cord for tumor, syrinx, and other intramedullary processes, minimizing the need for cord exploration.

Figure 10.4.   Gadolinium-enhanced Imaging Potential Pitfalls. A. Infiltration of the entire L-4 vertebral body on this unenhanced lumbar examination (*arrow*) is readily apparent. **B.** After contrast administration, the area involved with metastatic tumor (*arrow*) has enhanced to isointensity with the remaining normal vertebrae, and is far less conspicuous. The lesion still could be visualized with fat saturation or STIR techniques, despite the gadolinium, but why do things the hard way? Moral: always obtain a precontrast image when using gadolinium in the spine.

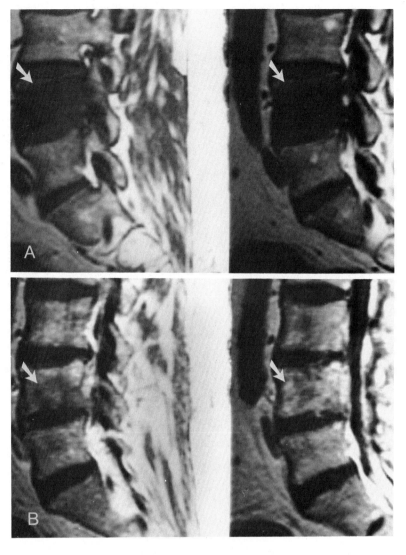

INFLAMMATION

This section focuses on inflammatory diseases that cause myelopathy, principally through direct involvement of the spinal cord (6–12). The mechanisms of many of these disorders is not fully understood, and they are sometimes lumped under the term "myelitis." Myelitis may be focal or diffuse. When both clinical and pathologic findings are confined to distinct level(s), the term "transverse myelitis" may be used. It must be recognized that this is not really a specific disease, but rather a category of diseases, and few agree on exactly what processes should be lumped under transverse myelitis. On the whole, it is better to carefully describe the imaging findings, and give specific differential diagnoses, than to invoke such nonspecific terms in MR reports. Strictly speaking, a distinction should be made between processes affecting the gray matter, termed poliomyelitis, and those affecting the white matter, or leukomyelitis. In practice, these terms are rarely heard, and poliomyelitis be-

come synonymous with the colloquial "polio," a specific syndrome caused by a specific picornavirus, against which we all hopefully have been vaccinated.

Multiple Sclerosis is the most common spinal cord "inflammatory" disorder. The epidemiology and pathophysiology of MS are reviewed in detail in Chapter 7. Multiple sclerosis of the brain and spinal cord are similar in terms of patient profile, with the hallmark of the disease being multiple neurologic deficits separated both anatomically and temporally. When spinal MS predominates, it tends to follow a progressive clinical course, as opposed to the relapsing/remitting pattern more characteristic with brain involvement. The majority of MS patients have "mixed" presentations, with both brain and spinal cord involvement. While imaging can be helpful, the diagnosis ultimately rests on clinical grounds.

Multiple sclerosis plaques appear as areas of increased signal in the white matter of the spinal cord, typically within the white matter of the anterior and posterior columns and lateral spinothalamic tracts. The best screening study is a gated sagittal T2-

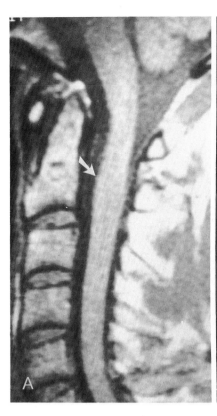
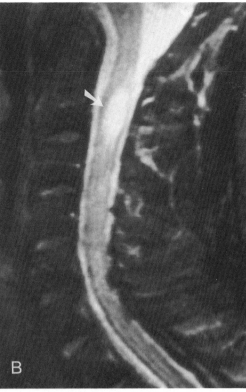

Figure 10.5. Multiple Sclerosis (MS). A. This solitary lesion shows subtle cord expansion on T1-weighted images, and **(B)** becomes bright on T2-weighted imaging (*arrow*), due to edema. Differential considerations included an intramedullary tumor, and the diagnosis of MS was supported by the confirmation of concomitant periventricular lesions classic for MS on brain MR.

weighted series, where MS plaques appear as areas of increased signal intensity, usually without significant change in cord diameter, which is why cord MS plaques are often occult myelographically. Occasionally, there may be subtle cord expansion in the acute phase because of edema, (Fig. 10.5) and "burnt out" MS plaques can present as myelomalacia (literally cord "softening" or atrophy).

As in the brain, plaque enhancement may be present, which correlates loosely with lesion activity (Fig. 10.6). Both edema and enhancement can appear to involve the central gray matter in addition to the white matter, probably because of perivenular inflammatory changes. Differentiation from a glial tumor may be difficult. When a small bright intramedullary lesion is seen on T2-weighted image, MR of the brain to search for concomitant MS plaques is a more useful next step than contrast administration. The brain and spinal cord are composed of the same tissue types, are physically connected, and share the CSF. Therefore, a good general rule is when presented with a diffuse spinal process, either intramedullary or leptomeningeal, remember to look "upstairs," because the same process may be involving the brain.

Lupus Erythematosis. Other CNS inflammatory processes are seen in both the brain and spinal cord. A classic example is systemic lupus erythmatosus, where a necrotizing arteritis leads to cord ischemia and injury. Antibodies may also damage neuronal elements directly. The white matter of both the brain and the spinal cord will show diffuse areas of increased signal intensity on T2-weighted images, sometimes with enhancement. (Fig. 10.7). These lesions are less well defined than the discrete plaques of MS, and may show dramatic improvement with corticosteriods. Multiple sclerosis plaques, in contrast, represent areas of focal myelin destruction, and although the symptoms improve with corticosteroids, the MR findings tend to show only mild improvement.

Rheumatoid Arthritis (RA) is another "collagen-vascular" disease that can compromise the spinal cord, although the mechanism is different. Focal inflammatory changes termed "pannus" destroy the transverse ligament of C-1, allowing the odontoid to slide posteriorly relative to C-1, and compressing the cord, particularly in flexion (Fig. 10.8). Therefore, the injury in RA is because of an extramedullary, extradural "mass" rather an intramedullary lesion. A soft-tissue mass at the C1-2 articulation with instablility does not necessarily imply RA; a fibrous pseudotumor has been described in the same location in association with os odontoideum, and can develop in response to any chronically unstable spinal anatomy.

The remaining list of inflammatory conditions of the spinal cord is long, and parallels the differential considerations in the brain. Chemotherapy, radiation, electrical burns, and lightning are physical factors that can injure the cord.

Figure 10.6. Multiple Sclerosis. Considerable swelling and enhancement of the spinal cord is noted on these postcontrast sagittal (**A**) and axial (**B**) images. Note how the central gray matter (*arrows*) is displaced posteriorly by the inflammatory changes in the anterior white matter.

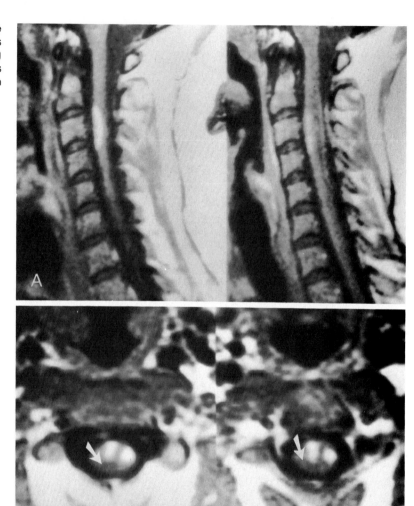

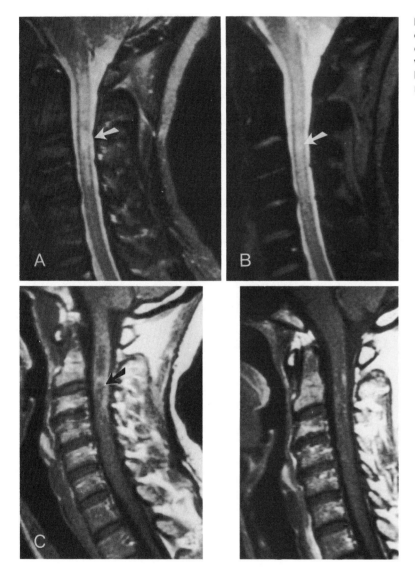

Figure 10.7.   Systemic Lupus Erythematosus. An MR in a 40-year-old patient with new myelopathy. The spinal cord shows ill-defined areas of edema on (**A**) T2-weighted image and (**B**) gradient echo image (*arrows*). Postcontrast images (**C**) show mild enhancement (*arrow*). The brain was free of abnormalities.

Figure 10.8. Rheumatoid Arthritis. A. This elderly patient had myelopathy due to atlantoaxial instability secondary to pannus (*arrows*), which has destroyed the transverse ligament of C-1. In extension, no cord impingement is seen. **B.** In flexion, the dens has borderline mass effect on the cord (*arrowheads*). The pannus enhances vigorously with contrast (*arrow*).

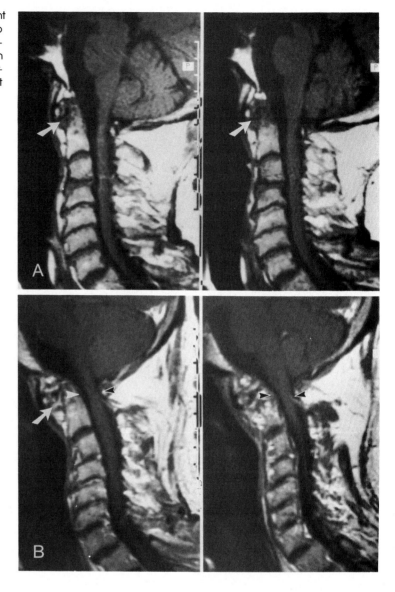

Radiation Myelitis is similar to radiation injury to the brain: peak incidence occurs roughly 6 to 12 months after initial treatment, with affected areas demonstrating increased signal intensity on T2-weighted images, with variable enhancement (Fig. 10.9). Radiation myelitis can lead to paralysis, and fear of this complication is usually the limiting factor in radiotherapy for vertebral body metastases. Radiation has a very characteristic effect on the vertebral bodies. The normal erythropoietic marrow is destroyed and replaced by fat, making the vertebrae very homogeneously bright on T1-weighted images (Fig. 10.10). In growing children, cellular repopulation of the vertebral marrow may occur, with stunted growth of the affected vertebrae because of radiation injury to the epiphyses being the main finding (Fig. 10.11).

Acute Viral Illnesses are associated with myelitis in a number of ways, some of which are well described, and others which are still poorly understood. The "po-lio" virus causes direct injury to the anterior horn cells. Herpes zoster is invisible to imaging when latent, but cord swelling and enhancement have been reported with acute "shingles" outbreaks, appearing at spinal levels corresponding to the dermatologic outbreak. Measles provokes an autoimmuine reaction that can damage the cord, which has been studied experimentally as a model for MS, and is termed subacute sclerosing panencephalitis. Acute disseminated encephalo-myelitis, described in Chapter 7, is a monophasic postviral syndrome, which also affects spinal cord as its name, "encephalo*myelitis*," suggests.

More mysterious still are patients who have sudden high fevers, presumably viral, although often never proven, and develop an acute paraplegia. This is a type of syndrome for which many neurologists reserve the catch-all term "transverse myelitis." It is unclear whether the injury is due to the virus, an autoimmune effect, ischemia, or other unknown factors. The imag-

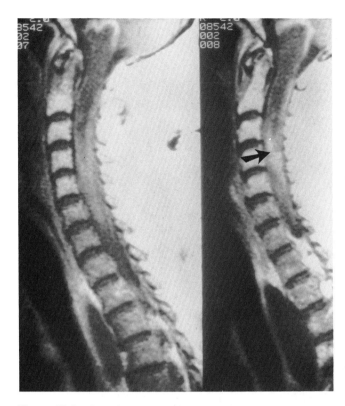

Figure 10.9. Radiation Myelitis. Intramedullary enhancement (*arrow*) is noted in this patient who received radiation therapy to the neck.

ing findings are rather nonspecific, and a focal area of cord edema may or may not be seen. Another puzzle is a myelopathy seen in patients with acquired immunodeficiency syndrome (AIDS), with vacuolar changes in the spinal cord. It is unclear whether this is due to the human immunodeficiency virus itself, or concomitant infections such as cytomegalovirus. The role of MR in these enigmatic syndromes is more to exclude other treatable conditions, such as unsuspected cord compression, than to make a highly specific diagnosis. However, it is important not to dismiss a case of noncompressive myelopathy with cord edema as idiopathic transverse myelitis until a thorough search for treatable causes, including spinal vascular malformations (see Fig. 10.53), has been performed.

Neurosarcoidosis. Inflammatory conditions involving pia and arachnoid have a similar differential diagnosis whether they involve cerebral or spinal leptomeninges. A classic example is neurosarcoidosis, which can present as diffuse leptomeningeal granulomatous nodules, which typically enhance (Fig. 10.12). This appearance is similar to that of carcinomatous and infectious meningitis, which will be discussed, and the distinction must be made on clinical grounds. Sarcoid can also present with intramedullary or vertebral body granulomatous changes.

Pantopaque Arachnoiditis. One "physical agent" that causes leptomeningeal irritation is Pantopaque, which was used in myelography. Patients can develop delayed arachnoiditis, which manifests itself as

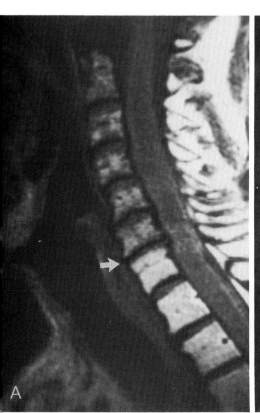

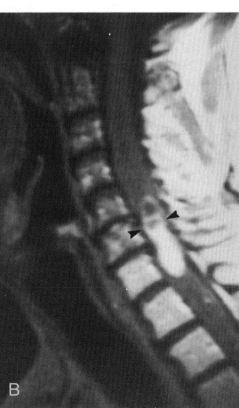

Figure 10.10. Acute Myelopathy—Intramedullary Metastasis. This patient, who had received radiation to the chest for an apical lung tumor, developed an acute myelopathy. **A.** The upper cervical vertebrae outside the field show normal marrow. The margin of the radiation port can be seen in the lower cervical spine (*arrow*). Below this margin, the cervical and upper thoracic vertebrae show a typical bright fat-replaced "postradiation appearance" on T1-weighted imaging. **B.** Postcontrast images show an enhancing lesion at the port margin (*arrowheads*) that proved to be an intramedullary lung metastasis. Note that the enhancement is much denser and more focal than seen with radiation myelitis in Figure 10.11.

A

B

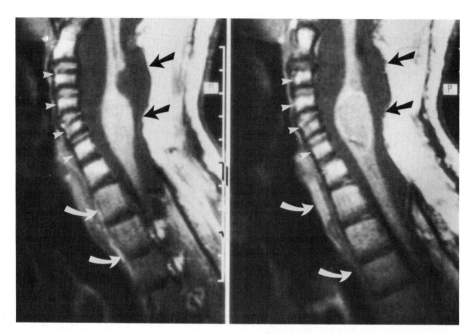

Figure 10.11.   Radiation Effect. This child is status postlaminectomy (*arrows*) and radiation for an intramedullary astrocytoma. Note the growth retardation of the vertebrae within the x-ray therapy field (*ar-*rowheads*), as compared with vertebrae left outside the field (*curved arrows*). The epiphyseal plates of vertebrae, like any other rapidly dividing tissue, are highly sensitive to radiation injury.

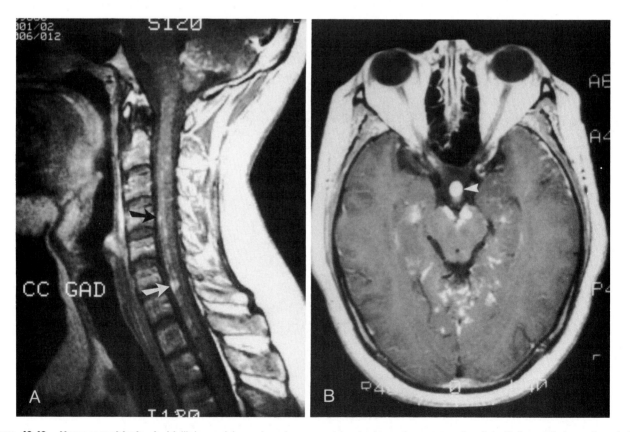

Figure 10.12.   Neurosarcoidosis. A. Multiple nodular enhancing areas are seen involving both the leptomeninges and the cord (*arrows*). **B.** A concomitant scan of the brain reveals similar findings in-volving leptomeninges, as well as the pituitary stalk (*arrowhead*). Accumulation of granulation tissue in this region is the source of the "suprasellar mass" associated with sarcoid.

Table 10.3. Imaging Evaluation of the Pathologic Vertebral Body

Criteria	Infection	Neoplasm	Osteoporosis
Number of vertebrae affected, and pattern	Single vertebral involvement rare Usually at least two vertebrae around an affected disc (pyogenic) or intact disc with subligamentous spread (tuberculosis/fungus)	Isolated or noncontiguous involvement common	Typically >1 vertebrae
Portions of vertebra affected	Destruction greatest at endplates Posterior elements relatively spared	Irregular vertebral body involvement Entire vertebra often infiltrated Pedicles typically affected	Anterior "wedge" deformity of the vertebral body Posterior elements spared
Marrow signal	Decreased on T1 Increased on T2 Abnormal marrow signal centered around disc in osteomyelitis/discitis complex	Decreased on T1 Increased on T2 Entire vertebral body usually infiltrated with pathologic compression fracture	Normal (unless acute) Portions of vertebral body retain normal marrow even with acute compression fracture
Disc integrity	Pyogenic: disc involved and enhances Nonpyogenic: disc spared	Discs typically spared (prostate cancer an exception)	Discs spared
Epidural component (if present)	Granulation tissue (best seen post-gadolinium) extends several levels above and below the affected vertebrae	Focal mass usually only at level of affected vertebra(e) Lymphoma an exception, with more extensive epidural mass	None, unless acute fracture with hematoma
Caveats	Discogenic vertebral sclerosis can mimic the osteomyelitis complex on T1-weighted images (but not on enhanced scans)	Gadolinium enhancement may obscure metastases, by reducing their conspicuity relative to fat	Acute compression fractures show marrow edema, and can be difficult to distinguish from pathologic fracture (although posterior elements are usually spared) A follow-up scan in 2-6 months helps make the distinction.

adhesions within the cauda equina. The normally free-layering roots become adherent to each other, or to the peripheral wall of the thecal sac, giving the sac a "bald" appearance on myelography or T2-weighted images. While this agent is rarely used today, keep this complication in mind in patients whose plain spine films show the telltale pearly white beads of residual Pantopaque. On MR, these droplets appear bright on T1-weighted images because of their lipid content.

INFECTION

Infections involving the spine can be classified according to the causative organism, or according to their anatomic location. Both approaches are useful. Certain infections, such as pediatric pyogenic meningitis, are so dramatic in their presentation that there is little need for imaging, with emergent lumbar puncture and CSF analysis being the cornerstone of diagnosis. Other processes, such as fungal osteomyelitis in the immunocompromised cancer patient, can be quite subtle, and imaging plays a crucial (if not always successful) role in differentiating spinal infection from tumor (13–16). Evaluation of the pathologic vertebral body is a constant challenge, and the many "rules of thumb" sprinkled throughout this chapter are summarized in Table 10.3.

In most spine infections, the organism is seeded via the arterial route, rather than transvenously, as was once believed. As is the case with most bacteremia, the source of the organism is usually the skin, gastrointestinal tract, or lungs. Exceptions are children with spinal dysraphism, or immediate postoperative patients, where a direct portal for infection exists.

Osteomyelitis/Discitis. In adults, the most common initial site of hematogenous infectious "seeding" is the vertebral body, particularly the anterior portions near the endplates, which have the richest blood supply. Vertebral osteomyelitis then develops (Fig. 10.13), which can be self-limiting. However, if pyogenic infection breaks through the endplates into the disc, discitis ensues, with inevitable infection of the adjacent vertebral body, creating an "osteomyelitis/discitis complex" (Fig. 10.14). This pattern is highly suggestive of infection, and unusual with neoplasms (Table 10.3). The epidural space can also be seeded hematogenously, but more often is involved by direct extension. Once the disc and epidural space are involved, extension into the paraspinous soft tissues, such as the psoas muscle, often occurs. The disc itself has a relatively poor blood supply in adults, but in children, blood vessels supply the growing disc and penetrate the endplate providing a route for hematogenous primary infection.

Epidural Abscess. The dura presents a relative barrier to infection, which tends rather to spread in a craniocaudad fashion within the epidural space, ex-

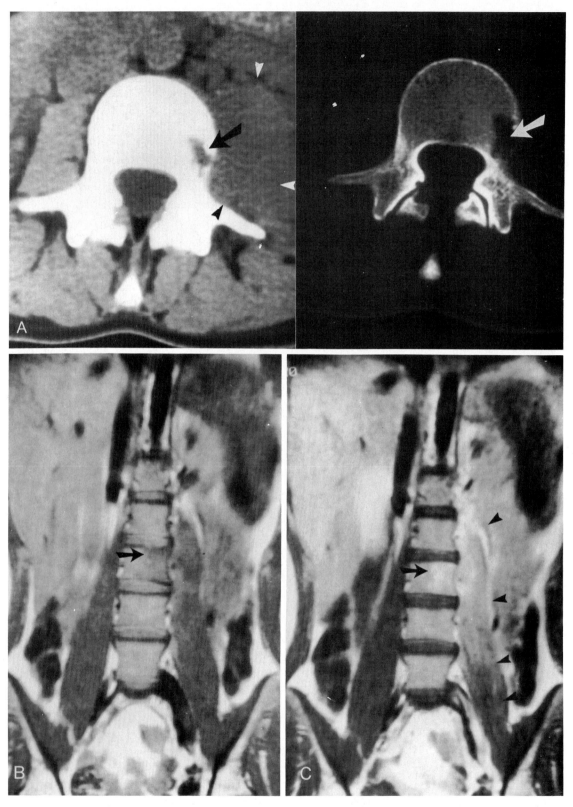

Figure 10.13. Early Osteomyelitis. This young athlete developed back pain, and a slightly elevated sedimentation rate, with negative blood cultures and negative plain films, and a bone scan showing increased uptake at L-3. **A.** A CT, filmed with different windows, shows a destructive process within the vertebral body (*arrow*), which extends into the left psoas muscle (*arrowheads*), which is enlarged. **B.** The unenhanced T1-weighted image in coronal plane shows decreased signal intensity within the left-sided marrow space of L-3,

consistent with edema (*arrow*). **C.** Postcontrast MR shows marked enhancement within the affected portion of L-3 (*arrow*) and the left psoas (*arrowheads*), which is enlarged and enhances all the way into the pelvis. This pattern would be unusual for a tumor. Biopsy yielded *S. Aureus*. The discs appear spared, which is atypical for *S. Aureus*. Note how well the coronal plane shows both the spine and paraspinous tissues over a large area. This plane is very effective in imaging of nondegenerative diseases, and is underutilized.

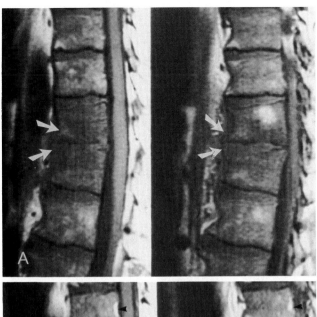

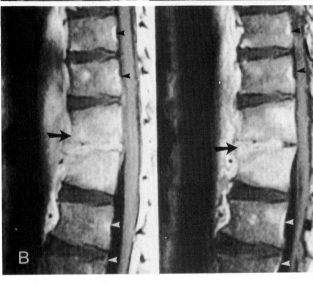

Figure 10.14. Osteomyelitis with Discitis. A. T1-weighted sagittal images show decreased signal in a pair of vertebral body endplates (*arrows*) centered around an abnormal disc. **B.** The disc (*arrow*) enhances intensely, confirming discitis. This "osteomyelitis/discitis complex" is classic for pyogenic infection, and virtually rules out neoplasm. Note basivertebral venous plexus (*arrowheads*), which normally becomes bright after gadolinium, due to normal venous enhancement. This basivertebral plexus enhancement confirms that gadolinium was given, much as nasal mucosal enhancement does in the head. Enhanced basivertebral veins should not be mistaken for epidural infection or tumor.

tending as many as three to four interspaces away from the vertebral abnormality, which is unusual with neoplasms (Table 10.3). Epidural abscesses have little room to expand axially, given the confines of the spinal canal, and can lead to cord compression (Fig. 10.15).

Subdural Empyemas are rare, and tend to be associated with surgery or other violation of the dura. This is fortunate, as subdural infections could rapidly spread through the arachnoid layer, resulting in meningitis. Infection of the subarachnoid space is termed meningitis, whether it is in the brain or spinal canal.

Indeed, the theory of a lumbar puncture is that there is continuous mixing of the CSF, with the fluid in the lumbar recesses being representative of the fluid bathing the brain. The clinical presentation of meningitis is discussed in detail in Chapter 6. Meningitis typically is because of direct hematogenous seeding, rather than contiguous spread of adjacent vertebral infection, unless there is a disruption of the leptomeninges on a congenital or acquired basis. Postcontrast MR is the most sensitive imaging examination for meningitis in both the brain and the spine, but the finding of leptomeningeal enhancement often appears relatively late in the infection's course, and sometimes not at all. Therefore, *a negative enhanced MR does not exclude meningitis—and should never delay or be a substitute for a lumbar puncture.*

Spinal Cord Abscesses are rare, and are usually the result of direct seeding of the cord from overwhelming sepsis. Given the difficulty of myelography in an acutely ill patient, and the relative insensitivity of the technique for small intramedullary lesions, the imaging literature on this topic is sketchy, with most data from autopsy reports. Magnetic resonance imaging, for the first time, allows a direct look inside the cord in these patients. Spinal cord pyogenic abscesses, not surprisingly, appear similar to those in the brain: bright on T2-weighted image, with rim enhancement (Fig. 10.16).

Plain films can not identify a spinal infection unless some disc or bone destruction has occurred, which may take 4–8 weeks, with the earliest sign being erosion of the vertebral endplates. Since older patients often have significant loss of vertebral body and disc height because of degenerative processes, evaluation of plain films in the setting of suspected infection is difficult, even after months of symptoms. Late in the infectious course, the endplates may become sclerotic bone as healing occurs, sometimes leading to fusion across the obliterated disc space. Technetium bone scans can turn positive in infection far sooner than plain films, but suffer from the same ambiguity: degenerative and nondegenerative processes can look the same. Indium-labeled white cell studies and gallium scans are more specific for infection, but relatively insensitive for small foci of vertebral osteomyelitis.

Computed tomography is useful for paraspinous disease, such as psoas infection, which may be associated with vertebral osteomyelitis and epidural abscess (Fig. 10.13). However, CT does not show the contents of the spinal canal adequately unless intrathecal contrast is used. Magnetic resonance imaging can demonstrate the initial replacement of the fatty marrow by osteomyelitis, and has therefore become the preferred technique of examination. Gadolinium-enhanced images are extremely helpful in confirming discitis. When evaluating the extent of epidural involvement,

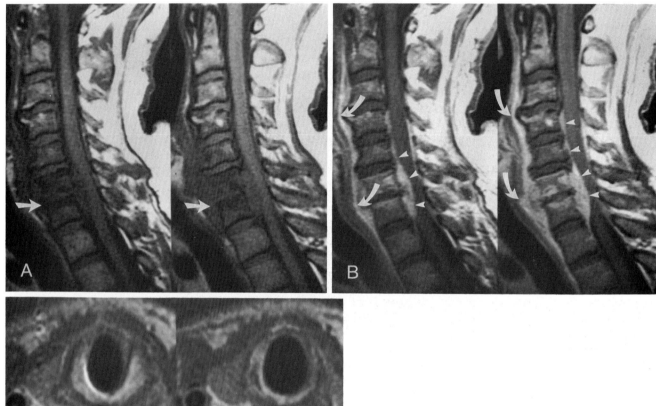

Figure 10.15. Osteomyelitis with Discitis and Epidural Abscess. T1-weighted sagittal images before (**A**) and after (**B**) contrast, show an osteomyelitis-discitis complex, centered around an abnormal enhancing disc (*arrow*). In this case, there is considerable enhancing tissue within the epidural space (*arrowheads*) as well as anterior to the spine, involving the anterior longitudinal ligament (*curved arrows*). Ligamentous involvement extending several vertebral bodies away from the area of infiltrated marrow favors infection, and is unusual for metastatic tumor. **C.** Axial images confirm compression of the cord (*arrows*).

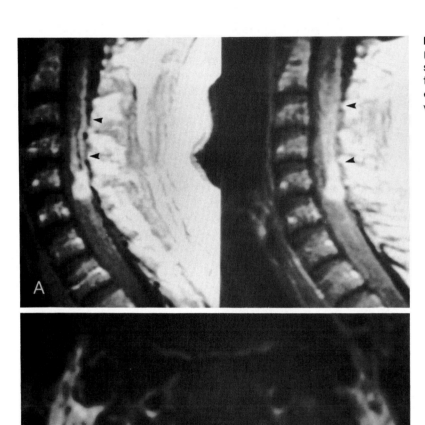

Figure 10.16.   Spinal Cord Abscess. (A) Sagittal and **(B)** axial enhanced images through the cervical spine show intramedullary enhancement in this patient with overwhelming sepsis, who developed myelopathy. Laminectomy (*arrowheads*) and biopsy revealed abscess.

fat suppression is a useful adjunct as the epidural fat is inherently bright (Fig. 10.17).

Pyogenic Infections

Staphylococcus aureus is by far the most common cause of spine infection in adults, followed by Gram-negative bacteria, particularly *Escherichia Coli, Pseudomonas,* and *Klebsiella. Salmonella* is seen in association with sickle cell disease. As already mentioned, the vertebrae are seeded hematogenously in most cases, resulting in osteomyelitis that then spreads to the disc space and adjacent vertebral body. This process typically results in severe back pain that unlike degenerative complaints, is unrelieved by any positional maneuvers. Fevers, chills, leukocytosis, and an elevated sedimentation rate may be present. However, the early and haphazard use of antibiotics for any "malaise" may mask these findings. Blood cultures are often negative, mandating disc biopsy, which also has a surprisingly low yield. *Staphylococcus aureus* produces enzymes that rapidly "digest" discs. This has led to the plain film "pearl" that destruction of the disc space implies pyogenic infection. Tuberculous spondylitis, in contrast, typically spares the disc.

On MR, however, the converse of this pearl does not always hold up, as *Staphylococcus* infections can be detected as early as the isolated osteomyelitis phase, as marrow edema with enhancement, before any discitis has developed (Fig. 10.13). Once the infection has broken through to the disc, intense contrast enhancement confirms the discitis (Fig. 10.14), and usually shows subligamentous spread to the vertebra on the other side of the disc. Infection can course along the anterior and posterior longitudinal ligaments, extending several vertebral body levels away from the affected disc. As the infection progresses, epidural involvement, with or without pathologic fracturing of the vertebra, can lead to cord compression (Fig. 10.15). Epidural infection can have a variable appearance, ranging from rounded rim-enhancing areas, which yield frank pus at surgery, to more oblong stretches of thickened granulation tissue.

Nonpyogenic Infections

The most important nonpyogenic infections of the spine are tuberculosis and fungal diseases. These disorders present a diagnostic challenge for several reasons. First, they typically have an indolent course and do not present with the acute pain and leukocytosis that are the hallmark of pyogenic infections. Second, the population most at risk for nonpyogenic infections, aside from certain endemic areas, is the immunosuppressed. Patients who are immunocompromised because of chemotherapy are at risk for metastases from their primary tumor, and AIDS pa-

tients are at risk for lymphoma involving the spine. In both settings, therefore, a pathologic fracture with mild epidural mass effect easily can represent either infection or neoplasm. The dichotomy of the potential treatments, antibiotics versus radiation, mandates a definitive diagnosis, often requiring biopsy. Sometimes, however, the radiologist can steer the work-up in such a way that invasiveness of this biopsy is minimized, or can detect findings so characteristic of a given disease that biopsy is not necessary (Table 10.3). Figure 10.18 illustrates such a case as it evolved, from plain films to CT, and finally MR.

Tuberculosis of the Spine, or Pott's disease, causes slow collapse of one or usually more vertebral bodies, spreading underneath the longitudinal ligaments (Fig. 10.19). The result is an acute kyphotic or "gibbus" deformity. This angulation, coupled with epidural granulation tissue and bony fragments, can lead to cord compression. Unlike pyogenic infections, the discs tend to be preserved. Psoas abscess without severe pain or frank pus is common, leading to the expression "cold abscess." As with other extrapulmonary tuberculosis, the chest film may be unrevealing, with the source being a primary lung lesion that is clinically silent. Unfortunately, the incidence of tuberculous spondylitis, as with other forms of tuberculosis, is on the rise, with new strains with multiple drug resistances. In many parts of the developing world, tuberculosis is the most common cause of vertebral body infection, with the majority of cases seen in patients under the age of 20. Tuberculosis can also affect the meninges of the spine, causing an intense pachymeningitis that enhances dramatically (Fig. 10.20).

Fungal Infections can be particularly difficult to differentiate from malignant processes, with the classic problem being *Candida* and *Aspergillus* in the oncology patient. Coccidioidomycosis and blastomycosis have specific endemic areas, but with widespread travel, geographic borders have less meaning. Coccidioidomycosis (Fig. 10.18) is common in the southwestern U.S., and blastomycosis in the southeast. Both are common in Africa and South America, with some variation in strains. Another distinction is that coccidioidomycosis, like tuberculosis, spares the discs, whereas blastomycosis, like actinomycosis, can destroy the discs and the ribs. *Cryptococcus*, usually associated with meningitis, also affects the vertebrae, with well-defined osteolytic changes.

Other infectious agents can occasionally involve the spine. Cysticercosis can involve the CSF pathways at any point, and has been described in the lumbar recesses. Recently, intramedullary toxoplasmosis has been described in AIDS patients. *Echinococcus* will occasionally affect the vertebral bodies. Viral and postviral syndromes are discussed under "Inflammation."

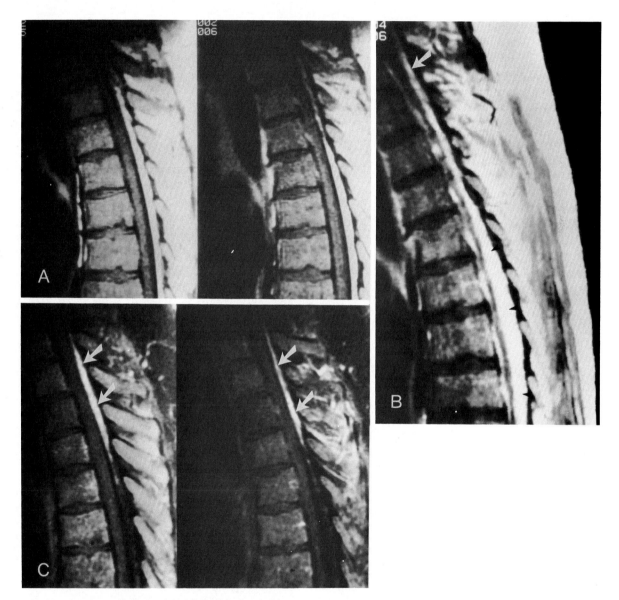

Figure 10.17.   Value of Fat Suppression on MR in Epidural Abscess. A. Unenhanced T1-weighted sagittal images are unremarkable in this immunosuppressed patient with infrascapular back pain. **B.** Postcontrast images, slightly motion-blurred and off midline, show enhancement posterior to the upper thoracic cord, where there is little epidural fat (*arrow*). However, in the middle and lower thoracic spine it is difficult to distinguish enhancement from normal epidural fat (*arrowheads*). **C.** Fat suppression images reveal the true extent of the epidural abscess (*arrows*).

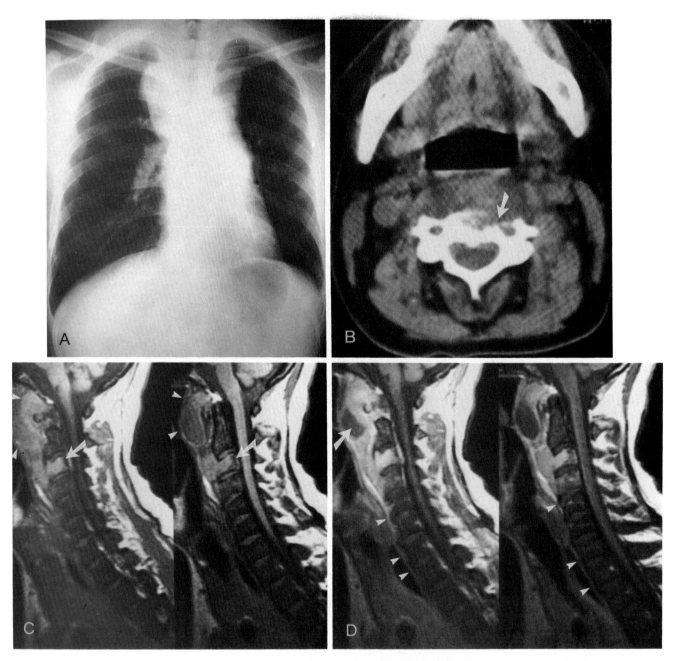

Figure 10.18.   Coccidioidomycosis Osteomyelitis with Prevertebral Abscess. A. This 26-year-old patient presented with 3 months of fevers, weight loss, and chills. Chest film shows an anterior mediastinal mass suspicious for lymphoma. **B.** An extensive CT was ordered, which confirmed mediastinal adenopathy, but destructive changes were seen in C-3 (*arrow*), atypical for lymphoma. **C.** T1-weighted images show abnormal low signal in all of the cervical vertebrae, due to anemia of chronic disease, likely accompanied by increased marrow iron. The C-3 vertebral body (*arrow*) is infiltrated with fluid. In a normal patient it would be the darkest vertebral body; here it is the brightest. A considerable anterior mass is noted, which is in the prevertebral space (*arrowheads*). **D.** After contrast, the prevertebral mass shows central low signal (*arrow*), consistent with necrosis or abscess. Note the dense enhancement of the anterior longitudinal ligament (*arrowheads*) well into the lower cervical spine, suggestive of infection. This proved to be coccidioidomycosis. **E.** Axial images prove that the mass is in the prevertebral space rather than the retropharyngeal space, as the longus colli muscles (*arrowheads*) are displaced forward.

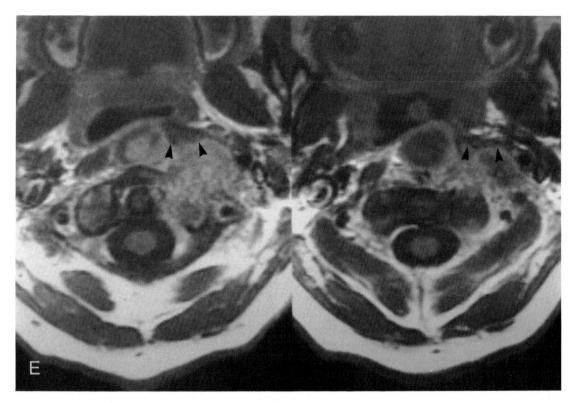

Figure 10.18. E.

NEOPLASMS

Magnetic resonance imaging is unique in its ability to detect nonexpansile tumors of the spinal cord, and is the only reliable noninvasive method for detection of tumors within the spinal canal that do not affect bone. When formulating the differential diagnosis for a spinal tumor, it is important to establish the location of the lesion as intramedullary, intradural extramedullary, or extradural, as described in "Myelography," and in Table 10.2. Having determined the "compartment," consider the patient's age when ranking the lesions occurring in that compartment in order of likelihood (16–21). In children, 38% of symptomatic spinal canal lesions are developmental. Meningiomas constitute a 25% of all intraspinal lesions in adults, but are rare in children. These figures exclude bony and epidural metastases, which are the most common neoplastic conditions involving the adult spine. Magnetic resonance imaging is also an excellent tool for evaluating these osseous metastases (Fig. 10.21). Signal alterations from tumor infiltration within the normal bright marrow fat on T1-weighted images usually precede any bony changes detectable on plain film or CT, and MR is probably the earliest reliable method (aside from bone marrow biopsy) for detecting the presence of metastatic disease of the spine. Technetium bone scanning, however, remains the most cost-effective tool for whole-body screening.

Intramedullary Masses

The classic plain film finding of an intramedullary mass, widening of the interpedicular distance due to slow expansile forces, is seen in less than 10% of cases. Plain CT is not useful for intramedullary tumors, as bony changes are relatively rare. Even with intrathecal contrast, the crucial internal details of the cord are not visualized. Astrocytomas and ependymomas are the two most common primary intramedullary tumors, but the distinction between them is difficult to make, even with high-quality MR. Both are expansile, low in signal intensity on T1-weighted images, bright on T2-weighted images, with variable enhancement. Both have an increased incidence in neurofibromatosis. While some guidelines, based on involvement of the entire cord diameter and longer cord segments (favors astrocytoma) and presence of cysts and hemorrhage (favors ependymoma), have been proposed to distinguish between the two types of tumors, in any single case they are rarely a substitute for biopsy. Gadolinium contrast is useful to identify tumor nidus, as well as to document spread of tumor along CSF pathways, or drop metastases.

Hemangioblastomas, on the other hand, are very distinctive, with a focal vascular blush at their nidus, with angiographic signs being virtually pathognomonic. Syringomyelia, while not a neoplasm, presents as an intramedullary mass on plain film myelogram, and is therefore traditionally included in this gamut.

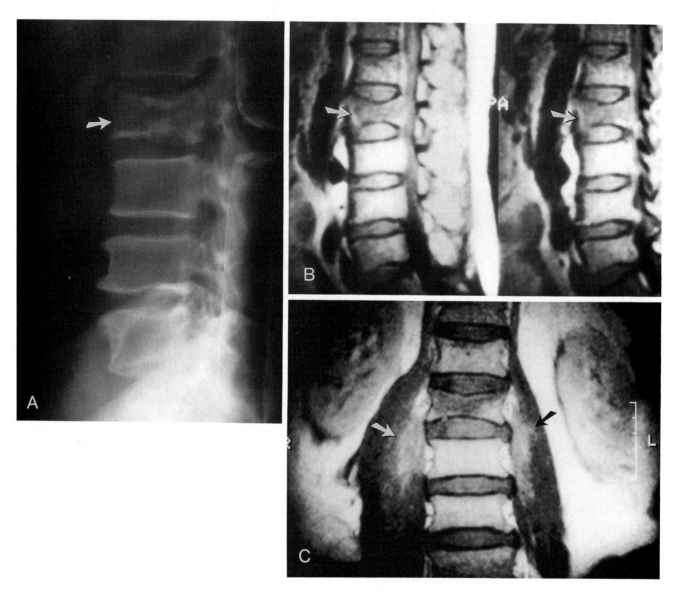

Figure 10.19.   Tuberculous Osteomyelitis. A. Plain films show loss of height of L-2 (*arrow*), with subtle sclerotic changes. **B.** Enhanced T1-weighted images show abnormal marrow throughout L-2 (*arrow*), consistent with a pathologic fracture, making neoplasm or infection prime suspects. Acute compression fractures usually show anterior "wedging," and chronic compression fractures have normal marrow. **C.** Coronal enhanced images reveal bilateral psoas infiltration (*arrows*), but normal discs, consistent with a nonpyogenic infection such as tuberculosis. Metastatic tumor rarely infiltrates the psoas in such a diffuse fashion.

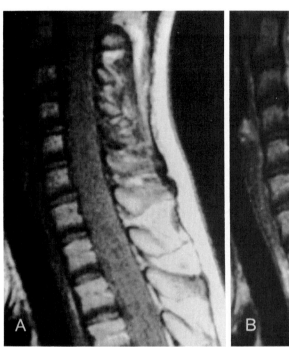
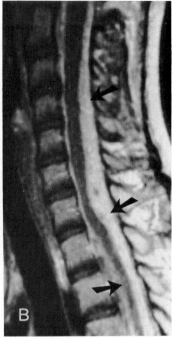

Figure 10.20. Tuberculous Meningitis. A. Sagittal T1 unenhanced image through the cervical spine shows relatively homogenous signal intensity tissue filling the spinal canal, making it difficult to decide if the process is intramedullary or extramedullary. **B.** Postcontrast image demonstrates enhancing granulation tissue filling the subarachnoid space (*arrows*). This patient had similar pachymeningitis surrounding the brain, yet was surprisingly intact clinically, typical for tuberculous meningitis, which is less angioinvasive, and consequently less destructive than pyogenic meningitis.

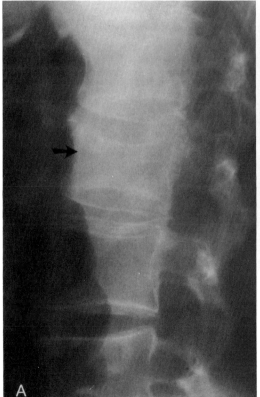
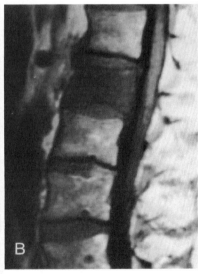
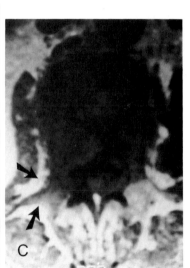

Figure 10.21. Prostate Metastasis. A. Plain films in this elderly male with acute lower back pain, revealed a compression deformity at L-1 (*arrow*), which could represent either a benign or pathologic compression fracture. **B** and **C.** T1 MR images reveal infiltration of the entire vertebral body marrow space, including the right pedicle (*arrows*), a pattern that is highly suspicious for metastasis. Biopsy revealed prostate carcinoma.

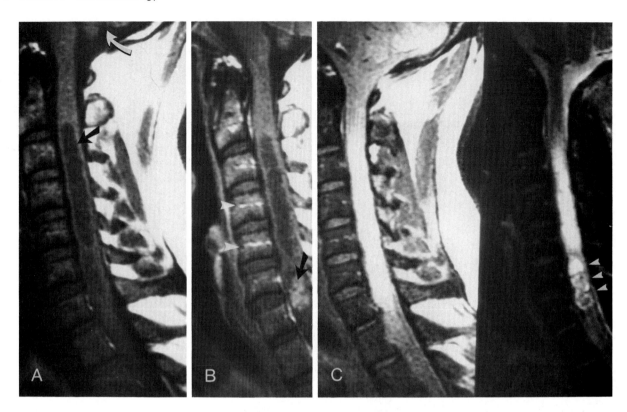

Figure 10.22.   Ependymoma. A. T1-weighted image shows a cavity (*arrow*) within the cervical cord, but the cerebellar tonsils (*curved arrow*) are normal in position, so this cannot be a Chiari I (contrast with Fig. 10.26). **B.** Postcontrast image shows an enhancing nodule (*arrow*) at the lower pole of the intramedullary cavity. Note the normal enhancement of the basivertebral plexus (*arrowheads*). **C.** T2-weighted images show blood breakdown products at the lower end of the cavity (*arrowheads*), suggestive of hemorrhage within the tumor.

Abscesses (Fig. 10.16), metastases (Fig. 10.10), lipomas (Fig. 10.58), and teratomas will present on rare occasions as intramedullary masses.

Ependymomas are the most common spinal cord tumor. Peak incidence is in the 3rd through 6th decades, with a male predominance. These slow-growing neoplasms arise from ependymal cells lining the central canal of the cord, or cell rests along the filum. Histologically, these tumors are usually benign, but a complete curative excision may be impossible with the intramedullary types. Sixty percent are seen within the conus and filum terminale. Associated hemorrhage can be seen, especially on MR, and cystic areas are common (Fig. 10.22). The filum terminale ependymomas typically have a myxopapillary histology, and because of their location a reasonably specific diagnosis can be made. These often can be excised completely, particularly if they are well encapsulated (Fig. 10.23).

Astrocytoma. Seventy-five percent of astrocytomas occur in the cervical and thoracic cord, and presentation in the conus and filum is rarer than with ependymomas. Fusiform cord widening, hyperintensity on T2-weighted MR, and contrast enhancement often extend over several vertebral body segments (Fig. 10.24). They generally have a lower histologic grade than astrocytomas in the brain. As in the brain, there is considerable histologic variability, and the unusual variants, such as protoplasmic astrocytoma, can also involve the spinal cord. Peak incidence is in the 3rd or 4th decade. They may be exophytic, and at times may even appear largely extramedullary. Brainstem gliomas will sometimes extend through the medulla into the rostral cervical spine.

Hemangioblastomas, discussed in detail in Chapter 5, occur in the spine as well as the posterior fossa. Both types have a high association with von Hippel-Lindau syndrome. These rare tumors, with their characteristic densely enhancing nidus, represent 2% of intraspinal neoplasms. Forty percent are extramedullary and 20% are multiple. The nidus shows vascular hypertrophy, and may be mistaken for an arteriovenous malformation (AVM). However, intramedullary AVMs do not typically show a related cyst or cord expansion (Fig. 10.25).

Syringohydromyelia. Hydromyelia refers to dilation of the central canal of the spinal cord, which is lined by ependyma. Syringomyelia, on the other hand, is a cavity outside the central canal lined by glial cells. Distinction between these two conditions is difficult on imaging studies, given that the lining of the cavity can not be examined histologically. The preferred generic term covering either, "syringohydromyelia," is a bit of a tongue-twister, and the abbreviated "syrinx" is often used for both conditions. The etiology of a syr-

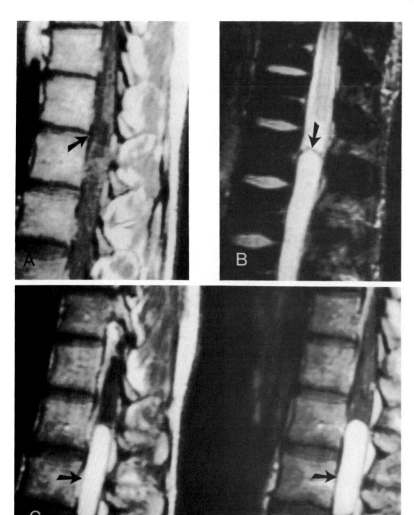

Figure 10.23. Myxopapillary Ependymoma of the Filum Terminale. A. This 29-year-old patient presented with lower extremity radicular complaints. T1-weighted sagittal images show an irregular appearance to the conus (*arrow*) and surrounding CSF, but no distinct mass. **B.** Sagittal gradient refocused echo images demonstrates a low signal "rim" (*arrow*), suggesting an intraspinal mass. **C.** Postcontrast images confirm an enhancing encapsulated intraspinal mass (*arrows*) abutting the conus. A complete resection was performed and the patient has done well.

inx can be developmental, such as in the Arnold-Chiari malformations, discussed in Chapter 8. However, trauma and tumors, as well as inflammatory and ischemic conditions, can also lead to a syrinx.

The preferred imaging method is T1-weighted images in the sagittal and axial planes, along with sagittal T2-weighted images. Be aware that high signal truncation (Gibbs) artifacts can superimpose themselves over the cord, mimicking a syrinx, particularly when a low resolution matrix, such as 128 × 128, is used. A syrinx cavity should have very well-defined margins, and its contents should follow CSF signal intensity. Always suspect tumor as a cause of unexplained syrinx. Unless definite benign etiology is apparent, such as prior history of cord contusion or the low cerebellar tonsils of a Chiari I (Fig. 10.26), give gadolinium to search for a tumor nidus. If the syrinx borders are indistinct and the signal is brighter than CSF on T1-weighted images and darker than CSF on T2-weighted images, you may be dealing with severe central cord edema. It is critical to establish the full extent of the cavity for potential shunting, so if on a

cervical spine examination a cord cavity extends into the thoracic spine, follow it down, or the patient will inevitably need to return to complete the examination. With CT myelography, contrast often enters into a syrinx cavity with delayed images. Occasionally, this technique is useful in establishing the degree to which a cord cavity communicates with the CSF.

Intradural/Extramedullary Masses

Meningioma is the most common intradural tumor in the thoracic region, and represents roughly 25% of all adult intraspinal tumors. Eighty percent occur in women, with an average age of 45. Multiple meningiomas, as in the brain, raise the question of neurofibromatosis. The usual location is extramedullary-intradural, although there can be an extradural component. Dense calcification can occur, as in the brain (Fig. 10.27). Computed tomography attenuation and MR signal characteristics are similar to that of intracranial meningiomas, with homogenous enhancement (Fig. 10.28). The main differential consid-

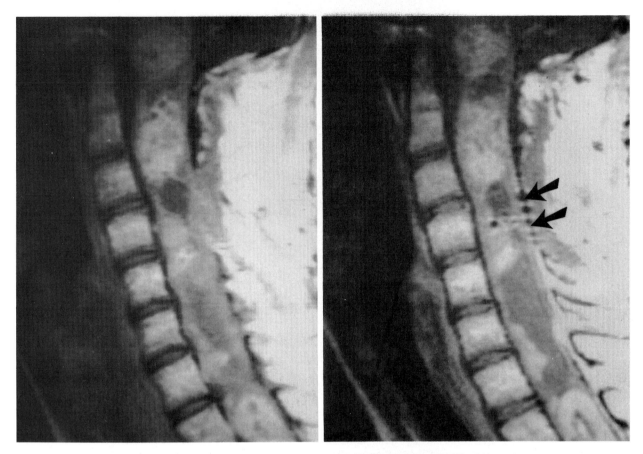

Figure 10.24.   Astrocytoma. Astrocytoma of the cervical spine in a child with NF-1. Patient is postlaminectomy (*arrows*) in an attempt at decompression.

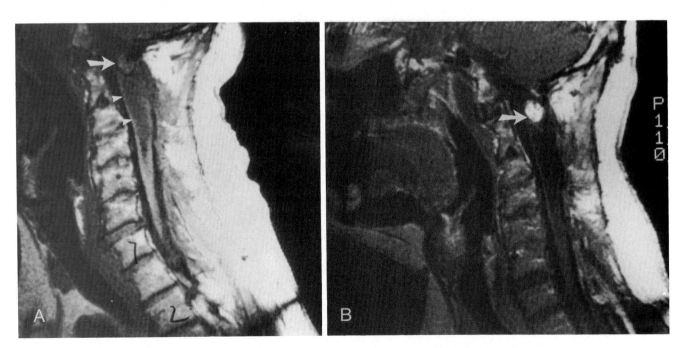

Figure 10.25.   Hemangioblastoma. A. Sagittal T1-weighted images show expansion of the upper cervical cord due to a low signal central mass (*arrow*), which has a darker inferior component suggestive of a cyst (*arrowheads*). This cavity must be investigated further, as it lacks sharp margins and does not follow CSF signal (compare to Fig. 10.26). **B.** Postcontrast image shows an intensely enhancing nodule (*arrow*) at the level of the foramen magnum, classic for a hemangioblastoma. (Courtesy of Dr. William P. Dillon, University of California, San Francisco.)

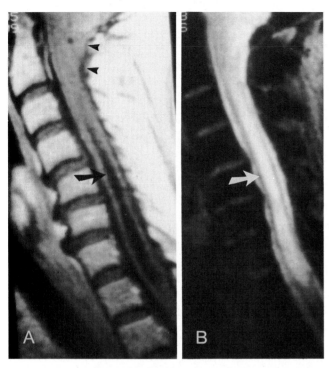

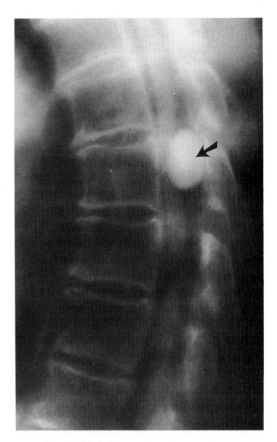

Figure 10.26. Syrinx. A. and **B.** This intramedullary lesion (*arrow*) shows the classic features of a benign syrinx: The margins of the intramedullary cavity are sharp and the intramedullary contents follow CSF signals on all sequences. The cause of the syrinx, the low cerebellar tonsils of the Chiari malformation (*arrowheads*), is also seen.

Figure 10.27. Meningioma. This myelogram was performed using air as contrast, a "pneumomyelogram." A densely calcified dorsal intradural extramedullary mass (*arrow*) is seen indenting the cord, which proved to be a meningioma. (Courtesy of Dr. Van Halbach, University of California, San Francisco.)

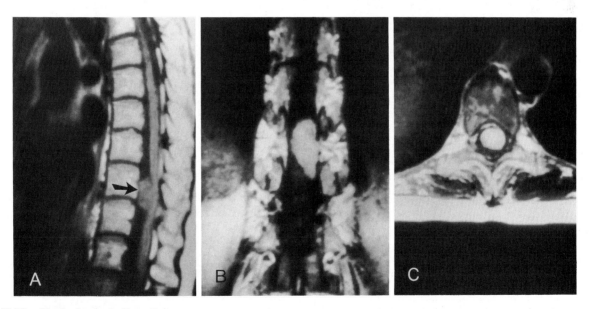

Figure 10.28. Meningioma. A. T1 sagittal images show a well-defined anterior extradural intraspinal mass, with a broad dural base (*arrow*). Coronal (**B**) and axial (**C**) images show dense enhancement, characteristic for a meningioma, as well as severe cord compression.

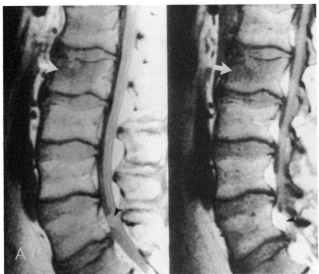

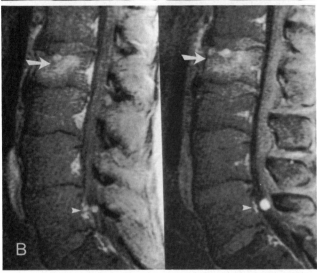

Figure 10.29. Schwannoma. A. This patient had acute focal back pain after an accident, resulting in an acute compression fracture of the superior aspect of L-2, which shows marrow edema (*arrow*). A small intraspinal mass was also noted at L-5 (*arrowhead*). **B.** This lesion enhanced with contrast (*arrowhead*). This was unchanged on follow-up examination, and likely represents a small schwannoma. Note enhancement of the L-2 compression fracture (*arrow*), which is highlighted on this fat saturation image.

eration is usually schwannoma, which often will extend out through a neural foramen, and lacks a broad dural base. Given that meningiomas and schwannomas are both relatively common, comprising together over half of intraspinal tumors, occasional mistakes are made in image interpretation. Luckily, these errors are of little consequence, as both types of lesions must be resected if causing symptomatic mass effect.

Nerve Sheath Tumors. These tumors include schwannoma (also known as neurinomas, neurolemmoma, neuroma) and neurofibromas. Schwannoma is the preferred term, because pathologically these tumors are composed of Schwann cells. They are the most common intraspinal mass, comprising 29% of the total. Schwannomas usually originate from the dorsal sensory nerve roots, but remain extrinsic to the nerve, causing symptoms by mass effect. Most are solitary, with a peak presentation in the 5th decade, although with MR more are being discovered as incidental findings in younger patients (Fig. 10.29). Extension into the neural foramen is a frequent finding, especially in the cervical and thoracic regions. Part of the tumor will be intraspinal, and part will be extraspinal, with the waist at the neural foramen, giving the classic "dumbbell" appearance (Fig. 10.30). In the lumbar region, schwannomas tend to remain within the dural sac (Fig. 10.29).

Spinal neurofibromas are almost always associated with neurofibromatosis (NF) type 1. They are less often multiple than the schwannomas of NF 2. Spinal neurofibromas can have a plexiform configuration, extending out through multiple adjacent neural foramina (Fig. 10.31). Pathologically, neurofibromas (unlike neurinomas) contain fibrous and myxoid tissue, infiltrate the nerve without encapsulated margins, and have a malignant potential. Radiographically, however, these two types of nerve sheath tumors are often indistinguishable. Both can be intradural or extradural in location. In patients with NF-1, look for the additional findings of kyphoscoliosis, rib dysplasia (ribbon ribs), and scalloping of the posterior vertebral body because of dural ectasia (Fig. 10.32). As in the brain, both schwannomas and neurofibromas enhance. Heterogeneous enhancement with areas of low signal is more characteristic of a neurofibroma.

Intrathecal (Drop) Metastases. The classic cause of spinal intradural extramedullary metastases is subarachnoid seeding of primary CNS tumors, such as posterior fossa medulloblastomas, ependymomas, and pineal region neoplasms. Tumor cells in the posterior fossa exfoliate into the CSF and "drop" down into the spinal canal, seed the arachnoid, and grow into small nodules, giving rise to the term "drop metastases" (Fig. 10.33). However, any tumor spreading via the CSF pathways of the brain can involve the spinal leptomeninges. Solid tumors, such as breast and lung carcinoma, can metastasize to the subarachnoid space. Leukemias, which will be discussed, probably have the highest rate of infiltration of the meninges of any non-CNS tumor. These leptomeningeal metastases can cause considerable inflammation, and patients can present with signs of meningeal irritation, leading to the term "carcinomatous meningitis." Systemic lymphoma (particularly T-cell lymphomas) and carcinomas can also spread to the CSF pathways.

Leptomeningeal metastases classically appear as multiple intradural nodules causing filling defects on myelography (Fig. 10.34) or CT myelograms. Good-

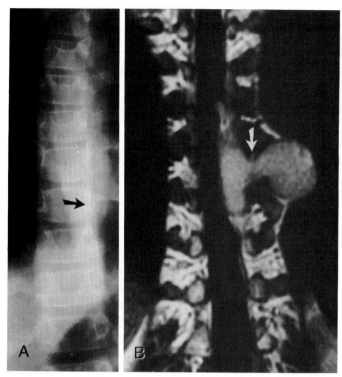

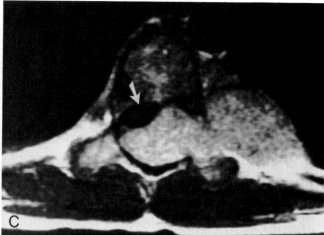

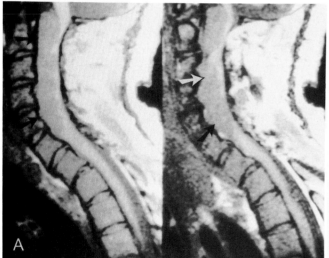

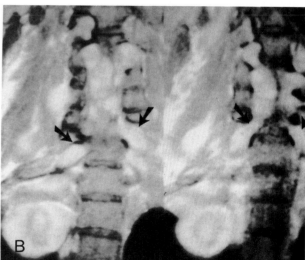

Figure 10.30.   Dumbell Neurofibroma. A. Plain thoracic antero-posterior film shows erosion of a left-sided pedicle (*arrow*). **B.** Coronal T1-weighted image demonstrates a huge neurofibroma with both intraspinal and extraspinal components in the classic dumbell configuration, with the waist at the neural foramen (*arrow*). **C.** Axial image is helpful in identifying the position of the spinal cord (*arrow*) and in assessing the degree of cord compression.

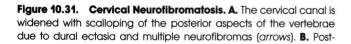

Figure 10.31.   Cervical Neurofibromatosis. A. The cervical canal is widened with scalloping of the posterior aspects of the vertebrae due to dural ectasia and multiple neurofibromas (*arrows*). **B.** Post-contrast coronal images reveal multiple enhancing intraspinal masses, consistent with neurofibromas, which extend out the neural foramina (*arrows*), consistent with a plexiform neurofibroma.

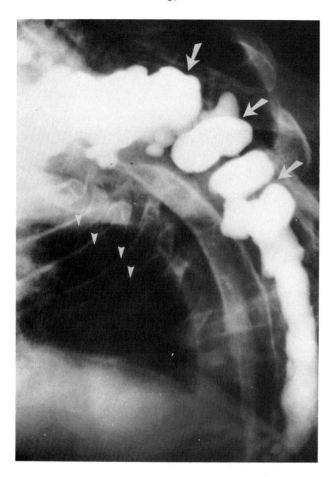

Figure 10.32. Neurofibromatosis. Myelogram shows severe dural ectasia due to NF (*arrows*). Note also the "ribbon ribs" (*arrowheads*).

quality MR with gadolinium enhancement is now the preferred method for screening, with myelography reserved for equivocal cases. Indeed, enhanced MR is probably better than myelography because thin, smooth sheets of intrathecal tumor cells, described by pathologists as "cake-frosting" on the cord and roots, may be difficult to detect on a myelogram since there is no discrete mass (Fig. 10.35). As these tumor layers thicken, widening of the cord contour may occur, mimicking an intramedullary mass from a myelographic standpoint. The differential diagnosis includes infectious meningitis, and in the immunocompromised patient, diffuse leptomeningeal enhancement requires CSF analysis to distinguish between tumor and infection.

Blood in the subarachnoid space may be bright on T1-weighted image, and in the immediate postoperative period it is essential to obtain pregadolinium images to ensure that trace methemoglobin is not mistaken for enhancing drop metastases. Subarachnoid and subdural blood in the spinal canal can cause leptomeningeal irritation and enhancement, further confusing the postoperative "rule out drop metasta-

sis" scan. These problems are easily avoided by obtaining a *preoperative* enhanced MR scan of the spine in any patient at risk for spinal drop metastases, such as a child with medulloblastoma. Once such a child has been sedated and contrast given for the brain, a complete spinal scan will only take another 15 minutes or so, and will save a lot of consternation postoperatively, when the case requires staging for adjunctive chemotherapy and radiation.

Extradural Masses

Metastases. Neoplasm is the second most common cause of extradural mass, after disc herniations and other degenerative processes; however, in immunosuppressed patients, and certain parts of the world, infections may outnumber neoplasms as a source of extradural mass effect. Primary vertebral tumors such as chordomas, giant cell tumors, hemangiomas, and sarcomas, discussed in Chapters 34 and 35, behave like any other extradural mass in terms of myelographic findings and must be kept in the differential diagnosis. The most common extradural neoplasm, however, is metastatic spread of solid tumors such as breast, lung, and prostate carcinoma. Most metastases, like infection, reach the vertebrae via arterial seeding, although prostate carcinoma may preferentially ascend to the lumbar region via Batson's venous plexus. The vertebral marrow space, like the liver and the lungs, "filters" a great deal of blood, and is a fertile ground for metastatic deposits.

As these deposits grow, they replace normal marrow, which contains considerable fat, and is bright on T1-weighted images. Metastases therefore appear as low signal areas on T1-weighted images, or high signal areas on T2-weighted images, because of their higher water content as compared with fat. Prostate cancer and other densely sclerotic metastases can be somewhat confusing on MR, unless one appreciates that areas of intensely sclerotic bone may be dark on all sequences (Fig. 10.36). Historically, T1-weighted images have been the mainstay of vertebral body evaluation. With gradient-refocused images the metastases should also be bright, but the susceptibility effects from the bony trabeculae reduce their conspicuity, making these sequences less useful. Short TR inversion recovery images are probably the most sensitive technique, but have until now been slow, with poor signal to noise. New faster versions of STIR hold great promise in this area (Fig. 10.37). As with other metastases, neovascularity develops to supply the expanding mass of intravertebral tumor cells, which is why vertebral metastases can enhance intensely, although this may reduce their conspicuity against background fat (Fig. 10.4).

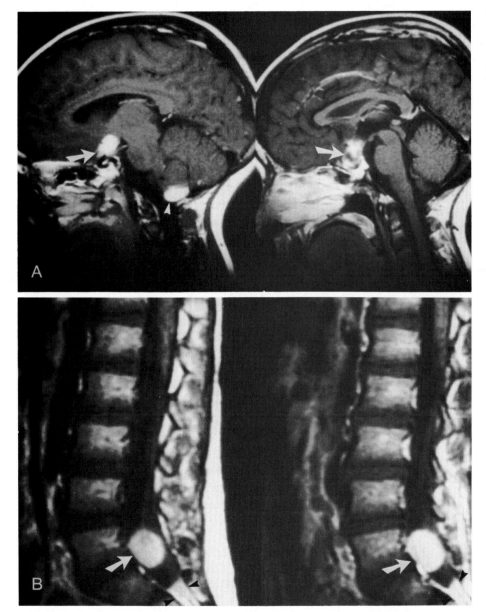

Figure 10.33. Central Nervous System Drop Metastases. A. Sagittal enhanced midline images through the brain show a suprasellar juvenile pilocytic astrocytoma (*arrow*), with a metastasis that has reached the cerebellar tonsils via the CSF (*arrowhead*). **B.** Sagittal enhanced lumbar images show a large intraarachnoid metastatic nodule posterior to L-5 (*arrow*). High signal tissue is also seen posterior to S-2 (*arrowheads*). If it were clinically necessary to confirm that this sacral area represents tumor rather than epidural fat, fat saturation images would be useful.

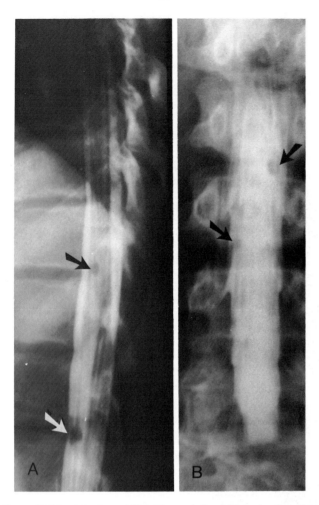

Figure 10.34.   Intrathecal Metastases. Lateral (**A**) and anteroposterior (**B**) myelographic images show multiple nodular filling defects within the subarachnoid space (*arrows*), consistent with nodular leptomeninigeal metastases, in this case of lung carcinoma. (Courtesy of Dr. Anton Pogany, Berkeley, CA.)

Once tumor has infiltrated the cortex, spread to the epidural space can occur, which along with compression fractures, may lead to cord compromise. As discussed in "Infection," there are certain signs (summarized in Table 10.3) that help determine whether a compression fracture is because of infection, tumor, or is merely secondary to osteoporosis (Fig. 10.38). In general, metastases differ from pyogenic infection in that they involve the vertebrae diffusely but noncontiguously, sparing the discs, with epidural mass and enhancement limited to the levels of the pathologic vertebrae (Fig. 10.39). Marked involvement of the pedicles is another sign of metastases (Fig. 10.40). Exceptions include disc-sparing nonpyogenic infections, notorious for mimicking tumor, and lymphoma, which may have extensive epidural infiltration, as will be discussed.

Direct Extension of Paraspinous Tumor.
Retroperitoneal and mediastinal tumors can invade the vertebral column and spinal canal by direct exten-

sion. Neuroblastoma, and its relatives ganglion-euroma and ganglioneuroblastoma, discussed in Chapter 45, arise from primitive paraspinous neural remnants, similar to fetal neuroblasts. These tumors frequently involve the spinal canal, infiltrating through the neural foramina (Figs. 10.41 and 10.42). Any paraspinous tumor can do likewise, including lymphomas, apical lung (Pancoast) tumors, and a variety of retroperitoneal and mediastinal carcinomas and sarcomas.

Hematologic malignancies affecting the spine include leukemia, myeloma, and lymphoma.

Leukemias change the appearance of the vertebrae in the characteristic fashion of diffuse, even replacement of the marrow with tumor (Fig. 10.43, also see 10.67). Solid leukemic infiltrates, or chloromas, can involve the epidural space and cause cord compression. Studies have been performed tracking the MR appearance of the marrow in these patients through induction chemotherapy, radiation, bone marrow transplantation and repopulation with normal marrow cells, which are referenced and worth reviewing when evaluating such cases (Fig. 10.44) (20).

Multiple myeloma can present as a diffuse and homogeneous low signal in the spine on T1-weighted images, but more typically shows multiple focal defects. Occasionally, a plasmacytoma is noted. Myelofibrosis will present as very dark marrow space on T1-weighted images, and remains dark on T2-weighted images since there is "dry" fibrous tissue rather than "wet" tumor replacing the marrow (Fig. 10.45). Such individuals, like patients with hemoglobinopathies such as sickle cell disease, may have areas of extramedullary hematopoiesis which are often paraspinous, and can infiltrate into the spinal canal, causing cord compression.

Lymphoma is a another "hematologic" tumor, with protean imaging manifestations that can serve as the topic for an entire monograph—and have! The classification schemes for lymphoma are complex, and not terribly helpful in understanding the presentations in the spine. Lymphomas may present as primary spinous or paraspinous lesions, with pathologic vertebral involvement and compression (Fig. 10.46). The related epidural and paraspinous mass is usually far more extensive than most metastatic disease from solid tumors. Lymphomas involving mediastinum and retroperitoneum can insidiously invade the spinal canal via the neural foramina. Given that CT remains the dominant technique for following lymphoma in the chest and abdomen, subtle intraspinous disease can easily be missed, and any lymphoma patient with back pain should be evaluated by MR (Fig. 10.47).

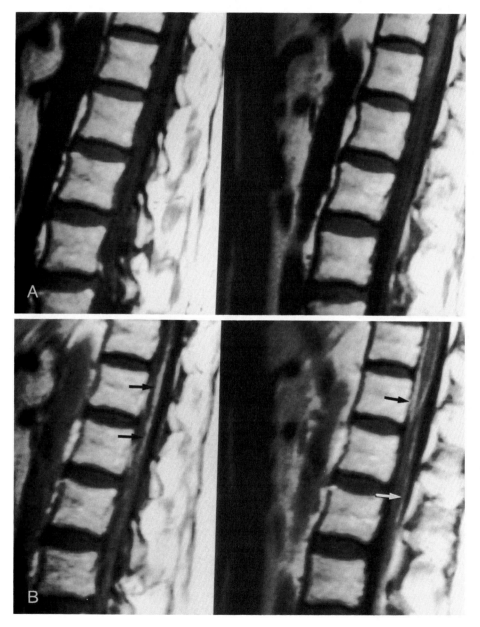

Figure 10.35.   Carcinomatous Meningitis.   A. Sagittal unenhanced T1-weighted images in this breast cancer patient are unremarkable. **B.** Enhanced images through the conus show fine sheets of enhancing tumor coating the distal cord and cauda equina (*arrows*). This thin diffuse cake-frosting type of leptomeningeal tumor involvement may be hard to detect myelographically.

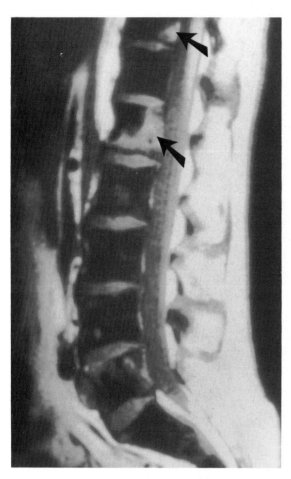

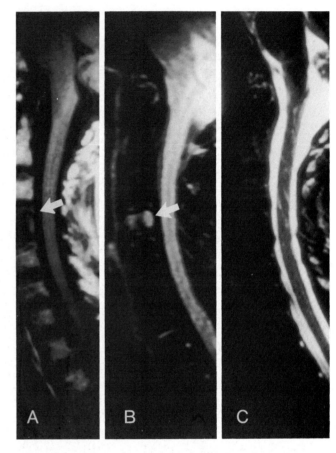

Figure 10.36. Prostate Cancer. The spine appears quite dark on these standard T1 sagittal images, with only occasional islands of normal marrow fat (*arrows*). The vertebrae remained dark on T2-weighted images (not shown). Plain films (not shown) showed dense bony sclerosis, consistent with the "ivory vertebrae" of prostate metastases.

Figure 10.37. Value of Inversion Recovery in the Evaluation of Metastases. This patient has breast carcinoma. **A.** Vertebrae C-2 and C-3 are bright consistent with radiation; C-4 (*arrow*) is quite dark, raising the question of metastasis; C-5 and below are intermediate in signal, and may or may not be normal. **B.** This STIR image shows high signal, consistent with metastasis limited to C-4 (*arrow*). **C.** Fast spin echo sequence with T2-weighting shows little useful information on the marrow, one of the shortcomings of this technique. (Courtesy of Dr. Rahul Metha, Stanford, CA.)

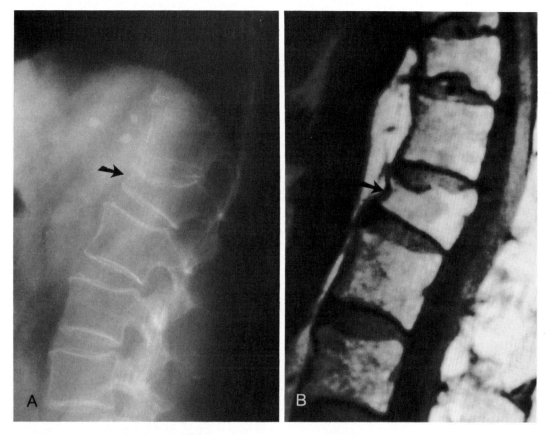

Figure 10.38. Benign Compression Fracture. A. Plain films show a compression fracture of L-1 (*arrow*). The vertebral body shows a classic wedge deformity, with greater loss of height anteriorly than posteriorly, with intact pedicles on the anteroposterior view (not shown). This configuration is suggestive of a benign compression fracture. **B.** T1 sagittal MR shows normal marrow signal in the affected vertebrae (*arrow*), confirming a benign cause of the compression fracture, such as osteoporosis.

Figure 10.39.   Metastatic Lung Carcinoma with Pathologic Fracture. A. Precontrast images show many of the features of metastatic involvement, such as complete infiltration of the affected vertebra and disc sparing. **B.** Postcontrast images demonstrate that the epidural involvement (*arrows*) is largely limited to the level of the affected vertebra, and there is no multisegment enhancement of the anterior and posterior longitudinal ligaments, as is often seen in infection. Contrast this case with Figure 10.15, which shows a typical epidural abscess.

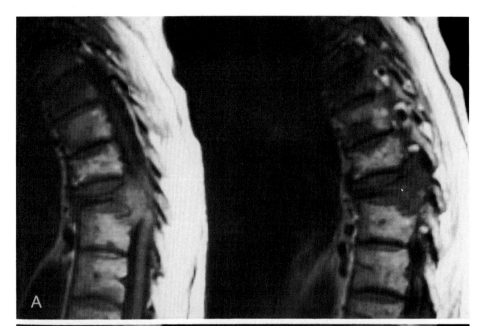

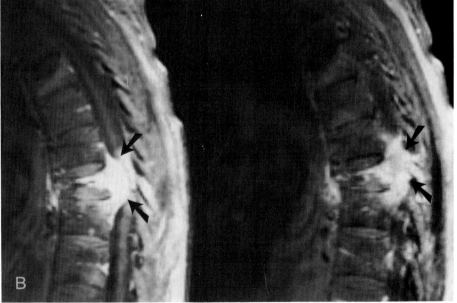

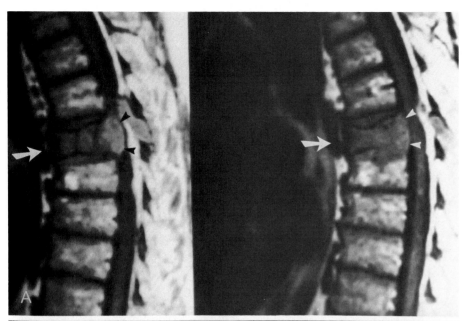

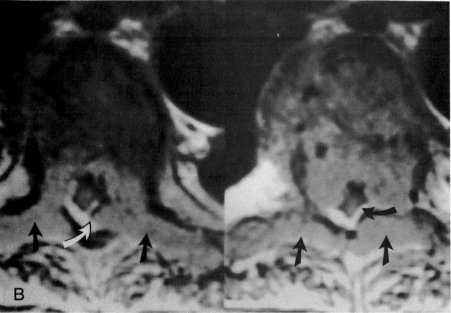

Figure 10.40. Multiple Myeloma. Sagittal (**A**) and axial (**B**) MR images demonstrate a midthoracic vertebra (*large arrows*) which shows several features associated with neoplastic infiltration. The affected vertebra is completely involved, the discs are spared, the epidural mass (*arrowheads*) is limited to the level of affected vertebra. The pedicles and lamina are infiltrated and expanded (*small arrows*) and the epidural fat (*curved arrow*) is displaced rather than infiltrated. None of these signs alone confirms a neoplastic process, but taken together they are highly suggestive of metastatic tumor.

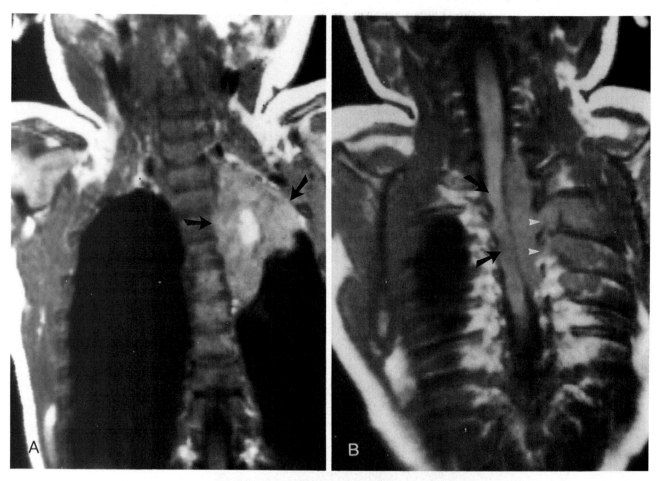

Figure 10.41.   Neuroblastoma. This patient presented with flaccidity of the lower extremities and an apical chest mass (*arrows*) on plain films and MR (**A**), which is paraspinous in location. **B.** The my-elopathy is easily explained by cord compression (*arrows*) due to the neuroblastoma infiltrating into the spinal canal via multiple neural foramina (*arrowheads*).

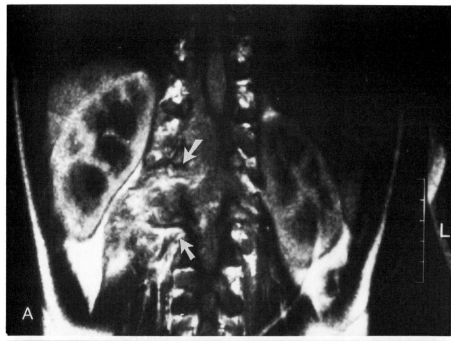

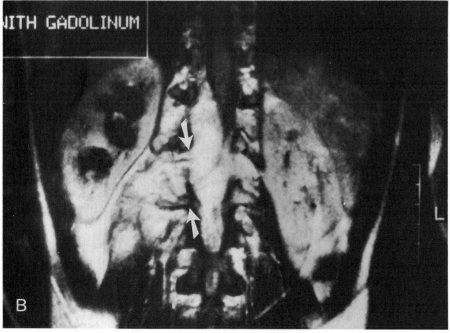

Figure 10.42. Ganglioneuroblastoma. A. This tumor is believed to represent a more "mature" or differentiated form of tumor of the sympathetic nervous system than neuroblastoma. It shares a similar paraspinous distribution, and tendency to dumbbell into the spinal canal (*arrows*) via the neural foramina. **B.** Note the diffuse enhancement with gadolinium.

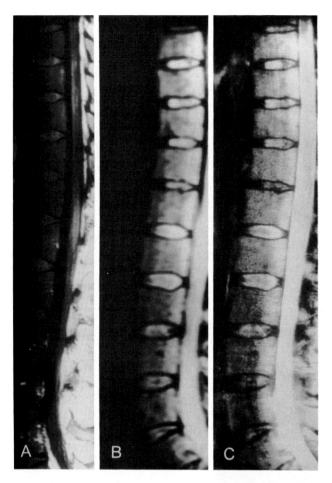

Figure 10.43.   Three MR Techniques for Evaluating the Marrow in Leukemia. A. T1-weighted image shows diffuse homogenous infiltration of the marrow, which is dark, as leukemic cells, high in water content, have replaced the normal marrow fat. Normal marrow should be brighter than the discs on T1-weighted spin echo images. **B.** Short TR inversion recovery images (STIR), make this "watery" marrow bright. **C.** "Fast inversion recovery" produces the same effect as conventional STIR in a fraction of the time. (Courtesy of Dr. Rahul Metha, Stanford, CA.)

VASCULAR DISEASES

Spinal Cord Infarction. Vascular diseases of the spine and spinal cord can be divided into cord infarctions and vascular malformations (22–24). Spinal "strokes" are quite rare compared with cerebrovascular accidents. The classic scenario is a patient who becomes paralyzed after major thoracic surgery, such as repair of a thoracic aortic aneurysm. The affected segments of the cord will appear bright on T2-weighted images, with enhancement, similar to a brain infarct, followed by the development of myelomalacia. The spinal gray matter in an infarct will enhance to a greater degree than the white matter, as is the case in the brain (Fig. 10.48). These findings were difficult to assess prior to MR, when the diagnosis was generally made solely on clinical grounds. Obviously, when a

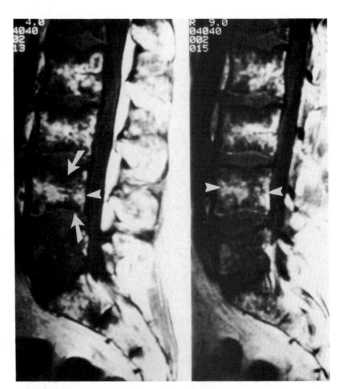

Figure 10.44.   Bone Marrow Transplantation. Marrow repopulation is occurring in this patient after bone marrow transplantation. The new hematopoietic marrow, dark on T1-weighted images, has settled in the areas of the vertebrae adjacent to the endplates (*arrow*), probably due to the rich arterial supply to these regions. The center of the vertebrae (*arrowheads*) shows less new active marrow ingrowth and more fat, and consequently, is bright on T1-weighted image.

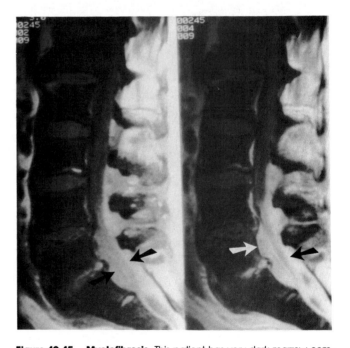

Figure 10.45.   Myelofibrosis. This patient has very dark marrow compartment on these enhanced T1-weighted images due to myelofibrosis, which has replaced the normal erythropoetic marrow. The marrow remained dark on T2-weighted imaging, as there is no increased water in this marrow condition. Note the enhancing epidural abscess (*arrows*).

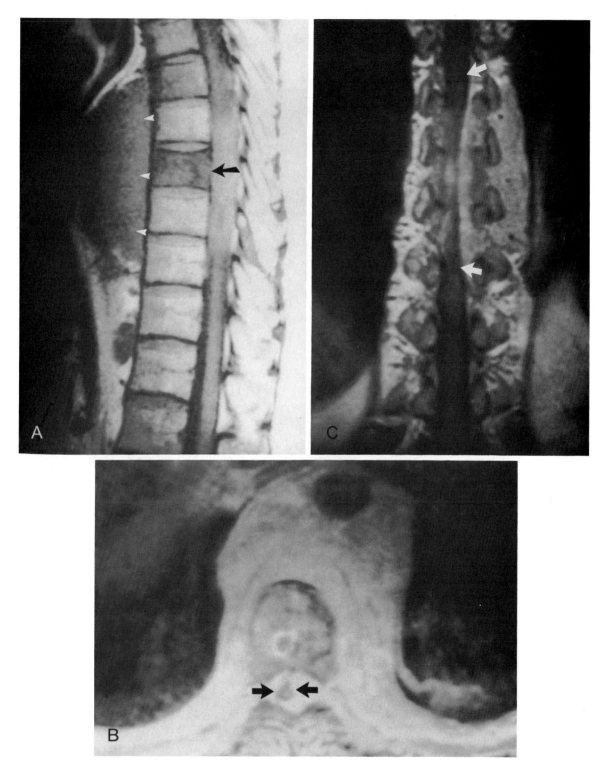

Figure 10.46. Lymphoma. A. Sagittal T1-weighted image shows a large posterior mediastinal mass (*arrowheads*), with infiltration of a midthoracic vertebral body (*arrow*). **B.** Axial images show the cord (*arrow*) and the degree of compression. **C.** A coronal image nicely shows the craniocaudal extent of spinal canal compromise (*arrows*). Lymphoma adjacent to the spine is always a threat for cord compression.

Figure 10.47. Lymphoma Infiltrating the Spinal Canal—Difficulty of CT Visualization. A. This patient with lymphoma was imaged for new back pain. Left renal involvement is obvious (*white arrow*), and left psoas infiltration is also noted (*arrowhead*). Spinal canal involvement (*curved arrow*), even in retrospect, is equivocal. **B.** The MR clearly demonstrates involvement of the spinal canal (*arrows*). Anytime a patient with paraspinous tumor presents with back pain, MR is the study of choice.

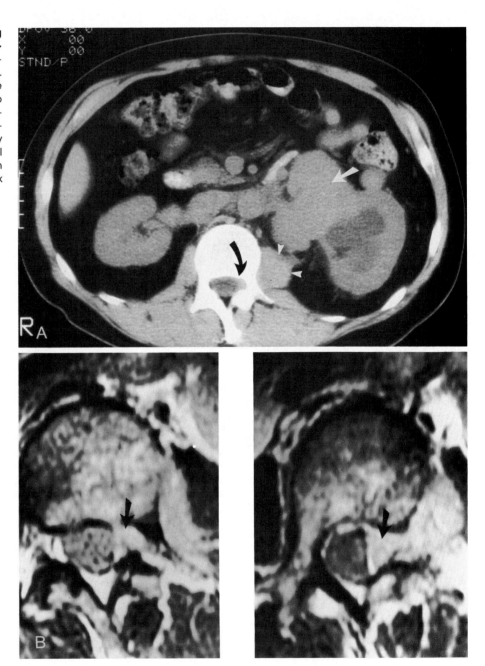

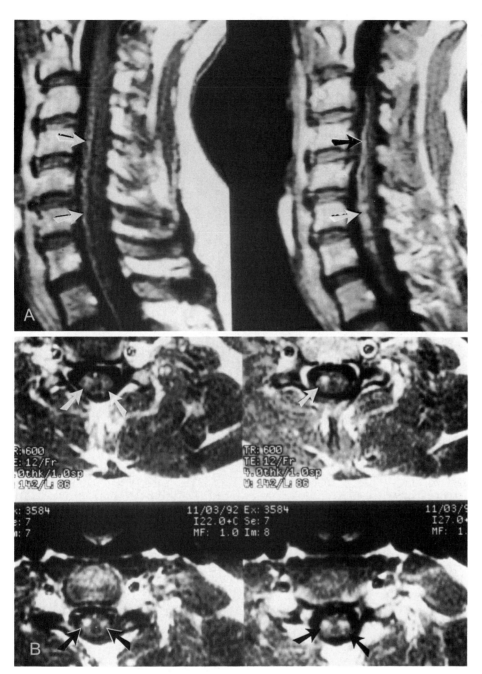

Figure 10.48. Spinal Stroke. This patient who presented with acute myelopathy, has increased signal in the cervical cord seen on T2-weighted imaging. Postcontrast sagittal (**A**) and (**B**) axial images show enhancement of the central gray matter (*arrows*), a finding highly suggestive of infarct.

patient in the recovery room after aortic surgery is paraplegic, it does not require great insight to consider a cord infarct. More subtle, however, are cases where atherosclerotic disease or severe degenerative disease leads to thromboembolic cord infarctions, and infarcts must be considered in the differential of unexplained myelopathy.

Spinal AVM. Spinal stroke can also be related to spinal AVMs. These lesions are an area of growing interest for two reasons. First, the development of superselective, interventional neuroangiographic, and microsurgical techniques has led to improved understanding and treatment of the lesions. Second, MR has allowed widespread screening of patients with un-

explained myelopathy, leading to the discovery of more patients with spinal AVMs.

"Arteriovenous malformation" is used here as a generic term to cover any abnormal vascular complex, which necessarily violates a number of rather complicated spinal AVM classification systems, where true AVMs represent a specific subtype. For a deeper discussion, the excellent article by Rosenblum is recommended (22). For a first pass at this topic, it is worth going back to the initial question one should ask about any spinal lesion: Is the location intramedullary, intradural extramedullary, or extradural? While an oversimplification, this approach provides a good initial analysis of spinal AVMs.

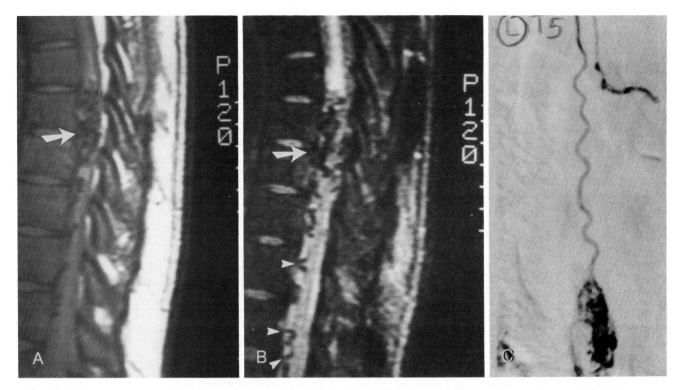

Figure 10.49. Intramedullary AVM. Proton density (**A**) and T2-weighted (**B**) sagittal images show multiple serpentine signal voids within the midthoracic spinal cord focally (*arrow*), consistent with an intramedullary AVM. A long draining vessel is also noted in the subarachnoid space (*arrowheads*). **C.** Spinal angiogram injecting the left T-5 intercostal artery confirms the MR findings. (Courtesy of Dr. Grant Hieshima, University of California, San Francisco.)

Intramedullary AVMs have a congenital "nidus" of abnormal vessels within the cord substance, which cause symptoms by hemorrhage or ischemia because of steal phenomenon. These typically present in young patients with hemorrhage, leading to acute paraparesis. Some are high flow, with visible signal voids within the cord substance (Fig. 10.49). Others escape detection even with angiography, and MR is the primary means for their identification, similar to occult vascular malformations in the brain (Fig. 10.50).

Extramedullary AVMs are located in the pia or the dura. When in the dura, they can be as far from the cord as the nerve root sleeves. The lesion is typically an arteriovenous fistula, a direct connection between an artery and vein without an intervening nidus. The direct arterial inflow into the local venous system through the fistula, undamped by the resistance of a capillary bed, raises pressure within the coronal venous plexus draining the spinal cord, which is valveless (Fig. 10.51). Spinal dural arteriovenous fistulas, or SDAVFs as they are known, cause symptoms through venous hypertension and congestion of the cord with edema. This edema can be detected on MR as increased signal on T2-weighted images, typically within an enlarged conus (see Fig. 10.53**A**), which often enhances. The reason for cord enhancement in SDAVFs is not fully understood, but probably results from breakdown of the blood-brain barrier because of either chronic infarction or some sort of capillary leak phenomenon secondary to venous hypertension. Regardless of the explanation, enhancement of the cord with SDAVFs is yet another reason why a postcontrast scan should be obtained in any patient with unexplained myelopathy.

The dilated vessels of the coronal venous plexus sometimes can be visualized by MR, but this is quite technique-dependent. With older imaging systems, normal CSF flow created tubular flow voids that mimicked vessels, leading to false-positive examinations (Fig. 10.52). Now, various motion suppression techniques have reduced this problem, but the sensitivity of MR for these small veins remains moderate at best. In the face of an equivocal MR, the best screening examination, short of spinal angiography, is supine thoracic high-dose plain film myelography. The dilated veins of the coronal venous plexus appear as serpentine filling defects in the dorsal subarachnoid space on myelography (Fig. 10.53**B**). An additional advantage of myelography is the potential to identify the primary arterialized vein fed by the fistula, a landmark that can greatly facilitate the angiographer's search for the arterial supply to fistula (Fig. 10.53**C**).

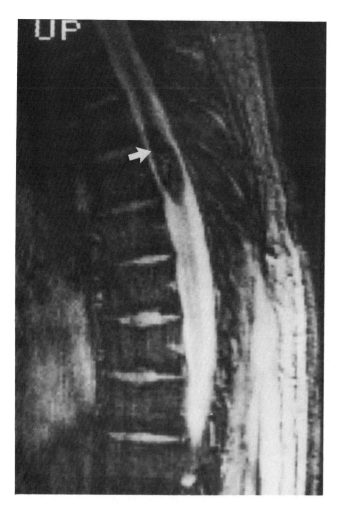

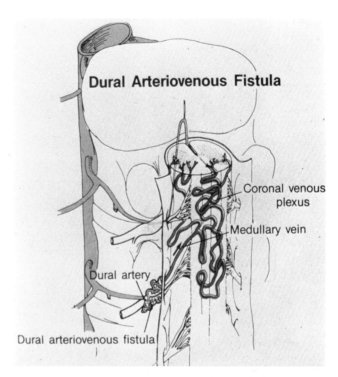

Figure 10.51. Anatomy of a Spinal Dural Arteriovenous Fistula. The fistula is an abnormal direct connection between an artery and a vein in the dura of the nerve root sleeve. The fistula results in reversal of flow in the draining vein (*arrow*), which in turn feeds the coronal venous plexus with arterial blood under high pressure. The coronal venous plexus dilates, becoming visible to imaging studies, and the cord has difficulty draining its blood because of this fistula-induced venous hypertension, and becomes edematous, and bright on T2-weighted imaging. (see Fig. 10.53). (From Rosenblum B, Oldfield EH, Doppman JL, et al. Spinal arteriovenous malformations: a comparison of dural arteriovenous fistulas and intradural AVMs in 81 patients. J Neurosurg 1987;67:796.)

Figure 10.50. Occult Vascular Malformation. This intramedullary area of decreased signal was present on all sequences, but was most prominent on this gradient series (*arrow*). No abnormal vessels were seen on MR or angiography, consistent with an occult vascular malformation, which was confirmed surgically.

CONGENITAL MALFORMATIONS

Magnetic resonance imaging has become the primary method for investigation of children born with neural axis defects, whether they involve the brain or the spine. Pediatric brain malformations, and the combined brain and spine malformation of the Chiari II syndrome, are discussed in detail in Chapter 8. The Chiari I syndrome was mentioned in the discussion of syringohydromyelia. This section briefly addresses the remaining range of congenital spine problems, emphasizing those that are not immediately apparent at birth, and may present in adulthood. The references listed are recommended for a more complete discussion of these disorders, which easily are as complex as the remaining topics of this chapter combined (25–27).

In the spine, neural tube defects that are open or have associated dermal defects are usually detected by prenatal ultrasound or at birth. Anomalies of neural tube closure where the covering skin is intact are more subtle, and range from asymptomatic nonfusion of the laminae and spinous processes to severe cord tethering with spinal lipomas (Fig. 10.54). A picture is worth a thousand words in understanding the range of presentations of spinal dysraphism, and Figure 10.55, adapted from Barkovich's text, serves as an introduction to this complex topic (25). It is worth remembering that developmental lesions are the most common cause of pediatric intraspinal masses, and T1-weighted images are preferred for evaluating fine anatomic detail, as well as the fat components that are seen in many of these disorders. The standard pediatric spine examination for congenital anomalies, therefore, includes T1-weighted sagittal and axial images; T2-weighted images are less critical.

Tethered Cord. When the cord is truly tethered, the conus will be low in position, although it is often difficult in such cases to determine the exact position of the conus, as the roots of the cauda

Figure 10.52. False-positive Dilated Spinal Veins. A. Sagittal T2-weighted images show multiple large tubular signal voids in the subarachnoid space (*arrows*), without cord edema. **B.** Axial images show flow voids that are most prominent in the lateral aspects of the spinal canal (*arrows*), areas of maximal velocity of CSF pulsation. All of the signal voids seen here are due to CSF pulsation rather than abnormal vessels in the subarachnoid space. The scan was repeated with cardiac gating and these "abnormalities" disappeared.

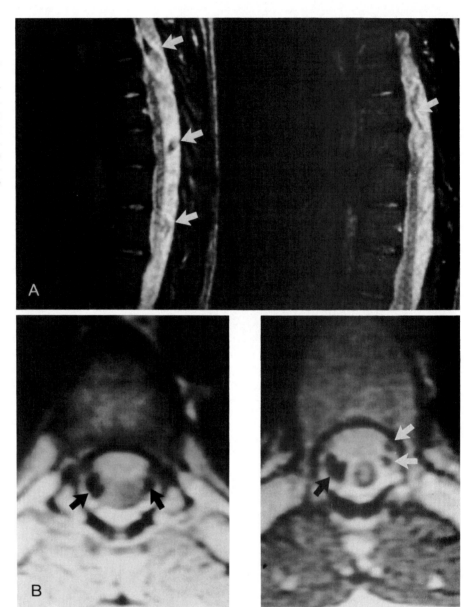

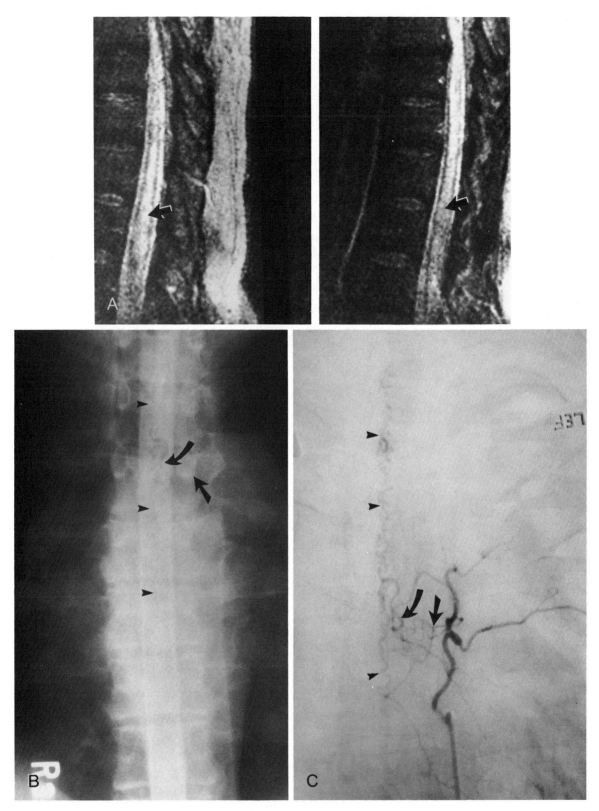

Figure 10.53. Spinal Dural Arteriovenous Fistula. A. This 45-year-old patient had progressive myelopathy, and this T2-weighted series showed increased signal in the conus (*arrow*), consistent with edema. Magnetic resonance was equivocal for abnormal vessels in the subarachnoid space. **B.** A supine thoracic myelogram demonstrates abnormal vessels causing filling defects in the contrast column posterior to the cord (*arrowhead*). The largest vessel (*curved arrow*) appears to exit the spinal canal just below the left T-5 pedicle (*arrow*), and represents the arterialized vein fed by the fistula. The myelogram, therefore, suggests a promising site to begin spinal angiography. **C.** A spinal angiogram demonstrates the dural fistula (*arrow*), and the arterialized vein with reversal of flow (*curved arrow*) that has led to dilation of the entire coronal venous plexus (*arrowheads*). Note how the subarachnoid vessels seen on the angiogram and myelogram are superimposable. Compare to the diagram shown in Figure 10.51.

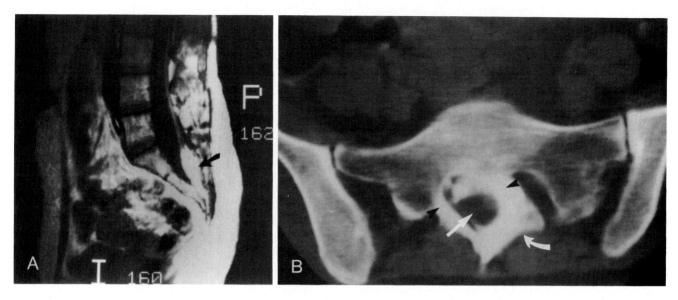

Figure 10.54.   Spinal Lipoma. A. T1 sagittal images show a dorsal intraspinal lipoma (*arrow*) at S-1. **B.** An axial CT myelogram demonstrates that the distal lipoma (*arrow*) is intrathecal, surrounded by enhanced CSF (*arrowheads*), with an incomplete posterior sacrum (*curved arrow*), consistent with spinal dysraphism. This defect is illustrated schematically in Figure 10.55**A.**

Figure 10.55.   Spinal Dysraphism. This series of drawings from Barkovich's text nicely illustrates the range of appearances of spinal dysraphism. In all of these conditions, there has been failure of the lips of the neural folds to close in the midline dorsally, forming a tube. The incompletely fused plaque of neural tissue is referred to as the neural "placode." When the placode is covered by intact skin and subcutaneous fat, without dorsal herniation of neural tissue, the defect (**A** and **B**) may be overlooked in the newborn examination, giving rise to the term "occult spinal dysraphism." **A.** Spinal lipoma. The dorsal spinal cord has failed to close, with an intradural lipoma situated between the lips of the unfused placode. The MR and CT appearance of this defect is shown in Figure 10.54. **B.** Lipomyelocele. The dorsal dura is incomplete. The subarachnoid space lies ventral to the placode, which is covered by pia and arachnoid on its internal surface. The subcutaneous fat is contiguous with a lipoma, which is adherent to the dorsal surface of the placode. **C.** Lipomyelomeningocele. This is similar to the lipomyelocele (**B**), except there the subarachnoid space is dilated, causing the placode to bulge posteriorly. In this drawing, the lipoma is asymmetric and extends into the canal on the left, rotating the placode and causing discrepancy in the length of the nerve roots, which complicates surgical repair. Lipomyelomeningoceles are seen in conjunction with rostral craniospinal abnormalities in the Chiari II syndrome, illustrated in Figure 8.20). **D.** Myelocele. The neural placode is contiguous with the skin, and will be obvious on newborn examination. The ventral aspect of the placode has the same anatomy as the lipomyelocele. **E.** Meningomyelocele. The ventral subarachnoid space is dilated, displacing the placode posteriorly (as in lipomyelomeningocele). Otherwise, the defect is identical to a myelocele. (From Barkovich AJ. Pediatric neuroimaging. New York: Raven Press, 1990:240, 248.)

equina, when tethered, form a taut mass in the posterior lumbar canal, obscuring the conus/cauda junction (Fig. 10.56). Not every lumbar intradural fatty deposit implies pathologic tethering, and small fibrolipomas of the filum terminale may be noted on MR examinations in patients with normal conus position and no symptoms of cord tethering (Fig. 10.57). A cohort of these patients needs to be followed throughout their lives before such fibroli-

pomas can be dismissed as incidental, since symptoms of cord tethering occasionally can present well into adulthood. Before describing the conus as low in position, recall that the conus in a newborn is normally at L-2, and typically ascends one to two vertebral segments as the child grows.

Intramedullary Lipomas can be seen in patients with normal or bifid spinal canals and, as with brain lipomas, may be discovered incidentally. These are

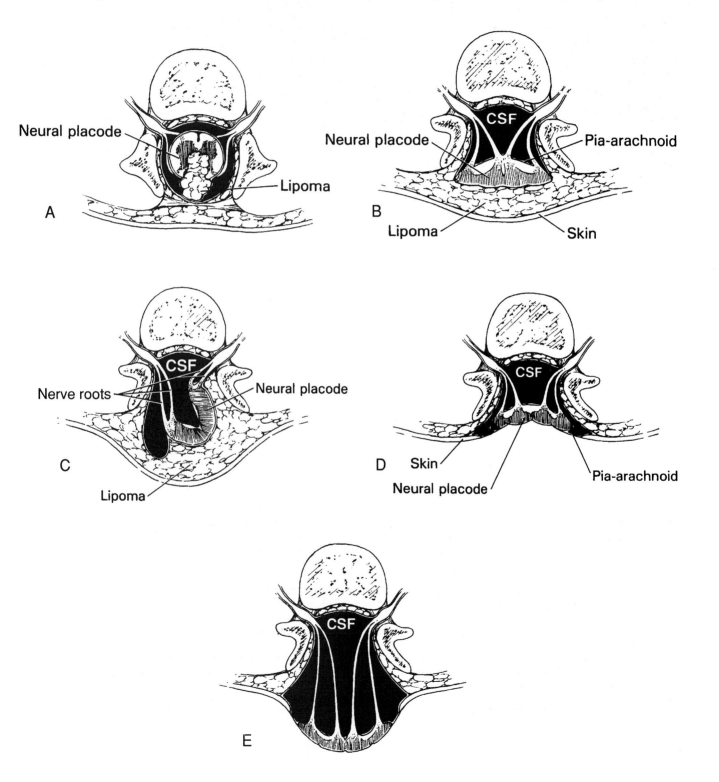

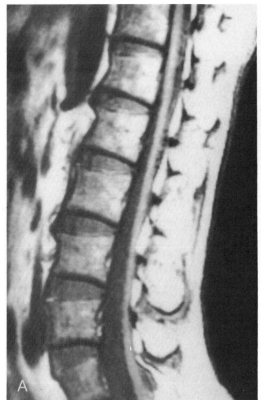

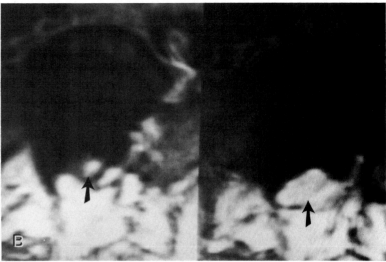

Figure 10.56. Adult Cord Tethering. This young adult presented with a gait disorder. **A.** It is difficult to be certain of the position of the conus on sagittal plane because of the clumping of the roots posteriorly, but it is definitely very low. **B.** Axial T1-weighted images demonstrate spinal dysraphism with a lipoma (*arrows*), consistent with cord tethering.

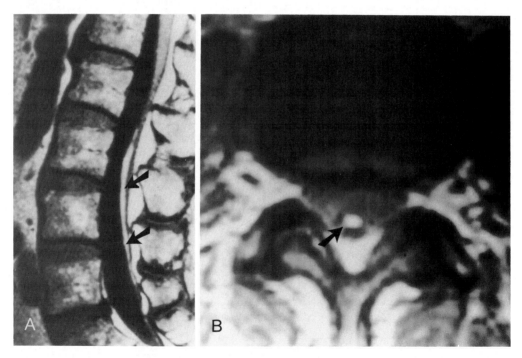

Figure 10.57. Fibrolipoma of the Filum Terminale. A. Sagittal T1-weighted images show that the conus is normal in position, but the filum terminale shows high signal consistent with fat (*arrows*). **B.** Axial T1-weighted image confirms the intrathecal position of the thickened fatty filum (*arrow*).

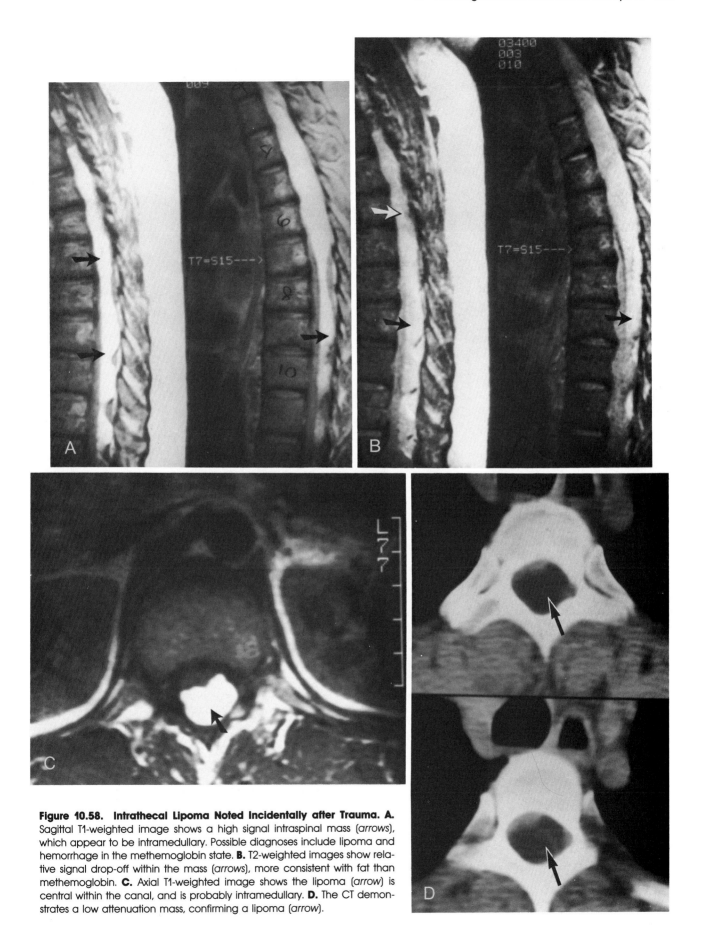

Figure 10.58. Intrathecal Lipoma Noted Incidentally after Trauma. A.
Sagittal T1-weighted image shows a high signal intraspinal mass (*arrows*),
which appear to be intramedullary. Possible diagnoses include lipoma and
hemorrhage in the methemoglobin state. **B.** T2-weighted images show relative signal drop-off within the mass (*arrows*), more consistent with fat than
methemoglobin. **C.** Axial T1-weighted image shows the lipoma (*arrow*) is
central within the canal, and is probably intramedullary. **D.** The CT demonstrates a low attenuation mass, confirming a lipoma (*arrow*).

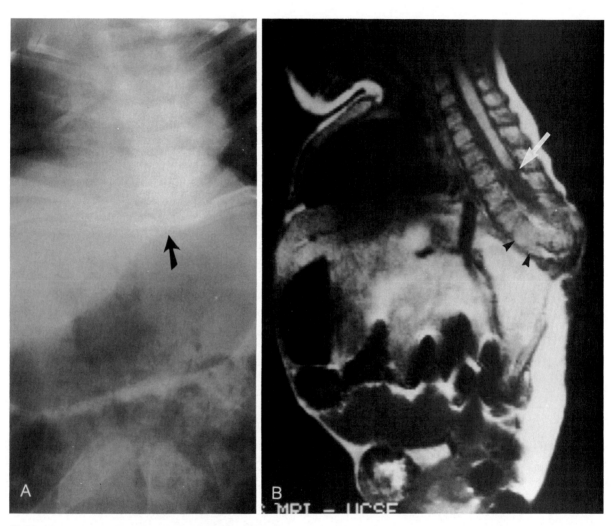

Figure 10.59. Severe Caudal Regression Syndrome. A. Plain film of the abdomen shows absence of the spinal column below T-8 (*arrow*). **B.** Sagittal T1-weighted image shows a characteristic blunted appearance of the distal cord (*arrow*), and fusion of the caudal vertebrae (*arrowheads*), the lowest of which is dysplastic. (From Barkovich AJ. Pediatric neuroimaging. New York: Raven Press, 1990:242.)

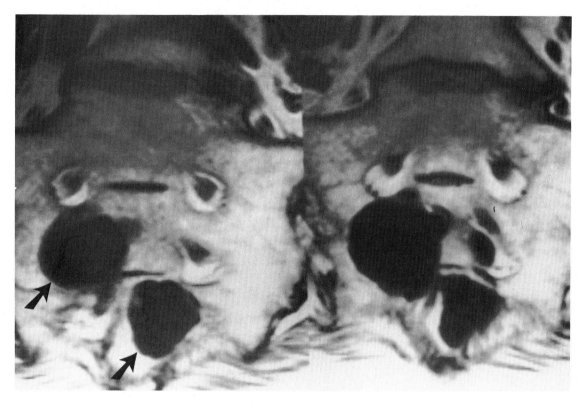

Figure 10.60. Sacral Cysts. Leptomeningeal-lined sacral cysts have been classified many different ways. The spectrum includes intrasacral meningoceles, anterior sacral meningoceles, and peri-neural (Tarlov's) cysts (*arrows*), shown here in this T1-weighted image through the sacrum. These are often asymptomatic, but can result in radicular compression.

Figure 10.61. Arachnoid Cyst. A. Sagittal T1-weighted images show a mass isointense to CSF (*arrow*) posterior to the proximal cauda equina, displacing it forward. **B.** This mass becomes brighter than the remainder of the CSF on the T2-weighted image (*arrow*). This proved to be an arachnoid cyst. These can be congenital or related to prior inflammation or injury.

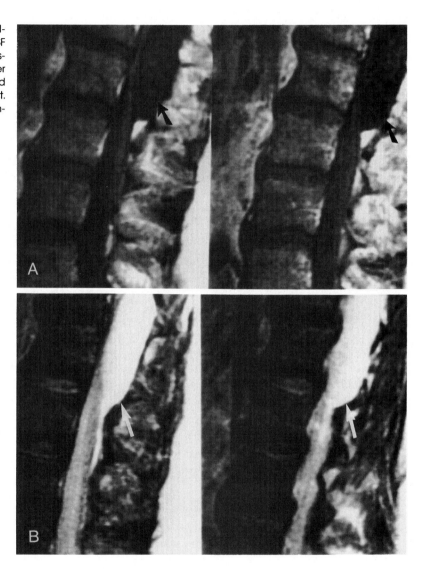

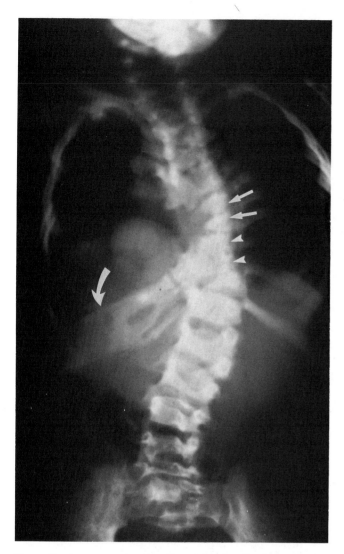

Figure 10.62. Congenital Scoliosis. This plain film shows hemivertebrae (*arrows*), block vertebrae (*arrowheads*), and fused ribs (*curved arrow*), leaving no doubt that this is congenital rather than idiopathic scoliosis. An MR would be valuable to evaluate the spinal cord for position and possible mass effect.

usually thoracic, more common in males, and when symptomatic, present with myelopathy in young adulthood (Fig. 10.58). If any cysts, hemorrhage, or debris are seen in association with the fat, suspect a teratoma. Dermoid and epidermoid tumors occur intraspinally, with imaging characteristics similar to their presentations in the brain. Both are associated with dorsal dermal sinus tracts. Intraspinal teratomas are a distinct entity from sacrococcygeal teratoma, a pediatric lesion with a high malignant potential, often associated with other anomalies.

Caudal Regression Syndrome. A number of other sacral anomalies have been grouped under the "caudal regression syndrome," where the distal spine and sacrum may be hypoplastic or absent and the conus has a blunted appearance (Fig. 10.59). Caudal regression is believed to be because of an in-

sult to the mesoderm during the 4th gestational week, and associated cardiac and renal anomalies are common. There is a high association with maternal diabetes. However, subtle forms, such as partial sacral agenesis, may not be discovered until adulthood. The distal spine is also the site of a number of CSF-filled, arachnoid-lined cystic lesions with associated bony deformity, ranging from small perineural (Tarlov's) cysts (Fig. 10.60) to huge anterior sacral meningoceles. The latter is distinct from posterior meningocele, which, like a myelomeningocele, results from failure of neural tube closure, rather than leptomeningeal diverticulation. Arachnoid cysts in the spine present as masses that are relatively isointense to CSF. As in the brain, the primary differential diagnostic consideration is an epidermoid. Either can occur in the lumbar spine as a rare complication of lumbar puncture (Fig. 10.61).

Many unsuspected spinal abnormalities present as curvature of the spine, or scoliosis. Most adolescents with curvature of the spine have idiopathic scoliosis, but when the onset is earlier or more severe, or plain scoliosis films show a vertebral anomaly (Fig. 10.62), MR is indicated to rule out an intraspinal abnormality. These cases are collectively known as "congenital scoliosis," and the primary cause, such as cord tethering, must be addressed before the spine undergoes mechanical straightening (Fig. 10.63).

TRAUMA

In the acute trauma patient, such as those who are involved in a motor vehicle accident, spine alignment must be evaluated immediately to rule out fractures. Unstable fractures can compromise the diameter of the spinal canal, leading to cord compression and paralysis. Plain films, therefore, are the study of choice in the emergency department, as they can be obtained quickly and inexpensively, without significant interruption of other recussitation efforts. When complex spine fractures are seen on plain films, CT studies are often helpful to define the relationship of the bone fragments. Computed tomography of the cervical spine is particularly useful in detecting injury to the foramen transversarium, which houses the vertebral artery, a vessel that can be compromised by cervical trauma. Spine fractures and their evaluation are critical topics for radiology residents and others responsible for emergency radiology to master, and are discussed in detail in Chapter 36.

Some discussion, however, is needed concerning the immediate and delayed consequences of vertebral trauma to the spinal cord and spinal nerves, that cannot properly be evaluated on plain films or with noncontrast CT. These include cord contusion, epidural hematoma (and their sequela, such as myelomalacia

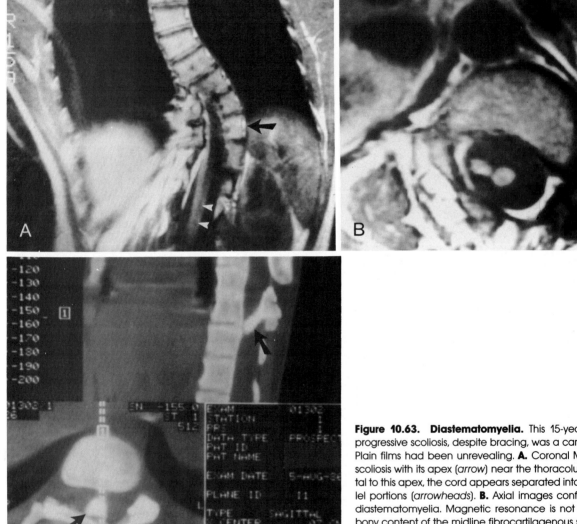

Figure 10.63. Diastematomyelia. This 15-year-old patient with progressive scoliosis, despite bracing, was a candidate for surgery. Plain films had been unrevealing. **A.** Coronal MR shows the levoscoliosis with its apex (*arrow*) near the thoracolumbar junction. Distal to this apex, the cord appears separated into two distinct parallel portions (*arrowheads*). **B.** Axial images confirm a split cord, or diastematomyelia. Magnetic resonance is not good at assessing bony content of the midline fibrocartilagenous spur. (**A** and **B** from Brant-Zawadzki M, Norman D. Magnetic resonance imaging of the central nervous system. New York: Raven Press, 1987.) **C.** A CT scan with sagittal reconstruction on a similar patient confirms a dense, bony midline spur (*arrows*). This spur was also visible on plain film.

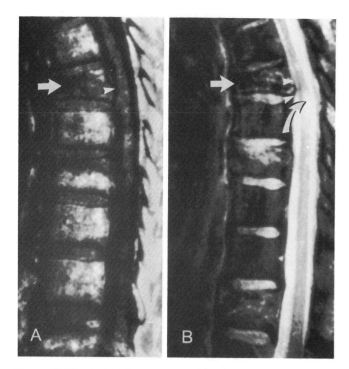

and syringohydromyelia), and nerve root avulsion (28–31).

Cord Contusion. The spinal cord, like the brain, lies suspended in a bath of CSF, contained by arachnoid membranes, dura, and bone. The cord, again like the brain, is subject to significant impact against its surrounding bony suit of "armor" during abrupt acceleration and deceleration. In the brain, contusions appear at the site of a blow and 180° opposite, in the classic coup-contrecoup pattern. Certain bony sites, such as the planum sphenoidale, tend to traumatize adjacent brain because of their irregular coutour. In the spine, contusions usually occur at sites of fractures, secondary to bony impingement and cord compression (Fig. 10.64). However, spinal cord contusions may occur in the absence of spinal fractures, because of hyperflexion or hyperextension, resulting in myelopathy (Fig. 10.65). The presence of cord edema, and particularly of cord hemorrhage, have been established as poor prognostic factors in spinal cord injury patients evaluated by MR. Therefore, T2-weighted or gradient-echo images are a critical portion of any MR protocol for spine trauma. Certain types of injury, such as sudden distraction forces along the long axis of the spine, can lead to cord avulsion (Fig. 10.66).

If the spinal cord is injured, myelomalacia results and further changes can occur because of CSF flow

Figure 10.64. Spinal Contusion. A. Compression fracture (*arrow*) with narrowing of the spinal canal (*arrowheads*) due to retropulsed bony fragments. **B.** Intramedullary edema (*curved arrow*), seen on this T2-weighted image, is a poor prognostic factor in this setting. The presence of a hematoma is associated with an even poorer outcome. Fortunately, none is evident.

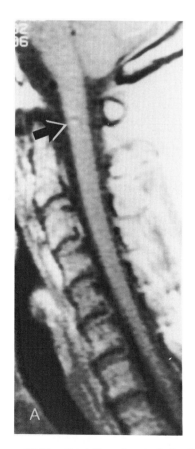
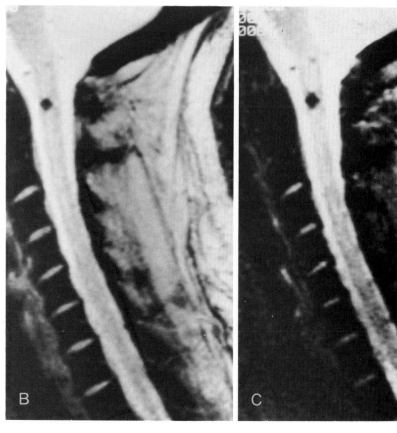

Figure 10.65. Cord Hematoma. A. Sagittal T1-weighted images show a tiny focus of methemoglobin with a dark rim (*arrow*) in the cord posterior to the dens. The dark rim "blooms" on the first (**B**) and second (**C**) echoes of the gradient refocused sequence, consistent with hemosiderin.

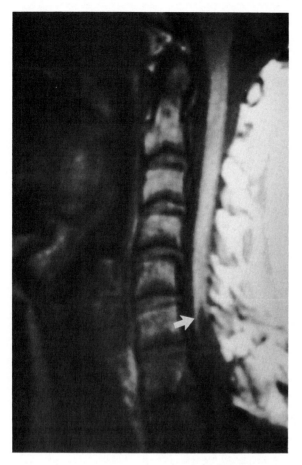

Figure 10.66.   Cord Avulsion. The junction of the cervical and thoracic cord is a weak point where tearing can occur in injuries that stretch the cord (*arrow*).

and evolve into a posttraumatic syrinx. The expanding syrinx can cause further neurologic deficit, and require shunting.

Epidural Hematoma. As in the head, extraaxial or, more appropriately, "extramedullary" hematomas can follow trauma, with certain important distinctions. Subdural hematomas are rare in the spine (and usually related to coagulopathies (Fig. 10.67)), while epidural hematomas are far more common. The reverse is true in the calvarium, as discussed in Chapter 3.

This distinction can be explained by differences in venous anatomy between the skull and the spine, as the majority of posttraumatic bleeding is venous. In the bony calvarium, the dura is functionally the periosteum, with no potential space between the dura and bone for low-pressure venous blood to accumulate. It takes bleeding under arterial pressure to create an epidural hematoma by stripping the dura away from the inner table. In the spine, the dura is separated from the bone by epidural fat. In the ventral spinal canal, the epidural space also contains a rich plexus of veins, which drains the vertebral bodies. Trauma, with or without vertebral fracture, can tear these veins, resulting in an epidural hematoma. These hematomas grow with time, leading to cord compression in the setting of normal plain films. Computed tomography may detect these epidural hematomas in the lumbar spine, where there is some fat to provide contrast, but generally will not demonstrate an epidural hematoma in the cervical or thoracic spine unless intrathecal contrast is given. Magnetic resonance is the study of choice, given its ability to image the contents of the spinal canal noninvasively and depict blood-breakdown products (Fig. 10.68).

patterns. An area of myelomalacia can enlarge with CSF entry, particularly if adhesions disturb CSF flow, and evolve into a posttraumatic syrinx. The ex-

Figure 10.67.   Spinal Hematoma. This spinal subdural hematoma (*arrows*) occurred spontaneously in this thrombocytopenic leukemia patient. Note the low marrow signal consistent with leukemia, and the constriction of the thecal sac (*curved arrow*) by the hematoma. The hematoma is difficult to distinguish from epidural fat (*arrowheads*) on the T1 image (**A**), but becomes more obvious as the epidural fat darkens on the T2 images (**B**).

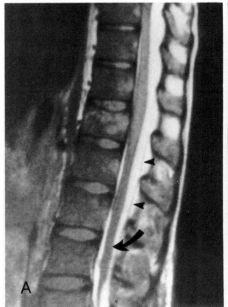
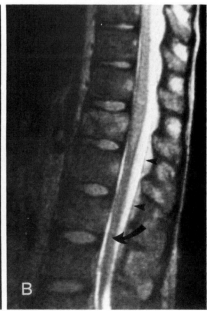

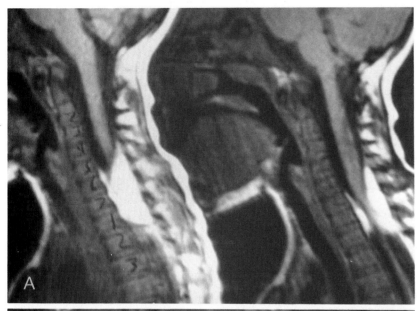

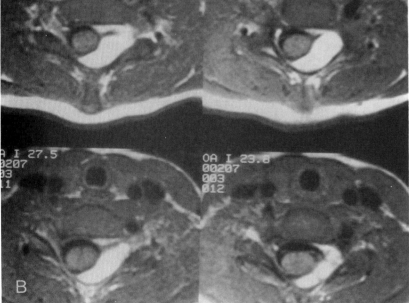

Figure 10.68. Epidural Hematoma. T1 sagittal (**A**) and axial (**B**) images show a bright epidural mass consistent with a hematoma in the methemoglobin stage. An epidural hematoma can occur in the face of normal plain films, and must be suspected if there is neurologic compromise.

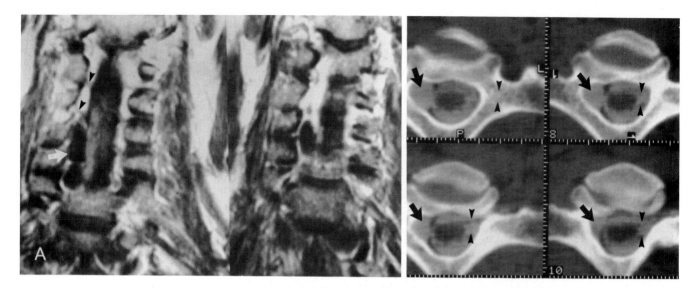

Figure 10.69.   Nerve Root Avulsion. A. Coronal T1 images show a low signal collection in the right epidural space in the midcervical spine (*arrow*), consistent with CSF that has leaked through avulsed nerve root sleeves. Intact spinal nerves (*arrowheads*) are seen in the upper cervical canal bilaterally traversing through the normal epidural fat. **B.** A CT myelogram confirms the absence of the right-sided nerve roots and the CSF leak (*arrow*). Note the normal roots on the left outlined by myelographic contrast (*arrowheads*).

Nerve Root Avulsion.   Most of these traumatic complications have been discussed in terms of their effects on the spinal cord. It should be remembered that epidural hematomas and contusions can also affect nerve roots and result in radicular complaints. An additional form of direct trauma to the spinal nerve roots is avulsion from their connection to the cord. In the spinal canal, the most common site for root avulsion is the cervical spine, probably because of its wide range of motion during accidents. The roots serving the brachial plexus and upper extremities are typically affected, with obvious neurologic deficits. The clinical diagnosis can be confirmed by MR or CT myelography. Typically, CSF will leak out into the epidural space through the rent in the arachnoid and dura from the missing nerve, as can be seen in Figure 10.69. The 12 paired thoracic spinal nerves and nerves of the lumbar cauda equina rarely undergo avulsion. Therefore, while MR is often not practical in the acute setting, it has become a superb noninvasive tool for evaluating the neurologic complications of trauma, and has increased our understanding of these entities.

References

1. Atlas S, ed. Magnetic resonance imaging of the brain and spine. New York: Raven Press, 1992.
2. Brant-Zawadzki M, Norman D. Magnetic resonance imaging of the central nervous system. New York: Raven Press, 1987.
3. Enzmann DR, DeLaPaz RL, Rubin JB, eds. Magnetic resonance imaging of the spine. St. Louis: Mosby, 1990.
4. Latchaw RE, ed. MR and CT of the head, neck, and spine. 2nd ed. St. Louis: Mosby, 1991.
5. Manlfe C, ed. Imaging of the spine and spinal cord. New York: Raven Press, 1992.
6. Aisen AM, Martel W, Ellis JH, et al. Cervical spine involvement in rheumatoid arthritis: MR imaging. Radiology 1987;165:159–163.
7. Larsson EM, Holtås S, Nilsson O. Gd-DTPA enhanced MR of suspected multiple sclerosis. AJNR 1989;10:1071–1076.
8. Friedman DP. Herpes zoster myelitis: MR appearance. AJNR 1992;13:1404–1406.
9. Merine D, Wang H, Kumar AJ, et al. CT myelography and MR imaging of acute transverse myelitis. J Comput Assist Tomogr 1987;11:606–608.
10. Petito CK, Navia BA, Cho ES, et al. Myelopathy pathologicly resembling subacute combined degeneration in patients with the acquired immunodeficiency syndrome. N Engl J Med 1985;312:874–987.
11. Provenzale J, Bouldin TW. Lupus related myelopathy: report of three cases and review of the literature. J Neurol Neurosurg Psychiatry 1992;55:830–835.
12. Wang PY, Shen WC, Jian SJ. MR imaging in radiation myelopathy. AJNR 1992;13:1049–1055.
13. Modic MT, Fieglin DH, Piraino DW, et al. Vertebral osteomyelitis: assessment using MR. Radiology 1985;157:157–166.
14. Post MJD, Sze G, Quencer RM, et al. Gadolinium-enhanced MR in spinal infection. J Comput Assist Tomogr 1990;14:721–729.
15. Smith AS, Weinstein MA, Mizushima A, et al. MR imaging characteristics of tuberculous spondylitis vs. vertebral osteomyelitis. AJNR 1989;10:619–625.
16. Scotti G, Scialfa G, Colombo N, et al. Magnetic resonance diagnosis of intramedullary tumors of the cord. Neuroradiology 1987;29:130–135.
17. Dillon WP, Norman DN, Newton TH et al, Intradural spinal cord lesions: Gd-DTPA-enhanced MR imaging. Radiology 1989;170:229–237.
18. Egelhoff JC, Bates DJ, Ross JS, et al. Spinal MR findings in neurofibromatosis types 1 and 2. AJNR 1992;13:1071–1077.
19. Sloof JL, Kernohan JW, MacCarty CS. Primary intramedullary tumors of the spinal cord and filum terminale. Philadelphia: WB Saunders, 1964.

20. Stevens SK, Moore SG, Amylon MD. Repopulation of marrow after transplantation : MR imaging with pathologic correlation. Radiology 1990;175:213–218.

21. Yuh WTC, Zachar CK, Barloon TJ, et al. Vertebral compression fractures: distinction between benign and malignant causes with MR imaging. Radiology 1989;172:215–218.

22. Rosenblum B, Oldfield EH, Doppman JL, et al. Spinal arteriovenous malformations: a comparison of dural arteriovenous fistulas and intradural AVMs in 81 patients. J Neurosurg 1987;67:795–802.

23. Friedman DP, Flanders AE. Enhancement of gray matter in anterior spinal infarction. AJNR 1992;13:983–985.

24. Mawad ME, Rivera V, Crawford S, et al. Spinal cord ischemia after the resection of thoracoabdominal aneurysms: MR findings in 24 patients. AJNR 1990;11:987–991.

25. Barkovich AJ, Naidich TP. Congenital anomalies of the spine. In: Barkovich AJ, ed. Pediatric euroimaging. New York: Raven Press, 1990.

26. Petterson H, Harwood-Nash DCF. CT and myelography of the spine and cord: techniques, anatomy and pathology in children. Berlin: Springer-Verlag, 1982.

27. Raghavan N, Barkovich AJ, Edwards MSB, et al., MR imaging in the tethered spinal cord syndrome. AJNR 1989;10:27–36.

28. Chakeres DW, Flickinger F, Bresnahan JC, et al. MR imaging of acute spinal cord trauma. AJNR 1987;8:5–10.

29. Flanders AE, Schaefer DM, Doan HT, et al. Acute cervical spine trauma: correlation of MR imaging findings with degree of neurologic deficit. Radiology 1990;177:25–33.

30. Petras AF, Sobel DF, Mani JR, et al. CT myelography in cervical nerve root avulsion. J Comput Assist Tomogr 1985;9:275–279.

31. Silberstien M, Tress BM, Hennessy O. Delayed neurologic deterioration in the patient with spine trauma: role of MR imaging. AJNR 1992;13:1373–1381.

11

Lumbar Spine: Disc Disease and Stenosis

Clyde A. Helms

Imaging Methods

Imaging the lumbar spine for disc disease and stenosis has evolved in the past 10 years from predominantly myelography-oriented examinations to plain computed tomography (CT) and magnetic resonance (MR) examinations. Multiple studies have shown that myelography is not as accurate as CT or MR (1–3), yet myelography continues to be performed. There is little justification for a lumbar myelogram to determine disc disease or stenosis in this era.

Although few differences between CT and MR have been noted concerning diagnostic accuracy in the lumbar spine, MR will give more information and a more complete anatomic depiction than will CT. It remains to be seen if the additional information afforded by an MR examination will prove to be clinically useful. For example, MR can determine if a disc is degenerated by showing loss of signal on T2-weighted images (Fig. 11.1). Computed tomography cannot give this information, but it hardly matters since no treatment is currently given solely for a degenerated disc. In fact, degenerative discs have been reported in asymptomatic children who deny a past history of back pain (4).

At present, MR is clearly superior to CT in imaging the lumbar spine in only one aspect: evaluating the back postoperatively. The use of gadolinium has greatly aided the differentiation of postoperative fibrosis from recurrent disc protrusion. The single area in which CT has been shown to be superior to MR in the lumbar spine is in diagnosing spondylolysis. Pars defects can be very difficult to appreciate with MR, yet they are easily seen with CT. Computed tomography and MR are seemingly diagnostically equivalent.

To achieve a high degree of accuracy it is imperative that the proper imaging protocols are observed. With CT scans, thin-section (3-5 mm) axial images should be obtained from the midbody of L-3 to the midbody of S-1 in a contiguous manner, i.e., no skip areas or gaps should be present (Fig. 11.2). One of the leading causes of failed back surgery is missed free fragments. Skip areas will often allow a free fragment to go undiagnosed. It is not necessary to angle the gantry parallel to the endplates, and image reformations are not helpful in the routine evaluation of disc disease and stenosis.

The MR imaging protocol is similar to that of CT in that thin-section axial images should be obtained from the midbody of L-3 to the midbody of S-1 (Fig. 11.3). Angling of the plane of imaging to be parallel to the endplates is not necessary, and contiguous

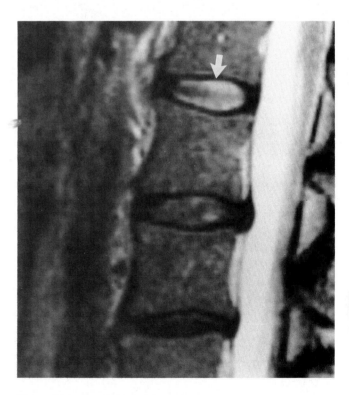

Figure 11.1. Dessicated Disc. A sagittal T2-weighted image (TR, 4000; TE, 102) shows the L2-3 and L3-4 discs to be abnormally low in signal, indicating disc dessication and degeneration. Compare with the normal L1-2 disc (*arrow*), which has high signal.

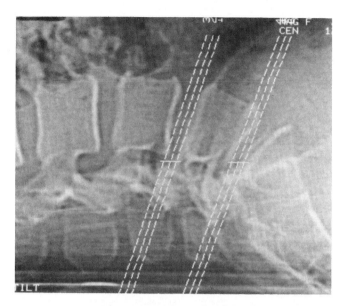

Figure 11.2. Inadequate Technique—Skip Areas. A CT scout film with cursors placed through the L4-5 and L5-S1 disc spaces. This allows large gaps or skip areas which can result in missed free fragments of discs. Also, the L3-4 disc space should be imaged.

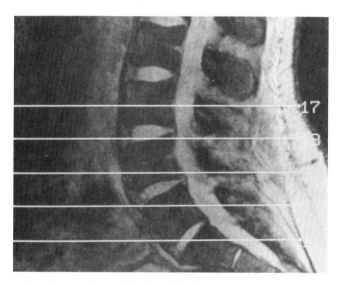

Figure 11.3. Proper MR Technique. This MR scout with cursors placed contiguously from the body of L-3 to S-1 allows complete coverage of the lower lumbar spine in the axial plane.

images without skip areas are considered mandatory. Even though sagittal images will be obtained, free fragments and areas of stenosis are often seen on the axial images to better advantage than on the sagittal images. Both T1 (or proton density)-weighted and T2 (or T2*)-weighted images should be obtained in the sagittal and the axial planes. Attempts to shorten the study by foregoing one of the T2 sequences are not recommended. The addition of T2 axial images will increase diagnostic accuracy as well as the diagnostic confidence of many diagnoses.

Disc Disease

DISC PROTRUSIONS

Terminology plays a large role in how radiologists describe disc bulges or protrusions. Since the advent of CT in the 1970s, disc bulges have been described by their morphology. A broad-based disc bulge has been said to be a bulging annulus fibrosus, while a focal disc bulge is a herniated nucleus pulposus. These interpretations are no more than 90% accurate. More significantly, most surgeons are not concerned with what name is applied to a disc bulge; they do not treat a bulging annulus differently than a herniated nucleus pulposus. They treat the patient's symptoms and have to decide if the disc bulge is responsible for those symptoms. It has been shown that 10–25% of asymptomatic young people have disc protrusions (5), hence; just seeing a disc bulge on CT or MR does not mean it is clinically significant.

Both CT and MR have a high degree of accuracy in delineating disc protrusions and showing if neural tissue is impressed (Fig. 11.4). The MR can also show if annular fibers of the disc are disrupted, a so-called extrusion. Although CT cannot be used to diagnose extrusions, clinicians treat extrusions the same way they treat protrusions (annular fibers intact).

FREE FRAGMENTS

A type of disc extrusion that is critical to diagnose is the free fragment or sequestration. Missed free fragments is one of the most common causes of failed back surgery (6). The preoperative diagnosis of a free fragment contraindicates chymopapain, percutaneous discectomy, and, for many surgeons, microdiscectomy. At the very least the presence of a free fragment means the surgeon needs to explore more cephalad or caudally during the surgery in order to remove the free fragment. As free fragments can be very difficult to diagnose clinically, imaging is critical in the evaluation of the spine for any patient contemplating surgery. At times it can be difficult to be absolutely certain as to whether or not a disc that has extruded is still attached to the parent disc or is really "free." So long as disc material is above or below the level of the disc space it really does not matter if it is attached or not; chymopapain and percutaneous discectomy would still be contraindicated and many surgeons would not perform a microdiscectomy. The key element is recognizing that disc material is present away from the level of the disc space.

Free fragments are diagnosed on CT by the presence of a soft tissue density with a higher attenuation value than the thecal sac (Fig. 11.5). A conjoined root (a normal variant of two roots exiting the thecal sac together; seen in 1–3% of the population (7)) (Fig. 11.6) or a Tarlov cyst (a normal variant referring to a

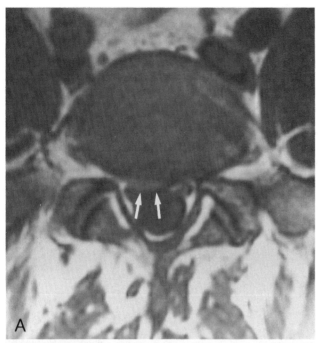

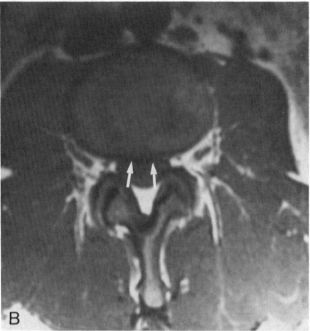

Figure 11.4.   Disc Protrusions. Axial T1-weighted images (TR, 800; TE, 20) show focal (**A**) (*arrows*) and broad-based (**B**) disc protrusions (*arrows*). Either of these could be a herniated disc or a bulging annulus fibrosis. Since these are both showing impression of the thecal sac, they could each cause symptoms.

dilated nerve root sleeve) can have a similar appearance to a free fragment, but will have attenuation values similar to the thecal sac.

Free fragments are diagnosed on MR by noting disc material that has moved away from the disc space (Fig. 11.7). Up to 80% of free fragments will have high signal on T2-weighted images even though the parent disc may be low signal (8). Free fragments migrate ei-

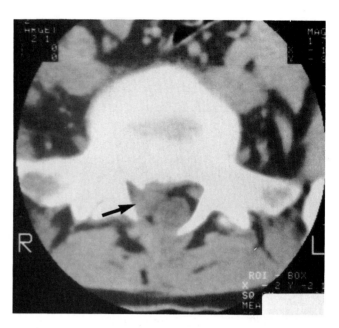

Figure 11.5.   Free Fragment (CT). A soft tissue mass is seen in the right lateral recess (*arrow*), which has a CT attenuation value of 24.1 Hounsfield units, while sampling of the thecal sac gave a measurement of only 4.6 CT units. Thus, the soft tissue mass is of higher density than the thecal sac and represents a free fragment of disc material, also called a sequestration.

ther cephalad or caudally, with no preference documented.

It is imperative to obtain contiguous axial images without large skip areas or gaps when imaging with both CT and MR in order to not miss free fragments.

LATERAL DISCS

Discs will occasionally protrude in a lateral direction, causing the nerve root that has already exited the central canal to be stretched (Fig. 11.8). Although not common (less than 5% of cases), these discs are frequently overlooked and are known to be a source of failed back surgery (9). Since they affect the already exited root they can clinically mimic symptoms of a disc protrusion from one level more cephalad (Fig. 11.9). For example, in a patient with multilevel disc disease and symptoms referable to the L3-4 disc, the disc protrusion is usually a posterior bulge that impresses the L-4 nerve root. However, a lateral disc at L4-5 could impress the L-4 nerve root and cause the same symptoms. If not noticed, surgery could be performed at the L3-4 disc, which is the wrong level. It is also important to notify the surgeon that the disc is lateral to the neuroforamen, as a standard surgical approach through the lamina might not allow removal of a lateral disc.

Lateral discs are best identified on axial images. Sagittal images will often show a lateral disc occluding a neuroforamen, but many times a lateral disc will not

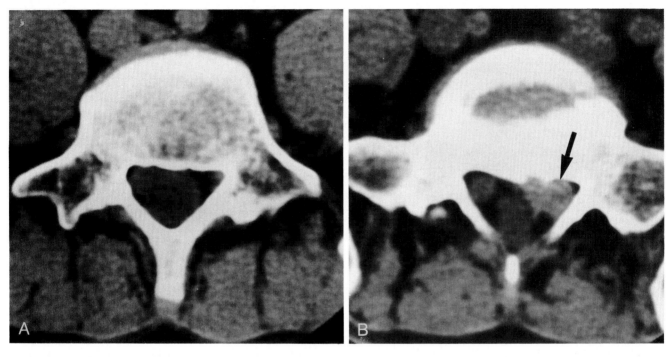

Figure 11.6.   Conjoined Root and Free Fragment. A. A soft tissue mass is seen in the right L-5 lateral recess, which has CT attenuation values identical to the thecal sac. This is a conjoined nerve root. **B.** In the same patient, a soft tissue mass is present in the left S-1 lateral recess (*arrow*) which has a density greater than the adjacent thecal sac. This is a free fragment.

Figure 11.7.   Free Fragment. A. A sagittal T1-weighted (TR, 500; TE, 20) MR image shows a large amount of disc material bulging posteriorly at the disc space (*arrows*). **B.** The adjacent slice shows disc material that has migrated cephalad (*arrows*) and now lies posterior to the L-5 vertebral body. This is a large free fragment.

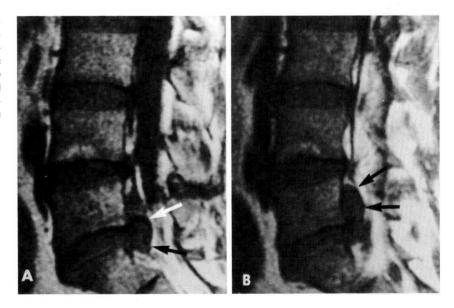

Figure 11.8. Lateral Disc (MR). A. A sagittal T1-weighted (TR, 600; TE, 30) MR image through the left neuroforamen shows a low signal structure in the L-4 neuroforamen (*arrow*) which is a lateral disc protrusion. **B.** Axial T1-weighted (upper) (TR, 600; TE, 30) and T2* image (lower) (TR, 600; TE, 30; 30°) show the lateral disc (*arrows*) in the left neuroforamen.

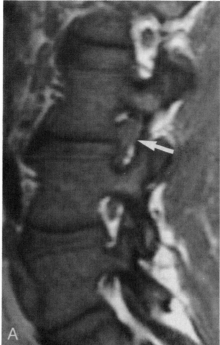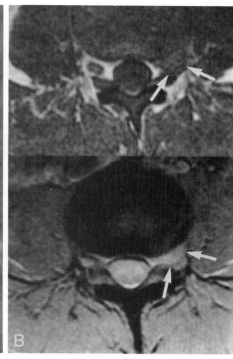

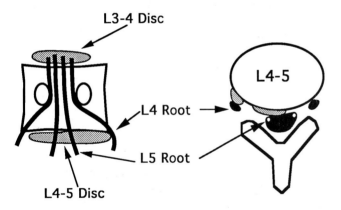

Figure 11.9. Schematic of Lateral Disc. This schematic illustrates how a posterior L4-5 disc protrusion affects the L-5 nerve root, yet a lateral L4-5 disc affects the L-4 root.

extend into the foramen and the sagittal images will appear normal.

SPINAL STENOSIS

By definition *spinal stenosis* is encroachment of the bony or soft tissue structures in the spine on one or more of the neural elements, with resulting symptoms. It is classically divided into congenital and acquired types; however, even the most severe forms of congenital stenosis do not cause symptoms unless a component of acquired stenosis (usually degenerative disease of the facets and the discs) is present. A more useful classification of stenosis is on an anatomic basis: central canal, neuroforaminal, and lateral recess.

It is important to realize that stenosis and disc disease are often present concomitantly, and it can be very difficult to clinically differentiate the two. As with disc disease, it is imperative that any imaging findings be matched with clinical findings. It is not unusual to have a patient with stenosis that appears severe on images, yet has no symptoms.

CENTRAL CANAL STENOSIS

Although at one time measurements were considered very useful in the determination of central canal stenosis, they are no longer felt to be a valid indicator of disease. Instead, simply noting whether the thecal sac is compressed or round will reliably serve to determine central canal stenosis (Fig. 11.10). A subjective assessment as to whether the compression (usually in an anteroposterior direction) is mild, moderate, or severe is all that is necessary for evaluating the central canal.

The most common cause of central canal stenosis is degenerative disease of the facets with bony hypertrophy that encroaches on the central canal (Fig. 11.11). This is also the most common cause of lateral recess stenosis. When the facets undergo degenerative joint disease (DJD) they often have some slippage, which results in buckling of the ligamentum flavum. This has been termed ligamentum flavum hypertrophy, and is a common cause of central canal stenosis (Fig. 11.12). Frequently, mild disc bulging is associated with minimal facet hypertrophy and ligamentum flavum hypertrophy. This combination can result in

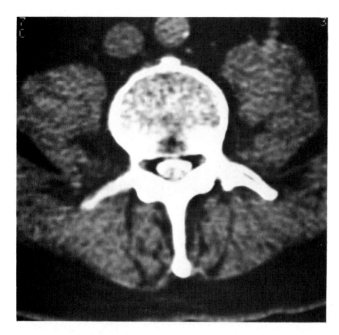

Figure 11.10. Central Canal Stenosis. A CT-myelogram demonstrates absence of the normally round thecal sac due to central canal stenosis. It is not necessary to perform a myelogram to see flattening of the thecal sac, a plain CT or MR will show this equally well.

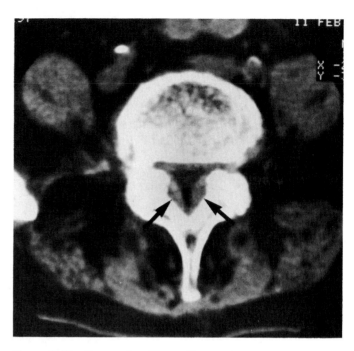

Figure 11.12. Ligamentum Flavum Hypertrophy. Inward bulging of the ligamentum flavum (*arrows*) is shown on this CT scan. Central canal stenosis from ligamentum flavum hypertrophy is common.

NEUROFORAMINAL STENOSIS

Degenerative joint disease of the facet with bony hypertrophy is the most common cause of neuroforaminal stenosis; however, encroachment on the nerve root in the neuroforamen can be seen with free disc fragments, postoperative scar, and from a lateral disc protrusion.

The neuroforamen are best evaluated on axial images, just cephalad to the disc space. The disc space lies at the inferior portion of the neuroforamen, and the exiting nerve root lies in the superior or cephalad portion of the neuroforamen. Although the neuroforamen can be clearly seen on sagittal MR images, care must be taken to evaluate the entire neuroforamen and not just the 4 or 5 mm of one sagittal image.

LATERAL RECESS STENOSIS

The lateral recesses are the bony canals in which the nerve roots lie after they leave the thecal sac and before they enter the neuroforamen. Hypertrophy of the superior articular facet from DJD is the most common cause of encroachment on the lateral recesses, although, as with the neuroforamen, disc fragments and postoperative scar can cause nerve root impingement.

SPONDYLOLYSIS AND SPONDYLOLISTHESIS

Defects in the bony pars interarticularis (spondylolysis) are commonly found in asymptomatic individuals, yet they can be a source of low back pain and

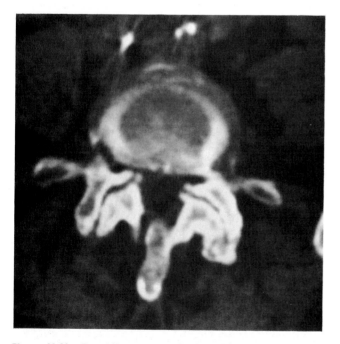

Figure 11.11. Facet Hypertrophy Causing Stenosis. This CT shows marked facet degenerative disease with hypertrophy of the facets causing lateral recess and central canal stenosis.

severe focal central canal stenosis. Both CT and MR will show these bony and soft tissue changes.

Less common causes of central canal stenosis include bony overgrowth from Paget's disease, achondroplasia, posttraumatic changes, and severe spondylolisthesis.

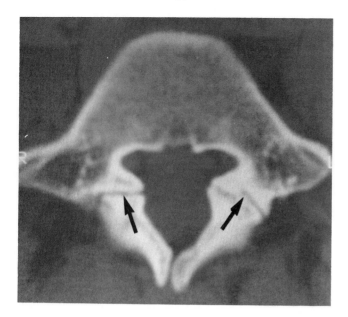

Figure 11.13. Spondylolysis (CT). A CT scan through the midvertebral body reveals a break bilaterally (*arrows*) in the bony lamina, which indicates bilateral spondylolysis.

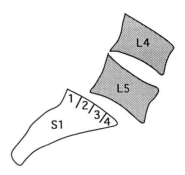

Figure 11.14. Schematic of the Spondylolisthesis Grading Scale. This schematic shows the grading scale used to gauge the degree of spondylolisthesis. This example would be a grade 2 spondylolisthesis since the posterior edge of the slipped L-5 vertebral body lies above the second quadrant of the S-1 vertebral body.

instability. Prior to disc surgery or other back surgery it is imperative that any spondylolysis is identified. Since spondylolysis can mimic back pain from other pathology, it is important that it is preoperatively assessed. If necessary, it can then be surgically addressed at the same time. Failure to note and evaluate spondylolysis is a known source of failed back surgery.

Computed tomography is superior to MR imaging at identifying spondylolysis (10). Although MR will show spondylolysis defects, they can be very difficult to see at times. As previously mentioned, this is the only area in which CT is reported to be clearly superior to MR in evaluating the lumbar spine. Spondylolysis is identified on the axial images through the midvertebral body as a break in the normally intact bony ring of the lamina (Fig. 11.13).

Spondylolisthesis (forward slippage of one vertebral body on a lower one) occurs from either slippage of two vertebral bodies following bilateral spondylolysis or from DJD of the facets with slippage of the facets. Bilateral spondylolysis can result in a large amount of slippage, whereas facet DJD will usually result in only minimal slippage. If spondylolisthesis is severe, it can result in central canal stenosis, neuroforaminal stenosis, or both.

A grading scale that is widely used to describe the degree of spondylolisthesis is the Meyerding grading scale. The more caudal vertebral body is divided into fourths, and the posterior corner of the more cephalad vertebral body is marked at the position where it has slipped forward. If it has slipped forward only into the first quarter of the more caudal vertebral body, it is a grade 1 spondylolisthesis; slippage into the second quarter is a grade 2, and so on (Fig. 11.14).

POSTOPERATIVE CHANGES

Failed back surgery is unfortunately common. It can occur from many causes including inadequate surgery (including missed free disc fragments), postoperative scarring, failure of bone grafting for fusion, and recurrent disc protrusion. Computed tomography is useful in evaluating bone grafts, but is not reliable for differentiating postoperative scar from disc material. However, MR has been shown to be particularly useful in distinguishing scar from disc material (11).

The use of intravenous gadolinium will allow virtual certainty in distinguishing scar tissue from a disc. Scar tissue will enhance following the administration of gadolinium, whereas disc material will have only some minimal peripheral enhancement, presumably due to inflammation (Fig. 11.15).

BONY ABNORMALITIES

Parallel bands of high or low signal adjacent to the vertebral body endplates are often seen in association with degenerative disc disease. The most common appearance is of high-signal bands on T1-weighted images that remain high on T2-weighted images (Fig. 11.16). This represents fatty marrow conversion. It was seen in 16% of cases in the first report in the literature (1) and was termed type 2. Type 1 changes are seen as low-signal bands parallel to the endplates on T1-weighted images that get brighter on T2-weighted images. This represents an inflammmatory or granulomatous response to degenerative disc disease. The type 2 changes were reported in 4% of cases, and must be distinguished from disc space infection. In disc space infection the disc should get bright on the T2-weighted images, whereas it is unusual for a de-

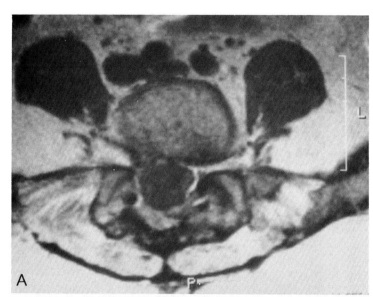

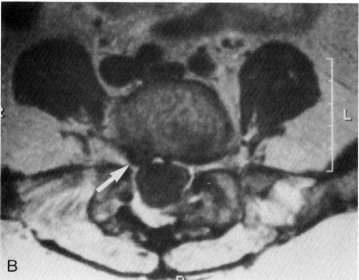

Figure 11.15. Postoperative Scar Enhancement with Gadolinium. A. A T1-weighted axial image (TR, 600; TE, 30) shows soft tissue around the thecal sac in this postoperative patient, which could represent scar, but makes evaluation for recurrent disc protrusion difficult. **B.** A T1-weighted axial image (TR, 600; TE, 30) through the same level following administration of gadolinium-pentetic acid (Gd-DTPA) intravenously shows enhancement of the scar tissue surrounding the thecal sac. In addition, a focal right-sided disc protrusion can be identified (*arrow*).

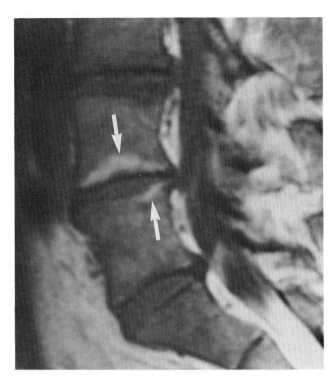

Figure 11.16.   Type 2 Marrow Changes. A sagittal T1-weighted image (TR, 600; TE, 11) in a patient with degenerative disc disease shows bands of fatty marrow parallel to the L4-5 endplates (*arrows*) which are type 2 marrow changes, seen often with degenerative disc disease.

generative disc to have high signal on T2-weighted images. Type 3 changes are parallel bands of low signal adjacent to the endplates on both T1- and T2-weighted images. Type 3 changes represent bony sclerosis seen on plain films.

Magnetic resonance imaging and CT have changed diagnostic imaging of the lumbar spine from a pain-ful, invasive study to a highly accurate, noninvasive study that gives a more complete anatomic depiction than plain films or myelography. Although MR has no ionizing radiation and is widely available, it can be much more expensive than CT and does not currently appear to increase the accuracy of diagnosis for disc disease or spinal stenosis.

References

1. Modic M, Masaryk T, Ross J, Carter J. Imaging of degenerative disk disease. Radiology 1988;168:177–186.
2. Hesselink J. Spine imaging: history, achievements, remaining frontiers. AJR 1988;150:1223–1230.
3. Sartoris DJ, Resnick D. Computed tomography of the spine: an update and review. CRC Crit Rev Diagn Imaging 1987;27:271–296.
4. Tertti M, Salminen J, Paajanen H, Terho P, Kormano M. Low-back pain and disk degeneration in children: a case-control MR imaging study. Radiology 1991;180:503–507.
5. Boden S, Davis D, Dina T, Patronas N, Wiesel S. Abnormal magnetic-resonance scans of the lumbar spine in asymptomatic subjects. J Bone Joint Surg 1990;72A:403–408.
6. Onik G, Mooney V, Maroon J, et. al. Automated percutaneous discectomy: a prospective multi-institutional study. Neurosurgery 1990;26:228–233.
7. Helms CA, Dorwart RH, Gray M. The CT appearance of conjoined nerve roots and differentiation from a herniated nucleus pulposus. Radiology 1982;144:803–807.
8. Masaryk T, Ross J, Modic M, Boumphrey F, Bohlman H, Wilber G. High-resolution MR imaging of sequestered lumbar intervertebral disks. AJR 1988;150:1155–1162.
9. Winter DDB, Munk PL, Helms CA, Holt RG. CT and MR of lateral disc herniation: typical appearance and pitfalls of interpretation. J Canad Assoc Radiol 1989;40:256–259.
10. Grenier N, Kressel HY, Schiebler ML, Grossman RI. Isthmic spondylolysis of the lumbar spine: MR imaging at 1.5 T. Radiology 1989;170:489–494.
11. Ross J, Masaryk T, Schrader M, Gentili A, Bohlman H, Modic M. MR imaging of the postoperative spine: assessment with gadopentetate dimeglumine. AJR 1990;155:867–872.

Section III   Chest

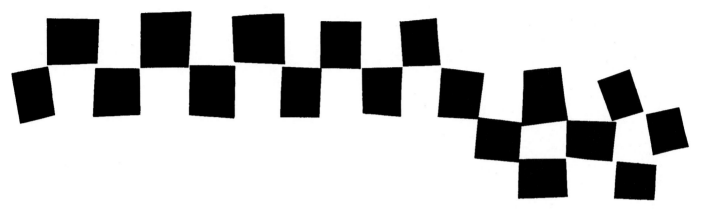

12

Methods of Examination and Normal Anatomy

Jeffrey S. Klein

Imaging Methods

There are many imaging techniques available to the radiologist for the evaluation of thoracic disease. The decision of which imaging procedures to perform depends upon many factors, the most important of which are the availability of various modalities and the type of information sought. While the indications for the utilization of certain modalities such as computed tomography (CT) and ventilation/perfusion lung scanning have been fairly well elucidated, the indications for other imaging techniques such as magnetic resonance imaging (MR) continue to evolve. Although the imaging algorithm for specific problems may seem relatively straightforward, a dogmatic approach to the individual patient should be discouraged. For example, a thin-section CT showing a suspicious solitary pulmonary nodule might be followed directly by a thoracotomy, or rather, in selected patients, by transthoracic needle biopsy. This type of flexible approach will often streamline the diagnostic workup and ultimately lead to better patient care.

Conventional Chest Radiographs. Posteroanterior (PA) and lateral chest radiographs are the mainstay of thoracic imaging. Conventional radiographs should be performed as the initial imaging study in all patients with thoracic disease. These films are obtained in most radiology departments on a dedicated chest unit capable of obtaining radiographs with a focus-to-film distance of 6 feet, a high kilovolt (peak) (i.e., 140 kVp) technique, a grid to reduce scatter, and a phototimer to control the length of exposure.

High kilovolt (peak) films provide adequate penetration of the cardiac and subdiaphragmatic tissues to allow visualization of the retrocardiac and posterior costophrenic regions of the lower lobes, respectively. With this technique, the normal mediastinal pleural reflections (junction lines, azygoesophageal recess), trachea, and main bronchi are visible within the mediastinum. In addition, a high kilovolt (peak) technique requires only a short exposure time, thereby diminishing cardiac and respiratory motion and allowing the cardiac margins, diaphragms, intrapulmonary vessels, and parenchymal opacities to appear sharp.

Both PA and lateral radiographs should be performed with the patient suspending respiration at total lung capacity. On the frontal radiograph, the chin should be raised off the anterior chest, and the scapulae rotated laterally to provide an unobscured view of the lungs. The anterior chest is placed squarely against the film cassette receiver to avoid kyphotic or lordotic projections.

The recognition of proper radiographic technique on frontal radiographs involves assessment of four basic features: penetration, rotation, inspiration, and motion. Proper penetration is present when there is faint visualization of the intervertebral disc spaces of the thoracic spine, and discrete branching vessels can be identified through the cardiac shadow. Rotation is assessed by noting the relationship between a vertical line drawn midway between the medial cortical margins of the clavicular heads and one drawn vertically through the spinous processes of the thoracic vertebrae. Superimposition of these lines (the former in the midline anteriorly and the latter in the midline posteriorly) indicates a properly positioned, nonrotated patient. An appropriate deep inspiration in a normal individual is present when the apex of the right hemidiaphragm is visible below the 10th posterior rib. Finally, the cardiac margin, diaphragm, and

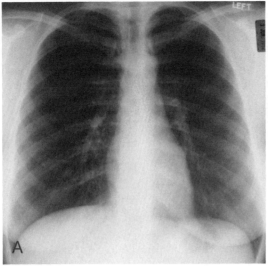

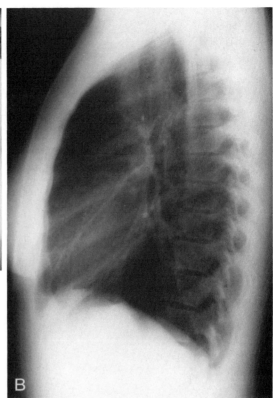

Figure 12.1.   Normal PA (A) and Left Lateral (B) Radiographs of the Chest.

pulmonary vessels should be sharply marginated in a completely still patient who has suspended respiration during the radiographic exposure (Fig. 12.1).

Portable Radiography. Portable frontal anteroposterior (AP) radiographs are obtained when patient transport to the radiology department and standing for PA radiographs is not feasible. This usually occurs in the critical care setting or the emergency department. Portable radiographs help monitor a patient's cardiopulmonary status, assess the position of various monitoring and life support tubes, lines, and catheters, and detect complications related to the use of these devices.

There are technical and patient-related limitations of kilovolt (peak) of portable bedside radiography. The limited maximal kVp of portable units requires longer exposures to obtain adequate radiographic penetration of cardiomediastinal structures, resulting in greater motion artifact, especially in ventilated patients and patients unable to hold their breaths. The short focus-to-film distance (typically 40 inches) and AP technique result in magnification of intrathoracic structures. This increases the apparent cardiac diameter by 15–20%; the upper limit of normal for the cardiothoracic ratio on AP radiographs is 57%. The supine position of critically ill patients makes it more difficult for the patient to inspire deeply, resulting in smaller lung volumes and compression of the lower lobes. The recognition of mild pulmonary venous hypertension is difficult in the supine patient because of the normal increase in pulmonary blood flow and the absence of gravitational effects that produce an even distribution of pulmonary blood flow from lung apex to base. The increase in systemic venous return to the heart produces a widening of the upper mediastinum or "vascular pedicle." The detection of small or moderate-sized pleural effusions may be difficult because of their posterior location in a supine patient. Similarly, a pneumothorax may be difficult to detect since free intrapleural air rises to a nondependent position, producing a subtle anteromedial or inferior radiolucency.

A device called the inclinometer has been developed that accurately records the position of the bedridden patient from Trendelenburg's to completely upright. This device, which clips onto the portable film cassette, allows the radiologist to precisely calculate the patient's position at the time of the radiograph, which helps assess the distribution of pulmonary blood flow and pleural effusions. As critically ill patients are difficult to position for portable radiographs, the patient is often rotated. Inaccuracies in directing the x-ray beam perpendicular to the patient lead to excessively kyphotic or lordotic radiographs. Lordosis foreshortens the height of the lung, increases cardiac magnification, and may cause obscuration of the left hemidiaphragm.

Lateral Decubitus Radiographs. Radiographs of the chest obtained with a horizontal x-ray beam while the patient lies in the decubitus position can demonstrate free-flowing pleural effusions (Fig. 12.2).

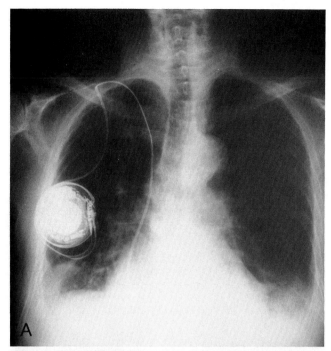

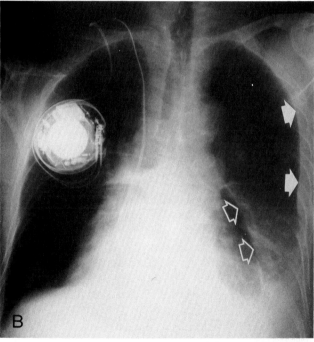

Figure 12.2. Lateral Decubitus Film for Diagnosis of Pleural Effusion. An upright radiograph (**A**) in a patient recovering from pulmonary edema shows blunting of both lateral costophrenic sulci. A left lateral decubitus film (**B**) demonstrates a free-flowing effusion laterally (*solid arrows*) and within the lateral aspect of an incomplete left major fissure (*open arrows*).

As little as 50 ml of fluid can be demonstrated by this technique. Decubitus films can be used to visualize the nondependent lung when a pleural effusion obscures the lower lobe. Similarly, a small pneumothorax can be seen on decubitus films in the nondependent lung when an upright film cannot be obtained.

Air trapping can be demonstrated in the dependent lung in patients with a check valve bronchial obstruction who are unable to cooperate for inspiratory/expiratory radiographs or fluoroscopy.

Expiratory Radiographs. Films obtained after maximal expiration to residual volume may be performed to detect focal or diffuse air trapping or to aid in the detection of a small pneumothorax. The increased sensitivity of expiratory films for pneumothorax is due to the increased density and decreased volume of the lung after exhalation. This creates a greater difference in radiographic density between air in the pleural space and the lung. The lung will also be displaced away from the chest wall, thereby aiding in recognition of the visceral pleural reflection.

Apical Lordotic Radiographs. Are usually performed to improve visualization of the lung apices, which are obscured on routine PA radiographs by the clavicles and first costochondral junctions. The lordotic film projects these anterior bony structures superiorly, providing an unimpeded view of the apices. This projection is also used occasionally to enhance the visualization of middle lobe atelectasis by placing the inferiorly displaced minor fissure in tangent with the x-ray beam, and by increasing the AP thickness of the atelectatic middle lobe.

Shallow Oblique Radiographs. Obtained by rotating the patient 5% in each direction from the PA projection, help localize focal opacities seen on frontal radiographs. This technique is useful for distinguishing a skeletal lesion (i.e., a bone island or healing rib fracture), nipple, or skin lesion from an intrapulmonary nodule.

Chest Fluoroscopy. Real-time visualization of the chest may be useful in several situations. In the evaluation of a nodular opacity seen on a frontal radiograph, the fluoroscopic observation of movement of the density with the chest wall, with spot films in oblique projections demonstrating the chest wall origin of the opacity, can obviate the need for CT. In a patient with an elevated diaphragm on a frontal radiograph, diaphragmatic movement can be assessed fluoroscopically to detect paralysis.

Digital Chest Radiography has followed from the digital techniques developed for ultrasound, CT and MR. There are several ways to produce a digital chest radiograph, from the digitization of an analog conventional chest film to direct analog-to-digital conversion of transmitted radiation. The main advantages of digital chest radiography are superior contrast resolution and the ability to transmit and view radiographs on a monitor where contrast levels and windows can be manipulated to enhance visualization of various regions in the chest. This latter feature helps compensate for the technical limitations of portable chest radiographs, where digital radiography has

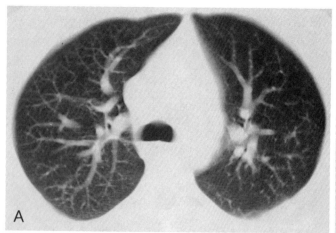
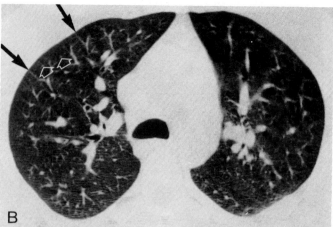

Figure 12.3.   Conventional versus High-Resolution CT of the lung. Ten-millimeter (**A**) and 1.5-mm (high-resolution)(**B**) scans obtained at the same level using a bone reconstruction algorithm and photographed at identical window level and width. Note that with 10-mm collimation (**A**), the vessel are seen along their course as continous branching structures from the hila peripherally. On HRCT at the same level (**B**), only a short portion of the vessels are seen, but the interfaces of the lung with bronchi, vessels, and pleura are sharper. In addition, the peripheral portion of the lung is seen in greater detail, with normal interlobular septa (*solid black arrows*) and centrilobular arteries (*open white arrows*) clearly visible.

had the greatest impact. In addition, dual-energy subtraction techniques allow for the detection of calcium within solitary pulmonary nodules. Disadvantages of this technique include limited spatial resolution and the high cost of most digital units.

Conventional Tomography in the evaluation of chest disease is now of historical interest only. Computed tomography has replaced conventional linear tomography for all situations in which chest tomography is indicated.

Computed Tomography and High-Resolution CT (HRCT).   Computed tomography has revolutionized the field of thoracic imaging. Routine chest CT is performed from the lung apices through the bases using contiguous 10-mm thick sections and a 2- or 3-second scan time. Each image is obtained during breath-holding at or near total lung capacity. More finely collimated scans (3–5 mm) are often used for evaluation of the hila, mediastinum, and central bronchi. The field of view for image reconstruction is determined by measuring the widest transverse diameter of the thorax as seen on the CT scout view. An edge-enhancing reconstruction computer algorithm that improves the resolution of parenchymal structures is used for both conventional and HRCT scans of the thorax (Fig. 12.3). Iodinated contrast agents administered intravenously are used to evaluate mediastinal vascular disease, to distinguish hilar lymph nodes from pulmonary vessels, to distinguish a central hilar mass from atelectatic lung, or to distinguish a peripheral parenchymal abnormality from pleural disease. Scans are recorded onto 14 x 17 film using a 12 on 1 format. Each image is photographed at a window width (WW) and window level (WL) that optimizes visualization of the mediastinum (WW = 400, WL = 40) or lung (WW = 1500, WL = −600).

The HRCT technique involves thinly collimated scans (1.0–2.0 mm) obtained through a nodule for performing densitometry or at spaced intervals through the thorax in the evaluation of parenchymal lung disease and bronchiectasis. As with all chest CT images, a high spatial frequency or edge-enhancing reconstruction algorithm is used. Because thin collimation reduces the quantity of transmitted photons, exposure factors (kilovolt [peak], milliamperes [mA]) are greater than with conventional scans to offset increased image noise due to quantum mottle. Scan time is limited to 2 seconds to minimize the effects of respiratory and cardiac motion.

The major advantages of CT are superior contrast resolution and the cross-sectional display. Superior contrast resolution allows for the detection of calcification within solitary pulmonary nodules and the depiction of mediastinal masses or lymph nodes within mediastinal fat. Intravenous contrast enhancement is an additional method of improving contrast resolution and identifying vascular structures. The cross-sectional display eliminates the superimposition of structures and allows visualization of parenchymal nodules as small as 3 mm. In addition, hilar or parenchymal masses seen only on a single view by conventional radiography are easily identified. Despite the many advantages of CT over conventional radiography, it should be remembered that the spatial resolution of CT is less than that of conventional radiography.

The clinical indications for thoracic CT will vary among institutions. A brief list of indications for conventional CT is shown in Table 12.1.

Table 12.1. Indications for Thoracic CT

Indication	Example
Evaluation of an abnormality identified on conventional radiographs	Densitometry of a solitary pulmonary nodule
	Localization and characterization of a hilar or mediastinal mass
Staging of lung cancer	Assess the extent of the primary tumor, and the relationship of the tumor to the pleura, chest wall, airways, and mediastinum
	Detect hilar and mediastinal lymph node enlargement
Detection of occult pulmonary metastases	Extrathoracic malignancies with a propensity to metastasize to the lung (osteogenic sarcoma, breast and renal cell carcinoma) or mediastinal lymph nodes (lymphoma); CT is the most sensitive imaging technique to detect subradiographic nodules or lymph node enlargement
Distinction of empyema from lung abscess	Contrast-enhanced CT can usually distinguish a peripheral lung abscess from loculated empyema

Magnetic Resonance Imaging involves the detection of emitted radio signal from tissues excited by radio frequency pulses. A discussion of the basic physics of MR may be found in Chapter 1. Routine thoracic MR involves spin echo, T1- and T2-weighted imaging sequences in the axial plane; coronal and sagittal planes are used in selected cases. Electrocardiographic gating should be used routinely for all thoracic MR studies to improve image quality. Respiratory gating is not performed, as this would significantly increase the time required for image acquisition. A technique termed reordering of phase encoding (ROPE) can reduce respiratory motion artifacts without prolonging image acquisition times by coordinating image acquisition with chest wall motion. Contrast-enhanced MR with intravenous injection of paramagnetic agents is not routinely performed.

The major advantages of MR are the superior contrast resolution between tumor and fat, the ability to characterize tissues based on T1 and T2 relaxation times, the ability to scan in direct sagittal and coronal planes, and the lack of need for intravenous iodinated contrast. The signal void produced by flowing blood in vascular structures helps identify the mediastinal and hilar vessels, detect vascular invasion by tumor, detect intraluminal tumor or thrombus, and distinguish vascular structures from nodes or masses without the need for intravenous contrast. In addition, the ability to obtain images along the long axis of the aorta and the advent of cine MR techniques have made MR the primary modality for the imaging of most congenital and acquired thoracic vascular disorders (Fig. 12.4).

Direct coronal scans are of benefit in imaging regions that lie within the axial plane and are therefore difficult to depict by CT. For this reason, superior sulcus tumors, subcarinal and aortopulmonary window lesions, and certain hilar masses are better depicted by MR than CT(2). Magnetic resonance imaging is superior to CT in the diagnosis of chest wall or mediastinal invasion because of the high contrast between tumor and chest wall fat and musculature, and tumor

Table 12.2. Indications for MR of the Thorax

Evaluation of thoracic aortic aneurysm
Evaluation of aortic dissection in stable patients
Assessment of superior sulcus tumors
Determination of vascular invasion by lung cancer
Evaluation of mediastinal and chest wall invasion of lung cancer
Staging of lung cancer patients unable to receive intravenous iodinated contrast
Evaluation of posterior mediastinal masses

and mediastinal fat, respectively. The characterization of tissues by their T1 and T2 relaxation times allows for the diagnosis of fluid-filled cysts, hemorrhage, and hematoma formation. The ability to distinguish tumor from fibrosis, based on their T1 and T2 relaxation times, has proven particularly useful in the follow-up of patients irradiated for Hodgkin's disease. Magnetic resonance imaging is currently unable to distinguish benign from malignant masses or lymph nodes.

The major disadvantages of thoracic MR are the limited spatial resolution, the inability to detect calcium, and the difficulties in imaging the pulmonary parenchyma. Magnetic resonance imaging is also more time-consuming and expensive than CT. These factors, along with the ability of CT to provide superior or equivalent information in most situations, have limited the use of thoracic MR for most noncardiovascular thoracic disorders. The primary indications for thoracic MR are listed in Table 12.2.

Ultrasound is now commonly used for the detection, characterization, and sampling of pleural, peripheral parenchymal, and mediastinal processes. The aspiration of small pleural effusions visualized on real-time ultrasound is preferable to blind thoracentesis. Similarly, sampling of visible pleural masses in patients with malignant effusions can diminish the number of negative pleural biopsies. The aspiration of pleural-based masses and abscesses can be safely performed by ultrasound-guided needle placement into the lesion through the point of contact between the mass and pleura. Large anterior medistinal masses

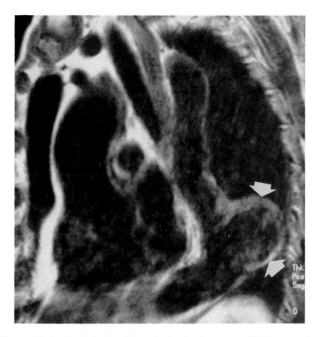

Figure 12.4. An MR of a Thoracic Aortic Aneurysm. Oblique sagittal MR (TR = 550, TE = 22) of a 63-year-old man with a left lower mediastinal mass demonstrates the flow void within a saccular aneurysm (*white arrows*) of the left posterolateral wall of the descending thoracic aorta.

that have a broad area of contact with the parasternal chest wall undergo biopsy without transgressing the lung.

Real-time ultrasound may be preferable to fluoroscopy in confirming phrenic nerve paralysis because of its lack of ionizing radiation, portability, and the ability to detect subpulmonic and subphrenic fluid collections that may cause diaphragmatic elevation.

Radionuclide Examination utilized in the evaluation of noncardiac thoracic disease are ventilation/perfusion lung scintigraphy and gallium scanning. Ventilation/perfusion scanning is used almost exclusively for the diagnosis of pulmonary embolism. Gallium-67 scanning of the chest is used in the detection of pulmonary infection (e.g., *Pneumocystis carinii* pneumonia in a patient with a normal radiograph) or inflammation (e.g., disease activity in idiopathic pulmonary fibrosis), and in the evaluation of suspected sarcoidosis.

Tracheography/Bronchography. Contrast tracheography, performed by anesthetizing the oropharynx, larynx, and upper trachea, instilling a sterile barium suspension, and obtaining spot radiographs during fluoroscopy, may be performed for the evaluation of tracheal pathology. Although CT is used to evaluate most tracheal disorders, contrast tracheography is occasionally performed for the preoperative measurement of segmental tracheal stenosis. Bronchography, the gold standard for detecting bronchiectasis and determining its extent, has been supplanted

by HRCT for this purpose. The only indication for bronchography is in the patient with presumed focal bronchiectasis on CT who is to undergo potentially curative resection, as the bronchographic detection of multifocal disease avoids unnecessary surgery.

Pulmonary Arteriography involves catheterization of the right heart via puncture of upper or lower extremity veins and fluoroscopically guided selective placement of a pigtail-tip catheter into the pulmonary arteries, followed by contrast injection and rapid filming. The main indication for pulmonary arteriography is the evaluation of suspected pulmonary embolism, particularly when ventilation/perfusion lung scanning is unable to provide a confident diagnosis. Additional indications include the evaluation of congenital pulmonary vascular disease, particularly pulmonary arteriovenous malformations, and, rarely, the detection of a pulmonary artery pseudoaneurysm in the patient with massive hemoptysis. Digital subtraction pulmonary angiography provides several advantages over conventional angiography. Improved contrast resolution allows for a decrease in the amount of contrast necessary to opacify pulmonary vessels. With the improved contrast resolution, contrast injection into the vena cava or right atrium can provide adequate opacification of the pulmonary vessels, thereby avoiding catheterization of the right heart and direct intrapulmonary arterial injection of contrast. Despite these advantages, the small field of view and limited spatial resolution outweigh the benefits, and this technique is not widely used in the evaluation of pulmonary arterial disease.

Thoracic Aortography involves the placement of a multihole catheter into the aorta via the femoral, axillary, or brachial artery followed by power injection of contrast and rapid filming. Many conditions previously evaluated with thoracic aortography, particularly congenital aortic anomalies and aortic dissection, are better evaluated presently with CT, MR, or ultrasound. However, there are several indications for this procedure. The most common indication is the detection of thoracic aortic or arch vessel injury following blunt chest trauma. Additional indications include the evaluation of selected patients for aortic dissection or aneurysm and the diagnosis of aortitis.

Bronchial Arteriography via a transfemoral arterial route with transcatheter arterial embolization is performed for the evaluation and treatment of massive or recurrent hemoptysis, most commonly from bronchiectasis or mycetomas.

Transthoracic Needle Biopsy guided by fluoroscopy, CT, or ultrasound is a diagnostic technique utilized in selected patients with pulmonary lesions or mediastinal masses.

Percutaneous Catheter Drainage of intrathoracic air or fluid collections, performed by imaging-guided placement of small-bore multihole catheters, is used for the treatment of pneumothorax, empyema, malignant pleural effusion, and other intrathoracic fluid collections (3).

Normal Lung Anatomy

Tracheobronchial Tree. The trachea is a cylindrical tube that extends vertically from the larynx to the main bronchi (Fig. 12.5A). It contains a series of U- or C-shaped cartilaginous rings that number two per centimeter. The rings are completed posteriorly by a flat band of muscle and connective tissue called the posterior tracheal membrane. The tracheal mucosa consists of a pseudostratified, ciliated columnar epithelium that contains scattered neuroendocrine cells. The submucosa contains cartilage, smooth muscle, and seromucous glands. The cervical trachea is a midline structure, while the intrathoracic trachea courses slightly to the right and posteriorly as it descends toward the carina. The left lateral wall of the distal trachea is indented by the transverse portion of the aortic arch. (4)

The trachea is approximately 12 cm long in adults, with an upper limit of normal coronal tracheal diameter of 25 mm in men and 21 mm in women. The trachea is a round or oval structure in cross-section, with a coronal-to-sagittal diameter ratio of 0.6:1.0. A ratio of <0.6 (coronal narrowing to sagittal widening) is seen with the saber sheath trachea.

On chest radiographs, the trachea casts a vertical lucency extending from the cricoid cartilage superiorly to the main bronchi inferiorly (Fig 12.1). The right lateral wall is marginated by the right paratracheal stripe. The paratracheal stripe is composed of the tracheal wall, a small amount of mediastinal fat, paratracheal lymph nodes, and the visceral and parietal pleural layers of the right upper lobe and any intervening pleural fluid. This stripe should be uniformly smooth and should not exceed 4 mm in width; thickening or nodularity reflects disease in any of the component tissues. The left lateral wall is surrounded by mediastinal vessels and fat and is not normally visible radiographically. The posterior tracheal stripe represents the thickness of the posterior tracheal wall and adjacent fat, and measures less than 3 mm in width. The presence of air in the esophagus produces the tracheoesophageal stripe, which represents the combined thickness of the tracheal and esophageal walls and intervening fat. This stripe should measure less than 5 mm; thickening is most commonly seen with esophageal carcinoma.

The bronchial system exhibits a branching pattern of asymmetric dichotomy, with the daughter bronchi of a parent bronchus varying in diameter, length, and the number of divisions. The main bronchi arise from the trachea at the carina, with the right bronchus

forming a more obtuse angle with the long axis of the trachea. The bronchi are composed of tissues that are similar to the trachea. The average width of the main bronchi (from tracheal carina to right upper lobe bronchus) is 15 mm on the right and 13 mm on the left. The right main bronchus is considerably shorter than the left (2.2 cm versus 5 cm, mean length). The main bronchi are readily visible on well-penetrated frontal radiographs; the intermediate bronchus is readily visible on lateral films. The lobar bronchi, which lie partly within the mediastinum and partly in the lung, are visible on frontal chest radiographs as tubular lucencies silhouetted by central pulmonary vessels, or as circular lucencies when seen end on surrounded by vessels on lateral radiographs. There are three right-sided (upper, middle, lower) and two left-sided (upper, lower) lobar bronchi (Fig. 12.5a). There are 10 segmental bronchi on the right (3 right upper, 2 right middle, and 5 right lower) and 8 on the left (4 left upper and 4 left lower). Those segmental bronchi that course horizontally (anterior segmental upper lobe, superior segmental lower lobe) may be seen as small circular lucencies within the pulmonary parenchyma when viewed end on. The tracheal and main, lobar, and segmental bronchial anatomy as seen on CT scans is shown in Figure 12.5B.

Lobar and Segmental Anatomy. The right lung is divided by invaginations of the visceral pleura (interlobar fissures) into three lobes (Fig. 12.6). The *right upper lobe* is marginated by the mediastinal pleura medially, costal pleura superiorly and laterally, the upper half of the major (interlobar) fissure posteriorly, and the minor (horizontal) fissure inferiorly. The right upper lobe is supplied by the right upper lobe bronchus and truncus anterior branch of the right pulmonary artery. In approximately 80% of individuals, the right upper lobe receives an accessory branch from the proximal interlobar pulmonary artery. The right upper lobe is further subdivided into three segments: anterior, apical, and posterior, each supplied by segmental branches of the right upper lobe bronchus and artery which run in unison. These segments are not marginated by pleura or connective tissue layers, and so their division is not easily recognizable. The *middle lobe* is a triangularly shaped structure marginated by mediastinal pleura medially, costal pleura laterally, the minor fissure superiorly, and the lower half of the major fissure posteroinferiorly. The middle lobe bronchus, which arises from the intermediate bronchus, and the middle lobe branch of the right interlobar pulmonary artery supply this lobe. The *right lower lobe* is marginated by costal pleura laterally and posteriorly, mediastinal pleura medially, diaphragmatic pleura inferiorly, and the lower half the major fissure anterosuperiorly. This lobe is supplied by the right lower lobe bronchus and pulmonary artery. It is subdivided into five seg-

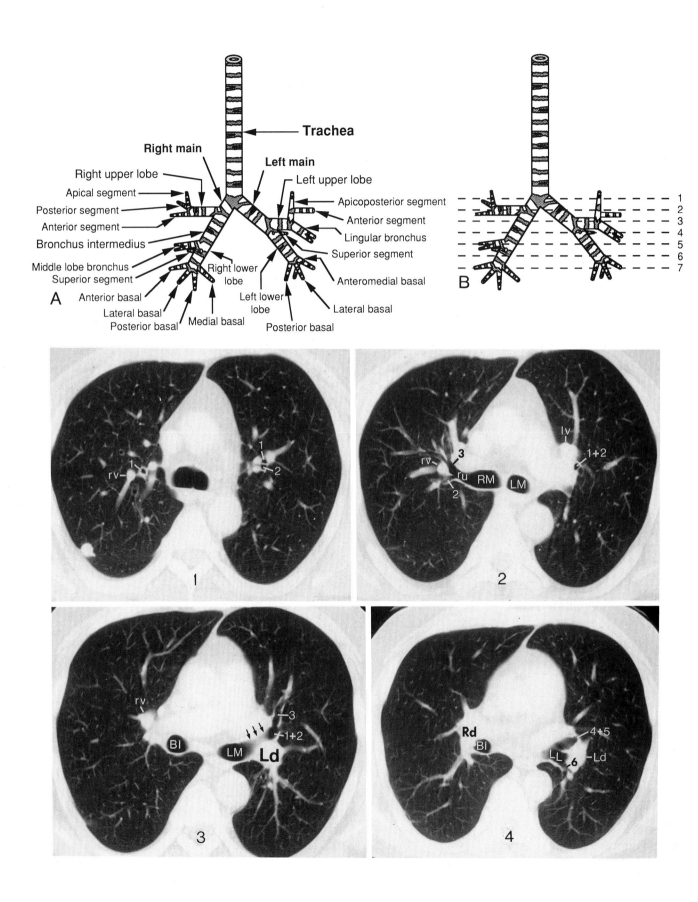

Trachea

Right main

Left main

Right upper lobe

Apical segment

Posterior segment

Anterior segment

Bronchus intermedius

Middle lobe bronchus

Superior segment

A

Anterior basal

Lateral basal

Posterior basal   Medial basal

Right lower lobe

Left upper lobe

Apicoposterior segment

Anterior segment

Lingular bronchus

Superior segment

Anteromedial basal

Lateral basal

Left lower lobe

Posterior basal

B   1 2 3 4 5 6 7

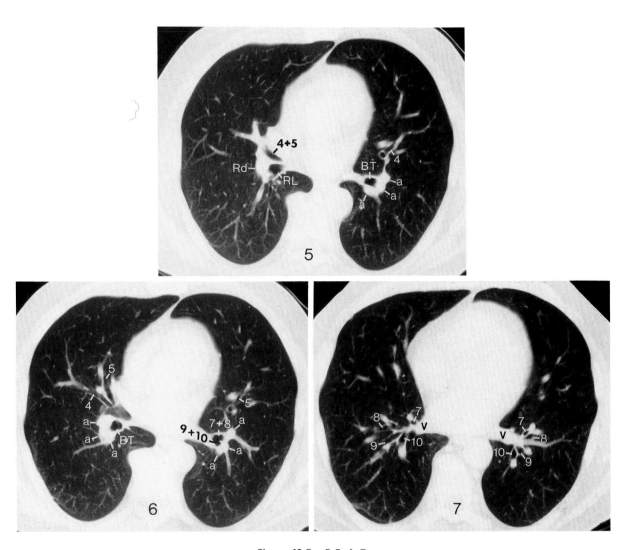

Figure 12.5. B 5, 6, 7.

Figure 12.5. Tracheobronchial and Hilar Anatomy. (A) Diagram of trachea and bronchi. **(B)** Diagram showing bronchial and hilar anatomy as depicted by CT. *1. Level of tracheal carina.* Right apical bronchus *(1)*, right superior posterior pulmonary vein *(rv)*; left apicoposterior bronchus *(1 and 2, on left)*. *2. Level of right upper lobe bronchus.* Right main bronchus *(RM)*, right upper lobe bronchus *(ru)*, right upper lobe anterior *(3)* and posterior *(2)* segmental bronchi, right superior pulmonary vein *(rv)*; left main bronchus *(LM)*, left apicoposterior segmental bronchus *(1 + 2)*, left superior pulmonary vein *(lv)*. *3. Level of left upper lobe bronchus, superior division.* Bronchus intermedius *(BI)*, right superior pulmonary vein *(rv)*; left main bronchus *(LM)*, superior division of left upper lobe bronchus *(small arrows)*, left upper lobe anterior *(3)*, and apicoposterior *(1 + 2)* segmental bronchi, left descending pulmonary artery *(Ld)*. *4. Level of left upper lobe bronchus, inferior (lingular) division.* Bronchus intermedius *(BI)*, right descending pulmonary artery *(Rd)*; lingular bronchus *(4 + 5)*; left lower lobe bronchus *(LL)*, left lower lobe superior segmen-

tal bronchus *(6)*, left descending pulmonary artery *(Ld)*. *5. Level of middle lobe bronchus.* Middle lobe bronchus *(4 + 5)*, right lower lobe bronchus *(RL)*, right descending pulmonary artery *(Rd)*; lingular superior segmental bronchus *(4)*, left lower lobe basal trunk *(BT)*, left lower lobe segmental arteries *(a)*. *6. Level of lower lobe basal trunks.* Lateral *(4)* and medial *(5)* segmental bronchi of the middle lobe, right lower lobe basal trunk *(BT)*, right lower lobe basal segmental arteries *(a, on right)*; lingular segmental bronchus *(5)*, left lower lobe anteromedial segmental bronchus *(7 + 8)*, left lower lobe lateral and basal posterior segmental bronchi *(9 + 10)*, left lower lobe basal segmental arteries *(a, on left)*. *7. Level of basal segmental bronchi.* Right lower lobe medial *(7, on right)*, anterior *(8, on right)*, lateral *(9, on right)*, and posterior *(10, on right)* basal segmental bronchi, right inferior pulmonary vein *(v, on right)*; left lower lobe medial *(7, on left)*, anterior *(8, on left)* lateral *(9, on left)* and posterior *(10, on left* segmental bronchi, left inferior pulmonary vein *(v, on left)*.

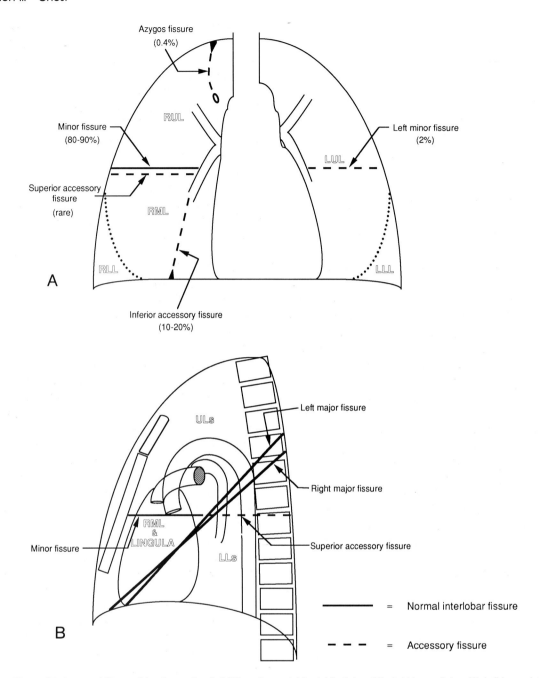

Figure 12.6. Normal Lobar and Fissural Anatomy: frontal (A) and lateral (B) views. *RUL,* right upper lobe; *LUL,* left upper lobe; *RML,* right middle lobe; *RLL,* right lower lobe; *LLL,* left lower lobe; *ULs,* upper lobes; *LLs,* lower lobes.

ments: superior (apical), anterior basal, lateral basal, posterior basal, and medial basal. Each of these segments has bronchoarterial supply from branches of the lower lobe bronchus and artery.

The left lung is divided into upper and lower lobes by the left major fissure. The *left upper lobe* is analogous to the combined right upper and middle lobes. The left upper lobe is marginated medially by mediastinal pleura, anteriorly and laterally by costal pleura, and inferoposteriorly by the entire major fissure. The left upper lobe is subdivided into four segments: the anterior and apicoposterior segments, and the supe-

rior and inferior lingular segments. Each of these segments is supplied by branches of the left upper lobe bronchus. Arterial supply to the anterior and apicoposterior segments parallels the bronchi, and is via branches of the upper division of the left main pulmonary artery. The superior and inferior lingular arteries are proximal branches of the left interlobar pulmonary artery, analogous to the middle lobe pulmonary artery. The *left lower lobe* is analogous to the right lower lobe, marginated by costal pleura laterally and posteriorly, mediastinal pleura medially, diaphragmatic pleura inferiorly, and the major fissure anter-

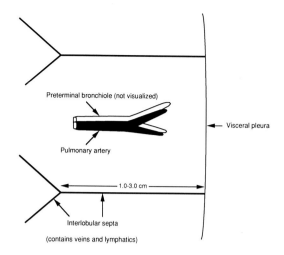

Preterminal bronchiole (not visualized)

Pulmonary artery

← Visceral pleura

1.0-3.0 cm

Interlobular septa

(contains veins and lymphatics)

Figure 12.7. Normal lobular anatomy as seen on HRCT.

osuperiorly. The left lower lobe is subdivided into four segments: the superior (apical) and the three basal segments—anteromedial, lateral, and posterior. Each basal segment receives bronchoarterial supply from the left lower lobe bronchus and artery.

Respiratory Portion of Lung. Distal to the terminal bronchioles, the bronchi lose their cartilage and become respiratory bronchioles. The respiratory bronchioles contain a few alveoli along their walls. They give rise to the gas-exchanging units of the lung: the alveolar ducts, alveolar sacs, and alveoli. The pulmonary alveolus is lined by two types of epithelial cells (pneumocytes). Type I pneumocytes are flattened squamous cells covering 95% of the alveolar surface area and are invisible by light microscopy. These cells are incapable of mitosis or repair. Type II pneumocytes are cuboidal cells that are visible under light microscopy and are capable of mitosis. Type II pneumocytes are the source of new type I pneumocytes, and provide a mechanism for repair following alveolar damage. These cells are also thought to be the source of alveolar surfactant, a phospholipid that lowers the surface tension of alveolar walls and prevents alveolar collapse at low lung volumes.

Pulmonary Subsegmental Anatomy. The secondary pulmonary lobule and the acinus, which comprise the functional gas-exchanging portion of the lung, are the basic units of lung structure. These structures are visible in life only on HRCT of the lung. The secondary pulmonary lobule is defined as that subsegment of lung supplied by three to five terminal bronchioles, which is separated from adjacent secondary lobules by intervening connective tissue (interlobular) septa. The lung subtended from a terminal bronchiole is termed a pulmonary acinus, and is composed of a series of respiratory bronchioles, alveolar ducts, sacs, and alveoli. Therefore, the secondary lobule is comprised of three to five pulmonary acini that are marginated by interlobular septa.

The typical secondary lobule is polyhedral in shape, with each side ranging from 1.0–2.5 cm in length (Fig. 12.7). The interlobular septa separating secondary lobules contain the pulmonary veins and lymphatic vessels. The interlobular septa are most prominent over the peripheral surface of the lung, and are readily visible on HRCT (Fig. 12.3B). At the surface of the lung, these septa are short, horizontal structures that are perpendicular to the pleural surface and completely separate adjacent lobules, whereas the more central interlobular septa incompletely marginate lobules and tend to be longer and obliquely oriented. The center or core of the secondary lobule comprises a pulmonary arteriole and an accompanying preterminal bronchiole, enveloped by the axial connective tissue of the lung. (5)

Fissures. The interlobar pulmonary fissures represent invaginations of visceral pleura deep into the substance of the lung (Fig. 12.6). These fissures may completely or incompletely separate the lobes from one another. An incomplete fissure has important consequences regarding interlobar spread of parenchymal consolidation, collateral air drift in patients with lobar bronchial obstruction, and the appearance of pleural effusion in the supine patient.

In the majority of individuals, there are two interlobar fissures on the right and one on the left. The right major fissure extends obliquely and courses posterosuperiorly from the level of the fifth thoracic vertebra to the anterior inferior portion of the right hemidiaphragm. The right major fissure is not a flat structure, nor does it face directly anteriorly. The upper half of the right major fissure has a concave anterior surface and faces slightly laterally. The lower half of the fissure similarly faces slightly laterally, but has a convex anterior surface. The right major fissure separates the right upper and middle lobes anteriorly from the right lower lobe posteriorly. The superior portion of the right major fissure, which separates the right upper from lower lobe, is incomplete in 70% of individuals, while the lower portion of the major fissure separating the middle from the lower lobe is incomplete in 50%. The minor fissure begins at the midportion of the major fissure and courses in a horizontal plane toward the anterior chest wall. As with the major fissure, the minor fissure is not flat but is usually a domed structure that is convex superiorly. The minor fissure, which separates the upper from the middle lobe, is incomplete in approximately 80% of individuals.

There is a single interlobar fissure on the left that separates the upper from the lower lobe. The left major fissure begins posterosuperiorly at the level of the fifth thoracic vertebra and extends anteroinferiorly to the anterior surface of the left hemidiaphragm. As on the right, the fissure is neither flat nor does it face directly anteriorly. The upper half of the left major fissure is a mirror image of the right, with a concave an-

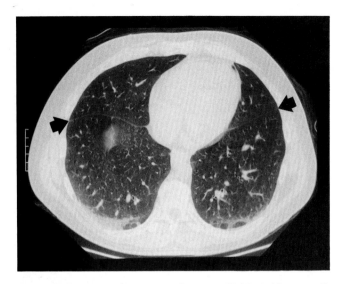

Figure 12.8. Major Fissures as Seen on HRCT. A 1.5-mm collimated scan through the lower thorax shows the major fissures as thin curvilinear lines (*arrows*) that are convex anteriorly.

terior surface that faces slightly laterally. The lower half of the fissure has a convex anterior surface, but in distinction to the lower half of the right major fissure, it faces slightly medially, giving the left major fissure the appearance of a propellor.

The major and minor fissures are best visualized on lateral radiographs. Variable portions of the major fissures are seen as obliquely oriented, thin, white lines coursing anteroinferiorly from back to front. The left major fissure usually begins more superiorly and has a slightly more vertical course than the right major fissure. Occasionally, the fissure is recognized as a sharp edge as it marginates a homogeneous air space filling process. At their points of intersection with the diaphragm, the inferior aspects of the major fissures often have a triangular configuration, with the apex of the triangle pointing toward the fissure. This appearance is due to the presence of a small amount of fat within the inferior aspect of the fissure. On frontal radiographs, the major fissures are not normally visualized because of their oblique orientation relative to the x-ray beam. Occasionally, the superolateral aspects of the major fissures are seen as curvilinear edges in the upper thorax with a ground glass opacity superolaterally and a lucency inferomedially. This appearance is caused by the intrusion of fat into the superolateral portion of the fissure. Rarely, the superolateral portion of the major fissure may be seen as a thin curvilinear line projecting superomedial to the hilar shadows. This latter appearance occurs when the upper portion of the major fissure is brought in tangent to the x-ray beam due to lordotic positioning or from lower lobe atelectasis.

The minor fissure projects at the level of the right fourth rib and is seen as a thin undulating line on frontal radiographs in approximately 50% of individuals. On lateral radiographs, the minor fissure is often seen as a thin curvilinear line with a convex superior margin extending anteriorly from the right major fissure. Not uncommonly, the posterior aspect of the minor fissure extends posterior to the margin of the right major fissure, an illusion explained by the concomitant visualization of the posterolateral aspect of the minor fissure and the anteromedial aspect of the undulating major fissure.

On sequential 10-mm collimated CT scans, the major fissures appear as broad avascular bands of decreased density separating the lower lobes from the upper or middle lobes. The oblique course of the major fissures within the scan section, which creates partial volume averaging of the fissure with the surrounding hypovascular lung, accounts for this appearance. The minor fissure is seen as a broad avascular region extending anteriorly from the midportion of the major fissure. The minor fissure is seen on only one or two contiguous axial images because of its horizontal orientation. High-resolution CT with its inherent 1.5–2.0 mm collimation and high spatial frequency reconstruction, depicts the major fissures as thin white curvilinear lines (Fig. 12.8). The upper concave and lower convex surface of both fissures is easily seen on HRCT. The apex of the minor fissure is typically seen as a thin circular density because of its convex superior contour.

The inferior accessory fissure is the most common accessory fissure, found in approximately 10–20% of individuals. This fissure, which separates the medial basal from the remaining basal segments of the lower lobe, is often incomplete (Fig. 12.6). It may be seen on frontal radiographs as a thin curvilinear line extending superiorly from the medial third of the hemidiaphragm toward the lower hilum. The inferior accessory fissure is often misidentified as the inferior pulmonary ligament, which is not seen on frontal chest radiographs since it lies in the coronal plane and is en-face to the x-ray beam. A small triangle of fat, seen at its point of insertion on the diaphragm, helps identify the inferior accessory fissure. An inferior accessory fissure can be seen on CT scans through the lower thorax, where it is identified as a curvilinear line extending anterolaterally from just in front of the inferior pulmonary ligament toward the major fissure.

The azygos fissure is seen in 0.5% of individuals (Fig. 12.6). It is composed of four layers of pleura (two visceral, two parietal) and represents an invagination of the right apical pleura by the azygos vein that has incompletely migrated to its normal position at the right tracheobronchial angle. The azygos fissure appears as a vertical curvilinear line, convex laterally, which extends inferiorly from the lung apex, ending in a teardrop, which is the azygos vein. The significance

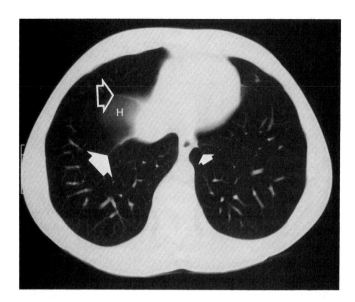

Figure 12.9. Inferior Pulmonary and Pericardiophrenic Ligaments. A CT scan of the chest just above the diaphragm demonstrates a thin line (*small solid arrow*) extending posterolaterally at the level of the esophagus that represents the intersublobar septum of the inferior pulmonary ligament. On the right, a curvilinear line (*large solid arrow*) extending from just lateral to the inferior vena cava represents the pericardiophrenic ligament containing branches of the phrenic nerve. More anteriorly, a thin line (*open arrow*) is seen just above the apex of the right hemidiaphragm (*H*), which represents fat within the inferior aspect of the major fissure.

of this fissure lies in its ability to limit the spread of apical segmental consolidation to the azygos lobe (that portion of the apical segment delineated by the azygos fissure) and in excluding pneumothorax from the apical portion of the pleural space. The superior accessory fissure separates the superior segment from the basal segments of the lower lobe. On the right side it may be distinguished from the minor fissure on lateral radiographs, as it extends posteriorly from the major fissure to the chest wall. The left minor fissure is a rarely seen normal variant that separates the lingula from the remaining portions of the upper lobe.

Ligaments. The inferior pulmonary ligament is a sheet of connective tissue that extends from the hilum to a level at or just above the hemidiaphragm. It is oriented in the coronal plane and is formed by an infolding of the visceral and parietal pleura of the infrahilar portions of the lower lobes; it is thus comprised of four pleural layers, two visceral and two parietal. The ligament contains the inferior pulmonary vein superiorly and a variable number of lymph nodes. The ligament is not visible on frontal radiographs, but is occasionally identified on lateral radiographs as a thin line extending a variable distance inferiorly from the hilum. The inferior pulmonary ligament is commonly seen on contiguous CT scans through the lower thorax as a short linear opacity extending laterally from the region of the esophagus (Fig. 12.9). The ligament may be seen on only one or

two sequential scans or may extend from the inferior pulmonary vein to reflect off the hemidiaphragm. The tethering effect of this ligament on the lower lobe accounts for the medial location and triangular appearance of lower lobe collapse. The ligament may also act as a barrier to the spread of pleural and mediastinal fluid, and may marginate medial pleural or mediastinal air collections to produce a characteristic appearance on radiographs.

The pericardiophrenic ligament appears as a triangular density extending toward the lung, which is seen along the posterior aspect of the right heart border on lung windows on chest CT (Fig. 12.9). It represents a reflection of pleura over the inferior portion of the phrenic nerve and pericardiophrenic vessels. It is distinguished from the inferior pulmonary ligament by its more anterior location and by its characteristic ramifications as branches of the nerve and vessel reflect over the hemidiaphragm.

Pulmonary Arteries. The pulmonary artery is an elastic artery that arises from the right ventricle anterior to the ascending aorta and courses superiorly, posteriorly, and toward the left before bifurcating into right and left main pulmonary arteries. The left pulmonary artery is a direct continuation of the main pulmonary artery. Within the left hilum, it envelopes the upper margin of the left main bronchus, at which point it divides into the upper and lower lobe arteries. The right pulmonary artery courses laterally toward the right from the main pulmonary artery. It then travels anterior to the tracheal carina and immediately posterior to the ascending aorta, and divides within the pericardium into the truncus anterior and interlobar arteries. The right and left pulmonary arteries are best visualized on the lateral chest radiograph (Fig. 12.1B). The upper and lower lobe divisions of the pulmonary arteries are best seen on frontal radiographs, particularly the interlobar arteries, which course inferolaterally and posteriorly, lying immediately lateral to the corresponding lower lobe bronchi (Fig. 12.1A).

The branches of the right and left pulmonary arteries accompany and divide in parallel with the corresponding lobar, segmental, and subsegmental bronchi. There are many accessory branches of the pulmonary artery. As the arteries divide, they diminish in caliber. At the same level that the bronchi lose their cartilage and become bronchioles, the elastic arteries lose their elastic lamina and become muscular arteries. At a diameter of 70–80 microns, the arteries lose their muscular layer and become arterioles. The capillary network of the pulmonary arterial circulation, which envelopes the alveoli, is the most prolific capillary system in the body. These capillaries are lined by endothelium and a basement membrane, which merges with the basement membrane of the alveolar epithelium to form the thin alveolocapillary membrane across which diffusion of oxygen and carbon dioxide occurs. Thickening of the alveolocapillary membrane from edema fluid or fibrosis impedes gas exchange and results in dyspnea and hypoxemia.

Bronchial Arteries. The bronchial arteries are the primary nutrient vessels of the lung. They supply blood to the bronchial walls to the level of the terminal bronchioles. In addition, several mediastinal structures receive a variable amount of blood supply from the bronchial circulation. These include the tracheal wall, midthird of the esophagus, visceral pleura, mediastinal lymph nodes, vagus nerve, pericardium, and thymus.

The origin of the bronchial arteries is quite variable. The bronchial arteries arise from the proximal descending thoracic aorta between the level of the third and eighth thoracic vertebral bodies. In the most common situation there is one right- and two left-sided arteries. The right bronchial artery usually arises from the posterolateral wall of the aorta in common with an intercostal artery as an intercostobronchial trunk. This artery typically arises at the T5-6 level, which corresponds radiographically to the level of the tracheal carina. The left bronchial arteries arise individually from the anterolateral aorta at or about the same level; the left bronchial arteries rarely arise from an intercostal artery. The anterior spinal artery, which originates from branches of the proximal vertebral arteries, supplies the anterior portion of the spinal cord. As the anterior spinal artery extends the length of the cord, it receives anterior radiculomedullary branches from intercostal and lumbar arteries. In the lower thoracic and lumbar region, the great anterior radicular artery (artery of Adamkiewicz) joins the anterior spinal artery. In approximately 5% of individuals the artery of Adamkiewicz originates from or receives a large branch from the right intercostobronchial artery.

Pulmonary Veins. The pulmonary veins arise within the interlobular septa from the alveolar and visceral pleural capillaries. The veins travel in connective tissue envelopes separate from the bronchoarterial trunks. The pulmonary veins, which may number from three to eight, drain into the left atrium. Approximately two-thirds of the blood from the bronchial arterial system returns to the pulmonary venous system via the bronchial veins. The remainder, which includes veins draining the large bronchi, tracheal bifurcation, and mediastinum, drain into the azygos or hemiazygos systems.

Pulmonary Lymphatic System. The lymphatic system of the lung helps clear fluid and particulate matter from the pulmonary interstitium. There are two major lymphatic pathways in the lung and pleura. The visceral pleural lymphatics, which reside in the vascular (innermost) layer of the visceral pleura, form a network over the surface of the lung that roughly parallels the margins of the secondary pulmonary lob-

ules. These peripheral lymphatics penetrate the lung to course centrally within interlobular septa along with the pulmonary veins toward the hilum. The parenchymal lymphatics originate in proximity to the alveolar septa ("juxtaalveolar lymphatics") and course centrally with the bronchoarterial bundle. The perivenous and bronchoarterial lymphatics communicate via obliquely oriented lymphatics located within the central regions of the lung. These communicating lymphatics and their surrounding connective tissue, when distended by fluid, account for the radiographic appearance of Kerley's A lines.

Pulmonary Interstitium. The pulmonary interstitium is the scaffolding of the lung, providing support for the airways and pulmonary vessels. It is a continuous structure that begins within the hilum and extends peripherally to the visceral pleura. (6) The interstitial compartment that extends from the mediastinum and envelopes the bronchovascular bundles is termed the axial or bronchovascular interstitium. Edema involving the axial interstitium is recognized radiographically as peribronchial cuffing or tramtracking. Once the bronchoarterial bundle and surrounding interstitium reach the level of the pulmonary acinus (terminal bronchiole), the interstitial tissues ramify along with the pulmonary arterioles and capillaries to provide support for the air-exchanging portions of the lung (i.e., respiratory bronchioles, alveolar ducts, sacs, and alveoli). This component of the interstitium has been termed the alveolar or parenchymatous interstitium. Pathologic involvement of the alveolar interstitium is difficult to discern radiographically, but may account for some cases of so-called ground-glass density on chest radiographs and HRCT scans. Thickening of portions of the alveolar intersitium are occasionally seen as intralobular lines on HRCT. Finally, the septa dividing secondary pulmonary lobules in the periphery of the lung are composed of pulmonary veins and lymphatics within the peripheral interstitium. This interstitial space is contiguous with the subpleural interstitial space, which is also called the vascular layer of the visceral pleura. Radiographically, edema of the peripheral and subpleural interstitium accounts for Kerley's B lines on frontal chest radiographs (or interlobular lines on HRCT) and "thickened" fissures on lateral radiographs, respectively.

Posteroanterior Chest Radiograph

A firm knowledge of the normal anatomy displayed on the frontal (usually PA) chest radiograph is the key to detecting and localizing pathologic conditions, and to avoid mistaking normal structures for pathologic findings (Fig. 12.1A).

Soft Tissues. The soft tissues of the chest wall consist of the skin, subcutaneous fat, and muscles.

The lateral edges of the sternocleidomastoid muscles are readily visible in most patients. The suprasternal fossa is a V- or U-shaped lucency seen in some asthenic individuals immediately above the manubrium, and is formed by air outlining the medial edges of the sterno-cleidomastoid muscles above their insertion at the clavicles. The visualization of normal fat in the supra-clavicular fossae and the companion shadows of skin and subcutaneous fat paralleling the clavicles helps exclude mass, adenopathy, or edema in this region. The inferolateral edge of the pectoralis major muscle is normally seen curving toward the axilla. Congenital absence of the pectoral muscle creates relative radiolucency on the affected side and should not be mistaken for a contralateral increase in density. Both breast shadows should be evaluated routinely to detect evidence of prior mastectomy or distorting mass. The soft tissues lateral to the bony thorax should be smooth, symmetric, homogeneous densities.

Bones. The thoracic spine, ribs and costal cartilages, clavicles, and scapulae are routinely visible on frontal chest radiographs. The bodies of the thoracic vertebrae should be vertically aligned, with endplates, pedicles, and spinous processes visualized. Twelve pairs of symmetric ribs should be seen; the upper ribs have smooth superior and inferior cortical margins, while the middle and lower ribs have flanged inferior cortices where the intercostal neurovascular bundles run. Ribs arising from cervical vertebra are identified in approximately 2% of individuals, and may be associated with symptoms of thoracic outlet syndrome. Companion shadows paralleling the inferior margins of the first and second ribs represent extrapleural fat, which may be abundant in obese individuals. Costal cartilage calcification is seen in a majority of adults, and increases in prevalence with advancing age. Men typically show calcification at the upper and lower margins, while the majority of women develop central cartilaginous calcification. The scapulae are visible in the upper outer portions of most chest radiographs. A winged scapula is seen when the nerve to the serratus anterior muscle is interrupted, and the scapula no longer contacts the posterolateral chest wall, producing a foreshortened appearance on frontal radiographs. A high-riding scapula (Sprengel's deformity) may be an isolated finding or part of the Klippel-Feil syndrome, in which the Sprengel's deformity is associated with an omovertebral bone and fused cervical vertebrae. The clavicles overlie the lung apices on frontal radiographs. They may be involved in congenital disorders such as cleidocranial dysostosis, in which portions of the clavicles are unossified, or in acquired disorders such as rheumatoid arthritis, scleroderma, and hyperparathyroidism, in which there is erosion of the distal clavicles.

Table 12.3. Normal Lung-Mediastinal Interfaces

Right-sided	Lateral margin of superior vena cava
	Anterior arch of the azygos vein
	Right paraspinal interface
	Azygoesophageal recess
	Lateral margin of right atrium
	Confluence of right pulmonary veins (right border of left atrium)
	Lateral margin of inferior vena cava
Left-sided	Lateral margin of left subclavian artery
	Transverse aortic arch
	Left superior intercostal vein ("aortic nipple")
	Aortopulmonary window interface
	Aortopulmonary interface
	Lateral margin of main pulmonary artery
	Preaortic recess
	Left paraspinal interface
	Left atrial appendage
	Left ventricle
	Epipericardial fat pad

Mediastinal Interfaces. A familiarity with the normal mediastinal interfaces is the key to the interpretation of frontal chest radiographs.

Lung-Mediastinal Interfaces. The lung-mediastinal interfaces (Table 12.3) are seen as sharp edges where the lung and adjacent pleura reflect off of various cardiovascular structures. The right lateral margin of the superior vena cava is commonly seen as a straight or slightly concave interface with the right upper lobe, extending from the level of the clavicle to the superior margin of the right atrium. Prominence or convexity of the caval interface may represent caval dilation or lateral displacement by a dilated or tortuous aortic arch or other mediastinal mass.

The anterior arch of the azygos vein creates an oval opacity as it curves forward from its paraspinal location at T4-T5 level to drain into the posterior aspect of the superior vena cava just anterior and to the right of the right tracheobronchial angle. The arch of the azygos vein indents the right upper lobe with a convex interface. Measurements for the azygos vein must take into account the position of the patient (i.e., supine or upright) and the intrathoracic pressure at the time the film was exposed. The measurement should be made through the midpoint of the azygos arch perpendicular to the right main bronchus. The supine position or performance of the Muller maneuver (forced inspiration against a closed glottis) will increase azygos venous diameter. In general, a diameter of >10 mm on a PA radiograph should raise the possibility of mass, adenopathy, or dilation of the azygos vein; the latter may be seen with right heart failure or obstruction of venous return to the heart. An increase in the diameter of the azygos vein from prior comparable radiographs is more important than the actual measurement.

The paraspinal interface is a straight, vertical interface extending the length of the right hemithorax and represents contact of the right lung with a small amount of tissue lateral to the thoracic spine. It is inconstantly visualized on the right side. A focal convexity of this interface suggests spinal or paraspinal disease.

The azygoesophageal recess interface is a vertically oriented interface between a crest of the right lower lobe known as the crista pulmonis and the esophagus or periesophageal tissues. This interface is seen overlying the thoracic spine and has an oblique orientation extending from the arch of the azygos vein superiorly to the diaphragm inferiorly (Fig. 12.1A). While normally straight or concave in contour, the midthird of the interface may have a slight rightward convexity at the level of the right inferior pulmonary veins. Convexity of the superior third of the interface should suggest subcarinal lymph node enlargement, left atrial enlargement, or a bronchogenic cyst, while convexity of the inferior third should raise the possibility of enlarged paraesophageal lymph nodes or a sliding hiatal hernia. When air is present in the distal portion of the esophagus and the azygoesophageal recess interfaces with the right lateral wall of the esophagus, a line (the right inferior esophagopleural stripe) rather than an edge is seen.

The right heart projects just to the right of the lateral margin of the thoracic spine on a normal PA radiograph. This portion of the heart is the lateral margin of the right atrium, which creates a smooth convex interface with the medial segment of the middle lobe. Individuals with pectus excavatum have leftward cardiac displacement and may not demonstrate this interface. In patients with right atrial dilation, this interface becomes more prominent, extending well into the right lung.

The confluence of right pulmonary veins or the right border of the left atrium may be seen as a convex interface visible through the shadow of the right atrium. Identification is usually possible if pulmonary veins are noted entering the lateral margin of the atrium. Pulmonary venous hypertension and left atrial dilation will enlarge and laterally displace this interface, producing a double density composed of the right lateral borders of both right and left atria.

The right lateral border of the inferior vena cava may be seen at the level of the right hemidiaphragm as a concave lateral interface. The inferior vena caval interface is best visualized on lateral radiographs. This interface may be absent in patients with azygos continuation of the inferior vena cava.

In the uppermost portion of the left mediastinum, one or more interfaces may be recognized cephalad to the aortic arch. The interface most often visualized is the subclavian artery medial to the anterior scalene muscle. The artery is concave and typically extends over the apex of the lung to exit the thorax. Less commonly, the interface of the left innominate vein and the upper portion of the paraspinal line may be seen paralleling the left subclavian interface.

The transverse portion of the aortic arch (aortic knob) creates a small convex indentation on the left lung in normal individuals. As the aorta elongates and dilates with age, this interface projects more laterally, and the lung may be seen to encircle a greater circumference of the knob.

In approximately 5% of individuals, the left superior intercostal vein may be seen on frontal radiographs as a rounded or triangular opacity that focally indents the lung immediately superolateral to the aortic arch. This density, termed the "aortic nipple," represents the superior intercostal vein as it arches anteriorly from its paraspinal position around the aortic arch to drain into the posterior aspect of the left innominate vein. This structure, which normally measures less than 5 mm, may enlarge with elevation of right atrial pressure or with congenital or acquired obstruction of venous return to the right heart.

Immediately inferior to the aortic arch, the left upper lobe contacts the mediastinum to produce the aortopulmonary window interface. This interface is usually straight or concave toward the lung; the latter appearance is seen with a tortuous aorta, emphysema, or congenital absence of the left pericardium. A convex lateral interface should suggest mass or lymph node enlargement in the aortopulmonary window.

A mediastinal-pleural interface, termed the aortopulmonary interface, is occasionally seen in the left upper mediastinum superimposed upon the aortic knob and extending inferiorly toward the main pulmonary artery. This interface represents the left upper lobe contacting mediastinal fat in a plane just anterolateral to the aortic arch and extending inferiorly toward the left hilum. Convexity or lobulation of this interface may be due to mediastinal lipomatosis, lymph node enlargement, or a mass in this region of the mediastinum.

Immediately inferior to the aortopulmonary window is the left lateral border of the main pulmonary artery. The interface of this structure may be convex, straight, or concave toward the lung. Enlargement of the main pulmonary artery is seen as an idiopathic condition in young women, due to poststenotic dilation in valvular pulmonic stenosis, or in conditions where there is increased flow or pressure in the pulmonary arterial system such as left-to-right intracardiac shunts.

The preaortic recess interface is seen in a small percentage of normal individuals as a reflection of the left lower lobe with the esophagus anterior to the descending aorta, extending vertically from the undersurface of the aortic knob for a variable distance toward the diaphragm. This interface is the left-sided analog of the azygoesophageal recess interface. As on the right side, the midthird of the preaortic recess in-

Table 12.4. Anterior and Posterior Junction Lines

Line	Features
Anterior junction line	Obliquely oriented from right superior to left inferior
	Extends from upper sternum to base of heart
Posterior junction line	Vertically oriented in the midline
	Extends from upper thoracic spine to level of azygos and aortic arches

terface may be interrupted by the confluence of left pulmonary veins. When there is air within the esophageal lumen, this interface is seen as a vertical line and is called the left inferior esophagopleural stripe.

The left paraspinal interface represents the reflection of the left lung from paraspinal soft tissues, which largely consist of fat but also contain the sympathetic chain, proximal intercostal vessels, intercostal lymph nodes, and hemiazygos and accessory hemiazygos veins. The left paraspinal interface, in contrast to the right paraspinal interface, is seen in a majority of individuals. The reason for this is that the left-sided descending thoracic aorta produces an interface between the left lower lobe and paraspinal soft tissues that is oriented in the sagittal plane. This interface lies farther lateral to the lateral margin of the spine than the right paraspinal reflection because of an increased amount of left paraspinal fat below the level of the aortic arch. Neurogenic tumors, hematoma, paraspinal abscess, lipomatosis, and medial pleural effusion can cause lateral displacement of this interface.

The left atrial appendage forms a concave interface immediately below the main pulmonary artery. Straightening or convexity of this interface is most commonly seen in rheumatic mitral valve disease, but may be seen in patients with left atrial enlargement of any cause.

The left ventricle comprises most of the left heart border. A gentle convex margin with the lingula is normal. Abnormalities of the left ventricular contour will be discussed in detail in the section on cardiovascular disease.

Fat adjacent to the cardiac apex may create a focal bulge in the left cardiac contour that obscures the heart border at the left cardiophrenic angle. This epipericardial fat pad is usually unilateral or more prominent on the left, and is most often seen in obese patients and those taking corticosteroids. A typical appearance on the lateral radiograph is usually diagnostic; CT is helpful in equivocal cases.

Lung-Lung or Lung-Air Interfaces produce lines when the aerated lung abuts the contralateral lung (Table 12.4) or the air-filled trachea or esophagus, respectively. The lung-lung interfaces are seen as thin vertical lines that overlie the thoracic spine. The *anterior junction line* is composed of four layers of pleura found be-

tween the right and left upper lobes as they meet anterior to the aorta and main pulmonary artery. The anterior junction line is a continuation of the reflections of the upper lobes from the innominate veins, which itself produces a triangular density at the level of the sternum. The anterior junction line continues inferiorly from the apex of this triangle and courses obliquely and to the left to end in a triangular reflection of fat over the base of the heart. The *posterior junction line* represents pleural layers between right and left upper lobes behind the esophagus and anterior to the spine. The posterior junction line is seen cephalad to the anterior junction line, beginning superiorly at the level of the upper thoracic vertebrae and continuing as a truly vertical linear density to reflect inferiorly off the azygos and aortic arches. Rarely, the right and left lower lobes meet behind the distal third of the esophagus and anterior to the aorta to produce an inferior posterior junction line (Fig. 12.10).

Along the right upper mediastinum, the right upper lobe contacts the right lateral tracheal wall in a majority of individuals. This produces the right paratracheal line or stripe, which represents the combined thickness of the right tracheal wall, paratracheal soft tissues and lymph nodes, and visceral and parietal pleural membranes. The thickness of this line, measured above the level of the azygos vein, should not exceed 4 mm. Thickening or nodularity of the paratracheal line is seen in abnormalities of the tissues comprising the line, including tracheal tumors, paratracheal lymph node enlargement, and right pleural effusion.

A line may be seen when air in the lower esophagus and air in the azygoesophageal recess of lung produce the right inferior esophagopleural stripe. More commonly, contact of the right lower lobe occurs with the collapsed esophagus to form the azygoesophageal recess interface.

It is rare for the left upper lobe to interface with the left lateral wall of the trachea to form the left paratracheal line, as the subclavian artery and adjacent fat usually intervene. The left inferior esophagopleural stripe is analogous to that on the right, and is formed by air in both the left lower lobe and distal esophageal lumen.

The Lungs. The density of the lungs as visualized radiographically is attributable solely to the presence of the pulmonary vasculature and enveloping interstitial structures. The intraparenchymal pulmonary arteries course vertically from the hilar pulmonary arteries, allowing distinction from the pulmonary veins, which are more horizontally oriented. The arteries have a characteristic tubular shape with a smooth dichotomous branching pattern. They gradually diminish in caliber as they travel distally in tandem with the bronchi, which are not visible radio-

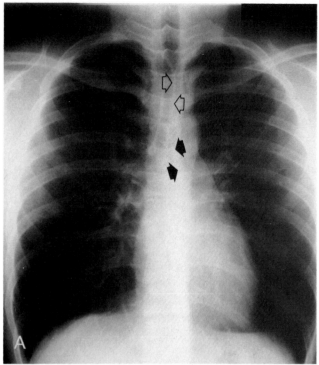

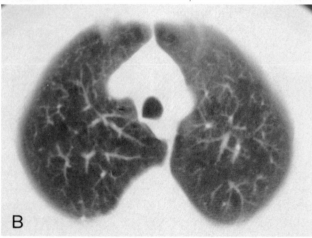

Figure 12.10. Anterior and Posterior Junction Lines. A PA chest film (**A**) shows both anterior (*solid arrows*) and posterior (*open arrows*) junction lines. Computed tomography through the upper thorax in another patient (**B**) shows the anterior junction line to lie in the retrosternal region while the posterior junction line lies between the esophagus anteriorly and the spine posteriorly.

graphically. The pulmonary veins can often be traced horizontally to the left atrium, but are otherwise indistinguishable from pulmonary arteries. In the upright individual, the lower lobe arteries and veins are larger in caliber than the upper lobe vessels because of the effects of gravity on pumonary blood flow. The normal dark gray density of the upper lungs increases inferiorly in females because of overlying breast tissue. The density of the lung may be increased by processes that render the interstitium or air spaces opaque, or decreased by any process associated with

diminished blood flow to the lung or destruction of parenchymal structures.

Diaphragm. The right and left portions of the diaphragm are smooth, domed-shaped structures. The right hemidiaphragm overlies the liver and the left hemidiaphragm overlies the stomach and spleen. On frontal radiographs exposed in deep inspiration, the apex of the right hemidiaphragm typically lies at the level of the sixth anterior rib, approximately one-half interspace above the apex of the left hemidiaphragm. A scalloped appearance to the right hemidiaphragm is not uncommon.

Upper Abdomen. Portions of the liver, spleen, and gastric fundus are routinely visualized on most frontal chest radiographs. Abnormalities of abdominal situs may be identified by noting the location and appearance of the liver, stomach, and spleen. Enlargement of the liver may cause right diaphragmatic elevation and right lateral compression of the stomach. Intrahepatic air may be seen within the biliary tree, portal vein, or a hepatic abscess. Calcified hepatic lesions such as echinococcal cysts or calcified gallstones overlying the lower portion of the liver may be visible. A mass arising within the gastric fundus can occasionally be seen as a soft tissue opacity protruding into a gas-filled gastric lumen. Splenomegaly may be identified by noting a soft tissue mass in the left upper quadrant that displaces the stomach medially and the splenic flexure of colon inferiorly.

Lateral Chest Radiograph

The normal lateral chest film is complex and difficult to interpret. Only small portions of both lungs are projected free of superimposed mediastinal structures, and the composite densities of the cardiomediastinal structures yield complex shadows (Fig. 12.1**B**). However, knowledge of normal lateral radiographic anatomy can greatly aid in detection and localization of parenchymal and cardiomediastinal processes (8, 9).

On well-penetrated lateral radiographs, the body of the sternum is readily visible. Posterior to the manubrium, the lung is indented by a broad-based bulge representing the left brachiocephalic vein as it traverses the retromanubrial area to join the right brachiocephalic vein to form the superior vena cava. Occasionally, a second, more inferior bulge behind the upper sternum is seen, caused by osteophytes that project posteriorly from the first costochondral junction. Immediately behind the body of the sternum, the lung interfaces with a small amount of retrosternal fat to produce the thin retrosternal stripe. Sternal fracture, infection, or tumor can distort or thicken this stripe. An undulating line seen immediately posterior to the anterior chest wall represents the contact of the lung with the costal cartilages of the anterior ribs, which produces the parasternal line.

This line is seen bilaterally in 90% of normal individuals. Enlargement of internal mammary lymph nodes (e.g., lymphoma or metastatic breast carcinoma) or arteries (e.g., coarctation of the aorta) produces masses seen projecting through the concavities seen between the costal cartilages. Inferiorly, the left lung may be excluded from contacting the anteromedial chest wall by a round or triangular density that represents the cardiac apex and adjacent epipericardial fat. This impression on the anterior surface of the lingula has been termed the cardiac incisura, and should not be mistaken for a mass. Computed tomography will prove helpful in equivocal cases.

The retrosternal space is composed of those portions of the upper lobes that meet behind the sternum and anterior to the ascending aorta to produce the anterior junction line seen on frontal radiographs. This space becomes more prominent in patients with a pectus carinatum deformity or a barrel chest from chronic obstructive pulmonary disease. A soft tissue mass may be produced in this region by tumors arising within the anterior mediastinum. These masses may not be visible on the frontal radiograph. The retrotracheal triangle is a radiolucent region composed of those portions of the upper lobes that meet to create the posterior junction line on frontal radiographs. It is marginated by the trachea anteriorly, the spine posteriorly, and the aortic arch inferiorly, with its apex pointing superiorly toward the thoracic inlet. Opacities in the upper lobes, retrotracheal masses (e.g., aberrant subclavian artery or posterior thyroid goiter), or esophageal masses may produce an abnormal density in this region. The posterior edge of the retrotracheal triangle may interface with a thin soft tissue stripe immediately anterior to the thoracic spine in this region. A thickness exceeding 3 mm should prompt an evaluation for spinal disease.

Posterior and inferior to the retrosternal space, the lung may be seen to outline the anterior aspect of portions of the ascending aorta, pulmonary outflow tract, and right ventricle in approximately 10% of individuals. The aortic arch may become visible on lateral radiograph in patients with tortuous aortic arches that protrude into the left lung to become outlined by air. If the descending aorta is similarly tortuous, its posterior and occasionally anterior margin may be followed to just above the diaphragm, where the aorta returns to a prespinal position to traverse the aortic hiatus and enter the abdomen. The superior margin of the arch of the azygos vein is rarely visible overlying the lower aspect of the aortic arch. In certain individuals, the posterior edges of the arteries arising from the aortic arch may be visible in relation to the tracheal air column. The innominate artery appears as a convex posterior curvilinear opacity projecting through the upper tracheal air column, while the left subclavian artery projects just behind the tracheal air column and has a straight posterior edge. The left common carotid artery is not normally visible as it is embedded in mediastinal fat and does not contact the left lung.

In approximately 20% of normal individuals, a thin curvilinear white line may be seen paralleling the anteroinferior cardiac margin. This line is visible when subepicardial fat and fat in the anterior mediastinum outline the inner and outer edges of the visceral and parietal pericardium, respectively. Normally less than 2 mm in thickness, thickening of this pericardial stripe suggests pericardial effusion or thickening.

The posterior aspect of the inferior vena cava is visible in the majority of individuals as a concave posterior or straight edge visible at the posteroinferior cardiac margin just above the diaphragm. In a small percentage of patients, the vena cava has a convex interface with the lung, which should not be mistaken for a mass or lymph node enlargement.

The trachea is seen on all properly penetrated lateral radiographs as a tubular lucency that extends from the neck through the thoracic inlet into the thorax, coursing inferiorly and slightly posteriorly through the level of the aortic arch (Fig. 12.1**B**). It is contacted posteriorly by the esophagus. The retrotracheal stripe, visible in approximately 50% of individuals, represents the thickness of the posterior tracheal wall and surrounding tissues. It is visible when the right upper lobe invaginates behind the trachea to contact its posterior wall and render it visible. As with the right paratracheal stripe, a thickness of greater than 4 mm may indicate disease of the tracheal wall, paratracheal soft tissue or lymph nodes, right pleural space, or an opacity in the right upper lobe in the region of contact with the posterior trachea. The tracheoesophageal stripe is seen when air in the esophagus produces a stripe behind the tracheal air column, which represents the combined thickness of the tracheal and esophageal walls. A thickness exceeding 4 mm implies tracheal, esophageal, or mediastinal pathology.

The thoracic spine is readily visualized on the lateral chest radiograph. The vertebral bodies should be aligned along their anterior and posterior cortical margins, forming a gradual kyphosis.

The anterior margins of the scapulae may be seen overlying the superior and posterior aspect of the thorax. They are identified by their location, bilaterality, and typical straight edge, which is obliquely oriented from superoposterior to anteroinferior.

Air outlining the anterior axillary folds may render the anterior edge of these skin folds visible, overlying the superior aspect of the thorax. The edges are seen as bilateral opacities that are concave anteriorly and

Table 12.5. Contents of the Thoracic Inlet and Mediastinum

Compartment	Contents
Thoracic inlet	Thymus
	Confluence of right and left internal jugular and subclavian veins
	Right and left carotid arteries
	Right and left subclavian arteries
	Trachea
	Esophagus
	Prevertebral fascia
	Phrenic, vagus, recurrent laryngeal nerves
Anterior mediastinum	Internal mammary vessels
	Internal mammary and prevascular lymph nodes
	Thymus
Middle mediastinum	Heart and pericardium
	Ascending and transverse aorta
	Main and proximal right and left pulmonary arteries
	Confluence of pulmonary veins
	Superior and inferior vena cava
	Trachea and main bronchi
	Lymph nodes and fat within mediastinal spaces
Posterior mediastinum	Descending aorta
	Esophagus
	Azygos and hemiazygos veins
	Thoracic duct
	Sympathetic ganglia and intercostal nerves
	Lymph nodes

can be followed through the level of the thoracic inlet to merge with the soft tissues of the arms.

The hemidiaphragms appear as parallel domed structures on lateral radiographs. At maximal inspiration the posterior portion lies at a more inferior level than the anterior portion, creating a deep posterior costophrenic sulcus and a more shallow anterior sulcus. There are several methods of distinguishing the right from left hemidiaphragm on the lateral view. The right hemidiaphragm is more commonly seen in its entire anteroposterior extent than the left, as the heart excludes the left lung from contacting the anterior aspect of the left hemidiaphragm. On a well-positioned left lateral chest radiograph, with the right side of the thorax farther from the x-ray cassette than the left, the right anterior and posterior costophrenic sulcus should project beyond the corresponding left-sided sulci because of x-ray beam divergence. Identifying the right and left costophrenic sulci should allow identification of the corresponding hemidiaphragms. The presence of air in the stomach or splenic flexure projecting above one hemidiaphragm and below another identifies the more cephalad structure as the left hemidiaphragm. Occasionally, when the right and left major fissures are distinguishable (the left is more vertically oriented than the right), tracing a major fis-

sure to its point of contact with the diaphragm will allow identification of that hemidiaphragm.

Anatomy of the Thoracic Inlet

The thoracic inlet is the junction between the neck and mediastinum proper (Table 12.5). It parallels the plane of the first rib, and therefore slopes upward from anterior to posterior (10). The anatomy of the thoracic inlet is best depicted by CT and MR (Fig. 12.11). The most anterior aspect of the thoracic inlet is occupied by the thymus gland. The thymus extends inferiorly into the anterior mediastinum, where it appears in adults as a triangular or bilobed fatty structure, with varied amounts of residual glandular tissue in younger adults. The right and left subclavian veins enter the thorax from the axillae anterior to the anterior scalene muscle to join the right and left internal jugular veins at the anterolateral aspect of the thoracic inlet to form the right and left brachiocephalic veins, respectively. The subclavian arteries occupy the lateral aspect of the thoracic inlet, behind the corresponding subclavian veins. They curve laterally to exit the thorax at a slightly higher level than the veins enter, coursing behind the anterior scalene muscles toward the axillae. The carotid arteries course vertically within the anterior portion of the thoracic inlet, anterolateral to the trachea, posteromedial to the subclavian and brachiocephalic veins, and immediately behind the thymus. The trachea occupies a midline position within the thoracic inlet, immediately surrounded anteriorly by the carotid artery, laterally by the subclavian arteries, and posteriorly by the upper esophagus. The esophagus lies in a prevertebral location immediately behind the posterior tracheal membrane. The thoracic duct lies to the left and posterolateral to the esophagus, arching forward above the left subclavian artery to enter the posterior aspect of the left internal jugular and subclavian veins at their confluence to form the left brachiocephalic vein. The right and left superior intercostal veins run vertically immediately anterolateral to the upper thoracic spine. The prevertebral fascia is a thin connective tissue membrane that is inseparable from the anterior longitudinal ligament of the upper thoracic spine. The phrenic and vagus nerves are not visible on CT scans, but run together in the space between the subclavian arteries and brachiocephalic veins. The recurrent laryngeal nerves lie on each side within the tracheoesophageal groove.

Normal Mediastinal Anatomy

The mediastinum is a narrow, vertically oriented space between the medial parietal pleural layers of the lungs that contains central cardiovascular and tracheobronchial structures, and the esophagus enveloped

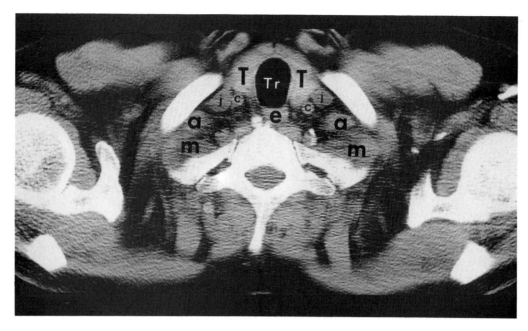

Figure 12.11. Normal Anatomy of the Thoracic Inlet. *Tr*, trachea; *T*, thyroid; *e*, esophagus; *j*, internal jugular vein; *c*, common carotid artery; *a*, anterior scalene muscle; *m*, middle scalene muscle.

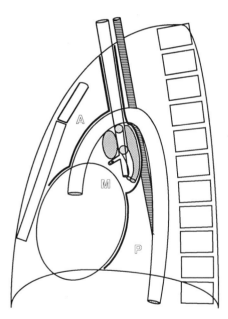

Figure 12.12. Mediastinal Compartments as Seen on Lateral View. *A*, anterior mediastinum; *M*, middle mediastinum; *P*, posterior mediastinum.

in fat with intermixed lymph nodes. Several schemes have been described to divide the mediastinum into separate compartments (Table 12.5). The most commonly utilized classification is an anatomic one, in which a line drawn through the sternal angle anteriorly and the fourth thoracic intervertebral space posteriorly divides the mediastinum into superior and inferior compartments. The inferior mediastinum is further subdivided into anterior, middle, and posterior compartments. This division of the mediastinum

is purely arbitrary, as there are no true anatomic boundaries between the three compartments. However, by using the most easily recognizable mediastinal structure, the heart, as the focal point, the relationship of mediastinal masses to the heart allows for simple and consistent compartmentalization. Furthermore, this division of the mediastinum corresponds to easily recognizable regions as seen on the lateral chest radiograph. A minor variation of the anatomic method, in which there is no superior and inferior division, and the anterior, middle, and posterior compartments extend vertically from the thoracic inlet superiorly to the diaphragm inferiorly, is most practical to radiologists and is used here (Fig. 12.12). Within each compartment are readily identifiable structures and a number of spaces, in free communication with one another, that contain fat and lymph nodes. The structures and spaces native to each compartment and their normal appearance are reviewed here.

Anterior Mediastinum. The anterior (prevascular) mediastinal compartment includes all structures behind the sternum and anterior to the heart and great vessels, and includes the internal mammary vessels and lymph nodes, thymus, and the brachiocephalic veins (Table 12.5). The internal mammary vessels reside within the parasternal fat and lie on either side of the sternum. Normal lymph nodes accompany the vessels but are not routinely visualized on CT. The interface of the retrosternal space with the anterior portion of right and left lungs may be visualized on lateral chest radiographs (see "Lateral Chest Radiograph"). The thymus is a triangular or bilobed

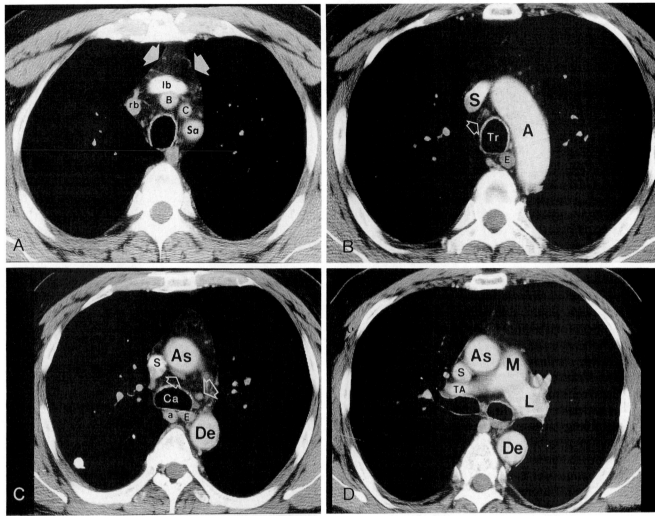

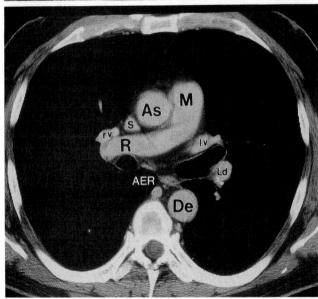

Figure 12.13. Normal Mediastinal and Hilar Anatomy on CT. A. Supraaortic level. A CT scan at the level of the crossing left brachiocephalic vein (*lb*) demonstrates the triangular appearance of the fatty thymus (*arrows*) occupying the anterior mediastinum. *rb*, right brachiocephalic vein; *B*, brachiocephalic artery; *C*, common carotid artery; *Sa*, left subclavian artery. **B.** Superior vena cava/aortic arch level. At this level, four main structures are identified: *A*, aortic arch; *S*, superior vena cava; *Tr*, trachea; *E*, esophagus. Normal-sized lymph nodes are seen in the retrocaval, pretracheal space (*open arrow*). **C.** Aortopulmonary window. The aortopulmonary window is seen to contain fat and small lymph nodes (*large open arrow*). The retroaortic portion of the superior pericardial recess is seen as a cresent-shaped fluid-filled structure (*small open arrow*). *As*, ascending aorta; *De*, descending aorta; *S*, superior vena cava; *Ca*, tracheal carina; *a*, azygos vein; *E*, esophagus. **D.** Main and left pulmonary artery. *As*, ascending aorta; *S*, superior vena cava; *De*, descending aorta; *M*, main pulmonary artery; *L*, left pulmonary artery; *TA*, truncus anterior branch of right pulmonary artery. **E.** Right pulmonary artery and azygoesophagel recess. *M*, main pulmonary artery; *R*, right pulmonary artery; *As*, ascending aorta; *De*, descending aorta; *S*, superior vena cava; *rv*, right superior pulmonary veins; *lv*, left superior pulmonary veins; *Ld*, left descending pulmonary artery; *AER*, azygoesophageal recess. **F.** Right ventricular outflow tract/atrial appendages. *RVOT*, right ventricular outflow tract; *RA*, right atrium; *LA*, left atrium, *rv*, right superior pulmonary vein; *As*, ascending aorta; *De*, descending aorta. **G.** Ventricles with intraventricular septum. *RA*, right atrium; *RV*, right ventricle; *LV*, left ventricle.

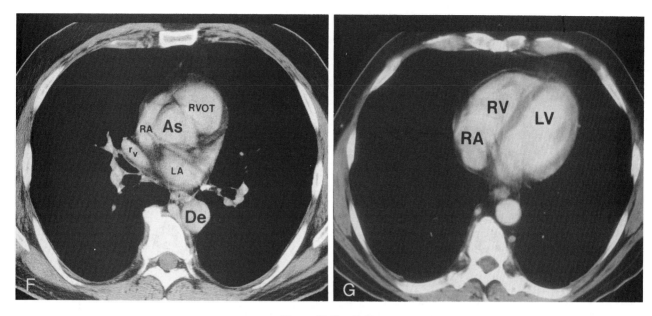

Figure 12.13. F, G.

structure that is maximal in size at puberty and then undergoes gradual fatty involution. In most individuals over the age of 35, the thymus is predominantly fatty, with little or no intermixed glandular (soft tissue) component (Fig. 12.13**A**). The margins of the gland in an adult should be flat or concave toward the lung. The left lobe is commonly larger than the right. Anatomically, the thymus lies in the prevascular space, which is continuous with the retrosternal space anteriorly. It lies immediately anterior to the superior vena cava, aortic arch and great vessels, the main pulmonary artery, and more inferiorly, the heart. The prevascular space generally retains the triangular configuration of the involuted thymus. Normal lymph nodes may be visible on CT within the fat of the prevascular space. Beginning at the level of the aortic arch in most individuals, the anterior portion of the prevascular space tapers to form a thin, vertically oriented linear density that represents the anterior junction line. The right and left brachiocephalic veins occupy the posterior aspect of the prevascular space at the level of the root of the great vessels. The right brachiocephalic vein is seen on CT as a rounded density because of its vertical orientation, while the crossing left brachiocephalic vein appears oval or tubular in configuration.

Middle Mediastinum. The middle (vascular) mediastinal compartment is composed of the pericardium and its contents, the aortic arch and proximal great arteries, central pulmonary arteries and veins, trachea and main bronchi, and lymph nodes (Table 12.5). The hila may be considered as extensions of the middle mediastinal compartment. Superiorly, at the level of the crossing left brachiocephalic vein, the brachiocephalic, left common carotid, and left sub-

clavian arteries surround the trachea with the large brachiocephalic artery directly anterior, the small left common carotid artery anterolateral, and the intermediate-sized subclavian artery directly lateral to the tracheal air column (Fig. 12.13**A**). More inferiorly, the superior vena cava and the oval-shaped, obliquely oriented aortic arch surround the trachea anteriorly (Fig. 12.13**B**).

Immediately below the aortic arch, through the level of the ascending and descending aorta, there are four middle mediastinal spaces that surround the trachea and carina (Fig. 12.13**C**) (11). The right paratracheal space, a narrow space that contains lymph nodes and a small amount of fat, appears as the right paratracheal stripe on frontal chest radiographs. This space extends from the thoracic inlet superiorly to the azygos vein inferiorly. At this level, the pretracheal space is seen between the trachea posteriorly and the posterior margin of the ascending aorta anteriorly. In addition to fat and small lymph nodes, this space, which is contiguous with the precarinal space inferiorly, contains the retroaortic portion of the superior pericardial recess. It is the pretracheal space that is traversed during routine transcervical mediastinoscopy. The retrotracheal space is highly variable in thickness in the anteroposterior dimension, depending upon the degree of invagination of the right upper lobe behind the upper trachea. To the left of the trachea lies the aortopulmonary window. The borders of the aortopulmonary window are the aortic arch superiorly, the left pulmonary artery inferiorly, the distal trachea, left main bronchus, and esophagus medially, the mediastinal pleural surface of the left upper lobe laterally, the posterior surface of the ascending aorta anteriorly, and the anterior surface of the proximal descending aorta posteriorly. This space contains fat, lymph nodes, the ligamentum arteriosum, and the left recurrent laryngeal nerve.

Continuing inferiorly, the main and left pulmonary arteries occupy the left anterolateral portion of the middle mediastinum (Fig. 12.13**D**). The tracheal carina forms the posterior margin of the middle mediastinum. The right upper lobe bronchus is seen just below the tracheal carina. More inferiorly, the right pulmonary artery is seen coursing toward the right and slightly posteriorly just behind the ascending aorta and anterior to the bronchus intermedius (Fig. 12.13**E**). The subcarinal space is outlined posteriorly by air in the azygoesophageal recess and anteriorly by the posterior aspect of the transverse right pulmonary artery. The left superior pulmonary vein lies immediately anterior to the left main and upper lobe bronchi.

The main pulmonary artery can be followed inferiorly to the level of the outflow tract of the right ventricle. At this level, the right and left atrial appendages and the top of the left atrium proper may be seen (Fig. 12.13**F**). Also at this level, the right superior pulmonary vein lies anterior to the middle lobe bronchus, which in turn lies immediately anterior to the right lower lobe bronchus. Inferiorly, the right atrium proper, right ventricle, and left ventricle are identified (Fig. 12.13**G**).

American Thoracic Society Nodal Stations. To provide greater uniformity in the nodal staging of bronchogenic carcinoma and thereby help guide diagnostic and therapeutic efforts in this disease, the American Thoracic Society has devised a standard classification scheme for mediastinal lymph nodes (see Chapter 13, Fig. 13.7).

Posterior Mediastinum. The posterior (postvascular) mediastinal compartment lies behind the pericardium and includes the esophagus, descending aorta, azygos and hemiazygous veins, thoracic duct, and intercostal and autonomic nerves (Table 12.5). The esophagus lies posterior or posterolateral to the trachea from the level of the thoracic inlet superiorly to the tracheal carina inferiorly. From the thoracic inlet to the level of the aortic arch, the right and left upper lobes of the lung meet behind the esophagus and anterior to the spine to form the narrow posterior junction line seen on CT scans through the upper thorax and appearing as a vertical line through the tracheal air column on frontal radiographs. The esophagus then maintains a constant relationship with the descending thoracic aorta, usually lying anteromedial to the aorta (Fig. 12.14) down to the level of the aortic hiatus, where the aorta is in a direct prevertebral position while the esophagus crosses the aorta anteriorly to exit the thorax via the esophageal hiatus.

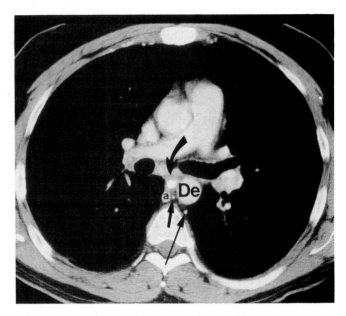

Figure 12.14. Postvascular (Posterior) Mediastinum. A CT scan shows a contrast-filled esophagus (*curved arrow*) anteromedial to the proximal descending aorta (*De*). Also visible within the posterior mediastinum are the azygos vein (*a*), hemiazygos vein (*long arrow*), and thoracic duct (*short arrow*).

There are lymph nodes about the descending aorta that are not normally visible. The descending aorta lies anterolateral to the thoracic spine at the level of the aortopulmonary window. In young adults the aorta maintains this position to the level of the aortic hiatus of the diaphragm, where it lies directly in the midline. In older patients and those with a tortuous or dilated aorta, the vessel lies more laterally and protrudes into the left lower lobe as it descends, carrying the esophagus with it before returning to a midline position at the level of the aortic hiatus. The azygos and hemiazygos veins lie on the right and left sides, respectively, posterolateral to the descending aorta within a fat-containing space that contains the thoracic duct and the sympathetic chains, structures that are not normally visible, and small lymph nodes (Fig. 12.14). Inferiorly, this space is continuous with the retrocrural space, and laterally with the paraspinal space, which contains the intercostal arteries, veins, and lymph nodes.

Normal Hilar Anatomy

Frontal View. The hilum represents the junction of the lung with the mediastinum, and is composed of pulmonary veins and branches of the pulmonary artery and corresponding bronchi (Fig. 12.15) (12). These are all enveloped by small amounts of fat with intermixed lymph nodes. The upper portion of the right hilum is composed of the right superior pulmonary vein, truncus anterior division of the right pulmonary artery, and the right upper lobe bronchus

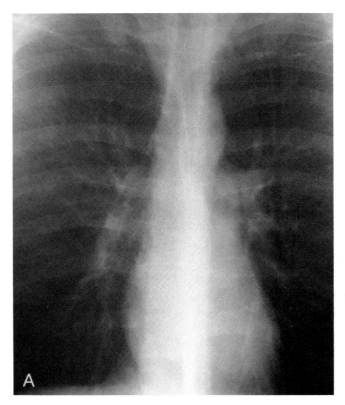

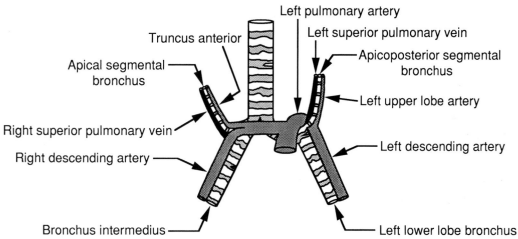

Figure 12.15. Normal Lateral Hilar Anatomy. A. Coned-down view of PA radiograph. **B.** Diagram of frontal hilar anatomy.

(Figs. 12.13**D** and 12.15). The right upper lobe pulmonary vein courses vertically, anterolateral to the truncus anterior. More inferiorly, it courses anterolateral to the distal main right pulmonary artery to empty into the right superolateral aspect of the left atrium just anteromedial to the origin of the middle lobe bronchus (Fig. 12.13**F**). The truncus anterior runs anterior to the right upper lobe bronchus, which lies superior and posterior to the proximal truncus anterior and distal main right pulmonary artery. The right upper lobe bronchus is an eparterial bronchus as it lies above the right pulmonary artery. The lower portion of the right hilum is composed of the right in-

terlobar pulmonary artery laterally and the bronchus intermedius and proximal right lower lobe bronchus medially (Fig. 12.15). The right inferior pulmonary vein courses horizontally to empty into the right lateral border of the left atrium at the lower margin of the hilum, medial to the right basal trunk bronchus (Fig. 12.5**B**7).

In the upper left hilum, the left superior pulmonary vein courses anterior to the left pulmonary artery and, more inferiorly, anterior to the left upper lobe bronchus to empty into the superolateral aspect of the left atrium. The left pulmonary artery arches posteriorly, superiorly, and to the left, over the left main and upper lobe bronchi, to bifurcate into upper and lower lobe arteries (Fig. 12.15**B**). The number and size of the branches of the upper division of the left pulmonary artery are variable. The left main and upper lobe bronchi are encircled anteriorly, superiorly, and posteriorly by the left main and proximal interlobar pulmonary artery, and are therefore hyparterial bronchi (Fig. 12.15). The lower portion of the left hilum is composed of the left interlobar artery which lies immediately behind the left lower lobe bronchus. The left inferior pulmonary vein courses horizontally at a level slightly behind that of the right inferior vein to empty into the left atrium just medial to the left basal trunk bronchus (Fig. 12.5**B**7).

As seen on frontal radiographs, the right and left pulmonary arteries comprise the predominant portion of the hilar density, with the superior pulmonary veins, lobar bronchi, bronchopulmonary lymph nodes, and a small amount of fat contributing little to the overall hilar density (Fig. 12.15**A**). In over 90% of normal individuals, the left hilar outline is higher than the right. This is because the left pulmonary artery, which comprises the predominant portion of the left hilum, ascends over the left main and upper lobe bronchus, whereas the right pulmonary artery lies inferior to the right upper lobe bronchus. In the remainder of individuals, the right and left hila lie at the same level; a right hilum that lies above the left suggests volume loss in the right upper or left lower lobe. The shape of the right hilum on frontal radiograph has been likened to a sideways V, with the opening pointing rightward. The upper portion of the V is composed primarily of the truncus anterior and the posterior division of the right superior pulmonary vein. The superior pulmonary vein forms the lateral margin of the upper portion of the right hilum. The anterior and posterior segmental divisions of the right upper lobe bronchus and artery are often seen at the superolateral margin of the upper right hilum. The right interlobar artery forms the lower half of the V as it descends lateral to the bronchus intermedius. The right inferior pulmonary vein crosses the lower right hilar shadow but does not contribute to its density.

The upper left hilar density is composed centrally of the distal left main pulmonary artery and more peripherally of one or more branches of its left upper lobe division and the posterior division of the left superior pulmonary vein. Either the superior pulmonary vein or apicoposterior branch of the artery may form the lateral margin of the upper hilar shadow. The left upper lobe bronchus is readily identified within the central aspect of the hilum as it is encircled by the left pulmonary artery. The anterior segmental bronchus and its accompanying artery may be seen end on at the lateral margin of the upper left hilum. The in-

terlobar artery forms the lower portion of the left hilar shadow as it descends behind the left heart. The adjacent left lower lobe bronchus is inconstantly visualized as it lies somewhat anterior and medial to the artery.

Left Lateral View. On the lateral radiograph, the right and left hilar outlines are superimposed, producing an oval opacity that represents a combination of the right and left pulmonary arteries and the superior pulmonary veins (Fig. 12.16). The anterior aspect of the hilar density is composed of the transverse portion of the right pulmonary artery, which produces a vertically oriented oval opacity projecting immediately anterior to the bronchus intermedius. The confluence of right superior pulmonary veins overlaps the lower portion of the right pulmonary artery and contributes to its density. Superiorly and posteriorly, the comma-shaped left pulmonary artery passes above and behind the round or oval lucency representing the horizontally oriented left upper lobe bronchus, and then descends behind the left lower lobe bronchus. The confluence of left superior pulmonary veins, which lies behind the level of the right superior pulmonary vein, creates an opacity that occupies the posteroinferior aspect of the composite hilar shadow. The avascular aspect of the composite hilar density, inferior to the density of the right pulmonary artery and veins and anterior to the descending left pulmonary artery and left superior vein, is called the inferior hilar window. This region is roughly triangular in shape, with its apex at the junction of the left upper and lower lobe bronchi and its base directed anteriorly and inferiorly. The right middle lobe and lingular veins cross the inferior hilar window but, because of their small size, do not contribute significant opacity to this area.

The vascular structures of the composite hilar density are suspended around the central bronchi (Fig. 12.16). Beginning superiorly, the right upper lobe bronchus is seen in approximately 50% of individuals as an end-on round lucency at the upper margin of the composite hilar density. Recognition of this bronchus when not visible on prior radiographs should suggest a mass or lymph node enlargement about the bronchus. The posterior wall of the bronchus intermedius (intermediate stem line) is a thin vertical line, 2 mm or less in thickness, extending inferiorly from the posterior aspect of the right upper lobe bronchus. The intermediate stem line is seen in 95% of patients and extends inferiorly to bisect the end-on lucency of the left upper lobe bronchus on a properly positioned lateral film. This structure is rendered visible because air within the intermediate bronchus anteriorly and lung within the azygoesophageal recess posteriorly outlines its posterior wall. Thickening or nodularity of this line

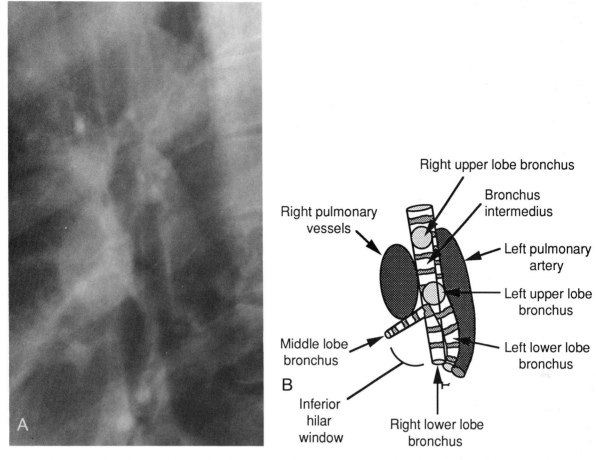

Figure 12.16. Normal Lateral Hilar Anatomy. A. Coned-down view of lateral radiograph. **B**. Diagram of lateral hilar anatomy.

is seen in bronchogenic carcinoma, pulmonary edema, or enlargement of azygoesophageal recess lymph nodes.

The left upper lobe bronchus, which is seen in 75% of individuals, lies no more than 4 cm directly inferior to the right upper lobe bronchus. This bronchus is visualized with greater frequency than the right upper lobe bronchus because it is silhouetted by the left pulmonary artery superiorly and posteriorly, the left superior pulmonary vein posteroinferiorly, and the superior aspect of the left atrium inferiorly, while the right upper lobe bronchus is contacted only by the right main pulmonary artery anteroinferiorly. The left upper lobe bronchus is identified by noting the concave anterior curvilinear density of the anterior wall of the left lower lobe bronchus extending inferiorly from its anteroinferior wall. The intersection of the posterior wall of the bronchus intermedius with the left upper lobe bronchus also helps identify the latter structure. Below the oval lucency of the left upper lobe bronchus, the basal trunk of the left lower lobe bronchus can sometimes be identified with its anterior wall visible as a white line, outlined by air in the bronchial lumen and air in the lung. The left lower lobe bronchus is

seen immediately below and continuous with the horizontal left upper lobe bronchus. The basal trunk bronchus of the right lower lobe lies slightly anterior to the left lower lobe bronchus and has a straight anterior wall. It may be seen extending inferiorly from the lucency of the right upper lobe bronchus, but is less commonly visualized than the left (8).

Pleural Anatomy

The pleura is a serosal membrane that envelopes the lung and lines the costal surface, diaphragm, and mediastinum. It is composed of two layers, the visceral and the parietal pleura, which join at the hilum. The parietal pleura is composed of a single layer of mesothelial cells that lies on a loose connective tissue containing systemic capillaries, lymphatic vessels, and sensory nerves. Deep to the parietal pleura is a dense connective tissue called the endothoracic fascia, composed of collagen and elastin, which lines the ribs and intercostal spaces. The visceral pleura is composed of five layers (beginning from the pleural space inward): (1) the mesothelial layer, (2) a thin connective tissue layer, (3) a strong connective tissue layer (the chief layer), composed of collagen and elas-

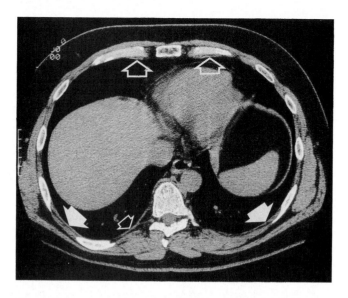

Figure 12.17. An HRCT of the Pleura. A 1.5-mm collimated HRCT scan through the lung bases demonstrates normal intercostal stripes (*solid arrows*) that are separated from the intercostal muscles by a layer of fat. An intercostal vein (*small open arrows*) is seen in the paravertebral region. Anteriorly, the transversus thoracic muscles (*large open arrows*) line the parasternal pleural surface.

tin, (4) a vascular (interstitial) layer, which contains blood vessels and lymphatics, and (5) the limiting membrane of the lung, which is connected to the strong connective tissue layer by collagen and elastin fibers. Blood supply to the parietal pleura is via the systemic circulation, while the visceral pleura is supplied by the pulmonary circulation. The parietal pleura is contiguous with the chest wall and diaphragm, and therefore extends deep posteriorly into the costophrenic sulci, while the visceral pleura is adherent to the surface of the lung. The pleural space is a potential space between the two pleural layers, and normally contains a small amount of fluid (<5 ml) that reduces friction during breathing.

The normal costal, diaphragmatic, and mediastinal pleura is not visible on plain radiographs or CT. On HRCT, a 1- to 2-mm stripe may be seen lining the intercostal spaces between adjacent ribs (Fig. 12.17). This "intercostal stripe" represents the combination of the two pleural layers, the endothoracic fascia, and the innermost intercostal muscle. Internal to the ribs, the normal pleura is not seen and the inner cortex of rib appears to contact the lung. The presence of soft tissue density between the inner rib and the lung, best appreciated on HRCT studies, indicates pleural thickening.

The normal radiographic and CT appearance of the fissures and the inferior pulmonary ligament was discussed earlier in this chapter in the sections on fissures and ligaments.

Chest Wall Anatomy

The radiographic anatomy of the soft tissues and bony structures of the chest wall were discussed in the section on the posteroanterior chest radiograph. Computed tomography provides detailed anatomic information about the normal chest wall and axillae. Although the bilateral symmetry of the chest wall on CT usually allows for the detection of pathologic conditions, a detailed knowledge of normal cross-sectional chest wall and axillary anatomy is the key to accurate localization and characterization of disease processes. The CT anatomy from six representative levels is shown in Figure 12.18.

Anatomy of the Diaphragm

The diaphragm is a musculotendinous membrane separating the thoracic and abdominal cavities. The diaphragmatic muscle arises anteriorly from the posterior aspect of the xiphoid process, anterolaterally, laterally, and posterolaterally from the 6th to 12th costal cartilages and ribs, and posteriorly from the upper 2 or 3 lumbar vertebrae and their transverse processes (Fig. 12.19). These muscles insert onto the central tendon of the diaphragm, which has right, left, and middle portions. The diaphragm has three normal and two potential gaps. The aortic hiatus lies in the midline immediately behind the diaphragmatic crura and anterior to the 12th thoracic vertebral body. The aorta, thoracic duct, and azygos and hemiazygos veins traverse this opening. The esophageal hiatus usually lies slighty to the left of midline, cephalad to the aortic hiatus, and transmits the esophagus and vagus nerves. The inferior vena cava pierces the central tendon of the diaphragm at the level of the eighth thoracic intervertebral disc space. The foramina of Morgagni are triangular gaps in the muscles of the anteromedial diaphragm. This cleft is normally occupied by fat and the internal mammary vessels; it is a site of potential intrathoracic herniation of abdominal contents. The foramina of Bochdalek are defects in the closure of the posterolateral diaphragm at the junction of the pleuroperitoneal membrane with the septum transversum. Hernias through the foramina of Morgagni and Bochdalek are discussed in Chapter 16.

The radiographic appearance of the diaphragms on frontal and lateral chest radiographs is discussed in preceding sections. The domes of the diaphragms appear as rounded densities on either side of the chest on CT scans at the level of the base of the heart. Inferiorly, the central portion of the diaphragm is intimately apposed to the liver on the right and the stomach and spleen on the left, while the lungs and pleural surfaces surround the diaphragms peripherally. At this level the diaphragm is most commonly seen as

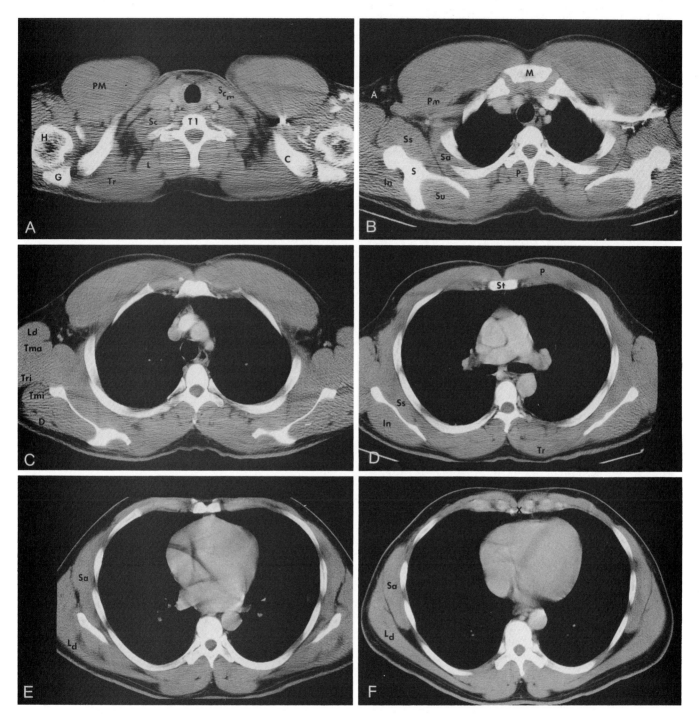

Figure 12.18. Normal Chest Wall Anatomy on CT. A. Level of thoracic inlet. *PM*, pectoralis major muscle; *Tr*, trapezius; *L*, levator scapulae muscle; *Sc*, scalene muscle; *Scm*, sternocleiodomastoid muscle; *H*, humeral head; *G*, glenoid; *C*, distal clavicle; *T1*, first thoracic vertebral body. **B**. Level of axillary vessels. *Pm*, pectoralis minor muscle; *Sa*, serratus anterior muscle; *Su*, supraspinatus muscle; *In*, infraspinatus muscle; *Ss*, subscapularis muscle; *P*, paraspinal muscles; *M*, manubrium of sternum; *S*, body of scapula; *A*, axilla with normal lymph nodes. **C**. Level of sternomanubrial joint. *Ld*, latissimus dorsi muscle; *Tma*, teres major muscle; *Tri*, long head of triceps muscle; *Tmi*, teres minor muscle; *D*, deltoid muscles. **D**. Level of body of sternum. *P*, pectoralis muscles; *Ss*, subscapularis muscle; *In*, infraspinatus muscle; *Tr*, trapezius muscle; *St*, body of sternum. **E**. Level of tip of scapula. *Ld*, latissimus dorsi muscle, *Sa*, serratus anterior muscle. **F**. Level of xiphoid process. *Ld*, latissimus dorsi muscle; *Sa*, serratus anterior muscle; *X*, xiphoid process of sternum.

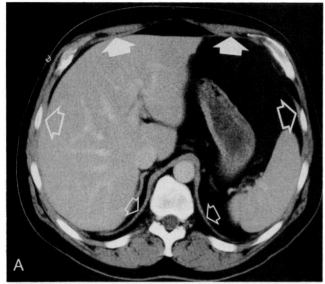

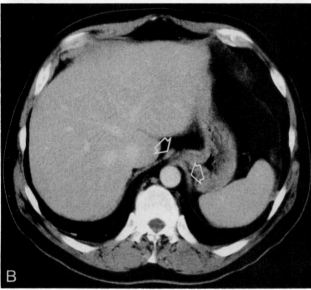

Figure 12.19. Normal Anatomy of the Diaphragm on CT. A scan through the upper abdomen (**A**) demonstrates the diaphragmatic crura posteriorly (*small open arrows*), the costal origins of the diaphragm laterally (*large open arrows*), and the costal cartilaginous origins anterolaterally (*solid arrows*). More inferiorly (**B**), the esophageal hiatus is seen between the crura (*open arrows*).

slips of diaphragmatic muscle. This appearance is seen with increasing frequency in older patients, and is more common on the left than the right. Posteriorly, the superior aspects of the diaphragmatic crura are seen. The crura are curvilinear densities that arise from the upper two to three lumbar vertebrae and transverse processes, coursing superiorly and anteriorly to insert onto the central tendon of the diaphragm (Fig. 12.19**A**). The esophageal and aortic hiatus and their contents are well visualized on CT (Fig. 12.19**B**). Continuing inferiorly into the upper abdomen, the inferior aspects of the diaphragmatic crura are seen arising from the upper lumbar vertebra. At this level, the crura may have a rounded appearance in cross-section and should not be mistaken for enlarged retrocrural lymph nodes. Review of contiguous CT images will allow for proper identification of these structures.

References

1. Lee JKT, Sagel SS, Stanley RJ. Computed body tomography with MR correlation. 2nd ed. New York: Raven Press, 1989: 5–8.
2. Webb WR, Sostrman HD. MR imaging of thoracic disease: clinical uses. Radiology 1992;182:621–631.
3. Klein JS, Schultz S. Interventional chest radiology. Curr Probl Diagn Radiol 1992;21:223–264.
4. Stark P. Radiology of the trachea. 1st ed. New York: Thieme, 1991:1–4.
5. Webb WR, Muller NL, Naidich DP. High-resolution CT of the lung. 1st ed. New York:Raven Press, 1992:15–22.
6. Weibel ER. Looking into the lung: what can it tell us? AJR 1979;133:1021–1031.
7. Woodring JH, Daniel TL. Mediastinal analysis emphasizing plain radiographs and computed tomograms. Med Radiogr Photogr 1986;62:2–46.
8. Proto AV, Speckman JM. The left lateral radiograph of the chest. Med Radiogr Photogr 1979;55:30–74.
9. Proto AV, Speckman JM. The left lateral radiograph of the chest. Med Radiogr Photogr 1980;56:38–63.
10. Heitzman ER. The mediastinum. 2nd ed. Berlin: Springer Verlag, 1988:45–74.
11. Gamsu G. The mediastinum. In: Moss AA, Gamsu G, Genant HK, eds. Computed tomography of the body with magnetic resonance imaging. Vol 1: thorax and neck. 2nd edition. Philadelphia: WB Saunders, 1992:51–56.
12. Fraser RG, Pare JAP, Pare PD, Fraser RS, Genereux GP. Diagnosis of diseases of the chest. Vol 1. 3rd ed. Philadelphia: WB Saunders,:86–127.

smooth, thin, curvilinear density. In some patients scanned on deep inspiration, the diaphragm has an undulating or nodular appearance from contraction of

13

The Mediastinum

Jeffrey S. Klein
Jeffrey L. Groffsky

This chapter will review the radiologic approach to mediastinal masses, disorders of the trachea and central bronchi, and diffuse mediastinal disease.

MEDIASTINAL MASSES

Localized mediastinal abnormalities are common diagnostic challenges for the radiologist. Patients with mediastinal masses tend to present in one of two fashions: with symptoms related to local mass effect or invasion of adjacent mediastinal structures (e.g., stridor in a patient with thyroid goiter), or incidentally with an abnormality on routine chest radiograph. Occasionally, a mediastinal mass is discovered in the course of an evaluation for known malignancy (e.g., a patient with non-Hodgkin's lymphoma) or for a condition such as myasthenia gravis, in which there is an association with thymoma.

Posteroanterior and lateral chest radiographs are the initial studies obtained in all patients. Mediastinal masses are recognized on frontal radiographs by the presence of a soft-tissue density that causes unilateral or bilateral displacement of the normal lung-mediastinal interface or displaces adjacent mediastinal structures. The lung-mass interface typically is well defined laterally where it is convex with the adjacent lung, and it creates obtuse angles with the lung at its superior and inferior margins. This latter characteristic is diagnostic of an extrapulmonary, intramediastinal lesion, although the occasional medial pleural mass may be indistinguishable from a mediastinal lesion. Lateral displacement of trachea or heart may be seen with large mediastinal masses, sometimes first recognized by displacement of an indwelling endotracheal tube, nasogastric tube, or intravascular catheter. The presence of calcification, fat, or, rarely, a fat-fluid level (as in a cystic teratoma) can limit the differential diagnosis of a mediastinal mass.

Virtually every patient with a mediastinal mass will have thoracic computed tomography (CT) or magnetic resonance imaging (MR) performed. Recent literature describes the use of transthoracic ultrasound in the evaluation of anterior mediastinal masses, but this is not used routinely at most institutions. These cross-sectional modalities provide invaluable information to the radiologist. Their utility in the evaluation of mediastinal masses is summarized in Table 13.1.

Table 13.1. Utility of CT and MR in the Evaluation of Mediastinal Masses

Indication for Study	Modalities[a]
Confirming the presence of a mass vs. tortuous vascular structures	CT = MR
Localization of mass to anterior, middle, or posterior compartment	CT = MR
Suspected aneurysm or vascular anomaly	MR >CT
Tissue characterization of mass	
Detection of fluid	CT = MR = US (for anterior masses)
Detection of calcium	CT
Distinction of tumor from fibrosis	MR
Relationship to adjacent structures	
Vascular invasion	CT = MR
Tracheal involvement	CT >MR
Involvement of spinal canal	MR >CT
Thoracic inlet lesions	MR >CT
Contraindication to iodinated contrast	MR >CT
Percutaneous biopsy of mediastinal mass	CT (US for anterior mediastinal masses)

[a]US, ultrasound.

Table 13.2. Thoracic Inlet Masses

Thyroid mass	Goiter
	Malignancy
	Thyromegaly due to thyroiditis
Parathyroid mass	Hyperplasia
	Adenoma
	Carcinoma
Lymph node mass	Lymphoma
	Hodgkin's disease
	Non-Hodgkin's
	Metastases
	Inflammatory
	Tuberculosis
Lymphangioma	

The two most important pieces of information that the radiologist can provide are whether the mass is of vascular origin and in which mediastinal compartment the predominant portion of the mass resides. The vascular origin of a mediastinal mass is readily appreciated on contrast-enhanced CT, MR, and occasionally, transthoracic or transesophageal ultrasound. As detailed in Chapter 12, many schemes have been proposed to divide the mediastinum into compartments. While recognizing that these divisions are arbitrary and do not represent actual anatomic barriers, and while acknowledging that most mediastinal masses do not lie solely within a single compartment, this division is useful in limiting the differential diagnosis and guiding further diagnostic evaluation. For example, most posterior mediastinal masses, particularly in children, are of neurogenic origin; not uncommonly, these masses will involve the spine. The identification of a posterior mediastinal mass on chest radiographs should lead to an MR study as the examination of choice. For the purposes of the following discussion, the mediastinum is divided into superior and inferior components, with the inferior mediastinum subdivided vertically into anterior, middle, and posterior compartments as described in Chapter 12.

Thoracic Inlet Masses

The thoracic inlet is the region of the upper thorax marginated by the first rib and represents the junction between the neck and thorax. Masses in this region commonly present as neck masses or with symptoms of upper airway obstruction due to tracheal compression. Thyroid masses, lymphomatous nodes, and lymphangiomas are the most common thoracic inlet masses (Table 13.2).

THYROID MASSES

In a small percentage of patients with a cervical thyroid goiter, a thyroid carcinoma, or an enlarged gland from thyroiditis, extension of the thyroid through the thoracic inlet into the superior mediasti-

num may occur. These lesions are usually discovered as incidental findings on chest radiographs; a minority of patients will present with complaints of dyspnea or dysphagia due to tracheal or esophageal compression by the mass. Thyroid goiters arising from the lower pole of the thyroid or the thyroid isthmus can enter the superior mediastinum anterior to the trachea (80%) or to the right and posterolateral to the trachea (20%).

On conventional chest radiographs, an antero-superior mediastinal mass typically deviates the trachea laterally and either posteriorly (anterior masses) or anteriorly (posterior masses) (Fig. 13.1). Coarse, clumped calcifications are common in thyroid goiters. Radioiodine studies should be performed as the initial imaging procedure, although false-negatives do occur. Computed tomography usually shows characteristic findings: (a) well-defined margins, (b) continuity of the mass with the cervical thyroid, (c) coarse calcifications, (d) cystic or necrotic areas, (e) baseline high CT attenuation (due to intrinsic iodine content), and (f) intense enhancement (>25 HU units due to the hypervascularity of most thyroid masses) and prolonged enhancement (due to active uptake of iodine from contrast media) following intravenous contrast administration (Fig. 13.1) (1).

LYMPHANGIOMAS

These uncommon masses are tumors comprised of dilated lymphatic channels. The cystic or cavernous form (cystic hygroma) is most commonly discovered in infancy and is often associated with chromosomal abnormalities including Turner's syndrome and trisomies 13, 18, and 21. In infants, these lesions tend to extend from the neck into the anterior mediastinum; less commonly they may arise primarily within the anterior mediastinum in older patients. Histologically these tumors are composed of cystic spaces lined by epithelium containing clear, straw-colored fluid. Although these lesions are benign histologically, they tend to insinuate themselves between vascular structures and the trachea. This makes complete surgical resection of lymphangiomas difficult, and they frequently recur. Computed tomography demonstrates a well-defined cystic mass within the thoracic inlet or superior mediastinum. Magnetic resonance typically shows the masses to have high signal intensity on T2-weighted images because of their fluid content.

Anterior Mediastinal Masses

There are a number of neoplasms and nonneoplastic conditions that arise in the anterior mediastinum and produce anterior mediastinal masses. These include thymic neoplasms, lymphoma, germ cell neo-

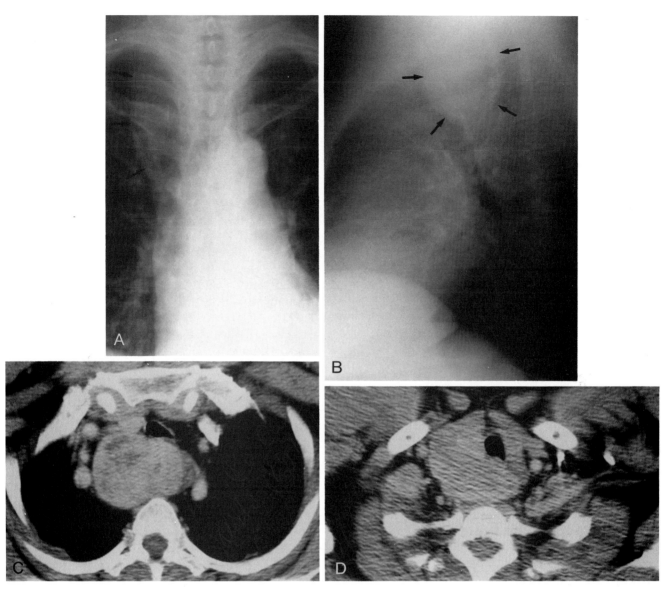

Figure 13.1. Thyroid Goiter. Posteroanterior (PA) (**A**) and lateral (**B**) radiographs shows a right superior mediastinal mass (*arrows*) compressing the tracheal air column posteriorly. Contrast-enhanced CT scan at the level of the sternoclavicular joints (**C**) shows an in-

homogeneously enhancing retrotracheal mass displacing the trachea and narrowing its lumen. Superiorly (**D**), the mass is contiguous with the right lobe of an enlarged thyroid gland.

plasms, and primary mesenchymal tumors (Table 13.3).

THYMIC MASSES

Thymoma is the second most common primary mediastinal neoplasm after lymphoma in adults. It is a neoplasm that arises from thymic epithelium and contains varying numbers of intermixed lymphocytes. The admixture of epithelial cells and lymphocytes, which varies with each tumor, gives rise to the histologic subtyping of thymoma as predominantly lymphocytic, mixed lymphoepithelial, and predominantly epithelial types. In the predominantly lymphocytic form, in which there are few interspersed epithelial tumor cells, the histologic differentiation from lym-

phoma may be difficult. There is no correlation between the histologic features of thymoma and malignant behavior; surgical and pathologic evidence of capsular and local invasion is the best predictor.

The average age at diagnosis of thymoma is 45–50; these lesions are rare in patients under the age of 20. While most often associated with myasthenia gravis, thymoma has been associated with other autoimmune diseases such as pure red cell aplasia and hypogammaglobulinemia. Ten to 28% of patients with myasthenia gravis have a thymoma, while a larger percentage of patients with thymoma (30–54%) have or will develop myasthenia.

On chest radiographs, thymomas are seen as round or oval, smooth or lobulated, soft-tissue masses

Table 13.3. Anterior Mediastinal Masses

Thymic masses	Thymoma
	Thymic cyst
	Thymolipoma
	Thymic hyperplasia
	Thymic neuroendocrine tumors
	Thymic carcinoma
	Thymic lymphoma
Lymphoma	Hodgkin's disease
	Non-Hodgkin's
Germ cell neoplasms	Teratoma
	Seminoma
	Embryonal cell carcinoma
	Endodermal sinus tumor
	Choriocarcinoma
Thyroid mass	Goiter
	Tumor
	Thyroiditis
Ectopic parathyroid mass	Hyperplasia
	Adenoma
	Carcinoma
Mesenchymal tumor	Lipoma
	Hemangioma
	Leiomyoma
	Liposarcoma
	Angiosarcoma

arising near the origin of the great vessels at the base of the heart (Fig. 13.2). Computed tomography is best for characterizing thymomas and detecting local invasion preoperatively. Cystic areas are not uncommon, and calcification is detected in 25% of cases (Fig. 13.2) (2). Invasion of tumor through the thymic capsule ("invasive" or "malignant" thymoma) is present in 33–50% of patients. In the majority of these patients, this determination cannot be made by CT or MR and may even be difficult to determine on examination of the resected specimen. Local invasion of pleura, lung, pericardium, chest wall, diaphragm, and great vessels occurs in decreasing order of frequency in approximately 10–15% of patients. Contiguity of a thymoma with the adjacent chest wall or mediastinal structures cannot be used as reliable evidence of invasion of these structures. Drop metastases to dependent portions of the pleural space are a recognized route of spread of thymoma that has invaded the pleura. Extrathoracic metastases are rare, although transdiaphragmatic spread of pleural tumor into the retroperitoneum has been described. For these reasons, it is important to image the entire thorax and upper abdomen in any patient with suspected invasive disease.

In patients with myasthenia gravis being evaluated for thymoma, CT can demonstrate tumors that are invisible on conventional radiographs. However, very small thymic tumors may not be distinguishable from a normal or hyperplastic gland with CT, particularly in younger patients with a large amount of residual thymic tissue.

Thymic Cysts may represent congenital or acquired lesions. Congenital thymic cysts contain thin or gelatinous fluid, and are characterized histologically by an epithelial lining with thymic tissue in the cyst wall. The latter feature distinguishes thymic cysts histologically from other congenital cystic lesions within the anterior mediastinum. Acquired thymic cysts have been associated with previous thoracotomy and concurrent or previously treated Hodgkin disease. Large cysts will be evident as soft-tissue masses on conventional radiographs, and CT or MR will demonstrate the cystic nature of the lesion. A history of Hodgkin's disease or confirmatory needle aspiration of the cyst will allow conservative management in most patients. If the distinction between a true thymic cyst and cystic degeneration of a thymoma, lymphoma, or germ cell neoplasm is impossible on clinical and radiographic grounds, the lesion should undergo biopsy or resection.

Thymolipoma is a rare, benign thymic neoplasm that consists primarily of fat with intermixed rests of normal thymic tissue. These masses are asymptomatic and therefore are typically large when first detected. Chest radiographs show a large anterior mediastinal mass that, because of its pliable nature, tends to envelope the heart and diaphragm. Computed tomography demonstrates a fatty mass with scattered soft-tissue densities. Resection is curative.

Thymic Carcinoid. Neuroendocrine tumors of the thymus are rare malignant neoplasms believed to arise from thymic cells of neural crest origin (APUD or Kulchitsky cells). The most common histologic type is carcinoid tumor that, as with similar lesions arising within the bronchi, ranges in differentiation and behavior from typical carcinoid to atypical carcinoid to small cell carcinoma. Approximately 25% of patients have Cushing's syndrome as a result of corticotropin secretion by the tumor; these patients tend to have smaller lesions at the time of diagnosis since they present early with signs of corticosteroid excess. The carcinoid syndrome is uncommon. This lesion is indistinguishable from thymoma on plain radiographs and CT scan.

Thymic Hyperplasia is defined as enlargement of a thymus that is normal on gross and histologic examination. This rare entity occurs primarily in children and is most likely a rebound effect in response to an antecedent stress, discontinuation of chemotherapy, or treatment of hypercortisolism. An association with Graves' disease has also been noted. The term "thymic hyperplasia" has been used incorrectly to describe the histologic findings of lymphoid follicular hyperplasia of the thymus found in 60% of patients with myasthenia gravis. In contrast to most cases of true thymic hyperplasia, lymphoid hyperplasia does not produce thymic enlargement. Most patients with

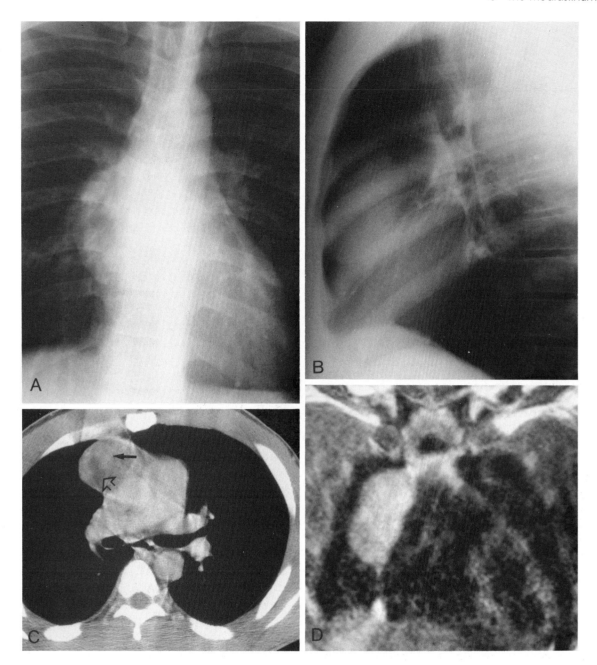

Figure 13.2.   Thymoma. Posteroanterior (**A**) and lateral (**B**) radiographs reveal a lower right anterior mediastinal mass. A CT scan (**C**) shows a mass with solid (*solid arrow*) and cystic (*open arrow*) components. Coronal MR (TR = 500, TE = 40) (**D**) shows a well-defined right-sided mass of intermediate signal intensity. This is a surgically proven noninvasive thymoma.

thymic hyperplasia have normal or diffusely enlarged glands on CT; occasionally, thymic hyperplasia will present as a mass that is radiographically indistinguishable from thymoma. Most cases can be resolved by noting a decrease in size on follow-up studies, thereby obviating the need for biopsy.

Thymic carcinoma is a rare malignant neoplasm of the thymus diagnosed when the epithelial elements of a thymic mass show characteristic findings of cellular atypia and numerous mitoses. This lesion is distinguished from invasive thymoma that, although malignant in behavior, lacks the histologic and cyto-

logic features of carcinoma. The most common histologic subtype is squamous cell carcinoma. Most thymic carcinomas are solid lesions that on CT or MR have invaded the mediastinum or lung at the time of diagnosis.

Thymic Lymphoma. The thymus is involved in 40–50% of patients with the nodular sclerosing subtype of Hodgkin's disease. The radiographic appearance is indistinguishable from other solid neoplasms arising within the thymus. The presence of lymph node enlargement in other portions of the mediastinum or anterior chest wall involvement, best seen on

T2-weighted MR images, should help suggest the diagnosis.

LYMPHOMA

Lymphoma, either Hodgkin's disease or non-Hodgkin's lymphoma (NHL), is the most common primary mediastinal neoplasm in adults. Hodgkin's disease involves the thorax in 85% of patients at the time of presentation. The majority (90%) of patients with intrathoracic involvement have mediastinal lymph node enlargement; this most commonly involves the superior mediastinal (prevascular and paratracheal), internal mammary, and hilar nodal groups. The superior mediastinum is the most frequent site of a localized nodal mass in patients with Hodgkin's disease, particularly those with the nodular sclerosing type (Fig. 13.3) (3). Enlargement of mediastinal nodes without

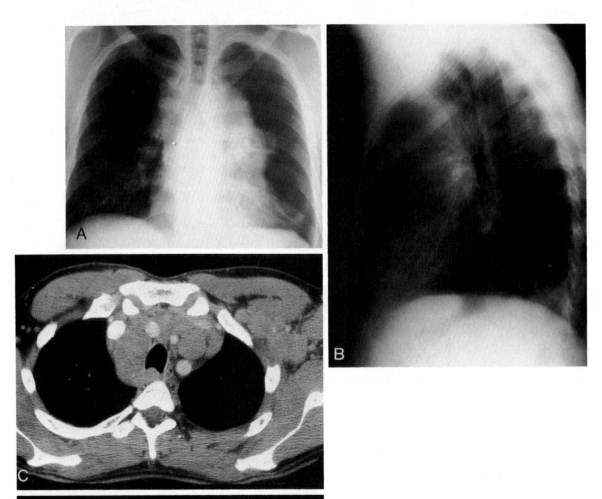

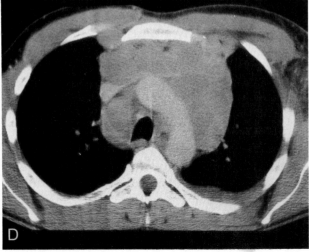

Figure 13.3.   Hodgkin's Lymphoma. Posteroanterior (**A**) and lateral (**B**) films in a 38-year-old male demonstrate a lobulated mass occupying both anterior and middle mediastinum and a small left pleural effusion. A CT (**C**) shows enlarged prevascular, paratracheal, and left axillary lymph nodes. More inferiorly (**D**) there is marked prevascular, internal mammary, and bilateral paratracheal lymph node enlargement.

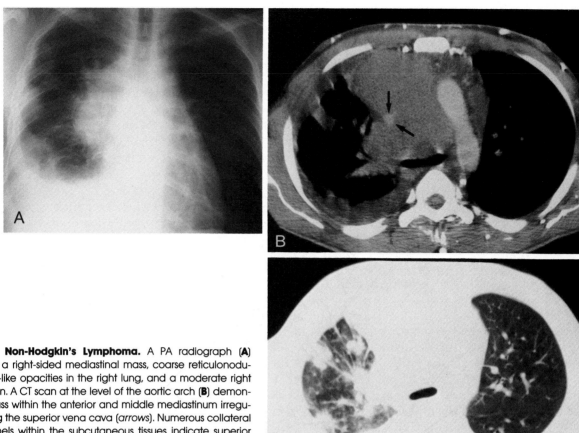

Figure 13.4. Non-Hodgkin's Lymphoma. A PA radiograph **(A)** demonstrates a right-sided mediastinal mass, coarse reticulonodular, and mass-like opacities in the right lung, and a moderate right pleural effusion. A CT scan at the level of the aortic arch **(B)** demonstrates the mass within the anterior and middle mediastinum irregularly narrowing the superior vena cava (*arrows*). Numerous collateral venous channels within the subcutaneous tissues indicate superior vena cava syndrome. A scan at a slightly higher level **(C)** viewed at lung windows shows linear and irregular nodular parenchymal opacities representing lymphomatous involvement of lung.

concomitant superior mediastinal disease should suggest an alternative diagnosis. Isolated mediastinal lymph node enlargement is seen in only 25% of all patients with Hodgkin's disease. Non-Hodgkin's lymphoma involves the thorax in 40% of patients at presentation. In contrast to Hodgkin's disease, only 50% of patients with NHL and intrathoracic disease have mediastinal nodal involvement; in only 10% of all patients with NHL is the disease limited to the mediastinum (Fig. 13.4). Lymphoma involving a single mediastinal or hilar nodal group is much more common in NHL than in Hodgkin's disease. Non-Hodgkin's lymphoma most commonly involves middle mediastinal and hilar lymph nodes; juxtaphrenic and posterior mediastinal nodal involvement is uncommon but is seen exclusively in NHL. Patterns of pulmonary parenchymal involvement in lymphoma are discussed in the section on parenchymal malignancies in Chapter 15.

While Hodgkin's disease spreads in a fairly predictable pattern from one nodal group to an adjacent group, NHL is believed to be a multifocal disorder where patterns of involvement are unpredictable. Localized intrathoracic Hodgkin's disease is usually treated with radiation therapy, with 90% response rates. More widespread Hodgkin's disease and NHL

are treated with chemotherapy, with better response rates for Hodgkin's disease than for NHL.

On plain radiographs, lymphoma involving the anterior mediastinum typically presents as a lobulated mass projecting to one or both sides (Fig. 13.4). Calcification in untreated lymphoma is extremely uncommon, and its presence within an anterior mediastinal mass should suggest another diagnosis. The plain film appearance of lymphoma is usually indistinguishable from thymoma or germ cell neoplasm. Involvement of other lymph nodes in the mediastinum or hila makes lymphoma more likely. An enlarged spleen displacing the gastric air bubble medially, seen in the upper abdominal portion of the frontal chest film, provides an additional clue to the diagnosis.

Computed tomography is performed in virtually all patients with lymphoma. The advantages of chest CT include the ability to better characterize and localize masses seen on chest radiographs; detection of subradiographic sites of involvement that can alter disease staging, prognosis, and therapy; guidance for transthoracic or open biopsy; monitoring response to therapy; and detecting relapse. The appearance of nodal involvement in lymphoma varies; most commonly, discrete enlarged solid lymph nodes or conglomerate masses of nodes are seen (Fig. 13.4**B**). Central necrosis, seen in 20% of patients, has no prognostic significance. Nodal calcification is rare in the absence of previous mediastinal radiation or systemic chemotherapy. Parenchymal involvement is usually the result of direct extranodal extension of tumor from hilar nodes along the bronchovascular lymphatics; this is better appreciated on axial CT images than on chest radiographs (Fig. 13.4**C**). Likewise, tumor extending from the mediastinum to the pericardium, subpleural space, and chest wall is best appreciated on CT or MR. On MR, untreated lymphoma appears as a mass of uniform low signal intensity on T1-weighted images, and uniform high signal intensity or intermixed areas of low and high signal intensity on T2-weighted images. The areas of low signal intensity on T2-weighted scans of untreated patients may be because of foci of fibrotic tissue in nodular sclerosing Hodgkin's disease.

Both CT and MR have been used to monitor the response of lymphoma to therapy. While CT can accurately assess tumor regression and detect relapse within nodal groups outside the treated region, the ability to distinguish residual tumor from sterilized fibrotic masses is limited. Residual soft-tissue masses have been reported in up to 50% of patients, most commonly with nodular sclerosing Hodgkin's disease, and are more common when the pretreatment mass is large. Some patients with residual masses on CT or MR will have tumor recurrence within 6–12 months following the completion of therapy. Recently, the MR signal characteristics of lymphomatous masses have been studied in an attempt to differentiate residual fibrotic masses from recurrent tumor. In general, the appearance of high signal intensity regions on T2-weighted images more than 6 months after treatment should suggest recurrence.

GERM CELL NEOPLASMS

Germ cell neoplasms, which include teratoma, seminoma, choriocarcinoma, endodermal sinus tumor, and embryonal cell carcinoma, arise from collections of primitive germ cells that arrest in the anterior mediastinum on their journey to the gonads during embryologic development. Since they are histologically indistinguishable from germ cell tumors arising in the testes and ovaries, the diagnosis of a primary malignant mediastinal germ cell neoplasm requires exclusion of a primary gonadal tumor as a source of mediastinal metastases. A key in distinguishing primary from metastatic mediastinal germ cell neoplasm is the presence of retroperitoneal lymph node involvement in primary gonadal tumors.

The most common benign mediastinal germ cell neoplasm is teratoma. Teratomas may be cystic or solid. Cystic or mature teratoma is the most common

type of teratoma seen in the mediastinum. In contrast to a dermoid cyst, which is an ovarian neoplasm containing only elements derived from the ectodermal germinal layer, a cystic teratoma of the mediastinum commonly contains tissues of ectodermal, mesodermal, and endodermal origins. For this reason, it is inaccurate to use the term "dermoid cyst" to describe cystic mediastinal germ cell neoplasms. Solid teratomas are usually malignant. Most germ cell neoplasms are detected in patients in the 3rd or 4th decade of life. While benign tumors have a slight female preponderance (female:male = 60:40%), malignant tumors are seen almost exclusively in men.

Radiographically, these tumors have a distribution similar to that of thymomas. While the majority are located in the anterior mediastinum, up to 10% are found in the posterior mediastinum. Benign lesions are often round or oval and smooth in contour; an irregular, lobulated, or ill-defined margin suggests malignancy. Calcification is present in 33–50% but is nonspecific unless in the form of a tooth. At CT, benign teratomas are usually cystic and may contain soft tissue, bone, teeth, fat or, rarely, fat-fluid levels. Seminoma, choriocarcinoma, and endodermal sinus (yolk sac) tumors are malignant lesions seen primarily in young men. Seminoma is the most common malignant germ cell neoplasm, accounting for 30% of these tumors. The radiographic findings are nonspecific. Computed tomography typically shows a large, lobulated, soft-tissue mass that may contain areas of hemorrhage, calcification, or necrosis (Fig. 13.5) (4). Elevated serum α-fetoprotein levels are present in virtually all patients with endodermal sinus tumors, and are useful markers for following tumor response. Similarly, two-thirds of patients with choriocarcinoma will have elevated levels of serum human chorionic gonadotropin. Clinical and CT evidence of gynecomastia are useful clues to the diagnosis.

THYROID MASSES

While masses arising from the thyroid can present as anterior and superior mediastinal masses, these lesions are best considered as thoracic inlet masses and have been discussed in the section by that name.

PARATHYROID MASSES

In approximately 2% of patients, the parathyroid glands fail to separate from the thymus in the neck and descend with the gland into the anterosuperior mediastinum. These glands can be found near the thoracic inlet in or about the thymus. This becomes important in the small percentage of patients with persistent clinical and biochemical evidence of hyperparathyroidism following routine neck exploration and parathyroidectomy. Most of these ectopic para-

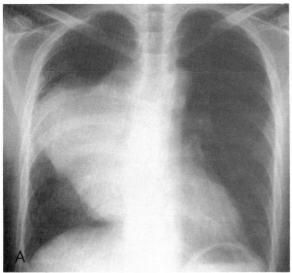
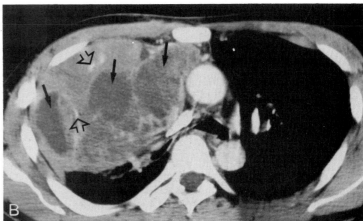

Figure 13.5. Malignant Teratoma. A PA chest radiograph (**A**) in a 31-year-old man demonstrates a large right mediastinal mass extending laterally to the chest wall and a small pleural effusion. A contrast-enhanced CT scan (**B**) shows a soft-tissue mass occupying most of the right upper thorax displacing and compressing the superior vena cava and right upper lobe bronchus. There are large areas of necrosis (*solid arrows*) and scattered foci of calcification (*open arrows*) within the mass. The surgical specimen revealed a malignant teratoma.

thyroid lesions are small (<3 cm) adenomas; they rarely represent hyperplastic glands or parathyroid carcinoma. While plain radiographs are usually normal, contrast-enhanced CT or MR can detect the majority of mediastinal parathyroid adenomas when ultrasound and nuclear medicine studies have failed to localize a lesion in the neck. Computed tomography typically shows a small, well-defined soft tissue nodule in the prevascular space. The MR features of parathyroid adenoma are fairly characteristic, with low signal intensity on T1-weighted images and a marked increase in signal on T2-weighted images.

MESENCHYMAL TUMORS

Benign and malignant tumors arising from the fibrous, fatty, muscular, or vascular tissues of the mediastinum may present as mediastinal masses, most commonly in the anterior mediastinum. Lipomas can occur in any location in the mediastinum but are most often anterior. The diagnosis is made by recognition of a well-defined mass of uniform fatty attenuation (< −50 HU). The presence of soft-tissue elements should raise the possibility of a thymolipoma or liposarcoma; the latter may show evidence of invasion of adjacent structures at the time of diagnosis. Fat within a mature teratoma or transdiaphragmatic herniation of omental fat is usually easily distinguished from a lipoma.

Hemangiomas are benign tumors composed of vascular channels that may be associated with the syndrome of hereditary hemorrhagic telangiectasia. A pathognomonic sign on chest radiographs is the recognition of phleboliths within a smooth or lobulated soft-tissue mass. Angiosarcomas are rare malignant vascular neoplasms that are indistinguishable from other invasive neoplasms arising within the anterior mediastinum.

Leiomyomas are rare benign neoplasms that arise from smooth muscle within the mediastinum. Similarly, fibromas and mesenchymomas (tumors that contain more than one mesenchymal element) can appear as anterior mediastinal masses.

Middle Mediastinal Masses (Table 13.4)

LYMPH NODE ENLARGEMENT AND MASSES

Most middle mediastinal lymph node masses are malignant, representing metastases from bronchogenic carcinoma, extrathoracic malignancy, or lymphoma. Benign causes of middle mediastinal lymph node enlargement include sarcoidosis, mycobacterial and fungal infection, angiofollicular lymph node hyperplasia (Castleman's disease), and angioimmunoblastic lymphadenopathy.

On plain radiographs, several findings can suggest that a middle mediastinal mass represents lymph node enlargement. The presence of multiple bilateral mediasinal masses that distort the lung-mediastinal interface is relatively specific for lymph node enlargement. Solitary masses resulting from lymph node enlargement tend to be elongated and lobulated rather than spherical, since usually more than a single node in a vertical chain of nodes is involved. Occasionally, calcification can be detected within enlarged lymph nodes on plain radiographs; CT is more sensitive in

Table 13.4.   Middle Mediastinal Masses

Lymph node masses	Malignancy
	Bronchogenic carcinoma
	Lymphoma
	Leukemia (CLL)
	Kaposi's sarcoma
	Extrathoracic malignancy
	Head and neck tumors (squamous
	cell carcinoma of skin, larynx,
	thyroid carcinoma)
	Genitourinary tumors (renal cell
	carcinoma, seminoma)
	Breast carcinoma
	Melanoma
	Infection
	Bacteria
	Anaerobic lung abscess
	Anthrax
	Plague
	Tularemia
	Tuberculosis
	Fungi
	Histoplasmosis
	Coccidioidomycosis
	Cryptococcosis
	Viral infection
	Measles
	Mononucleosis
	Idiopathic
	Sarcoidosis
	Castleman's disease
	Angioimmunoblastic lymphadenopathy
Foregut and mesothelial cysts	Bronchogenic cyst
	Pericardial cyst
Tracheal and central bronchial neoplasms	Malignant
	Carcinoid tumor (bronchi)
	Adenoid cystic carcinoma (trachea)
	Squamous cell carcinoma
Diaphragmatic hernias	Foramen of Morgagni hernia
	Traumatic hernia
Vascular lesions	Arterial
	Double arch/right arch
	Tortuous innominate/subclavian artery
	Aneurysm of the aortic arch
	Venous
	Dilated azygous vein
	Dilated hemiazygous vein
	Dilated superior vena cava
	Left-sided superior vena cava
	Dilated left superior intercostal vein
	Dilation of the main pulmonary artery

detecting nodal calcification and its distribution within lymph nodes, as will be described.

One of the prime indications for performing thoracic CT is to detect the presence of enlarged mediastinal lymph nodes. Computed tomography is most often obtained to confirm an abnormal chest radiographic finding or to evaluate a patient with suspected mediastinal disease despite normal radiographs (e.g., a patient with a suspicious solitary pulmonary nodule or with cervical Hodgkin's disease). The ability of CT to image in the axial plane and its inherent high-contrast reso-lution allows for the recognition of abnormally enlarged lymph nodes not evident on chest radiographs. In general, abnormal lymph nodes are seen as round or oval soft-tissue masses that measure more than 1.0 cm in their short axis diameter. However, CT is unable to distinguish between benign inflammatory nodes and those involved by malignancy based upon size criteria alone. Attempts at tissue characterization of enlarged mediastinal lymph nodes by MR have thus far proven unsuccessful. Magnetic resonance imaging is as sensitive as CT in detecting enlarged mediastinal lymph nodes. Advantages of MR include the absence of iodinated contrast, easy distinction between vascular and soft-tissue structures, exquisite contrast resolution between mediastinal nodes and fat on T1-weighted sequences, and the ability to image in the direct coronal or sagittal plane. The latter feature is an advantage in those mediastinal regions that parallel the axial plane (subcarinal space, aortopulmonary window) and therefore tend to suffer from partial volume averaging effects on CT (Fig. 13.6). The major disadvantages of MR at present are the inability to detect nodal calcification, high cost, and limited spatial resolution; the latter can result in an inability to distinguish between a group of normal-sized nodes and a single enlarged node, thereby leading to false-positive results.

A standardized classification system for hilar and mediastinal lymph nodes has recently been advanced by the American Thoracic Society (Fig. 13.7) (5). This scheme correlates with easily identifiable CT and anatomic landmarks, and is most important when reporting lymph node enlargement in patients with bronchogenic carcinoma.

In addition to detecting enlarged mediastinal lymph nodes, CT can also provide information about the internal density of these nodes. While this may not allow distinction between benign and malignant etiologies or provide a specific diagnosis, these characteristics help limit the differential diagnosis of lymph node enlargement. Central nodal calcification is most commonly seen in patients with tuberculosis or fungal infection; rarely, metastatic mucinous adenocarcinoma of the bowel can produce nodal calcification. Peripheral (eggshell) nodal calcification is seen predominantly in silicosis and sarcoidosis. Hypervascular lymph nodes as depicted on contrast-enhanced CT can be seen in carcinoid tumor, small cell carcinoma of lung, Kaposi's sarcoma, and metastases from renal cell or thyroid carcinoma. Nonmalignant conditions that can produce vascular nodal enlargement include Castleman's disease and sarcoidosis. Central necrosis within enlarged nodes is most often seen with mycobacterial infection; additional causes include metastatic squamous cell carcinoma, seminoma, and lymphoma (Fig. 13.8) (6).

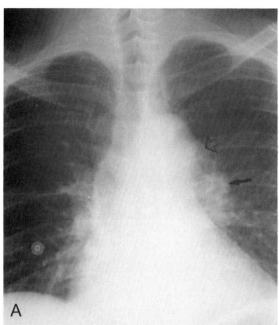

Figure 13.6. Enlarged Aortopulmonary and Peribronchial Lymph Nodes—CT versus MR. The frontal chest radiograph (**A**) in a 50-year-old man with hoarseness shows enlarged left hilar (*solid arrow*) and aortopulmonary (*open arrow*) lymph nodes. A CT scan at the level of the aortic arch (**B**) reveals enlarged aortopulmonary nodes without clear medial extension. A coronal MR (TR, 1333, TE, 30) (**C**) demonstrates enlarged aortopulmonary (*solid curved arrow*) and left peribronchial (*open curved arrow*) nodes.

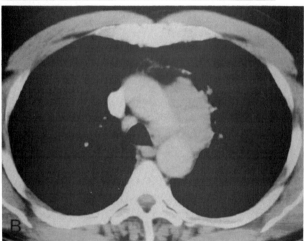

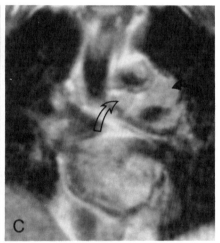

In addition to the detection and characterization of enlarged mediastinal nodes, CT can help guide diagnostic nodal tissue sampling. This is usually most helpful in the setting of suspected bronchogenic carcinoma, where accurate staging of mediastinal nodal disease is important for prognostic purposes and treatment planning. The recognition of enlarged subcarinal or pretracheal nodes on CT may suggest biopsy via transcarinal Wang needle or mediastinoscopy, respectively.

Lymphoma. As already mentioned, mediastinal lymph node enlargement is common in Hodgkin's disease and NHL. Lymphoma accounts for 20% of all mediastinal neoplasms in adults, and most patients with intrathoracic lymphoma have concomitant extrathoracic disease. In most patients, the nodal enlargement is bilateral but asymmetric. Nodular sclerosing Hodgkin's disease commonly results in lymph node enlargement predominantly within the ante-

rior mediastinum and thymus. Isolated posterior nodal enlargement is usually seen only in patients with NHL.

Leukemia, particularly the T-lymphocytic varieties, can cause intrathoracic lymph node enlargement. The lymph node enlargement is usually confined to the middle mediastinal and hilar nodes.

Bronchogenic Carcinoma is the most common source of metastases to middle mediastinal nodes. In the majority of patients, symptoms or plain radiographic findings suggest the presence of a primary tumor in the lung. In a small percentage of patients, particularly those with small cell carcinoma, the primary carcinoma may be inconspicuous or invisible on plain radiographs, with nodal metastases being the only visible abnormality. Lymph node enlargement is often unilateral on the side of the visible pulmonary or hilar abnormality. Paratracheal and aorticopulmonary nodes are most commonly involved. Since the accu-

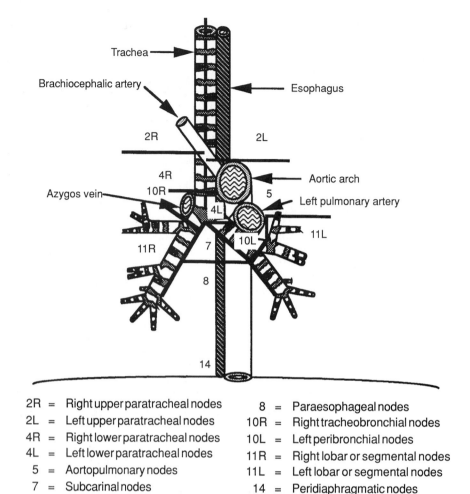

2R = Right upper paratracheal nodes
2L = Left upper paratracheal nodes
4R = Right lower paratracheal nodes
4L = Left lower paratracheal nodes
5 = Aortopulmonary nodes
7 = Subcarinal nodes

8 = Paraesophageal nodes
10R = Right tracheobronchial nodes
10L = Left peribronchial nodes
11R = Right lobar or segmental nodes
11L = Left lobar or segmental nodes
14 = Peridiaphragmatic nodes

Figure 13.7. Diagram of American Thoracic Society Nodal Stations.

racy of CT in predicting the presence or absence of mediastinal lymph node metastases is approximately 70–80%, biopsy of enlarged mediastinal lymph nodes should be performed before foregoing a possibly curative resection. A more thorough discussion of mediastinal nodal involvement in bronchogenic carcinoma may be found in the section on bronchogenic carcinoma in Chapter 14.

Lymph Node Metastases from extrathoracic malignancies can result in mediastinal node enlargement, either with or without concomitant pulmonary metastases. These mediastinal nodal metastases may result from inferior extension of neck masses (thyroid carcinoma, head and neck tumors), extension along lymphatic channels from below the diaphragm (testicular or renal cell carcinoma, gastrointestinal malignancies), or hematogenous (breast carcinoma, melanoma, Kaposi's sarcoma) (7).

Sarcoidosis. Mediastinal lymph node enlargement is very common in patients with sarcoidosis, occurring in 60–90% of patients at some stage of their disease. Nodal enlargement is typically bilateral, symmetric, and involves the hila as well as the mediasti-

num; this usually allows for differentiation of sarcoidosis from lymphoma and metastatic disease. In sarcoidosis, the enlarged nodes produce a lobulated appearance on chest radiographs and CT as the enlarged nodes do not coalesce (Fig. 13.9). This is in contrast to lymphoma and nodal metastases in which the intranodal tumor extends through the nodal capsule to form conglomerate enlarged nodal masses. Right and left paratracheal lymph nodes are typically involved; anterior or posterior mediastinal nodal enlargement has been described with greater frequency recently, likely because of the improved sensitivity of CT for detecting nodal involvement in these regions.

Infections. A variety of infections, most commonly histoplasmosis, coccidioidomycosis, cryptococcosis, and tuberculosis (Fig. 13.8) can cause mediastinal nodal enlargement. These patients typically have parenchymal opacities on chest radiographs, but isolated lymph node enlargement may be seen, particularly in children and young adults. Bacterial infections such as anthrax, bubonic plague, and tularemia are uncommon causes of lymph node enlargement. Typically, there will be symptoms and signs of acute

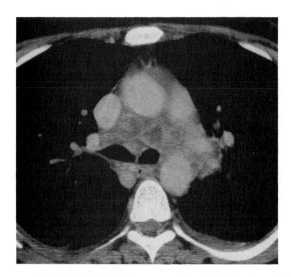

Figure 13.8. Tuberculous Lymph Node Enlargement. Contrast-enhanced CT scan at the level of the tracheal carina demonstrates enlarged precarinal and left peribronchial lymph nodes with peripheral enhancement and central necrosis. Stain and culture of nodes obtained at mediastinoscopy revealed infection by *Mycobacterium tuberculosis*.

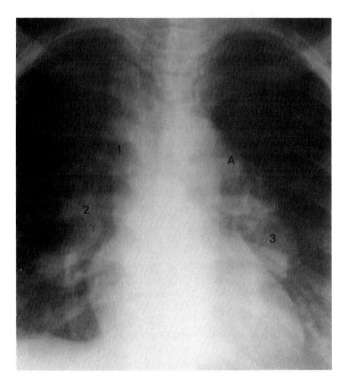

Figure 13.9. Bilateral Hilar Lymph Node Enlargement in Sarcoidosis. A PA radiography in a 56-year-old female with sarcoidosis reveals marked enlargement of paratracheal (1), right (2) and left (3) hilar, and aortopulmonary window (A) lymph nodes.

infection, and chest radiographs will show evidence of pneumonia. Bacterial lung abscesses also may

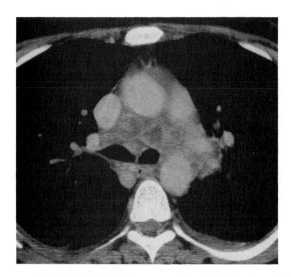

be associated with reactive lymph node enlargement. Hilar and mediastinal lymph nodes may be enlarged in patients with measles pneumonia and infectious mononucleosis.

Angiofollicular Lymph Node Hyperplasia (Castleman's Disease) is characterized by enlargement of hilar and mediastinal lymph nodes, predominantly in the middle and posterior mediastinal compartments. In the more common hyaline vascular type, the disease is localized to one lymph node region and presents as an asymptomatic mediastinal soft-tissue mass. Histologically, there is replacement of normal nodal architecture with multiple germinal centers and multiple small vessels with hyalinized walls that course perpendicularly toward the germinal centers to give a characteristic "lollipop" appearance on light microscopy. The vascular nature of these masses accounts for the intense enhancement seen on contrast-enhanced CT or angiography. Calcification within these masses has been described (Fig. 13.10). These lesions are cured by resection.

Angioimmunoblastic Lymphadenopathy is a rare disorder seen in older adults characterized by constitutional symptoms, lymphadenopathy, hepatosplenomegaly, and skin rash. Hemolytic anemia and hypergammaglobulinemia may be seen. Histologically, the enlarged nodes contain a chronic inflammatory infiltrate and are hypervascular. Chest radiographs and CT show hilar and mediastinal lymph node enlargement indistinguishable from other etiologies. As with Castleman's disease, the vascular nature of the involved lymph nodes accounts for the contrast enhancement seen on CT. These patients manifest signs of immunodeficiency similar to those associated with the acquired immunodeficiency syndrome with one-third developing high-grade lymphoma and many succumbing to opportunistic infections such as *Pneumocystis carinii* pneumonia and cytomegalovirus inclusion disease.

Foregut and Mesothelial Cysts are common mediastinal lesions that typically present as asymptomatic masses on routine chest radiographs in young adults. Computed tomography and MR show findings characteristic of the cystic nature of these lesions.

Congenital Bronchogenic Cysts result from anomalous budding of the tracheobronchial tree during development. To be characterized as bronchogenic in origin, the wall of the cyst must be lined by a respiratory epithelium with pseudostratified columnar cells and contain seromucous glands; some may contain cartilage and smooth muscle within their walls. It is often difficult to distinguish between bronchogenic and enteric cysts based upon their location and pathologic appearance; the term "foregut cyst" has been used to describe those lesions that cannot be specifically characterized. The majority of bronchogenic

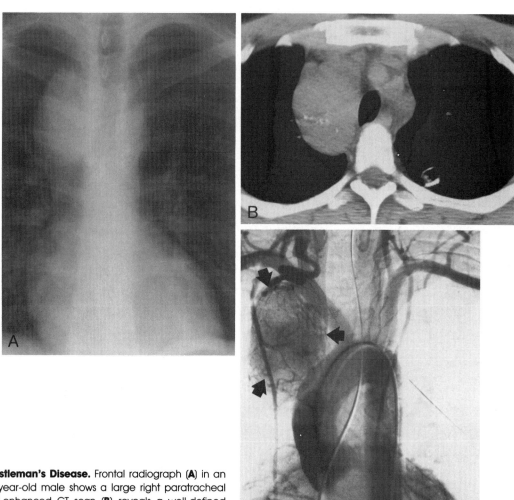

Figure 13.10. Castleman's Disease. Frontal radiograph (**A**) in an asymptomatic 26-year-old male shows a large right paratracheal mass. Noncontrast-enhanced CT scan (**B**) reveals a well-defined paratracheal soft-tissue mass with punctate calcifications. Uniform intense enhancement was seen after intravenous contrast administration. Subtraction image from the midphase of an aortogram (**C**) shows the mass (*arrows*) to be hypervascular. Resected specimen revealed Castleman's disease.

cysts (80–90%) arise within the mediastinum in the vicinity of the tracheal carina. Most mediastinal lesions are asymptomatic; occasionally, compression of the tracheobronchial tree or esophagus may produce dyspnea, wheezing, or dysphagia. Rarely, mediastinal cysts become secondarily infected after communication with the airway or esophagus, or cause symptomatic compression after rapid enlargement following hemorrhage.

Bronchogenic cysts are seen as soft-tissue masses in the subcarinal or right paratracheal space on frontal chest radiographs; less common sites of involvement include the hilum, posterior mediastinum, and periesophageal region. They appear as a single smooth, round or elliptical mass; a minority are lobulated in contour. Computed tomography is the method of choice for the diagnosis of a mediastinal cyst. If a well-defined, thin-walled mass of fluid density (0–10 HU) is seen that fails to enhance following

intravenous contrast administration, it can be assumed to represent a benign cyst. High CT numbers (>40 HU) suggesting a solid mass can be seen when the cyst is filled with mucoid material, milk of calcium, or blood. Calcification of the cyst wall has been described but is uncommon. Magnetic resonance shows characteristic low signal intensity on T1-weighted images and high signal intensity on T2-weighted images (Fig. 13.11). The presence of proteinaceous material within the cyst will shorten T1 relaxation times, yielding high signal intensity on T1-weighted images. In many patients, resection is required for definitive diagnosis. Recently, both transbronchoscopic and precutaneous needle aspiration and drainage has been used effectively for the diagnosis and treatment of these lesions.

Pericardial Cysts arise from the parietal pericardium and contain clear serous fluid surrounded by a layer of mesothelial cells. They most commonly arise

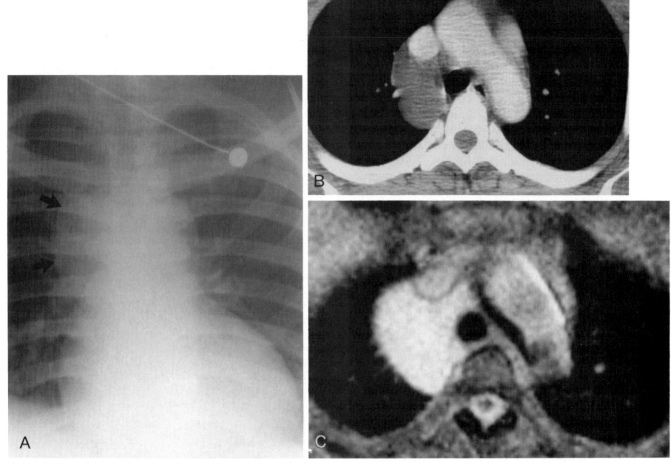

Figure 13.11. **Bronchogenic Cyst.** Anteroposterior portable radiograph (**A**) in a patient with malignant hypertension revealed an incidental right paratracheal mass (*arrows*). A contrast-enhanced CT scan (**B**) shows a well-defined paratracheal mass of low attenuation. Axial MR (TR = 967, TE = 20, flip angle, 15°) (**C**) shows high signal intensity within the mass equal to subarachnoid fluid, confirming its cystic nature.

in the anterior cardiophrenic angles, with right-sided lesions being twice as common as left; approximately 20% arise more superiorly within the mediastinum. These lesions usually present as incidental asymptomatic round or oval masses in the cardiophrenic angle. Their pliable nature can be demonstrated with a change in patient position. Computed tomography typically shows a unilocular cystic mass adjacent to the heart; MR or ultrasound via a subxiphoid approach show findings characteristic of a simple cyst. As with bronchogenic cysts, there have been reports of cysts with high attenuation on CT, which on resection are found to be filled with proteinaceous or mucoid material.

Tracheal and Central Bronchial Masses. commonly produce upper airway symptoms and rarely present as asymptomatic mediastinal masses, although they may be recognized radiographically when they distort the tracheal air column or mediastinal

contour. These masses are discussed in a separate section on disorders of the trachea and central bronchi.

Diaphragmatic Hernias. may present as pericardiac masses. They are discussed in Chapter 16.

Vascular Lesions. Congenital or acquired anomalies of the heart and great vessels are common middle mediastinal masses, and are discussed in Chapter 12.

Posterior Mediastinal Masses (Table 13.5)

NEUROGENIC TUMORS

Posterior mediastinal masses arising from neural elements are classified by their tissue of origin. Three groups have been recognized: tumors arising from intercostal nerves (neurofibroma, schwannoma), sympathetic ganglia (ganglioneuroma, ganglioneuroblas-

Table 13.5.   Posterior Mediastinal Masses

Neurogenic tumors	Peripheral (intercostal) nerves
	Neurofibroma
	Schwannoma
	Sympathetic ganglia
	Ganglioneuroma
	Ganglioneuroblastoma
	Neuroblastoma
	Paraganglion cells
	Chemodectoma
	Pheochromocytoma
Esophageal lesions	Duplication (enteric) cyst
	Diverticulum
	Neoplasm
	Leiomyoma
	Squamous cell carcinoma
	Esophageal dilation
	Achalasia
	Scleroderma
	Peptic stricture
	Carcinoma
	Paraesophageal varices
	Hiatal hernia
	Sliding
	Paraesophageal
Foregut cysts	Enteric
	Neurenteric
Vertebral lesion	Trauma
	Paraspinal hematoma
	Infection
	Paraspinal abscess
	Tuberculosis
	Staphylococcus
	Tumor
	Metastases (bronchogenic, breast, renal cell carcinoma)
	Multiple myeloma
	Lymphoma
	Degenerative disease (osteophytosis)
	Extramedullary hematopoiesis
Lateral thoracic meningocele	
Pancreatic pseudocyst	

toma, and neuroblastoma), or paraganglionic cells (chemodectoma, pheochromocytoma). Tumors in each of these three groups may be benign or malignant neoplasms (8). Although neurogenic tumors can occur at any age, they are most common in young patients. Neuroblastoma and ganglioneuroma are most common in children, whereas neurofibroma and schwannoma more frequently affect adults.

Histologically, both neurofibroma and schwannoma are comprised of spindle cells, which arise from the Schwann cell. While neurofibroma is an encapsulated tumor that contains interspersed neurons, schwannoma is not encapsulated and contains no neuronal elements. Both tumors are more common in patients with neurofibromatosis. Multiple lesions in the mediastinum, particularly bilateral apicoposterior masses, are virtually diagnostic of neurofibromatosis.

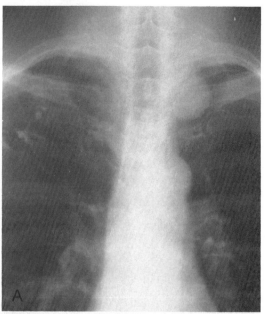

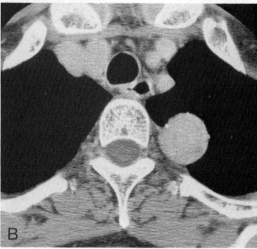

Figure 13.12.   Intercostal Neurofibroma. A coned-down view from a frontal radiograph (**A**) in a 52-year-old woman with a positive tuberculin skin test reveals fibrocalcific changes in the right upper lobe and an incidental left upper paraspinal mass. A CT scan (**B**) demonstrates a round mass that enhances uniformly after contrast administration. Thoracoscopic resection revealed a neurofibroma.

A small percentage of schwannomas (10%) are locally invasive (malignant schwannoma).

Radiographically, intercostal nerve tumors appear as round or oval paravertebral soft-tissue masses. Computed tomography shows a smooth or lobulated paraspinal soft-tissue mass that may erode the adjacent vertebral body or rib (Fig. 13.12). Computed tomography demonstration of tumor extension from the paravertebral space into the spinal canal via an enlarged intervertebral foramen is characteristic of a "dumbbell" neurofibroma. Magnetic resonance is the modality of choice for imaging a suspected neurofibroma. In addition to the occasional demonstration of both intra- and extraspinal canal components, MR of

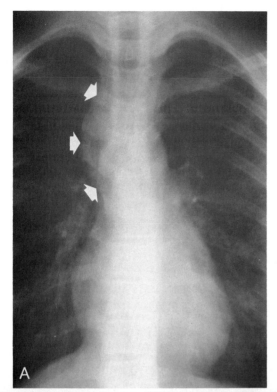

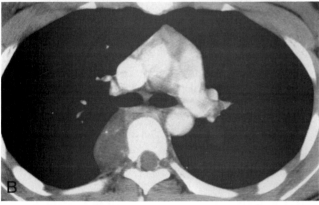

Figure 13.13. Ganglioneuroma. A PA radiograph in a 15-year-old female (**A**) reveals an oval, vertically oriented right-sided mediastinal mass (*white arrows*). Contrast-enhanced CT (**B**) shows a low attenuation posterior mediastinal mass with calcification. This is a surgically proven ganglioneuroma.

neurofibromas shows typical high signal intensity on T2-weighted images.

Tumors that arise from the sympathetic ganglia represent a continuum from the histologically benign ganglioneuroma found in adolescents and young adults to the highly malignant neuroblastoma seen almost exclusively in children under the age of 5. These tumors generally present as elongated, vertically oriented paravertebral soft-tissue masses with a broad area of contact with the posterior mediastinum (Fig. 13.13). These findings may help distinguish these lesions from neurofibromas, which usually maintain an acute angle with the vertebral column and posterior

mediastinum and therefore tend to show sharp superior and inferior margins on the lateral chest radiograph. Large masses may erode vertebral bodies or ribs. Calcification, seen in up to 25% of cases, is a helpful diagnostic feature of these tumors but does not help distinguish benign from malignant neoplasms. As these tumors often produce catecholamines, urinary levels of vanillylmandelic acid or metanephrines, which are byproducts of catecholamine metabolism, may be elevated. Prognosis depends upon the histologic features of the tumor and the patient's age and extent of disease at the time of diagnosis.

Paraganglionomas are tumors that arise in the aorticopulmonary paraganglia of the middle mediastinum or the aorticosympathetic ganglia of the posterior mediastinum. They are divided into nonfunctioning neoplasms (chemodectomas), which occur almost exclusively in or about the aortopulmonary window, and functioning neoplasms (pheochromocytomas), which are found in the posterior sympathetic chain or in or about the heart or pericardium. Approximately 2% of all pheochromocytomas arise in the mediastinum. The posterior mediastinum is the site of fewer than 25% of mediastinal paraganglionomas, with the majority arising in the anterior or middle mediastinum. Radiographically, these tumors are indistinguishable from other neurogenic tumors. However, most patients have hypertension and biochemical evidence of excess catecholamine production. Computed tomography and angiography demonstrate hypervascular masses; radionuclide M-iodobenzylguanioine scanning is diagnostic in functioning tumors.

ESOPHAGEAL LESIONS

As most of the intrathoracic esophagus is intimately associated with the thoracic spine and descending thoracic aorta, lesions in the middle or distal one-third of the esophagus may present as posterior mediastinal masses. Common presenting symptoms include dysphagia and aspiration pneumonia, although many patients will be asymptomatic.

Esophageal Carcinoma. The majority of esophageal neoplasms, excluding lesions arising at the esophagogastric junction, are squamous cell carcinomas. Unlike benign neoplasms of the posterior mediastinum, these lesions, when seen on chest radiographs, are rarely asymptomatic. These patients typically have a history of dysphagia and significant weight loss. Difficulty in detecting asymptomatic lesions and the absence of a serosa account for the advanced stage of most esophageal carcinoma at presentation and a 5-year survival rate of less than 20%. Most patients with esophageal carcinoma have abnormal plain radiographic findings, including an abnormal azygoesophageal interface, widening of the medi-

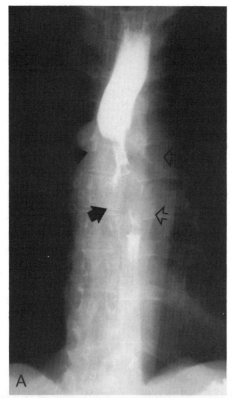

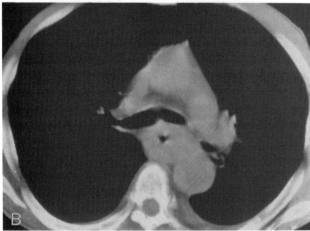

Figure 13.14. Esophageal Carcinoma. Upright spot film during barium esophagram (**A**) demonstrates an intraluminal mass with mucosal destruction and overhanging edges indicative of a carcinoma. Note the lateral displacement of the azygoesophageal (*solid arrows*) and preaortic (*open arrows*) recesses at the level of the mass. A nonenhanced CT scan at the level of the tracheal carina (**B**) reveals marked thickening of the esophageal wall with narrowing of the residual lumen.

astinum (because of the tumor itself or a dilated esophagus proximal to the obstructing lesion), abnormal thickening of the tracheoesophageal stripe, and tracheal deviation and compression. The diagnosis is usually made on barium esophagram and confirmed by endoscopic biopsy. Computed tomography scanning has proved accurate for staging esophageal carcinoma; findings include an intraluminal mass, thick-

ening of the esophageal wall, loss of fat planes between the esophagus and adjacent mediastinal structures (usually the trachea with upper esophageal lesions and the descending aorta with lower esophageal lesions), and evidence of nodal and distant metastases (Fig. 13.14).

Benign Esophageal Neoplasms, including leiomyoma, fibroma, and lipoma, can present as smooth, solitary mediastinal masses projecting laterally from the posterior mediastinum on frontal chest radiographs. They generally involve the lower third of the esophagus from the level of the subcarinal space to the esophageal hiatus. Initial evaluation is with barium studies, which show a smooth, broad-based mass forming obtuse margins with the esophageal wall. Computed tomography demonstrates a smooth, well-defined soft-tissue mass adjacent to the esophagus and without obstruction. The absence of esophageal dilation above the mass helps distinguish benign tumors from carcinoma.

Pulsion Diverticula arising at the cervicothoracic-esophageal junction or distal esophagus are false diverticula representing mucosal outpouchings through defects in the muscular layer of the esophagus. A large proximal pulsion diverticulum (Zenker's) may extend through the thoracic inlet and appear as a retroesophageal superior mediastinal mass containing an air-fluid level on upright chest radiographs. A distal pulsion diverticulum appears as a juxtadiaphragmatic mass with an air-fluid level projecting to the right of midline. Barium swallow is diagnostic.

Dilated Esophagus due to functional (achalasia, scleroderma) or anatomic (stricture, carcinoma) obstruction may produce a mass that courses vertically over the length of the mediastinum, projecting toward the right side on frontal chest radiograph. An air-fluid level on upright films is usually present. A completely air-filled, dilated esophagus appears as a thin curvilinear line along the medial right thorax because the right lateral wall of the esophagus is outlined by intraluminal air medially and the right lung laterally. Barium study or CT will confirm the diagnosis of a dilated esophagus; determination of the cause of obstruction often requires endoscopy or esophageal manometry.

Esophageal Varices may produce a round or lobulated retrocardiac mass in patients with portal hypertension. The diagnosis is usually made by endoscopic recognition of submucosal varices involving the distal esophagus. The varices are readily recognized on contrast CT, MR, or portal venography.

Hiatal Hernia. A common cause of a mass in the posteroinferior mediastinum is a hiatal hernia. This results from a separation of the superior margins of the diaphragmatic crura and stretching of the phrenicoesophageal ligament. The stomach is by far the most common structure in the hernia sac; the gastric cardia (sliding hernia) or fundus (paraesophageal hernia) may be involved. Rarely, omental fat, ascitic fluid, or a pancreatic pseudocyst herniates through the esophageal hiatus into the mediastinum. The characteristic location at the esophageal hiatus and the presence of a rounded density containing an air or air-fluid level on upright films is diagnostic. Barium swallow or a CT scan through the lower thorax will confirm the diagnosis.

ENTERIC/NEURENTERIC CYSTS

Enteric cysts are fluid-filled masses lined by enteric epithelium. Esophageal cysts usually arise intramurally or immediately adjacent to the esophagus. When an enteric cyst has a persistent communication with the spinal canal (canal of Kovalevsky) and is associated with congenital defects of the thoracic spine (anterior spina bifida, hemivertebrae, or butterfly vertebrae), it is termed a neurenteric cyst. Computed tomography or MR can confirm the cystic nature of these masses. If the cyst communicates with the gastrointestinal tract, it may contain air or an air-fluid level or opacify with contrast during an upper gastrointestinal series.

VERTEBRAL ABNORMALITIES

A variety of conditions that affect the thoracic spine may manifest as posterior mediastinal masses. These lesions typically produce lateral deviation of the paraspinal reflection on frontal radiographs. Often, the bony origin of these lesions is not obvious on the initial examination, making distinction from neurogenic tumors and other posterior mediastinal masses difficult.

Neoplastic, infectious, metabolic, traumatic, or degenerative processes of the thoracic spine may produce a paraspinal mass by one of four mechanisms: expansion of vertebral body or posterior elements (multiple myeloma, aneurysmal bone cyst); extraosseous extension of infection, tumor, or marrow elements (infectious spondylitis, metastatic carcinoma, extramedullary hematopoiesis, respectively) (Fig. 13.15), pathologic fracture and paraspinal hematoma formation (any destructive neoplastic or inflammatory process, trauma); or protrusion of degenerative osteophytes. Neoplastic processes are usually easily identified by expansion and destruction of vertebral bodies with sparing of intervertebral discs. Bronchogenic, breast, or renal cell carcinoma are the most common primary sites of thoracic spinal metastases (Fig. 13.15). Infectious spondylitis is distinguished from neoplastic processes by the presence of a paravertebral mass centered at the point of maximal bone destruction. In patients with a paravertebral abscess

secondary to tuberculosis or bacterial infection, narrowing of the adjacent disc space and destruction of vertebral endplates are important clues to the diagnosis. Extramedullary hematopoiesis is seen almost exclusively in conditions associated with ineffective production or excessive destruction of erythrocytes,

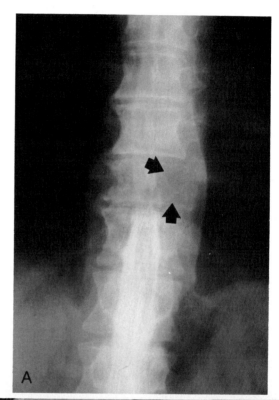

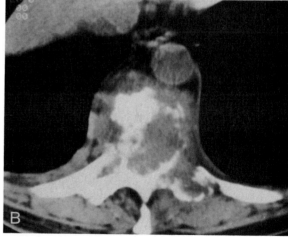

Figure 13.15. Metastatic Adenocarcinoma, Thoracic Spine. A coned-down anteroposterior view from a thoracic myelogram (**A**) shows a virtual complete block at the T-11 level. Note the lytic destruction of the body and left pedicle of T-11 (*arrows*) with bulging of the paraspinal interfaces. A CT scan at T-11 (**B**) shows bony destruction with tumor extending into the spinal canal and paraspinal soft tissues. The patient was a 56-year-old man who had undergone a left nephrectomy 1 year previously for renal cell carcinoma. Histologic examination of the tissue resected at laminectomy confirmed metastatic disease.

such as thalassemia major, congenital spherocytosis, and sickle cell anemia. It is recognized by noting expansion of the medullary space and cyst formation within long bones, ribs, and vertebral bodies with associated lobulated paraspinal soft-tissue masses. These masses represent hyperplastic bone marrow that has extruded from the vertebral bodies and posterior ribs. Traumatic injuries to the thoracic spine are usually obvious from the patient's history and recognition of spine fracture on conventional and CT studies of the spine. Degenerative disc disease may produce a localized paraspinal mass on frontal radiographs. Well-penetrated films will show the characteristic inferolaterally projecting osteophytes at the level of the mass, which are most commonly right-sided because of the inhibitory effect of the pulsating descending aorta on left-sided osteophyte formation.

Lateral Thoracic Meningocele represents an anomalous herniation of the spinal meninges through an intervertebral foramen, resulting in a paravertebral soft-tissue mass. Most meningoceles are discovered in middle-aged patients as asymptomatic masses. They are slightly more common on the right, and are multiple in 10% of cases. There is a high association between lateral thoracic meningoceles and neurofibromatosis. A meningocele is the most common posterior mediastinal mass in patients with neurofibromatosis; conversely, approximately two-thirds of patients with meningoceles have neurofibromatosis. Chest radiographs typically reveal a round, well-defined paraspinal mass that is indistinguishable from a neurofibroma. Additional clues to the diagnosis include rib erosion, enlargement of the adjacent neural foramen, vertebral anomalies, or kyphoscoliosis. When a lateral meningocele is associated with kyphoscoliosis, it is usually found at the apex of the scoliotic curve on the convex side. Magnetic resonance demonstration of a herniated subarachnoid space is the diagnostic technique of choice; conventional or CT myelography, which demonstrates filling of the meningocele with contrast, is reserved for equivocal cases.

Miscellaneous Conditions. As described earlier in the section "Hiatal Hernia," a pancreatic pseudocyst may rarely produce a posterior mediastinal mass by extending cephalad from the retroperitoneum through the esophageal or aortic hiatus of the diaphragm. The diagnosis relies on CT demonstration of continuity of a predominantly cystic mass with its retroperitoneal portion. The presence of a left pleural effusion is a further clue to the diagnosis. Hernias through the foramen of Bochdalek that produce a posterior mediastinal mass are discussed in Chapter 16.

Malignant lymph node enlargement may rarely produce a recognizable paraspinal mass. This is most often seen in NHL and metastatic lung cancer; other mediastinal or extrathoracic sites of involvement are invariably present.

Despite the advances in detection and characterization of mediastinal masses with cross-sectional imaging, most patients will require tissue sampling for definitive diagnosis. However, the radiologist can use the information provided by CT or MR to help limit the differential diagnosis and thereby guide the appropriate evaluation and treatment. In a large percentage of cases where tissue sampling is required, this can be accomplished by CT- or ultrasound-guided transthoracic biopsy.

TRACHEA AND CENTRAL BRONCHI
Congenital Tracheal Anomalies

Tracheal agenesis, cartilaginous abnormalities of the trachea, tracheal webs and stenosis, tracheoesophageal fistulas, and vascular rings and slings present as breathing and feeding difficulties in the neonatal and infancy period. These are uncommon congenital lesions and are discussed Chapter 12.

Tracheoceles are true diverticula that represent herniation of the tracheal fluid column through a weakened posterior tracheal membrane. These lesions occur almost exclusively in the cervical trachea as the pressure gradient from the extrathoracic trachea to the atmosphere with the Valsalva maneuver favors their formation in this region. These lesions are usually asymptomatic and easily recognized on fluoroscopy, CT, or contrast tracheogram.

Tracheal Bronchus or bronchus sus, so-called because it is the normal pattern of tracheal branching in pigs, consists of an accessory bronchus to all or a portion of the right upper lobe that arises from the right lateral tracheal wall within 2 cm of the tracheal carina. It is usually seen as an incidental finding on chest CT in 0.5–1.0% of the population. A tracheal bronchus most often supplies the apical segment of the right upper lobe. While it is usually an isolated and asymptomatic finding, there is an association with congenital tracheal stenosis and an aberrant left pulmonary artery.

Focal Tracheal Disease

Focal disorders of the trachea may produce narrowing or dilation of the tracheal lumen. Focal narrowing may be produced by extrinsic or intrinsic mass lesions, retraction, or inflammatory disorders of the tracheal wall (Table 13.6).

EXTRINSIC COMPRESSION/NARROWING

The most common causes of mass effect on the trachea are an intrathoracic goiter (Fig. 13.1) and a

Table 13.6. Focal Tracheal Disease

Narrowing	Extrinsic
	Thyroid goiter
	Paratracheal lymph node mass
	Asymmetric or unilateral upper lobe
	fibrosis
	Tuberculosis
	Histoplasmosis
	Intrinsic
	Tracheomalacia
	Endotracheal tube cuff
	Tracheostomy site
	Wegener's granulomatosis
	Sarcoidosis
	Infection
	Tuberculosis
	Fungus
	Histoplasmosis
	Coccidioidomycosis
	Aspergillosis
	Scleroma
Masses	Neoplasm
	Malignant
	Primary
	Squamous cell carcinoma
	Adenoid cystic carcinoma
	(cylindroma)
	Metastatic
	Direct invasion
	Laryngeal carcinoma
	Thyroid carcinoma
	Esophageal carcinoma
	Bronchogenic carcinoma
	Hematogenous (endobronchial)
	Breast carcinoma
	Renal cell carcinoma
	Colon carcinoma
	Melanoma
	Benign
	Chondroma
	Fibroma
	Squamous cell papilloma
	Hemangioma
	Granular cell myoblastoma
	Nonneoplastic
	Ectopic thyroid or thymus
	Mucus
Dilation	
	Tracheoceles
	Tracheomalacia
	Upper lobe fibrosis

large paratracheal lymph node mass. In older individuals, a tortuous or aneurysmal transverse portion of the aortic arch may cause right lateral deviation of the distal intrathoracic trachea. Extrinsic mass effect can also be seen with congenital vascular anomalies such as aberrant left pulmonary artery and aortic ring, or a large mediastinal bronchogenic cyst. Extrinsic masses tend to displace the trachea without narrowing its lumen, as the tracheal cartilage provides resiliency. Traction deformity of the trachea is generally seen in cicatrizing processes that asymmetrically af-

fect the lung apices, most commonly chronic tuberculosis and histoplasmosis. Occasionally, the distal trachea is narrowed in patients with sclerosing mediastinitis, although this disorder normally affects the central bronchi.

Focal Tracheal Stenosis. Focal tracheal or central (main and proximal lobar) bronchial narrowing may result from inflammatory disorders that affect the tracheal or central bronchial walls.

Tracheal Injury. Cartilaginous damage or the development of granulation tissue and fibrosis from the creation of a tracheostomy or at the site of a previously inflated endotracheal tube balloon cuff can lead to focal tracheal narrowing. The tracheal stenosis has a typical hourglass deformity on frontal radiographs. Those with tracheomalacia from cartilage damage may only manifest narrowing during phases of the respiratory cycle when extratracheal pressure exceeds intratracheal pressure. Therefore, those with extrathoracic tracheomalacia, most often at the site of prior tracheostomy, will demonstrate tracheal narrowing on inspiration, while those with intrathoracic tracheomalacia, usually from prior endotracheal intubation, will have tracheal narrowing on expiration. Postintubation stenosis is rare with the low-pressure, high-volume endotracheal tube cuffs in current use.

Wegener's Granulomatosis can produce a necrotizing granulomatous inflammation of the trachea and central bronchi leading to focal cervical tracheal narrowing or, in advanced disease, narrowing of the entire length of the trachea. The diagnosis of tracheal involvement by Wegener's granulomatosis is made by the radiographic demonstration of tracheal narrowing in association with upper airway and renal involvement, and characteristic findings on biopsy. Cyclophosphamide therapy administered early in the course of the disease may reduce inflammation and improve tracheal narrowing.

Sarcoidosis involving the central airways may rarely cause focal tracheal or bronchial stenosis.

Infectious Processes may result in tracheal or bronchial inflammation and stenosis. Endotracheal and endobronchial tuberculosis is usually associated with cavitary tuberculosis, where the production of large volumes of infected sputum predisposes to tracheal and central bronchial infection. Upper tracheal inflammation and stenosis may result from histoplasmosis and coccidioidomycosis. Invasive tracheobronchitis from aspergillus, candida, and mucormycosis infection has been described in immunodeficient patients. Tracheal scleroma is a chronic granulomatous disorder caused by infection with *Klebsiella rhinoscleromatis*. This disease is uncommon in the United States and is seen most commonly in people of lower socioeconomic standing in Central and South America and eastern Europe. The infection begins as an inflammation of the nasal mucosa and paranasal sinuses, extending inferiorly to involve the larynx, pharynx, and trachea in a minority of patients. In its chronic phase, intense granulation tissue and fibrosis lead to nasal cavity, pharyngeal, laryngeal, and upper tracheal stenosis; the latter is seen in less than 10% of patients. Radiographically, the upper trachea shows irregular, nodular narrowing that may extend to involve the length of the trachea. The diagnosis is made on biopsy, which reveals granulation tissue containing large foamy histiocytes filled with the causative organism (Mikulicz cells). Antibiotic treatment is effective if administered in the early phases of infection before extensive fibrosis has developed.

TRACHEAL MASSES

Intratracheal masses may be divided into neoplastic and nonneoplastic masses (9). Primary tracheal tumors are rare. However, 90% of all primary tracheal tumors in adults are malignant. The majority of primary tracheal malignancies arise from tracheal epithelium or mucous glands (90%) or from the mesenchymal elements of the tracheal wall (10%).

Squamous Cell Carcinoma is the most common primary tracheal malignancy, accounting for at least 50% of all malignant tracheal neoplasms. These tumors affect middle-aged male tobacco smokers and are associated with laryngeal, bronchogenic, or esophageal malignancies in up to 25% of cases. The majority arise in the distal trachea within 3—4 cm of the tracheal carina, with the cervical trachea the next most common site. Cough, hemoptysis, dyspnea, and wheezing are common presenting symptoms. Patients may be mistakenly treated for asthma before the correct diagnosis is made.

Adenoid Cystic Carcinoma (cylindroma) is a malignant neoplasm that arises from tracheal salivary glands and accounts for 40% of primary tracheal malignancies. The minor salivary glands from which these tumors arise are found at the junction of the cartilaginous and membranous portions of the proximal trachea, which accounts for the tendency of this neoplasm to involve the posterolateral wall of the proximal trachea.

The diagnosis of primary tracheal malignancy is rarely made prospectively on chest radiographs, although well-penetrated radiographs can demonstrate distortion of the tracheal air column by a mass. Computed tomography typically shows a lobulated or irregular soft-tissue mass that eccentrically narrows the tracheal lumen and has a variable extraluminal component. Masses greater than 2 cm in diameter are likely to be malignant, while those smaller than 2 cm

are more likely benign. Calcification is uncommon. Resectability of these lesions depends upon the length of tracheal involvement and the extent of mediastinal invasion at the time of diagnosis. Computed tomography is particularly well suited for this determination and has become the modality of choice for imaging tracheal neoplasms. The prognosis in patients with squamous cell carcinoma is poor, as up to 50% of patients have mediastinal extension of tumor at the time of diagnosis. While adenoid cystic carcinoma has a better prognosis, these slow-growing lesions are locally invasive and have a tendency toward late recurrence and metastasis.

A variety of other malignant lesions comprise the remainder of primary tracheal malignancies and include mucoepidermoid carcinoma, carcinoid tumor, adenocarcinoma, lymphoma, small cell carcinoma, leiomyosarcoma, fibrosarcoma, and chondrosarcoma. Chondrosarcoma arises from tracheal cartilage and is identified by the presence of calcified chondroid matrix within the tumor.

Secondary Malignancy. The trachea may become secondarily involved by malignancy either by direct invasion or hematogenous spread. Laryngeal carcinoma may extend below the vocal cords to involve the cervical trachea. There is also a tendency for tumor to recur at the tracheostomy site in patients who have undergone total laryngectomies for carcinoma. Papillary and follicular carcinoma are the most common types of thyroid malignancy to invade the trachea. Squamous cell carcinoma of the upper third of the esophagus can invade the posterior tracheal wall, and may produce a tracheoesophageal fistula. Bronchogenic carcinoma may involve the trachea by direct proximal extension from central bronchi, by extranodal spread of tumor from metastatic pre- or paratracheal lymph nodes, or by direct invasion of large right upper lobe tumors. Computed tomography is best at demonstrating tumor invasion of the tracheal wall and the extent of intraluminal mass. Extrathoracic primary tumors most often associated with hematogenous endotracheal metastases are carcinomas of the breast, kidney, and colon, and melanoma (Fig. 13.16). These lesions may appear on CT as irregular thickening of the tracheal wall or as well-defined, localized masses indistinguishable from benign tracheal tumors.

Benign Tumors. Chondroma, fibroma, squamous cell papilloma, hemangioma, and granular cell myoblastoma are the most common benign tracheal tumors in adults. A chondroma arises from the tracheal cartilage and produces a well-circumscribed endoluminal mass. Computed tomography may demonstrate stippled cartilaginous calcification within the mass. Fibromas are sessile or pedunculated fi-

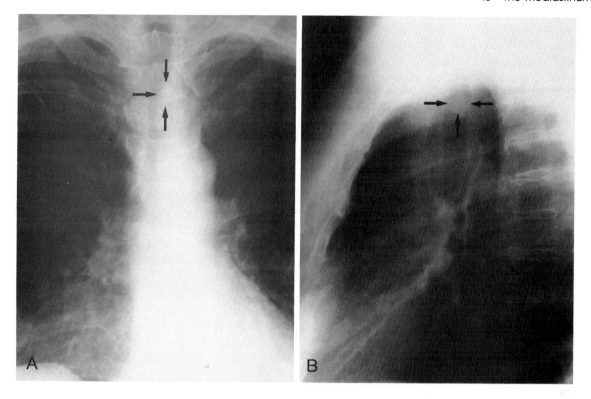

Figure 13.16. Endotracheal Metastasis from Melanoma. Posteroanteior (**A**) and lateral (**B**) radiographs in a patient with a cough 3 months after removal of a melanoma from the back. An intraluminal mass (*arrows*) projects into the tracheal air column on both views. Bronchoscopic biopsy revealed malignant melanoma.

brous masses arising in the cervical trachea. Squamous cell papilloma is a mucosal lesion caused by infection with human papilloma virus. Typically, this disease produces multiple laryngeal masses in children born to women with venereal warts (condylomata acuminata). The trachea, bronchi, and lungs may become involved over time. These lesions usually regress by adolescence and therefore are uncommon causes of a solitary tracheal lesion in adults. Similarly, hemangiomas are seen in the cervical trachea almost exclusively in infants and young children, appearing as focal masses on CT. Granular cell myoblastoma is a neoplasm that arises from neural elements in the tracheal or bronchial wall. These lesions usually involve the cervical trachea or main bronchi. Computed tomography shows a broad-based or pedunculated soft-tissue mass that may invade the tracheal wall and has a tendency toward local recurrence.

Nonneoplastic Intratracheal Masses from ectopic intratracheal thyroid or thymic tissue have been reported and are radiographically indistinguishable from intratracheal neoplasms. Intratracheal thyroid is seen in females with extratracheal goiters. The intratracheal tissue is likewise goitrous and most commonly found in the posterolateral wall of the cervical trachea, although any portion of the trachea may be involved. Mucus plugs may appear as intratracheal masses in patients with excess sputum production or diminished clearance mechanisms. They are typically low attenuation masses on CT that change position or disappear after an effective cough.

Primary malignant neoplasms of the central bronchi include carcinoma and bronchial adenoma. As most bronchogenic carcinomas produce a hilar mass as a result of the primary tumor or by metastases to regional bronchopulmonary lymph nodes, they will be discussed in detail in Chapter 14.

Bronchial Adenomas account for approximately 1% of all tracheobronchial neoplasms; 90% of these lesions arise in the bronchi or lung, while the remainder arise within the trachea. Carcinoid tumor accounts for nearly 90%; adenoid cystic carcinoma, 8%, and mucoepidermoid, 2% of all bronchial adenomas. This is opposite to the frequencies in the trachea, where adenoid cystic carcinoma accounts for 90% and carcinoid 10% of all adenomas. The use of the term "adenoma" to describe these lesions is misleading as these are malignant tumors that tend to locally invade and metastasize to regional lymph nodes.

Carcinoid tumors arise from neuroendocrine (APUD or Kulchitzky) cells within the airways. There is a spectrum of histologic differentiation and malignant behavior in tumors of Kulchitzky cell origin, ranging from the low-grade malignant typical carcinoid to atypical carcinoid to the highly malignant small cell carcinoma. Eighty percent of typical bronchial carcinoid tumors arise within central bronchi and present with cough, dyspnea, wheezing, recurrent episodes of atelectasis or pneumonia, or hemoptysis; the latter may be massive and is attributable to the highly vascular nature of these lesions. The average age at diagnosis is 50. Histologically, these tu-

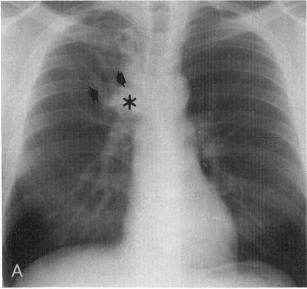

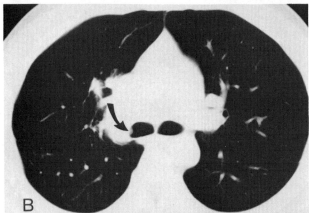

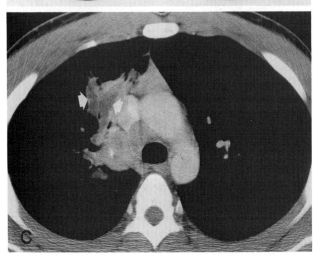

mors show sheets or trabeculae of uniform cells separated by a fibrovascular stroma. The cells may contain intracytoplasmic inclusions; immunohistochemistry will reveal a variety of neuroendocrine products including serotonin, vasoactive intestinal polypeptide, corticotropin and antidiuretic hormone. Carcinoid syndrome is seen in fewer than 3% of cases.

Radiologically, central bronchial carcinoids present with evidence of atelectasis or pneumonia secondary to large airway obstruction. A hyperlucent lobe or lung of diminished volume may result from incomplete obstruction or collateral airflow with reflex hypoxic vasoconstriction; this finding is also rarely seen in bronchogenic carcinoma. Carcinoids arising within the lung have a propensity to involve the right upper and middle lobes and appear as well-defined smooth or lobulated nodules or masses. Calcification or ossification is seen in 10% of pathologic specimens but is rarely visualized on plain radiographs. Computed tomography is ideally suited to demonstrate the relationship of the mass to the central airways. The typical appearance on CT is a smooth or lobulated soft-tissue mass within a main or lobar bronchus (Fig. 13.17). The presence of a small intraluminal and large extraluminal soft-tissue component has given rise to the term "iceberg tumor" to describe these lesions. Atypical carcinoids tend to have more irregular margins and inhomogeneous contrast enhancement, and are much more likely to be associated with hilar and mediastinal lymph node metastases. In some cases, the presence of small punctate peripheral calcifications or marked contrast enhancement on CT may allow distinction from bronchogenic carcinoma.

Prognosis in patients with typical bronchial carcinoid is excellent, with a 5-year survival rate of 90%. Regional lymph node metastases, seen in approximately 5% of operative specimens, lower the 5-year survival rate to 70%. Atypical carcinoids are associated with metastases in up to 70% of cases, although these may appear many years after discovery of the primary tumor. The 5-year survival rate in these patients is less than 50%.

Figure 13.17. Carcinoid Tumor. A PA radiograph (**A**) in a 25-year-old male with hemoptysis demonstrates a right upper hilar and paratracheal mass (*) associated with branching upper lobe tubular opacities (*solid arrows*) and volume loss (note elevation of the right hilum). A CT scan at the level of the right upper lobe bronchus (**B**) shows an endobronchial mass occluding the right upper lobe bronchus and protruding into the right main bronchus (*curved arrow*). A scan 3 cm above **B (C)** shows calcification within the paratracheal portion of the mass and dilated mucus filled anterior segmental bronchi (*white arrows*). Right upper lobectomy revealed a typical carcinoid tumor.

Pulmonary Hamartoma is a benign neoplasm comprised of disorganized tissue elements normally found in the bronchus or lung. Histologically, these lesions contain cartilage surrounded by fibrous connective tissue with variable amounts of fat, smooth muscle, and seromucous glands; calcification and ossification is seen in 30%. Ninety percent of these lesions arise within the pulmonary parenchyma; less than 10% are endobronchial. Endobronchial hamartomas are usually pedunculated lesions with fatty centers covered by fibrous tissue that contain little cartilage. Patients are usually diagnosed in the 5th decade. Central bronchial hamartomas present with cough or upper airway obstruction. Computed tomography typically shows a soft-tissue mass indistinguishable from bronchial carcinoid.

FOCAL TRACHEAL DILATION

Abnormal dilation of the tracheal lumen is caused by congenital or acquired abnormalities of the elastic membrane or cartilaginous rings of the trachea. Localized tracheal dilation may be seen with tracheoceles, acquired tracheomalacia related to prolonged endotracheal intubation, or as a result of tracheal traction from severe unilateral upper lobe parenchymal scarring.

Diffuse Tracheal Disease

Diffuse disorders of the trachea manifest as either narrowing or dilation of the tracheal lumen. Diffuse tracheal narrowing may be seen with saber-sheath trachea, amyloidosis, tracheobronchopathia osteochodroplastica, relapsing polychondritis, Wegener's granulomatosis, or tracheal scleroma (Table 13.7) (10). The latter two conditions may cause diffuse tracheal narrowing, but more commonly the involvement is limited to the cervical trachea. They were discussed in the section on focal tracheal narrowing.

DIFFUSE TRACHEAL NARROWING

Saber-Sheath Trachea is a fixed deformity of the intrathoracic trachea in which the coronal diameter is diminished to less than 60% of the sagittal diameter. The tracheal wall is uniformly thickened; calcification of the cartilaginous rings is present in most cases. This entity affects older males with functional, but not necessarily radiographic, evidence of chronic obstructive pulmonary disease. The tracheal narrowing likely reflects the chronic transmission of increased intrapleural pressure seen in obstructive lung disease and tracheal injury from chronic cough. The characteristic findings are seen on frontal radiographs and CT (Fig. 13.18).

Amyloidosis is characterized by the deposition of a fibrillar protein-polysaccharide complex in various

Table 13.7. Diffuse Tracheal Disease

Tracheal narrowing	Saber-sheath trachea
	Amyloidosis
	Tracheobronchopathia osteochondroplastica
	Relapsing polychondritis
	Wegener's granulomatosis
	Tracheal scleroma
Tracheal dilation	Tracheobronchomegaly (Mounier-Kuhn syndrome)
	Tracheomalacia
	Interstitial pulmonary fibrosis

organs. It may involve the airways as part of localized or systemic disease. Submucosal deposits in the tracheobronchial tree are more commonly a manifestation of localized disease, and may be associated with nodular or alveolar septal deposits in the lungs. Mass-like deposits which irregularly narrow the tracheal lumen are best demonstrated on CT and may cause recurrent atelectasis and pneumonia. Calcification of these deposits is common. The diagnosis is made by the presence of typical protein-polysaccharide deposits demonstrated on Congo red stains of tracheal or bronchial wall biopsy specimens.

Tracheobronchopathia Osteochondroplastica is a rare disorder characterized by the presence of multiple submucosal osseous and cartilaginous deposits within the trachea and central bronchi of elderly men. The lesions arise as enchondromas from the tracheal and bronchial cartilage, and project internally to produce nodular submucosal deposits that irregularly narrow the tracheal lumen and have a characteristic appearance and feel on bronchoscopy. The diagnosis is generally made on bronchoscopy and CT, where calcified plaques can be seen involving the anterior and lateral walls of the trachea. Sparing of the membranous posterior wall of the trachea, which lacks cartilage, is a helpful feature that distinguishes this entity from tracheobronchial amyloid. While usually asymptomatic, patients may have recurrent infection related to bronchial obstruction by the masses.

Relapsing Polychondritis is a systemic autoimmune disorder that commonly affects the cartilage of the earlobes, nose, larynx, tracheobronchial tree, joints, and large elastic arteries. Early in the disease, tracheal wall inflammation associated with cartilage destruction leads to an abnormally compliant and dilated trachea. Later in the disease, fibrosis leads to diffuse fixed narrowing of the tracheal lumen. Respiratory complications secondary to involvement of the upper airway cartilage accounts for nearly 50% of all deaths from this condition. The diagnosis is made by noting recurrent inflammation at two or more cartilaginous sites, most commonly the pinnae of the ear (producing cauliflower ears) and the bridge of the

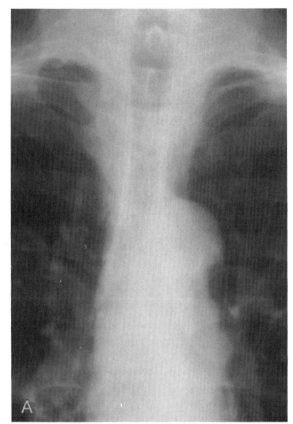

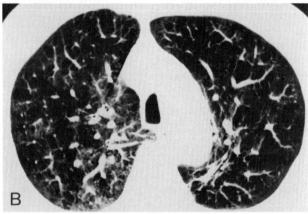

Figure 13.18.   Saber-sheath Trachea. A coned-down view of a PA radiograph (**A**) of a 65-year-old male smoker with chronic obstructive airways disease shows smooth narrowing of the intrathoracic trachea. A high-resolution CT scan (**B**) at the top of the aortic arch shows a thick-walled trachea with a coronal to sagittal diameter ratio of 0.5. Note the presence of extensive upper lobe emphysema.

nose (producing a saddlenose deformity). Radiographs and CT will show diffuse, smooth thickening of the wall of the trachea and central bronchi with narrowing of the lumen.

DIFFUSE TRACHEAL DILATION

Tracheobronchomegaly (Mounier-Kuhn syndrome) is a congenital disorder of the elastic and smooth muscle components of the tracheal wall. An

association with the Ehlers-Danlos syndrome, a congenital defect in collagen synthesis, and cutis laxa, a congenital defect in elastic tissue, has been reported. The disease is found almost exclusively in men under the age of 50. Abnormal compliance of the trachea and central bronchi leads to central bronchial collapse during coughing. The airways obstruction impairs mucociliary clearance, predisposing the patient to recurrent episodes of pneumonia and bronchiectasis. Symptoms are indistinguishable from those associated with chronic bronchitis and bronchiectasis. On frontal radiographs, the trachea and central bronchi measure greater than 3.0 cm and 2.5 cm, respectively, in coronal diameter. The trachea has a corrugated appearance because of herniation of tracheal mucosa and submucosa between the tracheal cartilages. The lungs are typically hyperinflated and may demonstrate bulla.

Tracheobronchomalacia with resultant diffuse tracheal and central bronchial dilation may result from a congenital or acquired defect of tracheal cartilage. The most common causes of acquired tracheomalacia are chronic obstructive pulmonary disease, chronic bronchitis, cystic fibrosis, and relapsing polychondritis. Symptoms and radiographic findings are similar to those in tracheobronchomegaly.

Diffuse Interstitial Fibrosis. In some patients with long-standing interstitial pulmonary fibrosis, diffuse tracheal dilation may be seen. The etiology of the tracheal dilation may relate to long-standing elevation in transpulmonary pressures because of diminished lung compliance or to chronic coughing.

Tracheal/Bronchial Injury

Injury to the trachea or main bronchi is most often seen with blunt chest trauma from a deceleration-type injury. Concomitant aortic laceration, great vessel injury, and rib (particularly an upper anterior rib), sternum, scapula, or vertebral fracture is the rule and may dominate the clinical picture. The mechanism of injury is forceful compression of the central tracheobronchial tree against the thoracic spine during impact. The fractures generally involve the proximal main bronchi (80%) or distal trachea (15%) within 2 cm of the tracheal carina; the peripheral bronchi are involved in 5% of cases. Horizontal laceration or transection parallel to the tracheobronchial cartilage is the most common form of injury.

The diagnosis of tracheobronchial injury is often first suggested on early posttrauma chest radiographs by the presence of pneumothorax and pneumomediastinum, particularly in a patient not receiving mechanical ventilation (Fig. 13.19). Typically, the pneumothorax fails to respond to chest tube drainage because of a large air leak at the site of airway interruption. The subtended lung remains collapsed

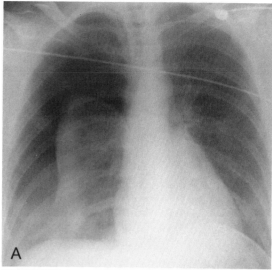

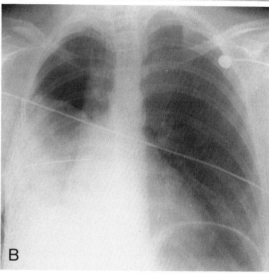

Figure 13.19. Transection of the Right Main Bronchus. In this 24-year-old woman struck by a car, an upright chest film (**A**) shows a broken right clavicle with a large right pneumothorax and pneumomediastinum. A film obtained following chest tube placement (**B**) shows a persistent pneumothorax and worsening pneumomediastinum. A large air leak was noted from the tube. Bronchoscopy revealed complete disruption of the right main bronchus, which was confirmed at thoracotomy.

against the lateral chest wall ("fallen lung" sign) (Fig. 13.19). An aberrant endotracheal tube or overdistended balloon cuff are further clues to the presence of an unsuspected tracheobronchial disruption. As many as one-third of tracheobronchial injuries have a delayed diagnosis; these patients may present with a collapsed lung or pneumonia secondary to bronchial stenosis. Definitive diagnosis is by bronchoscopy. Contrast bronchography may be useful in patients who develop bronchial occlusion or stenosis because of a delay in diagnosis.

Penetrating tracheal injuries usually involve the cervical trachea and result from gunshot or stab wounds to the neck. Injury to the intrathoracic trachea is usually associated with fatal penetrating cardiovascular injury.

MEDIASTINITIS

Mediastinal infection is an uncommon condition that may be divided into acute and chronic forms based upon etiology, clinical features, and radiologic findings. The distinction between acute and chronic infection is important, as there is a considerable difference in the treatment and prognosis.

Acute Mediastinitis

Acute mediastinitis is caused by bacterial infection, which most often develops following esophageal perforation or is a complication of cardiothoracic surgery. Esophageal perforation may complicate esophageal instrumentation (e.g., endoscopy, biopsy, dilation, or stent placement), penetrating chest trauma, esophageal carcinoma, foreign body or corrosive ingestion, or vomiting. Spontaneous esophageal perforation following prolonged vomiting is termed Boerhaave's syndrome. In this condition, a vertical tear occurs along the left posterolateral wall of the distal esophagus, just above the esophagogastric junction, leading to signs and symptoms of acute mediastinitis. Less commonly, acute mediastinitis may develop from intramediastinal extension of infection in the neck, retropharyngeal space, lungs, pleural space, pericardium, or spine.

The clinical presentation of acute mediastinitis is usually dramatic and is characterized by severe retrosternal chest pain, fever, chills, and dysphagia, often accompanied by evidence of septic shock. Physical examination may reveal findings associated with pneumomediastinum, with subcutaneous emphysema in the neck and an apical, systolic crunching sound on chest auscultation ("Hamman's sign").

The most common chest radiographic findings are widening of the superior mediastinum in 66% and pleural effusion in 50% of patients. Specific findings such as mediastinal air or air-fluid levels are less common. When mediastinitis occurs in association with Boerhaave's syndrome, pneumoperitoneum and left hydropneumothorax may be seen.

When esophageal perforation is suspected, an esophagram should be performed to detect leakage of contrast into the mediastinum and to localize the exact site of perforation. In a patient not at risk for aspiration, a water-soluble contrast agent is administered initially. Once gross contrast extravasation has been excluded, barium is then given for superior radiographic detail. The sensitivity of the esophagram for detecting contrast leakage is highest when the study is obtained within 24 hours of the perforation.

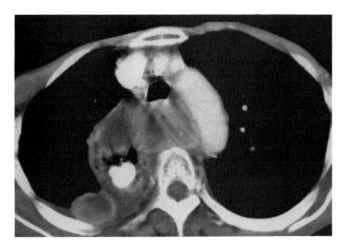

Figure 13.20. Mediastinitis with Abscess Formation. A CT scan in a patient with esophageal carcinoma demonstrates extraluminal contrast from a recent barium esophagogram with enhancing mediastinal fluid collections representing abscess formation.

Chest CT is the radiologic study of choice for the diagnosis of acute mediastinitis. Computed tomography findings include extraluminal gas, bulging of the mediastinal contours, and focal or diffuse soft-tissue infiltration of mediastinal fat. Localized fluid collections suggest focal abscess formation (Fig. 13.20) (11). Associated findings include mediastinal venous thrombosis, pneumothorax, pleural effusion or empyema, subphrenic abscess, and vertebral osteomyelitis.

While the clinical and radiographic diagnosis of mediastinitis is often straightforward, it may be difficult in postoperative patients who have undergone recent median sternotomy. In these patients, infiltration of mediastinal fat and focal air or fluid collections may be normal findings on postoperative CT scans performed days to weeks following the removal of intraoperatively placed mediastinal drains. In such patients, the progression of findings on follow-up CT scans will correctly identify the majority of those with postoperative mediastinal infection.

The prognosis for patients with acute mediastinitis varies with the underlying etiology and the extent of mediastinal involvement at the time of diagnosis. Esophageal perforation is associated with the poorest outcome, with the mortality approaching 50%. A delay in diagnosis and treatment of the mediastinal infection of greater than 24 hours is associated with a significant increase in overall morbidity and mortality.

In addition to its sensitivity in the diagnosis of mediastinitis, CT can be used to guide treatment and predict outcome. Those patients with evidence of extensive mediastinal infection, seen on CT as diffuse infiltration of the mediastinal fat without evidence of abscess formation, have a mortality approaching 50%. In contrast, patients with discrete mediastinal abscesses amenable to surgical or percutaneous drainage, or with small, localized abscesses amenable to antibiotic therapy alone, have a more favorable prognosis. In addition, patients with mediastinal abscesses and contiguous empyema or subphrenic abscess may respond favorably to drainage of these extramediastinal collections.

Chronic Sclerosing (Fibrosing) Mediastinitis

The hallmarks of chronic sclerosing mediastinitis are chronic inflammatory changes and mediastinal fibrosis. The most common cause of this rare condition is granulomatous infection, usually secondary to *Histoplasma capsulatum*. Tuberculous infection, radiation therapy and drugs (e.g., methysergide) are less common causes. Idiopathic mediastinal fibrosis, which is probably an autoimmune process, is related to fibrosis in other regions including the retroperitoneum, intraorbital fat, and thyroid gland.

Several theories have been advanced to explain the pathogenesis of sclerosing mediastinitis because of histoplasmosis. The most widely accepted theory suggests that affected patients develop an idiosyncratic hypersensitivity response to a fungal antigen that "leaks" from infected mediastinal lymph nodes.

Clinically, this condition occurs in adults and presents with a variety of symptoms that depend upon the extent of fibrosis and the mediastinal structures compromised by the fibrotic process. The superior vena cava is the most commonly affected structure, with involvement in over 75% of symptomatic patients. The superior vena cava syndrome manifests with headache, epistaxis, cyanosis, jugular venous distension, and edema of the face, neck, and upper extremities. The most serious and potentially fatal manifestation of sclerosing mediastinitis is obstruction of the central pulmonary veins producing pulmonary edema, which may mimic severe mitral stenosis. Patients with involvement of the tracheobronchial tree may have cough, dyspnea, wheezing, hemoptysis, and obstructive pneumonitis. Dysphagia or hematemesis can be seen with esophageal involvement. Less commonly, pulmonary arterial hypertension and cor pulmonale can develop from narrowing of the pulmonary arteries.

The most common finding noted on chest radiographs is asymmetric lobulated widening of the upper mediastinum, most often on the right (Fig. 13.21). When the process is secondary to granulomatous infection, enlarged calcified lymph nodes may be seen. Narrowing of the tracheobronchial tree may be evident. The sequelae of vascular involvement may be seen, including oligemia from pulmonary arterial compression or venous hypertension and pulmonary edema from involvement of the central pulmonary

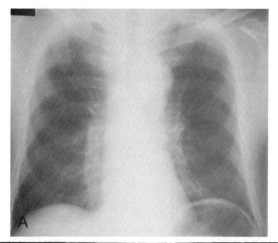

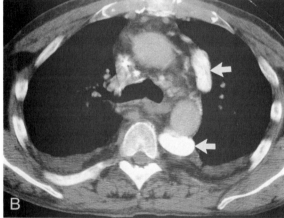

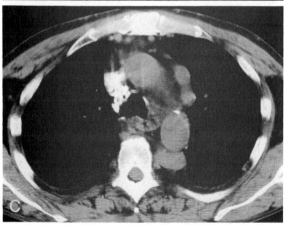

Figure 13.21. Sclerosing Mediastinitis from Histoplasmosis. A PA chest film (**A**) in an asymptomatic 68-year-old man shows lobulated widening of the upper mediastinum. Contrast-enhanced CT (**B**) reveals marked dilation of the left superior intercostal vein (*arrows*), high attenuation material in and around the superior vena cava, and numerous collaterals within the mediastinal fat. A noncontrast scan (**C**) at approximately the same level reveals mediastinal calcification obliterating the superior vena cava. The patient was a former resident of Ohio.

veins. Postobstructive atelectasis or consolidation may also be seen (12).

Computed tomography is the modality of choice for the diagnosis and assessment of chronic sclerosing

mediastinitis. Enlarged lymph nodes with calcification is the most common finding (Fig. 13.21**C**). The fibrotic infiltration of the mediastinal fat characteristic of this condition is seen as abnormal soft-tissue density replacing the normal mediastinal fat with obliteration of the normal mediastinal interfaces. Computed tomography delineates the degree of involvement of the mediastinal vessels, trachea, and central bronchi. In patients with significant superior vena cava involvement, collateral venous channels within the mediastinum and chest wall are well demonstrated (Fig. 13.21**B**).

Magnetic resonance is superior to CT in the assessment of vascular involvement. The ability to examine the mediastinal vessels in both axial and coronal planes without the need for intravenous contrast helps detect vascular compromise. A significant disadvantage of MR is the inability to detect nodal calcification, a finding which is key to the diagnosis. For this reason, MR is most often utilized as an adjunct to CT when findings of vascular involvement are equivocal.

A definitve diagnosis of chronic sclerosing mediastinitis and the establishment of the underlying etiology are difficult. Skin tests for histoplasmosis and tuberculosis may add additional information but are usually not helpful. The precise diagnosis, and more importantly the distinction from infiltrating malignancy, usually requires biopsy.

MEDIASTINAL HEMORRHAGE

Injury to mediastinal vessels resulting from blunt or penetrating thoracic trauma is the most common cause of mediastinal hemorrhage. Blunt chest trauma most often occurs in the setting of a motor vehicle accident, when rapid deceleration and thoracic cage compression produce shearing effects at the aortic isthmus. Iatrogenic trauma, usually from attempts at central line placement, can also cause mediastinal hemorrhage. Spontaneous hemorrhage may develop in patients with a coagulopathy, or with aortic rupture from aneurysm or dissection (Fig. 13.22). Chronic hemodialysis, radiation vasculitis, and bleeding into a mediastinal mass are rare causes of mediastinal hemorrhage.

In the nontraumatic setting, the symptoms and signs of mediastinal hemorrhage are often mild or absent. The patient may complain of retrosternal chest pain radiating toward the back. Rarely, superior vena cava compression may result in the superior vena cava syndrome. Extension of blood from the mediastinum superiorly into the retropharyngeal space may result in neck stiffness, odynophagia, or stridor.

The main radiographic finding in mediastinal hemorrhage of any cause is a focal or diffuse widening of the mediastinum that obscures the normal

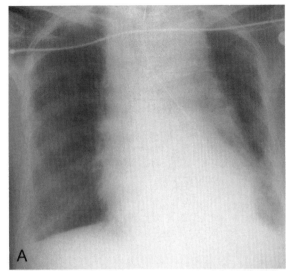

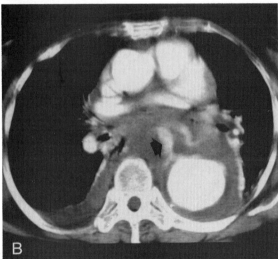

Figure 13.22. Mediastinal Hemorrhage from Ruptured Thoracic Aortic Aneurysm. Portable chest radiograph in a 83-year-old woman with chest pain (**A**) shows marked mediastinal widening. Contrast-enhanced CT (**B**) demonstrates aneurysmal dilation of the descending aorta with active bleeding (*arrow*) into a large mediastinal hematoma. The patient was not a surgical candidate and expired shortly after the study.

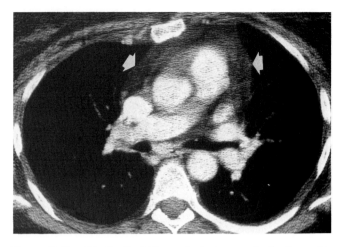

Figure 13.23. Mediastinal Lipomatosis. In a patient with a widened mediastinum on PA radiograph, a CT scan at the level of the right pulmonary artery demonstrates the characteristic low attenuation of mediastinal fat (*white arrows*).

mediastinal contours (13). In mediastinal hemorrhage, the mediastinum develops a flat or slightly convex outward contour, unlike the round, lobulated, or irregular contour seen with enlarged lymph nodes or a localized mediastinal mass. Blood extending from the mediastinum into the pleural or extrapleural space produces a free-flowing effusion or a loculated extrapleural collection, respectively. Rarely, extension of blood into the lungs via the bronchovascular interstitium produces interstitial opacities that mimic pulmonary edema. Serial radiographs may show rapid changes in mediastinal or pleural fluid collections in patients with persistent hemorrhage. Computed tomography demonstrates abnormal soft-tissue within the mediastinum that obliterates the normal interfaces between the mediastinal fat, vessels, and airways. Freshly clotted blood is high in attenuation, and rarely may be equal in attenuation to the opacified blood within adjacent vessels in the presence of active bleeding (Fig. 13.22**B**). Computed tomography is also superior to plain radiography in demonstrating the extramediastinal extent of hemorrhage.

MEDIASTINAL LIPOMATOSIS

Mediastinal lipomatosis is a benign, asymptomatic condition characterized by excessive deposition of fat in the mediastinum. Predisposing conditions include obesity, Cushing's disease, and corticosteroid therapy. However, this entity is unassociated with identifiable conditions in approximately 50% of patients.

On plain radiographs, the most common finding is smooth, symmetric widening of the superior mediastinum. If the amount of fat deposition is marked, the mediastinum may show lobulated margins. Unlike mediastinal tumor infiltration or hemorrhage, which usually causes tracheal deviation or narrowing, the trachea remains midline in position in mediastinal lipomatosis. Fat may also accumulate in the paraspinal regions, chest wall, and cardiophrenic angles; the latter produces enlargement of the epipericardial fat pads, which is a clue to the proper diagnosis.

Computed tomography provides a definitive diagnosis by demonstrating abundant, homogeneous, unencapsulated fat that bulges the mediastinal contours (Fig. 13.23). Displacement or compression of mediastinal structures, particularly the trachea, is notable by its absence. Heterogeneity within the fat suggests other primary or superimposed conditions

Table 13.8. Diffuse Mediastinal Widening

Smooth	Mediastinal lipomatosis
	Malignant infiltration
	Lymphoma
	Small cell carcinoma
	Adenocarcinoma
	Mediastinal hemorrhage
	Arterial bleeding
	Traumatic aortic arch/great vessel laceration
	Aneurysmal rupture
	Venous bleeding
	Superior vena cava/right atrial laceration
	Mediastinitis
	Acute (suppurative)
	Chronic (sclerosing) mediastinitis
	Histoplasmosis
	Tuberculosis
	Idiopathic
Lobulated	Lymph node enlargement (see Table 13.4)
	Thymic mass (see Table 13.3)
	Germ cell neoplasm (see Table 13.3)
	Vascular lesions
	Tortuosity of great vessels
	Superior vena cava occlusion (dilated venous
	collaterals)
	Malignancy
	Sclerosing mediastinitis
	Catheter-induced thrombosis
	Neurofibromatosis

such as neoplastic infiltration, infection, hemorrhage, or fibrosis.

Multiple Symmetric Lipomatosis is a rare entity that resembles simple mediastinal lipomatosis radiographically. The distinction between these two conditions is made by the distribution of abnormal fat and mass effect on mediastinal structures. In multiple symmetric lipomatosis, the cardiophrenic angles, paraspinal areas, and the anterior mediastinum are spared; periscapular lipomas may also be seen. The trachea is often compressed or displaced by fat in patients with this condition, whereas this is not seen in simple lipomatosis.

MALIGNANCY

Malignant involvement of the mediastinum is typically seen as discrete masses or lymph node enlargement. Rarely, diffuse soft-tissue infiltration of the mediastinal fat may occur, either alone or in association with focal lesions. Plain radiographs are nonspecific, usually demonstrating mediastinal widening. Computed tomography shows soft-tissue infiltration of the normal mediastinal fat and obliteration of the normal tissue planes. This pattern is most common with extracapsular spread of lymphoma or small cell carcinoma of lung. The latter disease has a high propensity to invade mediastinal structures, and therefore may present with symptoms of airway obstruction or superior vena cava syndrome.

DIFFERENTIAL DIAGNOSIS OF DIFFUSE MEDIASTINAL WIDENING

The diagnostic considerations in diffuse widening of the mediastinum are reviewed in Table 13.8.

PNEUMOMEDIASTINUM

Pneumomediastinum is the presence of extraluminal gas within the mediastinum. Possible sources of such gas include the lungs, trachea, central bronchi, esophagus, and extension of gas from the neck or abdomen (14).

Air from the lungs is the most common source of pneumomediastinum. The mechanism of pneumomediastinum formation involves a sudden rise in intrathoracic and intraalveolar pressure, which leads to alveolar rupture. The extraalveolar air first collects within the bronchovascular interstitium and then dissects centrally to the hilum and mediastinum (the Macklin effect). Less commonly, the air may dissect peripherally toward the subpleural interstitium and rupture through the visceral pleura to produce a pneumothorax.

Pneumomediastinum most commonly complicates mechanical ventilation in patients with adult respiratory distress syndrome because the combination of positive pressure ventilation and abnormally stiff lungs predisposes to alveolar rupture. Spontaneous pneumomediastinum can occur with deep inspiratory or Valsalva maneuvers during strenuous exercise, childbirth, weight lifting, and inhalation of drugs such as marijuana, nitrous oxide, and crack cocaine. Patients with asthma are prone to pneumomediastinum related to the airways obstruction, which characterizes this disease. Prolonged vomiting from any cause may lead to sufficiently high intrathoracic pressures to produce pneumomediastinum. In patients with diabetic ketoacidosis, the increased respiratory effort that accompanies attempts at correcting the underlying metabolic acidosis can lead to pneumomediastinum. Blunt chest trauma can result in pneumomediastinum because of an abrupt increase in intraalveolar pressure and shearing forces affecting the alveolar walls.

Pneumomediastinum arising from the tracheobronchial tree or esophagus usually results from traumatic disruption of these structures. The marked shearing forces that develop with blunt trauma may lead to fracture of the trachea or mainstem bronchi. Penetrating trauma to the tracheobronchial tree is usually iatrogenic and may follow endotracheal intubation, bronchoscopy, or tracheostomy. Rarely, neoplasms or inflammatory lesions (e.g., tuberculosis) may erode through the tracheal wall and into the peritracheal fat. Esophageal rupture is most often spontaneous, usually in the setting of severe, prolonged vomiting (Boerhaave's syndrome). In addition to pneumomediastinum, a left hydropneumothorax and pneumoperitoneum may be present in this condition. Spontaneous esophageal rupture may occur during childbirth, during a severe asthmatic episode, or with blunt chest trauma. Endoscopic procedures, stent placement, esophageal dilation, corrosive ingestion, and carcinoma may lead to esophageal perforation. Mediastinal gas may be produced by bacterial organisms in acute mediastinitis.

Air within the soft-tissues of the neck from penetrating trauma or laryngeal fracture may lead to pneumomediastinum by extending inferiorly through the retropharyngeal and prevertebral spaces, or along the sheaths of the great vessels. Deep space infections in the neck can spread along the same fascial planes and lead to mediastinitis. "Ludwig's angina" describes the substernal chest pain caused by the intramediastinal extension of such infections. Rarely, pneumomediastinum develops as air dissects superiorly from the retroperitoneum through the aortic hiatus or from the peritoneal cavity along the internal mammary vascular sheaths.

The symptoms associated with pneumomediastinum vary with the underlying etiology, extent of mediastinal air, and presence of mediastinitis. Mediastinal air without infection is generally asymptomatic and does not require treatment. In some patients with spontaneous pneumomediastinum, there may be substernal, pleuritic-type chest pain of sudden onset that can be related to a specific inciting incident such as vomiting or Valsalva maneuver. Dyspnea may be present. In adults, mediastinal air under pressure usually escapes into the neck, producing crepitus over the neck, supraclavicular regions, and chest wall. Rarely, mediastinal air under pressure may produce a tension pneumomediastinum in which the clinical findings are those of cardiac tamponade. Tube decompression of the pneumomediastinum is necessary in such cases. Patients with mediastinitis and pneumomediastinum are usually seriously ill with chest pain, high fevers, dyspnea, and signs of sepsis.

The diagnosis of pneumomediastinum is usually made by findings on conventional radiographs. Small amounts of extraluminal air appear as streaky or stippled radiolucencies within the confines of the mediastinum (Fig. 13.19). Larger collections may be seen outlining the cardiac silhouette, mediastinal vessels, tracheobronchial tree, or esophagus (Fig. 13.24). The most common finding is air outlining the left heart border, where a curvilinear lucency representing pneumomediastinum is paralleled by a thin curvilinear opacity representing the combined thickness of the visceral and parietal pleura of the lingula. Another sign of pneumomediastinum is the "continuous dia-

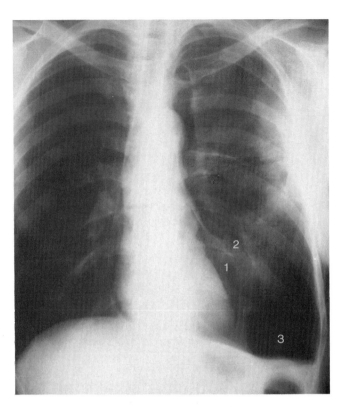

Figure 13.24. Pneumomediastinum and Pneumopericardium. A PA radiograph in a patient who sustained a stab wound to the left chest reveals (from central to peripheral) pneumopericardium (1), loculated hydropneumomediastinum (2), and a left basilar hydropneumothorax (3).

phragm" sign, in which air dissects between the pericardium above and central diaphragm below to allow visualization of the central portion of the diaphragm in contiguity with the right and left hemidiaphragms, each of which is outlined by air in the lower lobes, respectively. While this sign is fairly specific for pneumomediastinum, pneumopericardium may produce a similar finding. Small amounts of mediastinal air are often more easily appreciated on the lateral film, with air outlining the aortic root or main or central pulmonary arteries.

Pneumomediastinum should be distinguished from three entities that may mimic some of the radiographic findings and that have significantly different etiologies and therapeutic implications: pneumopericardium, medial pneumothorax, and Mach bands. Air in the pericardial sac is limited by the normal pericardial reflections and extends superiorly to the proximal ascending aorta and main pulmonary artery (Fig. 13.24). Additionally, pneumopericardium is often secondary to an infectious process with associated pericardial fluid and thickening, which will produce an air-fluid level on horizontal beam radiographs. Air within the pericardial sac will rise to a nondependent position on decubitus positioning, unlike mediastinal

Table 13.9.   Pneumomediastinum

Intrathoracic source	Alveoli
	Valsalva maneuver
	Positive pressure ventilation
	Esophagus
	Boerhaave's syndrome
	Endoscopic interventions (biopsy, dilation,
	sclerotherapy)
	Carcinoma
	Tracheobronchial tree
	Bronchial stump dehiscence
	Tracheobronchial laceration
	Fistula formation
	Tracheal/esophageal malignancy
	Infection (tuberculosis, histoplasmosis)
Extrathoracic source	Recent sternotomy/thoracotomy
	Pneumoperitoneum/pneumoretroperitoneum
	Subcutaneous emphysema in neck
	Stab wound
	Laryngeal fracture

air which is nonmobile. The differentiation of pneumomediastinum from a medial pneumothorax is also aided by decubitus views, as pleural air will rise nondependently along the lateral pleural space. In contrast to pneumothorax, pneumomediastinum may be seen to outline intramediastinal structures (e.g., pulmonary artery, trachea) and is often bilateral. However, the distinction between pneumomediastinum and pneumothorax may be impossible, and the two conditions often coexist, particularly in the neonatal period (Fig. 13.24). Paramediastinal lucent bands created by Mach effect are easily distinguished from pneumomediastinum. The lateral margin of lucent Mach bands consist of lung parenchyma as opposed to the thin pleural line seen with mediastinal air. These bands represent an optical illusion that disappears when the interface between mediastinal soft-tissues and lung is covered.

The differential diagnosis of pneumomediastinum is shown in Table 13.9.

References

1. Glazer GM, Axel L, Moss AA. CT diagnosis of mediastinal thyroid. AJR 1982;138:495–498.
2. Baron RL, Lee JKT, Sagel SS, et al. Computed tomography of the abnormal thymus. Radiology 1982;142:127–134.
3. Filly R, Blank N, Castellino RA. Radiographic distribution of intrathoracic disease in previously untreated patients with Hodgkin's disease and non-Hodgkin's lymphoma. Radiology 1976;120:277–281.
4. Levitt RG, Husband JE, Glazer HS. CT of primary germ-cell tumors of the mediastinum. AJR 1984;142:73–78.
5. Tisi GM, Friedman PJ, Peters RM, et al. Clinical staging of primary lung cancer. American Thoracic Society node mapping scheme. Am Rev Respir Dis 1983;127:659–669.
6. Naidich DF, Zerhouni EA, Siegelman SS. Mediastinum. In: Computed tomography and magnetic resonance imaging of the thorax. 2nd ed. New York: Raven Press, 1991:68–77.
7. McLoud TC, Kalisher L, Stark P, et al. Intrathoracic lymph node metastases from extrathoracic neoplasms. AJR 1978;131:403–407.
8. Reed JC, Haller KK, Feigin DS. Neural tumors of the thorax: subject review from the AFIP. Radiology 1978;126:9–17.
9. Felson B. Neoplasms of the trachea and main stem bronchi. Semin Roentgenol 1983;18:23–37.
10. Gamsu G. Trachea and central bronchi. In: Moss AA, Gamsu G, Genant HK, eds. Computed tomography of the body with magnetic resonance imaging. Vol 1: Thorax and neck. 2nd ed. Philadelphia: WB Saunders, 1992:12–24.
11. Carrol CL, Jeffrey RB, Federle MP, et al. CT evaluation of mediastinal infections. J Comput Assist Tomogr 1987;11:449–454.
12. Wieder S, Rabinowitz JC. Fibrous mediastinitis: a late manifestation of mediastinal histoplasmosis. Radiology 1977;125:305–312.
13. Woodring JH, Loh FK, Kryscio RJ. Mediastinal hemorrhage: an evaluation of radiographic manifestations. Radiology 1984;151:15–21.
14. Crylak D, Milne ENC, Imray TJ. Pneumomediastinum: a diagnostic problem. Crit Rev Diagn Imag 1984;23:75–117.

14
The Hila

Jeffrey S. Klein

The normal anatomy of the pulmonary hila as seen on posteroanterior (PA) and lateral chest radiographs has been reviewed in Chapter 12. Hilar abnormalities are first appreciated on conventional posteroanterior and lateral chest radiographs. Computed tomography (CT) and magnetic resonance imaging (MR) are used to confirm and characterize hilar masses or to detect subradiographic involvement of the hila; the latter most often in patients with bronchogenic carcinoma.

RADIOGRAPHIC FINDINGS OF HILAR ABNORMALITY (TABLE 14.1)
Enlarged (Prominent) Hilum

POSTEROANTERIOR RADIOGRAPH

Since the PA radiograph provides an unimpeded view of each hilum, hilar masses are best appreciated on this view. Signs of hilar abnormality on frontal films caused by enlarged bronchopulmonary lymph nodes or hilar mass include hilar enlargement, increased hilar density, lobulation of the hilar contour, and distortion of central bronchi (1). An abnormal hilum is most easily appreciated by comparison with the contralateral hilum and by review of prior chest radiographs. An enlarged right or left hilum appears as a widening of the hilar shadow with convexity or lobulation of its margins (Fig. 14.1). A left hilar mass may be difficult to detect on frontal radiographs as the lower portion of the left hilum is often obscured by the upper portion of the left cardiac shadow. Computed tomography will often show a left hilar mass not evident on plain radiographs. The normally sharp right hilar angle, formed by the intersection of the lower lateral aspect of the right superior pulmonary vein with the upper lateral aspect of the right interlobar pulmonary artery, is blunted or obscured by a right hilar mass. An increase in density of the hilar shadow is seen with a hilar mass that lies primarily anterior or posterior to the normal hilar vascular shadows. In such patients, the enlarged hilar nodes will produce an increase in density on frontal view and a lobulated appearance when viewed in profile on the lateral radiograph.

There are two common pitfalls in the detection of a hilar mass. An abnormally dense hilum due to an overlying intrapulmonary mass superimposed on the normal hilar shadow may be difficult to distinguish from an intrinsic hilar abnormality. The lateral radiograph or CT will clarify the abnormality. In addition, a well-penetrated radiograph will show a normal interlobar pulmonary artery in those with a mass superimposed on the hilar shadow, while an intrahilar mass obscures the shadow of the normal interlobar pulmonary artery. A mass in the lower right hilum on frontal radiographs may be simulated by the end-on projection of a horizontally oriented right interlobar artery. This is a common appearance that tends to be seen with low lung volumes or in patients with an exaggerated thoracic kyphosis. Comparison with prior radiographs will usually resolve the matter, with CT reserved for equivocal cases.

Table 14.1. Radiographic Findings of Hilar Abnormality

Imaging Method	Finding
Posteroanterior radiograph	Enlargement
	Increased density—mention hilum overlay pitfall
	Abnormal contour—lobulation, lateral convexity
	Abnormal bronchial air column
Lateral radiograph	Right upper lobe bronchus visualized anew
	Thickened intermediate stem line
	Soft tissue within the inferior hilar window
	Increased density and size of composite hilar shadow
Computed tomography	Abnormal mass-enhancing (pulmonary artery, aneurysm) vs. nonenhancing (nodes, mass, cyst)
	Lobulation/spiculation of hilar contour (best seen on lung windows)
	Distortion/invasion of bronchus by soft-tissue mass
	Thickening of bronchial wall
	Invasion of pulmonary artery or vein
	Abnormal soft tissue behind bronchus intermedius, behind left upper lobe bronchus (retrobronchial stripe), or lateral to apical segmental bronchi
Magnetic resonance	Intermediate signal mass(es) on spin-echo images
	Mass within signal void of bronchus/pulmonary artery
Small hilum (see Table 14.4)	

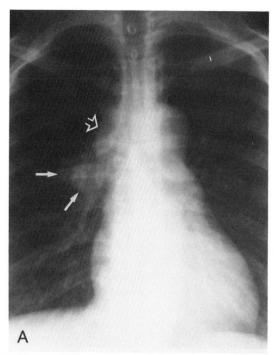

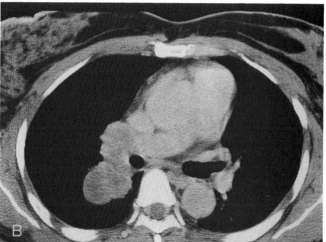

Figure 14.1. Hilar Lymph Node Enlargement on Frontal Radiograph. A. A PA radiograph in a 49-year-old woman with metastatic renal cell carcinoma demonstrates a lobulated enlargement and increased density of the right hilum (*solid arrows*) with concomitant paratracheal node enlargement (*open arrow*). **B.** A CT scan through the hila shows the lobulated soft-tissue mass within the right hilum surrounding the bronchus intermedius.

Bronchogenic carcinoma involving the lobar bronchi or bronchus intermedius may produce lumenal narrowing of the bronchi with enlargement of the hilar shadow. Occasionally, an endobronchial mass produces an abrupt cutoff of the bronchial air column, which is invariably associated with lobar atelectasis or obstructive pneumonitis. The walls of the right and left main and lobar bronchi are not seen on frontal radiographs as they are completely encircled by branches of the right and left pulmonary arteries and upper lobe pulmonary veins. In a small percentage of normal individuals, the right or left anterior segment upper lobe bronchi is visualized as an end-on ring shadows at the superolateral margin of the hila. The presence of a soft-tissue density greater than 5 mm in thickness lateral to an anterior segmental bronchus is suspicious for mass or adenopathy in this region, as the posterior division of the superior vein that lies immediately lateral to the anterior segmental bronchus should not exceed this thickness. Abnormal thickening of the walls of the main or lobar bronchi is a prominent feature of hilar abnormality on lateral chest films, as will be discussed.

Enlargement of the right or left hilar shadow from pulmonary artery dilation is produced by increased flow or increased pressure in the pulmonary arterial circulation. Pulmonary artery dilation is usually assessed by measurement of the right interlobar pulmonary artery on PA radiographs. The margins of this vessel are readily visible, with the lateral margin outlined by air in the lower lobe and the medial margin outlined by air in the bronchus intermedius. The upper limit of normal for the transverse diameter of the proximal right interlobar artery, measured on a PA radiograph at a level immediately lateral to the proximal portion of the bronchus intermedius, is 16 mm in

Figure 14.2.   Enlargement of Hilar Arteries. Posteroanterior (**A**) and lateral (**B**) radiographs in a 40-year-
old man with an atrial septal defect. The hilar enlargement is clearly attributable to dilated right and
left pulmonary arteries. Note the presence of right
heart enlargement, particularly on the lateral view,
indicating the development of cor pulmonale.

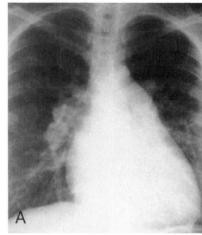

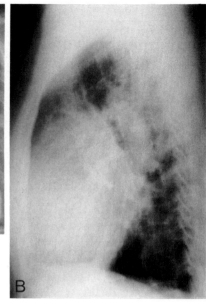

males and 15 mm in females. A dilated right pulmonary artery is most easily distinguished from a hilar
mass by noting smooth enlargement of the right hilar
shadow with concommitant left and main pulmonary
artery enlargement (Fig. 14.2). The enlarged right and
left pulmonary arteries produce a minimal increase in
hilar density without distortion of the adjacent bronchus intermedius or left lower lobe bronchus, respectively. An additional feature of arterial enlargement is
the ability to trace dilated intrapulmonary branches of
the interlobar artery proximally to the lateral margins
of the dilated interlobar vessel; this has been termed
the "'hilum convergence" sign by Felson.

LATERAL RADIOGRAPH

The lateral radiograph can confirm the impression
of hilar abnormality seen on frontal radiographs and
may demonstrate a mass when the frontal radiograph
is normal. A knowledge of the normal lateral hilar
anatomy enhances the ability to detect hilar masses
on the lateral radiograph, increasing the sensitivity of
plain radiographs for detecting hilar abnormalities.
Hilar masses that lie predominantly anterior or posterior to the hilar vessels are best visualized on the lateral view. As the lateral radiograph is a composite of
both hilar shadows, the cumulative density of bilateral hilar masses may produce a significant increase
in the normal density of the composite shadow, which
is more easily appreciated on the lateral than the frontal view.

The radiographic findings of a hilar mass on lateral
radiograph are similar to those seen on the frontal
view. These are an abnormal size of or a lobulated contour to the normal vascular shadows, the presence of
soft tissue in a region normally radiolucent, an increase in density of the composite hilar shadow, and

abnormalities of the central bronchi. An increase in
the size and density of the composite hilar shadow is
best appreciated by comparison with prior radiographs, and is usually seen with bilateral hilar lymph
node enlargement from sarcoidosis. Hilar lymph node
enlargement produces lobulation of the normally
smooth outlines of the right and left main pulmonary
arteries. There are additional findings unique to the
lateral radiograph that suggest the presence of a hilar
mass and may allow lateralization of the hilar abnormality. Since the right upper lobe bronchus is visualized on the lateral radiograph in only a minority of individuals, visualization of the right upper lobe
bronchial lumen, particularly if it was invisible on a
prior lateral radiograph, is strong evidence of mass or
adenopathy in the upper right hilum. The intermediate stem line, which represents the posterior wall of
the bronchus intermedius, is seen in a majority of
normal individuals as a thin vertically oriented line on
the lateral radiograph. A thickness of greater than 3
mm or lobulation of the wall indicates an abnormality
of the bronchus (bronchitis, bronchogenic carcinoma), edema of the axial interstitium (pulmonary
edema, lymphangitic carcinomatosis), or enlargement
of lymph nodes in the posterior aspect of the lower
right hilum.

A recently described finding of hilar mass on lateral radiographs is the presence of a soft-tissue mass
in the normally radiolucent region of the composite
hilar shadow known as the inferior hilar window.
The normal anatomy of the inferior hilar window has
been reviewed in Chapter 12. The identification of a
soft-tissue mass greater than 1 cm in diameter within
this radiolucent region is an accurate indicator of unilateral or bilateral hilar mass (2). Occasionally, the silhouetting of the anterior wall of the left

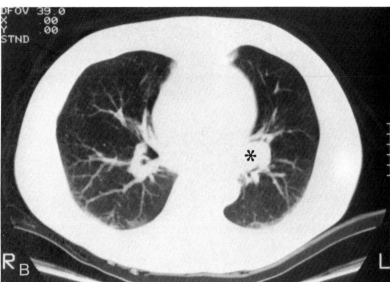

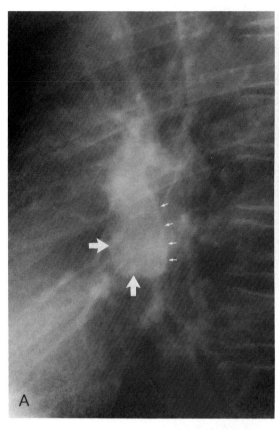

Figure 14.3. Hilar Mass Within the Inferior Hilar Window. A. A coned down view of a lateral radiograph in a patient subsequently found to have a plasmacytoma of the left hilum shows a mass (*large arrows*) within the inferior hilar window obliterating the anterior wall of the left lower lobe bronchus (*small arrows*). **B.** A CT scan through the lower hila confirms the presence of a left hilar mass (*).

lower lobe bronchus, recognized as a concave anterior curvilinear structure contiguous with the anterior aspect of the left upper lobe bronchus, allows lateralization of a mass to the left lower hilum (Fig. 14.3). The added opacity of a mass within the normally radiolucent inferior hilar window produces an oval opacity to the composite hilar shadow on lateral radiographs.

Dilation of the right and left main pulmonary arteries is recognized on lateral radiographs as an enlargement of the normal hilar vascular shadows (Fig. 14.2**B**). This is most easily appreciated on lateral radiographs obtained with the right chest rotated 10° anterior to the left chest.

COMPUTED TOMOGRAPHY AND MAGNETIC RESONANCE IMAGING

Computed tomography is the most sensitive method of detecting and localizing enlarged hilar (bronchopulmonary) lymph nodes and masses (3). Contrast enhancement of the hilar vessels allows for ready identification of enlarged vascular structures or nonenhancing enlarged nodes (defined as nodes that exceed 10 mm in short axis diameter) or masses. Hilar masses are seen on axial or coronal spin-echo MR as round masses of low or intermediate signal intensity, in distinction to the signal void of flowing blood within hilar vessels or of air in bronchi (4). Coronal

MR may be superior to CT in the detection of enlarged hilar lymph nodes since it displays the hilar vessels, which are oriented in the cephalocaudad direction, in length rather than in cross-section. Displacement or distortion of the hilar vessels provides indirect evidence of hilar disease. Tumor invasion of a branch of the pulmonary artery or vein within the hilum produces a filling defect within the vessel on contrast-enhanced CT or intraluminal signal on MR. The density characteristics of hilar masses on CT can help provide important information for differential diagnosis; for example, a round, cystic hilar mass with imperceptible walls in an asymptomatic young person is typical of a bronchogenic cyst.

Enlarged hilar lymph nodes can be detected by CT without the use of intravenous contrast. A detailed knowledge of the normal hilar vascular and bronchial anatomy as seen on CT is necessary for the identification of subtle hilar contour abnormalities. In those portions of the hilum where lung directly contacts a wall of a bronchus, thickening or lobulation of the normal thin linear shadow of the bronchial wall indicates hilar abnormality. This is particularly well seen where the right and left lower lobes contact the posterior walls of the bronchus intermedius and the left upper lobe bronchus, respectively (Fig. 14.4). Lymph node enlargement in these regions is obscured on frontal radiographs by the overlying cardiac and hilar vascular shadows. CT is more sensitive than plain ra-

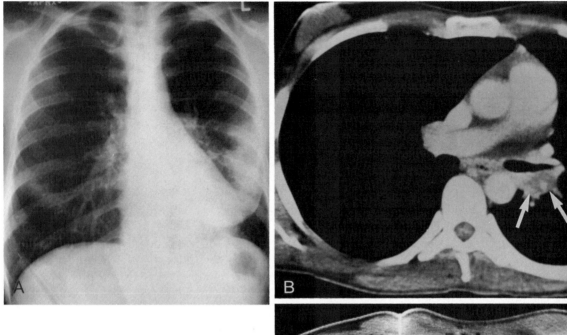

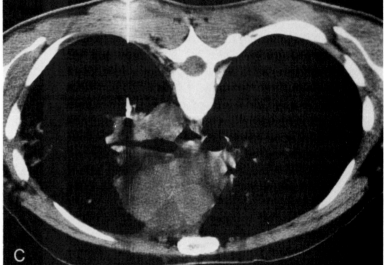

Figure 14.4. Enlarged Left Hilar Nodes Detected by CT. A. A frontal chest radiograph in a middle-aged woman with a nonproductive cough demonstrates patchy air-space opacity in the peripheral left lung. The left hilum is obscured by the heart. **B.** A CT scan through the hila shows a mass (*arrows*) behind the inferior division of the left upper lobe bronchus with extrinsic narrowing of the bronchial lumen. **C.** Cytologic examination of material obtained from a prone CT-guided transthoracic biopsy revealed squamous cell carcinoma.

diographs or MR in the detection of soft tissue masses within lobar or proximal segmental bronchi. In most patients with an endobronchial mass, a large extraluminal component produces a radiographically visible hilar soft tissue mass and obstructive atelectasis.

Enlarged hilar lymph nodes may have different appearances on CT. Enlargement of discrete lymph nodes, most commonly seen in sarcoidosis, appears as multiple, distinct, round masses. When tumor or an inflammatory process extends through the nodal capsule to involve contiguous nodes, a single large mass of confluent lymph nodes is produced that may be difficult to distinguish from a primary hilar bronchogenic carcinoma. This latter appearance is most often seen in hilar nodal metastases from small cell carcinoma of lung or lymphoma (Fig. 14.5).

As in enlargement of mediastinal lymph nodes, the CT density of enlarged hilar nodes can provide clues

to the diagnosis. Lymph nodes that enhance following the administration of intravenous contrast are usually hypervascular metastases from carcinoid tumor, small cell carcinoma of lung, or renal cell carcinoma. Enlarged hilar nodes with central low density suggest nodal necrosis related to *Mycobacterium* infection, nonsmall cell carcinoma of lung, or metastatic seminoma (Fig. 14.6). Calcification within enlarged hilar nodes suggests tuberculosis or fungal infection, sarcoidosis, silicosis, or treated Hodgkin's disease.

Small Hilum

An abnormally small hilum indicates a diminution in the size of the right or left pulmonary artery. The implications of this finding in one or both hila is discussed in a subsequent section.

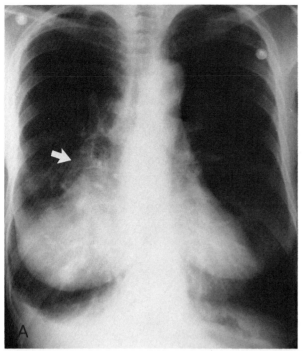

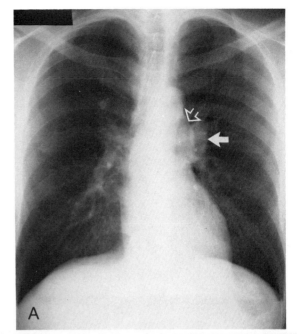

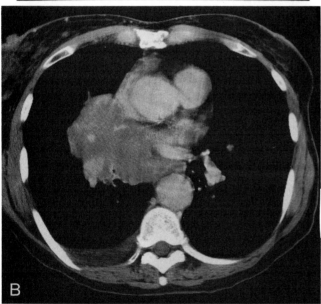

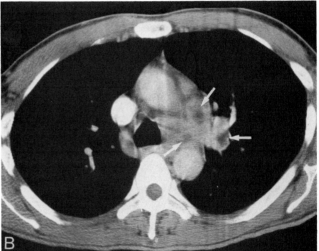

Figure 14.6. Necrotic Lymph Node Enlargement from Tuberculosis. A. A PA chest radiograph in a man with acquired immunodeficiency syndrome shows enlarged left hilar (*solid arrow*) and aortopulmonary window (*open arrow*) nodes. **B.** Contast-enhanced CT demonstrates enlarged nodes with central necrosis (*arrows*). Material aspirated by CT-guided transthoracic biopsy was positive for *Mycobacterium* tuberculosis.

Figure 14.5. Hilar Nodal Metastases from Small Cell Carcinoma of Lung. A. A frontal radiograph in a patient with small cell carcinoma of lung shows emphysema and a right hilar mass (*arrow*) producing middle lobe atelectasis and an associated pleural effusion. **B.** A CT scan demonstrates a large right hilar and mediastinal mass occluding the middle and lower lobe bronchi.

DIAGNOSTIC CONSIDERATIONS—UNILATERAL HILAR ENLARGEMENT (TABLE 14.2)

Malignancy

SQUAMOUS CELL CARCINOMA

A hilar mass usually represents bronchogenic carcinoma or confluent lymph node metastases. Unilat-

eral hilar enlargement may be the presenting radiographic feature of squamous cell carcinoma, where the hilar mass represents the central extension of an endobronchial tumor from its origin within a segmental bronchus (Fig. 14.7). Concomitant hilar lymph node involvement may contribute to the hilar enlargement in some of these patients. Approximately 20% of patients with squamous cell carcinoma have a hilar mass on chest radiograph. In contrast, a hilar mass from adenocarcinoma and large cell carcinoma is uncommon. These tumors more commonly present as a peripheral pulmonary nodule or mass. In many pa-

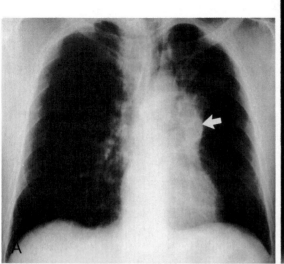

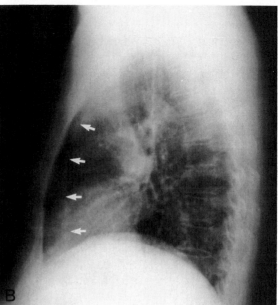

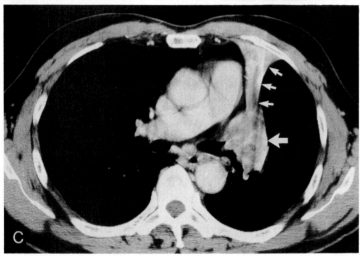

Figure 14.7. Squamous Cell Carcinoma with Obstructive Atelectasis. Posteroanterior (**A**) and lateral (**B**) radiographs demonstrate a left hilar mass (*large arrow*) with atelectasis of the left upper lobe (*small arrows*). **C.** A CT scan through the left upper lobe bronchus shows a left hilar mass (*large arrow*) with an endoluminal component and collapse of the left upper lobe anteriorly (*small arrows*). Bronchoscopic biopsy revealed squamous cell carcinoma.

Table 14.2. Unilateral Hilar Enlargement

Lymph node enlargement			Pulmonary artery enlargement	Valvular pulmonic stenosis
Malignancy	Bronchogenic carcinoma			Pulmonary artery aneurysm
	Lymph node metastases			Infection
	Bronchogenic carcinoma			Tuberculosis (Rasmussen's
	Head and neck malignancy			aneurysm)
	Squamous cell carcinoma of			Left-to-right shunts
	skin, larynx			Patent ductus arteriosis
	Thyroid carcinoma			Atrial and ventricular septal
	Breast carcinoma			defects
	Melanoma			Arteritis (see below)
	Genitourinary malignancy			Tetrology of Fallot
	Renal cell carcinoma			Central pulmonary embolus
	Testicular neoplasm			Chronic thromboembolic disease
	Lymphoma			Pulmonary arteritis
Infection	Tuberculosis			Behçet's disease
	Histoplasmosis			Hughes-Stovins syndrome
	Coccidioidomycosis			Takayasu's arteritis
	Pneumonic plaque		Cyst	Bronchogenic cyst
	Tularemia			
	Anaerobic lung abscess			
	Measles			
	Mononucleosis			

tients, the hilar mass may be obscured by adjacent lung collapse or obstructive pneumonitis.

METASTASES—SMALL CELL CARCINOMA

Unilateral hilar enlargement due to metastatic lymph node involvement is most often seen in small cell carcinoma (Fig. 14.5). The propensity of this tumor for early invasion of the bronchial submucosa and peribronchial lymphatics accounts for the high incidence of widespread hematogenous and hilar and mediastinal lymph node metastases at the time of diagnosis. Plain film evidence of enlarged hilar lymph nodes due to metastases from adenocarcinoma of lung or large cell carcinoma are seen in only 10–15% of patients. Contrast-enhanced CT or MR is more sensitive for detecting enlarged hilar nodes and should be performed in all patients to guide further staging procedures and for proper preoperative or treatment planning.

METASTASES—EXTRATHORACIC MALIGNANCY

Metastases to hilar and mediastinal lymph nodes from extrathoracic malignancies are uncommon, occurring in approximately 2% of patients. The malignancies that are most often associated with intrathoracic nodal metastases are genitourinary (renal and testicular), head and neck (skin, larynx, and thyroid), breast, and melanoma (5). In renal cell carcinoma and testicular carcinoma, lymphatic spread of tumor to retroperitoneal nodes and up the thoracic duct to the posterior mediastinum is the mode of spread to thoracic nodes. Although there is no direct communication between the thoracic duct and anterior mediastinal lymph nodes, reflux of tumor emboli through incompetent valves may allow tumor spread to hilar, paratracheal, and intraparenchymal lymphatics. Head and neck tumors reach the mediastinum via lymphatic spread from cervical lymph nodes. Intrathoracic nodal metastases from breast carcinoma are often seen late in the course of disease, often years after the initial diagnosis. Malignant melanoma is the extrathoracic neoplasm with the highest incidence of intrathoracic nodal metastases; these patients will almost invariably have radiographic evidence of parenchymal metastases.

LYMPHOMA

Although 75% of patients presenting with Hodgkin's disease have evidence of intrathoracic lymph node enlargement, isolated unilateral hilar lymph node enlargement is uncommon. The thoracic manifestations in non-Hodgkin's lymphoma differ in primary pulmonary lymphoma as compared with lymphoma that primarily involves extrathoracic sites with secondary pulmonary involvement. Thoracic involve-ment in primary pulmonary lymphoma is largely limited to parenchymal and pleural disease, whereas secondary pulmonary lymphoma generally manifests as intrathoracic lymph node enlargement, with 35% showing hilar or middle mediastinal lymph node enlargement, some as an isolated finding.

Infection

Unilateral hilar or mediastinal lymph node enlargement is a characteristic feature in primary pulmonary tuberculosis in distinction to postprimary tuberculosis; an exception is the severely immunocompromised patient with acquired immune deficiency syndrome. Isolated lymph node enlargement as a manifestation of primary tuberculosis is more common in children than in adults. There is almost always concomitant parenchymal disease in immunocompetent patients with lymph node enlargement. Fungal infections such as histoplasmosis and coccidioidomycosis may present with hilar lymph node enlargements typically associated with patchy or lobar air-space consolidation in the ipsilateral lung (Fig. 14.8). A variety of bacterial infections have been associated with unilateral hilar lymph node enlargement and include plague, tularemia, and anaerobic lung abscess. Tularemia (*Francisella tularensis*) causes parenchymal consolidation in association with hilar lymph node enlargement and pleural effusion.

The viral infections most commonly associated with hilar lymph node enlargement are infectious mononucleosis and measles pneumonia. The thorax is infrequently involved in mononucleosis, but hilar lymph node enlargement is the most common manifestation of intrathoracic disease. Lymph node enlargement may accompany the reticular interstitial opacities of typical measles pneumonia, or may be associated with nodular, segmental, or lobar opacities and pleural effusion in atypical measles pneumonia.

Pulmonary Artery Enlargement

Although unilateral hilar enlargement is most often due to a mass or enlarged lymph nodes, abnormal enlargement of the right or left pulmonary artery may cause hilar prominence. Vascular disorders producing unilateral pulmonary artery enlargement include poststenotic dilation from valvular or postvalvular pulmonic stenosis, pulmonary artery aneurysms, and distension of the pulmonary artery by thrombus or tumor. Patients with congenital valvular pulmonic stenosis may develop poststenotic dilation or aneurysms of the main and left pulmonary arteries from the jet effect of blood upon these vessels. Rarely, stenoses resulting from pulmonary artery vasculitis, congenital rubella, or Williams syndrome may lead to poststenotic dilation of a pulmonary artery. Aneurysms of

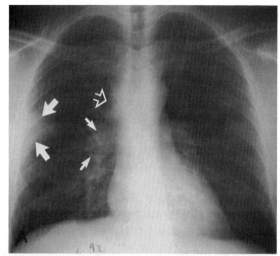

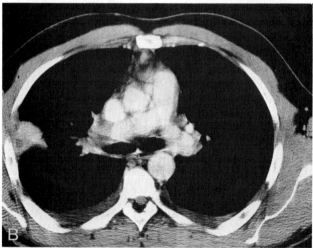

Figure 14.8. Hilar and Mediastinal Lymph Node Enlargement from Pulmonary Coccidioidomycosis. A. Frontal radiograph in a 42-year-old man reveals a pleural based wedge-shaped opacity in the peripheral portion of the right upper lobe (*large arrows*) with enlarged right hilar (*small arrows*) and paratracheal (*open arrow*) nodes. **B.** A CT scan confirms the presence of right hilar nodal enlargement and shows a small focus of necrosis within the parenchymal lesion. Fluoroscopic biopsy of the peripheral lung lesion revealed coccidioidomycosis.

the central pulmonary arteries are usually associated with congenital heart disease such as pulmonic stenosis and left-to-right shunts from ventricular septal defect and patent ductus arteriosis. Rare vasculitides such as Behçet's disease and the Hughes-Stovins syndrome may present with pulmonary artery aneurysms. A large pulmonary embolus lodging in the proximal portion of a pulmonary artery may cause proximal dilation. Obviously, these patients are symptomatic and will show characteristic findings on perfusion lung scan and pulmonary arteriography.

Bronchogenic Cyst

An uncommon cause of a hilar mass is a bronchogenic cyst. Computed tomography and MR will show a

Table 14.3. Bilateral Hilar Enlargement

Lymph node enlargement	Malignancy (see Table 14.2)
	Infection (see Table 14.2)
	Inflammatory disease
	Sarcoidosis
	Berylliosis
	Angioimmunoblastic
	lymphadenopathy
	Inhalational disease
	Silicosis
Pulmonary artery enlargement	Pulmonary arterial hypertension
	Left-to-right intracardiac shunt
	High output state
	Anemia
	Thyrotoxicosis
	Cystic fibrosis

round, smooth, thin-walled cyst, usually found in an asymptomatic young adult. Since the hilum is an unusual location for a bronchogenic cyst, and distinction from a necrotic tumor or lymph node mass cannot be made radiographically, these lesions should undergo biopsy or be removed.

DIAGNOSTIC CONSIDERATIONS—BILATERAL HILAR ENLARGEMENT (TABLE 14.3)

Bilateral hilar enlargement is due to either enlargement of the central pulmonary arteries or hilar lymph nodes.

Malignancy

The malignancies producing bilateral hilar lymph node enlargement are similar to those producing unilateral enlargement. In distinction to unilateral nodal enlargement, metastases are uncommon causes of bilateral hilar nodal enlargement. The most frequent solid tumors producing bilateral hilar disease are small cell carcinoma of lung and malignant melanoma.

Bilateral hilar lymph node involvement by lymphoma is more common in Hodgkin's disease than non-Hodgkin's lymphoma. Hilar involvement is virtually never seen without concomitant anterior mediastinal nodal enlargement in Hodgkin's disease, whereas non-Hodgkin's lymphoma may produce isolated hilar disease.

The most common chest radiographic manifestation of leukemic involvement of the thorax is hilar and mediastinal lymph node enlargement, which is seen in up to 25% of patients. Lymph node enlargement is much more common in the lymphocytic than the myelogenous form, particularly in chronic lymphocytic leukemia.

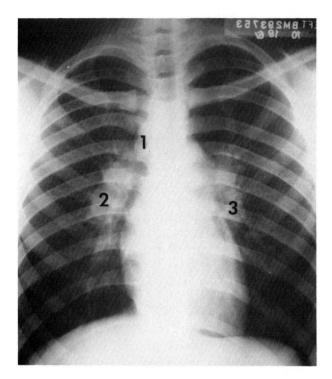

Figure 14.9. Bilateral Hilar Lymph Node Enlargement in Sarcoidosis. A PA radiograph in an asymptomatic 26-year-old man shows marked enlargement of right paratracheal (1), right hilar (2), and left hilar (3) lymph nodes characteristic of sarcoidosis.

Infection

Mediastinal and hilar lymph node enlargement from infection is most often seen in tuberculous and fungal infection with histoplasmosis and coccidioidomycosis. In these diseases, the lymph node enlargement may be unilateral or bilateral. With bilateral disease, the enlargement is asymmetric in distinction to sarcoidosis, which is typically symmetric. Bacterial infection from *Bacillus anthracis* (anthrax) and *Yersinia pestis* (plague) may produce bilateral hilar enlargement. In anthrax infection, the lymph node enlargement is often associated with lower lobe, patchy air space opacities. The bubonic form of plague may produce marked hilar and mediastinal adenopathy without pneumonia. Recurrent bacterial infection complicating cystic fibrosis is often associated with bilateral hilar lymph node enlargement, and distinction from pulmonary artery enlargement caused by the pulmonary hypertension may be difficult.

Sarcoidosis

Sarcoidosis is associated with bilateral hilar lymph node enlargement in 80% of patients (6). Most of these patients have concomitant paratracheal lymph node enlargement, and nearly half have concomitant radiographic parenchymal disease. The pattern of lymph node involvement in sarcoidosis has been

termed the 1-2-3 sign, with 1 being right paratracheal, 2 being right hilar, and 3 being left hilar lymph node enlargement. The enlarged nodes produce symmetric lobulated hilar masses on plain film since the enlarged nodes remain separate (Fig. 14.9). In 20% of patients, the involved lymph nodes will calcify; usually the calcifications are punctate in appearance, but occasionally peripheral "eggshell" calcification is seen. In some patients, the involved nodes can be seen to enhance after contrast administration on CT. In the majority of patients, the enlarged nodes resolve within 2 years of discovery; in a small percentage, the nodes remain enlarged for many years.

Berylliosis and Silicosis

The hilar and mediastinal lymph node enlargement of chronic berylliosis is radiographically indistinguishable from sarcoidosis. Similarly, silicosis can produce hilar and mediastinal lymph node enlargement; eggshell calcification of hilar nodes is highly suggestive of this entity, although peripheral nodal calcification may also be seen with sarcoidosis, histoplasmosis, or amyloidosis.

Pulmonary Artery Enlargement

Bilateral pulmonary artery enlargement is seen with increased flow or increased resistance in the pulmonary circulation.

PULMONARY ARTERY HYPERTENSION

Most often these entities are associated with pulmonary arterial hypertension (PAH), although in some patients with a left-to-right shunt, a drop in pulmonary vascular resistance early in the course of disease produces normal pulmonary arterial pressure. The diagnosis of PAH is usually evident from the clinical history, physical findings, and appearance on chest radiographs. Pulmonary artery hypertension is defined as a systolic pressure in the pulmonary circulation exceeding 30 mm Hg. This is usually measured directly by catheterization of the pulmonary artery or indirectly by echocardiography. The typical radiographic findings common to all causes of PAH are enlarged hilar and central (lobar and segmental) pulmonary arteries that taper rapidly toward the lung periphery (Fig. 14.2) (7). Occasionally, hypertension-induced atherosclerotic lesions in the large elastic arteries can produce mural calcifications on radiographs, a rare finding that is specific for PAH. A useful measurement for enlargement of the central pulmonary arteries, usually indicating PAH in the absence of a left-to-right shunt, is a transverse diameter of the proximal interlobar pulmonary artery on PA chest radiograph exceeding 16 mm. Another specific indicator of PAH is a transverse measurement of the main pulmonary artery on CT or MR that exceeds 28.6 mm. However, a normal measurement of the main or right interlobar pulmonary artery does not exclude PAH, as patients with mild or even moderate elevation of pulmonary artery pressure may have normal-sized arteries. Those patients with long-standing PAH will develop right ventricular hypertrophy, with eventual right ventricular dilation and failure ("cor pulmonale"). In addition, MR may also demonstrate intraluminal signal during the early diastolic phase of the cardiac cycle, a finding indicative of turbulent flow due to increased vascular resistance, sometimes seen with marked elevation of pulmonary artery pressure.

Increased Flow through the Pulmonary Circulation may be seen in any patient with a high cardiac output, such as anemia, thyrotoxicosis, or left-to-right shunts. The latter includes atrial and ventricular septal defect, patent ductus arteriosus, and partial anomalous pulmonary venous return. Early in the course of left-to-right shunts, the pulmonary artery pressure is normal or slightly elevated as pulmonary vascular resistance drops to compensate for the increased flow. In these patients, there is enlargement of both central and periphral pulmonary arteries, producing "shunt vascularity" on chest radiographs. Later, usually in young adulthood, the muscular pulmonary arterioles develop medial hyperplasia and intimal fibrosis, with resultant increased pulmonary vascular resistance. When this occurs, the chest radiograph demonstrates findings typical of PAH that is indistinguishable from PAH due to other etiologies.

An increase in resistance to pulmonary blood flow is the most common cause of PAH. The disorders producing increased pulmonary vascular resistance are pulmonary venous hypertension, parenchymal lung disease, chest wall deformity, diffuse pleural fibrosis, pulmonary arterial disease, and idiopathic pulmonary vascular disease. The most common cause of chronic elevation of pulmonary venous pressure is mitral stenosis, although any impedence to pulmonary venous return to the left heart can produce venous hypertension. Less common entities in this group include chronic left ventricular failure, atrial myxoma, cor triatriatum, and pulmonary vein stenosis or occlusion. In addition to the characteristic pulmonary arterial changes of PAH, patients may show left ventricular dilation in left ventricular failure or left atrial enlargement in mitral stenosis or cor triatriatum. The radiographic signs of pulmonary venous hypertension and pulmonary edema may be seen early in the course of these disorders, but are often absent by the time PAH has developed.

Parenchymal lung disease, particularly centrilobular emphysema and diffuse interstitial fibrosis, are common causes of PAH. The mechanisms by which these disorders produce increased vascular resistance include chronic hypoxemia and reflex vasoconstriction and the development of irreversible changes in pulmonary arteriolar caliber with widespread obliteration of the pulmonary vascular bed. The radiographic findings of emphysema and interstitial fibrosis are usually evident on plain radiographs by the time PAH has developed.

Chronic hypoxemia from alveolar hypoventilation is the likely mechanism for PAH, which complicates pleural fibrosis, kyphoscoliosis, and the obesity-hypoventilation syndrome. Pleural thickening and kyphoscoliosis are readily evident radiographically. The obesity-hypoventilation syndrome is usually associated with marked truncal obesity and lungs that are diminished in volume (mostly due to diaphragmatic elevation) but are normal in appearance.

Disorders of the pulmonary arteries producing PAH include pulmonary emboli, vasculitis, and the pulmonary arteriopathy resulting from long-standing increased pulmonary blood flow from left-to-right shunt. Occlusion of lobar and segmental vessels producing PAH can be the result of failure of pulmonary thromboemboli to lyse or completely recanalize. The diagnosis of large vessel thromboembolic pulmonary hypertension is usually made by demonstrating large mismatches on ventilation/perfusion lung scanning, with pulmonary arteriography showing occlusion or stenosis of multiple lobar or segmental pulmonary arteries. Radiographically, regions of peripheral oligemia may be seen, but more often the lungs are normal in appearance. Rarely, pulmonary vasculitis resulting from diseases such as rheumatoid lung disease or Takayasu's arteritis can produce obliteration of the pulmonary vasculature and lead to PAH.

Idiopathic or Primary Pulmonary Hypertension encompasses diseases of the pulmonary arterioles and venules that are not attributable to other etiologies and have characteristic histologic fndings. Plexogenic pulmonary arteriopathy, recurrent microscopic pulmonary embolism, and pulmonary veno-occlusive disease are the three diseases that comprise this category.

Plexogenic Pulmonary Arteriopathy is a disease of young women in whom medial hypertrophy and intimal fibrosis obliterate the muscular arteries. Dilated vascular channels within the periphery of the obliterated vessel produce the plexogenic lesions seen on biopsy in virtually all patients with this disease. Progressive dyspnea and fatigue develop with characteristic physical findings of PAH and cor pulmonale. In plexogenic pulmonary arteriopathy, pulmonary perfusion scans typically show normal perfusion or small, nonsegmental peripheral perfusion defects, allowing distinction from large vessel thromboembolic disease.

Microembolic Disease is clinically and radiographically indistinguishable from plexogenic arteri-

Table 14.4.   Small Hilum (Hila)

Unilateral	Absence or hypoplasia of the pulmonary artery
	Hypoplastic or hypogenetic lung
	Swyer-James syndrome
	Lobar atelectasis
	Lobar resection
	Compression/invasion of the pulmonary artery
	Cyst
	Neoplasm
	Fibrosing mediastinitis
Bilateral	Emphysema
	Obstruction to pulmonary flow
	Fibrosing mediastinitis
	Tetrology of Fallot
	Valvular pulmonic stenosis
	Ebstein's anomaly

opathy. In this entity, plexogenic lesions within arterioles are absent. Perfusion scans are more likely to show small perfusion defects in this disorder. The presence of small microemboli histologically is not a distinguishing feature, as in situ thrombosis within diseased arterioles can have a similar appearance.

Pulmonary Veno-occlusive Disease refers to the obliteration of small intrapulmonary venules which results in interstitial pulmonary edema. The transmission of increased pressure to the arterial side leads to medial hypertrophy and obliteration of vessel lumina with resultant arterial hypertension. Chest radiographs often show interstitial or air space pulmonary edema with a normal heart size. The radiographic signs of pulmonary venous hypertension are absent, and the pulmonary capillary wedge pressure is usually normal. Perfusion lung scanning is usually normal or shows small peripheral nonsegmental defects. The combination of pulmonary edema with a normal heart size, absent findings for pulmonary venous hypertension, normal pulmonary capillary wedge pressure, and the insidious onset of dyspnea should suggest this diagnosis rather than left heart failure, mitral valve disease, or large pulmonary venous occlusion. A definitive diagnosis can only be made by characteristic findings on open lung biopsy. The prognosis is universally poor, with most patients succumbing to their disease within 2 years of diagnosis.

DIAGNOSTIC CONSIDERATIONS—SMALL HILUM (HILA) (TABLE 14.4)

In an adult, this finding is usually unilateral, although bilaterally small hila can be seen in some patients with severe pulmonary overinflation from emphysema or in those with diminished pulmonary blood flow due to congenital pulmonary outflow obstruction (tetralogy of Fallot, Ebstein's anomaly). The most common cause of a small hilum is atelectasis or resection of a portion of lung, leaving a small residual hilar artery supplying the remaining lobe or lobes. Hy-

poplasia of the pulmonary artery, often with associated abnormalities of the ipsilateral lung (hypogenetic lung syndrome, Swyer-James syndrome), is another cause of a small hilum. Less commonly, invasion of the proximal pulmonary artery by mediastinal tumor, or obstruction of the pulmonary artery due to fibrosing mediastinitis can produce a diminutive hilar shadow. In any patient in whom a small hilum is a new radiographic finding, a CT scan should be performed to assess the mediastinum for central obstructing lesions. The left hilum can appear small in patients in whom the hilar shadow is obscured by the upper left heart margin or by fat in the region of the aortopulmonic interface. In these cases, the lateral radiograph will usually show a normal-sized left pulmonary artery.

BRONCHOGENIC CARCINOMA

Bronchogenic carcinoma is now the most common cause of death from malignancy in adult men and women. Although survival rates for lung cancer are poor, accurate radiographic diagnosis and staging remain important in the management of patients with lung cancer. This section will review the key pathologic, epidemiologic, and radiologic features of bronchogenic carcinoma, with particular emphasis on the radiologic staging of this disease.

Definition

Bronchogenic carcinoma is but one of several tumors that may arise within the lung. Epithelial tumors are the most common lung tumors. Benign epithelial tumors of the lung are rare in adults, and include squamous cell papilloma and pleomorphic adenoma (benign mixed tumor). Malignant epithelial tumors of the lung include bronchogenic carcinoma, carcinoid tumor, and tumors of mucus gland origin including adenoid cystic and mucoepidermoid carcinoma. In addition to those that arise from the pulmonary epithelium, tumors may rarely arise from mesenchymal or neural elements of the bronchial tree. Such tumors include lipoma, fibroma, leiomyoma, hemangioma, schwannoma, and granular cell myoblastoma. Malignant involvement of the lung in patients with Hodgkin's disease and non-Hodgkin's lymphoma is almost always associated with mediastinal or extrathoracic disease. Finally, there is a group of extremely rare malignant lung tumors that include pulmonary blastoma and primary malignant melanoma of lung.

Cytologic and Pathologic Features

Bronchogenic carcinoma is a malignant neoplasm that arises from bronchial or alveolar epithelium. Ninety-nine percent of malignant epithelial neoplasms of the lung arise from the bronchi or lung, while less than 0.5% arise from the trachea. Bronchogenic carcinoma is divided into four main histologic subtypes based on their gross and microscopic features: squamous cell carcinoma, adenocarcinoma, small cell carcinoma, and large cell carcinoma (8).

Squamous Cell Carcinoma is the most common subtype of bronchogenic carcinoma, accounting for 35% of all cases. This tumor arises centrally within a lobar or segmental bronchus. Grossly, these tumors are polypoid masses that grow into the bronchial lumen as they simultaneously invade the bronchial wall. The central location and endobronchial component of the tumor accounts for the presenting symptoms of cough and hemoptysis, and accounts for the common radiographic findings of a hilar mass with or without obstructive pneumonitis or atelectasis (Fig. 14.7). Central necrosis is common in large tumors; cavitation may be seen if communication has occurred between the central portion of the mass and the bronchial lumen. Histologically, squamous cell carcinoma is characterized by invasion of the bronchial wall by nests of malignant cells with abundant cytoplasm. The formation of keratin pearls and intercellular bridges, seen in well-differentiated tumors, is specific for squamous cell carcinoma.

Adenocarcinoma accounts for 25% of all bronchogenic carcinomas. These tumors arise from bronchiolar or alveolar epithelium in the lung periphery and have an irregular or spiculated appearance where they invade adjacent lung. Fibrosis in and about the tumor is common. These gross features produce an ill-defined pulmonary nodule on chest radiographs. Histologically, adenocarcinoma demonstrates gland formation and mucin production. A subtype of adenocarcinoma, bronchioloalveolar or alveolar cell carcinoma, has unique pathologic features. This tumor is characterized by growth along preexisting bronchiolar and alveolar walls without invasion or distortion of these structures. When localized, bronchioloalveolar cell carcinoma appears as a solitary pulmonary nodule. Diffuse disease, which represents either multifocal origin of disease or transbronchial spread of tumor, may present as air-space opacification simulating pneumonia or as diffuse bilateral nodular air-space opacities.

Small Cell Carcinoma accounts for 25% of bronchogenic carcinomas, equal in incidence to adenocarcinoma. These tumors arise centrally within the main or lobar bronchi. They are at the malignant end of the spectrum of neoplasms arising from bronchial neuroendocrine (APUD or Kulchitsky) cells, with atypical and typical carcinoid tumors representing progressively less aggressive malignant tumors, respectively. These tumors exhibit a small endobronchial component, invading the bronchial wall and peribronchial tissues early in the course of disease. This produces a hilar or mediastinal mass with extrinsic bronchial compression and obstruction. Invasion of submucosal and peribronchial lymphatics leads to local lymph node enlargement and hematogenous dissemination, which are almost invariable at the time of presentation (Fig. 14.5). Microscopically, tightly clustered malignant cells are seen that have nuclei molded together because of the scant amount of cytoplasm within the cells. Mitoses are invariably present, and help distinguish this lesion histologically from carcinoid tumor. Electron microscopy reveals the presence of intracytoplasmic neurosecretory granules.

Large Cell Carcinoma accounts for 15% of bronchogenic carcinomas, and is occasionally diagnosed when a non-small cell bronchogenic carcinoma is found that lacks the histologic characteristics of squamous cell carcinoma or adenocarcinoma. Histologic features include large cells with abundant cytoplasm and prominent nucleoli. This tumor tends to arise peripherally as a solitary mass and is often large at the time of presentation.

Epidemiology

Most patients with bronchogenic carcinoma are cigarette smokers in their 40s and 50s. Men are most commonly affected, although the percentage of lung cancer patients who are women has risen steadily in parallel with the increased prevalence of heavy cigarette smoking among women. The overall 5-year survival rate for all patients with lung cancer is 10–15%.

Well-recognized risk factors for the development of bronchogenic carcinoma include cigarette smoke, asbestos exposure, previous Hodgkin's disease, radon exposure, viral infection, and diffuse interstitial or localized lung fibrosis. The relationship between cigarette smoke and bronchogenic carcinoma is irrefutable. Lung cancer is uncommon in nonsmokers, and cigarette smoking is associated with a 10- to 30-fold increase in the incidence of bronchogenic carcinoma as compared with nonsmokers. Carcinogens in cigarette smoke produce cellular atypia and squamous metaplasia of the bronchiolar epithelium, which may precede malignant transformation. Squamous cell carcinoma and small cell carcinoma are the two histologic subtypes with the strongest association with cigarette smoking in men, while cigarette smoking in women is associated with an increased incidence of all histologic subtypes.

Asbestos exposure is associated with an increased incidence of bronchogenic carcinoma, malignant pleural mesothelioma, laryngeal carcinoma, and esophagogastric carcinoma. Bronchogenic carcinoma may follow prolonged exposure, usually 20 years or more, from the mining or processing of asbestos fibers. A long latency period from the initial asbestos exposure, generally 35 years or longer, is necessary for the development of bronchogenic carcinoma. While asbestos exposure alone is associated with a fourfold increase in the incidence of bronchogenic carcinoma, concomitant cigarette smoking, perhaps by acting as a co-carcinogen, is associated with a 40- to 50-fold increase in the incidence as compared to the nonexposed, nonsmoking individual.

Patients previously treated for mediastinal Hodgkin's disease with radiation, chemotherapy, or a combination of the two, have an eightfold increase in lung cancer beginning 10 years after treatment. Exposure to inhaled radioactive material, particularly radon, is associated with the development of small cell carcinoma of lung 20 years or more after the exposure.

The link between viral infection and bronchogenic carcinoma comes chiefly from the study of Jaagsietke, a disease of sheep that closely resembles alveolar cell carcinoma of the lung in humans. This disease is caused by a retroviral infection, leading to speculation that a similar pathogenesis exists in humans with this form of lung cancer.

It has been suggested that local lung scarring as a result of inflammation or infarction can induce the development of a "scar carcinoma," most commonly adenocarcinoma. As adenocarcinoma can produce fibrous tissue, it is unclear whether the scar is the result or cause of the carcinoma. Nevertheless, there are patients in whom a focal scar can be identified on prior radiographs in the region of a carcinoma. Diffuse interstitial fibrosis in patients with scleroderma has been associated with an increased incidence of bronchogenic carcinoma, particularly alveolar cell carcinoma. Similarly, adenocarcinoma occurs with greater than expected frequency in patients with interstitial fibrosis associated with rheumatoid lung disease.

Radiographic Findings in Bronchogenic Carcinoma

The chest radiographic findings in bronchogenic carcinoma depend largely upon the subtype of cancer and the stage of the disease at time of diagnosis. The most common finding is a hilar mass with or without bronchial obstruction. Since squamous cell carcinoma and small cell carcinoma arise from central bronchi, the majority of these types of bronchogenic carcinoma produce a hilar mass (Figs. 14.5 and 14.7). The hilar mass represents either the extraluminal portion of the bronchial tumor or hilar lymph nodes enlargement from metastatic disease. Extension of the hilar lesion into the mediastinum or the presence of mediastinal nodal metastases can produce a smooth or lobulated mediastinal mass. Marked mediastinal nodal enlargement producing a lobulated mediastinal contour is characteristic of small cell carci-

noma. Extensive replacement of the mediastinal fat by either primary tumor or extracapsular nodal extension may produce diffuse mediastinal widening, with loss of the mediastinal fat planes and compression or frank invasion of the trachea or central bronchi, esophagus, and mediastinal vascular structures as seen on contrast-enhanced CT or MR.

Obstruction of the bronchial lumen by the endobronchial component of a tumor can result in several different radiographic findings. The most common finding is resorptive atelectasis or obstructive pneumonitis of lung distal to the obstructing lesion. Resorptive atelectasis is recognized by the classic findings of lobar or whole-lung collapse, whereas obstructive pneumonitis results in minimal or no atelectasis, or occasionally an increase in the volume of the affected portion of lung. An abnormal increase in lobar or whole-lung volume is recognized radiographically by a bulging interlobar fissure marginating the obstructed lobe or by mediastinal shift, respectively, and is termed "drowned lung." Occasionally, the mass producing lobar atelectasis creates a central convexity in the normally concave contour of the collapsed lobe, producing the "S-sign of Golden." Most commonly, the opacity of the obstructed lung obscures the underlying central lesion. The lung with obstructive pneumonitis is not infected, but rather shows a chronic inflammatory infiltrate and alveolar filling with lipid-laden macrophages; the latter finding accounts for the descriptive terms golden or endogenous lipoid pneumonia.

Additional radiographic features of atelectasis that should suggest obstruction by tumor include obliteration of the main or proximal lobar bronchial air column, hilar mass, combined middle and lower lobe atelectasis, and atelectasis or opacification that persists beyond 3–4 weeks. Computed tomography confirms the presence of lobar atelectasis, and typically demonstrates mucus bronchograms within the lung distal to the obstructing lesion (Fig. 14.10). The central mass is readily distinguished from vascular structures, with narrowing or occlusion of the bronchial lumen best seen on images viewed at lung windows. The central tumor is usually distinguished from atelectatic lung by the contrast between the perfused but nonventilated enhancing lung and the low attenuation, nonenhancing central mass. An uncommon manifestation of bronchial obstruction by bronchogenic carcinoma is the development of mucoid impaction (mucocele). This represents mucus within dilated segmental bronchi distal to the obstructing neoplasm. Radiographic visualization of the mucocele requires collateral ventilation to the obstructed lobe or segment.

Tumors that arise from bronchiolar or alveolar epithelium, namely adenocarcinoma and large cell carci-

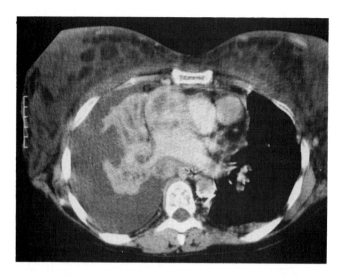

Figure 14.10. Mucus Bronchograms in Lung Distal to Obstructing Tumor. A contrast-enhanced CT scan in a woman with a large necrotic right hilar and mediastinal mass demonstrates tubular opacities within collapsed middle and right lower lobes representing mucus-filled bronchi distal to an obstructing squamous cell carcinoma.

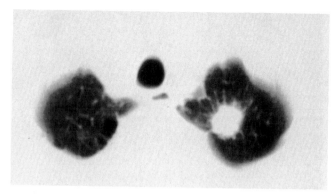

Figure 14.11. Spiculated Nodule in Adenocarcinoma of Lung. A CT scan in a patient with biopsy-proven adenocarcinoma shows a nodule with spiculated margins in the left lung apex.

noma, commonly produce a solitary pulmonary nodule or mass on chest radiograph. The radiographic evaluation of the solitary pulmonary nodule is reviewed in Chapter 15. A notched, lobulated, or spiculated margin to the nodule is common in bronchogenic carcinoma (Fig. 14.11). The radially spiculated appearance of a peripheral nodule has been termed "corona radiata." While it was initially believed to be pathognomonic for malignancy, the finding of a corona radiata is nonspecific and can be seen in granulomas. The edge characteristics of a solitary pulmonary nodule are best appreciated on thin-section high-resolution CT images through the lesion. Cavitation of solitary malignant nodules is uncommon, since adenocarcinoma infrequently cavitates. The walls of cavitating neoplasms tend to be thicker and more nodular than inflammatory lesions. Air bronchograms seen traversing a solitary pulmonary nodule are highly suspicious for adenocarcinoma, particularly bronchioloalveolar cell carcinoma. Eccentric calcification within nodules may represent dystrophic calcification of necrotic regions, granulomas engulfed by an enlarging tumor, or calcification of mucin or psammoma bodies secreted by tumor cells in adenocarcinomas. Masses greater than 3 cm in diameter seen in adults over 35 years of age are overwhelmingly malignant. The volume doubling time (equivalent to a 25% increase in diameter) for a malignant nodule usually ranges from 1 month (some squamous cell and large cell carcinomas) to 24 months (certain bronchioloalveolar cell carcinomas). However, this rule has exceptions and should only be used for retrospective evaluation of interval growth and not used to follow a newly discovered and potentially resectable lesion.

Pancoast's Tumor is a peripheral neoplasm arising within the superior sulcus of the lung, which is that portion of the lung apex indented superiorly by the subclavian artery. The majority of these lesions are squamous cell carcinomas or adenocarcinomas. Presenting symptoms relate to invasion of adjacent structures, with shoulder and arm pain attributable to brachial plexus involvement, Horner's syndrome from involvement of the sympathetic chain, and localized pain from chest wall invasion (Fig. 14.12). The plain radiographic diagnosis is difficult as an apical pleuroparenchymal fibrous cap is a common finding in older individuals. A thickness exceeding 5 mm, asymmetry of the apical opacities that exceeds 5 mm, enlargement on serial radiographs, or evidence of rib destruction should prompt further evaluation with CT or MR. The presence of a mass with an inferior convex margin toward the lung, or the presence of rib or vertebral body destruction are uncommon plain film findings. Computed tomography demonstrates the apical region to better advantage and is best for determining the extent of chest wall and vertebral invasion. Coronal and sagittal MR is useful for determining the relationship of the mass to the subclavian artery, brachial plexus, and spinal canal.

Air-space opacification caused by bronchogenic carcinoma is an uncommon radiographic finding in the absence of an obstructing endobronchial lesion. Bronchioloalveolar cell carcinoma may produce air-space opacification as malignant cells grow along the preexisting parenchymal lattice while producing large amounts of mucus. The majority (60–90%) of bronchioloalveolar cell carcinomas are localized and appear as solitary pulmonary nodules. Computed tomography often shows bronchi traversing the lesion and a pleural tail extending from the tumor toward the pleural surface. The diffuse form may present as lobar or multilobar air-space opacification, or as diffuse bilateral air-space nodules. These latter appearances may be indistinguishable from pneumonia or edema, al-

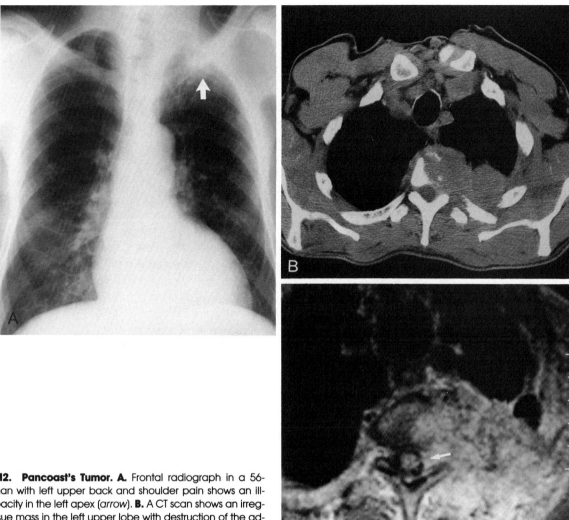

Figure 14.12. Pancoast's Tumor. A. Frontal radiograph in a 56-year-old man with left upper back and shoulder pain shows an ill-defined opacity in the left apex (*arrow*). **B.** A CT scan shows an irregular soft-tissue mass in the left upper lobe with destruction of the adjacent rib and vertebral body. **C.** Axial MR (TR = 1300, TE = 35) clearly shows the tumor extending into the spinal canal (*arrow*).

though the clinical findings, chronicity of the process, and cytologic examination of sputum and bronchoalveolar lavage specimens should provide the correct diagnosis. An additional finding on contrast-enhanced CT in patients with the diffuse form of bronchoalveolar cell carcinoma is the presence of a "CT angiogram" sign within consolidated areas. In these patients, filling of the air spaces with mucoid material produced by the malignant cells creates low density air space opacification surrounding the enhanced pulmonary arteries that traverse the consolidated regions.

The superior vena cava syndrome results from obstruction of the superior vena cava from compression or invasion by mediastinal tumor, particularly with small cell carcinoma. A discussion of the entity is found in Chapter 13.

A malignant pleural effusion is a bloody or exudative parapneumonic fluid collection in a patient with proven malignancy that shows malignant cytology on thoracentesis or tumor on closed pleural biopsy. Al-

though the presence of a pleural effusion in patients with bronchogenic carcinoma is associated with a poor prognosis, it is not synonymous with malignant pleural involvement since central lymphatic obstruction and postobstructive infection can produce benign effusions in patients with malignancy. Smooth or lobulated pleural thickening or a discrete pleural mass suggest malignant pleural involvement. Contrast-enhanced CT may demonstrate pleural thickening or mass obscured by pleural fluid on plain radiographs. The utility of CT in the diagnosis of pleural and chest wall invasion is discussed in "Radiographic Staging of Lung Cancer." Chest wall invasion is detected radiographically by the presence of an extrathoracic soft-tissue mass or rib destruction; CT is more sensitive in detecting subtle bone destruction, while MR is best for detecting invasion of chest wall fat or muscle, particularly in superior sulcus tumors. Diaphragmatic elevation and paralysis may be seen with malignant invasion of the phrenic nerve. Progressive enlargement of the cardiac silhouette may be seen in patients with a malignant pericardial effusion. Echocardiography and pericardiocentesis are diagnostic.

Lymphangitic carcinomatosis represents invasion of the lymphatic channels of the lung by tumor. Invasion of lymphatics or neoplastic involvement of hilar and mediastinal nodes leads to retrograde (centrifugal) lymphatic flow with dilation of lymphatic channels, interstitial deposits of tumor, and fibrosis. Radiographically, the typical findings are linear and reticulonodular opacities with peribronchial cuffing and subpleural edema or pleural effusion. In bronchogenic carcinoma, invasion and obstruction of lymphatic channels at the site of tumor may produce a segmental or lobar distribution of opacities. Lymphangitic spread to hilar and mediastinal lymph nodes produces unilateral lymph node enlargement with interstitial opacities, while hematogenous dissemination of tumor to the pulmonary capillaries leads to bilateral interstitial abnormalities. High resolution computed tomography show characteristic changes of smooth or beaded thickening of interlobular lines and the bronchovascular interstitium.

Diagnostic Evaluation in Bronchogenic Carcinoma

Efforts to diagnose lung cancer should also attempt to stage the patient whenever possible so that management decisions, particularly regarding resectability, can be made expeditiously. Cytologic examination of sputum or bronchoalveolar lavage fluid is simple and inexpensive and is most useful in central tumors. Bronchoscopy with endobronchial biopsy is useful for the visualization and biopsy of main or lobar bronchial lesions, with bronchoscopically guided transcarinal Wang needle biopsy used to sample subcarinal masses. Computed tomography- or fluoroscopically guided transthoracic biopsy of peripheral masses can establish a diagnosis in over 90% of patients with lung cancer. Radiologically guided sampling of hilar or mediastinal masses in patients with negative bronchoscopic examinations can provide material for cancer diagnosis and staging.

Computed tomography is obtained in all patients with possible bronchogenic carcinoma to guide efforts at tissue sampling. The detection of distal lesions in the adrenal gland, liver, or bones with biopsy of accessible lesions can provide both diagnostic and staging information. The relationship of the tumor to the central airways determines the utility of transbronchoscopic endobronchial or endotracheal biopsy, while the detection of large subcarinal nodes can direct transcarinal biopsy with a Wang needle. The pleura may be evaluated for thickening, masses, or effusions, suggesting that thoracentesis or closed pleural biopsy

is the appropriate initial diagnostic procedure. Thoracotomy with resection of a peripheral lesion is appropriate in suspicious solitary lesions lacking clinical or CT evidence of unresectable nodal, mediastinal, pleural, or extrathoracic metastases.

Radiographic Staging of Lung Cancer

The primary role of the radiologist in imaging the patient with bronchogenic carcinoma is to determine the anatomic extent or stage of the tumor (9). This has prognostic importance and determines the resectability of the lesion. In patients with small cell carcinoma, which is almost invariably not a surgically curable disease, patients are divided into two groups: those with disease limited to one hemithorax (limited disease) and those with extrathoracic spread (disseminated disease). The staging of nonsmall cell bronchogenic carcinoma is based on the extent of the primary tumor (T), the presence of nodal involvement (N), and evidence of distant metastases (M). Using this TNM classification scheme, lung cancer is divided into four stages. Traditionally, stage I or II disease was considered resectable for cure, while patients with stage III or IV disease did not benefit from surgery and were considered unresectable. Recently, the TNM scheme was modified to help identify patients with stage III disease who might benefit from resection using advanced and aggressive thoracic surgical techniques (Table 14.5). This modification of the TNM scheme allows further subdivision of stage III lung cancer into resectable (stage IIIa) and unresectable (stage IIIb) disease (Table 14.6). Stage IIIa disease is localized tumor invasion of the pleura, chest wall, diaphragm, or pericardium (T3), tumor extending into the proximal main bronchus with sparing of the tracheal carina (T3), or ipsilateral mediastinal or subcarinal nodal involvement (N2). The surgical techniques used for stage IIIa disease include en bloc resection of locally invaded chest wall, pleura, or pericardium, resection of proximal main bronchial tumors by resecting distal trachea and reimplanting the contralateral main bronchus into the proximal trachea, and mediastinal and subcarinal lymph node dissection with resection of the lung. Stage IIIb disease represents invasion of tracheal carina, mediastinum, major cardiovascular structures, esophagus, or vertebral body (T4), malignant pleural effusion (T4), or contralateral hilar or mediastinal, scalene or supraclavicular nodal involvement (N3). Stage IV disease indicates distant metastases (M1).

PRIMARY TUMOR (T)

Localized Invasion. Tumors invading the chest wall (including the superior pulmonary sulcus), dia-

Table 14.5.   The TNM Classification of Lung Cancer

Primary tumor (T)

Tx   Malignant cells in sputum without identifiable tumor
T0   No evidence of primary tumor
T1   Tumor <3.0 cm in diameter, surrounded by lung or visceral
       pleura, arising distal to a main bronchus
T2   Tumor >3.0 cm in diameter; any tumor invading the visceral
       pleura; any tumor with atelectasis or obstructive
       pneumonitis of less than an entire lung; the tumor must be
       >2 cm from the tracheal carina
T3   Any tumor with localized chest wall, diaphragmatic,
       mediastinal pleural or pericardial invasion; the tumor may
       be <2 cm from the carina but cannot involve the carina.
T4   Any tumor that invades the mediastinum or vital mediastinal
       structures including the heart, great vessels, trachea,
       carina, or vertebral body; presence of a malignant pleural
       effusion.

Nodal metastases

N0   No evidence of nodal metastases
N1   Metastasis to ipsilateral peribronchial or hilar nodes, including
       involvement by contiguous spread of tumor.
N2   Metastasis to ipsilateral mediastinal or subcarinal nodes
N3   Metastasis to contralateral mediastinal or hilar nodes, or
       scalene or supraclavicular nodes

Distant metastases (M)

M0   No evidence of distant metastases
M1   Distant metastases

Table 14.6.   Clinical Staging of Lung Cancer Based on TNM Classification

Stage	TNM
I	**T1** or **T2**N0M0
II	T1 or T2**N1**M0
IIIa	**T3**N0 or N1M0
	T1–T3**N2**M0
IIIb	T1–T3**N3**M0
	T4N0–N3M0
IV	T1–T4N0–N3**M1**

phragm, mediastinal pleura, pericardium, or proximal main bronchus are considered resectable by many surgeons and are classified as T3 lesions (Fig. 14.13). In superior sulcus tumors, local irradiation followed by en bloc resection of the tumor and chest wall has improved survival rates for affected patients compared with radiation alone.

Rib destruction or an extrathoracic soft-tissue mass are the only plain film findings specific for chest wall invasion; pleural thickening adjacent to a lung mass is nonspecific and need not indicate chest wall invasion. The CT diagnosis of chest wall invasion can be difficult, although CT should be obtained if this is suspected. Computed tomography findings suggestive of chest wall invasion are obtuse angles at the point of contact of the tumor and pleura, greater than 3 cm of contact between tumor and pleura, pleural thickening adjacent to the mass, and infiltration of extrapleural fat. Extrathoracic extension of the mass or rib destruction are specific but insensitive CT findings for

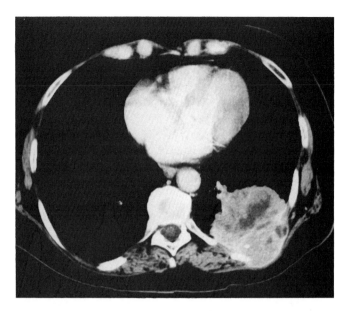

Figure 14.13.   A T3 Tumor with Localized Chest Wall Invasion. A. A CT scan through a large left lower lobe adenocarcinoma shows invasion of the posterior chest wall. A portion of the chest wall was removed en bloc with the tumor.

chest wall invasion (Fig. 14.13). Magnetic resonance imaging is equal to CT in its ability to diagnose chest wall invasion. T2-weighted images show excellent contrast between tumor and chest wall muscle and fat, and are used in selected cases to detect chest wall invasion. Magnetic resonance imaging also detects early obliteration of the high signal extrapleural fat that may be an early finding in chest wall invasion. Coronal MR images are useful in superior sulcus tumors to determine chest wall, brachial plexus, or subclavian artery involvement.

Mediastinal Invasion. Tumor invasion of the mediastinum with involvement of the heart, great vessels, trachea, or esophagus (T4 tumor) precludes resection. Localized invasion of the mediastinal pleura or pericardium (T3 tumor) does not prevent resection, although extensive invasion with replacement of mediastinal fat does.

On plain radiographs, a mediastinal mass, mediastinal widening, or diaphragmatic elevation (from phrenic nerve involvement) suggests invasion. As with the diagnosis of chest wall invasion, CT demonstration of tumor contiguous with mediastinal pleura or pleural thickening does not indicate mediastinal invasion, although tumors with extensive contact with the mediastinum (>3 cm) or the circumference of the aorta (>90°), and displacement and compression of mediastinal vessels are suggestive of mediastinal invasion. Replacement of mediastinal fat by soft-tissue density is specific for invasion (Fig. 14.14). Magnetic resonance imaging is at least as accurate as CT in the diagnosis of mediastinal invasion, particularly in the detection of vascular involvement (10).

Central Airway Involvement. Tumors extending into a main bronchus within 2 cm of the tracheal carina (T3 tumor) are resectable. While tracheal carinal involvement (T4 tumor) can be treated by carinal resection with end-to-side anastamosis of the remaining bronchus to the tracheal stump ("sleeve pneumonectomy"), most surgeons would consider this unresectable tumor. Although plain films can occasionally demonstrate a mass within the main bronchus or trachea, CT is more ac-

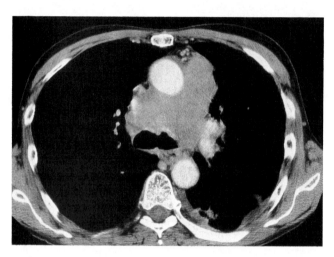

Figure 14.14. Mediastinal Invasion in Bronchogenic Carcinoma. A contrast-enhanced CT scan at the level of the aortopulmonary window in a patient with small cell carcinoma demonstrates a large soft-tissue mass replacing the normal mediastinal fat. The mass encircles the ascending aorta posteriorly and irregularly narrows the left main bronchus.

curate in assessing the relationship of the mass to the tracheal carina (Fig. 14.15). However, CT is known to underestimate the mucosal or submucosal extent of tumor as seen bronchoscopically. Therefore, any patient with a central lesion should undergo bronchoscopy to determine the proximal extent of tumor unless CT shows obvious carinal or tracheal invasion.

Pleural Effusion. Malignant pleural effusion (T4 tumor) precludes curative resection of tumor. There are no specific radiographic or CT features distinguishing benign from malignant effusions. As discussed previously, the detection of lobulated pleural thickening or discrete pleural masses on CT or MR are highly suggestive of malignant pleural invasion; thoracentesis and pleural biopsy will provide a diagnosis in most of these individuals.

LYMPH NODE METASTASES (N)

Selected patients with ipsilateral mediastinal or subcarinal node metastases are classified as N2 and are considered potentially resectable. Patients with N2 disease who have nonbulky intracapsular nodal metastases limited to one mediastinal nodal station or have negative preoperative mediastinoscopic examinations show the best 5-year survival rates following extensive mediastinal nodal dissection. Contralateral hilar or mediastinal, supraclavicular or infraclavicular node metastases represent N3 disease and are unresectable (Fig. 14.16).

The detection of a large mediastinal mass on chest radiograph in a patient with lung cancer requires mediastinoscopic or transthoracic biopsy confirma-

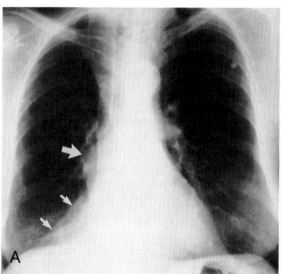
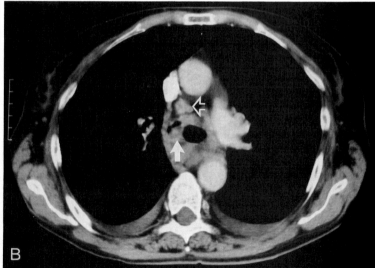

Figure 14.15. Tracheal Carinal Involvement in Squamous Cell Carcinoma. A. A frontal chest radiograph in a middle-aged woman with hemoptysis shows a mass in the lower right hilum (*large arrow*) with right lower lobe atelectasis (*small arrows*). **B.** A CT scan demonstrates a mass surrounding the main bronchi, with irregular narrow-

ing of the right main bronchial lumen and infiltration of the tracheal carina (*arrow*). An enlarged precarinal lymph node (*open arrow*) and small bilateral pleural effusions are also seen. Bronchoscopy revealed invasion of the tracheal carina by squamous cell carcinoma.

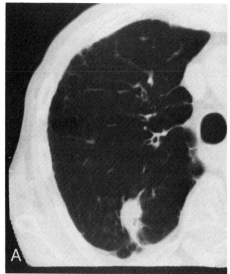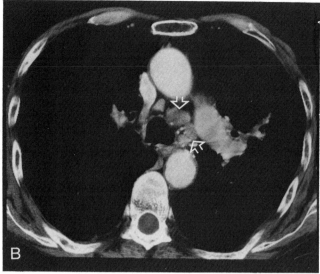

Figure 14.16. Contralateral Nodal Metastases from Adenocarcinoma. A. A coned-down view of a CT scan in a patient with severe emphysema shows a spiculated mass in the right upper lobe. **B.** A CT scan through the tracheal carina demonstrates enlarged left peribronchial lymph nodes (*open arrows*). Mediastinoscopic biopsy confirmed metastatic involvement of contralateral lymph nodes, indicating N3 disease.

tion of tumor invasion before rendering the patient unresectable. A normal chest radiograph or the suggestion of hilar or mediastinal adenopathy should prompt a chest CT to assess the status of the lymph nodes. There is no single measurement that allows completely accurate distinction of normal from malignant nodes. This is because malignant involvement does not always enlarge the lymph node (producing false-negative findings and reducing sensitivity), while enlarged nodes in patients with lung cancer may represent reactive hyperplasia rather than tumor replacement (producing false-positive findings and reducing specificity). If we choose a small nodal diameter (i.e., 5 mm) as the dividing point between benign and malignant, we will have excellent sensitivity but low specificity, whereas choosing a large nodal diameter (i.e., 2 cm) will increase specificity but decrease sensitivity. Most radiologists use a short axis nodal diameter of 1 cm as the dividing point, since this value seems to achieve the best compromise of sensitivity and specificity.

Recent studies have shown that CT is relatively inaccurate in determining the nodal status of the patient with lung cancer. Both sensitivity and specificity for nodal metastases, using a short axis diameter of 1 cm or greater as abnormal, are approximately 60–65% on a patient-by-patient basis, and may be even lower when looking at individual nodal stations. Although CT cannot be considered accurate enough to determine with certainty that mediastinal lymph nodes are or are not involved by tumor, it can provide information of value in guiding invasive staging procedures such as mediastinoscopy (Fig. 14.16), transcarinal Wang biopsy, and transthoracic or open biopsy.

In most institutions, mediastinoscopy plays a complementary role to CT in the nodal staging of lung cancer. Most patients with enlarged mediastinal nodes on CT that are accessible to transcervical mediastinoscopy (pretracheal, anterior subcarinal, and right tracheobronchial nodes) should have mediastinoscopy and biopsy. Whether patients with negative CT studies for nodal enlargement should have mediastinoscopy depends upon the local surgical practice. In patients with small, peripheral lung nodules, mediastinal metastases are uncommon and thoracotomy may be warranted without prior CT or mediastinoscopy, but this remains controversial. Patients with borderline pulmonary function would benefit most from mediastinoscopy, as a positive mediastinoscopic biopsy would almost certainly preclude any attempt at resection.

Magnetic resonance imaging has an accuracy equal to that of CT in the diagnosis of mediastinal lymph node metastases. There are specific advantages and disadvantages of MR in characterizing mediastinal lymph nodes. Clusters of normal-sized nodes may be mistaken for a single enlarged nodal mass because of the limited spatial resolution of MR. Magnetic resonance imaging is incapable of demonstrating calcification within nodes, which is diagnostic of benign lymph node disease. However, aortopulmonary window and subcarinal nodes are best demonstrated on coronal MR images, since CT demonstration of nodes in these regions is limited by partial volume averaging with adjacent cardiovascular structures. While the true promise of MR may be in the distinction of benign from malignant lymph nodes based on T1 and T2 relaxation values, this is not yet possible.

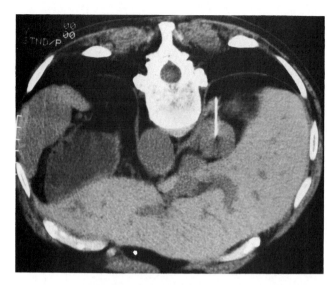

Figure 14.17. A CT-guided Biopsy of Adrenal Metastases from Bronchogenic Carcinoma (M1 Disease). Image obtained during a prone CT-guided biopsy of the left adrenal gland in a patient with a left upper lobe lung mass shows the biopsy needle within the mass. Cytologic examination revealed adenocarcinoma.

METASTATIC DISEASE (M)

Each patient with proven lung cancer should be carefully evaluated for the presence of distant metastases (M1). Unequivocal evidence of metastases can obviate an unnecessary thoracotomy. Common sites of extrathoracic spread in patients with lung cancer include lymph nodes, liver, adrenal gland, bone, and brain. Metastases to the opposite lung, although intrathoracic, are also considered in this category. Involvement of these sites probably represents hematogenous spread of tumor from the lung.

Virtually all patients evaluated for bronchogenic carcinoma will have chest and upper abdominal CT as part of their initial evaluation. This is adequate for assessing the liver, spleen, adrenal glands, and upper abdominal lymph nodes for evidence of metastases. Ultrasound may be used to distinguish soft-tissue hepatic masses from incidental cysts. Radionuclide bone scanning with technetium-99m methylene diphosphonate is used for patients with elevated serum alkaline phosphatase. Plain films are obtained to assess specific foci of abnormally increased bone tracer uptake or to evaluate localized bone pain.

Head imaging is routinely performed in patients with symptoms or signs suggesting brain metastases. This usually involves MR or contrast-enhanced head CT. Head scanning in patients without clinical evidence of central nervous system involvement is somewhat more controversial. Since virtually all patients with isolated or asymptomatic brain metastases are found to have adenocarcinoma or large cell carcinoma, patients with these subtypes of bronchogenic

carcinoma should have head CT scans regardless of the clinical findings in order to identify silent metastases. Patients with positive findings can be spared an unnecessary thoracotomy.

Approximately 60–65% of patients with small cell carcinoma have detectable M1 disease at the time of diagnosis. Since it is likely that all patients with small cell carcinoma have gross or microscopic metastatic foci at presentation, these patients are generally not candidates for curative surgical resection. However, accurate staging of these patients for extrathoracic involvement determines prognosis and allows for proper assessment of response to chemotherapy. An additional reason for extrathoracic staging of small cell carcinoma is the ability to manage localized bone or soft-tissue involvement with radiation or resection.

Adrenal masses are seen in approximately 10% of patients undergoing staging CT examinations for bronchogenic carcinoma. However, approximately 5% of normal individuals are known to have benign adrenal cortical adenomas. In fact, isolated adrenal masses in patients with nonsmall cell bronchogenic carcinoma are twice as likely to be adenomas than metastases. In many patients the adrenal mass is the only extrathoracic site of abnormality, making accurate diagnosis of the adrenal mass crucial in determining management. This usually requires tissue sampling of the adrenal mass via CT-guided percutaneous biopsy (Fig. 14.17).

The ratio of the signal intensity of adrenal mass to the signal intensity of liver on T2-weighted spin-echo MR has been used to differentiate benign adrenal adenomas from metastases, with low ratios (<1:2) seen in adenomas and high ratios (>1:4) seen in carcinoma and pheochromocytomas (11). Despite the initial encouraging results, most patients will require adrenal biopsy since the results have a profound impact on whether potentially curative thoracotomy and resection should be attempted.

References

1. Heitzman ER. The mediastinum. 2nd ed. Berlin: Springer-Verlag, 1988:318–349.
2. Park CK, Webb WR, Klein JS. Inferior hilar window. Radiology 1991;178:163–168.
3. Webb WR, Gamsu G, Glazer GM. Computed tomography of the abnormal pulmonary hilum. J Comput Assist Tomogr 1981;5:485–490.
4. Webb WR, Gamsu G, Stark DD, Moore EH. Magnetic resonance imaging of the normal and abnormal pulmonary hila. Radiology 1984;152:89–94.
5. McLoud TC, Kalisher L, Stark P, Greene R. Intrathoracic lymph node metastases from extrathoracic neoplasms. AJR 1978;131:403–407.
6. Kirks DR, McCormick VD, Greenspan RH. Pulmonary sarcoidosis: roentgenologic analysis of 150 patients. AJR 1973;117:777–786.
7. Armstrong P. Pulmonary vascular diseases and pulmonary edema. In: Armstrong P, Wilson AG, Dee P, eds. Imaging of

diseases of the chest. Chicago: Year Book Medical Publishers, 1990:373–383.

8. Haque AK. Pathology of carcinoma of lung: an update on current concepts. J Thorac Imaging 1991;7:9–20.

9. Klein JS, Webb WR. The radiologic staging of lung cancer. J Thorac Imaging 1991;7:29–47.

10. Webb WR, Gatsonis CA, Zerhouni EA, Heelan RT, Glazer GM, McNeil BJ. CT and MR imaging in staging non-small cell bronchogenic carcinoma: report of the Radiologic Diagnostic Oncology Group. Radiology 1991;178:705–713.

11. Reinig JW, Doppman JL, Johnson AR, Knop RH. Adrenal masses differentiated by MR. Radiology 1986;158:81–84.

15

The Lung

Jeffrey S. Klein
Nancy J. Fischbein

RADIOGRAPHIC FINDINGS IN PARENCHYMAL LUNG DISEASE

Parenchymal lung disease can be divided into those processes that produce an abnormal increase in density of all or a portion of the lung on chest radiographs (i.e., pulmonary opacity) and those that produce an abnormal decrease in lung density (i.e., pulmonary lucency) (1). The normal density of lung is due to the relative proportion of air to soft tissue (blood or parenchyma) in the ratio of 11:1. Therefore, it stands to reason that processes that increase the relative amount of soft tissue will create a significant decrease in this ratio and be more easily discernable than diffuse pro-

Table 15.1. Patterns of Parenchymal Opacity

Air space (alveolar) filling	
Interstitial opacities	Reticular
	Reticulonodular
	Nodular
	Linear
Nodule/mass	
Branching opacities	Mucoid impaction
Atelectasis	

Table 15.2. Radiographic Characteristics of Air Space Disease

Lobar or segmental distribution
Poorly marginated
Air space nodules
Tendency to coalesce
Air bronchograms
Bat's wing distribution
Rapidly changing over time

cesses that destroy blood vessels and parenchyma and cause little change in this ratio, thereby producing only small decreases in the overall lung density. Computed tomography (CT), by virtue of superior contrast resolution, is more sensitive to subtle decreases in overall radiographic density than is plain radiography.

Abnormal pulmonary opacities may be divided into air-space filling opacities, opacities resulting from atelectasis, interstitial opacities, nodular or mass-like opacities, and branching opacities (Table 15.1). These patterns have been shown to accurately represent pulmonary pathologic processes in correlative radiographic-pathologic studies, and are a practical means of generating a differential diagnosis based upon the known patterns of parenchymal involvement in a wide variety of pulmonary diseases.

PULMONARY OPACITY

Air Space Disease

RADIOGRAPHIC FINDINGS

The radiographic characteristics of air space disease are listed in Table 15.2. Air space patterns of opacity develop when the air normally present within the terminal air spaces of the lung is replaced by material of soft-tissue density such as blood, transudate, exudate, or neoplastic cells. A segmental distribution of disease may be seen in a process such as pneumococcal pneumonia, which begins in the terminal air spaces and spreads from involved to uninvolved air spaces via interalveolar channels (pores of Kohn) and channels bridging preterminal bronchioles with alveoli (canals of Lambert). Initially, the opacity is poorly marginated as the air-space filling process extends in an irregular fashion to involve adjacent air spaces, creating an irregular interface with the x-ray beam.

Not uncommonly, air space nodules, which are poorly marginated rounded opacities 6–8 mm in diameter, may be seen at the leading edge of an air space filling process. These nodules represent filling of acini or other sublobular structures, and are most often seen in diffuse alveolar pulmonary edema and transbronchial spread of cavitary tuberculosis.

A characteristic of air-space filling processes is the tendency of air space shadows to coalesce as they extend through the lung. When the air spaces are rendered opaque by the presence of intralveolar cellular material and fluid, the normally aerated bronchi become visible as tubular lucencies called air bronchograms. Occasionally, small intraacinar bronchi or groups of uninvolved alveoli may be visible within an air space nodule as air bronchiolograms or air alveolograms, respectively. Rarely, severe interstitial disease encroaching upon the air spaces may produce an air bronchogram; this is most typically seen in "alveolar" sarcoid. When the air-space filling process extends to the interlobar fissure, it is seen as a sharply marginated lobar opacity.

A pattern of parenchymal opacity that reliably represents an air-space filling process is the "bat's wing" or "butterfly" pattern of disease. In this pattern, dense opacities occupy the central regions of lung and extend laterally to abruptly marginate before reaching the peripheral portions of the lung, hence the term "bat's wing" (Fig. 15.1). To date, there is no explanation for this distribution of disease, which appears almost exclusively in patients with pulmonary edema or hemorrhage. Another feature of air-space filling processes is the tendency to rapidly change in appearance over short intervals of time. The development or resolution of parenchymal opacities within hours usually indicates an air-space filling process; prominent exceptions include atelectasis and interstitial pulmonary edema.

COMPUTED TOMOGRAPHY/HIGH-RESOLUTION CT (HRCT) FINDINGS

The CT and HRCT findings of air space disease are similar to those described on plain chest radiograph. These are: (*a*) lobar, segmental, and/or lobular distribution of disease, (*b*) poorly marginated opacities that tend to coalesce, (*c*) air space nodules, and (*d*) air bronchograms. A lobar or segmental distribution of disease is easily appreciated on cross-sectional imaging. Computed tomography and HRCT is further capable of showing individually opacified lobules, termed a "patchwork quilt" appearance, which is seen in many air space processes, most classically bronchopneumonia (Fig. 15.2). Coalescence of opacities, commonly seen in pulmonary edema and pneumonia, is best assessed on serial CT studies. With isolated air space disease, the interlobular septa are normal or ob-

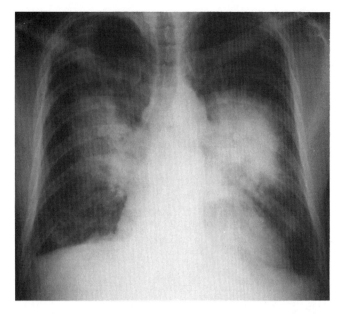

Figure 15.1. Bat's Wing Appearance of Pulmonary Edema. Frontal radiograph demonstrates dense bilateral perihilar air space opacities associated with cardiac enlargement and bilateral pleural effusions in this patient with pulmonary edema from idiopathic cardiomyopathy.

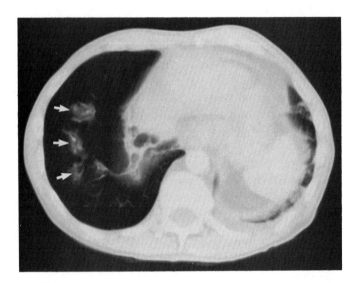

Figure 15.2. Lobular Distribution of Air Space Opacities in Bronchopneumonia. A CT scan through the base of the right lung shows multiple ill-defined air space opacities (arrows) within pulmonary lobules with intervening areas of normal lung. Sputum culture showed *Staphylococcus aureus* pneumonia.

scured. As with plain films, the presence of air space nodules provides further evidence of an air space process. On HRCT studies, these nodules are usually seen within the peribronchiolar (centrilobular) region of the pulmonary lobule. Air bronchograms or bronchiolograms are usually better appreciated on CT and HRCT than on plain radiographs because of the superior contrast resolution and the cross-sectional

Table 15.3. Types of Pulmonary Atelectasis

Type	Example
Obstructive (resorptive)	Bronchogenic carcinoma
Passive (relaxation)	Pleural effusion
Compressive	Bulla
Cicatricial	Postprimary TB
Adhesive	Respiratory distress syndrome of the newborn

nature of CT. This is particularly true in those regions of the lung where bronchi course in the transverse plane (i.e., anterior segments of upper lobes, middle lobe and lingula, and superior segments of the lower lobes).

Atelectasis

GENERAL PRINCIPLES AND MECHANISMS

Atelectasis literally means incomplete expansion. It is used to describe any condition in which there is loss of lung volume, and is usually but not invariably associated with an increase in radiographic density. There are four basic mechanisms of atelectasis (Table 15.3).

The most common form of atelectasis is obstructive or resorptive atelectasis and is secondary to complete endobronchial obstruction of a lobar bronchus with resorption of gas distally. Incomplete bronchial obstruction more often produces air trapping from a check-valve effect rather than atelectasis because air enters but cannot exit the lung. Complete obstruction of a central bronchus may not produce atelectasis if collateral air flow to the obstructed lung (via pores of Kohn, canals of Lambert, or incomplete interlobar fissures) allows the lung to remain inflated. An obstructed lobe or a lung containing 100% oxygen, as may be seen in some mechanically ventilated patients, will collapse more rapidly (sometimes within minutes) than a lung containing ambient air. This is due to the rapid absorption of oxygen from the alveolar spaces into alveolar capillaries. Bronchogenic carcinoma, foreign bodies, mucus plugs, and malpositioned endotracheal tubes are the most common causes of endobronchial obstruction and secondary resorptive atelectasis.

Passive or relaxation atelectasis results from the mass effect of an air or fluid collection within the pleural space on the subjacent lung. Since the natural tendency of the lung is to collapse when dissociated from the chest wall, pleural collections will produce atelectasis. The degree of atelectasis depends upon the size of the pleural collection, presence or absence of pleural adhesions, and the condition of the underlying lung. A large pleural collection in a normal pleural space will produce virtual complete

Table 15.4. Radiographic Signs in Lobar Atelectasis

Direct Signs	Indirect Signs
Displacement of interlobar fissure	Increased density of atelectatic lung
	Ipsilateral mediastinal shift
	Hilar elevation (upper lobe atelectasis) or depression (lower lobe atelectasis)
	Compensatory hyperinflation of adjacent lobe(s)
	Shifting granuloma
	Small hemithorax

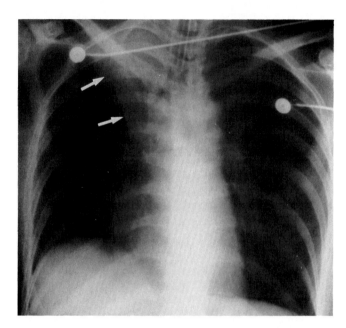

Figure 15.3. Atelectasis of right upper lobe. An AP radiograph in an intubated patient shows a sharply marginated homogeneous opacity in the right upper lung with a paucity of air bronchograms typical of right upper lobe atelectasis. The sharp inferior margin of the opacity (*arrows*) is formed by the superomedially displaced minor fissure, a direct radiographic sign of atelectasis. Note the presence of several indirect signs of upper lobe volume loss, including rightward shift of the trachea and heart, right hilar and diaphragmatic elevation, and hyperlucency of the middle and right lower lobes.

collapse of a normal lung, which will be seen as a small, dense, rounded opacity retracted to a perihilar location. Alternatively, if the underlying lung is abnormal (i.e., consolidated or has interstitial disease), it may show only minimal volume loss. A large pleural or chest wall mass or an elevated diaphragm can also produce passive atelectasis. Compressive atelectasis is a form of passive atelectasis in which an intrapulmonary mass compresses adjacent lung parenchyma; common causes include bullae, abscesses, and tumors.

Processes resulting in parenchymal fibrosis reduce alveolar volume and produce cicatricial atelectasis. Localized cicatricial atelectasis is most often seen in as-

sociation with chronic upper lobe fibronodular tuberculosis. The radiographic appearance is that of severe lobar volume loss with scarring, bronchiectasis, and compensatory hyperinflation of adjacent lung. Diffuse cicatricial atelectasis is seen in interstitial fibrosis of any etiology. An overall increase in lung density with reticular opacities and diminished lung volumes is characteristic of this condition.

Adhesive atelectasis occurs in association with surfactant deficiency. Type II pneumocytes, the cells responsible for surfactant production, may be injured as a result of general anesthesia, ischemia, or radiation damage. Surfactant deficiency causes increased alveolar surface tension and results in diffuse alveolar collapse and volume loss. Radiographs show a diminution in lung volume, which may be associated with an increase in density.

RADIOGRAPHIC SIGNS OF ATELECTASIS

Lobar Atelectasis (Table 15.4). The only direct radiographic finding of lobar atelectasis is the displacement of an interlobar fissure. There are several indirect findings of atelectasis, most of which reflect the attempts to compensate for the volume loss (Fig. 15.3). Diminished aeration results in increased density in the affected portion of lung. A shift of mediastinal and hilar structures toward the affected lung is a common finding in lobar atelectasis. Tracheal displacement and hilar elevation are common in upper lobe atelectasis, while hilar depression, cardiac shift, and elevation of the hemidiaphragm may be seen with lower lobe atelectasis. A shift of the entire mediastinum is typical of collapse of an entire lung. Compensatory hyperinflation represents an attempt by the normal portion of the lung to occupy a greater than normal portion of one or both hemithoraces in response to atelectasis. This mechanism usually develops with chronic volume loss and is not seen in acute collapse. It is seen as increased lucency with attenuation of pulmonary vascular markings. In complete lung or upper lobe atelectasis, the contralateral upper lobe may herniate across the midline, bowing the anterior junction line toward the affected side.

A characteristic but seldom seen plain radiographic finding of compensatory hyperinflation is the "shifting granuloma" in which a preexisting granuloma in an adjacent aerated lung changes position as it moves toward the collapsed lobe. In chronic atelectasis of a lung, a decrease in size of the hemithorax with approximation of the ribs may be seen. The absence of an air bronchogram helps distinguish resorptive lobar atelectasis from lobar pneumonia, particularly if the atelectatic lobe is only slightly diminished in volume. Compensatory hyperinflation in patients with long-

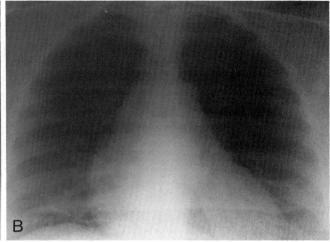

Figure 15.4. Subsegmental (Linear) Atelectasis. A. Frontal chest radiograph in a woman 1 day status/postcholecystectomy shows diminished lung volumes and numerous bilateral middle and lower zone linear opacities coursing perpendicular to the costal pleura representing areas of subsegmental atelectasis. **B.** A radiograph obtained 5 days postoperatively shows near complete resolution of the opacities with improvement in lung volumes.

standing atelectasis is best appreciated on CT because of its superior contrast resolution and cross-sectional nature.

Segmental Atelectasis. Atelectasis of one or several segments of a lobe is difficult to determine on plain radiographs. The appearance ranges from a thin linear opacity to a wedge-shaped opacity that does not abut an interlobar fissure. Segmental atelectasis is better appreciated on CT.

Subsegmental (Plate-like) Atelectasis. Band-like linear opacities representing linear atelectasis are commonly associated with disorders in which diaphragmatic movement is diminished. This is seen in patients with pleuritic chest pain, postoperative patients, or patients with massive hepatosplenomegaly or ascites. Subsegmental atelectasis tends to occur at the lung bases. The linear shadows are 2–10 cm in length and are typically oriented perpendicular to the costal pleura (Fig. 15.4). Pathologically these areas of linear collapse are deep to invaginations of visceral pleura formed by incomplete fissures or scars.

Round Atelectasis. This is an uncommon form of atelectasis in which the collapsed lung forms a round mass in the lower lobe. This condition is most closely associated with asbestos-related pleural disease, but may be seen in any condition associated with an exudative (proteinaceous) pleural effusion. The process develops when pleural adhesions form in the resolving phase of a pleural effusion and cause the adjacent lung to roll up into a ball as it reexpands. The round opacity is most often found along the inferior and posterior costal pleural surface adjacent to an area of pleural fibrosis or plaque formation. Plain radiographs reveal a well-defined pleural-based mass between 2 and 7 cm in size adjacent to an area of pleural thickening in the lower lung. The identification of a curvilinear bronchovascular bundle or "comet tail" entering the anterior inferior margin of the mass as seen on lateral radiographs or tomograms is characteristic. The CT appearance of round atelectasis is characteristic (Fig. 15.5). The round or wedge-shaped mass forms an acute angle with the pleura and is seen adjacent to an area of pleural thickening, usually in the inferior and posterior thorax. The comet tail of vessels and bronchi is seen curving between the hilum and the apex of the mass. The atelectatic lung enhances following intravenous contrast administration. When the characteristic CT findings are seen in a patient with a known history of asbestos exposure, the appearance is diagnostic and no further evaluation is necessary. However, if there is any doubt regarding the diagnosis, the lesion should undergo biopsy to exclude malignancy.

LOBAR AND SEGMENTAL ATELECTASIS

The characteristics of lobar atelectasis have been described. A triangular configuration with the apex at the pulmonary hilum is common to all types of lobar atelectasis. The displaced fissures typically assume a bowed configuration convex toward the collapse. The changes of lobar atelectasis are best appreciated on CT.

Right Upper Lobe Atelectasis. In right upper lobe atelectasis, the lung collapses superiorly and medially with superomedial displacement of the minor fissure and anteromedial displacement of the upper half of the major fissure, producing a right upper paramediastinal density on frontal radiographs (Fig. 15.3). An obstructing central mass may produce a central convexity along the interface of the collapsed

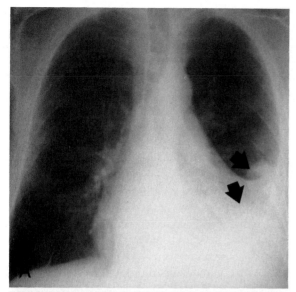

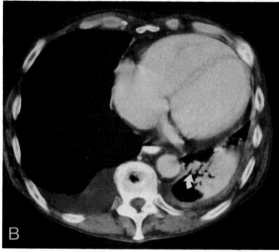

Figure 15.5.   Round Atelectasis. A. Frontal radiograph in a 56-year-old patient with exudative pleural effusions reveals two pleural-based masses (*arrows*) in the left lower lobe. **B.** Contrast-enhanced CT shows the inferior mass to represent enhancing atelectatic lung with the bronchovascular bundle entering the medial aspect of the mass (*arrow*).

lobe with the overinflated middle lobe. The continuity of a central convexity with the peripheral concave interface between the collapsed upper lobe and aerated lung produces the "S-sign of Golden." The trachea is deviated toward the right, and the right hilum and hemidiaphragm are elevated. "Tenting" or "peaking" of the diaphragm is occasionally seen and represents fat within the inferior aspect of a stretched inferior accessory fissure. The left upper lobe may herniate across the midline anteriorly toward the right. The lateral radiograph may reveal a triangular opacity with its apex at the hilum and base against the apicoposterior costal pleural surface. Compensatory hyperinflation of the middle and lower lobes may be seen in chronic atelectasis.

An atypical appearance of atelectasis, in which the collapsed right upper lobe maintains contact with the lateral costal pleural surface and collapses laterally rather than medially, has been described and is termed "peripheral right upper lobe atelectasis." In this form of atelectasis, the superior segment of the right lower lobe is interposed medial to the collapsed upper lobe, producing a well-marginated density laterally that mimics pleural disease on frontal radiographs. Scarring from tuberculosis, endobronchial tumor, and mucus plugging are common causes of right upper lobe atelectasis.

Middle Lobe Atelectasis produces inferior displacement of the minor fissure and superior displacement of the major fissure. Because of the minimal thickness of the collapsed middle lobe and the oblique orientation of the inferiorly displaced minor fissure, the detection of middle lobe atelectasis on frontal radiographs is difficult. The only finding on frontal radiographs may be a vague density over the right lower lung with obscuration of the right heart margin. The lateral radiograph shows a typical triangular density with its apex at the hilum (Fig. 15.6). A lordotic frontal radiograph, which projects the minor fissure tangent to the frontal x-ray beam, will depict the atelectatic middle lobe as a triangular opacity, which is sharply marginated superiorly by the minor fissure, with its apex directed laterally. Middle lobe atelectasis is most often cicatricial and follows middle lobe infection with secondary fibrosis and bronchiectasis.

Right Lower Lobe Atelectasis. The right lower lobe collapses toward the lower mediastinum because of the tethering effect of the inferior pulmonary ligament. This results in inferior displacement of the upper half of the major fissure and posterior displacement of the lower half, producing a triangular opacity in the right lower paravertebral space, which obscures the medial right hemidiaphragm on frontal radiographs. The lateral margin of this triangular opacity is formed by the displaced major fissure. The right hemidiaphragm may be elevated. The right interlobar pulmonary artery is obscured within the opaque collapsed lower lobe, a finding that helps distinguish the triangular opacity of right lower lobe atelectasis from a medial pleural effusion, which laterally displaces and does not obscure the interlobar artery. On lateral radiographs, a vague triangular opacity with its apex at the hilum and base over the posterior portion of the right hemidiaphragm and posterior costophrenic sulcus may be seen. Mucus plugs, foreign bodies, and endobronchial tumors are the most common etiologic agents.

Left Upper Lobe Atelectasis has a different appearance from right upper lobe atelectasis because of the absence of a minor fissure. The left upper lobe col-

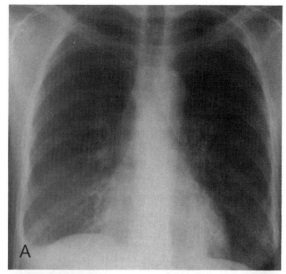

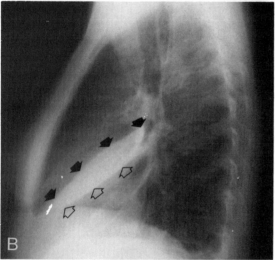

Figure 15.6. Middle Lobe Atelectasis. A. A frontal radiograph demonstrates a vague opacity in the right lower lung obscuring the right heart border, and a small right pleural effusion. **B.** The lateral radiograph shows the typical triangular opacity of middle lobe atelectasis overlying the cardiac shadow. The upper (*solid arrows*) and lower (*open arrows*) margins of the opacity represent the displaced minor and inferior portion of the right major fissure, respectively.

lapses anteriorly, maintaining a broad area of contact with the anterior costal pleural surface. The major fissure shifts anteriorly and is seen marginating a long, narrow band of increased opacity paralleling the anterior chest wall on lateral radiographs. The diagnosis on frontal radiographs may be difficult. There is a veil of increased opacity over the left upper thorax and obscuration of the left heart margin. The apex of the left hemithorax remains lucent because of hyperinflation of the superior segment of the left lower lobe. Leftward tracheal displacement, hilar and diaphragmatic elevation, and leftward bulging of the anterior junction line from an overinflated right upper lobe are additional clues to the diagnosis. An uncommon finding on the frontal radiograph in left upper lobe atelectasis is a

crescent of air ("Luftsichel") along the left upper mediastinum, which represents a portion of the overinflated superior segment of the left lower lobe interposed between the aortic arch medially and the collapsed upper lobe laterally. Postinflammatory cicatrization and endobronchial tumor are the common causes of left upper lobe atelectasis.

Left Lower Lobe Atelectasis is similar in appearance to atelectasis of the right lower lobe. A triangular opacity in the left lower paramediastinal region with loss of the medial retrocardiac diaphragmatic outline is seen on frontal radiographs. In addition, the left hilum is displaced inferiorly and the interlobar artery is obscured. The diaphragm may be elevated and the heart shifted toward the left. Compensatory hyperinflation of the left upper lobe may be seen. The left lower lobe commonly is atelectatic in patients with large hearts and in postoperative patients, particularly those who have had coronary bypass surgery.

Combined Middle and Right Lower Lobe Atelectasis may be seen with obstruction of the bronchus intermedius by a mucus plug or tumor. The radiographic appearance on the frontal radiograph is characteristic, with a homogeneous triangular opacity sharply marginated superiorly by the depressed minor fissure and obscuration both of the right heart border and the right hemidiaphragm. Cardiac and mediastinal shift toward the right is common.

Whole Lung Atelectasis. Collapse of an entire lung is most often seen with obstructing masses in the main bronchus. The lung is opacified with an absence of air bronchograms. The trachea and heart are shifted toward the side of collapse, with herniation of the contralateral anteromedial lung across the midline to widen the retrosternal space on lateral radiograph and bulge the anterior junction line on frontal radiograph. The chest wall may show approximation of the ribs in chronic collapse. Compensatory diaphragmatic elevation in left lung atelectasis may be recognized by noting superior displacement of the gastric air bubble or splenic flexure of colon.

Interstitial Disease

Interstitial opacities are produced by processes that thicken the interstitial compartments of the lung. Water, blood, tumor, cells, fibrous tissue, or any combination of these may render the interstitial space visible on radiographs. Interstitial opacities are usually divided into reticular, reticulonodular, nodular, and linear patterns on plain radiographs (Fig. 15.7) (2). The predominant pattern of opacity produced by an interstitial process depends upon the nature of the underlying disease and the portion of the interstitium affected.

Reticular

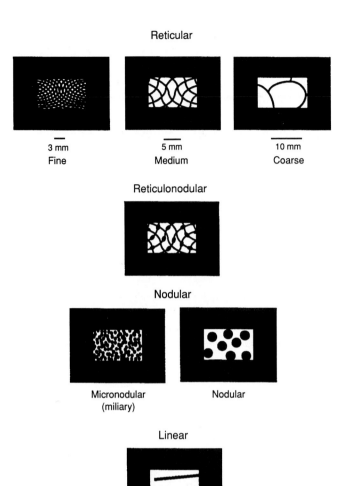

| 3 mm | 5 mm | 10 mm |
| Fine | Medium | Coarse |

Reticulonodular

Nodular

Micronodular (miliary)   Nodular

Linear

Figure 15.7. Patterns of Interstitial Opacity on Chest Radiographs.

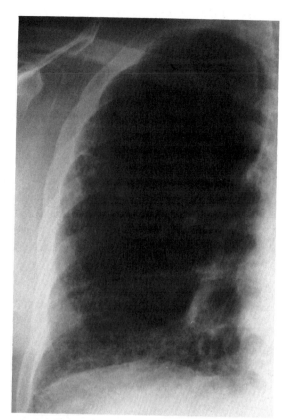

Figure 15.8. Honeycombing. A coned-down view of the right lung in a patient with end-stage rheumatoid lung disease demonstrates a medium reticular process with thin-walled cysts representing honeycomb lung. Note the predominant subpleural distribution of disease characteristic of idiopathic pulmonary fibrosis.

RADIOGRAPHIC FINDINGS

A reticular pattern refers to a network of curvilinear opacities that usually involves the lungs diffusely. The subdivision of reticular opacities into fine, medium, and coarse opacities refers to the size of the lucent spaces created by these intersecting curvilinear opacities (Fig. 15.7). A fine reticular pattern, also known as a ground-glass pattern, is seen in processes that thicken or line the parenchymal interstitium of the lung to produce a fine network of lines with intervening lucent spaces on the order of 1–2 mm in diameter. Diseases that most commonly produce this appearance include interstitial pulmonary edema and interstitial pulmonary fibrosis. Medium reticulation, also termed honeycombing, refers to reticular interstitial opacities where the intervening spaces are 3–10 mm in diameter. This pattern is most commonly seen in pulmonary fibrosis involving the parenchymal and peripheral interstitial spaces (Fig. 15.8). Coarse reticular opacities with spaces

greater than 1 cm in diameter are seen most commonly in diseases that produce cystic spaces as a result of parenchymal destruction. The most common interstitial diseases associated with coarse reticulation are idiopathic pulmonary fibrosis, sarcoidosis, and histiocytosis X of lung.

Reticulonodular opacities may be produced by the overlap of numerous reticular shadows or by the presence of both nodular and reticular opacities. In the latter situation, the nodules are usually because of granulomata or small tumor deposits in the interstitium. Sarcoidosis and lymphangitic carcinomatosis are diseases that may give rise to true reticulonodular opacities.

Nodular opacities represent small rounded lesions within the pulmonary interstitium. In contrast to air space nodules, interstitial nodules are homogeneous (i.e., they lack air bronchiolograms or air alveolograms) and are well defined, as their margins are sharp and they are surrounded by normally aerated lung. In addition, unlike air space nodules, which tend to be uniform in diameter (approximately 8 mm), interstitial nodules may be micronodular (<1 mm), small (1–5 mm), medium (5–10 mm) or large (>10 mm). A micronodular or miliary pattern is seen

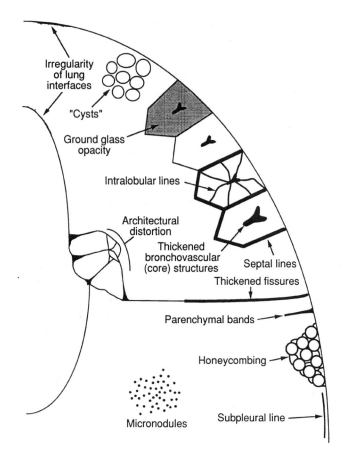

Irregularity
of lung
interfaces

"Cysts"

Ground glass
opacity

Intralobular lines

Architectural
distortion

Thickened
bronchovascular
(core) structures

Septal lines

Thickened fissures

Parenchymal bands

Honeycombing

Micronodules

Subpleural line

Figure 15.9.   Diagram of Interstitial Abnormalities as Seen on HRCT.

predominantly in granulomatous processes (e.g., miliary tuberculosis or histoplasmosis), hematogenous pulmonary metastases (most commonly thyroid and renal cell carcinoma), and pneumoconioses (e.g., silicosis). Medium and large nodules are most often seen in metastatic disease to the lung, commonly from breast carcinoma or colorectal malignancy.

A linear pattern of interstitial opacities is seen in processes that thicken the axial (bronchovascular) or peripheral interstitium of the lung. Since the axial interstitium surrounds the bronchovascular structures, thickening of this compartment produces parallel linear opacities radiating from the hila when visualized in length or peribronchial "cuffs" when viewed end on. A central distribution of linear interstitial disease is most often seen with interstitial pulmonary edema or "increased markings" emphysema. This pattern of interstitial disease may be impossible to distinguish from airways diseases, such as bronchiectasis and asthma, which primarily thicken the walls of airways. Thickening of the peripheral interstitium of the lung produces linear opacities that are either obliquely oriented 2–6 cm long, <1 mm thick lines that course through the substance of the lung toward the hila (Kerley's A lines) or shorter (1–2 cm), thin lines that

are peripheral and course perpendicular to and contact the pleural surface (Kerley's B lines). Kerley's A lines correspond to thickening of connective tissue sheets within the lung that contain lymphatic communications between the perivenous and bronchoarterial lymphatics, while Kerley's B lines represent thickened peripheral subpleural interlobular septa. A linear pattern of disease is seen in pulmonary edema, lymphangitic carcinomatosis, and acute viral or atypical bacterial pneumonia.

HIGH-RESOLUTION CT FINDINGS (Fig. 15.9)

Interlobular (Septal) Lines.   Septal thickening is most often seen as short, 1–2 cm lines that are oriented perpendicular to and intersect the costal pleura (3). These lines are best visualized in the subpleural and juxtadiaphragmatic regions of the lung where they outline the anterior and posterior margins of a secondary lobule. In the central regions of lung, the thickened septa can completely envelop lobules to produce polygonal-shaped structures. Although septa can be visualized in normal individuals, these lines are thicker (>1 mm) and more numerous in patients with diseases that thicken the interlobular septa, such as interstitial pulmonary edema, lymphangitic carcinomatosis, and idiopathic pulmonary fibrosis. Interlobular lines on HRCT are the equivalent of Kerley's B lines seen in the inferolateral portions of the lungs on frontal radiographs. Within the central regions of the lung, long (2–6 cm) linear opacities representing obliquely oriented connective tissue septa can be seen, which are the equivalent of radiographic Kerley's A lines.

Intralobular Lines.   In some patients, a lattice of fine lines is seen within the central portion of the pulmonary lobule radiating out toward the thickened lobular borders to produce a "spoke wheel" appearance. These lines are not normally visible, and represent thickening of the parenchymal interstitium. Intralobular lines are most commonly seen in patients with pulmonary fibrosis of any etiology.

"Thickened" Fissures and Bronchovascular (Core) Structures.   The apparent thickening of interlobar fissures in patients with interstitial lung disease is usually a direct extension of the thickening of interlobular septa to involve the subpleural interstitium of the lung. Small amounts of pleural fluid within fissures can give an identical appearance. Thickening of the bronchovascular structures of the lung results from thickening of the axial interstitium. This may produce apparent enlargement of perihilar vascular structures or cuffing or tram tracking of large bronchial walls. Involvement of the axial interstitium within the lobular core produces an abnormal prominence of the centrilobular "dot" or "Y." The apparent thickening of fissures and the axial interstitium are most commonly seen in pulmonary edema and lymphangitic carcinomatosis.

Subpleural Lines. These 5–10 cm long curvilinear opacities, found within 1 cm of the pleura and paralleling the chest wall, have been seen in patients with asbestosis, and less commonly, in patients with idiopathic pulmonary fibrosis. They are most often seen in the posterior portions of the lower lobes, usually in association with mild parenchymal fibrosis or honeycombing. These fixed abnormalities, which do not clear on nondependent positioning, probably represent an early phase of lung fibrosis.

Parenchymal Bands. These are linear, nontapering opacities 2–5 cm in length, extending from the lung to contact the pleural surface. These fibrotic bands can be distinguished from vessels and thickened septa by their length, thickness, course, absence of branching, and their association with regional parenchymal distortion. Parenchymal bands are usually seen in asbestosis, idiopathic pulmonary fibrosis, and sarcoidosis.

Honeycombing and Cysts. Small (6–10 mm) cystic spaces with thick walls, most common in the posterior subpleural regions of the lower lobes, represent end-stage pulmonary fibrosis of various etiologies. Most patients show additional signs of interstitial disease including thickened inter- and intralobular lines, parenchymal bands, irregularity of lung interfaces, and areas of ground-glass opacification.

Parenchymal cysts are a common manifestation of late stages of eosinophilic granuloma of lung (EG) and lymphangioleiomyomatosis (LAM). These cysts are slightly larger in diameter (10 mm) than honeycomb cysts, are more uniform in size, and have thinner walls. The cysts of EG and LAM are usually evenly distributed from central to peripheral portions of the upper lobes, with or without lower lobe involvement, while honeycombing tends to occur in the subpleural regions of the lower lobes. While normal lung may be found in the intervening spaces between the cysts of EG and LAM, honeycombing uniformly destroys lung and produces distortion of lung interfaces and traction bronchiectasis, features not found in EG and LAM.

Irregularity of Lung Interfaces. A common HRCT sign of interstitial disease, irregularity of the normally smooth interface between the bronchovascular bundles with the surrounding lung, reflects edema, fibrosis, or granuloma or tumor infiltration of the axial interstitium. Similarly, irregularity of the fissures or pleural surfaces with adjacent lung indicates peripheral interstitial disease. Pulmonary edema, idiopathic pulmonary fibrosis, and sarcoidosis are the most common causes of irregular interfaces.

Micronodules. These 1–3 mm sharply marginated round opacities demonstrated on HRCT represent conglomerates of granulomas or tumor cells and

are seen in sarcoidosis, histiocytosis X of lung, silicosis, miliary tuberculosis or histoplasmosis, metastatic adenocarcinoma, and lymphangitic carcinomatosis. They may be seen lining central bronchovascular bundles (sarcoidosis, histiocytosis X of lung), within interlobular septa or subpleural interstitium (sarcoidosis, lymphangitic carcinomatosis, silicosis), or within the substance of the pulmonary lobules (metastatic adenocarcinoma). On HRCT, it is often difficult to distinguish small vessels, particularly those in the upper and lower lobes that are vertically oriented, from interstitial nodules. Contiguous 10-mm scans obtained in addition to thin-section HRCT scans often help in distinguishing small vessels from micronodules.

Ground Glass or Hazy Increased Density. Multifocal areas of increased density can sometimes be identified in patients with diffuse interstitial lung disease. These regions, which often respect lobular borders, are distinguished from typical air space opacification by their granular appearance, the ability to visualize pulmonary vessels through the abnormal density, and by the absence of air bronchograms. These opacities are most often produced by thickening of the alveolar septa with or without lining of the alveolar spaces by inflammatory exudate or fluid. Diseases commonly associated with this appearance include the early, active phase of idiopathic pulmonary fibrosis, *Pneumocystis carinii* pneumonia, or interstitial pulmonary edema of any cause. The ground glass densities are occasionally confined to the immediate centrilobular regions of the pulmonary lobules, where they appear as fuzzy nodular densities that outline the normally invisible centrilobular bronchiole. This reflects involvement of the peribrochovascular interstitium and surrounding alveoli by an inflammatory process, and is seen in hypersensitivity pneumonitis, bronchiolitis obliterans organizing pneumonia, panbronchiolitis, and the early stages of idiopathic pulmonary fibrosis and histiocytosis X of lung. The presence of ground-glass opacities is important because it usually implies an active inflammatory process or edema that should be aggressively treated.

Distortion of Architecture. Processes that result in extensive parenchymal fibrosis can distort the normal architecture of the lung and the lung-mediastinal, lung-pleural, and lung-pulmonary vascular interfaces. Sarcoidosis is the disease most commonly associated with this finding. The parenchymal distortion seen in long-standing sarcoidosis is often better appreciated on HRCT than on plain radiographs.

Conglomerate Masses. In some patients with extensive pulmonary fibrosis, masses of fibrotic tissue develop in the perihilar regions of the upper lobes, often associated with bullous changes in the peripheral portions of the upper lobes. On CT and HRCT, these masses are seen to contain crowded bronchi and ves-

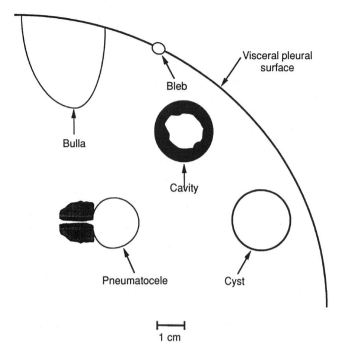

Figure 15.10. Diagram of Focal Lucent Pulmonary Lesions.

sels, and changes of traction bronchiectasis. These conglomerate masses are seen most often in patients with end-stage sarcoidosis, but may also be seen in complicated silicosis with progressive massive fibrosis, radiation fibrosis following treatment for Hodgkin's lymphoma or lung cancer, or rarely in the granulomatous fibrosis resulting from the parenchymal response to talc or starch mixed with intravenously administered narcotics.

Pulmonary Nodule

A pulmonary nodule refers to a discrete rounded opacity within the lung measuring less than 3 cm in diameter. A round opacity greater than 3 cm in diameter is termed a pulmonary mass. A solitary pulmonary nodule presents a common diagnostic dilemma that will be discussed in "The Solitary Pulmonary Nodule."

Branching Opacities

MUCOID IMPACTION

Branching tubular opacities that are distinguished from normal vascular shadows invariably represent mucus-filled dilated bronchi and are termed "bronchoceles" or mucoid impaction. Their appearance has been likened to that of a gloved finger or the shape of the letters V or Y, depending upon the length of airway and number of branches involved. When in a central perihilar location, these bronchoceles are caused by nonobstructive bronchiectasis, as in cystic fibrosis or allergic bronchopulmonary aspergillosis, or to postob-

structive bronchiectasis distal to an endobronchial tumor or a congenitally atretic bronchus. In the latter condition, a typical location immediately distal to the expected location of the apical segmental bronchus and a hyperlucent segment or lobe distal to the bronchocele because of collateral air drift should suggest the diagnosis. Peripheral bronchoceles are most often seen in cystic fibrosis and posttuberculous bronchiectasis.

PULMONARY LUCENCY

Abnormal lucency of the lung may be localized or diffuse. Focal radiolucent lesions of the lung include cavities, cysts, bullae, blebs, and pneumatoceles. These lesions are usually recognized by the identification of the wall that marginates the lucent lesion.

Focal Radiolucent Lesions (Fig. 15.10)

A *cavity* forms when a pulmonary mass undergoes necrosis and communicates with an airway, leading to gas within its center. The wall of a cavity is usually irregular or lobulated and, by definition, is greater than 1 mm in thickness. Lung abscess and necrotic neoplasm are the most common cavitary pulmonary lesions. A *bulla* is a gas collection within the pulmonary parenchyma that is greater than 1 cm in diameter and has a thin wall less than 1 mm thick. It represents a focal area of parenchymal destruction (i.e., emphysema) and may contain fibrous strands, residual blood vessels, or alveolar septa. An *air cyst* is a term used to describe any well-circumscribed intrapulmonary gas collection with a smooth thin wall greater than 1 mm thick. While some of these lesions will have a true epithelial lining (e.g., bronchogenic cyst that communicates with a bronchus), most do not and likely represent postinflammatory or posttraumatic lesions. A *bleb* is a collection of gas less than 1 cm in size within the layers of the visceral pleura. It is usually found in the apical portion of the lung. These small gas collections are not seen on plain radiographs, but may be visualized on chest CT where they are indistinguishable from paraseptal emphysema. Rupture of an apical bleb can lead to spontaneous pneumothorax. *Pneumatoceles* are thin-walled, gas-containing structures that represent distended air spaces distal to a check-valve obstruction of a bronchus or bronchiole, most commonly secondary to staphylococcal pneumonia. A *traumatic air cyst* results from pulmonary laceration following blunt trauma. These lesions generally resolve within 4–6 months. *Bronchiectatic cysts* are usually multiple, rounded, thin-walled lucencies found in clusters in the lower lobes, and represent saccular dilations of airways in varicose or cystic bronchiectasis.

Table 15.5.   Pulmonary Lucency

Localized	Cavity
	Cyst
	Bulla
	Bleb
	Pneumatocele
Diffuse	
Unilateral	Technical factors
	Grid cutoff
	Patient rotation
	Extrapulmonary disorder
	Soft-tissue abnormalities
	Absent pectoralis muscle
	Mastectomy
	Contralateral pleural effusion/thickening
	Pneumothorax
	Pulmonary disease
	Diminished pulmonary blood flow
	Hypoplastic lung/pulmonary artery
	Obstruction of pulmonary artery
	Pulmonary embolism
	Mediastinal/hilar tumor
	Fibrosing mediastinitis
	Diminished pulmonary blood flow and
	hyperinflation
	Lobar atelectasis/resection
	Swyer-James syndrome
	Endobronchial tumor/foreign body producing a
	check-valve effect
Bilateral	Technical factors
	Overpenetrated radiograph
	Diminished pulmonary blood flow
	Congenital pulmonary outflow obstruction
	Mediastinal tumor
	Pulmonary arterial hypertension
	Chronic thromboembolic disease
	Fibrosing mediastinitis
	Diminished pulmonary blood flow and hyperinflation
	Emphysema
	Asthma

Diffuse Pulmonary Hyperlucency (Table 15.5)

Unilateral Pulmonary Hyperlucency must be distinguished from differences in lung density because of technical factors or overlying soft-tissue abnormalities. Grid cutoff from a combination of lateral and near or far focus-grid decentering may lead to a graduated increase in density across the width of the chest film, simulating unilateral hyperlucency. Rotation of the patient will produce an increase in density over the lung rotated away from the film cassette, i.e., a left anterior oblique radiograph obtained with a posteroanterior beam will show increased density over the right hemithorax, simulating pleural disease on the right or hyperlucency on the left. Congenital absence of the pectoralis muscle (Poland's syndrome) or mastectomy can produce apparent hyperlucency.

True unilateral hyperlucent lung results from decreased blood flow to the lung. Diminished blood flow may be because of a primary vascular abnormality, to shunting of blood away from a lung, which traps air, or to a combination of the two. Hypoplasia of the right or left pulmonary artery produces a lung that is hyperlucent and diminished in size. A similar appearance may be produced by lobar resection or atelectasis, where the remaining lobe or lung hyperinflates to accommodate the hemithorax, thereby attenuating pulmonary vessels and producing hyperlucency. Pulmonary arterial obstruction may be secondary to extrinsic compression or invasion by a hilar mass or to pulmonary embolism. A check-valve effect from an endobronchial tumor or foreign body can produce air trapping, resulting in shunting of blood and unilateral hyperlucency. The Swyer-James syndrome or unilateral hyperlucent lung is a condition that follows adenoviral infection during infancy. An asymmetric obliterative bronchiolitis with severe air trapping on expiration and secondary unilateral pulmonary artery hypoplasia produces the hyperlucency in this condition. Finally, asymmetric involvement of lung by emphysema can produce a hyperlucent lung; this is most common with severe bullous disease.

Bilateral Hyperlucent Lungs may be simulated by an overpenetrated film or by a thin patient. As with unilateral hyperlucency, true bilateral hyperlucent lungs are the result of diminished pulmonary blood flow. This may be the result of congenital pulmonic stenosis, most commonly associated with the tetralogy of Fallot, or secondary to an acquired obstruction of the pulmonary circulation as in pulmonary arterial hypertension or chronic thromboembolic disease. Pulmonary emphysema results in hyperinflation with air trapping on expiration, destruction of the pulmonary microvasculature, and attenuation of lobar and segmental vessels, thereby producing bilateral hyperlucency. Asthma produces transient air trapping and diffuse bilateral vascular attenuation, resulting in both hyperinflation and hyperlucency.

PULMONARY EDEMA
Basic Principles

Under normal conditions, the interstitial space of the lung is kept dry by pulmonary lymphatics located within the axial and peripheral interstitium of the lung. The lymphatics drain the small amounts of transudated fluid that enters the interstitial spaces as an ultrafiltrate of plasma. Since there are no lymphatic structures immediately within the alveolar walls (parenchymal interstitium), filtered interstitial fluid is drawn to the lymphatics by a pressure gradient from the alveolar interstitium to the axial and peripheral interstitium. When the rate of fluid accumulation in the interstitium exceeds the lymphatic drainage capabilities of the lung, fluid accumulates first within the interstitial space. As the amount of extravascular

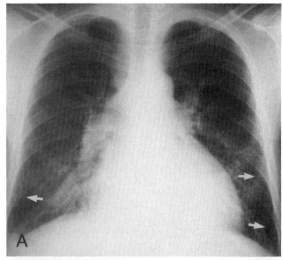

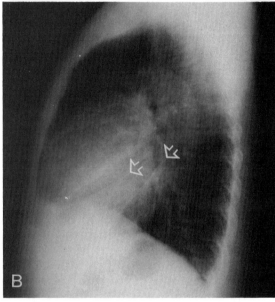

Figure 15.11. Interstitial Pulmonary Edema. Posteroanterior **(A)** and lateral **(B)** chest radiographs in a patient with congestive heart failure caused by cardiomyopathy. There is enlargement of the cardiac silhouette with redistribution of blood flow to the upper lobes, consistent with cardiac decompensation and secondary pulmonary venous hypertension. Indistinctness of the perihilar and lower zone vasculature with visible Kerley's B lines (*solid arrows*) is characteristic of interstitial pulmonary edema. A small right pleural effusion blunts the right lateral costophrenic sulcus; thickening of the oblique (major) fissures on the lateral view (*open arrows*) represents edema within the subpleural interstitial space.

fluid increases, fluid accumulates in the corners of the alveolar spaces. Progressive fluid accumulation eventually produces flooding of the alveolar spaces, resulting in air-space pulmonary edema. While interstitial edema may leave the gas-exchanging properties of the lung unaffected, flooding of the alveolar spaces leads to impaired oxygen and carbon dioxide exchange.

Excess fluid accumulation in the lung is caused by one of three basic mechanisms. The most common

mechanism involves a change in the normal Starling's forces that govern fluid movement in the lung. Since normal fluid movement is determined by the differences in hydrostatic and oncotic pressure between the pulmonary capillaries and surrounding alveolar interstitium, an imbalance in these forces may lead to pulmonary edema. Pulmonary edema is most commonly caused by increased capillary hydrostatic pressure from left heart failure, although diminished plasma oncotic pressure or diminished interstitial hydrostatic pressure may be contributing factors. Another mechanism involves an absence or obstruction of the normal pulmonary lymphatics, leading to the excess accumulation of interstitial fluid. Lastly, a wide variety of disorders can injure the capillary endothelium and alveolar epithelium, producing an increase in capillary permeability that allows protein-rich fluid to escape from the capillaries and into the pulmonary interstitium (4).

Radiographic Findings in Pulmonary Edema

The radiographic findings in pulmonary edema can be divided into interstitial and air space components. The radiographic appearance of interstitial pulmonary edema is because of thickening of the various components of the interstitial spaces by fluid. Thickening of the axial interstitium results in the loss of definition of the intrapulmonary vascular shadows, peribronchial cuffing, and tram tracking. Edema within alveolar septa is not discernable as discrete opacities but produces a ground glass opacification in the perihilar and lower lung zones, regions where fluid tends to accumulate in the early phases of edema. Involvement of peripheral and subpleural interstitial structures produces Kerley's lines and subpleural edema. Kerley's A and B lines represent thickening of central connective tissue septa and peripheral interlobular septa, respectively, while Kerley's C lines represent a network of thickened interlobular septa (Fig. 15.11). Subpleural edema is the accumulation of fluid within the innermost (interstitial) layer of the visceral pleura, and is best seen on lateral radiograph as smooth thickening of the interlobar fissures. The radiographic changes of interstitial pulmonary edema may progress to those of air space edema or, if successfully treated, resolve within 12–24 hours.

Air space pulmonary edema develops when progressive fluid accumulation in the interstitial spaces spills into the alveoli. The chest radiograph typically shows symmetric bilateral air space opacities that are confluent and predominate in the middle and lower lung zones. Air space nodules and the findings of interstitial edema (Kerley's B lines and subpleural edema) may be seen peripherally. An uncommon form of air space pulmonary edema, seen most commonly in left

Table 15.6.   Diffuse Confluent Air Space Opacities

Pulmonary edema	Cardiogenic
	Fluid overload/renal failure
	Noncardiogenic (ARDS) (see Table 15.8)
Pneumonia	*Pneumocystis carinii*
	Gram-negative bacteria
	Influenza
	Fungi
	Histoplasmosis
	Aspergillosis
Hemorrhage (see Table 15.9)	
Neoplasm	Bronchoalveolar cell carcinoma
	Lymphoma
Alveolar proteinosis	Acute silica inhalation
	Lymphoma
	Leukemia
	AIDS

heart failure or renal failure, is the bat's wing or butterfly distribution of disease. In this situation, the air space opacification is sharply confined to the central, parahilar regions of lung with sparing of the peripheral or subpleural regions (Fig. 15.1). The reason for this distribution of edema is unknown. As with interstitial edema, the air space opacities of alveolar edema tend to change rapidly, often within hours. The differential diagnosis of diffuse air space opacities is listed in Table 15.6.

Although not commonly used to image the patient with pulmonary edema, CT and HRCT demonstrate fairly characteristic findings in this disorder. Thickening of subpleural, septal, and bronchovascular structures are well depicted on HRCT. Mild parenchymal edema produces a ground-glass pattern around the hila. Early alveolar edema is seen as centrilobular air space nodules surrounding the arteries within the lobular core, while severe alveolar edema produces dense perihilar air space opacification. Cardiomegaly, pulmonary venous distension, and pleural effusions are associated findings in cardiogenic or fluid-overload edema.

Atypical Radiographic Appearances of Pulmonary Edema

There are several conditions that may give rise to atypical radiographic appearances of pulmonary edema. Since the distribution of edema is affected by gravity, it is not surprising that edema fluid accumulates posteriorly or unilaterally in patients maintaining a prolonged supine or decubitus position, respectively. The diagnosis of unilateral edema is suggested by typical radiographic and clinical findings of pulmonary edema in one lung that resolve rapidly or redistribute with changes in patient positioning (Fig. 15.12). Another cause of asymmetric or unilateral pulmonary edema is an interruption in the blood supply

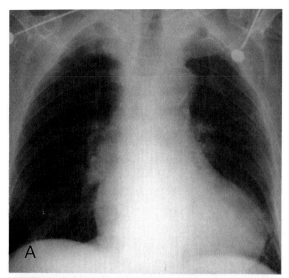

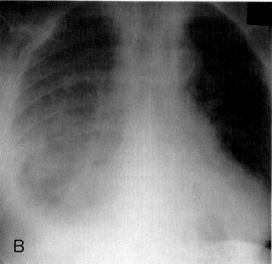

Figure 15.12.   Unilateral Pulmonary Edema. A. An AP portable radiograph in a patient with unstable angina demonstrates cardiomegaly and clear lungs **B.** A film obtained 10 hours later demonstrates opacification of the right lung and a right pleural effusion. The patient had been lying in the right lateral decubitus position in the interval between radiographs. The edema resolved with diuretic therapy.

to one lung. This may be seen in pulmonary artery hypoplasia or in an acquired obstruction to pulmonary arterial blood flow, such as central pulmonary embolus or extrinsic compression of the pulmonary artery from tumor or fibrosis. In these conditions, the lung with diminished pulmonary blood flow is "protected" from the transudation of fluid and the development of pulmonary edema. Bronchogenic carcinoma, lymphoma, or other causes of unilateral lymph node enlargement can impede normal lymphatic drainage and predispose to unilateral pulmonary edema. Similarly, unilateral pulmonary venous obstruction from tumor or fibrosing mediastinitis will predispose to edema on the affected side. Unilateral pulmonary edema may develop in the lung reexpanded by the rapid evacuation of a large pleural fluid collection or pneumothorax. This is known as reexpansion pulmonary edema and is discussed in "Reexpansion Pulmonary Edema."

Alveolar pulmonary edema localized to the right upper lung may be seen in patients with severe mitral regurgitation. The mechanism of edema formation is likely caused by preferential regurgitant flow of blood into the rightupper lobe pulmonary vein across the superiorly and posteriorly oriented mitral valve. These patients will usually have typical radiographic findings of interstitial edema elsewhere in the lungs.

Patients with pulmonary emphysema may have unusual appearances of alveolar edema. Areas of bulla, most commonly in the apical portions of the lungs, are spared from the development of alveolar edema because the pulmonary blood flow to these regions has already been obliterated by the emphysematous process. These emphysematous regions within adjacent areas of air space opacification can simulate cavity formation and may be difficult to distinguish radiographically from necrotizing pneumonia or pneumatocele formation. Comparison with previous radiographs and correlation with the clinical course will aid in the proper diagnosis.

Hydrostatic and Increased Permeability of Pulmonary Edema

HYDROSTATIC EDEMA

Hydrostatic (normal capillary permeability) pulmonary edema is the most common form of pulmonary edema. Patients with acute or chronic renal failure may develop pulmonary edema caused by increased pulmonary capillary hydrostatic pressure. The elevated hydrostatic pressure is because of a combination of hypervolemia and left ventricular dysfunction, with resultant pulmonary venous and capillary hypertension. Volume overload without renal failure may also produce pulmonary edema by a hydrostatic mechanism. Decreased capillary oncotic pressure, present in patients with hypoalbuminemia secondary to the nephrotic syndrome or liver failure, is not considered to be an independent risk factor for the development of pulmonary edema, but is a co-factor in several conditions.

Hydrostatic pulmonary edema is usually because of pulmonary venous hypertension secondary to congestive heart failure. Thus, identification of the radiographic findings of pulmonary venous hypertension and pulmonary edema will provide the diagnosis. Most of these patients will have left ventricular failure or mitral valve disease. A list of the causes of mechanical or functional obstruction to pulmonary venous return is found in Table 15.7.

Table 15.7. Pulmonary Venous Hypertension and Pulmonary Edema

Obstruction to left ventricular outflow	Aortic coarctation
	Aortic stenosis
	Hypoplastic left heart syndrome
Left ventricular failure	
Mitral valve disease	Mitral stenosis
	Mitral insufficiency
Left atrial myxoma	
Cor triatriatum	
Obstruction of pulmonary veins	
Central pulmonary veins	Fibrosing mediastinitis
	Pulmonary vein stenosis
Intrapulmonary veins	Pulmonary venous thrombosis
	Pulmonary venoocclusive disease

The radiographic findings of pulmonary venous hypertension are enlargement of pulmonary veins and redistribution of pulmonary blood flow to the upper lung zones. Pulmonary venous enlargement is seen as progressive dilation of horizontally oriented pulmonary veins on serial chest radiographs. The redistribution of pulmonary blood flow results from lower zone pulmonary venous constriction and increased resistance to lower zone blood flow with resultant preferential flow through upper lobe vessels. Therefore, in pulmonary venous hypertension in the upright patient, the upper zone vessels are equal to or greater in diameter than the lower zone vessels. This is the opposite of the normal appearance in which the lower zone vessels are larger than the upper zone vessels because of the normal gravitational effects on pulmonary blood flow. It should be noted that there are conditions other than pulmonary venous hypertension in which there is distension of upper zone pulmonary vessels, including left-right shunts and basilar lung disease. The association of upper zone vascular prominence with findings of left ventricular failure (cardiomegaly,pulmonary edema, and pleural effusion) usually allows for the correct diagnosis (Fig. 15.11).

The sequence of events following the development of pulmonary venous hypertension has been studied in patients with acute cardiac decompensation following myocardial infarction. Several studies have correlated the radiographic findings of pulmonary venous hypertension in the erect patient with measurements of pulmonary capillary wedge pressure (PCWP) using flow-directed balloon occlusion (i.e., Swan-Ganz) catheters. When PCWP is normal (8–12 mm Hg), the chest radiograph is normal. Mild elevation of PCWP (12–18 mm Hg) produces constriction of lower lobe vessels and enlargement of upper lobe vessels. Progressive elevation of PCWP (19–25 mm Hg) leads to the findings of interstitial pulmonary edema: loss of vascular definition, peribronchial cuffing, and Kerley's lines. A PCWP above 25 mm Hg produces alve-

Table 15.8. Etiologies of ARDS

Septicemia	Gram-negative bacteria
Shock	
Major surgery	
Burns	
Acute pancreatitis	
Disseminated intravascular coagulation	
Drugs	Narcotics
	Heroin
	Crack cocaine
	Aspirin
Inhalation of noxious fumes	Nitrogen dioxide (silo-filler's disease)
	Hydrocarbons
	Smoke
	Chlorine
	Phosgene
Aspiration of fluid	Fresh or salt water near drowning
	Gastric fluid aspiration (Mendelson's syndrome)
Fat embolism	
Amniotic fluid embolism	

olar flooding with radiographic findings of bilateral air space opacities in the perihilar and lower lung zones.

The causes of pulmonary venous hypertension may be divided radiographically into those associated with a normal heart size and those with cardiomegaly. Severe, long-standing obstruction to left ventricular outflow (e.g., aortic stenosis) is usually associated with a normal heart size unless the left ventricle has failed. Chronic left ventricular failure is invariably associated with cardiomegaly, although acute left ventricular decompensation, as in acute myocardial infarction or acute aortic regurgitation, may show a normal heart size. Obstruction or incompetence at the level of the mitral valve (e.g., mitral stenosis or regurgitation, left atrial myxoma) may only show left atrial enlargement without ventricular dilation. Obstruction of the central pulmonary veins (i.e., fibrosing mediastinitis, pulmonary vein thrombosis) is usually associated with the radiographic findings of pulmonary venous hypertension and pulmonary edema with a normal heart size. Intrapulmonary venous obstruction (i.e., pulmonary veno-occlusive disease) may show only pulmonary edema, but often the diagnosis is delayed until pulmonary arterial hypertension has developed (Table 15.7).

INCREASED PERMEABILITY EDEMA

Adult Respiratory Distress Syndrome (ARDS). Rapidly progressive respiratory failure because of leakage of protein-rich edema fluid into the lung resulting from damage to the pulmonary microcirculation may develop as a complication of a variety of systemic conditions. This clinical and radiographic condition is termed the adult respiratory distress syndrome (ARDS). The edema associated with this syndrome is called increased capillary permeability edema as compared with hydrostatic edema, which is associated with normal capillary permeability. A long list of pulmonary and nonpulmonary disorders has been associated with ARDS (Table 15.8); the most common are shock, severe trauma, burns, sepsis, narcotic overdose, and pancreatitis. Although the precise pathogenesis of capillary permeability edema has yet to be completely elucidated, current evidence suggests that recruitment and activation of neutrophils in the lung with release of enzymes and oxygen radicals are key factors in the development of capillary endothelial damage.

The pathologic changes associated with ARDS are those of diffuse alveolar damage and are common to all patients regardless of the underlying etiology. Within 12–24 hours following the initial insult, damage to capillary endothelium produces engorged capillaries and proteinaceous interstitial edema. Injury to type I pneumocytes leads to the flooding of alveoli with edema fluid. Within the 1st week, the proteinaceous and cellular debris forms hyaline membranes that line the distal airways and alveoli. Type II pneumocytes proliferate in an attempt to reline the denuded alveolar surfaces, and fibroblastic tissue proliferates within the air spaces. This fibroblastic tissue may resolve and leave minimal scarring or, particularly in those patients with severe disease and long-standing oxygen requirements, result in extensive interstitial fibrosis.

Radiographically, ARDS follows a predictable pattern. Chest radiographs demonstrating patchy peripheral air space opacities become abnormal 12–24 hours following the onset of dyspnea. These opacities coalesce over the next several days to produce confluent bilateral air space opacities with air bronchograms. Radiographic improvement in the opacities may be seen within the 1st week, but this is often because of the effects of increasing positive pressure ventilation rather than true histologic improvement. After 1 week, the air space opacities gradually give way to a coarse reticulonodular pattern that may resolve over the course of several months or remain unchanged, in which case the pattern represents irreversible pulmonary fibrosis (i.e., honeycombing). Pneumonia complicating ARDS is difficult to diagnose radiographically, but should be suspected when a focal area of air space opacification or a significant pleural effusion develops during the course of the disease. Likewise, the superimposition of left ventricular failure may be impossible to recognize but is suggested by rapid clinical and radiographic deterioration associated with changes in measured PCWP and edema fluid-protein content. Pneumomediastinum and pneumothorax may result as a complication of positive pressure ventilation to stiff lungs, and should be looked for on each chest radiograph.

The Radiographic Distinction of Hydrostatic from Permeability Edema

Beyond identifying the presence of pulmonary edema, the ability to distinguish between types of pulmonary edema has significant diagnostic and therapeutic import. Measurements of PCWP and transbronchial sampling of pulmonary edema fluid are techniques that accurately distinguish hydrostatic from increased capillary permeability edema. In hydrostatic edema, PCWP measurements are elevated and a protein-poor transudative edema fluid is present, while in increased capillary permeability edema, there is a normal PCWP and proteinaceous edema fluid is seen. Milne and colleagues (5) have described the findings on the chest radiograph used to distinguish cardiac and overhydration edema from increased capillary permeability edema. In pulmonary edema associated with chronic cardiac failure, the heart is usually enlarged with an inverted (redistributed) pulmonary blood flow pattern. The distribution of edema is even from central to peripheral over the lower lung zones. The vascular pedicle, which represents the mediastinal width at the level of the superior cava and left subclavian artery, is widened (>53 mm on posteroanterior PA radiograph), reflecting increased circulating blood volume. Lung volumes are diminished because of decreased pulmonary compliance from edema. Peribronchial cuffing, Kerley's lines, and pleural effusions represent interstitial and intrapleural transudation of fluid, respectively.

Overhydration or renal failure edema has some features in common with chronic cardiac failure and may be indistinguishable radiographically. Capillary permeability edema can sometimes be distinguished from hydrostatic edema. A more peripheral distribution of edema with a normal heart size and normal vascular pedicle width, the latter indicating normal circulating blood volume, are findings typical of capillary permeability edema.

It should be noted that there are factors that may render radiographic distinction of types of pulmonary edema difficult. Radiographs of supine patients will make evaluation of pulmonary blood flow distribution and vascular pedicle width difficult. The presence of severe alveolar edema will obscure the underlying vascular markings. Many patients with capillary permeability edema will be overhydrated in attempts to maintain circulating blood volume, producing complex radiographic findings.

Additional Types of Pulmonary Edema

Neurogenic Pulmonary Edema. Pulmonary edema following head trauma, seizure, or increased intracranial pressure is a complex phenomenon that appears to involve both hydrostatic and increased permeability mechanisms. Massive sympathetic discharge from the brain in these conditions produces systemic vasoconstriction and increased venous return with resultant increase in left ventricular diastolic pressure and hydrostatic pulmonary edema. However, the finding of protein-rich edema fluid and normal PCWP in some patients suggests that increased permeability may also be a contributing factor.

High Altitude Pulmonary Edema. This develops in certain individuals after rapid ascent to altitudes above 3500 m. Edema typically develops within 48–72 hours of ascent and appears to reflect a varied individual response to hypoxemia in which scattered areas of pulmonary arterial spasm result in transient pulmonary arterial hypertension. This produces an overflow of blood at high pressure to uninvolved areas, resulting in damage to the capillary endothelium and increased permeability edema, which is patchy in distribution. Rapid resolution, usually within 24–48 hours, occurs after the administration of supplemental oxygen or a return to sea level.

Reexpansion Pulmonary Edema. Rapid reexpansion of a lung after collapse of more than 48 hours may result in the development of unilateral pulmonary edema. Marked increases in negative pleural pressure following pleural tube placement, impaired pulmonary lymphatic drainage following prolonged lung collapse, and ischemia-induced surfactant deficiency resulting in the need for high negative pleural pressure to reexpand the collapsed lung are proposed mechanisms. Recent evidence points toward prolonged collapse producing ischemia and hypoxemia within the lung, which promotes anaerobic metabolism and free radical formation. Reperfusion of the lung upon reexpansion then leads to lung injury and permeability edema. Gradual reexpansion of the lung by slow removal of pleural air or fluid over a 24–48 hour period and supplemental oxygen administration help limit the incidence and severity of this complication.

Acute Upper Airway Obstruction. Pulmonary edema may be seen during or immediately following treatment of acute upper airway obstruction. The proposed mechanism involves the creation of markedly negative intrathoracic pressure by attempts to inspire against an extrathoracic airway obstruction, producing transudation of fluid into the lung. There are no distinguishing radiographic features.

Table 15.9. Pulmonary Hemorrhage

Spontaneous	Thrombocytopenia
	Hemophilia
	Anticoagulant therapy
Trauma	Pulmonary contusion
Embolic disease	Pulmonary embolism
	Fat embolism
Vasculitis	Autoimmune
	Goodpasture's
	Idiopathic pulmonary hemorrhage
	Wegener's granulomatosis
	Infectious
	Gram-negative bacteria
	Influenza
	Aspergillus
	Mucormycosis
Drugs	Penicillamine

Amniotic Fluid Embolism. A severe and often fatal form of pulmonary edema may develop in a pregnant woman when amniotic fluid gains access to the systemic circulation during labor. There is an association of this entity and fetal distress and demise, as the mucin within fetal meconium plays a key role in the pathogenesis of this disorder. Embolic obstruction of the pulmonary vasculature by mucin and fetal squamous cells within the amniotic fluid leads to sudden pulmonary arterial hypertension and cor pulmonale with decreased cardiac output and pulmonary edema. An anaphylactoid reaction and disseminated intravascular coagulation from factors within the amniotic fluid contribute to the shock state. Radiographically, there is bilateral confluent air space opacities indistinguishable from pulmonary edema of other etiologies. In severe cases, there is secondary enlargement of the central pulmonary arteries and right heart as a manifestation of cor pulmonale. The diagnosis can be confirmed premortem by identification of fetal squamous cells and mucin in blood samples obtained from indwelling pulmonary artery catheters.

Fat Embolism. The embolization of marrow fat to the lung is a common complication occurring 24–72 hours after the fracture of a long bone (e.g., femur). Within the lung, the fat is hydrolyzed to its component fatty acids, which causes increased pulmonary capillary permeability and hemorrhagic pulmonary edema. Radiographically, confluent air space opacities are seen that tend to be peripheral and have a lower zone predominance. The diagnosis is made by recognizing findings of systemic fat embolism (petechial rash, lipiduria, central nervous system depression) and pulmonary changes in the appropriate time period following trauma. Most patients have a mild course with minimal respiratory compromise, while a minority will develop progressive respiratory failure leading to death.

PULMONARY HEMORRHAGE

Hemorrhage or hemorrhagic edema of the lung can result from trauma, bleeding diathesis, infections (invasive aspergillosis, mucormycosis, *Pseudomonas* infection, influenza), drugs (penicillamine), pulmonary embolism, fat embolism, ARDS, and autoimmune diseases (Table 15.9). The autoimmune diseases that can cause pulmonary hemorrhage include Goodpasture's syndrome, idiopathic pulmonary hemorrhage, Wegener's granulomatosis, systemic lupus erythematosis (SLE), rheumatoid arthritis, and polyarteritis nodosa.

Autoimmune Diseases and Pulmonary Hemorrhage

Goodpasture's Syndrome is an autoimmune disease characterized by damage to the alveolar and renal glomerular basement membranes by a cytotoxic antibody. The antibody is directed primarily against renal glomerular basement membrane and cross-reacts with alveolar basement membrane to produce the renal injury and pulmonary hemorrhage characteristic of this disorder. Young adult males are most commonly affected and present with cough, hemoptysis, dyspnea, and fatigue. The pulmonary complaints usually precede clinical evidence of renal failure. Chest films show bilateral coalescent air space opacities that are radiographically indistinguishable from pulmonary edema (Fig. 15.13). Within several days, the air space opacities resolve, giving rise to reticular opacities in the same distribution. Complete radiographic resolution is seen within 2 weeks except in those patients with recurrent episodes of hemorrhage in whom the reticular opacities persist and represent pulmonary fibrosis. The diagnosis is made by immunofluorescent studies of renal or lung tissue, which show a smooth wavy line of fluorescent staining along the basement membrane. The overall prognosis is poor, although the use of immunosuppressive drugs and plasmapheresis has improved survival.

Idiopathic Pulmonary Hemorrhage. The pulmonary manifestations of idiopathic pulmonary hemorrhage are clinically and radiographically indistinguishable from those of Goodpasture's syndrome. In distinction to Goodpasture's syndrome, this disorder is most common in children, with an equal sex distribution. The diagnosis is one of exclusion, and is suggested when pulmonary hemorrhage and anemia are found in a patient with normal renal function and urinalysis, and absence of antiglomerular basement membrane antibodies.

Other Autoimmune Diseases and Pulmonary Hemorrhage. Wegener's granulomatosis, SLE, rheumatoid arthritis, and polyarteritis nodosa are autoimmune disorders associated with a systemic immune complex vasculitis. The development of pulmo-

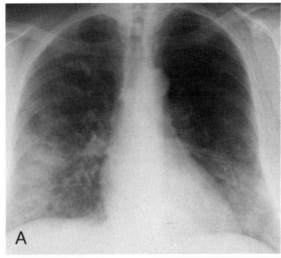

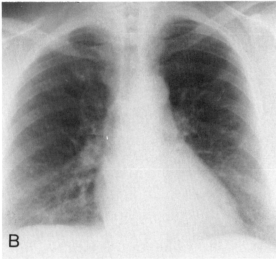

Figure 15.13. Goodpasture's Syndrome. A. Frontal radiograph in a 47-year-old woman with renal insufficiency and recurrent pulmonary hemorrhage demonstrates bilateral, predominantly middle and lower zone air space opacification. **B.** Follow-up film obtained 6 months later shows clearing of the air space opacities; minimal residual interstitial disease represents hemosiderosis and fibrosis from recurrent hemorrhage.

nary hemorrhage in these diseases is secondary to small vessel pulmonary arteritis, which results in spontaneous hemorrhage. The pulmonary manifestations of these diseases are discussed in subsequent sections.

The distinction of pulmonary hemorrhage from pulmonary edema or pneumonia may be difficult, particularly because many causes of pulmonary edema and pneumonia may have a significant hemorrhagic component. The rapid development of air space opacities associated with a dropping hematocrit and hemoptysis should suggest the diagnosis. Hemoptysis, however, is not always present. Associated renal disease, hematuria, or findings of a collagen vascular disorder or systemic vasculitis may provide additional clues. The distinction of pulmonary hemorrhage from

pneumonia is made by the absence of fever or purulent sputum, and the finding of a normal or elevated carbon monoxide diffusing capacity. This latter determination is directly related to the volume of gas-exchanging intra- and extravascular intrapulmonary red blood cells and is therefore elevated in pulmonary hemorrhage or hemorrhagic edema but decreased in pneumonia. The presence of hemosiderin-laden macrophages in sputum, bronchoalveolar lavage fluid, or tissue specimens is evidence of chronic or recurrent intrapulmonary hemorrhage. A rapid radiographic improvement of the air space opacities in pulmonary hemorrhage is common and may help in diagnosis.

PULMONARY EMBOLISM

In the United States over 600,000 cases of pulmonary embolism (P.E.) occur each year, with one-third of episodes causing or contributing to death. In patients surviving for 1 hour past the initial episode, 71% do not have P.E. diagnosed; this is associated with a 30% mortality rate. Alternatively, in the 29% of patients correctly diagnosed and treated for P.E., there is an 8% mortality rate. These data suggest that empiric treatment for all patients with suspected pulmonary embolism is warranted. However, the high (up to 30%) incidence of hemorrhagic complications associated with anticoagulant therapy requires that an accurate diagnosis of pulmonary embolism be made.

The radiologist plays a central role in the diagnostic evaluation of the patient with suspected pulmonary embolism (6). This section will review the nonimaging aspects of patient evaluation, and then detail the various imaging modalities available to the radiologist. A practical algorithm that serves as a useful guide to the workup of each patient with suspected P.E. will be provided.

Clinical and Laboratory Findings in Pulmonary Embolism

The majority of patients with pulmonary embolism have a variety of symptoms including dyspnea (84%), pleuritic chest pain (74%), anxiety (59%), and cough (53%). However, in certain groups of patients at high risk for P.E., asymptomatic embolization is known to occur. For example, in patients undergoing elective total hip or knee replacement, 4% will develop postoperative pulmonary embolism as documented on pulmonary angiography. Physical examination may reveal tachypnea (respiratory rate >16/min), rales, and a prominent pulmonary component of the second heart sound. Unfortunately, these findings are entirely nonspecific. Only 20% of patients presenting to an emergency department with pleuritic chest pain will be found to have P.E.

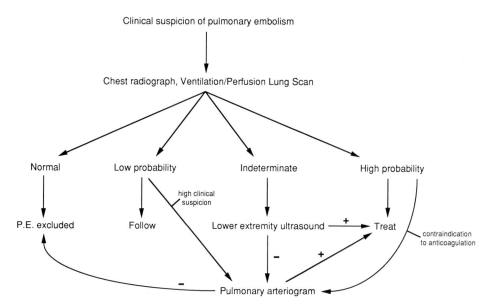

Laboratory tests commonly utilized in suspected pulmonary embolism include the measurements of PaO_2 and electrocardiography. Although <10% of patients with P.E. have a PaO_2 >90 mm Hg, hypoxemia is common in a variety of disorders and is therefore nonspecific. The electrocardiographic finding of an $S_1Q_3T_3$, right bundle branch block, right axis deviation, and right ventricular hypertrophy, all signs of cor pulmonale, are inaccurate for the diagnosis of P.E..

Radiologic Diagnosis of Pulmonary Embolism

A number of imaging techniques are routinely employed in the evaluation of the patient with suspected pulmonary embolism. These include the chest radiograph, ventilation/perfusion (V/Q) lung scintigraphy, and pulmonary angiography. Noninvasive methods of imaging deep venous thrombosis (DVT), such as compression and Doppler ultrasound, magnetic resonance imaging (MR) of the extremities and pelvis, and radiolabeled platelet scanning, are being used with greater frequency. The relatively noninvasive nature and high accuracy of these techniques to diagnose DVT and an increasing familiarity with their performance and interpretation among radiologists has led to their widespread use in the workup of pulmonary embolism. A practical algorithm for the radiologic evaluationof P.E. is shown in Figure 15.14.

CHEST RADIOGRAPH

The chest radiograph is the first examination obtained in all patients with suspected pulmonary embolism. Although the majority of patients with pulmonary embolism will have abnormal radiographs, a significant percentage of patients will have normal chest radiographs. The radiographic findings include cardiac, pulmonary arterial, parenchymal, pleural, and diaphragmatic changes.

Cardiac, or more precisely right heart enlargement, is an uncommon finding seen with massive or extensive pulmonary embolism producing cor pulmonale. Enlargement of the central pulmonary arteries from pulmonary arterial hypertension may also be seen, but is more commonly a late sequela of chronic embolic disease. The most common radiographic findings in embolism without infarction are localized peripheral oligemia with or without distended proximal vessels (Westermark's sign) and peripheral air space opacification or linear atelectasis. The air space opacification represents localized pulmonary hemorrhage produced by bronchial and pulmonary venous collateral flow to the obstructed region and is seen with peripheral but not central emboli. Volume loss in the lower lung from adhesive atelectasis because of ischemic injury to type II pneumocytes and secondary surfactant deficiency may produce diaphragmatic elevation and the development of linear atelectasis.

Less than 10% of all pulmonary emboli result in lung infarction. Collateral bronchial arterial and retrograde pulmonary venous flow prevent infarction in most patients. The distinction between embolism with and without infarction is usually impossible radiographically and is of limited importance as treatment is identical. Infarction from embolism occurs with greater frequency in patients with underlying heart failure because of limited collateral bronchial arterial flow to the ischemic region. In pulmonary embolism with infarction, the cardiac, pulmonary arterial, and peripheral vascular changes are indistinguishable from those seen in embolism without infarction. Radiographic features that suggest infarction include the presence of a small pleural effusion and the devel-

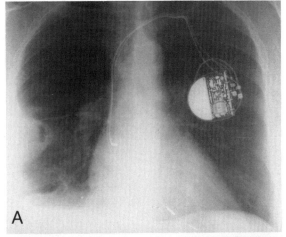

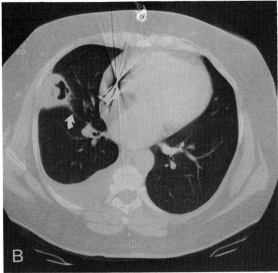

Figure 15.15. Pulmonary Infarct from Thromboembolism (Hampton's Hump). A. Frontal radiograph in a 56-year-old woman with cardiomyopathy, deep venous thrombosis, and pulmonary embolism shows a peripheral wedge-shaped opacity with cavitation in the right lower lung. **B.** A CT scan shows a smooth, cavitating, pleural-based mass representing infarcted lung, fed by a middle lobe pulmonary artery (*arrow*). There is an associated right pleural effusion, a common finding in pulmonary infarct.

opment of a pleural-based wedge-shaped opacity (Hampton's hump). This opacity, typically found in the posterior or lateral costophrenic sulcus of the lung, is wedge-shaped, homogeneous, and lacks air bronchograms. The blunted apex of the wedge points toward the occluded feeding vessel, while the base is against the pleural surface (Fig. 15.15). This wedge-shaped opacity is often obscured by surrounding areas of hemorrhage in the early phases following infarction, and becomes more obvious with time as the peripheral areas of hemorrhage resolve. A distinction between embolus with and without infarction is usually made by noting changes in the radiographic opacities with time. In embolism without infarction, the air space opacities should resolve completely within

7–10 days, while infarcts resolve over the course of several weeks or months and usually leave a residual linear parenchymal scar and/or localized pleural thickening.

None of the aforementioned radiographic findings, either alone or in combination, are useful in making a firm diagnosis of pulmonary embolism. Conversely, a completely normal radiograph may be seen in up to 40% of patients with emboli. The prime utility of the chest radiograph in the evaluation of P.E. is in the detection of conditions that mimic P.E. clinically, such as pneumonia or pneumothorax, and as an aid to the interpretation of the ventilation/perfusion lung scan.

VENTILATION/PERFUSION LUNG SCINTIGRAPHY

The intravenous administration of macroaggregates of albumin radiolabeled with technetium has given the radiologist a noninvasive method of assessing the patency of the pulmonary circulation. The sensitivity of this technique allows for the confident exclusion of pulmonary embolism when a technically adequate perfusion scan is normal. The addition of ventilation scanning increases the specificity of an abnormal perfusion scan, and is always performed in conjunction with the perfusion scan if possible. An extended discussion of lung scintigraphy is provided in Chapter 49.

Although V/Q scanning is commonly used in the evaluation of the patient with suspected P.E., there are limitations to its utility for the diagnosis of P.E. First, only a minority of patients undergoing V/Q studies will have either a normal or high probability study, results which clinicians can confidently rely upon to guide therapy. Second, there is significant interobserver variability in the interpretation of V/Q studies. Finally, there are few well-constructed prospective studies evaluating the accuracy of various patterns of V/Q abnormality in predicting the likelihood of pulmonary embolism.

Although it is often not definitive for the diagnosis or exclusion of pulmonary embolism, V/Q scanning does provide valuable information and should be performed whenever possible. Although uncommon, the finding of a normal perfusion study excludes embolism, whereas a high probability V/Q study, in the appropriate clinical setting, allows for a confident enough diagnosis of pulmonary embolism to initiate anticoagulant therapy. Additionally, the localization of regions of absent perfusion helps guide selective pulmonary angiography. While there is great interobserver variability in the interpretation of V/Q scans, a consensus of two viewers has been shown to significantly increase diagnostic accuracy.

Several diagnostic schemes have been proposed to assign a probability of pulmonary embolism (as deter-

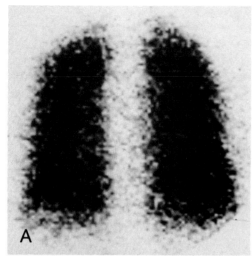

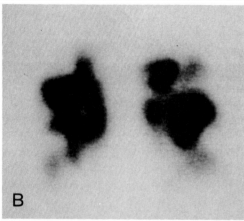

Figure 15.16. High-probability V/Q Scan in Acute Pulmonary Embolism. A. A posterior projection from a xenon-133 ventilation study in a 52-year-old woman with acute dyspnea and pleuritic chest pain demonstrates normal ventilation. **B.** The posterior perfusion study shows multiple, large, wedge-shaped pleural-based perfusion defects mismatched to the ventilation.

mined by pulmonary angiography) given specific combinations of ventilation, perfusion, and concurrent chest radiographic findings. The V/Q scan interpretation categories published with the results of the recently completed PIOPED (Prospective Investigation of Pulmonary Embolism Diagnosis) study has become the standard for radiologists interpreting V/Q studies (Table 49.1). This prospective, multiinstitutional study has confirmed several often-stated conclusions drawn from smaller, retrospective studies that lack adequate angiographic confirmation:

1. A minority of patients referred for V/Q studies have normal/near-normal (14%) or high probability (13%) scans.
2. A normal or near-normal V/Q study effectively excludes P.E. (positive predictive value = 4%).
3. Only 12% of patients with low probability V/Q studies have pulmonary embolism.

4. A high probability scan indicates pulmonary embolism with a high degree of certainty (positive predictive value = 88%; excluding those with previous P.E., the positive predictive value = 98%) (Fig. 15.16).
5. The predictive value of high or low probability scans improves when factoring in a high or low clinical suspicion for P.E., respectively.
6. The latter conclusion is an extension of Bayes' theorem, which states that the predictive value of a diagnostic test is a function of the prevalence of the disease in the population studied. For the diagnosis of P.E., this means that the predictive value of V/Q scintigraphy is a function of the prevalence of P.E. in the population referred for scanning (i.e., the pretest clinical suspicion of P.E.).

Patients with intermediate or indeterminate (because of extensive obstructive lung disease) probability scans have a 30–40% incidence of pulmonary embolism. These patients and those with V/Q scan results that are discordant with the clinical suspicion for pulmonary embolism should undergo noninvasive imaging of the deep venous system. Most patients with intermediate or indeterminate scan results will eventually be referred for definitive pulmonary angiography.

PULMONARY ANGIOGRAPHY

Pulmonary angiography is the gold standard in the diagnosis of pulmonary embolism. Selective film-screen pulmonary angiography can reliably detect pulmonary emboli at the segmental level. More sensitive techniques, such as balloon occlusion cineangiography and magnification angiography, can detect emboli as small as 2 mm in diameter. The accuracy of pulmonary arteriography in the diagnosis of P.E. is high. Based upon clinical follow-up of patients with negative studies, the sensitivity of pulmonary angiography is 98–99%, with almost 100% specificity for positive angiographic studies.

The indications for pulmonary angiography in the diagnosis of pulmonary embolism are listed in Table 15.10. The most common indication is a patient with an indeterminate or intermediate probability V/Q study who requires a definitive diagnosis. Although there are no absolute contraindications to pulmonary angiography, there are several conditions that place the patient at an increased risk from the procedure. These include a previously documented idiosyncratic reaction to contrast, right ventricular failure, renal insufficiency, and left bundle branch block. When any of these conditions exist in a patient referred for pulmonary angiography, an attempt at correcting these fac-

Table 15.10.   Indications for Pulmonary Angiography in Suspected Pulmonary Embolism

Patient with an indeterminate V/Q scan
Patient with a high clinical suspicion for pulmonary embolism and a low probability V/Q scan
Patient with a high probability V/Q scan and a relative or absolute contraindication to anticoagulation
Patient with diagnosis of pulmonary embolism who is considered for fibrinolytic therapy or embolectomy

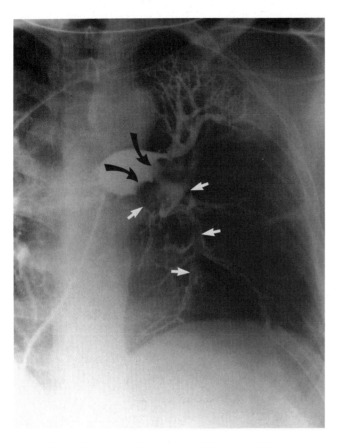

Figure 15.17.   Pulmonary Embolism on Pulmonary Arteriogram. A film from a left pulmonary arteriogram performed in the frontal projection shows a large intraluminal thrombus within the left main and descending pulmonary artery. Note the typical meniscus of contrast outlining the trailing edge of the clot (*curved black arrows*) and a rim of contrast around the body of the thrombus (*small white arrows*).

tors (e.g., premedication for contrast reaction or pacemaker placement for left bundle branch block) should be undertaken. Alternatively, these patients may undergo noninvasive imaging for proximal DVT using ultrasound, impedance plethysmography, or MR. Pulmonary angiography is discussed in detail in Chapter 20.

Pulmonary embolus is diagnosed on pulmonary angiography when an intraluminal filling defect or the trailing end of an occluding thrombus is outlined by contrast (Fig. 15.17). Secondary signs including a prolonged arterial phase, diminished peripheral perfusion, and delay in the venous phase are nonspecific and are not used to diagnose P.E.. Once thrombus is unequivocally identified, the study is terminated. The

only exception would be in a patient who is considered a candidate for surgical thrombectomy or thrombolytic therapy, where precise knowledge of the laterality, location, and extent of thrombus is required.

The overall complication rate of pulmonary angiography is 2–5%, and can be divided into those related to contrast administration and those secondary to cardiac catheterization and intrapulmonary arterial contrast injection. Many of these complications, such as myocardial and endocardial injury and cardiac perforation, were associated almost exclusively with the use of angled, sharp-tipped catheters. These traumatic complications are rare now that most angiographers use pigtail-tipped catheters. Mortality from pulmonary angiography is less than 0.5% and is usually related to sudden right ventricular failure from transient elevation of pulmonary artery pressure secondary to contrast injection. Death from pulmonary angiography is seen almost exclusively in critically ill patients and those with preexisting severe pulmonary arterial hypertension (pulmonary artery systolic pressure >70 mm Hg) or right ventricular dysfunction (right ventricular end diastolic pressure >20 mm Hg). However, there is no significant increase in the incidence of major, nonfatal reactions in patients with pulmonary arterial hypertension. In addition, the majority of patients with severe right ventricular dysfunction have uneventful studies. When one considers the added safety of selective contrast injections using nonionic contrast agents and the high mortality of untreated pulmonary embolism in this population, pulmonary angiography should be performed in these patients when indicated.

Digital subtraction angiography has been proposed as an alternative to conventional angiography for the diagnosis of pulmonary embolism. Its main advantage is that cardiac catheterization and intrapulmonary contrast injection, which are major factors associated with complications from conventional angiography, are obviated. Unfortunately, poor spatial resolution, motion artifact, and the inherent inability to selectively inject and thereby avoid overlap of vessels from the contralateral lung (which limits useful projections to the AP and shallow oblique views) have limited its usefulness. However, in certain situations, digital subtraction angiography may provide a useful alterna-

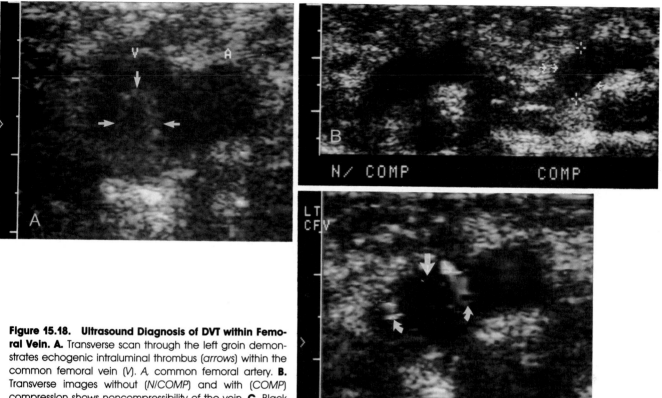

Figure 15.18. Ultrasound Diagnosis of DVT within Femoral Vein. A. Transverse scan through the left groin demonstrates echogenic intraluminal thrombus (*arrows*) within the common femoral vein (*V*). *A*, common femoral artery. **B.** Transverse images without (*N/COMP*) and with (*COMP*) compression shows noncompressibility of the vein. **C.** Black and white image of Doppler flow demonstrates flow (white regions with *curved arrows*) around the thrombus (*arrow*).

tive to conventional angiography. When right ventricular catheterization is dangerous (e.g., in a patient with malignant ventricular arrhythmias) or pulmonary arterial catheterization is impossible (e.g., a patient with tricuspid stenosis or huge right atrium) or hazardous (there is suspected large central embolus), a central venous or intraatrial injection with digital subtraction technique may be performed. Similarly, this technique may be employed in patients with severe pulmonary arterial hypertension and diastolic dysfunction, in whom an intrapulmonary arterial injection of contrast could prove deleterious.

NONINVASIVE IMAGING FOR DVT

The use of ultrasound and MR for the diagnosis of DVT has altered the conventional approach to the evaluation of pulmonary thromboembolic disease. Since 90% of pulmonary emboli arise from the lower extremities, and since the treatment for proximal (i.e., above the knee) DVT is identical to that for proven pulmonary emboli, a confident diagnosis of proximal DVT can provide an end-point in patient evaluation for thromboembolic disease. While contrast venography requires venipuncture and contrast administration and is associated with discomfort and possible thrombophlebitis, ultrasound and MR have no known associated risks. Ultrasound is utilized in the majority of patients with nondiagnostic V/Q stud-

ies that are referred for a diagnosis of pulmonary thromboembolism.

Most centers utilize compression ultrasound, discussed in Chapter 21, for the diagnosis of acute DVT. This technique relies on the ability of the normal venous lumen to collapse when external compression is applied. Deep venous thrombosis is diagnosed when the superficial or popliteal vein is noncompressible, shows no flow within its lumen, and when calf compression and elevation fail to augment flow on Doppler study (Fig. 15.18).

When performed by skilled personnel, compression ultrasound has a sensitivity of 90–95% and a specificity of 95–98% for the diagnosis of acute DVT when compared with contrast venography. False-negative studies occur when DVT is limited to the calf; this is not a serious limitation of the technique since these thrombi do not lead to significant pulmonary emboli. False-positive studies are seen most often in patients with prior DVT. Studies have shown that as many as 50% of patients with occlusive DVT have findings on follow-up compression ultrasound studies performed within 15 months of the acute episode that can mimic the findings of acute DVT. Pelvic masses compressing the iliac veins can make compression of the femoral vein difficult, thereby mimicking acute DVT on ultrasound examination. In addition to providing an accurate diagnosis of the presence of DVT, ultrasound offers the advantage of imaging the nonvenous structures in the leg, allowing the radiologist to find conditions that may simulate DVT clinically, such as Baker's cysts, enlarged lymph nodes, pseudoaneurysms, and pelvic masses compressing the iliac vein.

Although accurate for the diagnosis of proximal DVT, a negative compression ultrasound study does not exclude pulmonary embolus. Thus, patients with a negative ultrasound study should undergo pulmonary angiography.

Magnetic resonance imaging provides an alternative for the noninvasive diagnosis of DVT. Preliminary studies using conventional spin-echo and limited flip-angle gradient refocused MR have shown high sensitivity and specificity for the diagnosis of DVT as compared with contrast venography. Magnetic resonance imaging may provide the added benefit of determining the age of a thrombus based upon its T1 and T2 relaxation times, thereby allowing distinction between acute and chronic DVT. Evaluation of the iliac veins and superior vena cava is possible, as is the identification of pelvic masses that may compress the iliac vein and mimic DVT.

The use of radioisotopes for the diagnosis of DVT, discussed in Chapter 49, remains equivocal. Indium-111-labeled platelets have been used to successfully diagnose patients with venographically proven DVT. The problem with this agent is that it requires imaging at 24 hours to sensitively diagnose DVT, a delay that is unacceptable to most clinicians. Also, patients on heparin may have false-negative indium studies. More recently, ^{99m}Tc-labeled antifibrin antibodies in canines have shown promise in the accurate and rapid (within 3 hours) diagnosis of DVT. Clinical trials are needed to determine the utility of monoclonal antibodies in this setting.

INFECTION

The bronchopulmonary system is open to the outside world and, as such, is relatively accessible to microorganisms. Multiple host defense mechanisms exist at the level of the pharynx, trachea, and central bronchi. When these mechanisms fail, pathogenic organisms can penetrate to the small distal bronchi and the pulmonary parenchyma. Once the invading organisms penetrate the parenchyma, there is activation of both the cellular and humoral immune systems. This response may manifest clinically and radiographically as pneumonia, and in a normal host will often lead to eradication or at least suppression of the infecting organisms. If the immune response is impaired, a lower respiratory tract infection may lead to a very severe illness and often death, despite appropriate antibiotic therapy.

Pneumonia

Pneumonia is the most common life-threatening infectious disease. Organisms enter the lung and cause infection by three potential routes: via the tracheobronchial tree, via the pulmonary vasculature, or via direct spread from infection in the mediastinum, chest wall, or upper abdomen.

Infection via the tracheobronchial tree is generally secondary to inhalation or aspiration of infectious microorganisms and can be divided into three subtypes based on gross pathologic appearance and radiographic patterns: lobar pneumonia, lobular or bronchopneumonia, and interstitial pneumonia (7). As will be discussed in later sections, certain organisms will typically produce one of these three patterns, although there may be considerable overlap.

Bronchopneumonia is the most common pattern of disease, and is most typical of staphylococcal pneumonia. In the early stages of bronchopneumonia, the inflammation is centered primarily in and around lobular bronchi. As the inflammation progresses, exudative fluid extends peripherally along the bronchus to involve the entire pulmonary lobule. Radiographically, multifocal opacities that are roughly lobular in configuration produce a patchwork quilt appearance because of the interspersion of normal and diseased lobules (Fig. 15.2). While bronchopneumonia is the most common cause of multifocal patchy air space opacities, there are several differential diagnostic possibilities (Table 15.11). Exudate within the bronchi accounts for the absence of air bronchograms in bronchopneumonia. With coalescence of affected areas, the pattern may resemble lobar pneumonia.

Lobar Pneumonia is typical of pneumococcal pulmonary infection. In this pattern of disease, the inflammatory exudate begins within the distal air spaces. The inflammatory process spreads via the pores of Kohn and canals of Lambert and produces nonsegmental consolidation. If unchecked, the inflammation may eventually involve an entire lobe (Fig. 15.19). Because the airways are usually spared, air bronchograms are common and significant volume loss is unusual. The differential diagnosis of lobar opacification is listed in Table 15.12.

Interstitial Pneumonia, seen in viral and mycoplasma infection, is an inflammatory thickening of bronchial and bronchiolar walls and of the interstitial spaces of the lungs, producing a pattern of airways thickening and reticulonodular opacities. Air bronchograms are absent as the alveolar spaces remain aerated. Segmental and subsegmental atelectasis from small airways obstruction is common. The differential diagnosis of acute interstitial opacification of the lung includes infection and the entities listed in Table 15.13.

Table 15.11.   Multiple Ill-Defined Air Space Opacities

Infection	Bacteria
	Staphylococcus
	Gram-negative bacteria
	Pseudomonas
	Haemophilus
	Chlamydia
	Mycobacteria
	Tuberculosis (postprimary)
	Virus
	Influenza
	Mycoplasma
	Fungi
	Histoplasma
	Coccidioides
Vascular	Trauma
	Contusion
	Emboli
	Thromboemboli
	Septic
	Fat
	Vasculitis (see Table 15.9)
Neoplasm	Bronchoalveolar cell carcinoma
	Lymphoma
	Metastases (vascular tumors)
	Choriocarcinoma
	Renal cell carcinoma
Inhalation	Aspiration
	Lipoid pneumonia
Idiopathic	Eosinophilic pneumonia
	Bronchiolitis obliterans organizing pneumonia
	Sarcoidosis, alveolar form (rare)

Table 15.12.   Lobar Air Space Opacity

Pneumonia	Bacterial
	Pneumococcus
	Klebsiella
	Mycobacteria
	Tuberculosis
Hemorrhage	Pulmonary embolism
	Pulmonary contusion
Neoplasm	Bronchoalveolar cell carcinoma
	Lymphoma, pseudolymphoma
Inhalation	Aspiration
	Lipoid pneumonia
Lobar atelectasis	Mucus plug
	Endobronchial mass (obstructive pneumonitis)
	Bronchogenic carcinoma
	Carcinoid tumor
	Foreign body
	Extrinsic airway compression
	Enlarged hilar lymph nodes

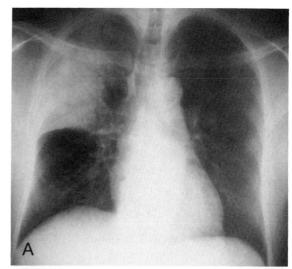
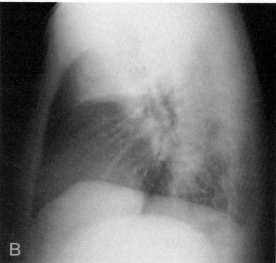

Figure 15.19.   Lobar Pneumonia from Pneumococcus. Posteroanterior **(A)** and lateral **(B)** radiographs in a 57-year-old man with fever, chills, and productive cough demonstrate air space opacification in the right upper lobe with air bronchograms. Sputum culture was positive for *Streptococcus pneumonia.*

Table 15.13.   Acute Interstitial Opacification

Pulmonary edema	Left ventricular failure
	Fluid overload/renal failure
	Noncardiogenic edema
	Drugs
	Nitrofurantoin
	Chemotherapeutic agents
Pneumonia	Viral
	Measles
	Mycoplasma
	Parasitic
	P. carinii
Inhalation	Extrinsic allergic alveolitis (hypersensitivity pneumonitis), acute phase

The spread of infection to the lung via the pulmonary vasculature usually occurs in the setting of systemic sepsis. The pattern of parenchymal involvement is patchy and bilateral. The lung bases are most severely involved, as blood flow is greatest in the dependent portions of the lungs. Pulmonary infection from direct spread usually results in a localized parenchymal process adjacent to an extrapulmonary source of infection. If an organism causes extensive parenchymal necrosis, abscess formation may result.

BACTERIAL PNEUMONIA—GRAM-POSITIVE BACTERIA

Streptococcal Pneumonia (Pneumococcus)

S. pneumoniae is a Gram-positive organism that may cause infection in healthy individuals but is much more commonly seen in the elderly, alcoholics, and other compromised hosts. Patients with sickle cell disease or who have undergone splenectomy are at particular risk for severe pneumococcal pneumonia. Of those patients with community-acquired pneumococcal pneumonia who require hospitalization, approximately one-quarter will have pneumococcal sepsis and one-quarter of these patients will die.

Pneumococcal pneumonia tends to begin in the lower lobes or the posterior segments of the upper lobes. Initially there is involvement of the terminal airways, but rather than remaining localized to this site, there is rapid development of an air-space inflammatory exudate. The spread of infection to contiguous air spaces via interalveolar connections accounts for the nonsegmental distribution and homogeneity of the resultant consolidation.

The typical radiographic appearance of acute pneumococcal pneumonia is lobar consolidation (Fig. 15.19). Air bronchograms are usually evident. Cavitation in pneumococcal pneumonia is rare, with the exception of infections because of serotype III. Uncomplicated parapneumonic effusion or empyema may be seen in up to 50% of patients. With appropriate therapy, complete clearing may be seen in 10–14 days. In older patients or those with underlying disease, complete resolution may take 8–10 weeks.

Patients with pneumococcal pneumonia occasionally present with atypical radiographic patterns of disease. Patchy lobular opacities similar to that seen with bronchopneumonia or, rarely, a reticulonodular pattern may be seen. In some patients, the atypical appearance may relate to the presence of preexisting lung disease (e.g., emphysema), partial treatment, or an impaired immune response (e.g., acquired immunodeficiency disease (AIDS)). In children, pneumococcal pneumonia may present as a spherical opacity ("round pneumonia") and simulate a parenchymal mass.

Staphylococcus aureus. Staphylococcal pneumonia is most common in hospitalized and debilitated patients. It may also develop following hematogenous spread to the lung in patients with endocarditis, indwelling catheters, and intravenous drug users. Community-acquired infection may complicate influenza or other viral pneumonias.

Staphylococcus aureus typically produces a bronchopneumonia and appears radiographically as patchy opacities (Fig. 15.2). In severe cases, the opacities may become confluent to produce lobar opacification. Because the inflammatory exudate fills the airways, air bronchograms are rarely seen. In adults, the process is often bilateral and may be complicated by abscess formation in 25–75% of patients. In patients who develop pulmonary infection from hematogenous seeding, one sees multiple bilateral poorly defined nodular opacities, which eventually become more sharply defined and cavitate. Parapneumonic effusion and empyema is common. Pneumatocele formation is common in children and may lead to pneumothorax. Pneumatoceles may be distinguished from abscesses by their thin walls, rapid change in size, and tendency to develop during the late phase of infection.

Streptococcus pyogenes. Acute streptococcal pneumonia is rarely seen today, though it can occasionally complicate viral infection or streptococcal pharyngitis. The radiographic appearance is similar to staphylococcal pneumonia, with lobular or segmental lower lobe opacities. The process may be complicated by abscess formation and cavitation; empyema is relatively common.

BACTERIAL PNEUMONIA—GRAM-NEGATIVE BACTERIA

Gram-negative bacteria are increasingly important causes of pneumonia in hospitalized patients, accounting for over 50% of nosocomial pulmonary infections. While Gram-negative organisms may be isolated from only a small percentage of healthy individuals, the isolation rate in hospitalized and severely ill patients ranges from 40–75%. The organisms most often responsible for pneumonia include members of the *Enterobacteriaceae* family (*Klebsiella, Escherichia coli, Proteus*), *Pseudomonas aeruginosa, Haemophilus influenzae,* and *Legionella pneumophila.*

The radiographic appearance of Gram-negative bacterial pneumonia varies from small, ill-defined nodules to patchy areas of opacification that may become confluent and resemble lobar pneumonia. Involvement is usually bilateral and multifocal, and the lower lobes are most frequently affected. Abscess formation and cavitation are relatively common. Parapneumonic effusion is common and is often complicated by empyema formation.

Klebsiella Pneumoniae occurs predominantly in older alcoholic males and debilitated hospitalized patients. Radiographically it appears as a homogeneous lobar opacification containing air bronchograms. There are three features that help distinguish it radiographically from pneumococcal pneumonia: (*a*) an increased volume of involved lobe caused by the exuberant inflammatory exudate, producing a bulging interlobar fissure, (*b*) the development of an abscess with cavity formation, which is uncommon in pneumococcal pneumonia, and (*c*) a higher incidence of pleural effusion and empyema. Pulmonary gangrene may be seen but is uncommon.

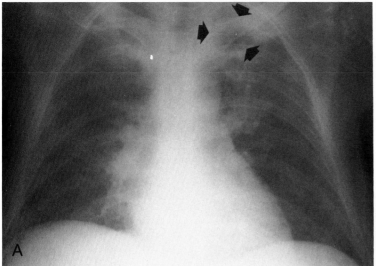

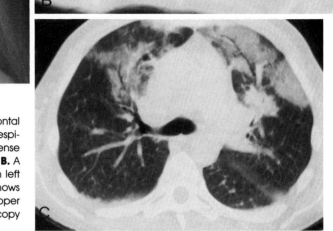

Figure 15.20. Pseudomonas aeriguinosa Pneumonia. A. Frontal radiograph in an HIV-positive male with fever and progressive respiratory symptoms shows multifocal air space opacities with dense opacification in the apices associated with cavitation (*arrows*). **B.** A CT scan through the apices shows air space opacification with left apical cavitation. **C.** A scan at the level of the tracheal carina shows air space disease in the anterior segments of right and left upper lobes with sparing of the dependent portions of lung. Bronchoscopy revealed *Pseudomonas*.

Haemophilus influenzae. In adults, *H. influenzae* infection is most common in patients with chronic obstructive pulmonary disease (COPD), alcoholism, diabetes mellitus, and those with an anatomic or functional splenectomy. It most often causes bronchitis, although it may extend to produce bilateral lower lobe bronchopneumonia.

Pseudomonas aeruginosa. *Pseudomonas* pneumonia most often affects debilitated patients, particularly those requiring mechanical ventilation. There is a high mortality rate associated with the disease. The radiographic pattern of parenchymal involvement depends upon the method by which the organisms reach the lung. Patchy opacities with abscess formation that mimic staphylococcal pneumonia are common when the infection reaches the lung via the tracheobronchial tree (Fig. 15.20). Diffuse, bilateral, ill-defined nodular opacities usually reflect hematogenous dissemination. Pleural effusions are common and are usually small.

Legionella pneumophila. Legionnaire's disease is caused by *L. pneumophila*, a Gram-negative bacillus commonly found in air conditioning and humidifier systems. It tends to affect older men. Community-acquired infection is seen in patients with COPD or malignancy, while nosocomial infection primarily affects immunocompromised patients or those with renal failure or malignancy.

The characteristic radiographic pattern is air space opacification that is initially peripheral and sublobar. In some patients, the air space opacities appear as a round pneumonia. The infection progresses to lobar or multilobar involvement despite the initiation of antibiotic therapy. At the peak of disease, the parenchymal involvement is usually bilateral. Pleural effusions are seen in approximately 30% of patients. Cavitation is not seen except in the immunocompromised patient. The radiographic resolution of pneumonia is often prolonged and may lag behind symptomatic improvement.

BACTERIAL PNEUMONIA—ANAEROBIC BACTERIA

The majority of anaerobic lung infections arise from aspiration of infected oropharyngeal contents. Approximately 25% of patients give a history of impaired consciousness, and many are alcoholic. The most common organisms responsible are the Gram-negative bacilli *Bacteroides* and *Fusobacterium*, although the majority of pulmonary infections are polymicrobial. All anaerobic pulmonary infections produce a similar radiographic appearance. The distribution of parenchymal opacities reflects the gravitational flow of aspirated material. When aspiration occurs in the supine position, the posterior segments of the upper lobes and superior segments of the lower lobes are predominantly involved, whereas aspiration in the erect position leads to involvement of basal segments of the lower lobes. The typical radiographic appearance is peripheral lobular and segmental air space opacities. Cavitation within areas of consolidation is relatively common, and discrete lung abscesses may be seen in up to 50% of patients. Hilar and/or mediastinal lymph node enlargement may be seen in those with lung abscesses. Empyema, with or without bronchopleural fistula formation, is a common complication and is seen in up to 50% of patients.

BACTERIAL PNEUMONIA—MISCELLANEOUS

Nocardia. *Nocardia* is a Gram-positive, branching filamentous bacillus which is weakly acid-fast. *Nocardia asteroides* is the most important cause of pulmonary disease. It is usually an opportunistic infection in patients on immunosuppressive therapy, those with lymphoma or leukemia, and patients with alveolar proteinosis.

The most frequent radiographic presentation is a homogeneous, nonsegmental air space opacity or a mass. Cavitation is frequent. Infection may extend into the pleural space and chest wall to produce empyema and osteomyelitis, respectively. Hilar lymph nodes may be enlarged. Treatment is with sulfur antibiotics.

Actinomycosis. *Actinomyces israelii* is an anaerobic gram-positive filamentous bacterium that is a normal inhabitant of the human oropharynx. It causes disease when it gains access to devitalized or infected tissues, which facilitate its growth. Actinomycosis most commonly follows dental extractions, manifesting as mandibular osteomyelitis or a soft-tissue abscess. The lungs may be infected by aspiration of infectious oral debris or, less commonly, by direct extension from the primary site of disease.

The typical pattern of acute actinomycosis consists of nonsegmental air space disease in the periphery of the lower lobes. In some cases, the infection manifests as a localized mass-like opacity that mimics bronchogenic carcinoma. If therapy is not instituted, a lung abscess may develop. Thoracic actinomycosis is characterized by its ability to spread to contiguous tissues without regard for normal anatomic barriers. Extension into the pleura will cause empyema, while chest wall involvement is characterized by osteomyelitis of the ribs and chest wall abscess. Involvement of the ribs is seen as wavy periosteal reaction or lytic rib destruction. If the pleuropulmonary disease becomes chronic, extensive fibrosis may be seen. Rarely, the disease is disseminated and a miliary pattern is seen.

Mycoplasma Pneumonia. *Mycoplasma pneumoniae* is an organism with both bacterial and viral characteristics and is considered as a separate group.

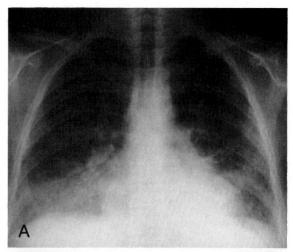
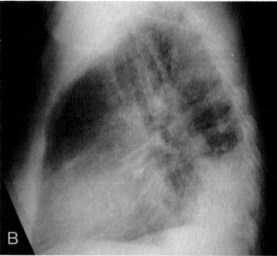

Figure 15.21. Mycoplasma Pneumonia. Posteroanterior **(A)** and lateral **(B)** radiographs in a 21-year-old woman demonstrate mixed diffuse interstitial and bibasilar air space opacities. Immunofluorescent staining of induced sputum samples revealed *M. pneumoniae*.

It is probably the most common nonbacterial cause of pneumonia and accounts for 10–30% of all community-acquired pneumonia. Affected patients usually have a subacute illness of 2–3 weeks' duration. Symptoms include fever, nonproductive cough, headache, and malaise. Unusual physical findings include bullous myringitis and rash.

In the early stages of infection, interstitial inflammation causes a fine reticular pattern on the chest radiograph. This may progress to patchy segmental air space opacities that may coalesce to produce lobar consolidation (Fig. 15.21). The process is often unilateral and tends to involve the lower lobes. Pleural effusion may be seen in the consolidative form of disease, and occurs most commonly in children. Lymph node enlargement is uncommon but may be seen in children. Radiographic resolution may require 4–6 weeks.

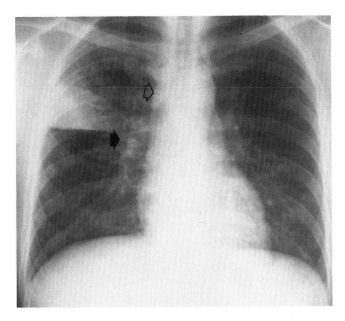

Figure 15.22. Primary TB. A PA chest radiograph in a 32-year-old homeless man shows air space disease within the anterior segment of the right upper lobe with right hilar (*solid arrow*) and paratracheal (*open arrow*) lymph node enlargement. Sputum stains and culture revealed *M. tuberculosis*.

MYCOBACTERIAL INFECTION

Mycobacterium tuberculosis is an aerobic acid-fast bacillus. Two principal forms of tuberculous pulmonary disease are recognized clinically and radiographically: primary tuberculosis (TB) and reactivation or postprimary disease. The inflammatory response to *M. tuberculosis* differs from the normal response to bacterial organisms in that it involves cell-mediated immunity (delayed hypersensitivity). Initially, droplet nuclei laden with bacilli are inhaled and implant in a subpleural location. In most patients, the bacilli are phagocytized and killed by alveolar macrophages. If the bacilli overcome host immune response, an inflammatory focus is established. The macrophages are then transformed into epithelioid cells, which aggregate to form granulomas. The granulomas are usually well formed by 1–3 weeks, coinciding with the development of delayed hypersensitivity. The granulomas typically demonstrate central caseating necrosis, thereby distinguishing them from the granulomas seen in sarcoidosis. Inflammation and enlargement of draining hilar and mediastinal lymph nodes are common in primary disease, particularly in children.

In primary infection, the parenchymal disease and adenopathy may completely resolve or there may be a residual focus of scarring or calcification. In some situations, usually in infants under the age of 1 year, local parenchymal disease progresses and is termed progressive primary TB. More commonly, the disease will be contained by the granulomatous response and

recur years later ("reactivation" or postprimary TB) in the setting of weakened host defenses from aging, alcoholism, diabetes, cancer, or human immunodeficiency virus (HIV) infection. Postprimary TB develops under the influence of hypersensitivity, with caseous necrosis seen histologically.

Primary Tuberculosis. Primary TB has classically been a disease of childhood, although the incidence of primary disease has increased because of the HIV epidemic. Most patients with primary TB are asymptomatic and have no radiographic sequelae of infection. In some patients a Ranke complex, consisting of a calcified parenchymal focus (the Ghon lesion) and nodal calcification, is seen. If the patient is symptomatic, a nonspecific focal pneumonitis occurs and is seen as small, ill-defined areas of segmental or lobar opacification (Fig. 15.22). In adults, there is a right-sided predominance. The parenchymal consolidation may mimic a bacterial pneumonia, but the clinical and radiographic course is much more indolent. Cavitation is relatively uncommon except in infants. The pulmonary focus may resolve completely or persist as a Ghon lesion or a Ranke complex.

Tuberculomas are discrete nodular opacities that may develop in primary TB but are much more common in postprimary disease. Unilateral pleural effusions are seen in 25% of cases and are usually associated with parenchymal disease. If a tuberculous empyema develops, it may break through the parietal pleura to form an extrapleural collection (empyema necessitans). Unilateral hilar or mediastinal lymph node enlargement is common, particularly in children, and may be the sole radiographic manifestation of infection. Bilateral hilar or mediastinal lymph node enlargement may be seen, but is uncommon and is almost invariably asymmetric in distinction to lymph node enlargement in sarcoidosis. During the primary tuberculous infection, there is hematogenous dissemination of the organism to regions with a high partial pressure of oxygen; these include the lung apices, renal medullae, and bone marrow. These microscopic foci are clinically silent and serve as a source of reactivation disease.

Postprimary TB. Patients with postprimary TB often present with cough and constitutional symptoms including chills, night sweats, and weight loss. Reactivation tends to occur in the apical and posterior segments of the upper lobes and the superior segments of the lower lobes. Ill-defined patchy and nodular opacities are commonly seen. Cavitation is an important radiographic feature of postprimary infection and usually indicates active and transmissable disease (Fig. 15.23). The cavitary focus may lead to transbronchial spread of organisms and result in a multifocal bronchopneumonia. Erosion of a cavitary focus into a branch of the pulmonary artery can produce an

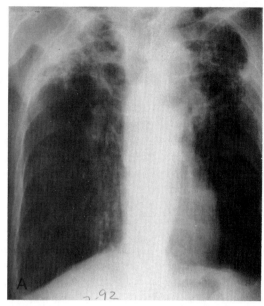

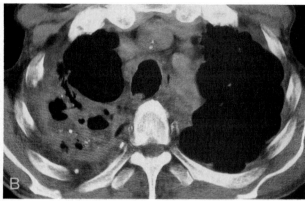

Figure 15.23. Postprimary (Reactivation) TB. A. Frontal chest film in a 69-year-old Asian immigrant with a cough and severe wasting reveals hyperinflation with marked fibrotic and cavitary disease in the upper lobes with severe volume loss. **B.** A CT scan through the lung apices demonstrate consolidative and cavitary changes with air-fluid levels and pleural and parenchymal calcifications. Sputum cultures were positive for *M. tuberculosis.*

There are several late complications of pulmonary TB. Interstitial fibrosis can cause pulmonary insufficiency and secondary pulmonary arterial hypertension. Hemoptysis may be secondary to bronchiectasis, mycetoma formation in an old tuberculous cavity, or erosion of a calcified peribronchial lymph node (broncholith) into a bronchus. Bronchostenosis is a result of healed endobronchial TB.

Miliary TB. Miliary TB may complicate either primary or reactivation disease. It results from hematogenous dissemination of tubercle bacilli and produces diffuse bilateral 2–3 mm pulmonary nodules (Fig. 15.24). Miliary disease is associated with a high mortality and requires prompt therapy.

Tuberculosis in HIV-infected Individuals. There has been a dramatic rise in the incidence of pulmonary and extrapulmonary TB in recent years, predominantly in HIV-infected individuals. Extrapulmonary TB in conjunction with HIV infection is an index diagnosis for AIDS. Pulmonary TB complicating HIV disease usually represents reactivation of prior pulmonary infection. When pulmonary TB develops relatively early in the course of HIV infection (CD4 counts >200 cells/mm^3), the radiographic manifestations are similar to those seen in patients not infected with HIV. These findings include upper lobe fibronodular opacities and cavity formation. As the patient's immunologic status deteriorates and the CD4 count falls below 200 CD4 cells/mm^3, the pattern of pulmonary involvement is that of primary or disseminated disease. Radiographic findings include lobar air space opacification, coarse reticulonodular opacities, pleural effusion, and centrally necrotic hilar and mediastinal lymph node enlargement on contrast-enhanced CT.

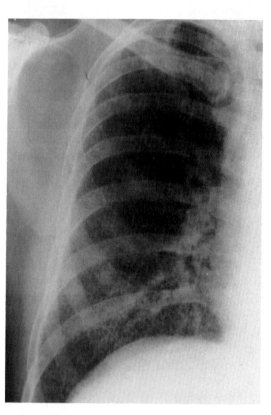

Figure 15.24. Miliary TB. A coned-down view of a frontal radiograph demonstrates innumerable micronodular opacities characteristic of micronodular (miliary) interstitial disease. Transbronchial biopsy demonstrated caseating granulomas containing acid-fast bacilli.

aneurysm (Rasmussen's aneurysm) and cause hemoptysis. With appropriate antimicrobial treatment, the disease is usually controlled by a granulomatous response. Parenchymal healing is associated with fibrosis, bronchiectasis, and volume loss (cicatrizing atelectasis) in the upper lobes.

Atypical Mycobacterial Infection. There are several nontuberculous mycobacteria that may cause pulmonary disease. Prior to the HIV epidemic, pulmonary disease secondary to atypical mycobacteria was seen primarily in elderly patients with underlying chronic lung disease. The most common organisms responsible for pulmonary disease are *M. avium-intracellulare* (MAI) or *M. kansasii*. The radiographic features are indistinguishable from reactivation TB, with chronic fibrocavitary opacities involving the upper lobes. While cavitation is common, pleural effusion, lymph node enlargement, and miliary spread are distinctly unusual. Although the disease caused by nontuberculous mycobacteria tends to be more indolent than that seen with *M. tuberculosis*, it is often difficult to treat effectively. The MAI infection in HIV-positive patients is most often extrapulmonary, with involvement of abdominal viscera, lymph nodes, and bone marrow. In the lung, MAI may cause focal or diffuse coarse reticulonodular opacities. Hilar and mediastinal lymph node enlargement is common. On CT, the enlarged nodes demonstrate central necrosis indistinguishable from *M. tuberculosis*.

VIRAL PNEUMONIA

Viruses are a major cause of upper respiratory tract and airways infection, although pneumonia is relatively uncommon. The diagnosis of viral pneumonia is often one of exclusion. Chest radiographic features are nonspecific and usually demonstrate a pattern of bronchopneumonia or interstitial opacities. Resolution is usually complete, but permanent sequelae may be seen, including bronchiectasis, bronchiolitis obliterans (which may produce the unilateral hyperlucent lung), and interstitial fibrosis.

Influenza. In adults, the most common cause of viral pneumonia is influenza. Outbreaks of influenza can occur in pandemics, epidemics, or sporadically. In most patients the disease is confined to the upper respiratory tract, but in elderly persons or those with underlying cardiopulmonary disease, a severe hemorrhagic pneumonia may develop. In adults with influenzal pneumonia, there is often bilateral lower lobe patchy air space opacification. In children, a diffuse interstitial reticulonodular pattern is more commonly seen. Bacterial superinfection with *Streptococcus* or *Staphylococcus* contributes to a fulminating course that may result in death. The development of lobar consolidation, pleural effusion, or cavitation suggests bacterial superinfection.

Respiratory Syncytial Virus is a major cause of severe bronchiolitis and bronchopneumonia in infants and young children. The chest radiograph shows hyperinflation and patchy areas of consolidation. Bronchial wall thickening and lobar atelectasis, indistinguishable from asthma, are common findings.

Adenovirus. Adenoviral pneumonia usually affects infants and young children, but may occur in epidemic form in adults, particularly in military personnel. The usual radiographic features are diffuse bilateral bronchopneumonia and severe hyperinflation. Lobar atelectasis and consolidation are not infrequent. In uncomplicated cases, the radiographic changes resolve within several weeks. Patients with invasive adenoviral pneumonia can develop bronchiectasis, bronchiolitis obliterans, and interstitial fibrosis.

Parainfluenza Virus. Parainfluenza virus is the most common cause of croup and bronchiolitis in children, but may also cause a bronchopneumonia. The radiograph findings are indistinguishable from other viral pneumonias and include bronchial wall thickening and patchy peribronchial consolidation.

Varicella-zoster Virus. The varicella-zoster virus, which causes chickenpox and shingles, may produce a severe pneumonia in adults. Patients on immunosuppressive therapy or with lymphoma are at greatest risk. Chest radiographs characteristically show diffuse, bilateral, ill-defined nodular opacities 5–10 mm in diameter. These opacities usually resolve completely, although in some patients they involute and calcify to produce innumerable small (2–3 mm) calcified nodules.

FUNGAL INFECTION

Fungal infections are now seen with increased frequency because of an increase in the incidence of disease caused by pathogenic fungi in healthy hosts and the emergence of opportunistic species in immunocompromised hosts. Fungi can cause pulmonary disease by several mechanisms. Some fungi, including *Histoplasma capsulatum*, *Coccidioides immitis*, and *Blastomyces dermatitidis*, are primary pathogens and most commonly infect healthy hosts. Other fungi, most notably *Aspergillus*, *Candida*, and *Cryptococcus*, are opportunistic pathogens in immunocompromised individuals. In all cases, the fungi elicit a necrotizing granulomatous reaction. The availability of effective antifungal therapy with amphotericin B has made the early and accurate diagnosis of fungal infection imperative. A number of serologic and histologic methods are available for the accurate diagnosis of fungal infection.

Histoplasmosis. *Histoplasma capsulatum* is endemic to certain areas of North America, most notably the Ohio, Mississippi, and St. Lawrence River valleys and Mexico. The overwhelming majority (95–99%) of infections because of *H. capsulatum* are asymptomatic. A routine chest film demonstrating multiple well-defined calcified nodules less than 1 cm in size, with or without calcified hilar or mediastinal lymph nodes, may be the only indication of prior infection.

Acute *Histoplasma* infection most often presents with the abrupt onset of flu-like symptoms. The chest radiograph in such patients may be normal or may show nonspecific changes including subsegmental air space opacities with or without associated hilar lymph enlargement. If the patient inhales a large inoculum of organisms, widespread fairly discrete nodular opacities 3–4 mm in diameter are seen with hilar adenopathy. Alternatively, acute histoplasmosis may result in a solitary, sharply defined nodular opacity <3 cm in diameter, termed a histoplasmoma. Histoplasmomas are most common in the lower lobes and frequently calcify.

Histoplasma capsulatum can also cause chronic pulmonary disease, usually in patients with underlying emphysema. Unilateral or bilateral upper lobe cicatrizing atelectasis with marked hilar retraction may mimic the radiographic findings seen in postprimary TB. Similarly, chronic upper lobe fibrocavitary disease may be seen. Involvement of the mediastinum by chronic granulomatous inflammation may lead to fibrosing mediastinitis.

Asymptomatic blood-borne dissemination of *H. capsulatum* is common, as judged by the frequency of calcified splenic granulomas in residents of endemic areas. Clinically apparent disseminated histoplasmosis, however, is extremely rare and is usually seen in infants or immunocompromised adults. The chest film most commonly shows widespread 2–3 mm nodules indistinguishable from those of miliary TB, though reticular opacities and patchy areas of consolidations may also be seen.

Coccidioidomycosis.
Coccidioides immitis is endemic to the southwestern United States and San Joaquin Valley of California. Primary coccidiodomycosis develops in 40% of infected adults. Affected individuals usually develop a self-limiting viral type illness, which is referred to as valley fever when associated with erythema nodosum and arthralgias. The chest radiograph may be normal or show focal or multifocal segmental air space opacities that resolve over several months. Hilar and mediastinal adenopathy and pleural effusions may be seen in association with parenchymal disease (Fig. 14.8).

Patients whose symptoms or radiographic abnormalities persist beyond 6–8 weeks are considered to have persistent coccidioidomycosis. The radiographic features of persistent pulmonary disease include coccidioidal nodules or masses (coccidioidomas), persistent areas of consolidation, and miliary nodules. Coccidioidal nodules are areas of round pneumonia, usually located in the subpleural regions of the upper lobes. These nodules tend to cavitate rapidly and produce characteristic thin-walled cavities. In chronic progressive disease, upper lobe fibrocavitary disease similar to postprimary TB and histoplasmosis is seen. Disseminated coccidioidomycosis is relatively rare and usually affects immunocompromised patients and non-Caucasians.

Cryptococcosis.
Seventy percent of individuals with clinical symptoms from cryptococcal infection are immunocompromised. In some of these patients, particularly those with AIDS, the organism disseminates from its portal of entry in the lung to involve the central nervous system, bones, and mucocutaneous tissues. The most common radiographic manifestation of cryptococcal pulmonary infection is a solitary well-defined pleural based mass 2–10 cm in diameter. Multiple masses are occasionally present. Cavitation and lymph node enlargement may occur and are more commonly seen in immunocompromised hosts. A less frequent radiographic appearance is segmental or nonsegmental air space consolidation; cavitation and adenopathy are less common with this pattern of disease. Pleural effusions are uncommon. A disseminated micronodular pattern resembling miliary TB may occur.

Blastomycosis.
North American blastomycosis, caused by *B. dermatitidis*, is a chronic systemic disease primarily affecting the lungs and skin. Its geographic distribution overlaps that of histoplasmosis, extending farther to the east and north. The pulmonary infection is often asymptomatic. Symptomatic infection resembles that of an acute bacterial pneumonia. The radiographic findings in pulmonary blastomycosis are nonspecific. The most common manifestation of disease is homogeneous, nonsegmental air space opacification with a propensity for the upper lobes. A less common presentation is single or multiple masses which cavitate in 15% of cases. Pulmonary masses tend to occur in patients with prolonged symptoms (>1 month) and may mimic bronchogenic carcinoma. A third pattern of disease is diffuse reticulonodular opacities. Pleural effusion and lymph node enlargement are uncommon. A disseminated miliary form may be seen in immunocompromised hosts.

Aspergillus.
Of the more than 300 species of *Aspergillus*, *A. fumigatus* is the most frequent pathogen in man. Respiratory involvement presents as a mass within a preexisting pulmonary cavity (aspergilloma), invasive aspergillosis, or allergic bronchopulmonary aspergillosis. The latter form of disease will not be discussed in this section.

An aspergilloma (mycetoma, fungus ball) is a ball of hyphae, mucus, and cellular debris that colonizes a preexisting bullae or a parenchymal cavity created by some other pathogen or destructive process. Invasion into adjacent lung parenchyma does not occur unless host defense mechanisms are compromised. The my-

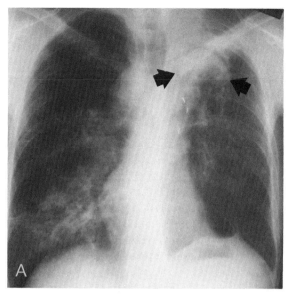

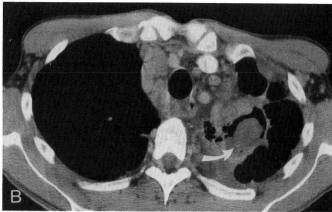

Figure 15.25. Aspergilloma. A. A PA chest radiograph in a 32-year-old man with long-standing bullous disease from sarcoidosis and prior left upper lobectomy for aspergilloma. A mass (*arrows*) is seen in the left upper lung capped by a crescent of air with adjacent apical pleural thickening. **B.** A CT scan shows a low-density mass representing a mycetoma (*curved white arrow*) within a pre-existing cavity. Sputum shows heavy *Aspergillus.*

cetoma is usually asymptomatic, but may cause hemoptysis that may be massive (>350 ml every 24 hours). An aspergilloma is seen as a solid round mass within an upper lobe cavity, with an "air crescent" separating the mycetoma from the cavity wall (Fig. 15.25). The mycetoma is usually free within the cavity and can be seen to roll dependently on decubitus radiographs or CT. Progressive apical pleural thickening adjacent to a cavity is a common radiographic finding and should prompt a search for a complicating mycetoma.

Invasive aspergillosis is usually seen in severely immunocompromised patients with neutropenia, most commonly those with leukemia or those receiving chemotherapy or corticosteroids. The radiographic manifestations range from large nodular opacities to diffuse parenchymal consolidation. The organism tends to invade blood vessels, and much of the observed opacity represents hemorrhage and edema. If pleural effusion develops, it usually indicates empyema. Cavitation, in the form of an air crescent, is not usually evident on chest films early in the course of disease, but characteristically develops when the patient's complement of circulating neutrophils returns to a normal level. Computed tomography, particularly HRCT, is useful for the early diagnosis of invasive aspergillosis. The demonstration of a zone of relative decreased attenuation surrounding a dense mass-like opacity has been termed the "CT halo sign," and is relatively specific for invasive aspergillosis in a neutropenic patient. The halo represents a region of edema and hemorrhage where an air crescent will develop separating the region of infected, necrotic lung from normal parenchyma.

Candidiasis. Candidal pneumonia almost always occurs in an immunocompromised host. Chest radiographs demonstrate a prominent interstitium and diffuse, bilateral, nonsegmental air space opacities. Miliary nodules may be seen with disseminated disease. Cavitation, adenopathy, and pleural effusion are uncommon features.

PARASITIC PULMONARY INFECTION

Parasitic infections of the lung are relatively uncommon in the United States. However, increasing travel to countries where parasites are endemic, the immigration of people from these regions to the United States, and an increasing number of immunocompromised patients requires a familiarity with these infections. In general, parasitic diseases of the thorax are manifested by either a direct invasion of lungs and pleura or, less commonly, a hypersensitivity reaction.

Pneumocystis carinii Pneumonia (PCP). *Pneumocystis carinii* infestation is common in humans, although this organism causes clinically significant pneumonia only in immunocompromised individuals. The *P. carinii* pneumonia is most prevalent and virulent in patients with AIDS, and is the most common AIDS-defining diagnosis in HIV-positive individuals. The disease affects approximately 70% of HIV-positive individuals at some point in their illness, and is a major cause of death in these patients. Organ transplant recipients on immunosuppressive drugs and patients with lymphoreticular malignancies are also at high risk.

The chest radiograph may be normal in the early phase of disease. In such patients, gallium scanning

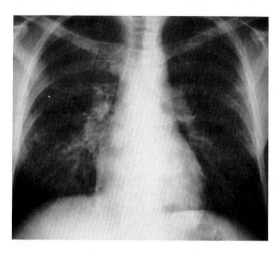

Figure 15.26. *Pneumocystis carinii* **Pneumonia.** Frontal radiograph in a 36-year-old man with HIV infection shows bilateral symmetric fine reticular or ground-glass opacities. Stains of induced sputum revealed *P. carinii.*

of the lung may provide evidence of subradiographic inflammation (see Chapter 54). As the disease progresses, a fine reticular or ground-glass pattern develops, particularly in the parahilar regions (Fig. 15.26). Although PCP produces a pattern of disease commonly attributed to interstitial involvement, it is predominantly an air space process pathologically with only a minor interstitial inflammatory component. This apparent discrepancy relates to a lining rather than a filling of the alveolar spaces by organisms and proteinaceous exudate, which produces interstitial opacities radiographically. The intraalveolar location of the inflammatory process explains the high yield of organisms from staining of induced sputum samples and bronchoalveolar lavage fluid. Progressive disease leads to confluent symmetric air space opacification. Pleural effusion or lymph node enlargement is distinctly uncommon (<5%) and should suggest an alternative or additional diagnosis.

There are several atypical radiographic features that have been described with PCP. Pneumocystis carinii pneumonia may manifest as single or multiple pulmonary nodules, simulating fungal infection or malignancy such as Kaposi's sarcoma. Patients receiving PCP prophylaxis with monthly inhalation of aerosolized pentamidine are prone to develop predominantly upper lobe PCP, which simulates postprimary TB. This atypical distribution of PCP likely results from asymmetric deposition of the inhaled drug to the gravity-dependent lung bases, which predisposes the upper lobes to infection. Patients on aerosolized pentamidine rather than systemic prophylaxis with Bactrim are also at risk for extrapulmonary pneumocystis infection. Systemic pneumocystis infection generally involves the liver, spleen, kidney, and lymph nodes, and appears on CT or ultrasound as microabscesses or punctate calcifications.

First-line treatment of PCP is with oral or intravenous trimethoprim-sulfamethoxazole (Bactrim, Septra). Intravenous pentamidine is reserved for treatment failures, drug allergies, or adverse reactions. While the majority of patients respond to antibiotic therapy, some have a progressive deteriorating course with the development of ARDS leading to death. In severely hypoxic patients with documented PCP, the clinical and radiographic pulmonary deterioration typically seen within 72 hours of the initiation of therapy can be blunted by the administration of corticosteroids. The development of pulmonary cysts or cavities during the treatment of PCP predisposes to spontaneous pneumothorax and bronchopleural fistula, particularly in mechanically ventilated patients.

Amebiasis. Symptomatic infection with *Entamoeba histolytica* is usually confined to the gastrointestinal tract and liver. If the infection remains confined to the subphrenic space, a right pleural effusion and basilar atelectasis may result from local diaphragmatic inflammation. The most common method of pleuropulmonary involvement by amebiasis is by the direct intrathoracic extension of infection from a hepatic abscess. This transdiaphragmatic spread of organisms may extend into the right pleural space to produce an empyema or may involve the right lower lobe to produce an amebic pneumonia or lung abscess. In rare instances pulmonary amebiasis is seen without evidence of hepatic involvement, with the organism reaching the lung by way of hemorrhoidal veins in lower rectal disease or via the thoracic duct.

Hydatid Disease (Echinococcosis) of the Lung. *Echinococcus granulosus* is the cause of most cases of human hydatid disease. The disease is endemic in sheep-raising areas and is relatively uncommon in the United States. Dogs are the usual definitive hosts, with sheep acting as intermediate hosts. When a human becomes an accidental intermediate host, disease may result. The larval organisms travel to the liver and lungs and, if they survive host defenses, encyst and gradually enlarge. Pulmonary echinococcal cysts are composed of three layers: an exocyst (chitinous layer), which is a protective membrane; an inner endocyst, which produces the daughter cysts; and a surrounding capsule of compressed, fibrotic lung known as the pericyst.

Pulmonary echinococcal cysts characteristically present as well-circumscribed, spherical soft-tissue masses. In distinction to hepatic cysts, lung cysts do not have calcified walls. The cysts range in size from 1–20 cm, with a predilection for the lower lobes and the right side. While most cysts remain asymptomatic, patients may present when the cyst develops a communication with the bronchial tree. If the pericyst ruptures, a thin crescent of air will be seen around the periphery of the cyst, producing the "meniscus" or "crescent" sign. If the cyst itself ruptures, the contents of the cyst are expelled into the airways producing an air-fluid level. On occasion, the cyst wall may be seen crumpled and floating within a noncollapsed pericyst, producing the pathognomonic "sign of the camalote" or "water lily" sign. Rarely, a cyst will rupture into the pleural space, producing a large pleural effusion.

Paragonimiasis results from infection with the lung fluke *Paragonimus westermani*. The organism is found predominantly in the Far East, and is usually acquired by eating raw crabs or snails. Infestation of the lung may be asymptomatic or may present with cough, hemoptysis, dyspnea, and fever. In 20% of affected patients, the chest radiograph is normal. The most common radiographic finding is multiple cysts with variable wall thickness. These cystic opacities may become confluent and are often associated with focal atelectasis and subsegmental consolidation. Dense linear opacities representing the burrows of the organisms may be identified. Since the flukes penetrate the pleura, effusions are common and may be massive.

Toxoplasmosis. *Toxoplasma gondii* is an obligate intracellular protozoan whose definitive host is the cat. Humans acquire the organism by ingestion of material contaminated by oocyst-containing stool. It has been estimated that toxoplasmosis exists in a chronic asymptomatic form in 50% of the population of the United States. Disease can be recognized in four clinicopathologic forms: congenital, ocular, lymphatic, and generalized. Pulmonary involvement is usually seen in the generalized form of the disease which affects immunocompromised hosts, including those with AIDS, organ transplant recipients, and patients with leukemia or lymphoma.

The radiographic findings in pulmonary toxoplasmosis include diffuse reticular opacities that resemble acute viral pneumonia. Less commonly, air space opacities with air bronchograms may be seen. Hilar and mediastinal lymph node enlargement is common, while pleural effusion is rare. With generalized disease, most often seen in patients with AIDS, diffuse, bilateral, small nodular opacities may be seen.

Schistosomiasis. Human schistosomiasis is caused by three blood flukes: *Schistosoma mansoni*, *S. japonicum*, and *S. haematobium*. It is one of the most important parasitic infestations of humans worldwide, although it is rarely acquired in the United States. The life cycle of the fluke is complex, with human infestation acquired through contact with infested water. The larvae penetrate the skin or oropharyngeal mucosa and travel via the venous circulation to the pulmonary capillaries. As the larvae pass through the lungs, an allergic response may develop that presents radiographically as transient air space opacities (eosinophilic pneumonia) that resolve spontaneously. The larvae then pass through the pulmonary capillaries into the systemic circulation. *Schistosoma japonicum* and *S. mansoni* eventually migrate to the mesenteric venules, while *S. haematobium* migrates to bladder venules. The mature flukes produce ova, which may embolize to the lungs where they implant in and around small pulmonary arterioles. The organism induces granulomatous inflammation and fibrosis, which leads to an obliterative arteriolitis resulting in pulmonary hypertension and cor pulmonale. Radiographically, a diffuse fine reticular pattern is most commonly seen in association with dilation of the central pulmonary arteries. Small nodular opacities resembling miliary TB may be seen as granulomata form around ova.

ASPIRATION PNEUMONIA

Aspiration pneumonia is a term generally used to describe the pulmonary inflammatory response to infectious material aspirated from the oropharynx. As was discussed earlier in this section, this form of pneumonia usually results from a mixed anaerobic infection and is seen in patients with poor oral hygiene. However, aspiration of oropharyngeal or gastric secretions may also occur in a "pure" form uncomplicated by anaerobic infection, leading to an "aspiration pneumonitis" that ranges greatly in severity.

Aspiration of oropharyngeal or gastric secretions, with or without food particles, is not an uncommon event. It is seen in debilitated patients with chronic diseases, in patients with tracheal or gastric tubes, in unconscious patients, and in those who have suffered strokes, seizures, or trauma. More chronic and less easily recognizable forms of aspiration may occur in patients with anatomic abnormalities of the upper gastrointestinal tract (e.g., Zenker's diverticulum, esophageal stricture) or functional disorders (e.g., gastroesophageal reflux, neuromuscular dysfunction).

Gastric fluid is highly irritating to the lungs and often stimulates explosive coughing and associated deep inspirations, which leads to widespread distribution of the fluid throughout both lungs and into the peripheral air spaces. The hydrochloric acid contained in gastric fluid causes direct damage to both the bronchiolar lining and the alveolar wall. When the aspirate includes admixed particulate material, the particles are distributed by gravity and may incite a granulomatous foreign body-type reaction.

Three basic radiographic patterns of aspiration pneumonitis have been observed. First, extensive bilateral air space opacification may be seen. Diffuse but discrete air space nodular opacities is a less common finding. Finally, one may see irregular parenchymal opacities that are not obviously air space filling in nature. Parenchymal involvement is most often bilateral, with a predilection for the basal and perihilar regions of lung. When a significant amount of admixed food is present, the opacities are usually posterior and segmental. Atelectasis is often present, presumably resulting from airways obstruction by food particles. The radiographic appearance may worsen over the first few days, but then demonstrates rapid improvement—a worsening of the radiographic appearance at this stage suggests development of a complicating infection, diffuse capillary permeability edema (ARDS), or pulmonary embolus.

CHRONIC INTERSTITIAL LUNG DISEASE

Chronic interstitial lung disease usually results from diffuse inflammatory processes that primarily affect the axial and parenchymal interstitium of the lung. A wide variety of disease processes can result in diffuse damage to the pulmonary interstitium (Table 15.14). Careful evaluation of all available radiologic studies and correlation with clinical findings and laboratory data are essential to the accurate diagnosis of chronic interstitial lung disease. However, the majority of patients with interstitial lung disease will require histologic examination of lung tissue for definitive diagnosis.

Chronic Intersitial Pulmonary Edema

Chronic elevation of pulmonary venous pressure may lead to increased interstitial markings on plain radiographs. The interstitial thickening is because of distension of pulmonary lymphatics and chronic interstitial edema, which may lead to fibrosis. This is seen most commonly in patients with long-standing mitral stenosis or left ventricular failure. Radiographically, peribronchial cuffing, tram tracking, poor definition of vascular markings, and linear or reticular opacities may be seen. Redistribution of flow to the upper lobes, a manifestation of pulmonary venous hypertension, and prominence of the fissures because of subpleural edema and fibrosis are concomitant findings. Honeycombing is not a feature of chronic pulmonary venous hypertension; its presence in a patient with cardiac disease should suggest other causes of pulmonary fibrosis (e.g., amiodarone lung toxicity).

Collagen Vascular Diseases

These disorders cause an immunologically mediated inflammation and damage to connective tissues throughout the body. The most common thoracic manifestations of this group of heterogeneous disorders are vasculitis and interstitial fibrosis, although the pleura, chest wall, diaphragm, and heart may also be affected (8).

Rheumatoid Lung Disease (Table 15.15). Rheumatoid arthritis produces a chronic arthritis of peripheral joints. Extraarticular manifestations are seen in up to 75% of patients. In contrast to the disease as a whole, pulmonary involvement is more common in men. The pleuropulmonary manifestations of rheumatoid disease typically follow the onset of joint disease, and tend to be seen in patients with high serum rhematoid factor titers and eosinophilia. However, in up to 15% of patients, pleuropulmonary involvement precedes the joint disease.

The most common radiographic manifestation of parenchymal lung involvement is an interstitial pneumonitis and fibrosis indistinguishable histologically from idiopathic pulmonary fibrosis. This begins as an alveolitis (inflammation of the alveolar interstitium), which is seen radiographically as fine reticular or ground-glass opacities with a lower zone predominance. There is gradual progression to end-stage pulmonary fibrosis with the development of a bibasilar medium or coarse reticular or reticulonodular pattern (honeycombing) (Fig. 15.8). The HRCT is more sensitive in detecting the earliest parenchymal changes than conventional radiographs, and is also more sensitive in depicting the development of interstitial fibrosis. Predominant upper lobe fibrosis and cavity or bulla formation is rare. This less common pattern of lung involvement is indistinguishable from that seen with ankylosing spondylitis, and must be distinguished from postprimary fibrocavitary TB by acid-fast staining of sputum.

Less common parenchymal manifestations of rheumatoid disease are lung nodules and changes attributable to bronchiolitis obliterans organizing pneumonia. Necrobiotic (rheumatoid) nodules in the lung can produce peripheral well-defined nodular opacities on chest radiographs that are indistinguishable from the subcutaneous rheumatoid nodules on the extensor surfaces of the elbows and knees, which are invariably present in these patients. The lung nodules commonly evolve into thick-walled cavities that tend to wax and wane in parallel with the flares of arthritis. Similar nodules may develop in the lungs of coal miners and silica or asbestos workers with rheumatoid arthritis as a hypersensitivity response to inhaled dust particles (Caplan's syndrome). Caplan's syndrome is usually indistinguishable radiographically from the necrobiotic nodules of simple rheumatoid disease, although the presence of the associated characteristic small nodular or irregular parenchymal opacities of simple pneumoconiosis helps make this distinction. Bronchiolitis obliterans with or without organizing pneumonia has been associated with rheumatoid disease. The clinical, functional, and radiographic findings are similar to idiopathic bronchiolitis obliterans or that associated with SLE, drugs, or viral infection.

Table 15.14.   Chronic Interstitial Opacities

PREDOMINANTLY LINEAR

Chronic interstitial edema
Lymphangitic carcinomatosis
Interstitial fibrosis of any etiology

PREDOMINANTLY RETICULAR OR RETICULONODULAR

Postinfectious scarring	Tuberculosis (postprimary)
	Histoplasmosis (chronic)
	Coccidioidomycosis (chronic)
	P. carinii
Chronic interstitial edema	Mitral valve disease
Collagen vascular disease	Rheumatoid lung
	Scleroderma
	Dermatomyositis/polymyositis
	Ankylosing spondylitis
	Mixed connective tissue disease
	Idiopathic pulmonary hemorrhage
Granulomatous disease	Sarcoidosis
	Eosinophilic granuloma (histiocytosis X)
Neoplasm	Lymphangitic carcinomatosis
	Lymphoma
	Lymphocytic interstitial pneumonitis
Inhalational	Asbestosis
	Silicosis
	Coal worker's pneumoconiosis
	Berylliosis
	Hypersensitivity pneumonitis (extrinsic allergic alveolitis), chronic phase
	Chronic aspiration
Drug reaction	Nitrofurantoin
	Chemotherapeutic agents
	Amiodarone
	Radiation pneumonitis (chronic)
Idiopathic	Idiopathic pulmonary fibrosis
	Lymphangioleiomyomatosis
	Tuberous sclerosis
	Neurofibromatosis
	Amyloidosis (alveolar septal form)

PREDOMINANTLY NODULAR

Miliary infection	Tuberculosis
	Fungi
	Histoplasmosis
	Coccidioidomycosis
	Cryptococcosis
	Virus
	Varicella (healed)
Pneumoconiosis	Silicosis
	Coal worker's pneumoconiosis
	Heavy metal dust
Granulomatous disease	Sarcoidosis
	Histiocytosis X
	Talc granulomatosis
Neoplasm	
Primary	Synchronous bronchogenic carcinoma
	Lymphoma
	Hodgkin's
	Non-Hodgkin's
	Lymphomatoid granulomatosis
Metastatic	Bronchogenic carcinoma
	Thyroid carcinoma
	Renal cell carcinoma
	Breast carcinoma
	Melanoma
	Choriocarcinoma
	Osteogenic carcinoma
Idiopathic	Alveolar microlithiasis
	Amyloidosis (nodular form)

Table 15.15. Manifestations of Rheumatoid Lung Disease

Manifestation	Radiographic Findings
Serositis	
Pleuritis	Pleural effusion, thickening
Pericarditis	Pericardial effusion
Interstitial pneumonitis	Pulmonary fibrosis (basilar predominance)
Necrobiotic nodules	Multiple peripheral cavitating nodules
Caplan's syndrome	Multiple peripheral cavitating nodules
Bronchiolitis obliterans	Hyperinflation
Pulmonary arteritis	Pulmonary arterial hypertension and right heart enlargement
	Pulmonary hemorrhage

Pleuritis is the most common thoracic manifestation of rheumatoid disease and is found in 20% of patients. As with pulmonary involvement, there is a male predilection for pleural disease. Unilateral or bilateral pleural effusions may be seen, which are exudative and have a characteristically low glucose concentration.

Enlargement of the central pulmonary arteries and right ventricular dilation may be seen on chest radiographs in those with pulmonary arterial hypertension. This is an uncommon manifestation of rheumatoid disease that usually develops secondary to diffuse interstitial fibrosis. Rarely, the pulmonary arteries are involved as a part of the systemic vasculitis seen in extraarticular rheumatoid disease. There are no parenchymal abnormalities associated with rheumatoid pulmonary arteritis.

Abnormalities that may be seen in the chest wall of individuals with rheumatoid arthritis include tapered erosion of the distal clavicles, rotator cuff atrophy with a high-riding humeral head, bilateral symmetric glenohumeral joint space narrowing with or without superimposed degenerative joint disease, and superior rib notching or erosion.

Systemic Lupus Erythematosis is a disease of young and middle-aged females that typically involves inflammation of multiple organs mediated by auto-antibodies and circulating immune complexes. The thorax is commonly affected and may be the initial site of involvement. The thoracic disease is often limited to the pleura and pericardium, although the lung, heart, diaphragm, and intercostal muscles are involved in as many as one-third of patients. In the pleura and pericardium, a fibrinous serositis produces painful pleural and pericardial effusions that are exudative in nature. Radiographically, the effusions are small or moderate in size and are unilateral or bilateral. The effusions usually resolve with corticosteroid therapy. Pleural fibrosis, seen in a majority of patients with long-standing disease, results in diffuse pleural thickening.

Pulmonary involvement may take the form of acute lupus pneumonitis or chronic interstitial disease. Acute lupus pneumonitis is characterized by rapid onset of fever, dyspnea, and hypoxemia which occasionally requires mechanical ventilation. These patients have pathologic changes indistinguishable from those seen in ARDS, with diffuse alveolar damage producing an exudative intraalveolar edema with hyaline membrane formation. Radiographically, rapidly coalescent bilateral air space opacities are seen that are difficult to distinguish from diffuse alveolar hemorrhage associated with pulmonary vasculitis, severe pneumonia related to immunosuppressive therapy, or pulmonary edema secondary to renal failure. The diagnosis is made by excluding pneumonia and pulmonary edema, and by noting an improvement following the initiation of immunosuppressive therapy. Radiographic evidence of interstitial pulmonary fibrosis, seen as basilar reticular opacities indistinguishable from the pattern seen in interstitial fibrosis associated with rheumatoid lung disease or scleroderma, is distinctly uncommon in SLE but is said to be present in one-third of patients pathologically. Therefore, the presence of severe interstitial fibrosis in patients with a collagen vascular disorder with features of lupus erythematosis should prompt consideration of a diagnosis of an overlap syndrome (e.g., mixed connective tissue disease). As with rheumatoid lung disease and scleroderma, HRCT is the most sensitive technique for demonstrating early interstitial disease.

Additional chest radiographic findings in SLE include elevation of the hemidiaphragms with decrease in lung volumes and resultant bibasilar areas of linear atelectasis. Diaphragmatic elevation is present in as many as 20% of patients and is the result of diaphragmatic weakness from a primary myopathy unrelated to corticosteroid therapy. Rarely, the central pulmonary arteries are enlarged from pulmonary arterial hypertension secondary to pulmonary vasculitis. Pulmonary embolism with or without infarction may produce peripheral parenchymal opacities and results from deep venous thrombosis which develops in the presence of a circulating lupus anticoagulant. Bronchiolitis obliterans organizing pneumonia has been described in patients with SLE, but is indistinguishable clinically and radiographically from lupus pneumonitis as both conditions produce parenchymal opacities that are steroid-responsive. Superior rib erosions may be seen, indistinguishable from similar findings in rheumatoid arthritis or scleroderma.

Scleroderma produces inflammation and fibrosis of the skin, esophagus, musculoskeletal system, heart, lungs, and kidneys in young and middle-aged females. The etiology and pathogenesis are unknown. The lungs are involved pathologically in nearly 90% of patients, although only 25% of patients have respiratory symptoms or radiographic evidence of pulmonary involvement. Pulmonary function testing is more sensitive than conventional radiography in the diagnosis of lung disease and shows the typical diminished lung volumes, preserved flow rates, and low diffusing capacity of interstitial pulmonary fibrosis. Pathologically, the sequence of parenchymal and radiographic changes is indistinguishable from rheumatoid lung disease and idiopathic pulmonary fibrosis. Severe pulmonary involvement is reflected radiographically as a coarse reticular or reticulonodular pattern involving the subpleural regions of the lower lobes. High-resolution CT is more sensitive than conventional radiographs at demonstrating the earliest changes. Progressive loss of lung volume is seen with advancing pulmonary fibrosis. The presence of large (1–5 cm) subpleural lower lobe lung cysts predisposes to the development of spontaneous pneumothorax.

Pulmonary arterial hypertension with enlarged central pulmonary arteries and right ventricular dilation is seen in up to 50% of patients with scleroderma, and may be seen in the absence of interstitial fibrosis. In these patients, thickening and obliteration of small muscular pulmonary arteries and arterioles are responsible for the development of pulmonary arterial hypertension. Pleural effusions are significantly less common in scleroderma than in rheumatoid disease or SLE, and may be a helpful distinguishing feature radiographically. Pleural thickening is more often attributable to extension of pulmonary interstitial fibrosis into the interstitial layer of the pleura than to pleuritis.

There are several additional chest radiographic findings that may be seen in patients with scleroderma. Eggshell calcification of mediastinal lymph nodes has been reported, though it is more common in silicosis and sarcoidosis. A dilated air-filled esophagus may be identified on upright chest radiographs and is a manifestation of esophageal dysmotility from smooth muscle atrophy and fibrosis. An air-fluid level within a dilated esophagus suggests secondary distal esophageal stricture formation from chronic reflux esophagitis. The functional or anatomic esophageal obstruction may result in aspiration with the development of lower lobe pneumonia. Since patients with scleroderma are at a greater risk for developing lung cancer, particularly alveolar cell carcinoma, the appearance of a mass or persistent air space opacity should raise this possibility. Patients with the CREST syndrome (subcutaneous *c*alcification, *R*aynaud's phenomenon, *e*sophageal dysmotility, *s*clerodactyly, and *t*elangiectasia), a variant of scleroderma, may have radiographically visible calcifications within the subcutaneous tissues of the chest wall. Superior rib notching or erosion may be seen.

Dermatomyositis/Polymyositis. These disorders involve an autoimmune inflammation and destruction of skeletal muscle that produces proximal muscle pain and weakness (polymyositis), occasionally associated with a skin rash (dermatomyositis). The thoracic manifestations of these diseases include respiratory and pharyngeal muscle weakness and an associated interstitial pneumonitis. Interstitial pneumonitis, indistinguishable from that associated with rheumatoid lung disease, SLE, scleroderma, or idiopathic pulmonary fibrosis, is seen in 5–10% of patients. A fine reticular interstitial pattern in acute disease leads to a chronic, coarse reticular or reticulonodular process that is predominantly basilar in distribution. Most patients with polymyositis and interstitial lung disease have clinical manifestations of rheumatoid arthritis or scleroderma, and these patients tend to respond favorably to corticosteroids. As with scleroderma, the early parenchymal changes may be subradiographic, but can be demonstrated on HRCT studies through the lower lobes. Additional chest radiographic findings in polymyositis reflect the involvement of skeletal muscle. Small lung volumes with diaphragmatic elevation and basilar linear atelectasis are secondary to diaphragmatic and intercostal muscle involvement. Pharyngeal and upper esophageal muscle weakness predispose to aspiration pneumonia. The chest radiograph should be examined carefully for lung masses, as bronchogenic carcinoma accounts for a significant percentage of the malignancies which are seen with a higher than normal frequency in patients with dermatomyositis or polymyositis.

Sjögren's Syndrome is an autoimmune disorder of middle-aged women characterized by the sicca syndrome of dry eyes (keratoconjunctivitis sicca), dry mouth (xerostomia), and dry nose (xerorhinia), which results from a lymphocytic infiltration of the lacrimal, salivary, and mucus glands, respectively. Most patients with the sicca syndrome have associated manifestations of other collagen vascular diseases such as rheumatoid arthritis, scleroderma, or SLE.

The chest is involved in approximately one-third of patients with Sjögren's syndrome, with or without associated collagen vascular disease. The most common manifestation is interstitial fibrosis indistinguishable from that seen with other collagen vascular disorders. Involvement of tracheobronchial mucus glands leads to thickened sputum with mucus plugging and recurrent bronchitis, bronchiectasis, atelectasis, and pneumonia. Pleuritis and pleural effusion are less common.

Patients with Sjögren's syndrome are at increased risk for developing lymphocytic interstitial pneumonitis and non-Hodgkin's lymphoma. The radiographic appearance of lymphocytic interstitial pneumonitis is lower lobe coarse reticular or reticulonodular opacities indistinguishable from interstitial fibrosis. The development of lymphoma in these patients should be suspected when nodular or alveolar opacities develop in the lung in association with mediastinal lymph node enlargement.

Ankylosing Spondylitis. Approximately 1–2% of individuals with ankylosing spondylitis develop pulmonary disease in the form of upper lobe pulmonary fibrosis. The fibrotic changes are commonly associated with the development of bullae and cavities, which are prone to mycetoma formation with *Aspergillus*. The diagnosis should be suspected in a young to middle-aged male with characteristic spine changes (kyphosis, spinal ankylosis) that are associated with abnormally increased lung volumes and upper lobe fibrobullous disease, the latter of which simulates postprimary fibrocavitary TB.

Overlap Syndromes and Mixed Connective Tissue Disease. Some patients with collagen vascular disease have features of more than one of the recognized syndromes discussed above. These patients are classified as having an overlap syndrome, with thoracic manifestations characteristic of the other disorders. Patients with a distinct form of overlap syndrome, called mixed connective tissue disease, have clinical features of SLE, scleroderma, and polymyositis and have serum antibodies to extractable nuclear antigen. The thoracic manifestations of mixed connective tissue disease include interstitial pulmonary fibrosis, pulmonary arterial hypertension because of plexogenic pulmonary arteriopathy, and pleural effusion and thickening from a fibrinous pleuritis typical of SLE.

Idiopathic Chronic Interstitial Lung Disease

Idiopathic Pulmonary Fibrosis (IPF) is the term used to describe a group of chronic interstitial diseases of unknown etiology that cause interstitial fibrosis. Other terms that have been used to describe this process include fibrosing alveolitis, usual interstitial pneumonia (UIP), desquamative interstitial pneumonia (DIP), and interstitial pulmonary fibrosis. In addition, the Hamman-Rich syndrome is the term used to describe an acute, aggressive form of idiopathic interstitial pneumonitis and fibrosis that is characterized by the rapid progression of pulmonary insufficiency that usually leads to death in less than a year.

Proposed etiologies for IPF include autoimmune disease, genetic disorders, and viral infection. Many patients with IPF present with symptoms, signs, and serologies suggesting an autoimmune process. There have also been reports of families with an autosomal dominant form of IPF. Evidence of a viral etiology emanates from the common association of a viral syndrome with the early stages of IPF, leading to speculation that viruses (in particular, the Epstein-Barr virus) may play a role in the pathogenesis of the disease.

The pathologic abnormalities seen in IPF represent a spectrum. The early stage of disease (desquamative intersititial pneumonitis or DIP) is characterized by marked proliferation of macrophages in the alveolar air aces associated with a mild and uniform thickening of the interstitium by mononuclear cells. The late changes of IPF (usual interstitial pneumonitis or UIP) is characterized by thickening of the alveolar interstitium by mononuclear inflammatory cells and fibrous tissue.

The prevalence of IPF is 3–5 persons per 100,000 population. The majority of patients are in their 40s or 50s, and there is a slight male preponderance. Clinical symptoms include progressive dyspnea, nonproductive cough, weight loss, and fatigue. Clubbing is common.

The radiographic manifestations of IPF parallel the pathologic changes. Early on, the chest radiograph may appear normal, though the patient may be clinically symptomatic and have abnormalities on pulmonary function testing. The earliest discernable changes consist of a fine reticular pattern with lower zone predominance. Small irregular areas of opacity representing air space involvement may be present. Areas of ground-glass opacity, predominantly at the bases, may be seen and correspond to areas of DIP pathologically. As the disease progresses, a coarse reticular or reticulonodular pattern develops in the lower lobes. Thick-walled cystic spaces ranging from 3–10 mm in diameter create a honeycomb pattern. Bullae may develop, and there may be findings of pulmonary arterial hypertension. The parenchymal abnormalities are associated with a progressive diminution of lung volumes, which is a helpful differential feature of end-stage IPF. Hilar lymph node enlargement and pleural effusions have been described but are rare; their presence should suggest an alternative diagnosis (i.e., sarcoidosis, rheumatoid lung disease) or superimposed infection. Pneumothorax may develop from rupture of a subpleural cyst or bulla.

The HRCT findings in IPF differ with the stage of the process and vary from one area of the lung to another. Patients with an active, inflammatory form of the disease, as demonstrated histologically by interstitial and intraalveolar inflammatory changes, show areas of ground-glass or air space opacification best demonstrated on HRCT. As fibrosis develops, the findings include irregular septal or subpleural thickening (in contrast to the smooth septal thickening seen with edema or lymphangitic spread of carcinoma), intralobular lines, parenchymal bands, honeycombing, and traction bronchiectasis. The changes are most severe peripherally in many patients, a finding that can be helpful in differential diagnosis (Fig. 15.27). However, the HRCT findings are not specific and can be seen in asbestosis and collagen vascular disorders.

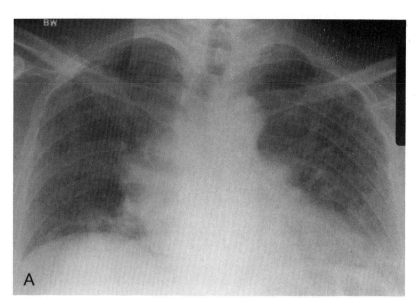

Figure 15.27. Idiopathic pulmonary fibrosis. A. A PA radiograph in a patient with idiopathic pulmonary fibrosis demonstrates bilateral coarse reticular opacities and diminished lung volumes. **B.** An HRCT through the midlungs shows honeycombing in a peripheral, subpleural distribution. Traction bronchiectasis is evident (arrow).

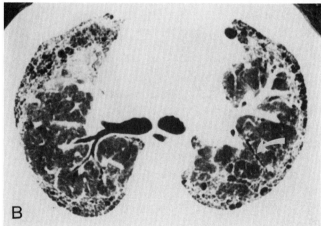

The diagnosis of IPF is made by noting characteristic clinical, radiologic, and functional abnormalities in a patient with typical histologic findings on open lung biopsy who lacks a known etiology for interstitial pulmonary fibrosis (e.g., asbestos). In most patients, the disease progresses inexorably with an overall mean survival of less than 5 years. Patients with early, active disease (positive gallium scan, ground-glass or air space opacities radiographically) may benefit from immunosuppressive therapy with corticosteroids or cyclophosphamide, while those with end-stage fibrosis (honeycombing) will not. Most patients succumb to respiratory failure, often precipitated by infection or cardiac disease. There is an increased incidence of bronchogenic carcinoma in patients with IPF; adenocarcinoma is the most common histologic type.

Neurofibromatosis *(NF)* is an autosomal dominant neurocutaneous syndrome that is divided into two types: type 1 or von Recklinghausen's disease, and type 2. The classic manifestations of NF 1 are cutaneous café au lait spots and neurofibromas of cutaneous and subcutaneous peripheral nerves and nerve roots. In addition, there is often involvement of the

skeletal, vascular, and pulmonary systems. The condition is also associated with a variety of neoplasms, including meningiomas, optic gliomas, neurofibrosarcomas, and pheochromocytomas.

Radiographically, there are several thoracic manifestations of NF 1. Cutaneous and subcutaneous neurofibromas may be seen along the chest wall or projecting over the lungs. The spine may show a kyphoscoliosis with scalloping of the posterior aspect of the vertebral bodies because of dural ectasia. "Ribbon rib" deformities and rib notching may be seen. Mediastinal masses in patients with NF 1 include neurofibromas, lateral thoracic meningoceles, and extraadrenal pheochromocytomas.

Parenchymal lung disease is seen in approximately 20% of patients with NF 1. The findings include diffuse interstitial fibrosis and bulla formation. The interstitial fibrosis is predominantly lower zone and symmetric bilaterally. Bullae usually develop in the upper zones and involve both lungs asymmetrically. Pulmonary symptoms are usually minimal or absent, with pulmonary function tests showing a mixed obstructive/restrictive pattern. A small number of patients will develop respiratory failure because of pulmonary fibrosis with secondary development of pulmonary arterial hypertension and cor pulmonale.

Tuberous Sclerosis *(TS)* is an autosomal dominant neurocutaneous syndrome with variable expression. The classical clinical triad of TS is seizures, mental retardation, and adenoma sebaceum. Additional manifestations include intracranial calcifications, cerebral cortical and periventricular hamartomas, renal angiomyolipomas, cardiac rhabdomyomas, retinal phakomas, and sclerotic bone lesions.

Pulmonary involvement in TS is rare and is seen in approximately 1% of cases. Patients with pulmonary TS tend to be older and have a lower incidence of seizures and mental retardation. The pulmonary involvement is indistinguishable clinically, pathologically, and radiographically from that seen in LAM. Pathologically, there is smooth muscle proliferation in the peribronchovascular and parenchymal interstitium of the lung. Small adenomatoid nodules measuring several millimeters in diameter may be seen scattered throughout the lungs.

Radiographically, there is symmetric bilateral reticular or reticulonodular opacities. In the later stages of disease, a pattern of coarse reticular or small cystic opacities may be seen. The cysts are uniform in size and less than 1 cm in diameter. High-resolution CT is best at depicting the presence of thin-walled pulmonary cysts and can help detect associated extrapulmonary abnormalities including renal angiomyolipomas and periventricular tubers. A helpful feature in distinguishing TS from other chronic interstitial lung diseases is the normal-to-increased lung volumes in patients with TS because of small airways obstruction and expiratory air trapping. In distinction to eosinophilic granuloma of lung and sarcoidosis, which have a predominant upper zone distribution of disease, pulmonary TS tends to affect the entire lung uniformly. Pneumothorax is common and results from the rupture of a subpleural cyst. Pleural effusions are uncommon. The pulmonary involvement often leads to pulmonary arterial hypertension and cor pulmonale, which are associated with a high mortality.

Lymphangioleiomyomatosis is an uncommon condition that is seen exclusively in women. The average age at diagnosis is 43 years. Although LAM shares many features with pulmonary tuberous sclerosis, it is not an inherited condition and lacks the extrapulmonary features of TS.

On gross pathologic examination, patients with advanced LAM show replacement of the normal lung architecture by cysts. These cysts, which range from 0.2 to 2.0 cm in diameter, are separated by thickened interstitium containing numerous interlacing bundles of smooth muscle. Smooth muscle proliferation is also seen within the walls of pulmonary veins, bronchioles, and lymphatics. The smooth muscle proliferation within lymphatic channels causes lymphatic obstruction and dilation, which may lead to the development of chylothorax, chyloperitoneum, or chylopericardium. Similarly, smooth muscle proliferation within mediastinal and retroperitoneal lymph nodes may result in nodal enlargement. The perilymphatic smooth muscle proliferation and nodal enlargement help distinguish LAM pathologically from the pulmonary involvement of TS.

The most common clinical presentation for LAM is a woman of childbearing age with progressive dyspnea or a spontaneous pneumothorax. In some pa-

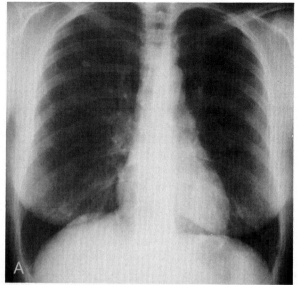

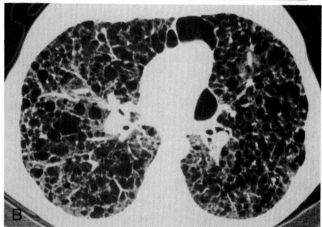

Figure 15.28. Lymphangioleiomyomatosis. A. A PA chest radiograph in a 36-year-old female patient demonstrates diffuse coarse reticular opacities with normal lung volumes. Open lung biopsy showed LAM. **B.** An HRCT in another patient with LAM shows almost complete replacement of the parenchymal by fairly uniform thin-walled cysts that are uniformly distributed from central to peripheral lung.

tients, hemoptysis may be seen, presumably related to pulmonary venous obstruction by the smooth muscle proliferation.

The chest radiograph may be normal early in the disease. Eventually, symmetric, bilateral, fine reticular or reticulonodular opacities are seen. The late radiographic pattern is one of cysts and honeycombing; the cysts tend to have thinner walls than those seen with idiopathic pulmonary fibrosis or NF (Fig. 15.28). As in TS, the lung volumes are typically normal or increased. Large, recurrent chylous pleural effusions may be unilateral or bilateral. Spontaneous pneumothorax is also a common finding and may be bilateral.

An HRCT demonstrates thin-walled cysts diffusely throughout the lungs. In less severely involved areas, the intervening lung is normal. Interlobular septal thickening is generally mild or absent. Although thin-walled cysts are seen in a variety of other diseases, most notably emphysema and eosinophilic granuloma, the HRCT findings, when seen in a patient with a characteristic history (a female with dyspnea, spontaneous pneumothorax, and chylous pleural effusions) are diagnostic.

The prognosis of patients with symptomatic LAM is poor, with approximately 70% of patients dying within 5 years. In some patients, the administration of antiprogesterone agents such as tamoxifen may slow the progression of disease.

Alveolar Septal Amyloid. Amyloidosis encompasses a group of diseases characterized by the extracellular deposition of insoluble fibrillary proteins termed amyloid. Amyloid represents a number of proteins that are distinctive biochemically but similar physically in that their polypeptide chains form β-pleated sheets. Amyloidosis has traditionally been divided into four forms: (*a*) primary, in which there is no associated chronic disease or in which there is an underlying plasma cell disorder; (*b*) secondary, in which an underlying chronic abnormality such as TB is present; (*c*) familial, which is very uncommon and usually localized to nervous tissue; and (*d*) senile, which affects many organs in patients over 70. More recently, a classification scheme has been developed that is based on the specific protein comprising amyloid. In this scheme, the most important forms are amyloid L, usually seen with plasma cell dyscrasias and associated with the deposition of immunoglobulin light chains, and amyloid A, occurring in patients with chronic inflammatory diseases such as familial Mediterranean fever and certain neoplasms including Hodgkin's disease.

There are three major patterns of amyloid deposition within the lungs and airways: tracheobronchial, nodular parenchymal, and diffuse parenchymal (alveolar septal). In most cases these patterns occur independently, but there can be overlap between them. The diffuse parenchymal form of pulmonary amyloidosis are discussed here; the tracheobronchial form is discussed in the section "Trachea" in Chapter 13.

In alveolar septal amyloidosis, the amyloid is deposited in the parenchymal interstitium and within the media of small blood vessels. Within the alveolar septa, amyloid deposits are located between the endothelial cells lining the septal capillaries and the alveolar epithelium; inflammatory cells are typically absent. This process is usually seen in older patients who have symptoms of chronic progressive dyspnea. Recurrent hemoptysis may also be seen and may be because of medial dissection of the involved pulmonary arteries.

Radiographically, patients with parenchymal alveolar septal disease show evidence of interstitial disease, with fine reticular or reticulonodular opacities that may become more coarse and confluent over time. The radiographic appearance simulates that seen in silicosis or sarcoidosis.

The diagnosis is made on lung biopsy by the identification of amorphous eosinophilic material thickening the alveolar septa that appears apple green in color when stained with Congo red and viewed under polarized light. There is no effective treatment.

Chronic Aspiration Pneumonia. Patients who repeatedly aspirate may develop chronic interstitial abnormalities on chest radiographs. With repeated episodes of aspiration over months to years, a residuum of irregular reticular interstitial opacities may persist, probably representing peribronchial scarring. A reticulonodular pattern may be seen because of granulomas forming around food particles. These chronic interstitial abnormalities can be observed in between episodes of acute aspiration pneumonitis.

GENERAL UTILITY OF HRCT IN THE EVALUATION OF CHRONIC INTERSTITIAL LUNG DISEASE

The HRCT characteristics of various interstitial lung diseases have been reviewed with the individual diseases. In addition to characterizing parenchymal abnormalities, HRCT may be used for biopsy planning, managing, and following patients with interstitial lung disease. In patients with undiagnosed diffuse interstitial lung disease undergoing open lung biopsy, HRCT can accurately localize areas of active inflammation (i.e., ground-glass or air space opacities) that are not evident on plain radiographs. This would avoid the indiscriminate sampling of nonspecific areas of honeycomb fibrosis, which would fail to provide a specific histologic diagnosis. Similarly, in patients with a diagnosis of idiopathic pulmonary fibrosis, HRCT can provide useful information regarding the utility of immunosuppressive therapy. Patients with idiopathic pulmonary fibrosis showing predominantly honeycombing with little or no ground-glass or air space opacification are unlikely to benefit from therapy. The high risk to benefit ratio of immunosuppressive therapy warrants only supportive care in these patients. Finally, the response of idiopathic pulmonary fibrosis to therapy is easily monitored on serial HRCT studies by noting stability of the abnormalities, resolution of ground-glass and air space opacities, or progression to areas of honeycombing.

Radiographic features that may help in distinguishing between the various chronic interstitial processes are reviewed in Table 15.16.

Table 15.16.   Differential Diagnostic Features in Chronic Interstitial Lung Disease

Upper zone distribution	Tuberculosis (postprimary)
	Chronic fungal infection
	Histoplasmosis
	Coccidioidomycosis
	Sarcoidosis
	Histiocytosis X
	Silicosis
	Ankylosing spondylitis
	Hypersensitivity pneumonitis (chronic)
	Radiation fibrosis from treatment of head and neck malignancy
Lower zone distribution	Idiopathic pulmonary fibrosis
	Asbestosis
	Rheumatoid lung
	Scleroderma
	Neurofibromatosis
	Dermatomyositis/polymyositis
	Chronic aspiration
Normal or increased lung volumes	Sarcoidosis
	Histiocytosis X
	Tuberous sclerosis
	Interstitial disease superimposed on emphysema
Honeycombing	Idiopathic pulmonary fibrosis
	Sarcoidosis
	Histiocytosis X
	Lymphangioleiomyomatosis
	Rheumatoid lung
	Scleroderma
	Pneumoconiosis
	Hypersensitivity pneumonitis
	Chronic aspiration
	Radiation fibrosis
Miliary nodules	Tuberculosis
	Fungi
	Histoplasmosis
	Coccidioiodomycosis
	Cryptococcosis
	Silicosis
	Metastases
	Thyroid carcinoma
	Renal cell carcinoma
	Bronchogenic carcinoma
	Melanoma
	Choriocarcinoma
	Sarcoidosis
	Histiocytosis X
Hilar/mediastinal lymph node enlargement	Sarcoidosis
	Lymphangitic carcinomatosis
	Lymphoma
	Hematogenous metastases
	Tuberculosis
	Fungal infection
	Silicosis
Pleural disease	Asbestosis (plaques)
	Lymphangitic carcinomatosis (effusion)
	Rheumatoid lung disease (effusion/thickening)
	Lymphangioleiomyomatosis (chylous effusion)
Abnormalities of soft tissues and bony thorax	Skin nodules
	Neurofibromatosis
	Subcutaneous calcifications
	Dermatomyositis
	Scleroderma
	Erosion of distal clavicles
	Rheumatoid lung
	Scleroderma
	Rib lesions

Table 15.16.—*continued*

INHALATIONAL DISEASE

Pneumoconiosis

The term "pneumoconiosis" is used to describe the nonneoplastic reaction of the lungs to inhaled inorganic dust particles. The inorganic dust pneumoconioses result from the inhalation and retention of asbestos, silica, or coal particles within the lung (9). With time, the accumulation of these particles leads to two types of pathologic reaction that may be seen alone or in combination: fibrosis, which may be focal and nodular or diffuse and reticular, and the aggregation of particle-laden macrophages. The organic dust inhalational syndromes, which are discussed at the end of this section, are not associated with the retention and accumulation of particles within the lungs. Instead, the organic dusts induce a hypersensitivity reaction known as hypersensitivity pneumonitis or extrinsic allergic alveolitis.

Asbestosis. Asbestos is the generic term for a group of fibrous silicates that are resistant to heat and various chemical insults. Asbestos is divided into two major subgroups, the serpentines and the amphiboles. The serpentines are curly, flexible and smooth; the only commercially important serpentine is chrysotile. The amphiboles have straight, needle-like fibers; this subgroup includes crocidolite and amosite. The different types of asbestos fibers vary in their potential to cause disease, with the amphiboles having a greater fibrogenic and carcinogenic potential than the serpentines. At present, more than 90% of the asbestos used in the United States is chrysotile.

Asbestos inhalation may cause disease of the pleura, parenchyma, airways, and lymph nodes. Pleural disease is the most common of these, and it usually manifests as parietal pleural plaques. Other pleural manifestations include pleural effusion, localized visceral pleural fibrosis, diffuse pleural fibrosis and mesothelioma. The pleural manifestations of asbestos exposure will be discussed in more detail in Chapter 16. The pulmonary parenchymal manifestations of asbestos inhalation include diffuse interstitial fibrosis (asbestosis), round atelectasis, and bronchogenic carcinoma.

Asbestosis is defined as a diffuse parenchymal interstitial fibrosis caused by the inhalation of asbestos fibers. The development of asbestosis depends upon both the length and severity of exposure, and clinical manifestations are usually not apparent for 20–40 years following initial exposure. Pathologically, a large number of "asbestos bodies" will be seen in lung tissue. This characteristic structure consists of a core composed of a transparent asbestos fiber surrounded by a variably thick coat of iron and protein. They are usually found within interstitial fibrous tissue or air spaces, but only rarely in pleural plaques. The number of asbestos bodies and fibers per gram of digested lung tissue is roughly proportional to the degree of occupational exposure and the severity of interstitial fibrosis. On gross examination of affected lungs, fibrosis is most prominent in the subpleural regions of the lower lobes. Microscopically, the appearance varies from a slight increase in interstitial collagen to complete obliteration of normal architecture and formation of thick fibrous (parenchymal) bands and cystic spaces (honeycombing).

The majority of patients with asbestos-related pleuropulmonary disease are asymptomatic. Patients beyond the early stages of interstitial fibrosis will often experience shortness of breath and a restrictive pattern on pulmonary function tests. These patients are also at risk to develop asbestos-associated neoplasia, especially bronchogenic carcinoma and pleural mesothelioma, and require close clinical follow-up.

The radiographic findings in asbestosis occur in two forms; small and large opacities. Small opacities may be reticular, nodular, or a combination of the two. The changes produced on chest radiographs are divided into three stages. The earliest finding is a fine reticulation predominantly in the lower lung zones and is a manifestation of early interstitial pneumonitis and fibrosis. With time, the small irregular opacities become more prominent, creating a coarse reticular pattern of disease. In later stages, the reticular opacities may extend into the middle and upper lung zones, with progressive obscuration of the cardiac and diaphragmatic margins and progressive diminution of lung volume. Large opacities, measuring more than 1 cm in diameter, are invariably associated with widespread interstitial fibrosis and pleural plaques. These large opacities show a lower zone predominance and may be well- or ill-defined and multiple.

High-resolution CT is a sensitive indicator of both the pleural and parenchymal changes associated with clinical asbestosis. Fixed thickening of core and septal lines, predominantly in the posterior subpleural regions of the lower lobes, is the most common HRCT finding in asbestos-exposed individuals. Subpleural lines, parenchymal bands, and honeycombing are also seen. The identification of intrafissural plaques, especially if they contain calcification, can also be made with HRCT. Certain HRCT features of focal lung masses in asbestos-exposed individuals may allow for conservative management of these lesions. For example, wedge-shaped masses adjacent to areas of focal pleural thickening, with evidence of lobar volume loss and a "comet tail" bronchovascular bundle entering the mass, can be confidently diagnosed as round atelectasis by HRCT.

Silicosis. Silica is an abundant mineral composed of regularly arranged molecules of silicon dioxide. It is ubiquitous in the earth's crust, and exposure to a high concentration may lead to pathologic and radiologic changes. Occupations associated with such levels of exposure include mining, quarrying, foundry work, ceramic work, and sandblasting.

There are two distinct histopathologic reactions to inhaled silica: silicotic nodules and silicoproteinosis. The silicotic nodule is made up of dense concentric lamellae of collagen. Silicotic nodules measure from 1 to 10 mm in diameter. They are typically most numerous in the upper lobes and parahilar regions of lung; calcification or ossification of the nodules is common. Coalescence of these nodules produces areas of progressive massive fibrosis (PMF). Progressive massive fibrosis may occupy an entire lobe, with areas of emphysema often seen adjacent to these masses. Focal necrosis is common within the central portions of these large conglomerate lesions, often the result of ischemia or superinfection by TB or anaerobic bacteria. Silicoproteinosis generally occurs in individuals exposed to very high concentrations of silica, and is characterized by filling of alveolar spaces with lipoproteinaceous material similar to that seen in idiopathic alveolar proteinosis. There is little collagen deposition associated with this reaction, and the well-defined collagenous nodule is not typically seen. Patients with both fibrotic silicosis and acute silicoproteinosis have an increased susceptibility to TB.

Ten to 20 years of exposure are usually required for the radiographic changes of silicosis to develop. The classic radiographic appearance is multiple well-defined nodular opacities ranging from 1–10 mm in di-

ameter. These nodules, which calcify in approximately 20% of cases, are diffuse and demonstrate an upper zone predominance. A reticular pattern of disease may be seen preceding or associated with the nodular pattern, and is sometimes the earliest radiographic finding. This pattern of reticulonodular opacities is often referred to as "simple" silicosis, in contrast to the large conglomerate opacities that characterize "complicated" silicosis. These conglomerate opacities represent areas of progressive massive fibrosis and most commonly develop in the peripheral portions of the upper and middle lung zones. The opacities tend to migrate toward the hila, leaving areas of emphysema between the pleural surface and the areas of progressive fibrosis. These conglomerate areas may cavitate, often in association with superimposed tuberculous infection. Hilar lymph node enlargement may be seen at any stage, and these hilar nodes often demonstrate peripheral eggshell calcification. A variant of the classic radiographic form of the disease is seen in patients with acute heavy exposure to silica, usually sandblasters, who develop acute silicoproteinosis. This appears radiographically as diffuse air space disease and is indistinguishable in appearance from idiopathic alveolar proteinosis. These patients are also predisposed to superinfection with *Nocardia*, which may produce mass-like consolidation and chest wall involvement.

Clinically, the diagnosis of silicosis is based on identification of a diffuse reticular, nodular, or reticulonodular pattern on the chest radiograph in a patient with an appropriate exposure history. Patients may be asymptomatic for many years, but may worsen functionally in conjunction with progression of the radiographic changes. The pulmonary fibrosis and associated restrictive functional impairment of silicosis may progress even after removing the individual from the offending environment.

Coal Worker's Pneumoconiosis. The inhalation of large amounts of carbon-containing inorganic material may lead to significant pulmonary disease. The exposure levels required to cause this disease occur almost exclusively in the workplace. Since the most common occupation producing this entity is coal mining, the resultant disease is termed coal worker's pneumoconiosis (CWP).

Coal worker's pneumoconiosis has two characteristic pathologic findings: the coal dust macule and PMF. The coal dust macule results from the deposit of carbonaceous material within the lung. Coal dust macules are round or stellate nodules ranging in size from 1 to 5 mm. They are composed of pigment-laden macrophages with minimal or absent collagen formation. They are found within the interstitium adjacent to respiratory bronchioles and are scattered throughout the lungs, with a predilection for the apices. The coal dust macule or nodule is the hallmark of simple CWP, and is generally not associated with functional impairment. In fact, radiographic abnormalities may be absent in simple CWP. Complicated CWP is characterized by the presence of PMF, which is defined as nodular or mass-like lesions exceeding 2 to 3 cm in diameter and composed of irregular fibrosis and pigment. Progressive massive fibrosis is most common in the posterior segments of the upper lobes and superior segments of the lower lobes. The conglomerate masses may cross interlobar fissures. Central cavitation is common, and is most often due to infarction from obliteration of pulmonary vessels by the fibrotic masses. Occasionally, superinfection of the masses by TB or fungus accounts for central necrosis and cavitation. The mass lesions of complicated CWP are similar to those seen in complicated silicosis. It should be noted that despite the definition, the lesions of PMF may not progress with time and are not necessarily massive in size.

Patients with CWP usually present with respiratory difficulties only when PMF has developed, as those with simple pneumoconiosis are generally asymptomatic. In complicated CWP, there is progressive dyspnea with cor pulmonale and right heart failure. Since many coal workers also smoke cigarettes, the development of centrilobular emphysema and chronic bronchitis may complicate the clinical picture.

Radiographically, "simple" CWP presents typically as upper zone reticulonodular or small nodular opacities. A purely reticular pattern may also be seen, especially in the early stages of the process. The nodules range from 1 to 5 mm in diameter and correspond to conglomerates of coal dust macules seen pathologically. The lesions are indistinguishable radiographically from the nodules of simple silicosis. In as many as 10% of coal miners, some of these nodules will calcify centrally. This is in distinction to the diffuse calcification of silicotic nodules. The nodular opacities of simple CWP do not progress once coal dust exposure has ceased. The lesions of complicated pneumoconiosis (PMF) range in size from 2 cm to an entire lobe and are seen in the upper portion of the lungs. Progressive massive fibrosis usually begins peripherally as a mass with a smooth, well-defined lateral border and an ill-defined medial border. Progressive massive fibrosis gradually "migrates" toward the hilum, creating a zone of emphysema between the opacities and the chest wall. These lesions may mimic primary carcinoma, particularly if a background of nodular opacities is not appreciated. The PMF seen with CWP may develop years after exposure to coal dust has ceased and may progress in the absence of further exposure.

Certain complicating factors may alter the radiographic appearance of CWP. Tuberculosis is relatively common in patients with CWP and may produce central cavitation in some patients with PMF. Caplan's syndrome or "rheumatoid pneumoconiosis", seen in coal workers with rheumatoid arthritis, is characterized radiographically by nodular opacities 0.5–5 cm in diameter that develop rapidly and tend to appear in crops. The nodules are more sharply defined and seen more peripherally than the masses of PMF. These lesions are not specific for CWP and may be seen in patients with silicosis or asbestosis.

Miscellaneous Pneumoconioses. A variety of inorganic dusts other than asbestos, silica, and coal dust can cause pleuropulmonary disease, but there are less common. Chronic berylliosis results in a granulomatous reaction that mimics sarcoidosis and has been discussed. Aluminum workers may develop disabling pulmonary fibrosis after years of exposure to aluminum dust, usually from bauxite mining. Radiographic changes include fine-to-coarse reticular or reticulonodular opacities distributed throughout the lungs with greatly diminished lung volumes and marked pleural thickening. Apical bullae may be seen that produce spontaneous pneumothorax. Hard-metal pneumoconiosis may result from exposure to cobalt and tungsten alloys and lead to interstitial pneumonitis with varying degrees of fibrosis. The chest radiograph demonstrates a reticulonodular pattern that may be very coarse and, if advanced, may be associated with small cystic shadows. Lymph node enlargement may be seen.

Hypersensitivity Pneumonitis

Hypersensitivity pneumonitis or extrinsic allergic alveolitis is an immunologic pulmonary disorder associated with the inhalation of antigenic organic dusts. These dusts must be of small particle size in order to penetrate into the alveolar spaces and incite a host inflammatory response. A wide variety of etiologic agents have been implicated, including many thermophilic bacteria, true fungi, and various animal proteins. Some of the more common disease entities include farmer's lung, which follows exposure to moldy hay; humidifier lung, which follows exposure to water reservoirs contaminated by certain thermophilic bacteria; and bird-fancier's lung, which results from exposure to avian proteins in feathers and excreta.

The development of hypersensitivity pneumonitis depends upon the size, number, and immunogenicity of the inhaled organic particles and the immune response of the host. There are two forms of the disease that are distinguished by their clinical presentation and immunopathogenesis. Acute disease develops 4 to 6 hours following exposure to the inciting antigen, and is mediated by a type III (immune complex) reaction. Typical symptoms include cough, dyspnea, and fever. Chronic disease is often insidious and commonly results in interstitial pulmonary fibrosis. Patients with chronic disease often have a chronic cough, malaise, and progressive dyspnea. This form of disease appears to be mediated by a type IV (cell-mediated) immune reaction.

The histopathologic features of the different types of hypersensitivity pneumonitis are usually indistinguishable, except in rare situations where antigenic material can be identified in the pathologic preparations. The pathologic features depend on the intensity of exposure to the allergen and on the stage of disease when tissue biopsy is obtained. Early findings include capillary congestion and inflammation within alveolar septae. In later stages of acute disease, bronchiolitis and alveolitis with granuloma formation is present. With repeated antigenic exposure, there is a progressive increase in interstitial fibrosis, which is initially patchy in distribution but may progress to diffuse interstitial fibrosis.

The radiographic changes of hypersensitivity pneumonitis parallel the pathologic findings. The chest radiograph may be normal early in the acute stage of disease. Within hours, fine nodular or ground-glass opacities develops, most often in the lower lobes; progressive air space opacification may simulate pulmonary edema. Within hours to days, the opacities resolve and the chest radiograph becomes normal. With continued or repeated exposures, the chest radiograph will remain abnormal between acute episodes. The chronic changes appear as diffuse coarse reticular or reticulonodular opacities with an upper zone predilection; a honeycomb pattern with loss of lung volume may be seen. The diagnosis of hypersensitivity pneumonitis should be considered when repeated episodes of rapidly changing ground-glass or air space opacification are seen in a patient with underlying coarse interstitial lung disease. Hilar or mediastinal lymph node enlargement and pleural effusion are uncommon findings in patients with hypersensitivity pneumonitis.

The diagnosis of hypersensitivity pneumonitis is made by eliciting a history that suggests a temporal relationship between the patient's symptoms and certain exposures. The intermittent exposure of susceptible persons to high concentrations of antigen leads to recurrent episodes that typically begin 4 to 6 hours following exposure. The symptoms usually persist for 12 hours and then resolve spontaneously if the exposure has been terminated. Repeated exposure to the inciting antigen will result in acute exacerbations with typical symptoms and radiographic findings. Chronic disease is more difficult to diagnose and develops when there is a continuous low level of exposure to the inciting antigen. The prognosis for patients whose disease is recognized at an early stage is good if the offending antigen can be removed from the environment (or vice versa). In the more insidious chronic form of disease, the diagnosis is often delayed and considerable interstitial fibrosis may be present at the time of diagnosis. These patients generally suffer from chronic respiratory insufficiency.

TRAUMATIC LUNG DISEASE
Pulmonary Contusion

Lung contusion usually follows blunt chest trauma and typically develops adjacent to the site of impact. Blood and edema fluid fill the alveoli of the lung within the first 12 hours after trauma, producing scattered areas of air space opacification that may rapidly become confluent and may be difficult to distinguish from aspiration pneumonia. The patient may have shortness of breath and hemoptysis; blood can usually be suctioned from the endotracheal tube. The typical radiographic course is stabilization of opacities by 24 hours and improvement within 2 to 7 days. Progressive opacities seen more than 48 hours after trauma should raise the suspicion of aspiration pneumonia or the development of ARDS.

Pulmonary Laceration (Traumatic Lung Cyst)

Pulmonary laceration is a common sequela of penetrating or blunt chest trauma; in the latter situation, it represents a shearing injury to the substance of the lung (10). The elastic properties of the lung quickly transform the linear laceration into a rounded air cyst. These cysts may be filled with varied amounts of blood as a result of laceration of pulmonary capillaries; those completely filled with blood are more appropriately termed "pulmonary hematomas." On radiographs, these cysts appear as thin-walled rounded lucencies that may contain air or an air-fluid level (Fig. 15.29). Initially, these cysts are often obscured by the adjacent contused lung, only to be recognized after resorption of the blood. The cysts tend to shrink gradually over a period of weeks to months. The term "traumatic air cysts" rather than pneumatoceles should be used for these lesions, the latter term being reserved for air cysts resulting from a check-valve overdistension of distal lung as seen in staphylococcal pneumonia.

CONGENITAL LUNG DISEASE
Bronchogenic Cysts

These cysts represent anomalous outpouchings of the primitive foregut that no longer communicate with the tracheobronchial tree (11). Bronchogenic cysts most commonly present as asymptomatic mediastinal masses and are considered in detail in Chapter 13.

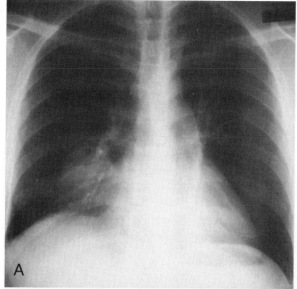

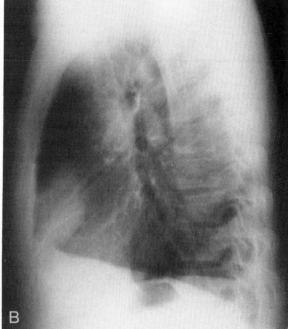

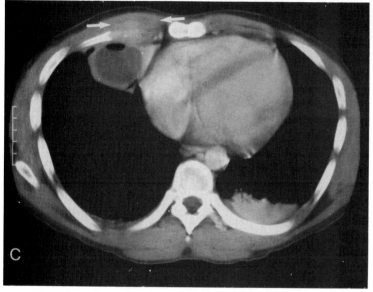

Figure 15.29. Traumatic Lung Cyst. Posteroanterior **(A)** and lateral **(B)** radiographs in a 26-year-old man who sustained a right parasternal stab wound 2 weeks previously. A well-defined mass with an air-fluid level is seen in the right middle lobe. A CT scan **(C)** demonstrates a thin-walled cystic lesion representing a pulmonary laceration. There is persistent swelling within the parasternal soft tissues (*arrows*).

Cystic Adenomatoid Malformation

Cystic adenomatoid malformation is a lesion usually seen in newborn infants, although it occasionally presents in childhood or early adulthood. The most common pathologic type shows one or several large cysts that are lined by respiratory epithelium with scattered mucus glands, smooth muscle, and elastic tissue in their walls. Multiple smaller cystic structures are present in the intervening lung between the larger cysts. Radiographically, these lesions most often appear as rounded air-filled masses exerting mass effect on adjacent lung and mediastinum. If seen in the left lower lobe, cystic adenomatoid malfunction may be difficult to distinguish from a congenital diaphragmatic hernia. Delayed clearance of fetal fluid in the newborn may give the radiographic appearance of an intrapulmonary soft-tissue mass. These lesions may be identified on prenatal ultrasound examination (see Chapter 33).

Bronchial Atresia

In this condition, a developmental stenosis or atresia of a lobar or segmental bronchus produces bronchial obstruction with resultant distal bronchiectasis. Most patients are asymptomatic and are first recognized by typical findings on frontal chest radiographs. These findings include a rounded, oval, or branching central lung opacity representing the obstructed mucus-filled dilated bronchus (mucocele) with hyperlucency in that portion of lung supplied by the atretic bronchus. The overinflated lobe or segment results from air trapping in the obstructed lung as air enters via collateral air drift on inspiration but cannot empty via the proximal tracheobronchial tree on expiration. The most common site of involvement is the apicopos-

Table 15.17. Intralobar vs. Extralobar Sequestration

Characteristic	Intralobar	Extralobar
Frequency	Not uncommon	Rare
Laterality	Left/right = 60%/40%	Left/right = 90%/10%
Associated anomalies	None (isolated finding)	Associated with other congenital anomalies (left diaphragmatic eventration/hernia)
Pleural covering	Within visceral pleura of lung	Separate visceral pleural lining
Arterial supply	Single large artery from aorta	Multiple small arteries from aorta and pulmonary artery
Venous drainage	Pulmonary vein (left-to-left shunt)	Systemic vein (left-to-right shunt)
Radiographic appearance	Cystic mass +/− air-fluid levels	Solid mass above or within diaphragm
Clinical findings	Pneumonia secondary to superinfection	Asymptomatic (incidental finding)

terior segment of the left upper lobe, followed by the segmental bronchi of the right upper and middle lobes. The combination of a central mucocele with peripheral hyperlucency in a young, asymptomatic patient is virtually diagnostic of this disorder.

Congenital Lobar Emphysema

Congenital lobar emphysema may develop from a variety of disorders that produce a check-valve bronchial obstruction. These include extrinsic compression by mediastinal bronchogenic cysts, anomalous left pulmonary artery, congenital deficiency of bronchial cartilage, and congenital or acquired bronchial stenosis. The bronchial obstruction leads to air trapping on expiration, with resultant overinflation of distal lung. In order of decreasing frequency, the left upper lobe, right middle lobe, and right upper lobe are the most common sites of involvement. Respiratory difficulties are usually evident within the first month of life, with a minority presenting later. Radiographically, hyperlucency of the affected lobe is seen, with compression of adjacent lung, diaphragmatic depression, and contralateral mediastinal shift. These findings are accentuated on expiratory films or on decubitus films obtained with the affected side down. Since many of these cases are not truly congenital but rather arise in the neonatal period from acquired abnormalities, and since overinflation of normal alveoli without destruction of alveolar walls is seen pathologically, the term "neonatal lobar hyperinflation" has been used to more appropriately describe this syndrome. Treatment is surgical for symptomatic patients, while relatively asymptomatic patients are observed for spontaneous resolution.

Bronchopulmonary Sequestration

This congenital abnormality results from the development of a detached portion of the tracheobronchial tree, which is isolated from the normal lung and maintains its fetal systemic arterial supply. Grossly, sequestered lung is cystic and bronchiectatic. These patients most often present with recurrent pneumonia from recurrent infection in the sequestered lung, although some are discovered as asymptomatic posterior mediastinal masses on routine radiographs.

Pulmonary sequestration is divided into intralobar and extralobar forms. Intralobar sequestration is found adjacent to and contained within the visceral pleura of the normal lung. Extralobar sequestration may be found adjacent to the normal lung or within or below the diaphragm, and is enclosed by its own visceral pleural envelope. The features that distinguish intralobar from extralobar sequestration are listed in Table 15.17. Most patients with intralobar sequestration present with pneumonia, while extralobar sequestration is usually asymptomatic and is seen as an incidental finding in a neonate with other severe congenital anomalies. Intralobar sequestration is more common than the extralobar type by a ratio of 3:1. While both forms are found in the lower lobes, extralobar sequestration is predominantly left-sided (90%), while one-third of intralobar sequestrations are right-sided. The major differentiating feature between the two types is the arterial supply to and venous drainage from the sequestered lung. An intralobar sequestration is supplied by a single large artery arising from the aorta just below the diaphragm, which enters the sequestered lung via the inferior pulmonary ligament. The venous drainage is to the pulmonary veins (Fig. 15.30). In contrast, extralobar sequestration receives several small branches from systemic and sometimes pulmonary arteries, with venous drainage into the systemic venous system (i.e., inferior vena cava, azygos or hemiazygos veins).

Radiographically, sequestration appears as a solid posterior mediastinal mass or as a single or multicystic air collection with or without air-fluid levels (Fig. 15.30). The latter appearance is seen when infection has produced communication of the sequestered lung with the normal tracheobronchial tree. The definitive diagnosis is made by the demonstration of abnormal systemic arterial supply to the abnormal lung, which is usually accomplished by thoracic aortography. More recently, contrast-enhanced CT and coronal MR and MR angiography have been used to demonstrate the feeding systemic artery, with arteriography re-

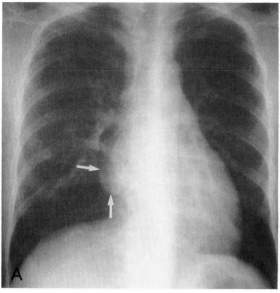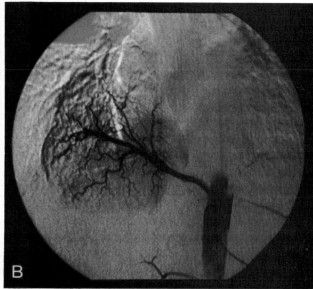

Figure 15.30. Intralobar Sequestration. A. Frontal chest film in a 19-year-old patient with recurrent right lower lobe pneumonia demonstrates a round mass in the infrahilar region with a hyperlucent region inferiorly (*arrows*). **B.** A digital subtraction aortogram shows a single large feeding artery from the upper abdominal aorta. At surgery, the infrahilar mass was found to represent a mucocele within the sequestered lung.

served for preoperative patients in whom precise demonstration of the origin and number of the systemic feeders is necessary.

Hypoplastic Lung

Hypoplastic lung is a developmental anomaly resulting in a small lung, which occurs secondary to congenital pulmonary arterial deficiency or from compression of the developing lung in utero from a variety of causes. Grossly, the lung is small with a decrease in the number and size of airways, alveoli, and pulmonary arteries. Radiographically, a small lung and hemithorax is associated with ipsilateral diaphragmatic elevation and mediastinal shift with anterior herniation of the hyperinflated contralateral lung toward the affected side. The radiographic appearance of hypoplastic lung can simulate total lung collapse, but can usually be distinguished on clinical grounds and review of prior radiographic studies, which show a small lung without evidence of pleural or parenchymal scarring.

Hypogenetic Lung—Scimitar Syndrome

This syndrome, a variant of the hypoplastic lung, is characterized by an underdeveloped right lung with abnormal venous drainage of the lung to the inferior vena cava just above or below the right hemidiaphragm. The systemic venous drainage of the lung produces an extracardiac left-to-right shunt. The anomalous vein, which drains all or most of the right lung, may be seen as a vertically oriented curvilinear density shaped like a scimitar in the medial right lower lung, thereby giving this syndrome its common name of scimitar syndrome (Fig. 15.31). Additional features include hypoplasia of the right pulmonary artery with systemic arterial supply to all or part of the lung (usually the lower lobe), bilateral left-sided (hyparterial) bronchial anatomy, eventration of the right hemidiaphragm, and cardiac anomalies including atrial septal defect, coarctation of the aorta, patent ductus arteriosus, and tetralogy of Fallot. The frontal chest radiographic findings are diagnostic and include a small right hemithorax with diaphragmatic elevation or eventration, dextroposition of the heart, and herniation of left lung anteriorly into the right hemithorax. The classic appearance of a solitary scimitar vein is seen in only one-third of cases, with the remainder having multiple small draining veins. Although plain film findings are usually diagnostic, CT or MR shows the abnormal draining vein and associated abnormalities. While most patients are asymptomatic, some may present with recurrent infection, symptoms related to a left-to-right shunt, or from associated cardiac anomalies.

Arteriovenous Malformation

Pulmonary arteriovenous malformations (AVMs) are abnormal vascular masses in which a focal collection of congenitally weakened capillaries dilate to become a tortuous complex of vessels fed by a single pulmonary artery and drained by a single pulmonary vein. Most pulmonary AVMs do not come to attention

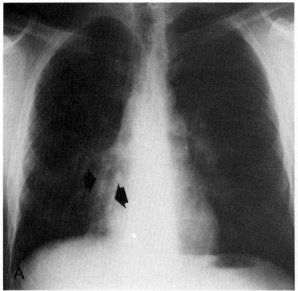

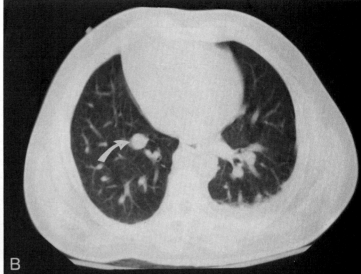

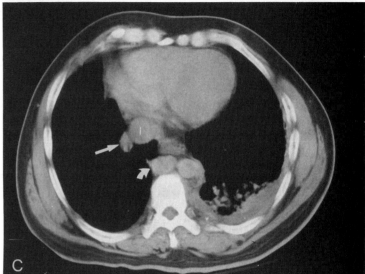

Figure 15.31. Scimitar Syndrome. A. Frontal chest film in a 36-year-old male with blunt chest trauma to the left chest wall demonstrates dextroposition of the heart with a vertically oriented structure barely visible behind the cardiac silhouette (*arrows*). **B.** A CT scan through the right lower lobe shows a round opacity (*curved arrow*) representing the vertically oriented anomalous vein in cross-section. **C.** More inferiorly, the vein (*arrow*) is seen draining into the inferior vena cava (*I*). Absence of the infrahepatic cava in this patient accounts for the dilated azygos vein seen on CT (*curved arrow* in **C**). A small left effusion is secondary to a fractured posterior rib (not shown).

until early adulthood. They are detected either incidentally, as part of a screening evaluation in patients with hereditary hemorrhagic telangiectasia (a condition that is present in approximately half of all patients with pulmonary AVMs), or because of a variety of symptoms. The most common pulmonary symptoms are hemoptysis and dyspnea, the latter attributable to the intrapulmonary right-to-left shunt with resultant hypoxemia. Nonpulmonary symptoms most often relate to central nervous system disease. Stroke may occur from paradoxical right-to-left cerebral emboli or from thrombosis, which is related to secondary polycythemia from chronic hypoxemia. Brain abscess may develop from paradoxical septic emboli.

The chest radiograph usually shows a solitary pulmonary nodule, most often located in the subpleural portions of the lower lobes. Approximately one-third of patients have multiple lesions. The lesion is often lobulated and has feeding and drainings vessels ema-

nating from the mass and extending toward the hilum (Fig. 15.32). These vessels are best demonstrated by dynamic contrast-enhanced CT or by MR. Angiography is reserved for preoperative evaluation and for those undergoing therapeutic transcatheter embolization with spring coils or detachable occlusion balloons. Transcatheter occlusion techniques have become the treatment of choice for patients with multiple AVMs.

AIRWAYS DISEASE
Chronic Obstructive Pulmonary Disease

Disorders of the trachea and main bronchi are discussed in Chapter 13. The diseases known collectively as COPD include asthma, chronic bronchitis, bronchiectasis, and emphysema. The common pathophysiology in this group of diseases is obstruction to expiratory airflow.

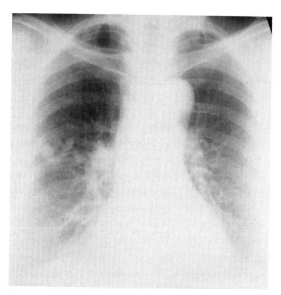

Figure 15.32. Pulmonary Arteriovenous Malformation. Frontal radiograph in a 66-year-old woman with dyspnea demonstrates a peripheral nodule with large feeding and draining vessels emanating from the hilum, characteristic of an AVM. The lesion was successfully treated by transcatheter coil embolization.

ASTHMA

Asthma is an airways disorder characterized by the rapid onset of bronchial narrowing with spontaneous resolution or improvement as a result of therapy. A wide variety of inciting factors and agents have been identified. Many patients have an allergic history and develop episodic bronchial constriction from excessive immunoglobulin-E production on exposure to antigenic stimuli. This results in bronchial smooth muscle contraction, bronchial wall inflammation, and excessive mucus production. These responses narrow the bronchial lumina and produce symptoms of coughing, wheezing, and dyspnea.

The radiographic findings in uncomplicated asthma are primarily the result of diffuse airways narrowing. Hyperinflation producing increased lung height, flattening or inversion of the diaphragm, attenuation of the peripheral vascular markings, and prominence of the retrosternal air space is the result of expiratory air trapping. Bronchial wall thickening appears radiographically as peribronchial cuffing and tram tracking. In some patients, the hila are prominent from transient pulmonary arterial hypertension caused by hypoxic vasoconstriction.

There are several reasons to obtain a chest radiograph in patients with asthma. Tracheal and central bronchial narrowing from extrinsic or intrinsic lesions may produce dysnea and wheezing and be mistaken for asthma. Bacterial pneumonia may induce airway hyperreactivity and present as an acute asthmatic attack. Complications of asthma may be de-

tected on chest radiographs obtained during and following the asthmatic episode. Mucus plugging can result in bronchial obstruction and resorptive atelectasis. Pneumonia can develop in these collapsed regions. Expiratory airflow obstruction with resultant alveolar rupture and dissection of air medially may produce pneumomediastinum. If the extralveolar air dissects peripherally to the subpleural space to form subpleural blebs, pneumothorax may result. Both pneumomediastinum and pneumothorax may be exacerbated in ventilated patients receiving high positive pressure ventilation.

CHRONIC BRONCHITIS

Chronic bronchitis is a clinical and not a radiographic diagnosis. It is defined as the excess production and expectoration of sputum that occurs on most days for at least 3 consecutive months in at least 2 consecutive years. Most individuals with chronic bronchitis are cigarette smokers. Morphologically, the lower lobe bronchi are most often affected, with thickening of their walls from mucus gland hyperplasia. The ratio of mucus gland thickness to bronchial wall thickness is known as the Reid index; an abnormally high index (>50%) correlates strongly with symptoms of excess mucus production. Fifty percent of patients with a history of chronic bronchitis have normal chest films. Some patients will show peribronchial cuffing or tram tracks when the thick-walled and mildly dilated bronchi are viewed end-on or in length, respectively. Still others are found to have a "dirty chest," in which the peripheral lung markings are accentuated. This radiographic appearance has no definite pathologic correlate, but may represent small airways disease or prominent pulmonary arteries from pulmonary arterial hypertension complicating associated centrilobular emphysema.

BRONCHIECTASIS

Bronchiectasis is defined as an abnormal permanent dilation of bronchi. Morphologically, bronchiectasis is divided into three groups: cylindrical, varicose, and saccular (cystic) bronchiectasis. Cylindrical bronchiectasis is characterized by mild diffuse dilation of the bronchi. Varicose bronchiectasis is diffuse cylindrical dilation interrupted by focal areas of cystic dilation, an appearance that has been likened to a string of beads. Cystic bronchiectasis is seen as clusters of bronchi with marked, localized saccular dilation. Bronchiectasis may be localized, most commonly as a result of prior TB or generalized, as seen in patients with cystic fibrosis. Patients usually have a history of chronic sputum production and recurrent

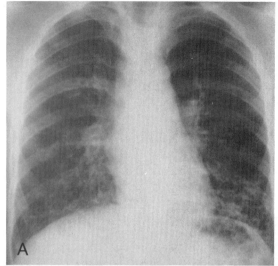

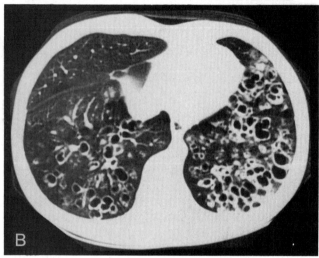

Figure 15.33. Cystic Bronchiectasis. A. A PA chest film in a 12-year-old Vietnamese immigrant with recurrent pulmonary infection shows innumerable small cystic lesions in the lower lobes, some of which contain air-fluid levels. **B.** A CT scan shows clustered, thin-walled cysts accompanying arteries diagnostic of cystic bronchiectasis.

lower respiratory infections. Hemoptysis associated with enlargement of bronchial arteries is common and may be massive and life-threatening.

The chest radiographic findings of bronchiectasis are typically nonspecific, with scarring, volume loss, and loss of the sharp definition of the normal bronchovascular shadows in affected regions. Parallel linear shadows that represent the walls of cylindrically dilated bronchi seen in length may be visualized. Cystic bronchiectasis has a characteristic appearance of multiple thin-walled cysts, with or without air-fluid levels, that are peripheral and tend to cluster together in the distribution of a bronchovascular bundle (Fig. 15.33) The findings tend to be peripheral in most cases of localized bronchiectasis; central bronchiectasis is seen only in allergic bronchopulmonary aspergil-

losis, cystic fibrosis, bronchial atresia, or acquired central bronchial obstruction.

Computed tomography has all but eliminated the need for contrast bronchography in the evaluation of bronchiectasis. The use of thin-section high-resolution scans obtained at regular intervals has been shown to have an accuracy exceeding 95%, compared with bronchography in the diagnosis of bronchiectasis. The CT appearance of bronchiectasis depends upon the site of involvement and the type of bronchiectasis. In the upper and lower regions, all bronchi are imaged in cross-section, and their luminal diameter can be directly compared with the accompanying pulmonary arteries. Cylindrical bronchiectasis in these regions appears as multiple-dilated thick-walled circular lucencies, with the adjoining smaller artery giving each dilated bronchus the appearance of a "signet ring." In the midlung regions, where the bronchi course horizontally, the appearance is that of parallel linear opacities or "tram tracks." Mucoid impaction within dilated upper or lower lung bronchi may be mistaken for lung nodules unless one observes the vertical nature of the opacity on sequential axial images. In the midlung regions, impacted bronchi sectioned in length are recognized as branching finger-like opacities. Cystic bronchiectasis in any region is easily recognized as clusters of rounded lucencies often containing air-fluid levels; this appearance has been likened to a "cluster of grapes" (Fig. 15.33**B**). Varicose bronchiectasis cannot be differentiated from cylindrical bronchiectasis unless sectioned longitudinally in the midlung regions, where the pattern of dilation simulates the contour of a caterpillar and has been described as a "string of pearls."

Bronchography remains the gold standard for the diagnosis of and evaluating the extent of bronchiectasis. However, its invasive nature and associated complications, particularly in patients with limited pulmonary reserve, preclude its routine use for evaluation of bronchiectasis. Computed tomography has replaced bronchography for the diagnosis of bronchiectasis because it is noninvasive and highly accurate. Scans obtained at 10-mm intervals with 1.5-mm collimation and a high spatial resolution reconstruction algorithm (HRCT) are used to detect the presence and extent of disease. Currently, bronchography is limited to those patients considered for curative resection who appear to have localized disease by CT examination.

Bronchiectasis is caused by a variety of disorders, all of which predispose the bronchi to chronic inflammation with resultant cartilage damage and dilation (Table 15.18).

Cystic Fibrosis is a hereditary disease of young Caucasians characterized in the lung by the production of abnormally thick, tenacious mucus. The thick

Table 15.18. Specific Causes of Bronchiectasis

Localized	Tuberculous scarring, upper lobes (postprimary disease)
	Bronchial disease
	Extrinsic compression
	Enlarged hilar nodes
	Bronchial stenosis/occlusion
	Bronchial atresia
	Tuberculosis
	Sarcoidosis
	Prior bronchial injury
	Endobronchial mass
	Carcinoid tumor
	Bronchogenic carcinoma
	Foreign body
Diffuse	Cystic fibrosis
	Dysmotile cilia syndrome
	Congenital immunodeficiency
	Postinfectious
	Adenovirus (Swyer-James)
	Measles
	Pertussis
	Chronic aspiration
	Allergic bronchopulmonary aspergillosis
	Interstitial pulmonary fibrosis (traction bronchiectasis)

mucus plugs the small airways, leading to bronchial obstruction and infection. A vicious cycle of recurrent infection, most often with *P. aeruginosa* or *S. aureus*, eventually leads to severe bronchiectasis. The bronchiectasis is associated with functional airways obstruction and dyspnea. Hemoptysis, sometimes massive, may complicate the bronchiectasis and may require treatment by transcatheter bronchial artery embolization. Chest radiographs in affected adults show hyperinflation with predominantly upper lobe bronchiectasis and mucus plugging. Distal atelectasis and obstructive pneumonitis are common findings. The pulmonary hila may be prominent from enlarged lymph nodes because of chronic infection or from vascular dilation associated with pulmonary arterial hypertension. The diagnosis rests on a positive family history and a sweat test with an abnormally high concentration of chloride. Improvements in antibiotic therapy and pulmonary toilet have increased long-term survival, but the overall prognosis remains poor, with most patients succumbing to respiratory insufficiency in young adulthood. Recently, inhaled recombinant DNAase used to reduce the viscosity of tracheobronchial secretions has brought symptomatic and functional improvement to a number of patients. Lung or heart/lung transplantation is an option in selected individuals.

Dysmotile Cilia Syndrome describes a disorder in which the epithelial cilial motion is abnormal and ineffective. A wide variety of structural cilial abnormalities may be found, the most common of which is an absence of the outer dynein arms of the peripheral microtubules of the cilia. The abnormality may result in rhinitis, sinusitis, bronchiectasis, dysmotile sper-matozoa and sterility, situs inversus, and dextrocardia. The triad of sinusitis, situs inversus, and bronchiectasis is known as Kartagener's syndrome. Chest radiographs show diffuse bronchiectasis and hyperinflation; situs inversus is seen in approximately 50% of patients (Fig. 15.34). The diagnosis is made on the basis of the clinical and radiographic findings, along with studies of cilial anatomy and motion on samples obtained from nasal biopsy.

Infection. A severe childhood pneumonia, usually the sequela of infection with adenovirus, measles, or pertussis (the latter two are seen not uncommonly in nonimmunized Asian immigrants), may cause severe bronchial damage and recurrent infection with resultant bronchiectasis (Fig. 15.33). In some patients, childhood bronchitis and bronchiolitis are associated with obstructive airways disease and an underdeveloped lung, the latter is known as the Swyer-James syndrome.

Allergic Bronchopulmonary Aspergillosis represents a hypersensitivity reaction to *Aspergillus* and is characterized clinically by asthma, blood eosinophilia, bronchiectasis with mucus plugging, and circulating antibodies to *Aspergillus* antigen. An immediate (type I) hypersensitivity reaction to *Aspergillus* antigen accounts for acute episodes of wheezing and dyspnea, while an immune complex-mediated (type III) hypersensitivity within the lobar bronchi leads to bronchial wall inflammation and proximal bronchiectasis. Affected patients invariably have an allergic history; there is a significant association with cystic fibrosis. Patients with this disorder have recurrent episodes of cough, wheezing, and expectoration of mucus plugs. The chest radiograph is diagnostic, with proximal, predominantly upper lobe bronchiectasis. The dilated bronchi may be seen as dilated air-filled tubules or as broad-branching opacities characteristic of mucoid impaction within the dilated bronchi. Computed tomography and HRCT are helpful in characterizing the opacities as dilated bronchi. Corticosteroids are the treatment of choice.

Bronchial Disease. Bronchiectasis can develop distal to an endobronchial obstruction because of neoplasm, atresia, or stenosis. Slow-growing central bronchogenic neoplasms that have a large endoluminal component (e.g., carcinoid tumor) may obstruct the distal bronchi and produce bronchiectasis with mucus plugging (mucoceles). Similarly, bronchial atresia or bronchostenosis from trauma or chronic bronchial infection, as is seen with endobronchial TB, can lead to distal bronchial dilation. The plain radiographic recognition of mucocele formation in patients with endobronchial obstruction rests upon adequate collateral ventilation to the lung supplied by the obstructed airway. Unfortunately, in most patients, collapse of lung around the dilated mucus-filled bronchi

Figure 15.34. Dysmotile Cilia (Kartagener's) Syndrome. A. A PA chest film shows bilateral lower lobe cystic bronchiectasis and thoracic situs inversus. The abdominal situs is ambiguous. **B.** A Water's view from a sinus series shows opacification of the maxillary sinuses, consistent with chronic sinusitis.

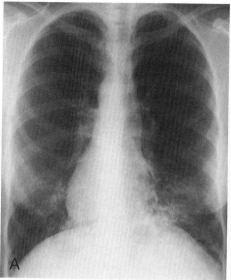
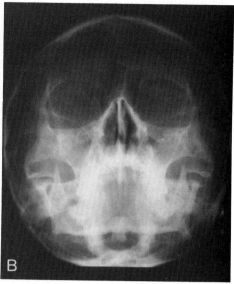

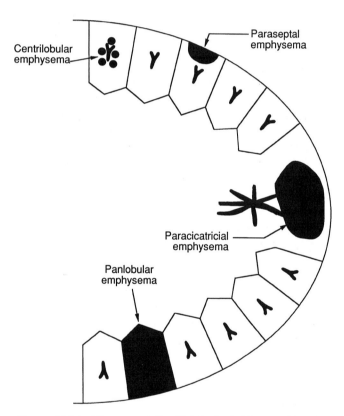

Figure 15.35. Diagram of the Histologic Subtypes of Emphysema.

precludes diagnosis on plain radiographs. Computed tomography will show the central airway obstruction and dilated mucus bronchograms, and can help guide bronchoscopic examination and biopsy.

Traction Bronchiectasis. Traction bronchiectasis is a term used to describe the effect of severe pulmonary fibrosis on the peripheral airways. Airways traversing regions of parenchymal fibrosis and honeycombing often become irregularly dilated as

their walls are retracted by the fibrotic process. This occurs most commonly in the upper lobes of the lung in patients with longstanding TB and in the subpleural regions of the lower lobes in patients with end-stage idiopathic pulmonary fibrosis. Because the accompanying fibrosis precludes visualization of the dilated bronchi radiographically, traction bronchiectasis is best appreciated on HRCT studies of the lung (Fig. 15.27**B**).

EMPHYSEMA

Definition and Subtypes. Emphysema is a pathologic diagnosis that is defined as an abnormal, permanent enlargement of the air spaces distal to the terminal bronchiole, accompanied by destruction of alveolar walls, and without obvious fibrosis. Emphysema is classified pathologically by the portion of the secondary pulmonary lobule that is primarily affected (Fig. 15.35) *Centrilobular emphysema* is the most common form and is characterized by air space distension in the central portion of the lobule centered about the proximal respiratory bronchioles, with sparing of the more distal portions of the lobule. This form of emphysema affects the upper lobes to a greater extent than the lower lobes. *Panlobular emphysema* results in uniform distension of the air spaces throughout the substance of the lobule from the central respiratory bronchioles to the peripheral alveolar sacs and alveoli. In contrast to centrilobular emphysema, this form has a predilection for the lower lobes. *Paraseptal emphysema* is seen as selective distension of peripheral air spaces adjacent to interlobular septa, with sparing of the centrilobular region. This form of emphysema is most often seen in the immediate subpleural regions of the upper lobes. Paraseptal emphysema may coalesce to form apical bullae; rupture of these bullae into the pleural space may give rise to spontaneous pneumothorax.

Etiology and Pathogenesis. The most common etiologic factor for the development of emphysema is cigarette smoking. This is associated predominantly with centrilobular emphysema, but may be a contributing factor in the development of panlobular emphysema. The pathogenesis of centrilobular emphysema is complex and has not been completely elucidated. It is known that cigarette smoke leads to excess neutrophil deposition in the lung. This causes the release of proteases (e.g., elastase) and antiprotease inhibitors, which in turn leads to destruction of alveolar septa. Inflammation and obstruction of small airways likely contribute to distal air distension and alveolar septal disruption. The association between deficiency of the serum protein α_1-antitrypsin (α_1-protease inhibitor) and the development of panlobular emphysema is well established. This disease is inherited as an autosomal recessive trait. Individuals homozygous for both recessive genes (ZZ phenotype) develop panlobular emphysema by middle age. Heterozygotes (MZ phenotype) have only a slightly increased incidence of emphysema. Cigarette smoking, by producing excess antiprotease inhibitors, can accelerate the development of emphysema in patients with the ZZ and MZ phenotypes.

Clinical Findings and Functional Abnormalities. As a definitive diagnosis of emphysema requires tissue, the diagnosis during life is based upon a combination of clinical, functional, and radiographic findings. Most patients with emphysema are long-term cigarette smokers. Symptoms associated with emphysema include dyspnea and a productive cough, the latter attributable to the presence of chronic bronchitis, which often accompanies centrilobular emphysema. The functional hallmarks of emphysema are decreased airflow on spirometry and decreased diffusing capacity. Expiratory airflow obstruction is expressed as a decrease in the volume of air expired in the first second of a forced expiratory maneuver from total lung capacity (FEV_1) and a decrease in the ratio of FEV_1 to the total volume of air expired during a forced expiratory maneuver (FEV_1/FVC). Airflow obstruction is secondary to increased airways resistance and decreased driving pressure (i.e., elastic recoil). In patients with moderate-to-severe emphysema, the predominant factor limiting expiratory airflow is the decreased elastic recoil that results from parenchymal destruction. Airflow obstruction, however, is not invariably present in patients with mild emphysema.

Diffusing capacity, measured by the diffusion of carbon monoxide from the alveoli into the bloodstream during a single breath hold ($DL_{CO}SB$), assesses the integrity and surface area of the alveolocapillary membrane within the lung. Emphysema decreases the diffusing capacity of the lung by diminishing the volume of pulmonary parenchyma available for gas exchange. A decreased $DL_{CO}SB$ due to emphysema correlates well with the severity of the emphysema. While an abnormal diffusing capacity is more sensitive than abnormal spirometry in diagnosing emphysema, it is nonspecific. Since $DL_{CO}SB$ depends predominantly on the surface area available for gas diffusion and the number and hemoglobin content of red blood cells within the pulmonary capillaries, any process affecting these factors can alter the measurement of $DL_{CO}SB$. For example, a decreased $DL_{CO}SB$ can be seen in any disease that diminishes the volume of pulmonary capillaries available for gas diffusion (e.g., pulmonary embolism), interferes with gas exchange across the alveolocapillary membrane (e.g., interstitial pulmonary fibrosis), or produces airway obstruction, thereby diminishing the gas-exchanging air spaces (i.e., cystic fibrosis). Furthermore, some patients with mild-to-moderate morphologic emphysema can have a normal $DL_{CO}SB$.

Radiologic Evaluation. Frontal and lateral chest radiographs are the initial radiographic examinations obtained in patients with suspected emphysema. The plain radiographic findings of emphysema are listed in Table 15.19. Hyperinflation is the most important plain radiographic finding and reflects the loss of lung elastic recoil; it is the radiographic equivalent of an abnormally increased total lung capacity (TLC). The abnormal increase in lung volume is best detected by noting inferior displacement and flattening of the normally convex superior hemidiaphragms, right or obtuse angles to the normally acute-angled costophrenic sulci, and an increase in the AP chest diameter, best appreciated by noting an increase in the depth of the retrosternal clear space. Absent or attenuated peripheral vascular markings results from parenchymal destruction and obliteration of peripheral pulmonary arteries traversing emphysematous areas (Fig. 15.36). When the characteristic thin walls of bullae are seen marginating the peripheral avascular regions, emphysema can be diagnosed with certainty. Increased radiolucency of the lungs on radiographs due to pulmonary hyperinflation and attenuation of peripheral vascular markings is difficult to detect because it is subject to various patient and technical factors and therefore is an inaccurate indicator of the presence of emphysema.

The effects of emphysema and chronic hypoxemia on the right heart may be appreciated as enlargement of the central pulmonary arteries and right ventricle in those with complicating pulmonary arterial hypertension and cor pulmonale (12). The use of the term COPD to describe patients with the plain radiographic findings of emphysema is inaccurate and should be

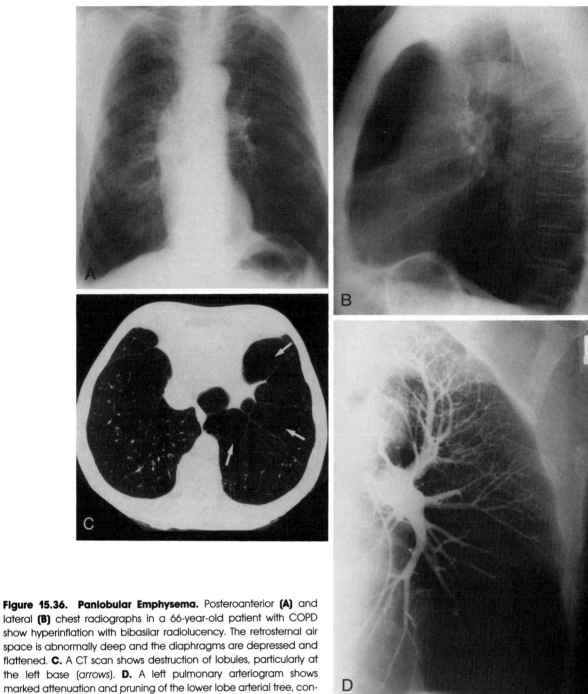

Figure 15.36. Panlobular Emphysema. Posteroanterior **(A)** and lateral **(B)** chest radiographs in a 66-year-old patient with COPD show hyperinflation with bibasilar radiolucency. The retrosternal air space is abnormally deep and the diaphragms are depressed and flattened. **C.** A CT scan shows destruction of lobules, particularly at the left base (*arrows*). **D.** A left pulmonary arteriogram shows marked attenuation and pruning of the lower lobe arterial tree, consistent with arterial deficiency (panlobular) emphysema.

Table 15.19. Radiographic Findings in Pulmonary Emphysema

Finding	Explanation
Diffuse hyperlucency (panlobular)	Destruction of pulmonary capillary bed and alveolar septa
Flattening and depression of the hemidiaphragms; increased retrosternal air space (panlobular > centrilobular)	Hyperinflation due to loss of elastic recoil of lung
Bulla (panlobular > centrilobular)	Thin-walled region of confluent emphysematous destruction
Enlarged central pulmonary arteries; right heart enlargement (centrilobular)	Loss of pulmonary capillary bed; associated chronic hypoxemia causes increased pulmonary vascular resistance
Increased peripheral vascular markings (centrilobular)	? Small airways disease
	? Increased pulmonary vascularity

discouraged. Chronic obstructive pulmonary disease is a functional diagnosis, while the chest radiograph depicts anatomy only. In fact, patients with radiographic findings of hyperinflation and vascular attenuation, while invariably having emphysema morphologically, rarely can lack functional evidence of airflow obstruction and therefore do not have COPD.

It is well recognized that many patients with severe centrilobular emphysema have minimal or absent hyperinflation on chest radiographs, and tend to show increased lung markings rather than peripheral vascular attenuation. These observations have led to the description of two major groups of patients with emphysema, each with distinctive radiographic patterns. Patients with predominant panlobular emphysema show hyperinflated lungs with peripheral vascular attenuation and a normal-sized heart and central pulmonary vessels. Bullae are common in this form of emphysema. This pattern of emphysema has been termed "arterial deficiency" emphysema. Clinically, these patients are described as "pink puffers" because of their tachypnea and normal partial pressure of oxygen. Those with centrilobular emphysema show mild hyperinflation and increased linear parenchymal markings that likely represent the small airways thickening of chronic bronchitis seen concomitantly in these patients. Bullae are uncommon in this form of emphysema. This radiographic pattern of emphysema has been termed "increased markings" emphysema. As a result of chronic hypoxemia, these individuals develop secondary polycythemia and are described as "blue bloaters." Although most patients do not fit neatly into one or the other category either clinically or radiographically, familiarity with these two patterns will allow for the correct diagnosis in the majority of patients with moderately severe or severe centrilobular or panlobular emphysema.

While widespread, extensive emphysema may be accurately diagnosed on chest radiographs, mild disease is often not evident radiographically. The use of chest CT has allowed for the diagnosis of emphysema in the absence of chest radiographic findings of hyperinflation or parenchymal abnormalities. Computed tomography, due to its cross-sectional nature and high-contrast resolution, is ideally suited to the diagnosis of emphysema. Early reports on the use of CT to diagnose emphysema depended upon the recognition of either large avascular areas or regions with abnormally low Hounsfield attenuation numbers. More recently, improvements in detectors, shorter scan times, and the ability to perform HRCT have allowed for better characterization of centrilobular emphysema. Centrilobular emphysema is now seen as discrete, well-defined areas of abnormally low attenuation lacking definable walls and situated centrally within the secondary pulmonary lobule adjacent to

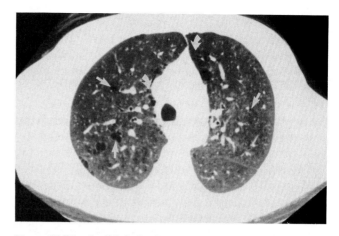

Figure 15.37. Centrilobular Emphysema on HRCT. An HRCT scan through the upper lobes in a 56-year-old cigarette smoker demonstrates well-defined regions of low attenuation that lack definable walls (*straight arrows*) centered around pulmonary arteries, diagnostic of centrilobular emphysema. Paraseptal emphysema (*curved arrows*) is also seen.

the bronchovascular bundle. The HRCT, with its thin collimation technique and high spatial resolution, can detect mild centrilobular emphysema that may be missed on conventional, 10-mm collimated CT due to partial volume averaging of small emphysematous areas within the thickness of the scan section (Fig. 15.37).

Bullous Lung Disease

Bullae are thin-walled cystic spaces exceeding 1 cm in diameter that are found within the lung parenchyma (Fig. 15.10). Bullae represent confluent areas of emphysematous lung and may be seen in a variety of disorders in which there is no functional evidence of COPD. The increased lung weight and chronic elevation of transpleural pressure in patients with lower lobe interstitial pulmonary fibrosis predispose to bullae formation. Bullae may also be seen in diseases causing chronic upper lobe fibrosis, including sarcoidosis, pulmonary histiocytosis X, and ankylosing spondylitis. In these diseases, chronic bronchiolar obstruction leads to distal air space distension, alveolar septal disruption, and development of bullae.

There is a group of disorders in which bullae are isolated lesions without intervening areas of emphysema or interstitial lung disease (primary bullous disease) (Table 15.20). Primary bullous lung disease has been found in families, in association with Marfan's or Ehlers-Danlos syndromes, in intravenous drug users, in HIV infection, and in the vanishing lung syndrome, which is an accelerated form of paraseptal emphysema seen in young adult males (Fig. 15.38). Most patients are asymptomatic unless large bullae compress normal parenchyma, resulting in compressive atelectasis and dyspnea. Radiographically, iso-

Table 15.20.   Primary Bullous Lung Disease

Familial
Vanishing lung disease
Marfan's syndrome
Ehlers-Danlos syndrome
Intravenous drug use
HIV infection

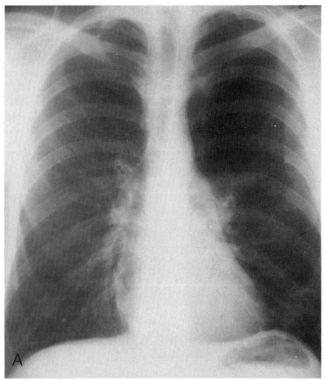

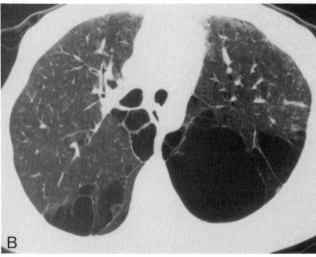

Figure 15.38.   Primary Bullous Lung Disease. A. Frontal radiograph in an asymptomatic 29-year-old man demonstrates biapical bullous disease that is most severe in the left upper lobe. **B.** A CT scan demonstrates peripheral upper lobe bulla with normal adjacent lung.

lated bullae tend to have an upper lobe distribution and appear as rounded, thin-walled lucencies of vary-

ing size. These lesions can become huge as a result of air trapping, causing depression of the ipsilateral lung and hemidiaphragm and even producing contralateral mediastinal shift. Computed tomography is useful in evaluating the extent of bullous disease and the amount of compressed pulmonary tissue.

Spontaneous pneumothorax is a complication of the rupture of a subpleural bulla into the pleural space. Patients with this condition may be difficult to manage; persistent air leaks lead to prolonged and often unsuccessful closed tube drainage of the pleural space and reexpansion of the lung. If a bulla becomes secondarily infected, chest radiographs or CT will demonstrate an air-fluid level within the bulla that resolves over several weeks with the administration of antibiotics. Rarely, cancer develops within the wall of a bulla. Symptomatic patients and those with enlarging bullae should be considered for bullectomy. Radioisotope lung perfusion studies may be performed preoperatively to assess the amount of perfused and potentially functional lung parenchyma compressed by the bulla (see Chapter 49).

Bronchiolitis, Bronchiolitis Obliterans, and Bronchiolitis Obliterans Organizing Pneumonia (BOOP)

Bronchiolitis and Bronchiolitis Obliterans. Bronchiolitis refers to an inflammation of the small, noncartilaginous airways. Infectious bronchiolitis, a disease of young children caused by respiratory syncytial virus or adenovirus, produces respiratory distress and radiographic hyperinflation indistinguishable from asthma. Bronchiolitis in adults is a subacute disorder that is most often idiopathic but may be seen in a variety of disorders. It is characterized pathologically by a mononuclear cell inflammatory process within the walls of respiratory bronchioles that leads to the formation of granulation tissue that plug small airways; hence the term "bronchiolitis obliterans." This disease causes dyspnea and functional airways obstruction. As discussed in "Chronic Interstitial Lung Disease," bronchiolitis obliterans with or without organizing pneumonia may be secondary to viral infection, toxic fume inhalation, collagen vascular disorders, organ transplantation, and chronic aspiration.

Bronchiolitis obliterans in the adult may be the result of an early childhood lower respiratory infection with adenovirus, in which case it is known as unilateral hyperlucent lung or the Swyer-James syndrome. In the Swyer-James syndrome, the bronchiolitis causes diffuse small airways obliteration, air trapping, and destruction of alveolar walls and emphysema due to overdistension of peripheral air spaces. Since bronchiolitis obliterans tends to occur during

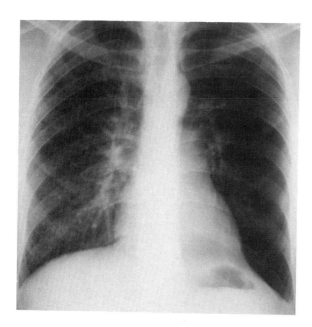

Figure 15.39. Swyer-James Syndrome. A PA radiograph in a 27-year-old man demonstrates a hyperlucent left lung with diminished vasculature. Air trapping in the left lung was evident on fluoroscopy. The patient had a history of multiple childhood pulmonary infections.

the time of continued lung growth and development, the lung is usually small and the ipsilateral pulmonary artery hypoplastic. This process is asymmetric, involving one lung solely or predominantly, producing a unilateral hyperlucent lung for which this disease is named. Most patients with the Swyer-James syndrome are asymptomatic, while others complain of dyspnea or repeated lower respiratory tract infections. If the inflammatory process and granulation tissue of bronchiolitis obliterans extend to involve the alveolar spaces adjacent to the affected bronchioles, it is termed BOOP; BOOP is more common than bronchiolitis obliterans and is discussed in this section.

The chest radiograph in patients with pure bronchiolitis obliterans may be normal despite the presence of severe dyspnea and functional evidence of airflow obstruction. The most common radiographic abnormality in this disorder is diffuse reticulonodular opacities with associated hyperinflation. Central bronchiectasis has been described, particularly in those with bronchiolitis obliterans developing as a complication of heart-lung transplantation. In patients with the Swyer-James syndrome, the affected lung is normal or small in volume (Fig. 15.39); marked unilateral air trapping is seen on fluoroscopy or expiratory films. The air trapping is due to bronchiolar obstruction with collateral air drift to the distal air spaces on inspiration that cannot escape on expiration. The ipsilateral hilum is small and the pulmonary vasculature reduced, accounting for the hyperlucency seen radiographically. Perfusion lung scanning

shows decreased perfusion of the affected lung, while the xenon ventilation study shows decreased ventilation with markedly delayed radioisotope washout. This latter finding helps distinguish the Swyer-James syndrome from primary central pulmonary artery occlusion or hypoplastic lung in which ventilation is maintained.

Bronchiolitis Obliterans Organizing Pneumonia. Bronchiolitis obliterans organizinq pneumonia (BOOP) is characterized by the widespread deposition of granulation tissue (fibroblasts, collagen, and capillaries) within small airways and peribronchiolar air spaces. Most cases are idiopathic but a number of conditions have been associated with this disorder, including viral infection (influenza, adenovirus, measles), toxic fume inhalation (sulfur dioxide, chlorine), collagen vascular disorders (rheumatoid arthritis and SLE), organ transplantation (bone marrow and heart-lung), drugs, and chronic aspiration.

Pathologically, a mononuclear cell exudate in the bronchioles and surrounding alveoli organizes to form intrabronchiolar and intraalveolar granulation tissue. A characteristic of this disease is the uniformity of the histologic changes and the absence of parenchymal distortion and fibrosis; these features help distinguish BOOP from idiopathic pulmonary fibrosis, which can have similar clinical, functional, and radiographic features.

Patients with BOOP often have a subacute illness characterized by a nonproductive cough and dyspnea of several weeks or months in duration. The physical examination may reveal rales or wheezes. Pulmonary function tests usually show a restrictive pattern of disease with diminished lung volumes and normal-to-increased flow rates. Airways obstruction is uncommon in BOOP, but is invariably present in patients with pure bronchiolitis obliterans. The diffusing capacity is significantly decreased.

Radiographic examination in patients with BOOP reveals patchy bilateral air space or ground-glass opacities, with some patients showing scattered nodular opacities. These opacities represent areas of organizing pneumonia centered about the affected bronchioles. The air space and ground-glass opacities tend to be peripheral in distribution, a feature best appreciated on CT scans.

The diagnosis of BOOP can be made only by recognizing the characteristic histologic changes on open lung biopsy. The distinction of BOOP from idiopathic pulmonary fibrosis may be difficult but is important as BOOP has a more favorable prognosis and usually responds rapidly to corticosteroid therapy. Bronchiolitis obliterans organizing pneumonia complicating heart-lung transplantation generally has a worse prognosis but may respond favorably to immunosuppressive therapy.

Broncholithiasis

Broncholithiasis, the presence of calcified material within the tracheobronchial tree, develops from erosion of a calcified peribronchial lymph node into the bronchial lumen. Most calcified lymph nodes result from granulomatous lymph node inflammation due to histoplasmosis or TB. Broncholiths may occlude the airway and lead to bronchiectasis, obstructive atelectasis, or pneumonia. Patients are often asymptomatic but may have cough productive of stones or calcified material (lithoptysis). Hemoptysis may develop from erosion of the broncholith into a bronchial vessel.

DRUG-INDUCED LUNG DISEASE

Drugs can induce a variety of adverse effects in the lung (13). The majority of cases of drug-induced lung disease are iatrogenic, though accidental or intentional drug overdoses may result in severe pulmonary disease. The changes are often difficult to distinguish from infection, cardiogenic or fluid overload pulmonary edema, or a pulmonary manifestation of the disease being treated. The pleuropulmonary effects of drugs can be divided by category of drug, mechanism of the adverse effects, or by acute or chronic disease.

Mechanisms of Drug Reaction

ACUTE REACTIONS

There are a limited number of ways for drugs to produce acute pulmonary disease. An acute pulmonary reaction may involve a hypersensitivity response to a metabolite of the drug combined with an endogenous protein. Antibody production directed against this haptene-protein complex leads to antibody-mediated immediate or immune complex hypersensitivity reactions. In the lung, this produces bronchospasm or eosinophilic pneumonia, usually associated with fever, skin rash, and blood eosinophilia. Radiographically, fleeting peripheral patchy air space opacities are seen, which develop hours to days after the initiation of drug therapy (Fig. 15.40). The opacities often respond to corticosteroid therapy. The penicillin and sulfonamide antibiotics are the drugs most often associated with hypersensitivity reactions.

The other common acute lung reaction to administered drugs is a capillary leak pulmonary edema that is histologically identical to the early changes seen in ARDS. Heroin and crack cocaine are commonly associated with this reaction. Radiographically, the lungs show acute interstitial or air space opacities that are indistinguishable from those of cardiogenic pulmonary edema, although the heart size is usually normal. Characteristically, the edema clears as rapidly as it appeared.

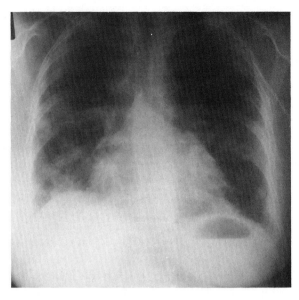

Figure 15.40. Bleomycin Lung Toxicity. A PA radiograph in a 42-year-old woman with 3 weeks of shortness of breath following completion of chemotherapy for Hodgkin's disease with bleomycin. There are bilateral, predominantly peripheral air space opacities with a lower lobe predominance. Open biopsy showed changes consistent with bleomycin lung toxicity.

Acute pulmonary hemorrhage and infarction may occur secondary to drug-induced pulmonary vasculitis, while diffuse hemorrhage may complicate anticoagulation therapy with Coumadin (warfarin) or following intensive chemotherapy administered prior to bone marrow transplantation. Penicillamine therapy has been associated with pulmonary hemorrhage in patients with rheumatoid arthritis via an unknown mechanism. Affected individuals typically have hemoptysis and a falling hematocrit, which is associated with the rapid development of diffuse bilateral air space opacities. The diagnosis is usually confirmed by noting bloody fluid return on bronchoalveolar lavage, with an increased percentage of alveolar macrophages containing hemosiderin deposits. The opacities of diffuse pulmonary hemorrhage clear completely without residual scarring, while the focal opacities of pulmonary infarcts may leave pleuroparenchymal scars.

CHRONIC REACTIONS

Chronic pulmonary or pleural disease generally develops weeks to months after initial exposure to the offending drug, but can be delayed for years. The most common form of chronic lung toxicity from drugs is that of a chronic interstitial pneumonitis, with the subsequent development of pulmonary fibrosis seen in the healing phase of this disorder. The drugs most commonly implicated in this form of lung disease are the chemotherapeutic agents cyclophosphamide, bleomycin, and methotrexate, amiodarone, and nitrofurantoin. Radiographically, there are bilateral, predominantly lower lobe, coarse reticular and linear opacities with diminished lung volumes. These findings in patients undergoing chemotherapy for malignancy are difficult to distinguish from lymphangitic carcinomatosis, pulmonary hemorrhage, or opportunistic pneumonia, while pulmonary edema is the major differential diagnosis in patients on amiodarone therapy. The diagnosis is usually made by excluding one of these other processes. Unusually, pulmonary nodules are seen as a manifestation of chronic lung injury from bleomycin or cytoxan, which is indistinguishable radiographically from pulmonary metastases from solid tumors.

A number of drugs have been associated with a lupus-like syndrome that is often indistinguishable from SLE. The drugs most commonly producing a lupus-like reaction are procainamide, hydralazine, and isoniazid. Pleural and pericardial effusions are common. Basilar interstitial disease has been described, but is uncommon.

A chronic granulomatous vasculitis may develop as a response to particulate substances such as talc or starch mixed with illicit intravenous drugs. This can lead to obliteration of the pulmonary vasculature, producing pulmonary hypertension and right ventricular failure. Radiographically, the lungs may show an interstitial pattern of disease, with enlargement of the central pulmonary arteries and right heart. Rarely, the radiographs may show central conglomerate masses indistinguishable from those seen in the progressive massive fibrosis of silicosis or end-stage sarcoidosis.

Enlargement of hilar and mediastinal lymph nodes on chest radiographs is an uncommon manifestation of drug toxicity. Dilantin (phenytoin) and methotrexate are the main drugs associated with this complication. The lymph node enlargement is usually part of a systemic hypersensitivity reaction, and regresses with removal of the offending agent.

SPECIFIC DRUG TOXICITIES

Nitrofurantoin is an oral antibiotic widely used in the treatment of urinary tract infections. There are two distinct patterns of nitrofurantoin-associated pulmonary reaction: acute and chronic. The acute form, seen in approximately 90% of cases, most likely represents a hypersensitivity reaction; the chest film demonstrates interstitial or mixed alveolar/interstitial infiltrates with a basal predominance, often accompanied by small pleural effusions. The chronic form only becomes manifest after weeks to years of continuous therapy and is probably due to direct toxic damage. Pathologically, interstitial pneumonitis and fibrosis indistinguishable from idiopathic pulmonary fibrosis is usually seen. The chest radiograph demonstrates a diffuse reticular pattern with relative basal predominance; lung volumes are usually reduced.

Bleomycin is a cytotoxic antibiotic used in the treatment of lymphoma, squamous cell carcinoma, and testicular cancer. The development of bleomycin-induced lung disease is related to the cumulative dosage of the drug. Free oxygen radicals within the lung are believed to play a major role in the lung injury, accounting for the deleterious effects of supplemental oxygen administration in patients with bleomycin toxicity. Radiographically, a reticular pattern is seen which often progresses to patchy or widespread air space opacification. The opacities have a basal predominance. An unusual radiographic appearance of bleomycin lung toxicity is that of a solitary or multiple pulmonary nodules indistinguishable radiographically from pulmonary metastases; the lesions generally disappear following cessation of the drug.

Alkylating Agents. Drugs such as busulfan, which is used in the treatment of myeloproliferative disorders, and cyclophosphamide, used widely in the treatment of malignancies and autoimmune disease, can cause clinically recognizable pulmonary toxicity in 1–4% of patients. Pathologic findings include organizing intraalveolar exudate, fibrosis, and the presence of large atypical type II pneumocytes. Radiographically, a diffuse reticular pattern with basal predominance is seen; air space opacities may be present and are more common with busulfan than from cyclophosphamide.

Methotrexate is an antimetabolite used for the treatment of malignancy and autoimmune disease such as rheumatoid arthritis and psoriasis. In contrast to bleomycin and the alkylating agents, methotrexate usually causes reversible pulmonary disease resulting from a hypersensitivity reaction rather than direct toxic damage to the lung. However, diffuse alveolar damage leading to restrictive lung disease is seen in approximately 10% of cases and appears radiographically as a diffuse reticular pattern.

Amiodarone. This antiarrhythmic agent is an important cause of drug-induced pulmonary damage, affecting approximately 5% of individuals on chronic therapy. Amiodarone is concentrated in the lung and has a long tissue half-life. The exact mechanism of lung damage is unknown, but relates to the accumulation of phospholipids that disturb metabolic functions in the lung. Pathologically, there is inflammation and fibrosis of the alveolar septae, with an accumulation of lipid-laden alveolar macrophages and hyperplasia of type II pneumocytes.

Pulmonary toxicity begins months to years after the initiation of therapy. Patients typically present with dyspnea or a nonproductive cough that may be difficult to distinguish from congestive heart failure or pneumonia. The chest film typically shows a diffuse reticular pattern due to interstitial fibrosis. In addition, multiple peripheral air space opacities may be seen, often with an upper lobe predominance. Gallium lung scanning is often used to detect subradiographic pulmonary involvement from amiodarone toxicity and to distinguish this from pulmonary edema. Amiodarone should be withdrawn or the dose diminished at the earliest sign of toxicity as the drug has an extraordinarily long half-life (approximately 90 days). The cessation of therapy at an early stage of toxicity, with occasional use of corticosteroids, usually provides relief.

RADIATION-INDUCED LUNG DISEASE

The pulmonary effects of external irradiation, most commonly administered for palliation of unresectable bronchogenic carcinoma or the treatment of mediastinal Hodgkin's lymphoma, depend upon several variables. The volume of lung treated will affect the incidence of radiation injury; the greater the volume irradiated, the more likely radiation injury will ensue. Most radiation treatment is limited to less than one-third to one-half of the lung, as an equivalent dose administered to an entire lung or both lungs would cause serious lung injury. The total dose and the method of fractionation will affect the incidence of radiation injury. Doses of less than 2000 rads rarely produce lung injury, while doses exceeding 3000 rads have a significant incidence of radiation pneumonitis. Administration of a single large dose is more deleterious than fractionation of a similar total dose over the course of several weeks. There is variation in the susceptibility to radiation among individuals; a given dose may cause pneumonitis in one patient while another remains unaffected. The concomitant use of chemotherapeutic agents, particularly bleomycin, or the withdrawal of corticosteroid therapy may accentuate the deleterious effects of radiation.

The mechanism of radiation-induced lung injury is not completely understood, but the acute effects involve injury to capillary endothelial and pulmonary epithelial cells that line the alveoli. This diffuse alveolar damage produces a cellular, proteinaceous intraalveolar exudate and hyaline membranes that are indistinguishable histologically from ARDS. These changes develop 4–12 weeks following the completion of therapy. While most patients with acute radiation pneumonitis are asymptomatic, dyspnea and a nonproductive cough may be present. Radiographically, a sharply marginated, localized area of air space opacification is seen that does not conform to lobar or segmental anatomic boundaries and directly corresponds to the radiation portal. Adhesive atelectasis of the involved portion of lung is common as the radiation pro-

duces a loss of surfactant by damaging type II pneumocytes. Small pleural and pericardial effusions may be seen but are uncommon. The pneumonitis may resolve completely with or without the administration of corticosteroids, or may progress to pulmonary fibrosis. Pulmonary fibrosis corresponds histologically to a reparative phase with regeneration of type II pneumocytes, reorganization of the parenchyma, ingrowth of granulation tissue, and eventually interstitial fibrosis. The fibrosis usually appears as coarse linear opacities or occasionally as a homogeneous parenchymal opacity with severe cicatrizing atelectasis of the involved portion of lung. The sharp margination of the parenchymal fibrotic changes may be difficult to appreciate on plain radiographs but is usually obvious on cross-sectional CT or MR studies (Fig. 15.41). Fibrotic tissue is characteristically low signal on T2-weighted spin-echo MR sequences, a finding that is helpful in distinguishing fibrosis from recurrent tumor, which is typically high signal on T2-weighted sequences. The parenchymal changes are usually stable by 1 year following radiation therapy. Pleural thickening due to fibrosis is a common finding.

The diagnosis of radiation pneumonitis is usually made by the exclusion of infection or malignancy as a cause of the patient's symptoms and the presence of typical radiographic findings following a course of radiation therapy to the chest. This distinction may require bronchoalveolar lavage and transbronchial biopsy. The demonstration of an increased number of lymphocytes in bronchoalveolar lavage fluid and the absence of malignant cells help confirm the diagnosis. The demonstration of air space opacification on CT that conforms to a known portal of radiation is usually sufficient for the diagnosis. Gallium scanning may be used to detect subradiographic radiation-induced lung inflammation.

GRANULOMATOUS DISEASES
Sarcoidosis

Sarcoidosis is a multisystem granulomatous disease of unknown etiology characterized histologically by noncaseating granulomas that may progress to fibrosis. The disease is seen more commonly in blacks than whites and is rare in Asians. Black American women are at particular risk for this disease. Most patients are 20–40 years of age at the time of diagnosis. However, since patients with this disease are often asymptomatic, many cases are never identified.

ETIOLOGY AND PATHOGENESIS

The etiology of sarcoidosis is unknown, although an inhaled infectious agent such as *Mycobacterium*,

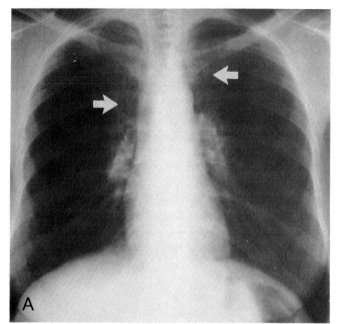

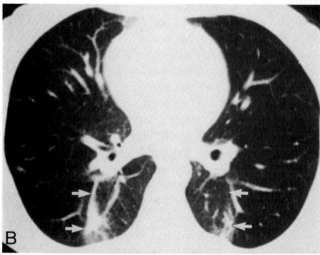

Figure 15.41. Radiation Pulmonary Fibrosis. A. A PA chest film in a 29-year-old woman who received mediastinal radiation for Hodgkin's disease at age 23. There are bilateral, coarse, vertically oriented linear opacities (*arrows*) in the paramediastinal portions of the upper lobes. **B.** A CT scan shows sharply defined fibrotic areas posteriorly (*arrows*), characteristic of radiation fibrosis.

Yersinia, or a virus has been suggested. Whatever the etiologic agent, the underlying pathogenesis involves the activation of pulmonary macrophages that in turn recruit mononuclear cells to the pulmonary interstitium leading to the formation of granulomas. The activated macrophages also stimulate proliferation of T helper lymphocytes in the lung, which induces an overactivity of B lymphocytes, resulting in the hypergammaglobulinemia characteristically seen in this disease. The excess number of T helper lymphocytes in the lung may be detected in bronchoalveolar lavage fluid of patients with sarcoidosis, and is helpful in the differential diagnosis of this condition.

PATHOLOGIC FINDINGS

The pathologic changes of sarcoidosis follow a fairly predictable pattern. The earliest changes involve the pulmonary interstitium, with the development of a nonspecific lymphocytic and histiocytic infiltrate. This progresses to the formation of microscopic granulomas. The granulomas contain palisading epithelioid histiocytes with intermixed multinucleated giant cells, and in contrast to tuberculous granulomas, are typically noncaseating. The giant cells within the granulomas may contain dark-staining lamellated structures within their cytoplasm, called Schaumann's bodies, which are characteristic of sarcoidosis. The granulomas are found most commonly within the axial (peribronchovascular) and peripheral or subpleural interstitium of the lung, but may involve the parenchymal (alveolar) interstitium and airway mucosa; the airway lesions may be visualized bronchoscopically. Involvement of the axial interstitium of the lung accounts for the high (approximately 90%) diagnostic yield of blind transbronchial biopsy in sarcoidosis, since this technique usually provides samples of the bronchial wall, the surrounding axial interstitium, and adjacent air spaces. The small granulomas usually resolve after months or years. In some patients, the microscopic granulomas coalesce to form larger nodules. Rarely, these nodules grow to form large, well-defined masses or poorly marginated opacities that contain air bronchograms and simulate an air space filling process. In this "alveolar" form of sarcoidosis, the air spaces are not filled with material but rather are compressed and obliterated by the exuberant granuloma formation within the surrounding interstitium.

In approximately 20% of patients, fibrous tissue is deposited at the periphery of the granulomas and eventually grows inward to replace the granulomas, resulting in interstitial fibrosis. The fibrosis tends to progress over time, with the development of broad bands of fibrous tissue extending from the hilar regions toward the lung apices, producing hilar elevation and distortion of the hilar vessels and upper mediastinum. Masses of fibrous tissue may develop in the perihilar regions of the upper lobes with peripheral areas of emphysema or cyst formation. These cysts predispose to spontaneous pneumothoraces and provide a site for mycetoma formation.

Lymph node involvement in sarcoidosis is characterized by replacement of the normal nodal architecture with granulomas indistinguishable from those found in the pulmonary parenchyma. As with parenchymal involvement, these may regress, coalesce, or undergo fibrosis.

CLINICAL FINDINGS AND FUNCTIONAL ABNORMALITIES

The clinical presentation may be dominated by pulmonary or extrapulmonary manifestations of the disease, but a considerable percentage of patients are asymptomatic and are identified by incidental findings on chest radiographs. Pulmonary symptoms are present in 25% of patients and include dyspnea and a nonproductive cough. Common extrapulmonary findings include fever, malaise, uveitis, and erythema nodosum. In a minority of patients, involvement of liver, heart, kidneys, or central nervous system may dominate the clinical picture.

Common laboratory findings in sarcoidosis include hypercalcemia, hypergammaglobulinemia, and elevated serum angiotensin-converting enzyme levels. Cutaneous anergy to PPD (purified protein derivatives) reflects an abnormality of delayed hypersensitivity found in these patients. Pulmonary function tests vary from normal in those with minimal or no parenchymal disease to a severe restrictive pattern with low diffusing capacity in patients with end-stage pulmonary fibrosis.

RADIOGRAPHIC FINDINGS

Lymph Node Enlargement. Enlargement of mediastinal and hilar lymph nodes is found in 80% of patients with sarcoidosis, and is associated with radiographically normal lungs in slightly more than half of these patients. The typical appearance on chest radiographs is right paratracheal and bilateral symmetric hilar lymph node enlargement (Figs. 13.9, 14.9). The symmetric enlargement is a key feature that allows distinction from malignancy and TB, conditions that usually produce unilateral or asymmetric lymph node enlargement. Left paratracheal lymph node enlargement is common, as determined by CT, though enlargement of these nodes is usually not appreciated on radiographs since this region is obscured by the aorta and great vessels on frontal radiographs. The enlarged nodes tend to have a lobulated contour as the individual nodes remain discrete. Mediastinal (i.e, paratracheal) lymph node enlargement without concomitant hilar enlargement is uncommon and should suggest lymphoma or metastatic disease. Similarly, unilateral hilar nodal enlargement is unusual, seen in only 5% of individuals. Involvement of anterior mediastinal, posterior mediastinal, subcarinal, and aortopulmonary lymph nodes occurs with greater frequency than previously believed, because of the ability of CT to detect nodes in regions that are invisible on plain radiographs. Involved nodes may show contrast enhancement.

The enlarged lymph nodes regress within 2 years in 75% of patients. A small percentage of patients will have persistent lymph node enlargement for years.

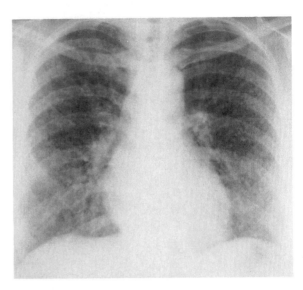

Figure 15.42. Sarcoidosis. A PA chest film in a 39-year-old black female with minimal shortness of breath shows extensive bilateral reticulonodular opacities. Transbronchial biopsy showed noncaseating granulomas typical of sarcoidosis.

The development of parenchymal opacities concomitant with the resolution of lymph node enlargement is a helpful feature in differentiating sarcoidosis from lymphoma, in which enlarged lymph nodes do not regress when parenchymal abnormalities develop. Calcification of involved lymph nodes is common, seen in up to 20% of patients, and may involve only the periphery of the node (eggshell calcification).

Lung Disease. The lung is involved radiographically in only 40–50% of patients with sarcoidosis, despite the nearly 90% yield from transbronchial biopsy of the lung (14). The earliest finding is a diffuse micronodular pattern identical in appearance to miliary TB, which represents the superimposition of microscopic granulomas. This pattern, which is rarely identified radiographically, may precede the development of hilar lymph node enlargement. The most common parenchymal abnormality is bilateral symmetric reticulonodular opacities that have a predilection for the middle and upper lung zones (Fig. 15.42). The reticulonodular opacities represent the combination of granulomas and fibrosis. Computed tomography shows most nodules lie predominantly in a peribronchovascular and subpleural location. The appearance of reticulonodular opacities never precedes the enlargement of hilar and mediastinal lymph nodes.

In approximately 10% of patients, the coalescence of granulomas can produce one of two unusual radiographic manifestations of parenchymal sarcoidosis. Exuberant interstitial granulomas can obliterate adjacent air spaces, producing poorly defined air space opacities that may contain air bronchograms. In some cases, intraalveolar inflammation and granulomas contribute to the alveolar pattern of disease. These air

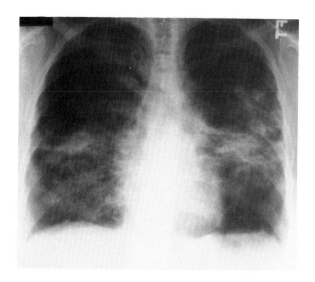

Figure 15.43. Bullous Changes in Sarcoidosis. In a 49-year-old woman with long-standing sarcoidosis, a PA chest film shows extensive middle and lower zone coarse interstitial opacities and biapical bullous disease.

Table 15.21. Radiographic Staging of Sarcoidosis

Stage	Radiographic Findings
0	Normal chest radiograph
1	Bilateral hilar lymph node enlargement
2	Bilateral hilar lymph node enlargement and parenchymal disease
3	Parenchymal disease only
4	Pulmonary fibrosis

space opacities are primarily seen in the peripheral portions of the midlung zone, thereby simulating eosinophilic pneumonia radiographically. The presence of reticulonodular opacities elsewhere in the lung or concomitant symmetric hilar and mediastinal lymph node enlargement, best seen on CT and HRCT, provide important clues to the diagnosis.

Nodular or mass-like sarcoidosis develops in a manner similar to alveolar disease. These masses can be quite large and typically have a sharp margin. Air bronchograms are often demonstrated on CT and HRCT; cavitation is extremely rare.

Pulmonary fibrosis develops in 20% of patients with long-standing parenchymal involvement. The chest radiograph shows coarse linear opacities extending obliquely from the hila toward the upper and middle lung zones. There is considerable distortion and elevation of the hila, scalloping of the lung-mediastinal interface. Occasionally, conglomerate masses of fibrosis form in the upper perihilar regions, which simulate the progressive massive fibrosis of complicated silicosis. On CT, these masses contain air bronchograms with traction bronchiectasis. Distortion and obstruction of the airways from fibrosis can lead to secondary air trapping, with resultant alveolar septal disruption and bullae formation. An increase in radiographic lung volumes may accompany these cystic changes, a finding characteristic of bullous sarcoidosis (Fig. 15.43). Mycetomas can develop within the cysts and lead to massive hemoptysis from erosion into bronchial arteries. Cysts may also rupture into the pleural space and produce spontaneous pneumothoraces.

Pleural Changes. Pleural thickening or effusion occurs in approximately 7% of patients with sar-

coidosis, and is caused by a granulomatous inflammation of the visceral and parietal pleura.

Miscellaneous Findings. Endobronchial granulomas can result in fibrosis of the bronchial wall and bronchostenosis. Pulmonary arterial hypertension is an uncommon finding and is usually secondary to long-standing pulmonary fibrosis.

HIGH-RESOLUTION CT FINDINGS IN SARCOIDOSIS

The HRCT is clearly more sensitive that chest radiographs in detecting the parenchymal abnormalities in sarcoidosis. A variety of HRCT findings have been described in this disease, which represent both the granulomatous and fibrotic response seen histologically. The most frequent finding is the presence of interstitial nodules, 3 mm to 1 cm in diameter, seen as nodular thickening of the peribronchoarterial (axial) interstitium and interlobular septa, or as subpleural nodules. The nodules correlate closely with the coalescing noncaseating granulomas seen microscopically on tissue specimens. Septal thickening, thickening of bronchovascular bundles, architectural distortion, lung cysts, honeycombing, and central conglomerate masses with crowded, ectatic bronchi are findings indicative of fibrosis from long-standing disease. Segmental or mass-like air space opacities, termed "alveolar" sarcoid, usually indicate active disease and resolve with corticosteroid therapy. Likewise, the finding of patchy areas of ground-glass density have been shown to correlate with increased uptake on gallium scans and may be indicative of an active alveolitis. Several recent published reports have shown good correlation between conventional and HRCT findings and pulmonary function tests.

RADIOGRAPHIC STAGING OF SARCOIDOSIS

The chest radiographic manifestations of sarcoidosis have been divided into five stages (Table 15.21). These stages generally parallel the course of disease, and are useful for prognostic purposes. Stage 1 disease is associated with a 75% rate of resolution, whereas only 30% of patients with stage 2 and 10% of patients with stage 3 disease resolve.

The diagnosis of sarcoidosis is usually based upon the histologic demonstration of noncaseating granulomas involving multiple organs. Tissue is most often obtained by bronchoscopically guided transbronchial biopsy, which provides a diagnosis in up to 90% of patients. Biopsy of organs likely to be involved in this disease, such as the liver and scalene lymph nodes, will provide a diagnosis in a majority of patients. Percutaneous needle biopsy can provide diagnostic tissue specimens in those with mass-like pulmonary lesions. In certain situations, the diagnosis of sarcoidosis is made on a constellation of chest radiographic findings and characteristic eye or skin changes. In such patients, gallium scintigraphy showing a pattern of increased uptake in the hilar lymph nodes, lung, and salivary glands may be used as a confirmatory test. Gallium scanning has also been used to assess the degree of disease activity.

Berylliosis

Although berylliosis is actually an inhalational lung disease, it is discussed here because of the clinical, pathologic, and radiographic similarities to sarcoidosis. This uncommon disease produces noncaseating granulomas in multiple organs, with primary lung involvement. The radiographic features of berylliosis are indistinguishable from sarcoidosis. Hilar and mediastinal lymph node enlargement and bilateral reticulonodular opacities are the most common findings. As with sarcoidosis, progression to end-stage interstitial fibrosis with honeycombing or upper lobe bullous disease may occur, with the latter predisposing the patient to aspergilloma formation and spontaneous pneumothorax.

Histiocytosis X (Eosinophilic Granuloma) of Lung

This entity includes three disorders with similar pathologic features that differ in the age at the time of diagnosis, mode of presentation, specific organs involved, and prognosis. These diseases are believed to be related to an acquired immunologic defect. Eosinophilic granuloma (EG) is the form of this disease affecting adults, with predominant involvement of lung and bones. The disease most commonly affects young adults without a sex predilection. There is a very high association between pulmonary involvement and cigarette smoking.

PATHOLOGIC FINDINGS

Pathologically, EG of lung demonstrates multiple small nodules that are found predominantly in the axial interstitial tissues of the upper and middle lung zones around small bronchioles. The nodules represent granulomas composed predominantly of cells with eosinophilic cytoplasm previously called histio-

cytosis X cells and now known as Langerhans cells. These cells are normally found in the skin and appear to proliferate in the lung and other organs in response to an unidentified antigenic stimulus. In some patients, the nodular phase of disease may be preceded by an exudative phase with filling of the alveolar spaces with a cellular exudate containing the Langerhans cells. The small peribronchiolar nodules may coalesce to form larger nodules that may cavitate, or they may extend to infiltrate the alveolar septa and induce an interstitial inflammatory reaction. The nodules may resolve completely, but in most patients, the central portions of the nodules undergo fibrosis, producing a stellate nodular lesion characteristic of pulmonary EG histologically. In the late stages, characteristic findings include fibrosis and the development of small, uniform, thin-walled cysts. Larger peripheral cysts or bullae may develop in the apical regions, presumably as a result of bronchiolar obstruction by fibrosis with distal air trapping.

CLINICAL FINDINGS AND FUNCTIONAL ABNORMALITIES

Pulmonary symptoms are present in two-thirds of patients with EG of lung at presentation. Cough and the gradual onset of dyspnea are the most common complaints. Pleuritic chest pain may indicate the development of a spontaneous pneumothorax from rupture of a subpleural cyst. The physical examination is typically unremarkable. Pulmonary function tests reflect the fibrosis and cystic changes seen in this disorder, with characteristic restrictive and obstructive patterns of disease and a diminished diffusing capacity.

RADIOLOGIC FINDINGS

The radiographic findings in EG of lung usually follow a predictable pattern. Although the earliest changes in EG of lung are associated with filling of alveoli, the radiographic demonstration of air space opacities is uncommon. The earliest findings are small to medium-sized nodular opacities that tend to have an upper and middle lung zone distribution (Fig. 15.44**A**). In some cases the nodules coalesce to form larger nodules or masses that rarely cavitate. The nodular pattern may resolve completely or be replaced by a predominantly reticulonodular or reticular pattern, which represents the fibrotic phase of the disease. Late stages of the disease are characterized by a coarse reticular pattern with intermixed thin-walled cysts (Fig. 15.44**B**). These cysts account for the relative preservation or increase in lung volumes typical of EG which is a distinguishing feature of this disease. The parenchymal changes of EG are best demonstrated on HRCT. Hilar or mediastinal lymph node enlargement is distinctly uncommon, a feature which

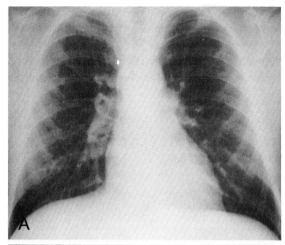

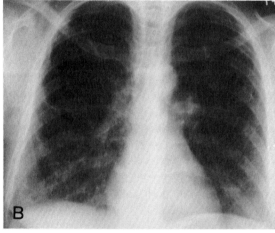

Figure 15.44. Eosinophilic Granuloma of Lung (Histiocytosis X).
A. A PA film in a 17-year-old male with biopsy-proven EG shows a micronodular pattern with a middle and upper zone predominance. **B.** In another patient with longstanding EG, there is upper lobe cystic disease, representing late-stage disease.

helps distinguish EG from sarcoidosis. Pneumothorax from rupture of a cyst or bulla is the presenting finding or develops during the course of disease in up to 25% of patients. Pleural effusion in the absence of a pneumothorax is rare. Extrapulmonary manifestations include well-defined lytic lesions in the ribs or vertebral bodies.

High-resolution CT in patients with EG and a relatively short duration of symptoms (<6 months) shows well-defined interstitial nodules of varying size, sometimes with cavitation, and cyst formation in the upper lungs. More long-standing disease is characterized by larger cysts and honeycombing. The distinguishing features between EG and emphysema are the presence of nodules (with or without cavitation) and thin-walled cysts in EG that lack a constant relationship to the centrilobular core structures. The HRCT distinction of EG from LAM in a female is more difficult; an upper zone distribution and the presence of nodules favors EG.

The diagnosis of EG of lung is made by noting the characteristic stellate nodular lesions with Langerhans cells on open lung biopsy specimens. The treatment for symptomatic patients is corticosteroid therapy, although more than half of the patients with lung disease stabilize or improve spontaneously.

Wegener's Granulomatosis

This is a systemic autoimmune disorder characterized pathologically by a necrotizing granulomatous vasculitis involving the upper and lower respiratory tracts and kidneys. The characteristic lesions in the lungs are discrete nodules or masses of granulomatous inflammation with central necrosis and cavitation. The lesions involve pulmonary vessels, accounting for the high incidence of central necrosis and for the occasional presentation with pulmonary hemorrhage. Mucosal and submucosal lesions may be present in the tracheobronchial tree and are seen almost exclusively in females.

Most patients with Wegener's granulomatosis are middle-aged, with a slight male predominance. The respiratory tract is affected in 100% of patients, with symptoms usually dominated by the sinus and nasal mucosal involvement. Pulmonary involvement may be asymptomatic or manifested by cough, dyspnea, or chest pain. Presentation with pulmonary hemorrhage and hemoptysis may mimic other pulmonary-renal syndromes such as Goodpasture's and idiopathic pulmonary hemorrhage. Renal involvement usually follows involvement of the respiratory tract and is seen in almost 90% of patients.

The characteristic chest radiographic features of lung involvement in Wegener's granulomatosis are multiple sharply marginated nodules or masses; solitary lesions are seen in up to one-third of patients. Irregular, thick-walled cavitary lesions are seen in 50% of patients during the course of disease. Localized or diffuse areas of air space opacification may be seen, representing either hemorrhage or pneumonia, the latter often due to complicating *S. aureus* infection. Tracheal or bronchial lesions may be present and are usually best appreciated on CT, where they appear as calcified mucosal or submucosal deposits producing irregular narrowing of the airway lumen. The airway lesions are usually unassociated with parenchymal disease, but endobronchial lesions may produce distal atelectasis. Pleural effusion from pleural involvement is not uncommon. Pneumothorax may result from rupture of a cavitary lesion into the pleural space. Lymph node enlargement is not seen in this disease.

The diagnosis of Wegener's granulomatosis should be made on biopsy of involved tissues, usually nasal

Table 15.22. Eosinophilic Lung Disease

Idiopathic	Simple pulmonary eosinophilia (Loeffler's syndrome)
	Chronic eosinophilic pneumonia
	Hypereosinophilic syndrome
Known etiology	Drugs
	Antibiotics
	Penicillins
	Nitrofurantoin
	Nonsteroidal antiinflammatory agents
	Aspirin
	Chemotherapeutic agents
	Bleomycin
	Methotrexate
	Parasites
	Filaria
	Strongyloides
	Ascaris
	Hookworm
Autoimmune disease	Wegener's granulomatosis
	Sarcoidosis
	Rheumatoid lung disease
	Polyarteritis nodosa
	Allergic angiitis and granulomatosis (Churg-Strauss syndrome)

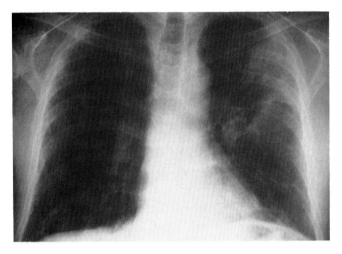

Figure 15.45. Eosinophilic Pneumonia. An AP chest film in a 64-year-old man with nonspecific pulmonary symptoms demonstrates bilateral peripheral air space opacities that are most severe in the left upper lobe. The patient had peripheral eosinophilia and responded dramatically to corticosteroids. (Case courtesy of John D. Murao, M.D., El Camino Hospital, Mountain View, California.)

mucosa or lung, which show the granulomatous inflammation and vasculitis characteristic of this disease. The pathologic changes in the kidneys are often nonspecific, and therefore renal biopsy is often nondiagnostic. This disease usually responds dramatically to cyclophosphamide therapy. Untreated patients invariably die of renal failure or, less commonly, progressive respiratory disease. High serologic titers for the presence of antineutrophil cytoplasmic antibody are specific for the diagnosis of Wegener's granulomatosis, although a negative test does not exclude the diagnosis, particularly in patients with limited or inactive disease.

Eosinophilic Lung Disease

This term refers to a heterogeneous group of allergic diseases that are characterized by excess eosinophils in lung and occasionally blood. Recently, Fraser and Pare (13) have classified these diseases into three groups: idiopathic, those of known etiology, and autoimmune or collagen vascular disorders (Table 15.22).

IDIOPATHIC EOSINOPHILIC LUNG DISEASE

The idiopathic disorders associated with eosinophilic lung disease include simple pulmonary eosinophilia, chronic eosinophilic pneumonia, and the hypereosinophilic syndrome.

Simple Pulmonary Eosinophilia, also known as Loeffler's syndrome, is a transient pulmonary process characterized pathologically by pulmonary infiltration with an eosinophilic exudate. Most patients have a history of allergy, most commonly asthma. Radiographically, the characteristic findings are peripheral, homogeneous, ill-defined areas of air space opacification that may parallel the chest wall; this latter feature is best appreciated on CT (Fig 15.45). The opacities in Loeffler's syndrome have been described as fleeting, since the tendency is for rapid clearing in one area along with new involvement in other areas. A dry cough, dyspnea, and peripheral blood eosinophilia are common but are not invariably present. The diagnosis is based on the combination of pulmonary symptoms, blood eosinophilia, and characteristic radiographic findings. Most patients having a self-limiting illness that resolves spontaneously within 4 weeks.

Chronic Eosinophilic Pneumonia. Patients with symptoms and radiographic abnormalities that last more than 4 weeks are considered to have chronic eosinophilic pneumonia. The clinical and radiographic features are similar to Loeffler's syndrome, although there is a distinct predilection for women. Patients are usually symptomatic with fever, malaise, and dyspnea. The pulmonary symptoms and radiographic opacities respond dramatically to corticosteroid therapy and improve within 4 to 7 days, although relapse upon discontinuation of treatment is common.

Hypereosinophilic Syndrome is a systemic disorder with a male predominance that is characterized by multiorgan damage from eosinophilic infiltration of tissues. Blood eosinophilia is prolonged and marked in this condition. The major chest radiographic findings are associated with cardiac involvement and secondary congestive heart failure and include cardiomegaly, pulmonary edema, and pleural effusions.

Pulmonary parenchymal infiltration with eosinophils may produce interstitial or air space opacities.

EOSINOPHILIC LUNG DISEASE OF IDENTIFIABLE ETIOLOGY

Pulmonary eosinophilia of known etiology includes drug- and parasite-induced eosinophilic lung disease. Drugs associated with pulmonary eosinphilia include nitrofurantoin and the penicillins. The parasitic infections most commonly responsible are filaria and the roundworms *Ascaris lumbricoides* and *Strongyloides stercoralis*. These parasites may produce pulmonary eosinophilia as they migrate through the alveolar capillaries and into the alveoli during their tour of the body. These disorders are usually indistinguishable clinically and radiographically from Loeffler's syndrome.

AUTOIMMUNE DISEASE

A number of autoimmune disorders are associated with eosinophilic pulmonary infiltrates. These include Wegener's granulomatosis, sarcoidosis, rheumatoid lung disease, polyarteritis nodosa, and allergic angiitis and granulomatosis. The first three disorders have a variety of thoracic manifestations and are discussed elsewhere. The predominant chest radiographic findings seen in polyarteritis nodosa represent hemorrhage due to a vasculitis involving the bronchial arterial circulation; this condition is discussed in "Pulmonary Hemorrhage." Allergic angiitis and granulomatosis (Churg-Strauss syndrome) is a multisystem disorder in which asthma, blood eosinophilia, necrotizing vasculitis, and extravascular granulomas are invariable features. Pulmonary involvement, as seen radiographically or pathologically, is indistinguishable from chronic eosinophilic pneumonia.

THE SOLITARY PULMONARY NODULE
General Considerations

The radiologic evaluation of the solitary pulmonary nodule (SPN) is one of the most common and most difficult diagnostic dilemmas in thoracic radiology (15). Before embarking on a detailed diagnostic evaluation of a SPN, one must determine if the nodular opacity seen on the chest radiograph is real or artifactual. A small, poorly defined opacity warrants repeat films, preferably using a different film cassette and after overlying garments have been removed. If the opacity is judged to represent a real lesion, the radiologist must then determine whether he or she is dealing with a SPN. First, is the lesion truly solitary? Not uncommonly, a dominant pulmonary nodule on chest radiographs is associated with smaller nodules or

nodules that are obscured by the heart or the hemidiaphragms. A careful search on PA and lateral chest radiographs will identify most of these patients, although CT may be necessary to identify additional subradiographic nodules. Multiple pulmonary nodules of similar size and appearance are almost always metastases or granulomas and require a different evaluation from that of a solitary lesion.

Second, is the lesion intrapulmonary? Intrapulmonary lesions are discrete opacities that are completely circumscribed by aerated lung on both frontal and lateral radiographs. A pleural or mediastinal lesion may be outlined by lung when it projects inward. However, the base of the lesion, which forms obtuse angles with the lung, is not outlined by lung where it arises from the pleura or mediastinum. On lateral films, pleural and mediastinal lesions will be difficult to see as they are seen en face with little of the interface between the lesion and the lung tangent to the x-ray beam. Skin or chest wall lesions can also mimic intrapulmonary nodules as they project outward to be outlined by air, but these are not completely circumscribed where they arise from the chest wall (the breast is a good example). Some skin lesions are completely circumscribed by air, but a careful physical examination of the patient, usually following the chest radiograph, will reveal the surface lesion responsible for the "nodule" seen on chest film. One of the most troublesome skin "lesions" to distinguish from a true pulmonary nodule is the nipple shadow. This is usually readily identified by the typical position and bilaterality, although in some patients only a single nipple shadow is seen on frontal radiographs. By obtaining films in the PA, lateral, and 5° oblique (from the PA) projections with nipple markers, or by performing chest fluoroscopy, these will be properly identified. A sclerotic bone lesion or healing rib fracture can simulate a new pulmonary nodule; oblique radiographs or fluoroscopy will often help localize these lesions to a rib. Occasionally, CT will be necessary for confident localization of a nodular density seen on plain radiographs.

Finally, is the lesion a nodule? A nodule is a discrete round or oval opacity; linear or angular opacities are not nodules and represent scars or areas of linear atelectasis. When a focal opacity is seen in the lung apices, an apical lordotic film or CT scan may be necessary to distinguish a linear from a nodular opacity. A round opacity greater than 3 cm in diameter is termed a mass. Since the majority of lung masses in patients over the age of 35 represent bronchogenic carcinoma, these lesions are not considered SPNs.

Once a SPN has been identified, the radiologist should initiate a series of investigations in an attempt to determine whether the nodule is definitely benign or if it is still suspicious for malignancy (i.e., indeter-

Figure 15.46. Algorithm for Approach to the SPN. *Ca,* calcification; *TNB,* transthoracic needle biopsy, *CXR,* chest x-ray.

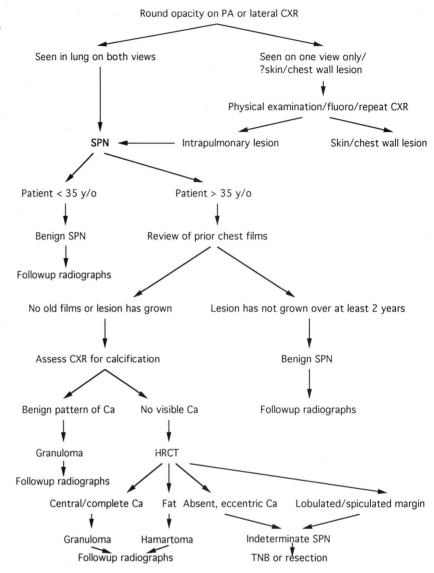

minate). This stepwise approach is summarized in Figure 15.46.

Clinical Factors

Before considering the radiologic characteristics used to distinguish benign from indeterminate nodules, there are important clinical factors that may be helpful in making this distinction. In a patient under the age of 35, particularly a nonsmoker, a SPN is invariably a granuloma, hamartoma, or inflammatory lesion. Asymptomatic patients under the age of 35 with SPNs can be followed with plain radiographs to confirm the benign nature of these lesions. Patients over the age of 35 have a significant incidence of malignant SPNs, with approximately 50% of noncalcified SPNs in those over 50 years of age found to be malignant at thoracotomy. Therefore, as a rule, a SPN in a patient over 35 years of age should never be followed radiographically without tissue confirmation unless a benign pattern of calcification or the presence of intralesional fat is identified on radiographs or HRCT, or there has been radiographically documented lack of growth over a minimum of 2 years. However, there are exceptions to this rule. A history of cigarette smoking or asbestos exposure or both raises the level of concern for malignancy in a patient with a SPN. Alternatively, if the patient is from an area where histoplasmosis or TB is endemic, the possibility of the SPN being a granuloma is higher. In a patient with a newly discovered noncalcified, smoothly marginated nodule <2 cm in diameter who is newly PPD positive, a trial of antituberculous therapy and careful radiographic follow-up may be appropriate. Finally, the finding of a SPN in a patient with an extrathoracic malignancy raises the possibility of a solitary pulmonary metastasis. If the lung is the sole site of metastatic disease, distinguishing between a primary bronchogenic carcinoma and a pulmonary metastasis is usually unimportant as many surgeons will resect a solitary pulmonary metastases. A SPN that arises more than 2 years after the diagnosis of an extrathoracic malignancy is virtually always a primary lung tumor rather than a metastasis; breast carcinoma and melanoma are notable exceptions to this rule.

Growth Pattern

Pulmonary malignancies grow at a relatively predictable rate. The growth rate of a SPN is usually expressed as the doubling time, or the time it takes for a nodule to double its volume. For a sphere, this corresponds to a 25% increase in diameter. Although some benign lesions (mostly hamartomas and histoplasmomas) may exhibit a growth rate similar to that of malignant lesions, the absence of growth or an extraordinarily slow or rapid rate of growth is reliable evidence that a SPN is benign. Studies have shown that bronchogenic carcinoma has a doubling time of between 1 month and 2 years. Therefore, a doubling time of less than 1 month or greater than 2 years reliably characterizes a lesion as benign. Infectious lesions and rapidly growing metastases from choriocarcinoma, seminoma, or osteogenic sarcoma comprise the majority of rapidly growing solitary nodules, while lack of growth or a doubling time exceeding 2 years is seen in hamartomas and histoplasmomas. However, there are exceptions to this rule. Giant cell carcinoma, a subtype of large cell carcinoma, may have a doubling time of less than 1 month, and any malignancy that hemorrhages into its substance will appear to enlarge rapidly. Alternatively, some pulmonary malignancies such as the occasional adenocarcinoma or carcinoid tumors may have a doubling time of greater than 2 years. There are two important caveats to using the growth rate of a SPN to determine benignity. The first is that the growth rate of a SPN that is not visible on prior radiographs cannot be estimated, since noncalcified nodules less than 1 cm in diameter are not usually visible on conventional radiographs. Most importantly, with few exceptions, a patient over the age of 35 with a noncalcified SPN should never be evaluated prospectively to determine benignity by following the growth rate on serial chest radiographs. The use of growth rate to determine benignity should only be used retrospectively in comparing the size of a SPN with prior radiographs from at least 2 years previously.

Size

Although size does not reliably discriminate benign from malignant SPNs, as a rule the larger the lesion the more likely it is to be malignant. Masses exceeding 4 cm in diameter are usually malignant. However, the converse does not hold true; many pulmonary malignancies are less than 2 cm in diameter at the time of diagnosis.

Margin (Border) Characteristics

The appearance of the edge of a SPN is a helpful sign in determining the nature of the lesion. The edge characterisitics are best evaluated on thin-section HRCT as this technique is considerably more accurate than plain radiographs. A round, smoothly marginated nodule is most likely a granuloma or hamartoma, although a rare primary pulmonary malignancy such as a carcinoid tumor, adenocarcinoma, or a solitary metastasis may have a perfectly smooth margin. A notched or lobulated margin is strongly suggestive but not diagnostic of malignancy. Pathologic examination has shown that the lobulated edge of a malignant nodule represents mounds of tumor extending into the adjacent lung. The presence of a spiculated margin in a SPN is highly suspicious for malignancy. The term "corona radiata" as been used to describe this appearance, in which linear densities radiate from the edge of a nodule into the adjacent lung. Pathologically, these linear radiations represent reoriented connective tissue (interlobular) septa drawn into the tumor by the cicatrizing (scarring) nature of many malignant lung tumors. Tumor extension from the nodule, or fibrosis and edema of these connective tissue septa may thicken these linear densities. However, it has been shown that spiculation is not specific for malignancy since a variety of benign processes that produce cicatrization can have an identical appearance. Benign lesions that may show a spiculated margin include lipoid pneumonia, organizing pneumonia, tuberculomas, and the mass lesions of PMF in complicated silicosis. A peripherally situated pulmonary nodule may contact the costal pleura or interlobar fissure via a linear opacity known as a "pleural tail." As with the corona radiata, the recognition of this line, while suggestive of malignancy (particularly bronchioloalveolar cell carcinoma), is not specific and may be seen in peripheral granulomas.

There are two additional characteristics of the border of a SPN that help identify the nature of the lesion. The presence of small "satellite" nodules around the periphery of a dominant nodule is strongly suggestive of benign disease, particularly in the proper clinical setting. However, since a "scar" carcinoma can arise within an area of preexisting granulomatous disease, and since some malignancies grow by discontiguous spread into the adjacent lung, the identification of satellite nodules is not definitive evidence of a benign lesion. The identification of feeding and draining vessels emanating from the central portion of a SPN is pathognomonic of a pulmonary AVM. Administration of intravenous contrast and dynamic CT scanning through the nodule or MR is diagnostic. Similarly, a posttraumatic pulmonary artery pseudoaneurysm will show marked contrast enhancement and contiguity with the feeding artery on CT. Pulmonary arteriography is performed in most patients with AVMs or pulmonary artery aneurysms prior to therapeutic embolization with endovascular coils or balloons.

Non-calcified (indeterminate) SPN

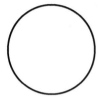

Complete calcification

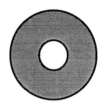

Central calcification

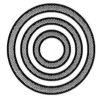

Laminated calcification

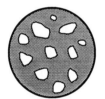

"Popcorn" calcification

Figure 15.47. Benign Patterns of Calcification within a SPN.

Density

The internal density of a SPN is probably the single most important factor in characterizing the lesion as benign or indeterminate. In general, lesions that are calcified are benign. Specifically, there are four patterns of calcification that have been recognized as reliably indicating the benignity of a SPN (Fig. 15.47). These patterns may be identified on plain chest radiographs, but more often thin-section HRCT is necessary to detect and characterize the calcification. The visualization of complete or central calcification within a SPN is specific for a healed granuloma from TB or histoplasmosis. Similarly, concentric or laminated calcification indicates a granuloma and allows confidently exclusion of neoplasm. The presence of popcorn calcification within a nodule is diagnostic of a pulmonary hamartoma in which the cartilaginous component has calcified (Fig. 15.48).

It is important to remember that the presence of calcification within a SPN is synonymous with a benign lesion only if the calcification follows one of the four patterns of benign calcification shown in Figure 15.47. A small percentage of SPNs that are malignant will contain calcification on CT. A bronchogenic carcinoma that arises in an area of previous granulomatous infection may engulf a preexisting calcified granuloma as it enlarges. In this situation, the calcification will be eccentric in the nodule, allowing distinction from a centrally calcified granuloma. Small or microscopic calcification may also be found from dystrophic calcification of malignant pulmonary neoplasms, particularly adenocarcinomas that produce mucin or psammoma bodies. The rare solitary pulmonary metastasis from osteosarcoma or chondrosarcoma may contain calcium, but the diagnosis in these patients will usually be obvious clinically.

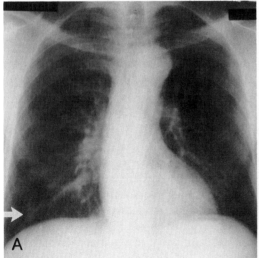

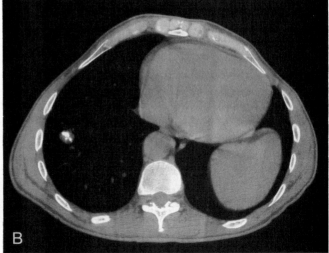

Figure 15.48. Hamartoma. Routine chest radiograph (**A**) in a 48-year-old man demonstrates a well-defined nodule in the right lower lobe (*arrow*) with calcification. HRCT (**B**) shows a smoothly margi-nated nodule containing coarse "popcorn" calcifications typical of a pulmonary hamartoma.

Although benign patterns of calcification may be detected on plain radiographs or HRCT, some benign nodules contain microscopic calcifications that are not readily evident on visual inspection of the images. This has led to the use of quantitative CT nodule densitometry to detect the presence and distribution of microscopic calcification within SPNs. This technique is performed by comparing the CT density of the SPN with that of a reference nodule containing a benign quantity of calcium placed in a chest phantom, or by evaluation of the absolute CT numbers of a SPN by obtaining a computer-generated pixel display of a region in the center of the nodule. If at least 10% of the pixels contained within a nodule demonstrate a mean CT value exceeding 200 HU, there is reliable evidence of the presence of benign calcification. As with visible calcification, the calcification detected by densitometry must be either central or evenly distributed throughout the nodule to be considered benign. The use of nodule densitometry has significantly reduced the percentage of patients considered to have indeterminate SPNs by visual inspection alone, thereby decreasing the number of thoracotomies performed for benign lesions.

The identification of fat within a SPN is diagnostic of a pulmonary hamartoma. A discussion of the radiographic and CT features of a pulmonary hamartoma can be found in the section "Neoplastic and Nonneoplastic Lesions Presenting as SPNs."

It is important to remember that not all SPNs require CT densitometry. A nodule that on plain radiographs or CT has a diameter greater than 2 cm, shows lobulated or spiculated margins, or is cavitary, has such a high likelihood of malignancy regardless of its internal density that the results of HRCT densitometry could only be misleading. Likewise, the demonstration of an air bronchogram within a SPN is highly suspicious for adenocarcinoma, particularly bronchoalveolar cell carcinoma. Such SPNs, along with those small, well-defined solid lesions lacking benign calcification or fat on HRCT, are suspicious enough for malignancy to be considered indeterminate.

Patients with indeterminate SPNs should undergo biopsy or resection of the lesion. When the lesion is likely to be malignant, it is reasonable to forego biopsy and proceed directly to thoracotomy and resection. However, there are several reasons to perform a preoperative biopsy on an indeterminate SPN; the primary reason is to make the diagnosis of a benign lesion, thereby avoiding an unnecessary thoracotomy. This would only benefit the patient if there was a reasonable likelihood that the SPN is benign. The factors suggesting benignity have been discussed: age under 35, nonsmoker, patient from an area endemic for TB or histoplasmosis, patient with a small nodule with smooth margins who has recently converted to a positive PPD, nodule <2 cm with smooth margins, and a doubling time of less than 30 days or more than 2 years. The other major indication for the biopsy of an indeterminate SPN is a patient with severe pulmonary functional abnormalities who is a poor surgical candidate for pulmonary resection. In these patients, a biopsy can provide a diagnosis and guide nonoperative therapy. As most SPNs are peripherally situated in the lung, transthoracic needle biopsy is the procedure of choice for tissue sampling. Patients with SPNs that are centrally situated with a large bronchus entering the mass should undergo transbronchoscopic biopsy.

A SPN that is judged benign based on patient age, growth rate, presence of benign calcification, or those with a specific benign diagnosis provided by transthoracic needle biopsy should be followed carefully with radiographs for a minimum of 2 and preferably 3 years to confirm their benign nature. The radiographic follow-up consists of PA and lateral chest radiographs.

In summary, the following questions must be answered when evaluating a SPN:

1. Is the opacity real or artifactual?
2. If the opacity is real, does it fit the criteria of a solitary pulmonary nodule? Is it solitary on CT? Could the opacity represent a skin, chest wall, or rib lesion on physical examination, oblique radiographs, chest fluoroscopy, and CT? Is it a nodule?
3. Is the patient under 35 years of age?
4. If dealing with a SPN, is it present on previous radiographs and if so, has it grown in size? If yes, is the doubling time <30 days or >2 years?
5. Is the nodule calcified, and if so, is it a benign pattern on HRCT?
6. Is there fat within the nodule on HRCT?
7. Are there feeding and draining vessels on CT, MR or pulmonary angiography?
8. Is the nodule larger than 2 cm?
9. Is the margin of the nodule lobulated or spiculated on HRCT?

Neoplastic and Nonneoplastic Lesions Presenting as SPNs

The differential diagnosis of a SPN is shown in Table 15.23. In addition to bronchogenic carcinoma (particularly adenocarcinoma) and granulomas (e.g., TB and histoplasmosis), there are a number of entities that may produce a SPN. Many of these entities are discussed elsewhere in the text.

Carcinoid Tumors. While carcinoid tumors may present as SPNs, the majority (80%) are central endobronchial lesions that present with atelectasis or

Table 15.23. Solitary Pulmonary Nodule or Mass

Neoplasm	Bronchogenic carcinoma
	Hamartoma
	Bronchial adenoma
	Granular cell myoblastoma
	Mesenchymal neoplasms
	Leiomyoma/leiomyosarcoma
	Fibroma
	Lipoma
	Neurofibroma
	Lymphoma
	Solitary metastasis
	Colon carcinoma
Infection	Septic embolus
	Staphylococcus
	Round pneumonia
	Pneumococcus
	Legionella
	Nocardia
	Fungi
	Lung abscess
	Infectious granuloma
	Tuberculosis
	Histoplasmosis
	Coccidioidomycosis
	Cryptococcosis
	Parasitic
	Echinococcal cyst
	Amebic abscess
Collagen vascular disease	Necrobiotic nodule (rheumatoid lung)
	Wegener's granulomatosis
Vascular	Infarct
	AVM
	Pulmonary artery aneurysm
	Hematoma
Airways	Congenital foregut malformations
	Bronchogenic cyst
	Sequestration
	Mucocele
	Infected bulla
Miscellaneous	Amyloidoma
	Round atelectasis

obstructive pneumonitis. A detailed discussion of carcinoid tumors can be found in Chapter 13.

Pulmonary Hamartoma. A pulmonary hamartoma is a benign neoplasm composed of an abnormal arrangement of the mesenchymal and epithelial elements found in normal lung. Histologically, these lesions contain cartilage surrounded by fibrous connective tissue with variable amounts of fat, smooth muscle, and seromucous glands; calcification and ossification is seen in 30% of cases. These tumors are seen most commonly in the 4th–5th decade of life. Approximately 90% of hamartomas arise within the pulmonary parenchyma, accounting for approximately 5% of all solitary pulmonary nodules.

These lesions usually present as incidental findings on chest radiographs (Fig. 15.48). While the diagnosis is often suggested on plain radiographs, CT is obtained in most patients. A confident diagnosis of hamartoma can be made when HRCT shows a nodule <2.5 cm in diameter, demonstrates a smooth or lobulated borders, and contains focal fat. Calcification, when present, is in the form of multiple clumps of calcium dispersed throughout the lesion ("popcorn" calcification) (Fig. 15.48**B**). While hamartomas tend to grow slowly, the presence of characteristic HRCT findings allows for observation alone. Rapid growth, pulmonary symptoms, or a size >2.5 cm warrants biopsy or resection.

Granular Cell Myoblastoma is a benign neoplasm arising from neural elements in the central airways or parenchyma. The skin is the most common site for these tumors. These tumors may present as endobronchial masses or as SPNs.

Leiomyoma/Leiomyosarcoma, Fibroma, Neurofibroma. Arising from the smooth muscle of the airways or pulmonary vessels, leiomyomas and leiomyosarcomas are rare neoplasms that present with equal frequency as endobronchial or intrapulmonary lesions. Radiographically, the parenchymal lesions are sharply marginated, smooth or lobulated nodules or masses. The histologic distinction of benign from malignant lesions is difficult. Similarly, fibromas and neurofibromas appearing as SPNs lack distinguishing radiographic features.

Lipoma is a rare intrapulmonary lesion, arising more commonly within the tracheobronchial tree to produce atelectasis. The demonstration of fat attenuation on CT is diagnostic.

Hemangiopericytoma is a connective tissue tumor that arises within the lung from the pericyte, a cell associated with the arteriolar and capillary endothelium. On chest radiographs, these lesions are seen as SPNs and are indistinguishable from bronchogenic carcinoma.

Plasma Cell Granuloma (Inflammatory Pseudotumor) of Lung refers to a localized chronic inflammatory process in the lung that represents an inflammatory response to an unknown agent. It is characterized histologically by an abundance of plasma cells. There are no distinguishing radiographic features.

Lipoid Pneumonia. The inadvertent aspiration of mineral oils ingested by elderly patients to treat constipation may produce a localized pulmonary lesion. Patients with gastroesophageal reflux or disordered swallowing mechanisms are at particular risk. Radiographically, a focal area of air space opacification or a solid mass may be seen in the lower lobes of the lung. A spiculated appearance to the edge of the mass is not uncommon as the oil may produce a chronic inflammatory reaction in the surrounding lung that leads to fibrosis. While CT can demonstrate fat within the lesion, most patients with the mass-like form of this entity require resection for definitive diagnosis.

Bronchogenic Cyst. Fluid-filled cystic lesions of the lung may produce a SPN. Intrapulmonary bronchogenic cysts are uncommon causes of SPNs as the majority of these lesions are found in the middle mediastinum. The characteristic finding is a sharply marginated cyst on CT or MR in a young patient are seen, although distinction from an infected bullae, solitary echinococcal cyst, mucocele, or thin-walled lung abscess may be impossible. Superinfection of a lung bulla may produce a SPN or mass. In such patients, the radiographic or CT appearance of an intraparenchymal air-fluid level within a thin-walled, localized air collection (usually in an upper lobe), with typical bullous changes in other portions of lung, usually allows for the proper diagnosis.

PULMONARY NEOPLASMS
Benign Neoplasms

Benign pulmonary neoplasms are discussed in the sections on endobronchial masses and SPNs.

Malignant Neoplasms

BRONCHOGENIC CARCINOMA

Bronchogenic carcinoma commonly produces radiographic findings in the lungs as well as hilar, mediastinal, and pleural abnormalities. A discussion of the pulmonary parenchymal findings in bronchogenic carcinoma is found in Chapter 14. Likewise, carcinoid tumors can produce atelectasis or obstructive pneumonitis when arising within central bronchi (see the chapter on the mediastinum), or appear as a SPN when arising from peripheral airways within the parenchyma.

METASTATIC PULMONARY NEOPLASM

The spread of extrapulmonary neoplasm to the lung may occur by direct invasion of the pulmonary parenchyma or as a result of hematogenous dissemination to the lung, with the latter mechanism much more common. Rarely, a tumor can disseminate throughout the lungs via the tracheobronchial tree, as in laryngotracheal papillomatosis and some cases of bronchoalveolar carcinoma.

Direct invasion of the lung may occur with mediastinal, pleural, or chest wall malignancies. The most common mediastinal malignancies to invade the lung are esophageal carcinoma, lymphoma, and malignant germ cell tumors, or any malignancy metastasizing to mediastinal or hilar lymph nodes. Malignant mesothelioma and metastases to the pleura or chest wall can extend through the pleura to invade the adjacent lung.

Hematogenous metastases to the lung may be seen with any tumor that gains access to the superior or inferior vena cava or the thoracic duct as the pulmonary artery is the final common pathway for these channels. Although only a minority of tumor emboli survive within the pulmonary interstitium, those that do survive produce one of two morphologic and radiographic appearances: pulmonary nodules or lymphangitic carcinomatosis (LC).

Pulmonary Nodules. Multiple pulmonary nodules are the most common manifestation of hematogenous metastases to the lung. They are most commonly seen in carcinomas of the lung, breast, kidney, thyroid, colon, uterus, and head and neck. Although most patients have multiple nodules, metastasis can present as a solitary pulmonary nodule. Solitary pulmonary nodules due to metastasis are typically smooth in contour, while primary bronchogenic tumors tend to be lobulated or spiculated. The likelihood that a SPN in a patient without a synchronous extrathoracic malignancy represents a solitary metastasis is slightly less than 50%, while SPNs in patients without prior malignancies are almost always primary bronchogenic tumors or granulomas. However, the site of the primary tumor may affect the likelihood that a SPN is a metastasis. Carcinoma of the rectosigmoid colon, osteogenic sarcoma, renal cell carcinoma, and melanoma are more likely to give solitary pulmonary metastases. It should be cautioned that what may appear as a solitary metastasis on plain radiographs may be only one of multiple pulmonary nodules as shown by chest CT.

Nodular pulmonary metastases are usually smooth or lobulated lesions found in greater numbers in the peripheral portions of the lower lobes because of the greater pulmonary blood flow to these regions. Computed tomography is the modality of choice for the evaluation of pulmonary metastases as it is considerably more sensitive than plain radiographs or conventional whole-lung tomography in detecting lung nodules. Although there are no characteristic features of nodular metastases that allow distinction between different primary neoplasms, there are certain features that may prove helpful in the differential diagnosis. These are listed in Table 15.24. Similarly, the distinction between metastases and granulomas is usually impossible, although there are three findings on CT that may help in this regard. First, the demonstration of a feeding vessel entering the central aspect of a well-defined peripheral pulmonary nodule strongly suggests hematogenous metastases; however, this may be seen in other blood-borne pulmonary processes such as pulmonary infarcts and septic emboli. Second, the demonstration of calcification within multiple pulmonary nodules, in the absence of a history of a primary bone-forming neoplasm such as osteogenic sarcoma or chondrosarcoma, is diagnostic of granulomas. Although primary mucinous adenocarcinomas

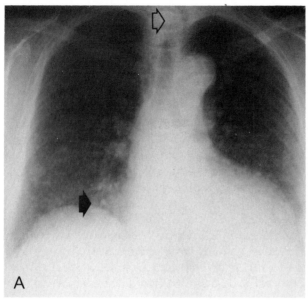

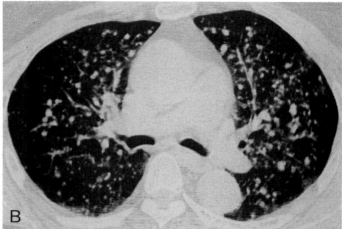

Figure 15.49. Metastastic Thyroid Carcinoma. A. A PA chest film in a middle-aged woman demonstrates innumerable small lung nodules with a larger nodule in the right paracardiac region (*arrow*). Note the presence of a right paratracheal mass deviating the tra- chea leftward (*open arrow*). **B.** A CT scan confirms the micronodular pattern, with nodules ranging in size from 1 to 6 mm. The CT-guided biopsy of the right paracardiac nodule revealed metastatic adeno- carcinoma of the thyroid.

Table 15.24. Differential Characteristics of Nodular Pulmonary Metastases

Radiographic finding	Malignancy
Cavitation	
Thin walled	Head and neck squamous cell carcinoma
Thick walled	Head and neck squamous cell carcinoma
	Cervix
	Colon carcinoma
Calcification	Osteogenic sarcoma
	Chondrosarcoma
Ill-defined margins	Renal cell carcinoma
	Thyroid carcinoma
	Choriocarcinoma
	Colon carcinoma
Miliary nodules	Renal cell carcinoma
	Thyroid carcinoma
	Melanoma
	Choriocarcinoma
	Bronchogenic carcinoma
Snowstorm appearance	Thyroid carcinoma
Cannonball lesions	Thyroid carcinoma
	Renal cell carcinoma
	Colon carcinoma
	Melanoma
	Seminoma
Spontaneous pneumothorax	Sarcoma
	Osteogenic sarcoma

of the colon and ovary may rarely produce calcification within pulmonary metastases, these microscopic cal- cifications are usually too small to be detected even on CT. Finally, in patients with miliary nodular opaci- ties, the presence of one or more larger nodules inter- spersed with uniformly sized miliary nodules is highly suggestive of metastases from melanoma or carci- noma of the lung, thyroid, or kidney (Fig. 15.49).

The diagnosis of nodular pulmonary metastases is usually presumptive. It is based on the demonstration of multiple pulmonary nodules in a patient with a known malignancy that has a propensity for lung me- tastases who lacks evidence of a granulomatous pro- cess. In some patients, particularly those with solitary pulmonary nodules who lack evidence of additional sites of metastases or those with a history of a prior localized malignancy, a biopsy of the nodule should be performed. In selected patients, resection of a solitary pulmonary metastasis or several peripheral metasta- ses may be undertaken. Computed tomography is the best imaging modality to follow the response of metas- tases to chemotherapy, with resolution of nodules in- dicating a positive response. An important caveat is that persistent nodular opacities representing steril- ized tumor deposits may be seen following successful treatment of metastatic choriocarcinoma or semi- noma. In these patients, follow-up CT scans will dem- onstrate a lack of growth of the nodules.

Lymphangitic Carcinomatosis. While direct parenchymal lymphatic invasion and obstruction of hilar and mediastinal lymph nodes by bronchogenic carcinoma is the most common cause of unilateral LC, extrapulmonary malignancies may invade pulmo- nary lymphatics after hematogenous dissemination to both lungs to produce interstitial deposits of tumor.

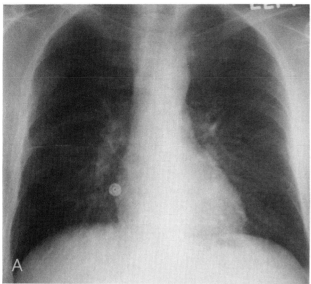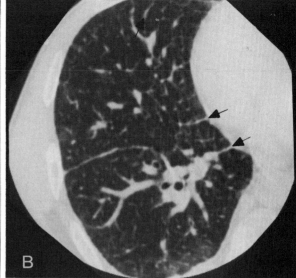

Figure 15.50.   Lymphangitic Carcinomatosis. A. A PA chest film in a 54-year-old patient with squamous cell carcinoma of the neck reveals bilateral linear interstitial opacities. **B.** The HRCT recon-structed to the right lung demonstrates thickening of interlobular septa (*straight arrows*) characteristic of LC. The diagnosis was confirmed by transbronchial biopsy.

In LC, the tumor cells invade the lymphatic vessels within the peribronchovascular and peripheral interstitium, resulting in lymphatic dilation, interstitial edema, and fibrosis. The most common extrathoracic malignancies to produce LC are carcinomas of the breast, stomach, pancreas, and prostate. Occasionally, LC will present in a patient without a known primary malignancy. Most patients with LC will have slowly progressive dyspnea and a nonproductive cough.

The chest radiographic findings in LC complicating extrathoracic malignancy correlate with the involvement of the peribronchovascular and peripheral interstitium seen pathologically. Peribronchial cuffing and linear opacities, particularly Kerley's B lines, are characteristically seen (Fig. 15.50). Coarse reticulonodular opacities may also be present. Concomitant hilar and mediastinal lymph node enlargement need not be present.

The predominant HRCT findings in LC are thickening of interlobular septa and the subpleural interstitium (Fig. 15.50**B**). While nodular thickening of the septa, reflecting tumor nodules, is characteristic of LC, it is seen in only a minority of patients. The thickened septal lines do not produce distortion of the lobule, a feature that helps distinguish LC from interstitial fibrosis, which characteristically distorts the normal lobular shape. Visibility of the intralobular bronchioles or prominence of the centrilobular vessel is frequently seen, as is thickening of the peribronchovascular interstitium within the central (parahilar) portions of the lung. The findings may be unilateral or even limited to one lobe, particularly

when LC occurs secondary to bronchogenic carcinoma. Since most patients have pathologic involvement of the peribronchovascular interstitium, the diagnosis is best made by transbronchial biopsy. In a patient with the appropriate history, the HRCT appearance of lymphangitic spread may be specific enough to obviate the need for transbronchial biopsy. Occasionally, the HRCT study will demonstrate the typical findings of LC when the plain radiograph is normal or equivocal.

NONEPITHELIAL PARENCHYMAL MALIGNANCIES AND NEOPLASTIC-LIKE CONDITIONS

Lymphoma. Parenchymal involvement in Hodgkin's disease is two to three times more common than in non-Hodgkin's lymphoma. The parenchymal abnormalities in Hodgkin's lymphoma usually take the form of linear and coarse reticulonodular opacities that directly extend into the lung from enlarged hilar lymph nodes. Extensive areas of parenchymal involvement can produce mass-like opacities and areas of air space opacification. Atelectasis in Hodgkin's disease is never due to extrinsic nodal compression of the bronchi, but rather develops from obstructing endobronchial tumor. Extension into the subpleural lymphatics may produce subpleural plaques or masses visible only by CT. While parenchymal involvement in Hodgkin's disease does not occur in the absence of hilar and mediastinal nodal disease (excluding patients who have undergone mediastinal irradiation), non-Hodgkin's lymphoma may involve the parenchyma without concomitant nodal disease in up to 50% of patients. The parenchymal involvement most often appears as masses or air space opacities (Fig. 13.4**C**); the latter may simulate lobar pneumonia. Coarse reticulonodular opacities may be seen and, rarely, a SPN is the sole manifestation of intrathoracic disease.

Pseudolymphoma is the term is used to describe a localized nonneoplastic reactive proliferation of lymphocytes in the lung. Histologically, the distinction from well-differentiated lymphoma may be difficult; the demonstration of a polyclonal population of lymphocytes with multiple germinal centers and the absence of lymph node enlargement is necessary for the diagnosis. A more appropriate term for this disorder is "nodular lymphoid hyperplasia" as it produces a sharply marginated pulmonary nodule or mass radiographically. The mass may contain air bronchograms as alveoli are compressed by large numbers of interstitial lymphocytes. Pseudolymphoma is usually associated with a good prognosis.

Lymphocytic Interstitial Pneumonitis, or diffuse lymphoid hyperplasia, is a pulmonary interstitial infiltration by mature lymphocytes that is histologically indistinguishable from nodular lymphoid hyperplasia. Patients with Sjögren's syndrome, hypogammaglobulinemia, and AIDS are at particular risk for this condition. Radiographically, a predominantly lower zone reticulonodular and linear pattern of disease is seen, often with intermixed areas of air space opacification. Some patients with this disorder develop frank pulmonary lymphoma or interstitial fibrosis; others resolve with the administration of corticosteroids.

Lymphomatoid Granulomatosis was originally believed to represent a distinct histologic entity, but has recently been reclassified as a form of pulmonary lymphoma. Histologically, there are multiple round nodules containing lymphocytes that infiltrate small vessels to produce an obliterative vasculitis. These findings are similar to those in Wegener's granulomatosis, although well-formed granulomas are rare in lymphomatoid granulomatosis. Central nervous system and skin involvement are common, while renal failure is not seen in this condition. Radiographically, there are multiple nodular opacities with a lower lobe predilection. Cavitation is common and results from ischemic necrosis. This condition is a lymphatic malignancy and is treated with chemotherapy. The prognosis is poor, with 50% of patients developing frank lymphoma. Overall 5-year survival is approximately 20%.

Leukemia. While leukemic involvement of the lung is found in approximately one-third of patients at autopsy, clinical or radiographic evidence of parenchymal infiltration is uncommon during life. The majority of pulmonary disease in leukemic patients is due to the associated immunosuppression, cardiac disease, or thrombocytopenia. Parenchymal involvement in leukemia usually takes the form of interstitial infiltration by leukemic cells, with resultant peribronchial cuffing and reticulonodular opacities on chest radiograph. Focal accumulation of leukemic cells can produce a chloroma and the radiographic appearance of a SPN. An unusual pulmonary manifestation of leukemia is pulmonary leukostasis, which is seen in acute leukemia or those in blast crisis in whom the peripheral white blood cell count exceeds $100,000-200,000/cm^3$. In this condition, the white cell blasts clump within the pulmonary microvasculature to produce dyspnea. Approximately half of affected patients will have normal radiographs, while the remainder will have a diffuse reticulonodular pattern of disease.

Kaposi's Sarcoma of lung is a common complication of AIDS. Pulmonary involvement almost invariably follows skin, oropharyngeal, and/or visceral involvement. The histologic features are characteristic; clusters of spindle cells with numerous mitotic figures are separated by thin-walled vascular channels containing red blood cells. The tumor involves the tracheobronchial mucosa and the peribronchovascular, alveolar, and subpleural interstitium of the lung. Radiographically, Kaposi's sarcoma produces small to medium-sized poorly marginated nodular and coarse linear opacities that extend from the hilum into the middle and lower lung zones. Computed tomography shows the typical peribronchovascular location of the opacities and may demonstrate air bronchograms traversing mass-like areas of confluent disease (Fig. 15.51). A bloody pleural effusion is present in up to 50% of patients and can be attributed to the presence of lesions within the subpleural interstitium of the lung. Hilar and mediastinal lymph node enlargement is less common, found in only 20% of patients. Important diagnostic features of pulmonary Kaposi's sarcoma are the slow rate of progression of disease (usually over many months) and the absence of fever or pulmonary symptoms despite the presence of extensive parenchymal disease. Bleeding from endobronchial or parenchymal lesions may produce focal or diffuse air space opacities that are difficult to distinguish from complicating bacterial pneumonia or *P. carinii* infection.

The diagnosis of pulmonary Kaposi's sarcoma is usually made indirectly by the visualization of typical endobronchial lesions in a patient with characteristic chest radiographic findings. Recently, combined thallium and gallium lung scanning has been used successfully to distinguish Kaposi's sarcoma from pneumonia and non-Hodgkin's lymphoma. While pneumonia is both gallium- and thallium-avid, lym-

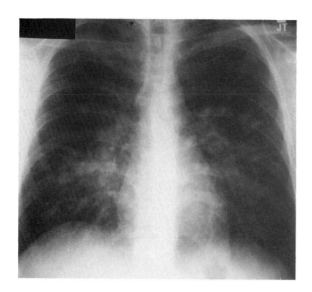

Figure 15.51. Kaposi's Sarcoma of Lung. PA chest film in a 34-year-old homosexual man with AIDS and extensive endobronchial Kaposi's sarcoma. There are bilateral ill-defined nodular and linear opacities typical of pulmonary Kaposi's sarcoma with probable hilar lymph node enlargement.

phoma is gallium-avid only and Kaposi's sarcoma is thallium-avid only.

Pulmonary Blastoma is a rare malignant tumor affecting children and young adults. These tumors arise from primitive pulmonary cells capable of forming both connective tissue and epithelial portions of lung, thereby simulating the development of the fetal lung. Pulmonary blastomas are difficult to distinguish histologically from carcinosarcomas. Radiographically, these tumors tend to be extremely large at presentation. Diagnosis is made by resection of the lesion.

There are a variety of other rare neoplasms and nonneoplastic tumors that may affect the lung. Since many of these present as a nodule or mass on chest radiographs, they are discussed in "The Solitary Pulmonary Nodule."

MISCELLANEOUS PULMONARY DISORDERS
Alveolar Microlithiasis

This is a rare disorder characterized by the deposition of minute calculi within the alveolar spaces of the lung. The underlying abnormality responsible for the formation of these calculi, known as calcispherytes, is unknown. While alveolar microlithiasis can affect individuals of any age without sex predilection, there is a very high incidence of this disease in siblings. Pathologically, small, less than 1 mm in diameter, calculi composed of calcium phosphate are found within normal alveoli; interstitial fibrosis may develop in long-standing disease. The radiographic findings are specific: confluent, bilateral, dense micronodular opacities are seen that, because of their high intrinsic

density, produce the so-called "black pleura sign" at their interface with the chest wall. Apical bullous disease is common and may lead to spontaneous pneumothorax. The diagnosis is made by a history of disease in a sibling of an affected individual and typical radiographic findings; biopsy is usually unnecessary. The majority of patients are asymptomatic at presentation despite the marked radiographic abnormalities, a feature that is characteristic of this disorder. Most patients develop progressive respiratory insufficiency, although some remain well for years. There is no effective treatment.

Pulmonary Alveolar Proteinosis (PAP)

This is a rare disease in which the lipoproteinaceous material surfactant deposits in abnormal amounts within the air spaces of the lung. Pulmonary alveolar proteinosis has a predilection for males in their 20s to 40s, although the disease has been reported in children. In adults, PAP has been associated with acute exposure to large amounts of silica dust (acute silicoproteinosis), most commonly in sandblasters, and with an immunocompromised state as is seen in patients with lymphoma, leukemia, or AIDS. These conditions produce an acquired defect of alveolar macrophages that fail to phagocytize the surfactant produced by type II pneumocytes, resulting in the accumulation of surfactant within the alveolar spaces. Pathologically, the alveoli are filled with a lipoproteinaceous material that stains deep pink with periodic acid-Schiff. The interstitium is usually uninvolved, but some patients have chronic interstitial inflammation and fibrosis.

Patients with PAP are often asymptomatic, although some complain of progressive dyspnea and a nonproductive cough. The absence of orthopnea is an important clinical feature distinguishing PAP from pulmonary edema secondary to congestive heart failure.

The typical radiographic finding in alveolar proteinosis is bilateral symmetric perihilar air space opacification indistinguishable in appearance from pulmonary edema (Fig. 15.52). Air space nodules are commonly seen at the periphery of the confluent opacities. Cardiomegaly, pleural effusions, and evidence of pulmonary venous hypertension are notably absent. Interstitial opacities may be seen following bronchoalveolar lavage in regions of previous air space opacification, but are usually more evident on HRCT scans.

Patients with PAP are particularly prone to superinfection of the lung with *Nocardia*. *Appergillus*, *Cryptococcus*, and atypical *Mycobacteria*. The factors responsible for this propensity may include macrophage dysfunction and the favorable culture medium of intraalveolar lipoproteinaceous material. Infection by one of these organisms should be suspected in any

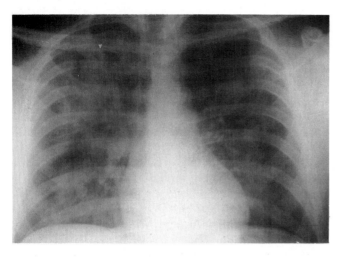

Figure 15.52. Pulmonary Alveolar Proteinosis. Frontal radiograph in a 36-year-old man with slowly progressive shortness of breath shows bilateral confluent air space opacities. Open lung biopsy revealed alveolar proteinosis.

patient with PAP who develop symptoms of pneumonia or radiographic findings of focal parenchymal opacification or cavitation and pleural effusion. Computed tomography helps in the early detection of opportunistic infection since pneumonia or abscess formation may be obscured by the underlying process on plain radiographs.

Prior to the advent of bronchoalveolar lavage, one-third of patients died from respiratory failure or opportunistic infections, while the remaining two-thirds either stabilized or resolved spontaneously. Repeated bronchoalveolar lavage with saline has significantly reduced the mortality from this disease. The duration of treatment with bronchoalveolar lavage varies; some patients require repetitive long-term therapy, while others resolve after only a single treatment.

References

1. Pare JAP, Fraser RG. Roentgenologic signs in the diagnosis of chest disease. In: Synopsis of diseases of the chest. 1st ed. Philadelphia: WB Saunders, 1983:164–235.
2. Genereux GP. Pattern recognition in diffuse lung disease. A review of theory and practice. Med Radiogr Photogr 1985;61:2–31.
3. Webb WR, Muller NL, Naidich DP. HRCT findings of lung disease. In: High-resolution CT of the Lung. 1st ed. New York: Raven, 1992:24–40.
4. Putman CE. Cardiac and noncardiac edema: Radiologic approach. In: Goodman LR, Putman CE, eds. Critical care imaging. Philadelphia: WB Saunders, 1992:107–127.
5. Milne EN, Pistolesi M, Miniati M, Giuntini C. The radiographic distinction of cardiogenic and noncardiogenic edema. AJR 1985;144:879–894.
6. Alderson PO, Martin EC. Pulmonary embolism: diagnosis with multiple imaging modalities. Radiology 1987;164:297–312.
7. Armstrong P, Wilson AG, Dee P. Infections of the lung and pleura. In: Imaging of diseases of the chest. 1st ed. Year Book, 1990:152–248.
8. Fraser RG, Pare JAP, Pare PD, Fraser RS, Genereux GP. Diseases of altered immunologic activity. In: Diagnosis of diseases of the chest. Vol 2. 3rd ed. Philadelphia: WB Saunders, 1989:1189–1240.
9. Armstrong P, Wilson AG, Dee P. Inhalational diseases of the lung. In: Imaging of diseases of the chest. 1st ed. Year Book, 1990:405–462.
10. Wagner RB, Crawford WO Jr, Schimpf PP. Classification of parenchymal injuries of the lung. Radiology 1988;167:77–82.
11. Heitzman ER. Embryology of the lung and pulmonary abnormalities of developmental origin. In: Heitzman ER, ed. The lung. 2nd ed. St. Louis: CV Mosby, 1984:13–41.
12. Thurlbeck WM, Henderson JA, Fraser RG, Bates DV. Chronic obstructive pulmonary disease: a comparison between clinical, roentgenologic, functional, and morphologic criteria in chronic bronchitis, emphysema, and bronchiectasis. Medicine 1970;49:81–145.
13. Fraser RG, Pare JAP, Pare PD, Fraser RS, Genereux GP. Drug- and poison-induced pulmonary disease. In: Diagnosis of diseases of the chest. Vol 4. 3rd ed. Philadelphia: WB Saunders, 1991:2417–2447.
14. Kirks DR, McCormick VD, Greenspan RH. Pulmonary sarcoidosis: roentgenologic analysis of 150 patients. AJR 1973;117:777–786.
15. Webb WR. Radiologic evaluation of the solitary pulmonary nodule. AJR 1990;154:701–708.

16

Pleura, Chest Wall, and Diaphragm

Jeffrey S. Klein
Scott R. Schultz

This chapter will review the diagnostic approach to and imaging characteristics of disorders affecting the pleura, chest wall, and diaphragm. The chest radiograph often provides the initial clue to disease involving these structures; as with mediastinal disease, computed tomography (CT) and magnetic resonance imaging (MR) play key roles in the radiologic evaluation of these disorders.

PLEURA

Pleural Effusion

PLEURAL FLUID PHYSIOLOGY AND PATHOPHYSIOLOGY

The normal volume of fluid in each pleural space is approximately 2 ml. Pleural fluid is formed by filtration from systemic capillaries in the parietal pleura and is resorbed by pulmonary capillaries within the visceral pleura. The formation and absorption of pleural fluid follows Starling's law and therefore depend upon the balance of hydrostatic and oncotic forces in the pleural capillaries and pleural space (Fig. 16.1) (1). The net effect of these forces results in the flow of pleural fluid from the parietal pleura into the pleural space and the resorption of this fluid at the visceral pleura.

Pleural effusions may be classified by their gross appearance (bloody, chylous, purulent, serous), the causative disease (Table 16.1), or by the pathophysiology of abnormal pleural fluid formation (transudative versus exudative). This latter differentiation is made by measuring the protein lactate dehydrogenase (LDH), and glucose concentration within pleural fluid obtained by thoracentesis. Conditions associated with an elevation of plasma hydrostatic pressure or a decrease in plasma oncotic pressure will produce a transudative pleural effusion characterized by (*a*) pleural/serum protein ratio of <0.5, (*b*) pleural/serum LDH ratio of <0.6, and (*c*) pleural LDH of <200 IU/liter. Left heart failure is the most common cause of pleural effusion resulting from an increase in hydrostatic pressure, which in turn results from pulmonary venous and capillary hypertension. Fluid overload from renal failure or pregnancy and constrictive pericarditis are additional causes of hydrostatic pleural effusion. The hypoproteinemia associated with liver disease is the most common cause of a transudative effusion secondary to decreased plasma oncotic pressure; additional causes are the nephrotic syndrome, severe malnutrition, and protein-losing enteropathy. An exudative pleural effusion, characterized by (*a*) pleural/serum protein ratio of >0.5, (*b*) pleural/serum LDH ratio of >0.6, and (*c*) pleural LDH of >200 IU/liter, is the result of an increase in pleural capillary permeability. Peripheral pulmonary or pleural processes that inflame the pleura (pneumonia, serositis) or directly invade the pleura (malignancy) are the commonest causes of pleural exudates.

RADIOGRAPHIC APPEARANCE OF PLEURAL EFFUSION

The radiographic appearance of pleural effusions depends upon the amount of fluid, the patient's position during the radiographic examination, and the presence or absence of adhesions between the visceral and parietal pleura (2). Small amounts of pleural fluid initially collect between the lower lobe and diaphragm in a subpulmonic location. As more fluid accumulates, it spills into the posterior and lateral costophrenic sulci. A moderate amount of pleural fluid (>175 ml) in the erect patient will have a characteristic appearance on the frontal radiograph, with a homogeneous lower zone opacity seen in the lateral costophrenic sulcus with a concave interface toward the lung. This concave margin, known as a pleural menis-

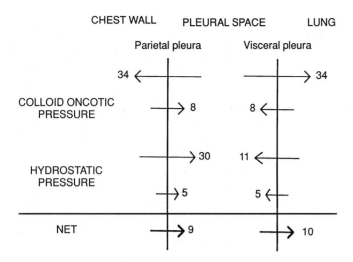

Figure 16.1. Physiology of Pleural Fluid Formation.

Table 16.1. Etiology of Pleural Effusions

Infectious	Bacterial/mycobacterial
	Viral
	Fungal
	Parasitic
Cardiovascular	Heart failure
	Pericarditis
	Superior vena cava obstruction
	Postcardiac surgery
	Myocardial infarction
	Pulmonary embolism
Neoplastic	Bronchogenic carcinoma
	Metastases
	Lymphoma
	Pleural or chest wall neoplasms (e.g., mesothelioma)
Immunologic	SLE
	Rheumatoid arthritis
	Sarcoidosis (rare)
	Wegener's granulomatosis
Inhalational	Asbestos
Trauma	Blunt or penetrating chest trauma
Abdominal disease	Cirrhosis
	Pancreatitis
	Subphrenic abscess
	Acute pyelonephritis
	Ascites (from any cause)
	Splenic vein thrombosis
Miscellaneous	Drugs
	Myxedema

cus, appears higher laterally than medially on frontal radiographs because the lateral aspect of the effusion, which surrounds the costal surface of the lung, is tangent to the frontal x-ray beam. Similarly, the meniscus of pleural fluid as seen on lateral radiographs peaks anteriorly and posteriorly (Fig. 16.2).

In patients with suspected pleural effusion, a lateral decubitus film with the affected side down is the most sensitive technique to detect small amounts of fluid. With this technique, pleural fluid collections as small as 5 mm may be seen layering between the lung and lateral chest wall. While a moderate-sized free-flowing collection should be obvious on upright radiographs, a large pleural effusion can cause passive atelectasis of the entire lung, producing an opaque hemithorax. It may be difficult to distinguish the latter condition from collapse of an entire lung. While a massive effusion should produce contralateral mediastinal shift, a collapsed lung without pleural effusion will show shift toward the opaque side. In some patients, CT or ultrasound may be necessary to distinguish pleural fluid from collapsed lung.

Computed tomography is quite sensitive in the detection of free pleural fluid. On axial scans, pleural fluid layers posteriorly with a characteristic meniscoid appearance and has a CT attenuation value of 0–20 Hounsfield units (HU). Small effusions may be difficult to differentiate from pleural thickening, fibrosis or dependent atelectasis, and decubitus scans are useful in this distinction. The pleural and peritoneal spaces are oriented in the axial plane at the level of the diaphragm. This may cause some difficulty in localizing the fluid to one or both spaces. Fluid in either the pleural or peritoneal space can displace the liver and spleen medially, away from the chest wall. A key to distinguishing ascites from pleural fluid on axial CT scans is to observe the relationship of the fluid to the diaphragmatic crus. Pleural fluid in the posterior costophrenic sulcus will lie posteromedial to the diaphragm and displace the crus laterally. In contrast, peritoneal fluid lies within the confines of the diaphragm and therefore will displace the crus medially.

Another useful distinguishing feature is the quality of the interface of the fluid with the liver or spleen. Intraperitoneal fluid will show a distinct, sharp interface with the liver and spleen as it directly contacts these organs, whereas pleural effusions will have a hazy, indistinct interface with these viscera due to the interposed hemidiaphragms. Since the peritoneal space does not extend posterior to the bare area of the liver, right-sided fluid extending posteromedially must be pleural. A large effusion will allow the inferior edge of adjacent atelectatic lower lobe to float in the fluid, creating a curvilinear opacity that can be misinterpreted as the diaphragm separating pleural fluid from ascites. This "pseudodiaphragm" is recognized as a broad band that does not extend far laterally or anteriorly and is contiguous superiorly with atelectatic lung containing air bronchograms (Fig. 16.3). Ultrasound is particularly useful in detecting free-flowing pleural effusions, which are usually seen as anechoic collections at the base of the pleural space surrounding atelectatic lung (3).

Pleural fluid may become loculated between the pleural layers to produce an appearance indistinguishable from a pleural mass. Fluid loculated within the costal pleural layers appears as a vertically ori-

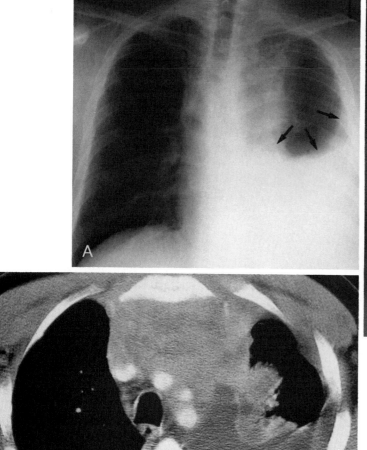

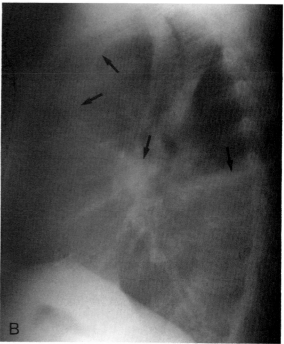

Figure 16.2. Chylous Effusion Due to Hodgkin's Disease. Posteroanterior (**A**) and lateral (**B**) radiographs demonstrate a left pleural effusion with typical meniscoid appearance (*arrows*). A computed tomography scan at the level of the superior mediastinum (**C**) reveals enlarged prevascular lymph nodes associated with the effusion. Chylous fluid was obtained at thoracentesis.

ented elliptical opacity with a broad area of contact with the chest wall, producing a sharp convex interface with the lung when viewed in tangent. Computed tomography is commonly utilized to detect and localize loculated pleural fluid collections. The characteristic finding is a sharply marginated lenticular mass of fluid attenuation, conforming to the concavity of the chest wall, which forms obtuse angles at its edges and compresses and displaces the subjacent lung. Multiple fluid locules can mimic pleural metastases or malignant mesothelioma radiographically; CT or ultrasound can confirm the fluid characteristics of these pleural "masses."

Pleural fluid may extend into the interlobar fissures, producing characteristic findings. Free fluid within the minor fissure is usually seen as smooth, symmetric thickening on frontal radiograph. Fluid within the major fissure is normally not visible on frontal radiographs as the fissures are viewed en face. An exception is fluid extending into the lateral aspect of an incomplete major fissure, which produces a cur-

vilinear density extending from the inferolateral to the superomedial aspect of the lung. Fluid loculated between the leaves of visceral pleura within an interlobar fissure results in an elliptical opacity oriented along the length of the fissure. These loculated collections of pleural fluid are termed "pseudotumors," and are most often seen within the minor fissure on frontal radiographs in patients with congestive heart failure. The tendency for these opacities to disappear rapidly with diuresis has led to the term "vanishing lung tumor." Although a characteristic appearance on plain radiographs is usually sufficient for diagnosis, the CT demonstration of a localized fluid collection in the expected location of the major or minor fissure is confirmatory.

An uncommon appearance of pleural effusion is seen when fluid accumulates between the lower lobe and diaphragm, which is termed a "subpulmonic effusion." While small amounts of pleural fluid normally accumulate in this location, it is uncommon for larger effusions to remain subpulmonic without spilling into

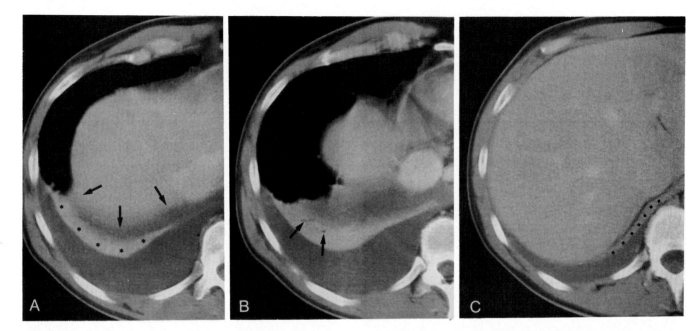

Figure 16.3. Subpulmonic Pleural Effusion on CT. A. A CT scan through the lower chest shows fluid surrounding an enhancing broad curvilinear structure (*asterisks*). The fluid creates an ill-defined interface with the liver (*arrows*). **B.** A scan 1 cm image 16.3A above shows that the curvilinear density represents the tip of an atelectatic right lower lobe containing air bronchograms (*arrows*). **C.** More inferiorly, the crus of the diaphragm (*dotted structure*) is displaced laterally by posteromedial pleural fluid.

the posterior and lateral costophrenic sulci. A subpulmonic effusion may be difficult to appreciate on upright chest radiographs as the fluid collection mimics an elevated hemidiaphragm. Clues to its presence on frontal radiographs include apparent elevation of the diaphragm, which is new; lateral peaking of the hemidiaphragm, which is accentuated on expiration; a minor fissure, which is close to the diaphragm (right-sided effusions); and an increased separation of the gastric air bubble from the base of the lung (left-sided effusions). Despite the atypical subpulmonic accumulation of fluid with the patient upright, the effusion will layer dependently on lateral decubitus radiographs (Fig. 16.4).

The radiographic detection of pleural effusion in the supine patient can be difficult as fluid accumulates in a dependent location posteriorly. The most common finding is a hazy opacification of the affected hemithorax with obscuration of the hemidiaphragm and blunting of the lateral costophrenic angle. Fluid extending over the apex of the lung may produce a soft-tissue cap with a concave interface inferiorly, while medial fluid may cause an apparent mediastinal widening.

SPECIFIC CAUSES OF PLEURAL EFFUSION

Congestive Heart Failure is the condition most commonly associated with a transudative pleural effusion. The effusions are usually bilateral, with the right-sided collection larger than the left. An isolated right effusion is twice as common as an isolated left effusion.

Parapneumonic Effusion and Empyema. A parapneumonic effusion is defined as an effusion associated with pneumonia. Peripheral parenchymal infection can cause visceral pleural inflammation and increased pleural capillary permeability, producing an exudative pleural effusion. Inflammatory thickening of the pleural membranes with lymphatic obstruction may be a contributing factor. Extension of the infection into the pleural space leads to empyema formation. The parenchymal infections that typically result in empyema formation are bacterial pneumonia, septic emboli, and lung abscess. Fungal, viral, and parasitic infection are uncommon causes of empyema. Less commonly, infection may extend into the pleural space from the spine, mediastinum, and chest wall.

Bacterial pneumonia. Forty percent of bacterial pneumonias have associated pleural effusion. *Staphylococcus aureus* and Gram-negative pneumonias are the most common cause of parapneumonic effusion and empyema. The natural history of parapneumonic effusions may be divided into three stages. Stage 1 is an exudative stage, with visceral pleural inflammation causing increased capillary permeability with resultant accumulation of pleural fluid. Most of these sterile exudative effusions resolve with appropriate antibiotic therapy. A stage 2 parapneumonic effusion is a fibrinopurulent pleural fluid collection containing bacteria and neutrophils. Fibrin deposition on the visceral and parietal pleura impairs fluid resorption and produces loculations (Fig. 16.5).

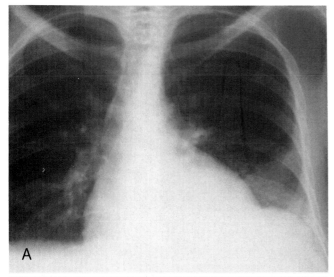

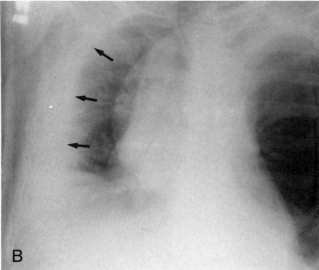

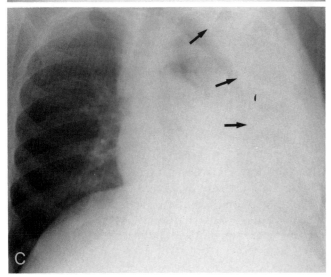

Figure 16.4. Bilateral Subpulmonic Pleural Effusions. A posteroanterior radiograph (**A**) in a 41-year-old woman with ascites demonstrates apparent elevation of both hemidiaphragms. Right (**B**) and left (**C**) lateral decubitus films demonstrate dependent layering of the subpulmonic pleural fluid (*arrows*).

If the infection is not treated, the loculations will impair attempts at closed pleural fluid drainage. A stage 3 parapneumonic effusion, which develops 2 to 3 weeks after initial pleural fluid formation, is characterized by the ingrowth of fibroblasts over the pleura, producing pleural fibrosis, which entraps the lung. Dystrophic calcification of the pleura may develop following resolution of the pleural infection.

Tuberculous pleural effusion or empyema resulting from the rupture of subpleural caseating granulomas may complicate pulmonary infection or occur as the primary manifestation of disease. Effusions in tuberculosis are more common in young adults with pulmonary disease and in human immunodeficiency virus-positive individuals with severe immunodeficiency. The pleural fluid is characteristically straw-colored with more than 70% lymphocytes and a low glucose concentration.

Empyema most often appears radiographically as a loculated pleural fluid collection. On CT, it is elliptical in shape and is seen most commonly within the posterior and inferior pleural space. The collection conforms to and maintains a broad area of contact with the chest wall. The distinction of empyema from peripheral lung abscess has important therapeutic implications, as empyemas require external drainage while lung abscesses usually respond to postural drainage and antibiotic therapy. Contrast-enhanced chest CT is most useful in making this distinction. *Lung abscesses* are round, fluid-filled masses with irregular margins that form acute angles with the adjacent chest wall. Since they destroy parenchyma, there is minimal compression of the adjacent lung. In contrast, empyemas are elliptical fluid collections that create obtuse angles with the chest wall and displace and compress adjacent lung. While the wall of an abscess is typically thick and enhances with contrast, the inflamed pleural layers encompassing an empyema are thin, smooth, and enhance homogeneously, producing the "split pleura" sign, which is helpful in diagnosis (Fig. 16.6) (4). The detection of an empyema may be difficult when there is extensive parenchymal consolidation. In these cases, CT and ultrasound are useful in detecting parapneumonic fluid collections and guiding diagnostic thoracentesis and pleural drainage.

Neoplasms. Pleural effusion may be seen with benign or malignant intrathoracic tumors. The tumors most commonly associated with pleural effusion are, in order of decreasing frequency, lung carcinoma, breast carcinoma, pelvic tumors, gastric carcinoma, and lymphoma. Pleural fluid formation may result from pleural involvement by tumor or from lymphatic obstruction anywhere from the parietal pleura to the mediastinal nodes. The effusions are exudative and may be bloody. The demonstration of malignant cells

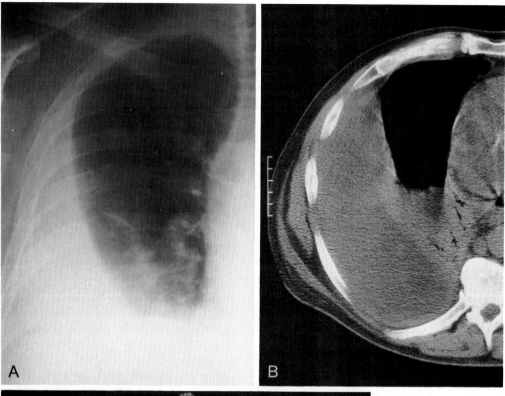

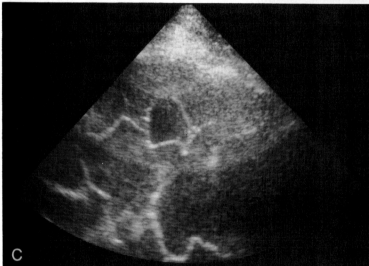

Figure 16.5.   Stage 2 Parapneumonic Effusion: CT vs. Ultrasound. A. A coned-down view of the right thorax in a patient with right lower lobe pneumonia reveals a large right pleural effusion with typical meniscoid appearance. **B.** A CT through the right base shows an apparently unilocular parapneumonic fluid collection with passive lower lobe atelectasis. **C.** Transthoracic ultrasound shows multiple septations within the pleural fluid. Diagnostic thoracentesis yielded only a small amount of exudative fluid with an elevated white blood cell count.

on cytologic examination of pleural fluid obtained at thoracentesis is necessary for the diagnosis of a malignant effusion. Closed or pleuroscopically guided biopsy is reserved for patients with negative cytologic examination. Clues to the presence of a malignant pleural effusion include smooth or lobulated pleural thickening, mediastinal or hilar lymph node enlargement or mass, or a solitary or multiple parenchymal nodules. Computed tomography is useful in demonstrating pleural masses or underlying parenchymal lesions in those with large effusions.

Trauma. Blunt or penetrating trauma to the chest, including iatrogenic trauma from thoracotomy, thoracostomy, or placement of central venous cathe-

ters, may result in a hemothorax. The hemothorax may arise from lacerated vessels within the lung, mediastinum, chest wall, or diaphragm. Intrapleural blood coagulates rapidly, and septations form early. In some individuals, the clotted blood will lyse as pleural motion causes defibrination. In the acute setting, pleural fluid of high CT attenuation (>80 HU) may be seen; associated rib fractures or subcutaneous emphysema should suggest the diagnosis. An acute hemothorax is treated with thoracostomy tube drainage, while thoracotomy is generally reserved for persistent bleeding or hypotension. Esophageal perforation from prolonged vomiting (Boerhaave's syndrome) or as a complication of esophageal dilation may produce a

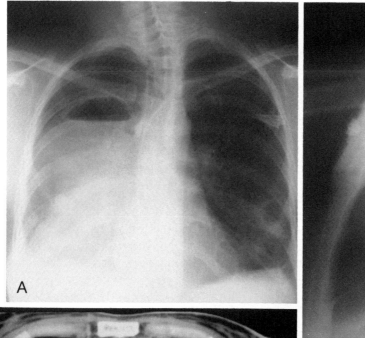

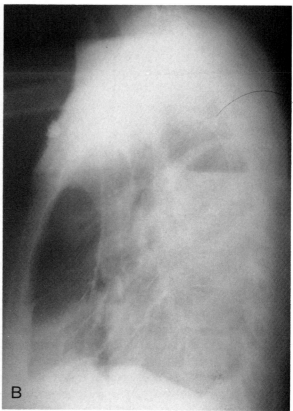

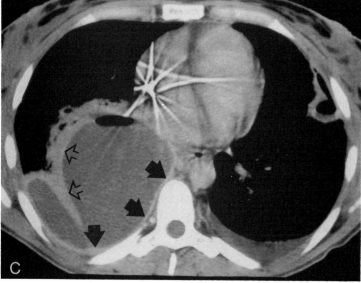

Figure 16.6. Bronchopleural Fistula and Empyema. Posteroanterior (**A**) and lateral (**B**) radiographs in a 31-year-old woman with endocarditis and septic pulmonary emboli reveals a large air and fluid collection occupying the posterior aspect of the right hemithorax. A CT scan (**C**) prior to thoracentesis shows a large air and fluid collection conforming to the posterior chest wall and mediastinum, which compresses and displaces the lower lobe anteriorly and demonstrates enhancement of visceral (*open arrowheads*) and parietal (*solid arrowheads*) pleura, producing a split pleura sign. Note the septic embolus in the lingula associated with a loculated pneumothorax. It is likely that a right-sided embolus ruptured into the pleural space to produce a bronchopleural fistula and empyema.

pleural effusion, most commonly on the left. Extravascular placement of a central line can lead to a hydrothorax when intravenous solution is inadvertently infused into the pleural or extrapleural space.

Collagen Vascular and Autoimmune Disease. Systemic lupus erythematosus (SLE) has a reported incidence of pleural effusions ranging from 33 to 74%. The effusions usually result from pleural inflammation, and patients present with pleuritic chest pain and an exudative pleural effusion. In some cases, nephrotic syndrome associated with SLE may produce transudative effusions. Cardiomegaly is a common chest radiographic finding, and may be due to pericardial effusion, hypertension, renal failure, or lupus-associated endocarditis or myocarditis.

Pleural effusion is the most common intrathoracic manifestation of rheumatoid arthritis, most fre-

quently seen in male patients following the onset of joint disease. Rheumatoid effusions occur independent of pulmonary parenchymal involvement but may develop following intrapleural rupture of peripheral rheumatoid nodules. The effusions of rheumatoid arthritis are exudative, with a lymphocytosis, low glucose concentration, and low pH (<7.2). Rheumatoid effusions may persist unchanged for years.

Autoimmune syndromes producing pleural and pericardial effusions have been described following myocardial infarction (Dressler's syndrome) or cardiac surgery (postpericardiotomy syndrome). Both are characterized by fever, pleuritis, pneumonitis, and pericarditis developing within days to weeks of the precipitating event. The radiographic findings include enlargement of the cardiac silhouette, pleural effusions, and parenchymal air space opacities. A serosanguinous exudative pleural effusion is seen in over 80% of patients. Treatment with nonsteroidal antiinflammatory agents usually results in symptomatic and radiographic improvement.

Abdominal Disease. As demonstrated by radioisotope studies, peritoneal fluid may enter the pleural space via transdiaphragmatic lymphatic channels or through defects in the diaphragm. The lymphatic channels are larger on the right than the left, accounting for the higher incidence of right-sided effusions associated with ascites.

Either acute or chronic pancreatitis can cause pleural effusion, which is most often left-sided because of the proximity of the pancreatic tail to the undersurface of the left hemidiaphragm. The effusion associated with acute pancreatitis is typically exudative and may be bloody. Pleural effusion from chronic pancreatitis may cause pleuritic chest pain and shortness of breath. Rupture of the pancreatic duct can lead to pancreaticopleural fistula formation. A high amylase concentration in the pleural fluid should suggest the pancreas as the etiology of the effusion, although an elevated amylase may be seen in effusion because of malignancy or esophageal perforation.

Subphrenic abscesses complicating abdominal surgery or perforation of a hollow viscus can cause diaphragmatic paresis, basilar atelectasis, and pleural effusion. Patients with a pleural effusion associated with upper abdominal pain, fever, and leukocytosis should have CT or ultrasound examination and, when feasible, percutaneous catheter drainage of the abscess.

An association between benign pleural effusions and pelvic tumors has long been recognized. First described with ovarian fibroma (Meigs' syndrome), a number of pelvic and abdominal tumors including pancreatic and ovarian malignancy, lymphoma, and uterine leiomyomas have been found to cause pleural effusion. The effusions in Meigs' syndrome are usually transudative and resolve after removal of the pelvic tumor.

Chylothorax refers to a pleural fluid collection containing suspended lipids in the form of chylomicrons. It results from a thoracic duct perforation that communicates with the pleural space. The thoracic duct originates from the cisterna chyli at the level of the first lumbar vertebra and ascends along the right paravertebral space, entering the thorax via the aortic hiatus. The duct crosses from right to left at the level of the sixth thoracic vertebra to lie alongside the upper esophagus. At the level of the left subclavian artery, the duct arches anteriorly to empty into the confluence of the left internal jugular and subclavian veins. A disruption of the upper duct, resulting from direct trauma or obstruction with rupture, will produce a left chylothorax, while injury to the lower in-

trathoracic duct produces a right chylothorax. The most common causes of chylothorax are malignancy, iatrogenic trauma, and tuberculosis (Fig. 16.2). The radiographic appearance is indistinguishable on plain radiographs and CT from other causes of free-flowing effusions.

Pulmonary Embolism. Infarction complicating pulmonary embolism is a well-recognized cause of pleural effusion. The effusion may be associated with elevation of the ipsilateral diaphragm and peripheral wedge-shaped opacities (Hampton's hump). The pleural effusion is typically a small, unilateral, serosanguinous exudate.

Drugs may cause pleural effusions as a result of pleural inflammation (e.g., methysergide) or by producing a lupus-like syndrome (e.g., phenytoin, isoniazid, hydralazine, procainamide). Nitrofurantoin administration has been associated with an immunologic reaction that causes pleuropulmonary disease with eosinophilia.

Bronchopleural Fistula

A bronchopleural fistula represents a communication between lung and the pleural space, most often originating from a peripheral airway. A bronchopleural fistula from a bronchus often results in an empyema, while an air leak from peripheral air spaces may cause an intractable pneumothorax. Bronchopleural fistulas most often develop from dehiscence of a bronchial stump following lobectomy or pneumonectomy, or as the result of a necrotizing pulmonary infection. Presenting symptoms include fever, cough, and dyspnea; large air leaks may be noted in patients with pleural drains. Radiographically, a bronchopleural fistula presents as a loculated intrapleural air and fluid collection (Fig. 16.6). The development of an air-fluid level in the postpneumonectomy space or a drop in the air-fluid level during the early postoperative period, associated with shift of the mediastinum back toward the midline, should suggest the diagnosis. Computed tomography is useful in evaluating patients with suspected bronchopleural fistula and empyema; it can distinguish a hydropneumothorax from a peripheral lung abscess, and occasionally demonstrates the actual fistulous communication.

Postpneumonectomy Space

Following pneumonectomy, the residual space gradually fills with fluid and appears radiographically as an opaque hemithorax with ipsilateral mediastinal shift. The radiographic findings suggesting bronchopleural fistula formation complicating pneumonectomy are described in the previous section. Computed tomography and MR are useful in evaluating the postpneumonectomy space for evidence of tumor recur-

Table 16.2. Etiology of Pneumothorax

Trauma	Iatrogenic	
		Thoracic/abdominal surgery
		Percutaneous interventional procedures
		Lung/pleural biopsy
		Thoracentesis
		Central line placement
		Aberrant feeding tube placement
		Mechanical ventilation
		Esophagoscopic biopsy/dilation
		Bronchoscopic biopsy
	Noniatrogenic	
		Penetrating injury
		Stab wound
		Gunshot wound
		Blunt injury
		Tracheobronchial disruption
		Esophageal rupture
		Rib fractures
Spontaneous	Primary (idiopathic)	
	Secondary	
		Obstructive airways disease
		Asthma
		Emphysema
		Infection
		Cavitating pneumonia
		Lung abscess
		Septic emboli
		Pneumatoceles
		Pulmonary infarction (rare)
		Neoplasm
		Bronchogenic carcinoma
		Pleural or chest wall neoplasm
		Metastases
		Cystic lung disease
		Sarcoidosis
		Eosinophilic granuloma
		Cystic fibrosis
		Tuberous sclerosis
		Lymphangioleiomyomatosis
		Catamenial pneumothorax
		Connective tissue disorders
		Marfan's syndrome
		Ehlers-Danlos syndrome
		Cutis laxa

rence, and may help in the diagnosis of postoperative bronchopleural fistula and empyema.

Pneumothorax

Pneumothorax results from air entering the pleural space, and may be traumatic or spontaneous. Spontaneous pneumothorax is further subdivided into a primary form, which has no identifiable etiology, and a secondary form associated with underlying parenchymal lung disease (Table 16.2). Pneumothoraces typically present with the sudden onset of dyspnea and pleuritic chest pain.

Traumatic Pneumothorax. Trauma is the most common cause of pneumothorax. Penetrating injuries can produce pneumothorax by introducing air from the atmosphere into the pleural space or by laceration of the visceral pleura, resulting in an air leak from the lung. Gun shot and knife wounds to the chest and upper abdomen, central line placement, thoracentesis, transbronchial biopsy, and percutaneous needle biopsy are common penetrating injuries that cause traumatic pneumothorax. Blunt chest trauma may cause pneumothorax by acutely increasing intrathoracic pressure. This results in extraalveolar interstitial air because of alveolar disruption, which tracks peripherally and ruptures into the pleural space. In addition, tracheobronchial laceration can produce a pneumothorax with a large bronchopleural fistula. In patients with rib fractures, the free edge of the fractured ribs can project inward to lacerate the lung and cause pneumothorax.

SPONTANEOUS PNEUMOTHORAX

Primary Spontaneous Pneumothorax most often occurs in young or middle-aged men. A familial incidence and a propensity for taller individuals has been noted. While the exact pathogenesis of primary spontaneous pneumothorax remains unclear, affected patients are often found to have blebs or bullae within the lung apices, which are likely responsible for the development of the pneumothorax.

Secondary Spontaneous Pneumothorax has been associated with multiple entities. Most of these disorders have associated blebs, bullae, cysts, or cavities, although in some patients the lungs are intrinsically normal. In the majority of the latter, there is usually a history of sudden increases in intrathoracic pressure. Chronic obstructive pulmonary disease is the most common predisposing disease. Acute obstruction to expiration from bronchoconstriction (i.e., asthma) or the performance of the Valsalva maneuver (e.g., crack cocaine or marijiuana smoking, transvaginal childbirth) may cause spontaneous pneumothorax. Pneumothorax may complicate cystic lung changes in sarcoidosis, histiocytosis X of lung, and lymphangioleiomyomatosis. Necrotizing pneumonia or lung abscess due to Gram-negative or anaerobic bacteria, tuberculosis, or *Pneumocystis carinii* pneumonia can lead to pneumothorax, particularly in the mechanically ventilated patient (Fig. 16.7). A peripheral bronchogenic carcinoma rarely presents with pneumothorax. Metastases to the lung are an infrequent cause of pneumothorax, and rarely are a presenting feature of disease. Pneumothorax develops when necrotic subpleural metastases rupture into the pleural space. Sarcomas, particularly osteogenic sarcoma, lymphoma, and germ cell malignancies, are the most common primary malignancies to produce spontaneous pneumothorax. Marfan's syndrome is the most common connective tissue disease producing pneumothorax, which usually results from the rupture of apical bullae. Other connective tissue diseases

Figure 16.7. Bilateral Pneumothoraces Caused by Necrotizing P. carinii Pneumonia. An anteroposterior radiograph in a patient with severe P. carinii pneumonia shows dense opacification with cavity formation (*arrows*) associated with bilateral pneumothoraces.

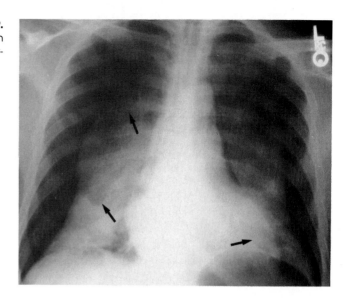

that can produce pneumothorax are Ehlers-Danlos syndrome and cutis laxa.

Mechanically ventilated patients are particularly at risk for pneumothorax development because of the administration of positive pressure, underlying or complicating necrotizing pneumonia or emphysema, and frequent line placements and other invasive procedures. Not uncommonly, patients with adult respiratory distress syndrome develop small peripheral cystic air spaces that can rupture into the pleural space. When these are seen to develop on serial chest radiographs, impending pneumothorax can be suggested.

A particularly rare type of recurrent pneumothorax that occurs with menstruation is catamenial pneumothorax. This condition affects women in their 4th decade, and is most likely caused by the cyclic necrosis of pleural endometrial implants that create an air leak between the lung and pleura. Rarely, air entering the peritoneal cavity during menstruation gains access to the pleural cavity via diaphragmatic defects. The predilection for right-sided pneumothoraces in this disorder indicates a key role for right-sided diaphragmatic defects. The pneumothoraces tend to be small and resolve spontaneously. Catamenial pneumothorax is managed by preventing menstruation with the administration of oral contraceptives.

Tension Pneumothorax is a critical condition that most often results from iatrogenic trauma in mechanically ventilated patients. Tension pneumothorax results from the development of a pleural defect that allows air to enter but not exit the pleural space. This leads to a pleural air collection that has a pressure exceeding atmospheric pressure, causing complete collapse of the underlying lung and impairing venous return to the heart. Clinically, patients present with tachypnea, tachycardia, cyanosis, and hypotension. Radiographically, the involved hemithorax will be expanded and hyperlucent, with a medially retracted lung, ipsilateral diaphragmatic depression or inversion, and contralateral shift of the mediastinum. While the radiographic findings are suggestive, tension pneumothorax remains a clinical diagnosis. Immediate evacuation of the pleural space should be performed with a needle, catheter, or large-bore thoracostomy tube.

RADIOGRAPHIC APPEARANCE OF PNEUMOTHORAX

The classic radiographic finding of pneumothorax on upright chest films is visualization of the visceral pleura as a curvilinear line that parallels the chest wall, separating the partially collapsed lung centrally from pleural air peripherally (Fig. 16.8). An expiratory radiograph aids in the detection of a small pneumothorax because the volume of intrapleural air increases relative to the lung, thereby displacing the visceral pleural reflection away from the chest wall.

The detection of a pneumothorax is difficult when chest films are obtained in the supine position (5). Approximately 30% of pneumothoraces present on supine radiographs go undetected. Since many portable radiographs are obtained with the patient supine, the recognition of a pneumothorax on a supine film is particularly important in the critically ill patient who is at high risk from iatrogenic trauma or barotrauma. In a supine patient, the most nondependent portion of the pleural space is anterior or anteromedial. Small pneumothoraces will initially collect in these regions and will fail to produce a visible pleural line. The affected hemithorax may appear hyperlucent. Anteromedial air may sharpen the borders of mediastinal soft-tissue structures, resulting in improved visualization of the cardiac margin and aortic knob. The lateral costophrenic sulcus may appear abnormally deep and hyperlucent, a finding known as the "deep sulcus" sign. Visualization of the anterior costophrenic

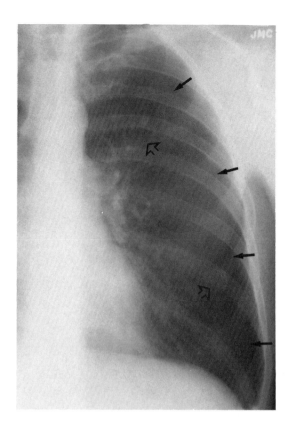

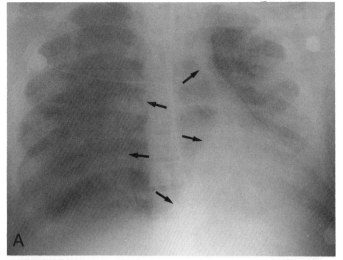

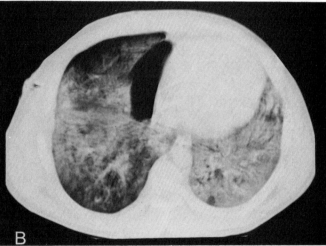

Figure 16.8. The Visceral Pleural Line in Pneumothorax. A coned-down view of a posteroanterior radiograph in a patient with a spontaneous pneumothorax demonstrates the curvilinear visceral pleural line (*solid arrows*) separating the lung medially from the chest wall laterally. Note the thin-walled cysts (*open arrows*) from *Coccidioides* infection, which are most likely responsible for the pneumothorax.

Figure 16.9.   Pneumothorax in Supine Patient. A. A supine radiograph in a patient with adult respiratory disease syndrome demonstrates a localized collection of gas over the medial right thorax (*arrows*). **B.** A CT scan from the same day reveals an anteromedial pneumothorax.

sulcus due to anterior and inferior air produces the "double diaphragm" sign, as the dome and anterior portions of the diaphragm are outlined by lung and pleural air, respectively. When an anterior pneumothorax is suspected on a supine radiograph, an upright film, lateral decubitus film with the affected side up, or a CT scan should be obtained (Fig. 16.9).

Subpulmonic pneumothoraces are rare. Radiographically, a localized area of hyperlucency is seen inferiorly with the visceral pleural line paralleling the hemidiaphragm. Loculated pneumothoraces develop as the result of adhesions between visceral and parietal pleura, and may be found anywhere in the pleural space. Computed tomography is often necessary for diagnosis.

There are several entities that produce a curvilinear line or interface or hyperlucency on chest radiographs that must be distinguished from a pneumothorax. Skin folds resulting from the compression of redundant skin by the radiographic cassette can produce a curvilinear interface that simulates the visceral pleural line. A skin fold produces an edge or interface with atmospheric air, in distinction to the visceral pleural line seen in a pneumothorax. The interface produced

by a skin fold rarely continues over the lung apex, and is often seen to extend beyond the chest wall. Pulmonary vascular opacities may be followed peripheral to the skin fold interface. Bullae may simulate pneumothorax by producing localized or unilateral hyperlucency. They are marginated by thin curvilinear walls that are concave rather than convex to the chest wall. The distinction of pneumothorax from bullous disease may be difficult but is usually evident by the clinical presentation. However, since this distinction has important therapeutic implications, certain patients may require CT.

Computed tomography is more sensitive than conventional radiographs in the detection of pneumothorax because of its cross-sectional nature and superior contrast resolution. The CT demonstration of linear parenchymal bands of tissue traversing large avascular areas helps distinguish bullae from localized pneu-

Table 16.3.   Focal Pleural Disease

Opacities that mimic focal pleural thickening	Apical cap
	Companion shadows of first and second ribs
	Subpleural deposits of fat
Thickening	Pneumonia
	Pulmonary infarct
	Trauma
	Asbestos exposure (bilateral)
Calcification	Visceral pleura
	Hemothorax
	Empyema (tuberculosis)
	Parietal pleura
	Asbestos exposure (bilateral)
Pleural/extrapleural mass	Neoplasm
	Benign
	Fibroma
	Lipoma
	Neurofibroma
	Malignant
	Metastases (usually multiple)
	Mesothelioma (usually diffuse pleural thickening)
	Loculated pleural effusion/empyema
	Hematoma

mothoraces. Computed tomography may be used to detect and drain loculated pneumothoraces in critically ill patients.

Focal Pleural Disease

Focal pleural disease may be divided into localized pleural thickening, pleural calcification, or pleural mass (Table 16.3).

LOCALIZED PLEURAL THICKENING

Localized pleural thickening from fibrosis is usually the end result of peripheral parenchymal and pleural inflammatory disease, with pneumonia the most common cause. Additional causes include pulmonary embolism with infarction, asbestos exposure, trauma, prior chemical pleurodesis, and drug-related pleural disease.

Radiographically, localized pleural thickening is seen as a flat, smooth, slightly raised soft-tissue opacity extending over one or two intercostal spaces that displaces the lung from the innermost cortical margin of the ribs when viewed in tangent. Localized pleural thickening viewed en face is usually undetectable radiographically as the lesion does not significantly attenuate the x-ray beam and does not present a raised edge to be recognized as a distinct opacity. Focal areas of pleural fibrosis are best appreciated on conventional and high-resolution CT (HRCT) scans. They are distinguished from deposits of subpleural fat by their CT density (Fig. 16.10).

There are two additional radiographic findings that mimic the appearance of focal pleural thickening. The apical cap is a curvilinear subpleural opacity less than

5 mm thick with a sharp or slightly irregular inferior margin that represents nonspecific fibrosis of the apical lung and adjacent visceral pleura. While it is usually bilateral and symmetric, slight asymmetry in thickness is not uncommon. Any growth of the opacity, significant asymmetry, inferior convexity of the opacity, rib destruction, or symptoms should prompt a CT or MR examination followed by biopsy to exclude an apical neoplasm (i.e., Pancoast's or superior sulcus tumor). The companion shadows of the inferior aspects of the first and second ribs are smooth apical linear opacities that parallel the lower cortical margins of the first two ribs and represent the pleural layers and subpleural fat viewed in tangent. These are seen most prominently in obese individuals and should not be mistaken for pleural fibrosis.

PLEURAL CALCIFICATION (TABLE 16.3)

Pleural calcification is most often unilateral and involves the visceral pleura. It is usually the result of prior hemothorax or empyema (e.g., tuberculous), although pleural thickening of any cause may calcify. Asbestos exposure can cause bilateral calcified parietal pleural plaques. Visceral pleural calcification from pleural hemorrhage or infection are indistinguishable radiographically. Initially, the calcification is punctate, but it often progresses to become sheet-like. Computed tomography is particularly useful in detecting pleural calcification (Fig. 16.11). The presence of fluid within calcified pleural layers seen on CT should suggest an active empyema; this is most often seen in patients with prior tuberculosis. The use of CT and HRCT in the evaluation of asbestos-related fo-

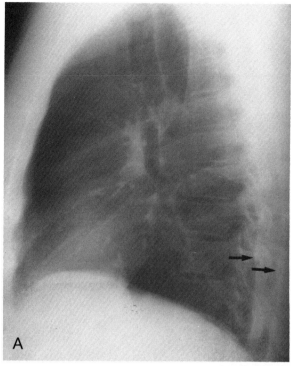

A

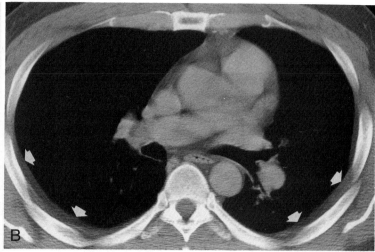

B

Figure 16.10. Subpleural Fat Mimicking Focal Pleural Thickening or Plaque Formation. A. A lateral radiograph demonstrates bilateral focal pleural or extrapleural opacities (*arrows*). **B.** A CT scan reveals subpleural deposits of fat (*arrows*) accounting for the pleural opacities on the radiograph.

cal pleural disease and calcification is discussed in "Asbestos-related Pleural Disease."

PLEURAL MASS

Focal pleural masses are usually benign neoplasms such as fibromas and lipomas; loculated pleural fluid can mimic a pleural mass radiographically.

Lipomas of the thorax may arise in the chest wall or subpleural fat, the latter producing a pleural mass. Lipomas, because of their pliable nature, can change shape during respiration or with changes in patient positioning. Homogeneous fatty attenuation on CT scan (-30 to -100 HU) is diagnostic.

Pleural Fibromas, also known as benign mesotheliomas or localized fibrous tumors, are rare benign pleural tumors (Fig. 16.12) (6). They appear as well-defined, spherical or oblong masses that arise from the visceral pleura in 80% of cases. Uncommonly, these tumors are attached to the pleura by a narrow pedicle, a finding that is virtually pathognomonic and accounts for changes in intrapleural location seen with changes in patient positioning in some individuals. An association between pleural fibroma and hypertrophic pulmonary osteoarthropathy and hypoglycemia is recognized. Unlike malignant mesothelioma, there is no association between benign mesothelioma and asbestos exposure.

The shape and margins of a peripheral opacity as seen on conventional radiographs help define the opacity as parenchymal, pleural, or extrapleural. Pleural masses form obtuse angles with the adjacent normal pleura, in distinction to peripheral lung lesions that usually contact the normal pleura at acute angles. Pleural and extrapleural masses are usually vertically orientated elliptical opacities. Pleural lesions tend to have smooth, well-defined margins as they compress normal lung. These smooth margins are best appreciated on radiographic projections with the x-ray beam tangent to the interface between the mass and the lung. Another feature of pleural lesions is the clarity of the margin of the lesion on frontal and lateral radiographs; a mass sharply outlined by lung on one view but poorly marginated on the orthogonal view should suggest a pleural or extrapleural process. In distinction, intraparenchymal lesions are surrounded by air and will have similar margins on both views. Pleural lesions, unlike parenchymal lesions, do not change position with respiratory motion. Lung disease is often confined to a lobe, while pleural disease may extend across fissures. Pedunculated pleural lesions such as fibromas are rare but can present with radiographic features of both pleural and parenchymal lesions.

Despite the just-mentioned features, the distinction of pleural from peripheral parenchymal lesions may be difficult. This distinction has important diagnostic implications; while parenchymal processes are best evaluated by examination of expectorated sputum or by bronchoscopy, pleural lesions will require thoracentesis or pleural biopsy. Computed tomography is often used to help distinguish between pleural and parenchymal disease (see "Parapneumonic Effusion and Empyema"). A peripheral lesion that is completely surrounded by lung on CT is intraparenchy-

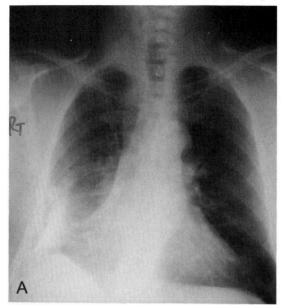

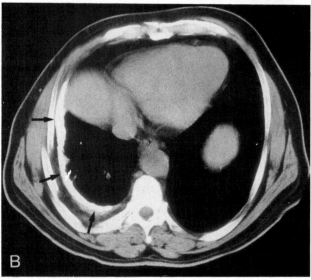

Figure 16.11.   Pleural Calcification Due to Tuberculosis. A. Poster-oanterior chest radiograph in a 61-year-old man with prior tuberculosis demonstrates a small right hemithorax and a dense opacity inferiorly. **B.** A CT scan through the lung bases shows a thick rind of pleural calcification (*arrows*) surrounding a contracted lung.

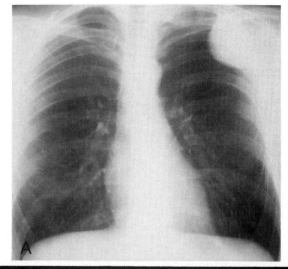

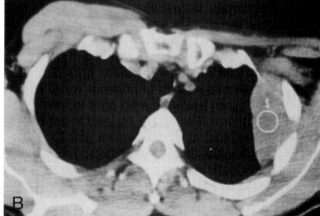

Figure 16.12.   Pleural Fibroma. A. Posteroanterior radiograph in a 37-year-old man reveals a superolateral pleural mass **B.** A CT scan shows a sharply defined soft tissue mass forming obtuse margins with the lung. Note the incidental finding of absence of the left pectoralis major muscle. Thoracotomy revealed a benign fibrous pleural tumor.

mal, the exception being the rare pleural lesion arising within an interlobar fissure. Peripheral lung masses generally have irregular margins and may contain air bronchograms. Those parenchymal lesions that contact the pleura will form acute angles with the chest wall, as on plain films. The CT appearance of pleural and extrapleural or chest wall lesions are similar. Both pleural and extrapleural lesions are sharply defined and form obtuse angles with the chest wall (Fig. 16.12); rib destruction or subcutaneous mass are the only findings that localize an extrapulmonary lesion to the chest wall. When a peripheral parenchy-

mal lesion invades the pleura, determining the origin of the mass may be impossible.

Computed tomography can further characterize peripheral lesions by their density; a smooth fatty mass is almost certainly a pleural lipoma, whereas a homogeneous pleural or extrapleural soft-tissue mass is most likely a fibroma or neurogenic tumor (Fig. 16.12**B**). The signal intensity on T1- and T2-weighted spin-echo MR images may be useful in the characterization of focal pleural masses. On T1 and T2 weighting, loculated fluid collections will show homogeneous low and high signal, respectively. Lipomas will show homogeneous high signal intensity on T1 weighting and intermediate signal intensity on T2 weighting, while fibromas are typically of intermediate and high-signal intensity, respectively, because of the high cellularity of these tumors.

Table 16.4. Diffuse Pleural Disease

Smooth thickening	Pleural fibrosis
	Hemothorax
	Prior empyema or exudative effusion (including asbestos exposure)
	Interstitial pulmonary fibrosis
	Pleural effusion (particularly on supine radiographs)
Lobulated	Primary
	Mesothelioma
	Metastastatic
	Adenocarcinoma of lung, breast, ovary, kidney, gastrointestinal tract
	Invasive thymoma
	Lymphoma (subpleural deposits)
	Multiloculated pleural effusion/empyema

Diffuse Pleural Disease

Diffuse pleural disease represents either diffuse pleural fibrosis (fibrothorax), pleural malignancy, or multiloculated pleural effusion (Table 16.4); the latter has been discussed in "Pleural Fluid."

Diffuse Pleural Fibrosis (Fibrothorax) is defined as pleural thickening extending over more than one-fourth of the costal pleural surface. Fibrothorax most commonly results from the resolution of an exudative pleural effusion, (including asbestos-related effusions), empyema, or hemothorax. It may also be seen as a subpleural extension of diffuse interstitial fibrosis. The fibrothorax can encompass the entire lung and produce entrapment. When this results in a restrictive ventilatory defect, pleurectomy (decortication) may be necessary to restore function to the underlying lung.

Radiographically, fibrothorax appears as a thin, smooth band of soft tissue with a sharp internal margin seen immediately beneath and parallel to the inner margin of the ribs and intercostal spaces. It is usually unilateral and extends over large areas of the dependent (i.e., posterior and inferior) portions of the pleural space. Anterior or posterior costal pleural thickening creates a veil-like opacity without sharp margins when viewed en face on frontal radiographs. Blunting of the lateral costophrenic sulcus may be seen on frontal radiographs, while sparing of the posterior costophrenic sulcus and an absence of layering fluid on decubitus positioning help distinguish pleural fibrosis from a small effusion. Fibrothorax tends to spare the interlobar fissures and mediastinal pleura. Computed tomography and HRCT are more sensitive than conventional radiographs in the detection of pleural thickening. The diminished volume of the affected hemithorax seen with extensive fibrothorax is more easily appreciated on axial CT images than on frontal radiographs (Fig. 16.11). Computed tomography and HRCT provide an unimpeded view of the un-

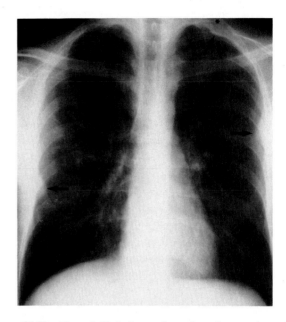

Figure 16.13. Pleural Metastases from Lymphoma. A posteroanterior radiograph in a 41-year-old man with acquired immunodeficiency syndrome and non-Hodgkin's lymphoma demonstrates multiple pleural masses (*arrows*), representing pleural metastases. The left apical lesion has destroyed the undersurface of the left second rib (*asterisk*), indicating local chest wall invasion.

derlying lung in patients with diffuse pleural thickening, allowing detection of associated interstitial pulmonary fibrosis. This is important in evaluating patients with suspected asbestosis and in assessing the extent of pulmonary disease in patients being considered for pleurectomy.

Pleural Malignancy. Metastatic disease to the pleura commonly causes irregular or lobulated pleural thickening, usually in association with a pleural effusion. The malignant tumors with a propensity to metastasize to the pleura include adenocarcinomas of the lung, breast, ovary, kidney, and gastrointestinal tract. Malignant mesothelioma is seen almost exclusively in asbestos-exposed individuals.

Malignant pleural disease (either metastatic adenocarcinoma or mesothelioma) usually presents radiographically as multiple discrete pleural masses or lobulated pleural thickening (Fig. 16.13). However, in many patients the pleural lesions are obscured by an associated malignant pleural effusion. Contrast-enhanced CT can distinguish solid pleural masses from loculated pleural fluid, and can show discrete pleural masses or thickening in patients with large effusions. In contrast to benign pleural thickening, malignant pleural disease is more likely when CT shows pleural thickening that is circumferential and nodular, greater than 1 cm in thickness, and/or involves the mediastinal pleura. Mesothelioma is radiographically indistinguishable from metastatic pleural disease and will be discussed in "Asbestos-related Pleural Disease." Chest wall invasion by pleural tumor, seen as rib destruction or soft-tissue infiltration of the subcutaneous fat and musculature, is better appreciated on CT or MR than on plain films. The diagnosis of malignant pleural disease is made by cytologic examination of fluid obtained at thoracentesis, closed or thoracosopically guided pleural biopsy, or by thoracotomy.

Asbestos-Related Pleural Disease

Prolonged exposure to the inorganic fibers generically known as asbestos can result in a variety of pleural and pulmonary disorders. Benign pleural disease is the most common thoracic manifestation of asbestos inhalation and includes pleural plaques, pleural effusions, and diffuse pleural fibrosis. Malignant asbestos-related pleural disease is manifested as malignant mesothelioma.

BENIGN ASBESTOS-RELATED PLEURAL DISEASE

Pleural Plaques are the most common benign manifestation of asbestos inhalation. The plaques develop 20 to 30 years after the initial asbestos exposure, and are more frequent with increasing length and severity of exposure. Asbestos plaques are found on the parietal pleura, most commonly over the diaphragm and lower posterolateral chest wall. Characteristically, they spare the mediastinal pleural surface and costophrenic sulci. The plaques are discrete, bilateral, slightly raised (2–10 mm in thickness) foci of pleural thickening that are pearly white and shiny in gross appearance. Histologically, the plaques are comprised of dense bands of collagen. Punctate or linear calcification within the plaques is common, and is more frequent as the plaques enlarge. Asbestos bodies (short, straight asbestos fibers coated with iron and protein) are not seen within the plaques. Visceral pleural plaques, seen as discrete flat regions of pleural thickening within the major fissures on HRCT, are most commonly associated with interstitial fibrosis. Most patients with isolated asbestos-related pleural plaques are asymptomatic, as discrete plaques do not result in restrictive lung disease.

The detection of pleural plaques on conventional radiographs is best with 45° oblique views that profile the anterolateral and posterolateral plaques. When viewed en face, the calcified plaques appear as geographic areas of opacity that have been likened to a holly leaf. Computed tomography and HRCT studies are highly sensitive in detecting calcified and noncalcified pleural plaques in asbestos-exposed individuals (Fig. 16.14). In addition, CT and HRCT can distinguish pleural plaques and diffuse pleural fibrosis from subpleural fat deposits that can mimic pleural disease on conventional radiographs (Fig. 16.10). Although plaques are invariably bilateral on gross examination of the pleural space in affected individuals, it

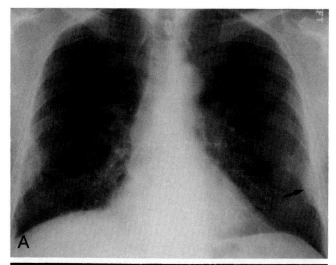

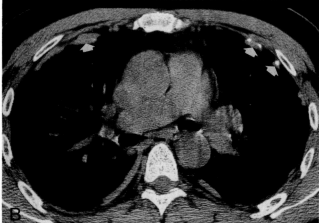

Figure 16.14.   Pleural Plaques from Asbestos Exposure. A. Posteroanterior radiograph in a 57-year-old former shipyard worker demonstrates multiple poorly circumscribed peripheral opacities (*arrows*). **B.** A CT scan demonstrates typical pleural plaques, some of which are calcified (*arrows*).

is not unusual to see unilateral plaques (most often left-sided) on conventional radiographs or HRCT studies of the chest.

Pleural Effusion is the earliest manifestation of asbestos-related pleural disease, occurring 10–20 years after the initial exposure. The effusions are usually small, unilateral or bilateral, exudative in nature, and may be bloody. The development of asbestos-related effusions appears to be dose-related. The diagnosis of a benign asbestos pleural effusion is one of exclusion and, in addition to a history of exposure, requires the exclusion of tuberculosis or pleural malignancy (i.e., mesothelioma or metastatic adenocarcinoma). A long latent period between the initial exposure and the development of pleural effusion (i.e., >20 years) should prompt a diagnostic evaluation for malignant mesothelioma. While most asbestos pleural effusions resolve spontaneously, as many as one-third recur and some result in diffuse pleural fibrosis.

Diffuse Pleural Thickening or fibrosis may follow asbestos pleural effusion or result from the confluence of pleural plaques. Diffuse asbestos pleural thickening is defined as smooth, flat pleural thickening extending over one-fourth of the costal pleural surface. In distinction to pleural plaques, which affect the parietal pleura alone, diffuse pleural fibrosis involves both the parietal and visceral pleura. Radiographically, diffuse pleural thickening is seen as a smooth thickening of the pleura involving the lower thorax with blunting of the costophrenic sulci. Computed tomography and HRCT are useful for determining the extent of pleural thickening, involvement of the interlobar fissures, and for detecting underlying fibrotic or emphysematous lung disease. Diffuse pleural fibrosis can result in symptomatic restrictive lung disease.

MALIGNANT ASBESTOS-RELATED PLEURAL DISEASE

Malignant Mesothelioma is a rare malignant pleural neoplasm associated with asbestos exposure, which, unlike other pleural and parenchymal manifestations of asbestos, does not appear to be dose-related. Mesothelioma most often occurs 30–40 years after the initial exposure. Although the incidence increases with heavy exposure, mesothelioma may develop after minimal exposure, unlike benign asbestos pleural disease in which the relationship between the dose of asbestos exposure and the development of disease is linear. Crocidolite is the fiber type most often implicated in the development of malignant mesothelioma. The tumor grows by contiguous spread from the pleural space into the lung, chest wall, mediastinum, and diaphragm; distant metastases are not uncommon.

Malignant pleural mesothelioma most often appears radiographically as thick (>1 cm) and lobulated diffuse pleural thickening (7). Calcification is seen in only 20% of tumors, although calcified pleural plaques may be seen in uninvolved areas of pleura. Most patients have an associated pleural effusion that, if large, may obscure the pleural tumor. Malignant involvement of the mediastinal pleural surface may prevent contralateral mediastinal shift despite extensive pleural tumor volume and effusion, a finding that may help distinguish mesothelioma from metastatic disease. Computed tomography is the imaging modality of choice in the evaluation of malignant mesothelioma, and depicts the extent of pleural involvement and invasion of the chest wall and mediastinum (Fig. 16.15). Diaphragmatic invasion by tumor, best assessed by coronal MR scans, is important only in those considered for resection. Adenopathy is seen in the ipsilateral hilum and mediastinum in approximately 50% of patients. While the radiologic findings may be highly suggestive of mesothelioma,

metastatic pleural malignancy can have a similar appearance, and histologic confirmation is necessary.

The diagnosis of malignant mesothelioma is made on examination of histologic specimens and often requires the use of special stains. The malignant cells may be of the spindle or epithelial type or a combination of both. The epithelial type of malignant mesothelioma may be indistinguishable from adenocarcinoma on light microscopy. Periodic acid-Schiff staining of the cellular cytoplasm following diastase digestion of the tissue specimen detects the presence of intracellular neutral mucins, and is found in 80% of patients with metastatic adenocarcinoma to the pleura. Alternatively, Alcian blue staining of the cytoplasm following tissue pretreatment with hyaluronidase detects the presence of intracellular acid mucins and is diagnostic in 50% of patients with the epithelial type of malignant mesothelioma. Positive keratin staining will help diagnose the spindle cell type of mesothelioma and distinguish this form of mesothelioma from fibrosarcoma.

While surgical resection by pleurectomy or extrapleural pneumonectomy may benefit selected patients with limited disease and good pulmonary reserve, the median survival from the time of diagnosis is only 6–12 months.

CHEST WALL

Disorders of the soft tissues or bony structures of the chest wall may come to attention because of local symptoms or physical findings, during evaluation of pulmonary or pleural disease, or as an incidental finding on radiographic studies (Table 16.5).

Soft Tissues

Congenital Absence of the Pectoralis Muscle will result in hyperlucency of the affected hemithorax on frontal radiographs. Poland's syndrome is an autosomal recessive disorder characterized by unilateral absence of the sternocostal head of the pectoralis major (Fig. 16.13**B**), ipsilateral syndactyly, and rib anomalies. There may be associated aplasia of the ipsilateral breast. Patients who have had a mastectomy will also show unilateral hyperlucency. In those who have undergone a modified radical mastectomy, the horizontally oriented inferior edge of the hypertrophied pectoralis minor muscle may be identified on frontal radiographs.

Skin Lesions. A variety of skin lesions including moles, nevi, warts, neurofibromas, and accessory nipples may produce a nodular opacity on frontal radiographs mimicking a solitary pulmonary nodule. Examination of the skin surface should be performed in any patient with a new nodular opacity seen on chest radiographs; repeat radiographs obtained with a radi-

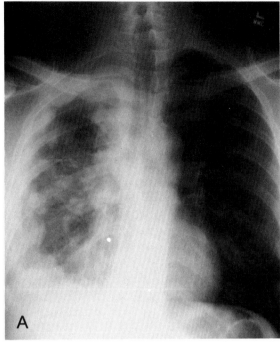

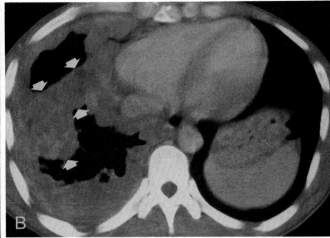

Figure 16.15. Malignant Mesothelioma. A. Posteroanterior chest radiograph in a 34-year-old man evaluated for a positive PPD reveals a lobulated pleural opacity encompassing the right lung. **B.** A CT scan through the lung bases demonstrates a circumferential pleural soft tissue process traversing the major fissure (*arrows*). Ultrasound-guided cutting needle biopsy of the pleura revealed malignant mesothelioma.

Table 16.5. Chest Wall Lesions

Tumors	Benign
	Mole
	Nevus
	Wart
	Neurofibroma
	Lipoma
	Hemangioma
	Desmoid
	Malignant
	Fibrosarcoma
	Liposarcoma
	Metastases
	Melanoma
	Bronchogenic carcinoma
Infection (abscess)	*Staphylococcus*
	Tuberculosis
Trauma	Hematoma

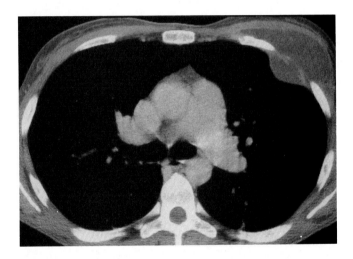

Figure 16.16. Staphylococcal Abscess of the Chest Wall. A CT scan demonstrates a fluid collection with minimal rim enhancement that is beneath the left pectoralis major muscle and protrudes into the thorax. Forty milliliters of purulent fluid was removed by incision and external drainage.

opaque marker over the skin lesion will confirm the nature of the opacity and avoid unnecessary follow-up radiographs and chest CT scans.

Chest Wall Abscesses may present as localized, painful, fluctuant subcutaneous masses. *Staphylococcus* and tuberculosis are the most common organisms responsible. The diagnosis is usually obvious clinically. Chest radiographs demonstrate a poorly defined opacity on frontal radiograph when the abscess involves the anterior or posterior chest wall. Computed tomography shows a localized fluid collection with an enhancing wall, and is used to determine the exact location and extent of the collection prior to open drainage (Fig. 16.16).

Soft-tissue Neoplasms of the chest wall are rare. They are most often detected clinically as a mass pro-

truding from the chest wall and appear as nonspecific extrathoracic soft-tissue masses on chest radiographs. The most common benign neoplasm of the chest wall is a lipoma. Lipomas may be intrathoracic, extrathoracic, or project partially within and outside the thorax (dumbbell lipoma). Computed tomography will show a sharply circumscribed mass of fatty density, while MR will show characteristic high and intermediate signal intensity on T1- and T2-weighted sequences, respectively. A desmoid tumor is a rare fibroblastic tumor arising within striated muscle; it is histologically benign but has a tendency for local invasion. Desmoid tumors are most common in the abdominal wall muscu-

Table 16.6. Rib Lesions

Congenital disease	Fusion anomalies
	Cervical rib
	Ribbon ribs
	Rib notching
	Inferior
	Coarctation of the aorta
	Tetralogy of Fallot
	Superior vena caval obstruction
	Blalock-Taussig shunt (unilateral right)
	Neurofibromatosis
	Superior
	Paralysis
	Collagen vascular disease
	Rheumatoid arthritis
	SLE
Trauma	Healing rib fracture
Nonneoplastic tumors	Fibrous dysplasia
	Eosinophilic granuloma
	Brown tumor
Neoplasms	Benign
	Osteochondroma
	Enchondroma
	Osteoblastoma
	Malignant
	Primary
	Chondrosarcoma
	Osteogenic sarcoma
	Fibrosarcoma
	Metastatic
	Multiple myeloma
	Metastases
	Breast carcinoma
	Bronchogenic carcinoma
	Renal cell carcinoma
	Prostate carcinoma
Osteomyelitis	*S. aureus*
	Tuberculosis
	Actinomycosis
	Nocardiosis

lature of multiparous women, but may arise in the chest wall musculature following local trauma. Hemangiomas are uncommon chest wall tumors. While often indistinguishable from other soft-tissue tumors radiographically, the recognition of phleboliths, hypertrophy of involved bones, or the identification of vascular channels on contrast-enhanced CT or MR studies should suggest the diagnosis.

The most common malignant soft-tissue neoplasms of the chest wall in adults are fibrosarcomas and liposarcomas. Malignant tumors often present with symptoms of localized chest wall pain and a visible, palpable mass. Patients who have received chest wall radiation are at particular risk for developing sarcomas. Radiographically, these appear as soft-tissue masses associated with bony destruction. Computed tomography best depicts the bone destruction and intrathoracic component of tumor, while MR shows the extent of tumor and delineates tumor from surrounding muscle and subcutaneous fat (8).

Bony Structures of the Thorax

RIBS (TABLE 16.6)

Congenital Anomalies. The most common congenital anomalies of the ribs are bony fusion and bifid ribs, both of which have no clinical significance. Intrathoracic ribs are extremely rare congenital anomalies where an accessory rib arises from a vertebral body or the posterior surface of a rib and extends inferolaterally into the thorax, usually on the right side. Osteogenesis imperfecta and neurofibromatosis may be associated with thin wavy "ribbon" ribs. A relatively common congenital anomaly is the cervical rib, which arises from the seventh cervical vertebral body. Cervical ribs are usually asymptomatic, although in a minority of individuals with the thoracic outlet syndrome, the rib or associated fibrous bands can compress the subclavian artery and produce secondary ischemic symptoms or compress the subclavian vein and brachial plexus producing pain, weakness, and swelling of the upper extremity. Surgical resection of the cervical rib can relieve the symptoms in selected patients.

Rib Notching is seen in a wide variety of pathologic conditions. Inferior rib notching is much more common than superior rib notching, and is due to enlargement of one or more of the structures that lie in the subcostal grooves (intercostal nerve, artery, or vein). The notching predominantly affects the posterior aspects of the ribs bilaterally and may be narrow, wide, deep, or shallow.

The most common cause of bilateral inferior rib notching is coarctation of the aorta distal to the left subclavian artery. In this condition, blood circumvents the aortic obstruction by traversing the subclavian, internal mammary, and intercostal arteries to reach the descending aorta. The increased blood flow through the intercostal arteries produces tortuosity and dilation of these vessels, which then erode the inferior margins of the adjacent ribs. In addition to coarctation, other causes of aortic obstruction that can lead to inferior rib notching include aortic thrombosis and Takayasu's aortitis. Congenital heart disease associated with decreased pulmonary blood flow may lead to rib notching as the intercostal arteries enlarge in an attempt to supply collateral flow to the oligemic lungs. Superior vena cava obstruction can cause increased flow through intercostal veins and produce rib notching.

Patients with aortic coarctation develop rib notching gradually; it is most common in adolescents and is rare in children under the age of 7. The first two ribs are uninvolved since the first and second intercostal arteries arise from the superior intercostal branch of the costocervical trunk of the subclavian artery, and therefore do not communicate with the descending thoracic aorta. Coarctation may produce unilateral left rib notching when the aortic narrowing occurs proximal to an aberrant right subclavian artery. Unilateral right-sided notching occurs when the coarctation is proximal to the left subclavian artery. Additional causes of unilateral inferior rib notching include subclavian artery obstruction and surgical anastamosis of the proximal subclavian artery to the ipsilateral pulmonary artery (Blalock-Taussig procedures).

Multiple intercostal neurofibromas in neurofibromatosis type I is the major nonvascular cause of inferior rib notching. The neurofibromas appear as multiple extrapleural soft-tissue masses, most often seen in the upper paravertebral regions. Other thoracic bony manifestations of neurofibromatosis include ribbon ribs, thoracic kyphoscoliosis, and scalloping of the posterior aspect of the vertebral bodies caused by dural ectasia.

Superior rib notching is much less common than inferior rib notching. The pathogenesis of superior rib notching is unknown, although a disturbance of osteoblastic and osteoclastic activity and the stress effect of the intercostal muscles are proposed mechanisms. Paralysis is the most common condition associated with superior rib notching. Other etiologies include rheumatoid arthritis, SLE, and, rarely, marked tortuosity of the intercostal arteries from severe, long-standing aortic obstruction.

Trauma.   Rib fractures may result from blunt or penetrating trauma to a normal rib cage or from minimal trauma to abnormal ribs such as those affected by metastases. An acute rib fracture is seen as a thin, vertical lucency; occasionally malalignment of the superior and inferior cortices of the rib segments is the only radiographic finding. The tendency to affect the posterolateral aspects of the ribs explains the utility of obtaining ipsilateral posterior oblique radiographs for suspected fracture, as this projection best displays the fracture line. In any patient with an acute rib fracture, a careful search should be made for associated pneumothorax, hemothorax, or pulmonary contusion or laceration. Since the first three ribs are well protected by the clavicles, scapulae, and shoulder girdles, fracture of these ribs indicates severe trauma and should prompt a careful evaluation for associated great vessel and visceral injuries. Fracture of the 10th, 11th, or 12th ribs may be associated with injury to the liver or spleen. Severe blunt trauma to the rib cage in which multiple contiguous ribs are fractured in more than one place is termed a "flail chest." This results in a free segment of the chest wall that moves paradoxically inward on inspiration and outward on expiration. Healing rib fractures will demonstrate callus formation, which may be exuberant in patients receiving corticosteroids. Multiple contiguous healed rib fractures, particularly if bilateral, should suggest chronic alcoholism or a prior motor vehicle accident.

Nonneoplastic Lesions.   The ribs are the most common site of involvement by monostotic fibrous dysplasia. The typical appearance is an expansile lesion of the posterior aspect of the rib with a lucent or ground-glass density; rarely, the lesion is sclerotic. Multiple rib involvement from polyostotic fibrous dysplasia can result in severe restrictive pulmonary disease. Eosinophilic granuloma can cause lytic lesions in patients under the age of 30. These are usually solitary lytic lesions that can be expansile but do not have sclerotic margins; this latter feature helps distinguish these lesions from fibrous dysplasia. Brown tumors from hyperparathyroidism can also produce lytic rib lesions.

Neoplasms.   Primary osteochondral neoplasms or metastatic disease can involve the ribs. Osteochondromas are the most common benign neoplasm of ribs, followed in relative frequency by enchondromas and osteoblastomas. Primary malignant neoplasms of the ribs in adults are uncommon. Chondrosarcoma is the most common primary rib malignancy, with osteogenic sarcoma and fibrosarcoma less common (Fig. 16.17). Rib involvement from multiple myeloma or metastatic carcinoma can produce multiple lytic lesions and is much more common than primary tumors. Myeloma can also produce a solitary rib lesion or permeative bone destruction indistinguishable from severe osteoporosis. The diagnosis of myeloma is made by identification of a monoclonal spike on serum protein electrophoresis and typical findings of abnormal aggregates of plasma cells on bone marrow biopsy. The most common metastatic lesions to ribs are from bronchogenic and breast carcinoma, which produce multiple lytic lesions when dissemination is hematogenous, or localized rib destruction when invasion is by direct contiguous spread. Expansile lytic rib metastases are seen most commonly from renal cell and thyroid carcinoma (Fig. 16.18). Sclerotic rib metastases are most commonly seen in breast and prostate carcinoma.

Infection.   Chest wall infection and osteomyelitis of the ribs usually develops from spread of infection from contiguous sites in the lung, pleural space, and vertebral column. Less commonly, infection complicates penetrating chest trauma or spreads to the ribs hematogenously. Pleuropulmonary infections that may traverse the pleural space and produce a chest wall infection include tuberculosis, actinomycosis, and nocardiosis. Radiographs may demonstrate bone destruction, periostitis, and subcutaneous emphysema; bone scans can detect subradiographic bone involvement. Computed tomography can demonstrate bone destruction, soft-tissue swelling, and abscesses within the chest wall. Additionally, CT may show in-

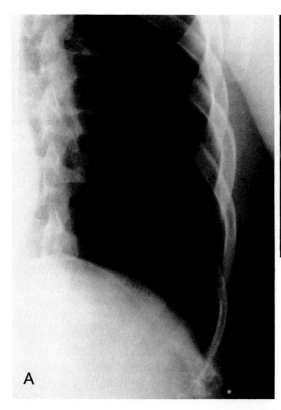

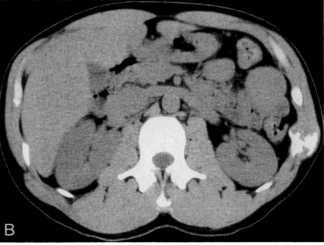

Figure 16.17. Chondrosarcoma of the Rib. A. Coned-down view of an oblique chest radiograph of the left lower thorax in a patient with a palpable left chest wall mass. A radiographic marker has been placed over the lesion that demonstrates chondroid calcification. **B.** A CT scan through the lesion shows an exophytic lesion with soft-tissue and calcific components arising from the 11th rib. The resected specimen revealed chondrosarcoma.

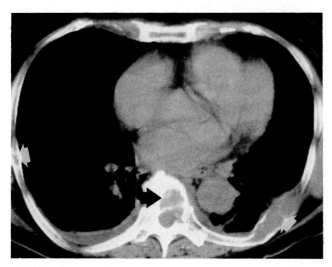

Figure 16.18. Lytic Metastases from Thyroid Carcinoma. A CT scan in a 68-year-old woman demonstrates expansile lytic lesions of the ribs (*white arrows*) and thoracic vertebral body and pedicle (*black arrow*), representing metastases from papillary carcinoma of the thyroid.

volvement of the adjacent portions of the pleural space, lung, sternum, or vertebral column.

COSTAL CARTILAGES

Ossification of the costal cartilages is a normal finding on frontal chest radiographs in adults. Female costal cartilage ossification involves the central portion of the cartilage, extending from the rib toward the sternum in the shape of a solitary finger, while male costal cartilage ossification involves the peripheral portion of the cartilage and has the appearance of two fingers ("peace" sign). These typical patterns of male and female costal cartilage ossification are seen in 70% of patients and do not apply to the first rib.

SCAPULA

Scapular abnormalities visible on frontal radiographs include congenital, posttraumatic, and neoplastic lesions. Sprengel's deformity is a congenital anomaly in which the scapula is elevated and hypoplastic. The association of Sprengel's deformity with an omovertebral bone, fused cervical vertebrae, hemivertebrae, kyphoscoliosis, and rib anomalies is termed the Klippel-Feil syndrome. Scapular fractures may result from direct trauma to the upper back and shoulder or from impaction of the humeral head into the glenoid. A winged scapula is identified when the scapula is superiorly displaced from its normal position and the inferior portion is posteriorly displaced from the chest wall, thereby foreshortening its appearance on the frontal radiograph. The deformity develops secondary to an interrupton in the innervation of the serratus anterior muscle, which maintains the scapula against the chest wall. Metastatic disease to the scapula is recognized by the presence of lytic destructive lesions; bronchogenic and breast carcinomas are the most common primary malignancies.

CLAVICLE

The clavicle is involved in cleidocranial dystostosis, in which there is partial or complete aplasia of the clavicle. The clavicle is commonly fractured in blunt trauma and usually involves the distal third. Rheumatoid arthritis and hyperparathyroidism are associated with erosion of the distal clavicles. Whereas in rheumatoid arthritis the distal clavicle tapers to a point and is sharply defined, it is often widened and irregular in hyperparathyroidism. An additional finding in rheumatoid arthritis is narrowing of the glenohumeral joint with a high-riding humeral head due to rotator cuff atrophy. Primary malignant neoplasms of the clavicle include Ewing's or osteogenic sarcoma. Metastases to the clavicle are usually associated with lesions in other portions of the bony thorax. Osteomyelitis of the clavicle is uncommon and is most often seen in intravenous drug users.

THORACIC SPINE

Disorders of the thoracic spine are discussed in Section 8, "Bones and Joints." A variety of thoracic spine abnormalities are visible on chest radiographs. Congenital anomalies including hemivertebrae, butterfly vertebra, spina bifida, and scoliosis can be seen on well-penetrated frontal radiographs. Vertebral compression fractures caused by trauma, osteoporosis, or metastases are best seen on lateral radiographs and may produce an exaggerated kyphosis. Large bridging osteophytes may mimic a paraspinal mass on frontal radiographs or a pulmonary nodule on lateral films. Vertebral osteomyelitis is seen as destruction of vertebral bodies and intervertebral discs, often associated with a paraspinal abscess. Chronic anemia in patients with thalassemia major or sickle cell disease may have pre- or paravertebral masses of extramedullary hematopoiesis, which represent herniated hyperplastic bone marrow.

STERNUM

Developmental sternal deformities include pectus excavatum (funnel chest), pectus carinatum (pigeon breast), and abnormal segmentation (9).

Pectus Excavatum. In pectus excavatum, the sternum is inwardly depressed and the ribs protrude anterior to the sternum. It often has an autosomal dominant pattern of inheritance but may occur sporadically. Pectus excavatum is commonly associated with congenital connective tissue disorders such as Marfan's syndrome, Poland's syndrome, osteogenesis imperfecta, and congenital scoliosis. Most patients are asymptomatic. A clinically insignificant systolic murmur may result from compression of the right ventricular outflow tract, although some patients with

pectus deformities and systolic murmurs have mitral valve prolapse. On frontal chest radiograph, pectus excavatum has a characteristic appearance. The heart is displaced to the left and the combination of the depressed soft tissues of the anterior chest wall and the vertically oriented anterior ribs results in loss of the right heart border. The findings on frontal radiographs may be mistakenly attributed to middle lobe opacification from pneumonia or atelectasis. On lateral chest radiographs, the typical inward depression of the middle and lower sternum is seen. Computed tomography helps define the deformity and its effect upon the heart and mediastinal structures.

Pectus Carinatum is an outward bowing of the sternum that may be congenital or acquired. The congenital form is seen more commonly in boys and in families with a history of chest wall deformities or scoliosis. Congenital atrial or ventricular septal defects and severe childhood asthma account for the majority of the acquired cases of pectus carinatum. Affected patients are asymptomatic. The characteristic outward bowing of the sternum with deepening of the retrosternal air space is seen on lateral radiographs.

Trauma. Severe blunt trauma to the chest, most often associated with deceleration injury from a motor vehicle accident, can result in sternal fracture or dislocation. Sternal body fracture and sternomanubrial dislocation are associated with a 25–45% mortality from concomitant injuries to the aorta, diaphragm, heart, tracheobronchial tree, and lung. Sternal films or lateral radiographs will show the fracture and often demonstrate a retrosternal hematoma; CT may be useful in those with normal plain films and a high suspicion of sternal disruption.

Prior Median Sternotomy is the most common sternal abnormality seen on conventional radiographs and chest CT. Circular wires that encompass the width of the sternum are seen spaced along its length within the interspaces between costal cartilages. The vertical lucency representing the sternotomy may heal, but in many patients bony union does not occur. In the early postoperative period, a retrosternal hematoma may be seen that normally resolves within the first several weeks postoperatively. The radiologist plays a key role in the evaluation of possible sternal wound infection. Plain film evidence of bony destruction or air in the sternal incision appearing days to weeks after sternotomy are specific but insensitive findings for osteomyelitis. Bone scans are not particularly useful as there will be increased radionuclide uptake for months following sternotomy. Computed tomography is the modality of choice in the evaluation of sternal wound infection. The CT findings of sternal osteomyelitis include bone destruction and peristernal soft-tissue mass, enhancing fluid collection,

Table 16.7. Unilateral Diaphragmatic Elevation

Eventration	
Diminished lung volume	Congenital
	Hypoplastic lung
	Aquired
	Lobar/lung atelectasis
	Pulmonary resection
Paralysis	Idiopathic
	Iatrogenic phrenic nerve injury
	Phrenic crush (tuberculosis)
	Intraoperative
	Malignant invasion of phrenic nerve
	Bronchogenic carcinoma
	Inflammation of diaphragmatic muscle
	Pleuritis
	Lower lobe pneumonia
	Subphrenic abscess
Upper abdominal mass	Hepatomegaly or mass
	Splenomegaly
	Gastric/colonic distention
	Ascites (usually bilateral)
	Diaphragmatic hernia[a]
	Subpulmonic pleural effusion[a]

[a]Apparent diaphragmatic elevation.

and gas. The extent of infection, specifically associated mediastinitis, can also be determined.

DIAPHRAGM
Abnormalities of Diaphragmatic Position

DIAPHRAGMATIC ELEVATION

Unilateral Diaphragmatic Elevation. The differential diagnosis of unilateral diaphragmatic elevation is shown in Table 16.7. Eventration of the diaphragm is a congenital absence or underdevelopment of diaphragmatic musculature. This usually produces a localized elevation of the anteromedial portion of the right hemidiaphragm on frontal radiographs in older individuals, indistinguishable from the rare foramen of Morgagni hernia. Total diaphragmatic eventration is usually left-sided and is indistinguishable radiographically from diaphragmatic paralysis.

Unilateral diaphragmatic paralysis is usually due to surgical injury or neoplastic involvement of the phrenic nerve, which affects the right and left hemidiaphragms with equal frequency. Idiopathic phrenic nerve dysfunction as a result of a viral neuritis is a common cause of diaphragmatic paralysis in males and is usually right-sided. A fluoroscopic or ultrasonographic sniff test is diagnostic.

A chronic effect of loss of lung volume is diaphragmatic elevation, particularly from collapse or resection of the lower lobe. This is also a common sequela of chronic cicatrizing atelectasis of the upper lobe from tuberculosis.

An enlarged liver or hepatic mass can produce right hemidiaphragmatic elevation by direct pressure on the undersurface of the hemidiaphragm. Similarly, an enlarged spleen, gas-distended stomach, or enlarged splenic flexure of colon can produce an elevated left hemidiaphragm. Irritation of the superior surface of the hemidiaphragm by a pleural or pleural-based parenchymal process (e.g., infarct, pneumonia), or of the undersurface of the diaphragm by a subphrenic abscess, hepatitis, or cholecystitis may cause the diaphragm to become flaccid, leading to elevation. A subpulmonic effusion may simulate an elevated hemidiaphragm; the radiographic recognition of a subpulmonic effusion was discussed in "Pleural Effusion."

Bilateral Diaphragmatic Elevation that is not effort-related may be a result of a neuromuscular disturbance or intrathoracic or intrabdominal disease. Radiographically, the diaphragms are elevated on both frontal and lateral views. Bibasilar linear atelectasis or passive lobar or segmental lower lobe atelectasis may be seen.

An impedance to bilateral phrenic nerve stimulation or intrinsic diaphragmatic muscular disease will produce bilateral diaphragmatic paralysis and elevation. Common disorders include cervical cord injury, multiple sclerosis, and the myopathy associated with SLE. In these patients, fluoroscopic or real-time ultrasound imaging of the diaphragms reveals characteristic paradoxical superior movement of the diaphragms with sniffing (positive sniff test), which results from the effects of negative intrathoracic pressure on a flaccid diaphragm during inspiration.

Lung restriction due to interstitial fibrosis, bilateral pleural fibrosis, or chest wall disease (most commonly from obesity) can produce bilateral diaphragmatic elevation. An increase in intraabdominal volume, most often from ascites, hepatosplenomegaly, or pregnancy, can restrict diaphragmatic motion. These conditions may be distinguished from bilateral paralysis by observing normal but diminished inferior excursion of the diaphragms on fluoroscopy, ultrasound, or inspiratory/expiratory radiographs.

DIAPHRAGMATIC DEPRESSION

Depression and flattening of one hemidiaphragm is seen with unilateral overinflation of a lung, usually as a compensatory mechanism when the contralateral lung is small, or as a result of a large pneumothorax. Distinction between these two entities is usually possible by the clinical history and by characteristic findings in patients with pneumothorax. A tension pneumothorax may cause inversion of the hemidiaphragm. Bilateral diaphragmatic depression is either a permanent finding as a result of abnormally increased lung compliance in patients with emphysema, or is a transient finding in those with asthma and expiratory air trapping.

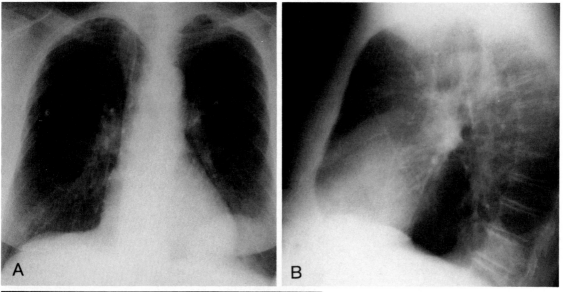

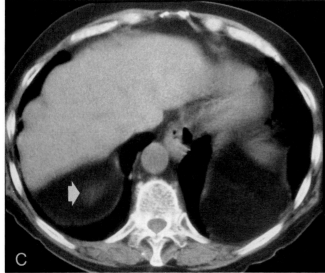

Figure 16.19.   Foramen of Bochdalek Hernia. Posteroanterior (**A**) and lateral (**B**) chest radiographs in an asymptomatic 82-year-old man show a mass arising from the posterolateral aspect of the left hemidiaphragm. A CT scan through the diaphragm (**C**) shows fat herniating through bilateral Bochdalek hernias. Note the top of the right kidney within the herniated fat (*arrow*).

DIAPHRAGMATIC HERNIAS

Hiatus Hernia.   The most common is the esophageal hiatal hernia, which represents herniation of stomach through the esophageal hiatus. These are usually seen as incidental asymptomatic masses on chest radiographs, although some patients may have symptoms of gastroesophageal reflux or, rarely, severe pain from strangulation of the herniated stomach. Hiatal hernias are seen on frontal chest radiographs in the immediate supradiaphragmatic region of the posterior mediastinum, projecting behind the heart. An air-fluid level may be seen in the hernia. An esophagram is confirmatory. Computed tomography shows widening of the esophageal hiatus and depicts the contents of the hernia sac, which often include stomach, omental fat, and, rarely, ascitic fluid.

Foramen of Bochdalek Hernia.   As described in Chapter 12, the foramen of Bochdalek represents a

defect in the hemidiaphragm at the site of the embryonic pleuroperitoneal canal. Large hernias through Bochdalek's foramen present in the neonatal period with hypoplasia of the ipsilateral lung and respiratory distress. In adults, small hernias through this foramen are common and are predominantly seen on the left side, presumably because of the protective effect of the liver, which prevents herniation of right infradiaphragmatic fat through the right foramen of Bochdalek. The hernia typically appears as a posterolateral mass above the left hemidiaphragm, although it can occur anywhere along the posterior diaphragmatic surface. Computed tomography shows the diaphragmatic defect with herniation of retroperitoneal fat, omentum, spleen, or kidney (Fig. 16.19).

Foramen of Morgagni Hernia.   A defect in the parasternal portion of the diaphragm, the foramen of Morgagni, is the least common type of congenital diaphragmatic hernia. A Morgagni's hernia is almost in-

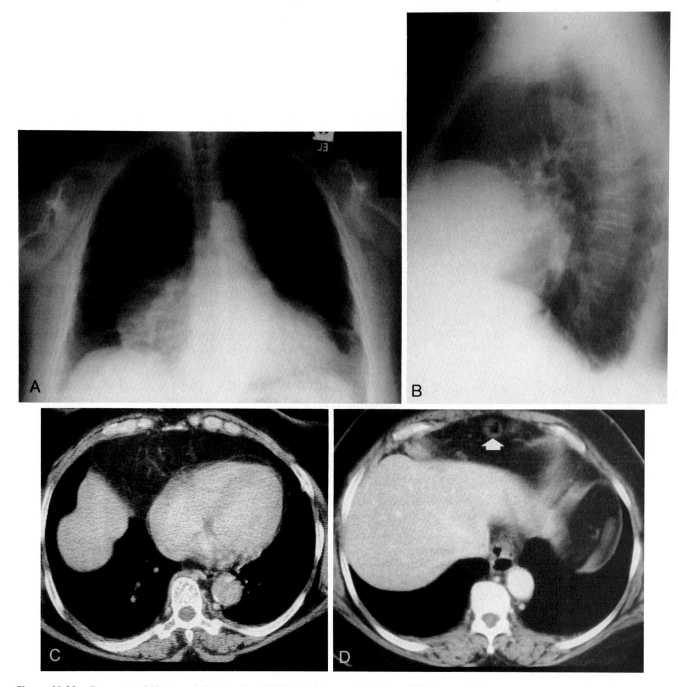

Figure 16.20.   Foramen of Morgagni Hernia. Frontal (**A**) and lateral (**B**) chest radiographs in a 60-year-old woman reveals a large mass in the right cardiophrenic angle. A CT scan at the level of the diaphragm (**C**) shows a fatty pericardiac mass containing omental vessels. A more inferior scan (**D**) demonstrates an abnormally high transverse colon (*arrow*), which is characteristic of this entity.

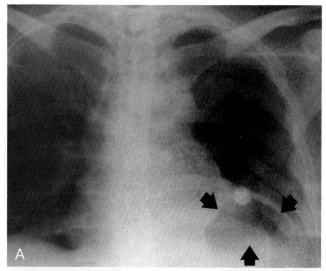

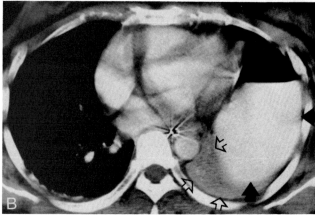

Figure 16.21. Traumatic Diaphragmatic Hernia. A. An upright chest radiograph shows an abnormally high gastric fundus (*arrows*). **B.** A CT scan after oral contrast administration reveals the stomach (*solid arrows*) within the left lower thorax with adjacent left lower lobe atelectasis (*open arrows*).

variably right-sided and appears as an asymptomatic cardiophrenic angle mass. The diagnosis is made by noting herniation of omental fat, liver, or transverse colon through the paracardiac portion of the right hemidiaphragm on CT scans through the lung bases. The presence of omental vessels within a fatty paracardiac mass is diagnostic (Fig. 16.20). Coronal MR or ultrasound can demonstrate the diaphragmatic defect, distinguishing this entity from partial eventration of the hemidiaphragm.

Traumatic Herniation of abdominal contents through a tear or rupture of the central or posterior aspect of the hemidiaphragm may follow blunt thoracoabdominal trauma or penetrating injury (10). The left side is affected in over 90% of cases, as the liver dissipates the traumatic forces and protects the right hemidiaphragm from injury. Radiographically, the diagnosis should be suspected when the left hemidiaphragmatic contour is indistinct or elevated, or when gas-filled loops of bowel or stomach are seen in the left

lower thorax following severe trauma. Early diagnosis is often difficult as associated thoracic and abdominal injuries may obscure the clinical and radiographic findings. The diagnosis is often made long after the traumatic episode, with symptoms due to intestinal obstruction with strangulation (pain, vomiting, fever) or compression of the left lung (cough, dyspnea, chest pain). In addition to stomach, small intestine, and colon, the omentum, spleen, kidney, and left lobe of liver can herniate through the defect. The diagnosis is usually made by upper or lower gastrointestinal contrast studies demonstrating bowel herniating into the thorax through a constricting diaphragmatic defect. The resultant narrowing or "waist" of the herniated intestine as it traverses the diaphragmatic defect helps differentiate a hernia from simple diaphragmatic elevation. Large diaphragmatic defects may be demonstrated on CT, which can also characterize the herniated tissues and detect associated visceral injuries (Fig. 16.21).

DIAPHRAGMATIC TUMORS

Primary diaphragmatic tumors are rare, with an equal incidence of benign and malignant lesions. Benign lesions include lipomas, fibromas, Schwannomas, neurofibromas, and leiomyomas. Echinococcal cysts and extralobar sequestrations may be found within the diaphragm. Fibrosarcomas are the most common primary malignant diaphragmatic lesions. Radiographically, they appear as focal extrapulmonary masses obscuring all or part of the hemidiaphragm, and are indistinguishable from masses arising within the diaphragmatic pleura. Computed tomography may show the origin of the mass, although the relationship of the mass to the diaphragm is best appreciated on coronal MR images or transabdominal ultrasound. Direct invasion of the diaphragm by lower lobe bronchogenic carcinoma, mesothelioma, or a subphrenic neoplasm is much more common than primary diaphragmatic malignancy.

References

1. Light RW. Pleural diseases. 2nd ed. Philadelphia: Lea and Febiger, 1990:9–19.
2. Vix VA. Roentgenographic manifestations of pleural disease. Semin Roentgenol 1977;12:277–286.
3. McLoud TC, Flower CDR. Imaging the pleura: sonography, CT, and MR imaging. AJR 1991;156:1145–1155.
4. Naidich DF, Zerhouni EA, Siegelman SS. Pleura and chest wall. In: Computed tomography and magnetic resonance imaging of the thorax. 2nd ed. New York: Raven Press, 1991:420–422.
5. Tocino IM, Miller MH, Fairfax WR. Distribution of pneumothorax in the supine and semirecumbent critically ill patient. AJR 1985;144:901–905.
6. Dedrick CG, McLoud TC, Shepard JO, et al. Computed tomography of localized pleural mesothelioma. AJR 1985;144:275–280.

7. Wechsler RJ, Rao VM, Steiner RM. The radiology of malignant mesothelioma. CRC Crit Rev Diagn Imaging 1984;20: 283–310.

8. Jafri SZH, Roberts JL, Bree RL, et al. Computed tomography of chest wall masses. Radiographics 1989;9:51–68.

9. Lester CW. Pectus carinatum, pigeon breast and related deformities of the sternum and costal cartilages. Arch Paediatr 1960;77:399–405.

10. Ball T, McGory R, Smith JO, et al. Traumatic diaphragmatic hernia: errors in diagnosis. AJR 1982;138:633–638.

Section IV   **BREAST RADIOLOGY**

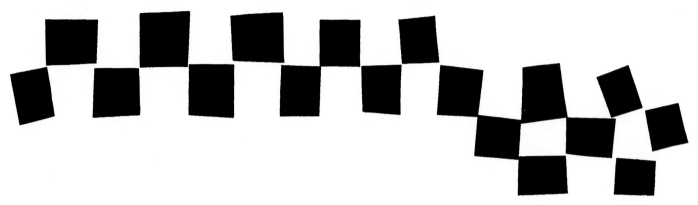

17   Breast Imaging

17

Breast Imaging

Karen K. Lindfors

Breast imaging is utilized for two purposes. The first purpose is to screen asymptomatic women for early breast cancer. The second purpose is to evaluate breast abnormalities in symptomatic patients or patients with indeterminate screening mammograms. Screening is accomplished with standard two-view mammography, but diagnostic evaluation often requires the additional use of special mammographic views, breast ultrasound, and interventional procedures.

SCREENING FOR BREAST CANCER

Breast cancer survival is influenced by the size of the tumor and the lymph node status at the time of diagnosis. Small tumors with negative axillary lymph nodes have survival rates well above 90%. Such cancers are detected far more often with screening mammography than with physical examination. It follows that screening mammography should lower mortality from breast cancer. Several randomized clinical trials have proven the efficacy of this technique.

In 1963 the Health Insurance Plan of New York (HIP) invited 31,000 women aged 40–64 to participate in four annual screenings for breast cancer by mammography and physical examination. This study group was compared with a control group of women who received routine medical care. Nine years after beginning the study there was a 29% reduction in breast cancer mortality in the group receiving annual screening (1).

Several other breast cancer screening trials were begun in Europe in the 1970s. In Sweden, the WE or Two County Study was a randomized population-based trial of screening for breast cancer with single-view mammography alone. The screening intervals were from 24 to 33 months. Eight years after the initiation of the program, breast cancer mortality in the screened group was reduced by 31% (2).

Even greater benefits were shown in two Dutch case-control studies. In Nijmegen, women who died from breast cancer were half as likely to have undergone mammographic screening as women who did not die from this disease (3). In Utrecht, the relative risk of dying from breast cancer in the screened group compared with the control group was 0.3 (4). These studies suggest that mortality from breast cancer can be reduced by 50–70% with screening.

Not all studies have shown significant reductions in breast cancer mortality with mammographic screening. In Malmö, Sweden, a population-based randomized trial was performed, including 42,000 women. After 9 years, no significant difference between the study and control groups was evident (5). It is difficult to understand why such differences exist between the Malmö study and the WE study. Hypotheses include a higher rate of mammography among the controls and a lower compliance with screening among the study population in Malmö, as well as questions about technical quality.

When the results of the screening studies are stratified by age, the evidence suggests a clear benefit in women aged 50–69. There is still debate over the benefit of screening mammography in the 40- to 49-year-old age group. In the HIP study, a significant mortality reduction was not initially evident in the 40- to 49-year-old study group, but at the 18-year followup a 25% reduction in mortality was noted in the screened group aged 40–49 at entry (6). It is thought that a significant reduction in mortality was not evident initially in the younger group because of the small number of women in this age group and because of the even smaller numbers of breast cancers diagnosed. It is also possible that technical limitations in the equipment used in the 1960s may have made mammographic diagnosis in this age group more difficult.

None of the European trials could conclusively demonstrate a significant reduction in breast cancer mortality with screening in the younger age group. Although the actual data from the recent Canadian National Breast Screening Study have not yet been published, preliminary results suggest that no significant reduction in mortality from breast cancer will be seen in the screened group aged 40–49 in this study either.

A variety of hypotheses have been offered to explain this lack of mortality reduction in the 40- to 49-year-old age group. Many experts believe that breast cancer can be a more aggressive disease in younger women. As such, the biennial mammographic screening utilized in some trials will only detect less aggressive tumors. The faster growing breast cancers will occur between screenings, causing increased mortality in the screened group (7). Annual screening might lead to a significant reduction in mortality in the screened group.

To be effective, mammography screening must be performed in a technically adequate manner and must be interpreted by a skilled radiologist. In the Canadian trial, 50% of the mammograms completed during the first 2 years of the study were technically unsatisfactory (8). Review of over 5000 Canadian mammograms by outside expert radiologists also demonstrated a significant number of studies that were misinterpreted by the Canadian radiologists (9). These factors have led to serious questions regarding the validity of the results obtained in this most recent study.

Although there are little firm scientific data showing a reduction in breast cancer mortality in the 40- to 49-year-old age group, the only deterrents to screening are the cost and inconvenience of mammography. In the past there were also questions about the radiogenic breast cancer risk from the procedure for all women.

Radiation Risk

An increased susceptibility to breast cancer has been documented among women exposed to high doses of radiation (1–20 Gy). The survivors of the atomic bomb explosions in Japan, patients undergoing radiation therapy, and sanatoria patients undergoing multiple chest fluoroscopies for monitoring of tuberculosis therapy are all groups having an increased incidence of breast cancer. Such data raised questions about the risk incurred from the low doses of radiation received during screening mammography (approximately 2 mGy).

A controlled study of the effects of low doses of radiation such as those received during mammography would require large numbers of women in both the study and control groups. Close to 100 million patients in each group would be required in order to provide statistically significant data. Clearly, this would not be practical or possible. As such, estimates or risk have been hypothesized by extrapolation from data obtained at higher doses using a linear dose-response model.

The latest follow-up data from the Japanese atomic bomb survivors have shown progressively decreasing radiation risk with increased age at exposure. Women exposed in their youth and teens suffered the highest increase in risk. No increased risk was demonstrable for women aged 40 or older at exposure. Studies of the other populations sustaining significant breast radiation exposure have also supported a diminished risk with advancing age at exposure.

Estimated lifetime risk of breast cancer death from a single mammogram in the age group from 40 to 49 years is approximately 2 in 1 million. In women aged 50–59, this risk is reduced to less than 1 in 1 million; progressive reductions in risk are seen at older ages (10).

These theoretical risks should be weighed against the risk of dying from spontaneous breast cancer, which would be approximately 700 per million in women aged 40–49 and 1000 per million in women aged 50–59. This risk increases steadily with advancing age.

Screening Guidelines

After publication of the favorable results in the HIP trial, the American Cancer Society (ACS) and the National Cancer Institute began an effort to disseminate information on breast cancer screening to the public and to physicians. By 1975 there were 29 Breast Cancer Detection Demonstration Project (BCDDP) centers throughout the United States. Women were voluntarily enrolled in a screening program utilizing physical examination, mammography, and, initially, thermography. The use of thermography was later discontin-

Table 17.1. American Cancer Society Guidelines for Breast Cancer Screening

Age	Clinical Examination	Mammography
20–39	Every 3 years	Not recommended
40–49	Annually	Every 1–2 years
50 and over	Annually	Annually

ued when no benefit to its use could be demonstrated. The BCDDP was not a controlled study; however, some important data did emerge; these data have played an important role in shaping the ACS guidelines for breast cancer screening. Approximately one-third of cancers diagnosed in the BCDDP occurred in women aged 35–49. The majority of these cancers were of an early stage, noninvasive, or not involving regional lymph nodes. Most of these early cancers were found by mammography and not by physical examination (11). These data and those from the screening trials previously discussed have led to the establishment of current screening guidelines (12).

American Cancer Society guidelines for breast cancer screening among asymptomatic women are shown in Table 17.1. Both clinical examination and mammography are essential components of a screening program. Over 90% of cancers are seen on mammograms, but the remainder are not seen. These are diagnosed by physical examination. The ACS also recommends the practice of monthly breast self-examination by all women.

The variable interval for the 40- to 49-year-old age group is based mainly on economic grounds. The incidence of breast cancer is lower in this age group and so screening is not as cost-effective. Many experts caution that breast cancer can be more aggressive in younger women and they feel that mammography should be performed yearly in this age group. Others suggest that women at high risk have annual mammograms, while those with no risk factors undergo biennial mammography. Certain factors are known to increase a woman's risk of getting breast cancer. These include a close family history of the disease, precancerous lesions diagnosed on breast biopsy, first child born after age 30, nulliparity, and obesity.

When adopting a screening policy, the physician must remember that all women are at risk for developing breast cancer. The ACS estimates that one women in every nine will develop the disease. The majority of women who contract breast cancer will not have histories that place them at higher risk.

Screening Outcomes

What are the expected outcomes in a group of 1000 asymptomatic women undergoing bilateral screening

mammography for the first time? Approximately 100 of these women will be recalled for additional studies. These may include magnification or other special mammographic views and ultrasound. Biopsy will be recommended in about 20 of these women, and cancer will be found in about 7 of them. With subsequent screenings of the same women, the numbers of cancers found will decrease and the positive predictive value, or percentage of women undergoing biopsy who actually have cancer, should increase.

Our goal in screening asymptomatic women is to find breast cancer in its earliest stages when survival is greatest. In a well-established screening program, over 30% of cancers will be minimal; minimal cancers are defined as those that are noninvasive or invasive, but less than 1 cm in size with negative nodes. Over 70% of breast cancer discovered by screening mammography should be node-negative (13).

Optimal effectiveness of a breast cancer screening program requires the use of physical examination in addition to mammographic screening. Although 88% of the cancers detected during the BCDDP were seen on mammography and nearly 42% were diagnosed by mammography alone, there were still approximately 9% of cancers that were not visualized mammographically; these cancers were discovered on physical examination (11). The minimum size of breast cancers that can be felt on physical examination averages between 1.5 and 2 cm.

False-negative mammograms can occur for a variety of reasons. The palpable abnormality may not be included on a film. Dense breast parenchyma may obscure visualization of a mass. The filming technique may be suboptimal for visualization of an abnormality. The particular tumor type may not be visible mammographically or there may be observer error in the interpretation of the mammogram. It must be emphasized that a negative mammogram should not deter further diagnostic evaluation of a clinically palpable mass.

Some breast cancers will arise in the interval between screening examinations. The number of such cancers will depend on the frequency of screening. Interval cancers tend to be more advanced at diagnosis when compared with those diagnosed at screening (7); they may be biologically more aggressive. Additionally, a previous negative mammogram or the knowledge that screening will be performed regularly may be a disincentive for patients to perform breast self-examination or to seek immediate medical care for a breast mass found in the interval between screens. Physicians must stress that any breast mass requires immediate attention, regardless of whether the patient has had a recent negative mammogram.

The Use of Other Imaging Modalities for Breast Cancer Screening

Mammography is the only imaging modality with proven capability to screen asymptomatic women for breast cancer. Other modalities have been investigated for their potential in screening, but as yet none can approach the sensitivity and specificity of mammography.

In the mid-1970s when there were questions regarding the radiation risk from mammography, ultrasound was investigated as a screening technique. Ultrasound units that would scan the entire breast were developed; however, studies revealed that up to 42% of all breast cancers were not visualized by ultrasound. The results were even worse for cancers smaller than 1 cm; in one study, 92% of these were not seen sonographically (14). Furthermore, in follow-up studies of patients who had suspicious abnormalities by ultrasound, but negative mammograms and normal physical examinations, no cancers were found (15). These data have led to the conclusion that there is no role for ultrasound in screening for breast cancer. Ultrasound is useful only in diagnosis or further characterization of a specific lesion detected by mammography or physical examination; its primary utility is in distinguishing simple cysts from solid masses in the breast. Such distinction is of great importance, as simple cysts are invariably benign.

Thermography and transillumination are two other imaging techniques that have been studied for use as potential screening modalities. Neither has proven efficacious in screening or in diagnosis of breast cancer.

Recent technical advances have led to increasing interest in magnetic resonance imaging (MR) as a possible detection technique for breast cancer in certain populations. Preliminary data suggest that MR can reveal lesions that are missed by conventional mammography in radiographically dense breasts. The cost of MR, as well as the time it takes to perform, will probably prohibit its use as a general screening tool, but the technique may prove useful as an adjunct to mammography in specific cases.

Other technologies, such as positron-emission tomography, are also being explored for use in breast cancer detection and diagnosis. For the present, however, mammography remains the single best test for early detection of breast cancer; it is the "gold standard" by which all other potential screening modalities must be measured.

EVALUATION OF THE SYMPTOMATIC PATIENT

Bilateral mammography should be the first imaging study performed in patients over the age of 30 who present with breast masses that are suspicious for carcinoma. The mass should be indicated by placing a radiopaque marker over the site. This will assist the radiologist in a targeted mammographic evaluation of this area and will also assure that the palpable abnormality corresponds to the mammographic abnormality, if one is visualized. Such correlation is important in assuring that the surgical biopsy of a palpable abnormality will encompass the mammographically suspicious area.

The primary reason for performing mammography in a patient with a suspicious palpable mass is to assess the affected breast for multifocal disease and the contralateral breast for suspicious abnormalities that should be biopsied concurrently. Mammography may also be helpful in definitively diagnosing the palpable abnormality as benign, thus avoiding biopsy.

Mammography should be performed before any intervention. A hematoma, resulting from percutaneous fine-needle aspiration biopsy (FNAB), can look similar to a small carcinoma. When such procedures have been performed prior to mammography, it is best to perform a follow-up mammogram 4 to 6 weeks later.

If mammography is negative in a patient with a clinically evident mass and dense breasts, ultrasound is often suggested as a subsequent imaging study. Ultrasound can determine whether the mass represents a simple cyst. Simple cysts are virtually never malignant. Ultrasound cannot provide a definitive diagnosis of a solid or complex mass.

Alternatively, definitive diagnosis of a palpable mass can usually be made by performing a fine-needle aspiration of the mass. When a simple cyst is present, the aspiration is both diagnostic and therapeutic, as all of the fluid can be withdrawn. In solid or complex masses a cytologic examination of the cells removed at aspiration will yield the diagnosis. Ultrasound is usually unnecessary in cases where fine-needle aspiration of a palpable mass is going to be performed.

In younger patients who present with breast masses, mammography must be used more judiciously. This more cautious approach is based on data from the atomic bomb survivors in Japan showing an excess risk of breast cancer in younger women exposed to high doses of radiation. These data combined with the low incidence of breast cancer in young women (less than 1% of breast cancer occurs in women under 30) suggest that a restricted use of mammography is prudent. Some experts also believe that dense breast tissue, which is more common in younger women, limits the sensitivity of mammography, but studies have shown that mammography can demonstrate up to 90% of cancers in women under 35 (16).

Women under the age of 30 who have a focal suspicious palpable abnormality are frequently first evaluated with ultrasound. If the ultrasound is negative and the patient is over age 20, a single oblique view of the affected breast is performed to assess for suspicious microcalcifications, which are not visualized by ultrasound. Women under age 20 should not undergo mammography.

If fine-needle aspiration is available it may be used in lieu of imaging studies when young patients have suspicious palpable masses. In the extremely rare circumstance of a diagnosis of carcinoma, mammography can be performed subsequently. The radiologist should be aware that a previous needle aspiration may confound the mammographic assessment of the affected area, but it will not compromise assessment of surrounding or contralateral tissues.

Increased awareness of breast cancer has led many clinicians to request more imaging studies in young women. Breast imaging cannot replace careful clinical evaluation of the breasts. If there is no suspicious focal abnormality, imaging studies will not be helpful; they may subject the patient to unnecessary risk.

TECHNICAL CONSIDERATIONS IN BREAST IMAGING

Because both high-contrast and high-spatial resolution are needed for optimal mammography, standard radiographic equipment cannot be utilized for this examination. Mammography must be performed on a unit dedicated to this purpose. Mammographic equipment and technique differ from standard radiography in several ways. The anode material utilized to generate the x-rays in most dedicated mammography units is molybdenum. This allows the production of lower energy x-rays, which in turn produces greater contrast between soft tissue structures. The structures of the breast do not differ greatly in their inherent contrast, so these low kilovolt or "softer" photons are extremely important in producing a high contrast image. Some newer units also have rhodium anodes that can be used to increase the contrast in denser breasts, while keeping radiation dose and time of exposure low.

The radiologist must be able to discern tiny microcalcifications on mammograms; some of these calcifications may be 0.1 mm or less in size. The small focal spot size used in mammography units, a longer distance from the x-ray source to the image, and special high resolution, single intensifying screens used with single emulsion film, contribute to the creation of images with high resolution.

All mammographic units are equipped with compression paddles that squeeze the breast against the film holder. Good compression of the breast is essential to high-quality mammography for several reasons. Compression spreads overlapping breast structures so that true masses can be differentiated from summation shadows that occur because of overlapping soft tissues. The breast is immobilized during compression so motion unsharpness or blurring due to patient movement is minimized. Geometric unsharpness, caused by the finite focal spot dimension, is minimized by bringing the breast structures closer to the film. Compression renders the breast nearly uniform in thickness so the film density of tissues near the nipple will be similar to those near the chest wall. Radiation dose can be reduced by good compression; a thinner breast requires fewer photons for penetration. Beam attenuation is also reduced.

Some women find breast compression uncomfortable, but most can tolerate it once the benefits are explained. During routine mammography the breast is compressed for a few seconds while each film is taken. Many units are equipped with automated compression devices so the technologist can release the tension immediately after the film is exposed.

Other factors are also important to consider in the production of high quality mammograms. These include other equipment features such as type of x-ray generator, beam filtration, grid use, as well as film-intensifying screen combinations and the film processing system. All of these factors are interrelated and must be optimized to produce technically acceptable films of the breast.

Mammographic Positioning for Screening

Mammography can be performed with the patient seated or standing. Most screening practices prefer the standing position because it allows faster throughput and is less cumbersome. Patients are able to lean into the unit to a greater degree when standing, thus allowing more of the posterior breast tissues to be imaged. Recumbent imaging is possible, but quite difficult; its use should be restricted to problem-solving situations.

Two views of each breast are generally utilized for screening mammography in the United States. Several European countries utilize a single mediolateral oblique view for screening examinations, but authorities in this country have shown that one-view examinations would lead to an excessive number of patients being called back for additional views. Asking large numbers of patients to return for such views would result in unacceptable levels of patient anxiety and cost. The standard views for screening mammography are the mediolateral oblique (MLO) view and the craniocaudal (CC) view.

The MLO view, when properly positioned, depicts the greatest amount of breast tissue. It is the most useful view in mammography. In those countries using single-view screening, the MLO view is preferred. To perform an MLO view, the x-ray tube and film

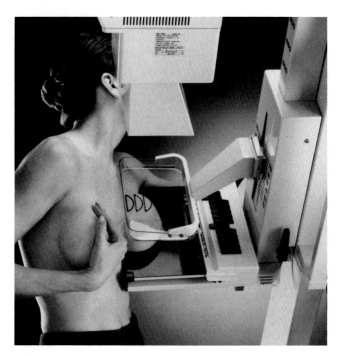

Figure 17.1. Patient positioning for a MLO view. (Reproduced with permission from General Electric Medical Systems, Milwaukee, Wisconsin.)

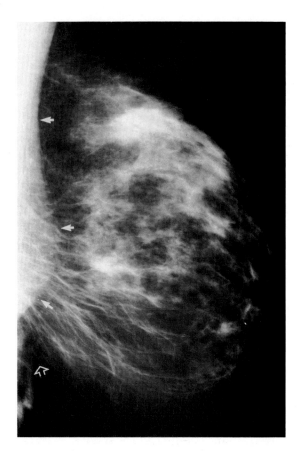

Figure 17.2. Normal MLO view of left breast. The pectoralis muscle (*white arrows*) is seen from the axilla to below the level of the nipple. The inframammary fold (*open arrow*) is well seen, and the nipple is in profile.

holder, which are fixed with respect to one another, are moved to an angle that parallels the orientation of the patient's pectoralis major muscle. The technologist is given flexibility in choosing the angle so that the greatest amount of breast tissue possible can be imaged. The angle is generally between 40° and 60° from the horizontal.

The patient is asked to relax her arm and chest muscles and to lean into the machine. The breast is placed on the film holder and compression is applied from the superomedial direction, the same direction from which the x-rays will be generated. The breast must be pulled anteriorly and spread in a superior-inferior direction as much as possible to minimize overlapping structures and to maximize the amount of tissue imaged. The nipple should be in profile. Compression must be applied vigorously (Fig. 17.1). By convention in the MLO view a marker indicating the side (left or right) and type of view is placed near the superior axillary tissues of the breast.

A properly positioned MLO mammogram should show the pectoralis major muscles down to the level of the nipple. The nipple should be in profile so that the subareolar area can be adequately evaluated. The intramammary fold should be visible to ensure that the inferior portion of the breast has been imaged (Fig. 17.2).

For the CC view, the unit is placed in the vertical position so that the x-ray tube is perpendicular to the floor. Photons will travel from the anode, located superior to the breast, to the film underneath the breast.

The breast is placed on the film holder, pulled anteriorly, and spread horizontally before the compression plate is applied to the superior skin surface (Fig. 17.3). The nipple should again be in profile. The chest wall should rest against the film holder. The markers indicating the side imaged and type of view should be placed near the skin close to the lateral aspect of the breast.

The curvature of the chest wall can hinder imaging of some of the most lateral or medial tissues in the CC projection. Some authorities recommend a slight exaggeration of the CC view so that more lateral tissues are imaged since breast cancer is more common laterally. Others recommend slight medial exaggeration because the upper outer quadrant is so well-imaged on the MLO view and there is a possibility that some of the medial tissues could be omitted on that view. The best compromise is probably centering the nipple and attempting to place as much medial and lateral tissue on the film holder as possible.

When evaluating a CC mammogram, optimal positioning can be assured when pectoralis muscles are seen centrally on the film and the nipple is in profile (Fig. 17.4).

Interpreting the Mammogram

For interpretation, CC and MLO mammograms should each be hung together in a mirror image configuration. This will allow the radiologist to scan the breasts for symmetry. Viewing conditions are extremely important to optimal mammographic film reading. The room must be darkened. All adjacent view box light should be blocked out. Dedicated mammography film alternators and view boxes can do this automatically. If standard view boxes or alternators are used, exposed blackened film can be cut to mask out unwanted light.

A magnifying lens should be used to examine each film thoroughly. All visible parenchyma should be scanned systematically with magnification. This will allow visualization of tiny microcalcifications and it will ensure that the radiologist has examined all parts of the breast in detail.

If previous mammograms are available they should be compared to the current study so that the radiologist can evaluate the examination for any changes in the mammographic appearance of the breasts. In turn, current questionable areas can be evaluated for their stability.

In most practices, patients are asked to complete a brief history form that includes questions relevant to breast health and cancer risk. Knowledge of the patient's history will be helpful in assessing the malignant potential and likely diagnosis of a particular mammographic finding. The risk of malignancy is much greater in a 60-year-old woman than in a 30-year-old woman. A woman with a personal or family history of breast cancer is at greater risk for development of malignancy, and the interpretation of mammographic findings should be tailored accordingly. Other information such as previous surgical biopsies or hormone intake must also be taken into account during interpretation of the mammogram.

Correlation with the physical examination is also extremely important so that false-negative reports can be minimized. All palpable lesions should be marked and assessed mammographically. Special views can image palpable lesions that occur in locations not included on standard mammography. The mammographer can also be certain that the mass felt corresponds to the mammographic abnormality. Areas of asymmetric tissue seen mammographically can be assessed for palpable abnormalities, which may render them more suspicious for malignancy.

Classic mammographic signs of malignancy are spiculated masses or pleomorphic clusters of microcalcifications; however, only about 40% of all occult breast carcinoma presents in these ways (17). In the remainder of cases, more subtle or indirect signs of malignancy are present. The radiologist must look at

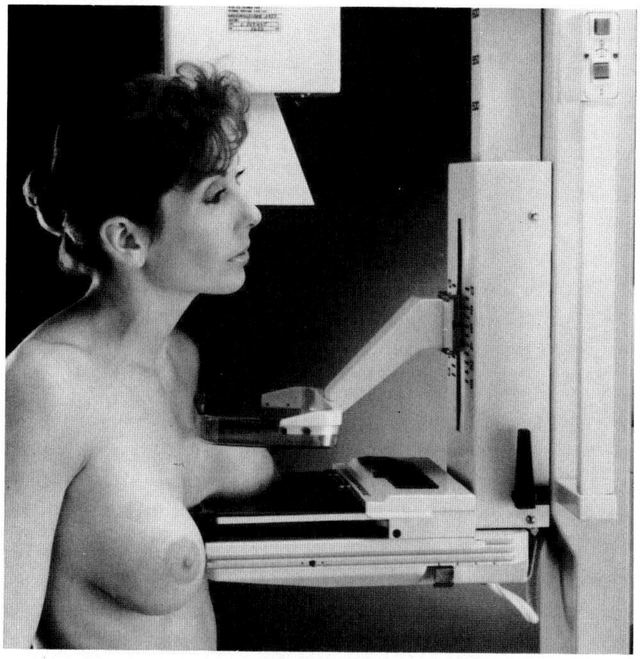

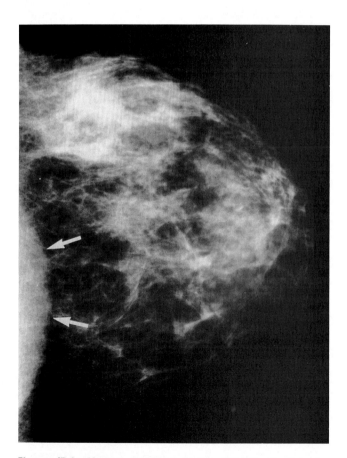

Figure 17.3. Patient positioning for the CC view. (Reproduced with permission from General Electric Medical Systems, Milwaukee, Wisconsin.)

Figure 17.4. Normal CC view of the left breast. Note the pectoralis muscle (*arrows*) centrally indicating optimal visualization of breast tissue.

each mammogram with great care, utilizing all available diagnostic techniques so that false-negative diagnoses are minimized. This charge must be balanced against the need to minimize false-positive diagnoses. Each time a woman is subjected to a surgical biopsy, financial and emotional costs as well as risks are incurred.

Diagnostic Evaluation of the Indeterminate Mammogram

In the majority of cases a two-view screening mammogram will provide a conclusive interpretation, but when the results of mammography are indeterminate, further evaluation is necessary; additional mammographic views or ultrasound may be required for clarification. The workup must be tailored to the specific situation.

Projections other than the standard CC and MLO views may help to visualize a lesion that is seen only in one standard view or that is obscured by surrounding parenchyma. Tangential views of the skin can be used to establish a dermal location for calcifications or superficial masses. Dermal abnormalities do not represent breast cancer.

Further characterization of an abnormality can be accomplished with spot compression and magnification views. The compression plate used is much smaller than that used in standard views, therefore greater force can be applied, which results both in further spreading of any overlying tissue and in bringing the abnormality closer to the film for increased detail. Magnification also produces finer detail, which allows more accurate assessment of the morphology of microcalcifications and the borders of masses.

Well-defined or partially obscured masses can be evaluated with ultrasound. A high frequency (5–10 MHz), hand-held linear array transducer is most commonly used. A targeted evaluation of the mammographically visible abnormality is performed. Simple cysts are easily distinguishable from complex or solid masses. This differentiation is extremely important as simple cysts are always benign and require no further workup, whereas noncystic masses may represent cancers.

ANALYZING THE MAMMOGRAM
Masses

Complete assessment of a mammographically visible, potentially malignant mass requires several steps. First the radiologist must decide whether the mass is real. The left and right breasts must be compared in each view.

Most women have reasonably symmetric parenchyma; however, at least 3% of women have areas of asymmetric, but histologically normal breast tissue.

When attempting to distinguish asymmetric normal breast tissue from a true abnormality, the radiologist must look for the mammographic features of a mass. Masses have convex borders and become denser toward the center. They distort the normal breast architecture. True masses are seen in multiple projections and can still be visualized when focal compression is utilized (Fig. 17.5).

Asymmetric breast parenchyma has an amorphous quality. On spot compression the tissue spreads apart and fat can be seen interspersed with the denser breast structures in a pattern of normal architecture (Fig. 17.6). The appearance of asymmetric tissue varies significantly from one mammographic projection to another.

When evaluating the breast for a possible mass, it is important to correlate the mammographic findings with the physical examination. When a suspicious palpable abnormality corresponds to the area of asymmetry seen on mammography a biopsy should be undertaken. In a recent series of 221 patients with mammographically visible asymmetries, only 3 patients had malignancies and all 3 had suspicious, palpable abnormalities corresponding to the visualized asymmetries (18).

Summation shadows that resemble masses on mammography can be produced by overlapping breast tissue. They are visible in only one view and usually disappear when focal compression spreads the tissues apart.

Once the radiologist has concluded that a mass is present, its margins, density, location, and size should be assessed. The number of mammographically visible masses and their similarities or differences should be analyzed. Previous films should be compared with the current study to look for new masses or an increase in the size of a mass. It is impossible to evaluate one characteristic independent of the others.

Margins

The margins of a mass are probably the most important characteristics to be assessed. Overlying breast parenchyma often obscures margin analysis, but liberal use of magnification compression views, in multiple projections, will aid the radiologist.

Ill–Defined Margins

Breast Carcinoma classically appears as a spiculated mass on mammography (Fig. 17.7); however, less than 20% of nonpalpable cancers present as such (17). Most spiculated-appearing breast cancers will be infiltrating ductal carcinoma; however, tubular and lobular carcinomas can present as such. Tubular carcinomas are more well-differentiated histologically

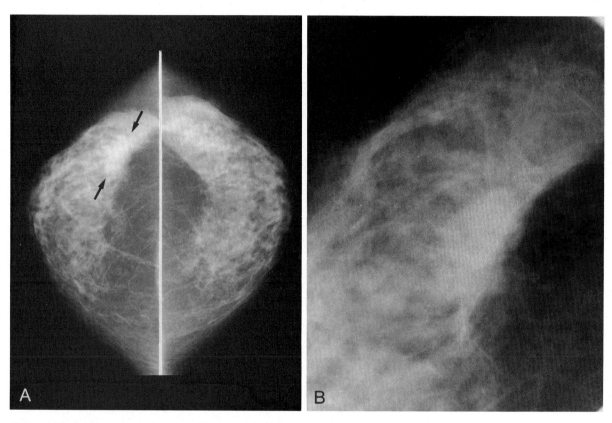

Figure 17.5.   Infiltrating Duct Carcinoma. A. Craniocaudal views of both breasts, showing an asymmetric area of increased density in the outer aspect of the right breast (*arrows*). **B.** Magnification compression view shows this to be a true mass with defined, convex borders and increasing density toward its center.

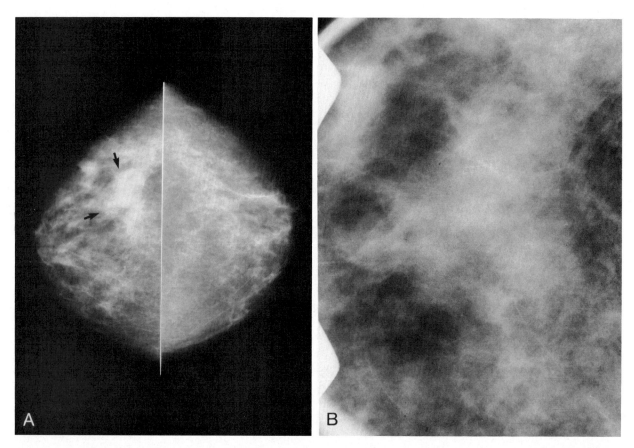

Figure 17.6. Asymmetric Breast Parenchyma. A. Craniocaudal views of both breasts in an asymptomatic woman. There is an area of asymmetric density in the outer aspect of the right breast (*arrows*). **B.** Compression magnification view demonstrates normal breast ar-chitecture in the area of increased density. These findings are con-sistent with histologically normal, but asymmetric mammary paren-chyma.

Figure 17.7. Classic Breast Carcinoma. This spiculated breast mass is an infiltrating duct carci-noma.

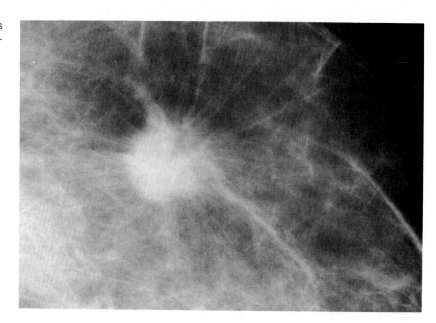

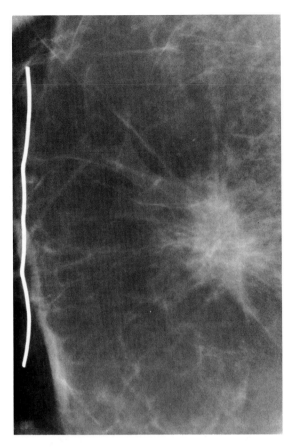

Figure 17.8. Postsurgical fat necrosis. This spiculated mass had been stable for 7 years. The radiopaque wire indicates the scar on the patient's skin from the previous lumpectomy.

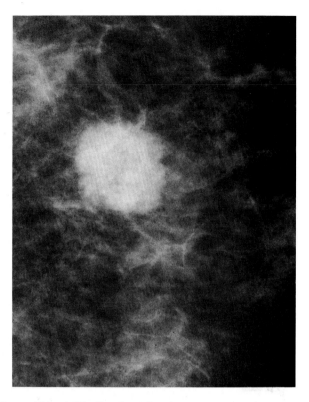

Figure 17.9. Infiltrating Duct Carcinoma presenting as a round mass with indistinct, microlobulated borders.

and carry a better prognosis. Lobular carcinomas comprise about 10% of all invasive carcinomas. They are not mammographically distinguishable from invasive ductal carcinomas, although they are frequently more subtle. Single rows of lobular cancer cells can infiltrate surrounding tissues, so they generally cause less tissue distortion.

A very limited differential exists for a spiculated mass.

Fat Necrosis from a previous surgical biopsy can appear spiculated (Fig. 17.8).

Scars from previous breast surgery should be carefully marked with radiopaque wires. Comparison should be made with previous films, both to determine the location of the abnormality that underwent biopsy and to assess for any increase in size of the presumed scar. Many scars will regress with time, but others will be stable in appearance and size. Any increase in size should be viewed with suspicion and biopsy should be undertaken.

A Complex Sclerosing Lesion or a radial scar can also present as a spiculated lesion. These are spontaneous lesions that are benign and consist histologically of central sclerosis and varying degrees of epithelial proliferation, represented by strands of fibrous connective tissue. Histologic differentiation of these lesions from carcinoma is mandatory.

Breast carcinoma can also present as a round mass with fuzzy or indistinct borders (Fig. 17.9). Benign lesions that can present as such include abscess, hematoma, and focal fibrosis.

Breast Abscesses are most commonly seen in a subareolar location in lactating women (Fig. 17.10). Clinically, there is associated pain, swelling, and erythema.

Spontaneous Hematomas are seen in women on anticoagulant therapy or in those with blood dyscrasias. They can, of course, also be secondary to trauma, needle aspiration, or surgery. Correlation with the patient's history and physical examination will be helpful in discerning whether a lesion represents a hematoma. If doubt persists as to the nature of a possible hematoma, short-interval followup mammograms to demonstrate resolution will be helpful (Fig. 17.11).

Well-Circumscribed Margins

Well-circumscribed masses are almost always benign; however, up to 5% of masses that appear well circumscribed on conventional mammograms may represent carcinomas (19). The "halo sign," which is a partial or complete radiolucent ring surrounding a mass, is not helpful in determining benignity. Magni-

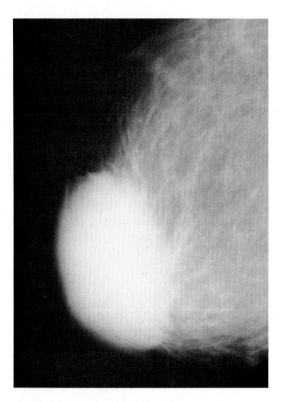

Figure 17.10.   A Large Subareolar Abscess. The indistinct borders of the mass are the result of surrounding inflammation.

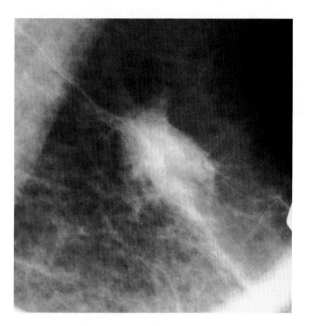

Figure 17.11.   Infiltrating Duct Carcinoma. Magnification view of a palpable abnormality in the upper outer quadrant. The patient had undergone a negative FNAB the previous day; the mammographic differential diagnosis included hematoma and carcinoma. Follow-up mammogram 6 weeks later demonstrated no resolution. Surgical biopsy showed infiltrating duct carcinoma.

fication compression views will be of great assistance in clarifying the nature of borders of an apparently well-circumscribed mass. Often, masses that appear well circumscribed on conventional views will be shown to have indistinct, fuzzy, or microlobulated margins on compression magnification views (20).

Cysts are the most common well-circumscribed masses seen in women between the ages of 35 and 50 (Fig. 17.12). They are rare after menopause. They can be accurately diagnosed by ultrasound and are virtually never malignant. A high-frequency (generally 5–10 MHz) ultrasound transducer is utilized in a targeted examination of the mass in question. On sonography, cysts are round or oval, smooth-walled, anechoic, and produce enhanced through transmission of sound. They can frequently be deformed with gentle pressure from the transducer. It is essential that the focal zone and gain of the ultrasound unit be optimally adjusted for the lesion so that cysts can be accurately diagnosed sonographically. The cyst must be thoroughly examined in two projections to rule out any irregularities or masses emanating from the walls.

Fibrosis is another manifestation of fibrocystic change that can be seen mammographically. It can be quite focal, giving it the appearance of a well-defined mass on the films. Such areas of focal fibrosis may also present with ill-defined borders, making them difficult to differentiate from carcinomas.

Fibroadenomas are the most common well-defined solid masses seen on mammography (Fig. 17.13). They are homogenous, but frequently show large, coarse calcifications. They may have a lobulated contour, but there are usually only a few large lobulations. If a fibroadenoma is not calcified it cannot be distinguished from a cyst by mammography. Sonography will allow this distinction as fibroadenomas will be solid hypoechoic masses. The peak age of patients with clinically detected fibroadenomas is 20 to 30 years; however, fibroadenomas are seen into the 8th decade. They rarely appear or grow after menopause.

Primary Breast Malignancies to be considered when a well-defined density is visualized on mammography are *infiltrating duct carcinoma, papillary carcinoma, mucinous carcinoma,* and *medullary carcinoma.*

Lymphoma, either primary or metastatic, may also present as a well-circumscribed mass.

Metastatic Disease to the breast from other sources may present as a well-circumscribed nodule. The most common primary cancer to produce breast metastases is melanoma, but a large variety of other primary sites have also been reported to metastasize to the breast. When these malignancies are encountered, magnification compression views of the abnormality often demonstrate some irregularity to the contour of the mass (Fig. 17.14).

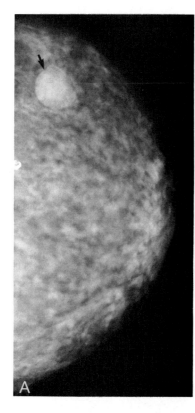

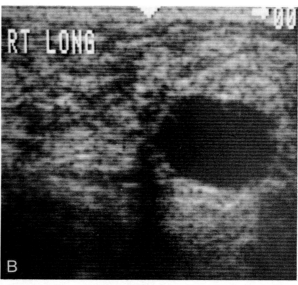

Figure 17.12. Simple Breast Cyst. A. Craniocaudal mammogram demonstrates a 1.5-cm mass in a 47-year old-woman (*arrow*). The mass is at least partially well circumscribed. **B.** Ultrasound of the mass demonstrates a round, anechoic structure with well-defined margins and enhanced through transmission of sound. These features are diagnostic of a simple cyst. (From Kline TS, Kline IK. Guides to aspiration biopsy breast. New York: Igaku-Shoin, Medical Publishers, 1989:204.)

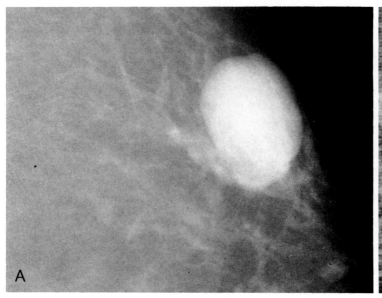

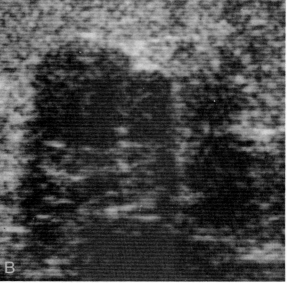

Figure 17.13. Fibroadenoma. A. Craniocaudal view of a 1.8-cm fairly well-circumscribed mass. **B.** Ultrasound demonstrates a solid hypoechoic mass with posterior acoustical shadowing.

Density

Density is relevant to analysis of mammographically detected masses when these masses contain lucent areas indicative of fat. Breast masses that clearly contain fat are benign. The assessment of density in homogeneous nonfatty masses is not, however, useful in the prediction of benignity or malignancy.

Fat Density. Benign breast lesions that are purely fat density include oil cysts from fat necrosis, lipomas, and sometimes galactoceles. **Oil cysts** are generally the result of trauma (Fig. 17.15). They are round lucent lesions surrounded by a thin capsule; often they are multiple and can demonstrate rim calcifications. **Lipomas** are similar to oil cysts in appearance; they are also lucent with a surrounding capsule. The sur-

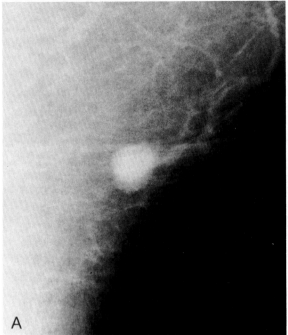

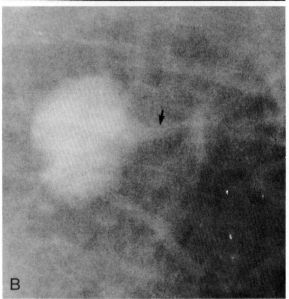

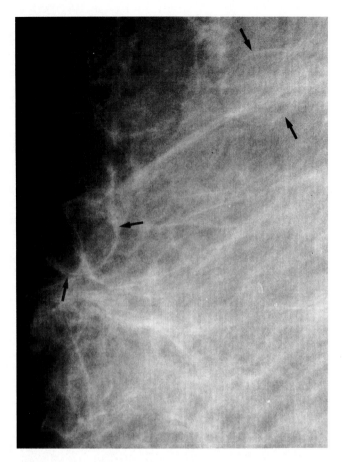

Figure 17.15. Oil Cysts. Multiple lucent masses with thin capsules (*arrows*) are characteristic of oil cysts. The patient had suffered trauma to the breast.

Figure 17.14. Infiltrating Duct Carcinoma. A. A well-circumscribed, 8-mm mass that had increased in size compared with a study done 1 year previously. **B.** Magnification view shows a spiculation anteriorly (*arrow*). Infiltrating duct carcinoma was proven at biopsy.

rounding breast architecture may be distorted because of the mass effect of the lipoma. *Galactoceles* usually occur in lactating or recently lactating women and are probably the result of an obstructed duct. If the inspissated milk is of sufficient fat quantity, these lesions will appear lucent; however, they can also be of mixed or water density.

Mixed Fat and Water Density. Other benign masses that are mixed fat and water density are **hamartomas,** which are rare benign tumors, and in-

tramammary lymph nodes. ***Intramammary lymph nodes*** are frequently seen on mammograms. They are located in the upper outer quadrant in the posterior three-fourths of the breast parenchyma. They normally contain a fatty center or a lucent notch, representing fat in the hilus of the node (Fig. 17.16).

Location

Breast cancers can occur in any location within the breast. As such, the location of a lesion is helpful in mammographic diagnosis in only two situations. The first occurs when the mammographer is considering an intramammary lymph node in the differential. The second occurs when a lesion can be localized to the skin.

Intramammary Nodes visualized on mammograms are always located in the upper outer quadrant of the breast. Although they have been noted in other locations in autopsy series, there are no reports of visualization of these masses by mammography in any location other than the upper outer quadrant.

Skin Lesions. If a lesion is located only on the skin, it does not represent a breast carcinoma. Frequently, however, skin lesions project over the paren-

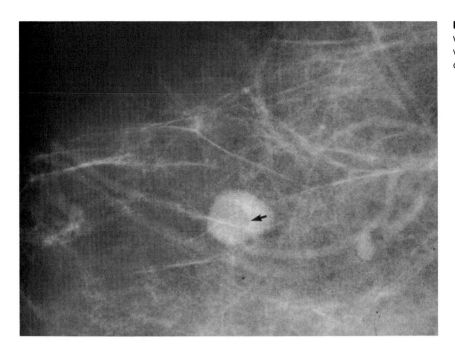

Figure 17.16. Intramammary Lymph Node with a characteristic lucent center (*arrow*) and well-circumscribed margins. The node was located in the upper outer quadrant.

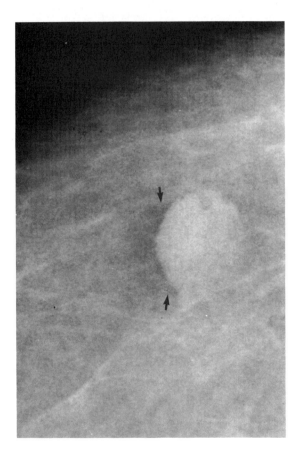

Figure 17.17. Skin Nevus. The dark halo produced around one edge is the result of air trapping (*arrows*).

chyma and can appear to be within the breast. Such lesions are usually recognizable by air trapping around the edges or in the interstices. This air trapping can produce a dark halo around one edge (Fig.

17.17). Air trapping will not, however, be evident with flat, pigmented skin lesions or sebaceous cysts.

It is helpful to examine the patient and place a radiopaque marker on any skin lesions or possible sebaceous cysts. The technologist can then perform a repeat film in the projection that the lesion was visualized. If necessary, this view can be followed by a tangential view to demonstrate that the lesion is located in the skin.

Size

By itself, the size of a mammographically discovered mass is not particularly helpful in determining its etiology. A spiculated or ill-defined mass should undergo biopsy no matter what its size. However, when the mammographer is dealing with a well-circumscribed, rounded mass that has a much lower chance of being malignant, size will play a role in determining the next step in the workup. Ultrasound is not usually helpful when lesions are less than about 5 to 7 mm in size. Frequently, patients with small, well-defined round lesions, under 1.5 cm in diameter, will be asked to return in 6 months for a follow-up study to assess for interval growth. If the lesion increases in size, further investigation with ultrasound and possible biopsy can be performed. After the first 6-month follow-up, such lesions should be followed at yearly intervals for a minimum of 3 years.

Number of Masses

Multiple Masses. In many cases, multiple well-defined round masses will be seen on mammography. When evident, such masses are also frequently bilat-

Figure 17.18.   Multiple Benign Masses. Bilateral CC views show multiple large round masses in both breasts. The patient was asymptomatic. Differential diagnosis was cysts or fibroadenomas.

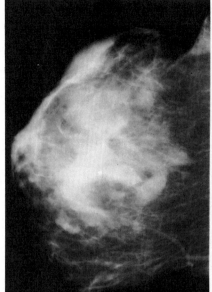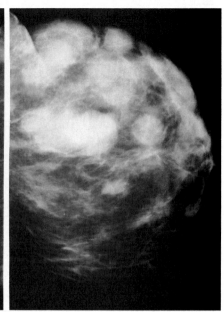

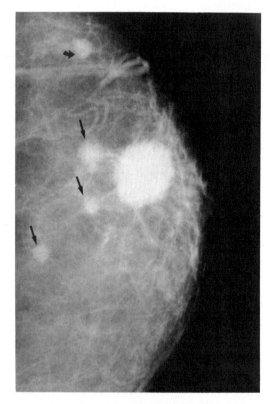

Figure 17.19.   Multifocal Carcinoma, Craniocaudal view. The largest mass was palpable. The others were discovered by mammography (*straight arrows*). The more well-defined nodule (*curved arrow*) probably represented an intramammary lymph node.

eral. Multiple, bilateral round masses are usually benign. They most often represent **cysts** or **fibroadenomas** (Fig. 17.18). In patients with a history of previous malignancy, however, **metastasis** may also be considered, although metastatic disease is much more commonly unifocal.

All lesions should be evaluated carefully. Benign and malignant lesions can coexist in the same breast. A lesion with a different, suspicious morphology should prompt a biopsy.

When evaluating the patient with similar appearing multiple, bilateral, rounded breast masses, it is not generally advisable to utilize ultrasound. Ultrasound is confusing and frequently demonstrates hypoechoic areas that, although disconcerting to the radiologist, do not prove to be malignant.

Multifocal primary breast cancers generally present as obvious, ill-defined or stellate lesions that are suspicious in appearance (Fig. 17.19).

Calcifications

Malignant Calcifications.   Clustered, pleomorphic microcalcifications, with or without an associated soft tissue mass, are a primary mammographic sign of breast cancer. Such calcifications are seen in more than half of all mammographically discovered cancers; about one-third of all nonpalpable cancers are manifest by calcifications alone, without an associated mass (17).

The calcifications associated with malignancy are dystrophic; they are the result of abnormalities in the tissues. Some malignant calcifications occur in necrotic tumor debris; others are the result of calcification of stagnant secretions that are trapped in the cancer (21).

Calcifications are a frequent finding on mammographic examinations. In the majority of cases, such calcifications will be benign and their origin, as such, will be easily identifiable. There is, however, a significant overlap in the appearance of benign and malignant calcifications. Only 25–35% of all calcifications that undergo biopsy will be malignant.

The importance of technically optimal mammography cannot be overstated when calcifications are being studied. The film exposure must be appropriate; an underexposed film can hide calcifications in a background of white breast tissue. Slight overpenetration of films is optimal for detection of calcifica-tions. Magnification views will be extremely helpful for assessing the malignant potential of a group of calcifications.

Careful analysis of the form, size, distribution, and number of calcifications, as well as any association with other soft tissue structures, will allow the radiologist to determine which calcifications are unequivocally benign and which require biopsy or follow-up studies.

Form

Benign Calcifications. Some shapes of calcifications can be easily identified as benign. Any calcification with a lucent center should not cause concern. Calcifications with lucent centers are often located in the skin. A skin marker can be placed over the calcifications and a subsequent tangential view taken to confirm their location in the skin (Fig. 17.20). Calcifications with lucent centers are also seen as a result of fat necrosis. Such calcifications can be smooth and round or they can be eggshell-type calcifications in the walls of an oil cyst (Fig. 17.21).

Calcifications that layer into a curvilinear or linear shape on 90° lateral films, yet appear as smudged clusters on CC views, are also representative of a benign process (Fig. 17.22). Such calcifications represent sedimented calcium ("milk of calcium") within the fluid of tiny breast cysts. Similar benign calcifications can also be seen within larger cysts and oil cysts. Sedimented calcium is a common finding in approximately 5% of women presenting for mammography.

Other benign calcifications that are easily recognizable by their form include arterial calcifications, the calcifications in a degenerating fibroadenoma, and calcifications associated with secretory disease. Arterial calcifications generally present as tubular parallel lines of calcium (Fig. 17.23). Occasionally, early arterial calcification can present a diagnostic problem,

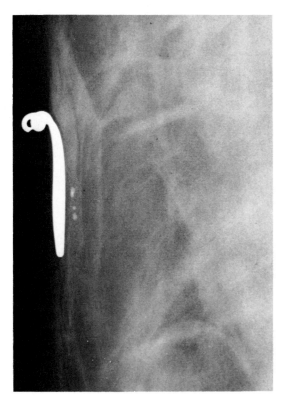

Figure 17.20. Skin Calcifications. Tangential view showing calcifications to be in the skin. A radiopaque marker had been placed on the skin at the site of the calcifications. This was done to facilitate positioning for the tangential view.

Figure 17.21. Eggshell Calcifications in Oil Cysts. These are large calcifications with lucent centers that are benign.

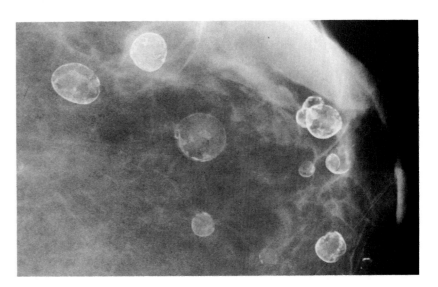

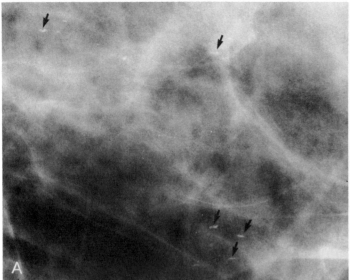

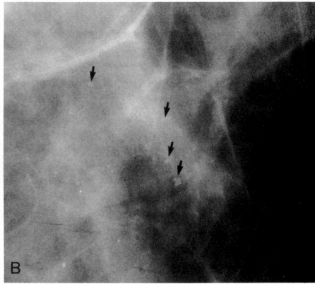

Figure 17.22.   Milk of Calcium in Breast Cysts. A. Magnification of a 90° lateral mammogram showing diffuse linear calcifications (*arrows*). **B.** Craniocaudal magnification view of the same area showing smudged, rounded calcifications (*arrows*). This change in configuration between views is typical of sedimented calcium. The calcium is layering in the bottom of microcysts so it appears as a line or meniscus when viewed from the side in the lateral projection. When viewed from the top, these calcifications simply appear smudged and rounded.

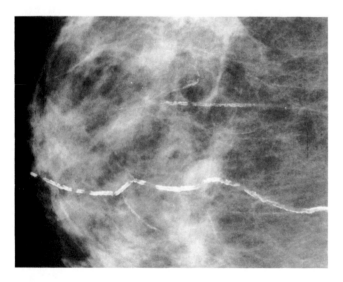

Figure 17.23.   Arterial Calcifications. Arterial calcifications in the breast are identified by their location in the wall of a tortuous vessel.

but this can usually be resolved by looking for soft tissue of the vessel in association with the calcification. Magnification in multiple projections can be helpful (Fig. 17.24).

Fibroadenomas can calcify in various patterns. Sometimes the calcifications are indeterminate, but the classic calcifications, associated with an atrophic fibroadenoma, are large, coarse, and irregular in shape (Fig. 17.25).

Secretory Disease. The calcifications associated with secretory disease are smooth, long, thick linear calcifications that radiate toward the nipple in a generally orderly pattern (Fig. 17.26). These calcifi-

cations are located in ectatic ducts. When periductal inflammation has occurred, these calcifications may appear more lucent centrally since calcium is deposited in the tissues adjacent to the ducts.

Malignant Calcifications. Calcifications that are associated with malignancy vary in shape and size (Fig. 17.27). The margins of the calcifications are jagged and irregular. Malignant calcifications are often branching. Ductal carcinoma in situ (DCIS), or noninvasive breast cancer, is most often detected mammographically as a result of such calcifications. Groups of pleomorphic calcifications that appear more linear of "dot-dash" in appearance are more commonly associated with the comedocarcinoma type of intraductal carcinomas (Fig. 17.28). The cribriform and micropapillary types are often manifest by more punched out or granular appearing calcifications. The morphology of the calcification cannot, however, be used to predict the subtype of DCIS since there is considerable overlap in the forms of the calcification associated with each subtype. In the comedocarcinomas, the calcifications can be an approximate indication of the size of the tumor, although the extent of disease is often greater than mammographically predicted. In the noncomedo varieties, correlation is even poorer. The biological behavior of these subtypes also differs; comedocarcinomas are the most likely to recur (22).

Pleomorphic microcalcifications in association with a malignant soft tissue mass can also indicate areas of extensive intraductal component within or adjacent to the invasive tumor. It is especially important to recognize malignant calcifications occurring

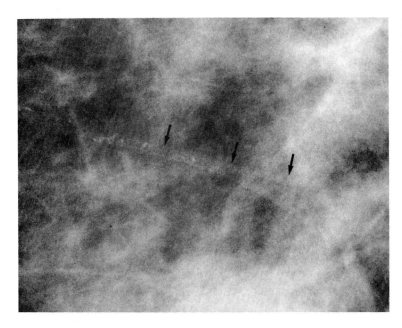

Figure 17.24.   Early Arterial Calcification. Magnification view. The calcification can be seen clearly in the walls of an artery (*arrows*). The soft tissue of the artery was difficult to appreciate on the conventional views.

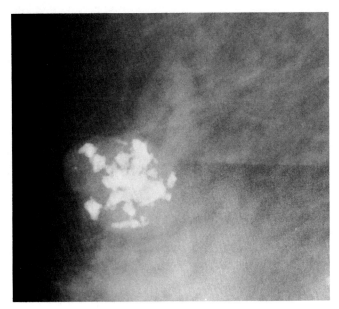

Figure 17.25.   Fibroadenoma. Typical large, coarse, irregular calcifications are seen in a fibroadenoma.

in tissues surrounding invasive cancers so they can be excised with the invasive tumor. Such extensive intraductal component-positive cancers also have a greater tendency to recur.

Indeterminate Calcifications. Morphologically indeterminate calcifications account for the majority of mammographically generated surgical biopsies of calcifications (Fig. 17.29). Such calcifications are most often associated with fibrocystic change. Diagnoses included under the general category of fibrocystic disease are fibrosis adenosis, sclerosing adenosis, epithelial hyperplasia, cysts, apocrine metaplasia, and atypical hyperplasia. Occasionally, biopsy of indeterminate calcification will yield a diagnosis of lobular carcinoma in situ (LCIS), also called lobular neoplasia. Although not an invasive cancer, LCIS places a woman at higher risk for development of invasive breast cancer. Mammographically, LCIS has no distinct features. If it is clinically occult it is most often found serendipitously adjacent to a focus of mammographically indeterminate, but histologically benign, calcifications.

Distribution

Calcifications that are widely scattered and seen bilaterally are usually indicative of a benign process, such as sclerosing adenosis or adenosis. Multiple, bilateral clusters of calcifications that appear morphologically similar are also generally benign. Careful analysis with a magnifying lens is essential in these cases so that a morphologically dissimilar cluster is not overlooked. Such calcifications should be thoroughly examined with magnification views.

Malignant calcifications usually occur in tight clusters within a small volume of tissue, but DCIS can produce calcifications that encompass large areas of the breast. Calcifications that are morphologically suspicious or indeterminate and occupy a segment of the breast should undergo biopsy.

Size

Malignant calcifications are generally less than 0.5 mm in size. Because the calcifications associated with carcinoma are so small, they are frequently referred to

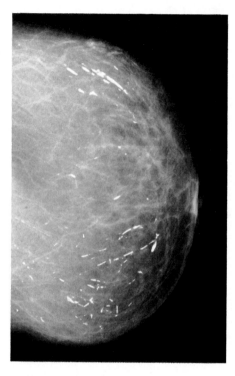

Figure 17.26. Secretory Calcifications. Craniocaudal view demonstrates long and thick calcifications in ectatic ducts that radiate toward the nipple.

Figure 17.27. Malignant Calcifications. Magnification view of infiltrating ductal carcinoma. Note the irregular forms as well as the variety of sizes and shapes.

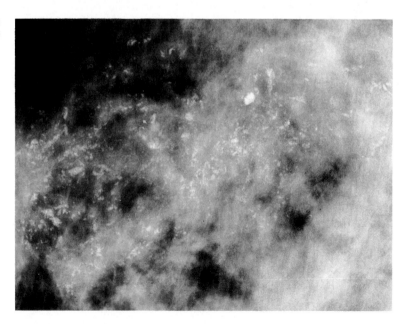

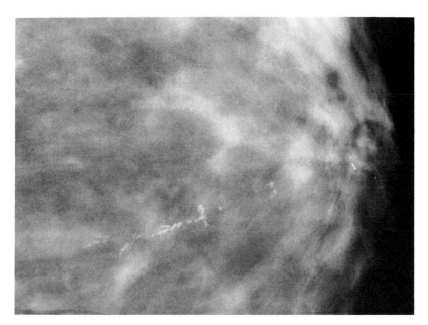

Figure 17.28. Malignant Calcifications. Dot-dash or "casting" calcifications of the comedo subtype of DCIS. Note the pleomorphism in the size and shape of the calcifications. (From Kline TS, Kline IK. Guides to aspiration biopsy breast. New York: Igaku-Shoin, Medical Publishers, 1989:201.)

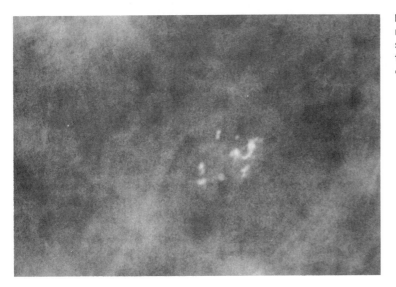

Figure 17.29. Indeterminate Calcifications. Magnification view of cluster of calcifications. There is some irregularity in shape and variation in size, but these calcifications were benign. They were associated with fibrocystic change.

as microcalcifications. Within a cluster there will be a variety of sizes.

Benign calcifications are often larger. When benign disease produces clusters of calcifications, the size of these calcifications is usually similar.

Number

Calcifications associated with malignancy are generally quite numerous. The greater the number of calcifications the more likely they are associated with malignant disease. Establishing the lower limit of the number of calcifications in a cluster that would require biopsy is extremely difficult. Assessment of the morphology of these calcifications by magnification views will influence this decision. Clusters composed of small numbers of smoothly rounded calcifications can be followed for stability. A unilateral 6 month follow-up examination followed by a bilateral examination in 6 months, and yearly follow-up thereafter, can be used to follow low-suspicion calcifications.

Architectural Distortion

Breast cancer is occasionally heralded by distortion in the normal architecture of the breast (Fig. 17.30). Differential diagnosis includes fat necrosis related to scarring from previous surgery and a complex sclerosing lesion, also known as radial scar. On close inspection, fat may be seen interspersed with fibrous elements in the center of fat necrosis or complex sclerosing lesions, but this appearance is not specific for benignity. Similar findings can be seen in malignant lesions.

Figure 17.30. Architectural Distortion Representing Breast Carcinoma. Note how the cancer pulls the surrounding parenchyma toward it (arrows).

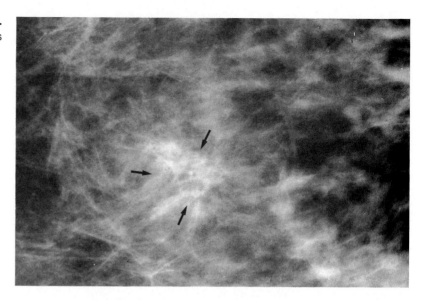

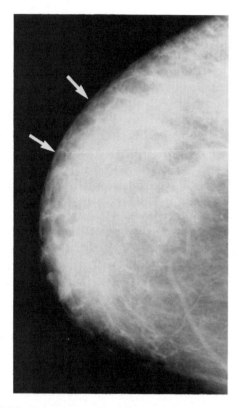

Figure 17.31. Inflammatory Carcinoma. Craniocaudal view demonstrates a diffuse increase in parenchymal density, along with skin thickening laterally (arrows).

Increased Density of Breast Tissue

Hormone Therapy. Increasing parenchymal density of breast tissue can be bilateral or unilateral. Bilateral increased density is usually the result of estrogen replacement therapy in postmenopausal women. Such hormone therapy can give the breasts a more glandular, premenopausal appearance. Intrinsic hormonal fluctuations in premenopausal, pregnant, or lactating women may cause similar changes in the density of the breasts. Hormonally related changes in breast density are not associated with skin thickening.

Inflammatory Carcinoma. A unilateral increase in breast density with associated skin thickening may result from several processes. The most ominous of these is inflammatory carcinoma of the breast (Fig. 17.31). Clinically, this disease is manifest by a warm, erythematous, firm, tender breast. Histologically, the dermal lymphatics are diffusely involved. Mammographically, a focal mass may be seen within the dense tissue, but often the breast appears homogeneously dense. Inflammatory carcinoma of the breast is a locally advanced disease that carries a poor prognosis.

Radiation Therapy. A unilateral increase in parenchymal density with skin thickening can also be seen in patients who have undergone radiation therapy to the breast. Radiation changes are most pronounced during the first 6 months following therapy. They usually resolve gradually over a period of years.

Diffuse Mastitis can produce a generalized skin thickening and increase in breast density. Clinical differentiation from inflammatory carcinoma is usually possible.

Obstruction to the Lymphatic or Venous Drainage from metastatic disease, surgical removal, or thrombosis can produce a unilateral increase in breast density with skin thickening due to edema. The anasarca associated with congestive heart failure, renal failure, cirrhosis, or hypoalbuminemia most often presents as bilateral increased breast density with skin thickening; however, asymmetric involvement of the breasts can occur.

Correlation of physical examination findings and history will usually allow differentiation of the various causes of an increase in breast density.

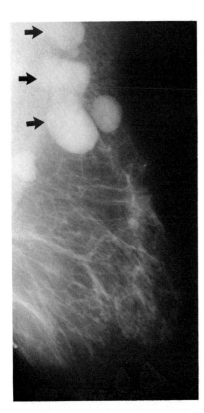

Figure 17.32. Lymphoma. Hodgkin's disease involves the axillary lymph nodes. The nodes are homogeneous, dense, and enlarged (*arrows*).

Axillary Adenopathy

Axillary lymph nodes are frequently visualized on the MLO mammogram. Normally they are less than 2 cm in size and have lucent centers or notches resulting from fat in the hilum. Fatty infiltration of the nodes themselves can cause lucent enlargement and replacement.

Pathologic axillary nodes are homogeneously dense and enlarged. A variety of processes can result in replacement of normal nodal architecture. Malignant involvement of axillary nodes can be the result of primary breast cancer, metastatic disease, or lymphoma (Fig. 17.32). Axillary nodes can also become pathologically enlarged because of inflammation. Patients with rheumatoid arthritis, systemic lupus erythematosus, scleroderma, and psoriasis may also have axillary adenopathy.

Coarse calcifications in axillary nodes may reflect granulomatous disease. Microcalcifications are occasionally seen in nodes involved with metastatic breast cancer. Gold deposits, seen in patients being treated for rheumatoid arthritis, are occasionally seen in axillary nodes and may be confused with calcifications.

The Augmented Breast

More than 1.5 million women in the United States have undergone augmentation mammoplasty. Imaging of the augmented breast poses unique challenges. Special techniques must be employed both to screen for breast cancer and to evaluate the patient for possible complications related to the implant.

Various types of implants have been used in augmentation procedures. They include silicone envelopes filled with saline or with viscous silicone gel, as well as double-lumen implants containing an inner core of silicone gel surrounded by an outer envelope filled with saline. Silicone is more radiopaque than saline, although neither allows adequate visualization of immediately surrounding tissue.

Implants can be placed either anterior (subglandular) or posterior (subpectoral) to the pectoralis muscle. Patients having subglandular implants are subject to a greater risk of fibrous and calcific contractures around the implant. Such contractures are not only painful and deforming, but they also make mammography more difficult.

Screening mammography in the woman with implants requires the use of at least two extra views of each breast. Standard MLO and CC views are performed. Then the implants are displaced posteriorly against the chest wall while the breast tissue is pulled anteriorly and vigorously compressed (Fig. 17.33). The compression paddle keeps the implant from migrating into the field. Greater compression of anterior tissues allows more optimal imaging (Fig. 17.34). Both MLO and CC views are repeated using this technique. These modified views are generally called displacement views or Eklund views, after the radiologist who first described them (23).

Displacement views are more difficult to accomplish in patients having subglandular implants with associated contractures. The implants are not easily displaced, and so less of the anterior breast tissue is depicted on the modified views. In such cases, a 90° lateral view may also be helpful in screening.

Although some breast tissue may be obscured in patients with implants, these women, when in the appropriate age groups, deserve the same careful screening examinations at the same intervals as patients without implants. The indeterminate mammogram in an implant patient should be evaluated in a manner similar to that in a patient without implants.

Women who have undergone augmentation mammoplasty may also present with abnormalities related to their implants. These include capsular contractures, herniations of the implant through rents in the capsules, implant rupture with free or contained silicone, and deflation of saline implants. Many patients will present for breast imaging subsequent to noticing a change in implant contour or size (Fig. 17.35). Mammography is generally the first examination performed if the woman is over the age of 30. Special

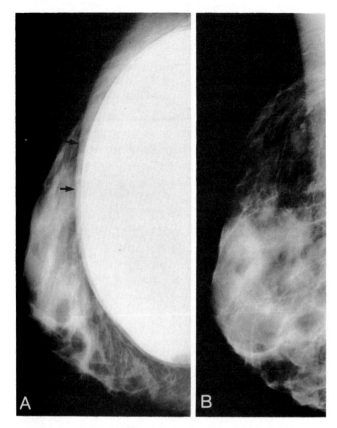

Figure 17.33.   Breast Implants. A. Standard MLO view of a patient with a subpectoral implant. Note the pectoralis muscle (*arrows*) anterior to the implant. **B.** Mediolateral oblique Eklund view on the same patient. The implant has been displaced posteriorly, out of view, while the compression has been applied anteriorly.

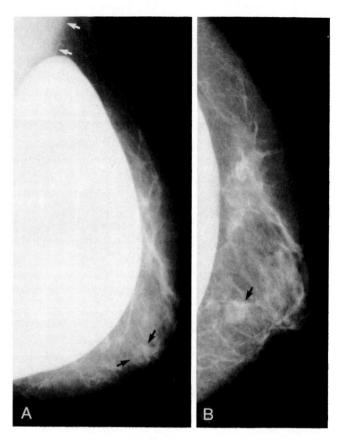

Figure 17.34.   Infiltrating Duct Carcinoma. A. Standard MLO view in a patient with subglandular implants. Note the pectoralis muscle (*white arrows*) extending posterior to the implant. A poorly defined 1-cm mass (*black arrows*) was noted in the subareolar tissues. **B.** Mediolateral oblique Eklund view in the same patient. The subareolar mass (*black arrow*) is more clearly defined because of greater compression of the tissues anterior to the implant. Histologic examination of the mass showed infiltrating duct carcinoma.

views, such as tangential, spot compression, and magnification views, are frequently required.

Other modalities are currently under study for assessment of implant complications. Preliminary data suggest that MR may be effective in identifying silicone implant rupture in localizing free silicone (24). Ultrasound may also be helpful in evaluating breast masses in implant patients, particularly when the mass is suboptimally visualized on mammography. Ultrasound has also been helpful in distinguishing true breast lesions from palpable irregularities of the implant.

The Male Breast

The most common indication for breast imaging in men is a palpable asymmetric thickening or mass. Gynecomastia is usually the cause. Breast cancer is rare, but can occur.

Normal Male Breast appears on mammography as a mound of subcutaneous fat without glandular tissue (Fig. 17.36). The nipple is small.

Gynecomastia generally appears as a triangular or flame-shaped area of subareolar glandular tissue that points toward the nipple. There is fat inter-

spersed with parenchymal elements. A gradual merging of the more glandular elements with the fat occurs at the deep margin (Fig. 17.37). Gynecomastia can be unilateral or bilateral. When bilateral, it is most frequently asymmetric. Many causes have been reported, including ingestion of a variety of drugs, such as reserpine, cardiac glycosides, cimetidine, and thiazides, as well as marijuana. Testicular, adrenal, and pituitary tumors are associated with gynecomastia. Chronic hepatic disease, by virtue of reduced ability to clear endogenous estrogens, can also cause male breast enlargement.

Male Breast Cancer is mammographically similar to that found in women. it can have a variety of appearances, including an ill-defined, spiculated, or circumscribed mass (Fig. 17.38). Microcalcifications can occur.

Comparison with Previous Films

The importance of comparing current mammograms with previous films cannot be overstated. In

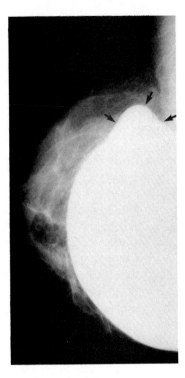

Figure 17.35. Ruptured Implant. Standard MLO view of a patient with subglandular implants. The patient had noted a new mass superolaterally in her breast. The mammogram shows a contained rupture of the implant (*arrows*) that corresponded to the palpable abnormality.

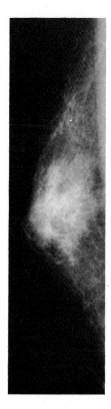

Figure 17.37. Gynecomastia. Mediolateral oblique view of a male with breast enlargement. There is glandular tissue in the subareolar area; this tissue gradually intersperses with the fat and does not appear as a mass.

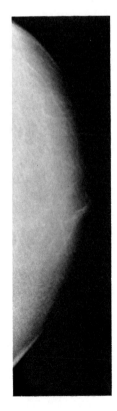

Figure 17.36. Male Breast. Relatively normal male breast, which is a mound of subcutaneous fat. Note the lack of glandular tissue.

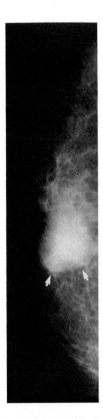

Figure 17.38. Male Breast Cancer. Mediolateral oblique view of the breast in a male. The mass has a defined interface with the surrounding fat (*arrows*). (Courtesy of Patricia Bell, M.D., Auburn, California.)

one series, developing densities accounted for 6% of nonpalpable breast carcinomas (17). Comparison with previous films will allow detection of subtle changes, in turn suggesting the need for further evaluation of such areas at an earlier time than might be possible if no comparison had been made (Fig. 17.39). It must, of course, be remembered that benign masses may appear or enlarge over time. In fact, in the majority of cases, interval change will be benign, but such changes should be fully evaluated by correlation with the history and physical examination, as well as the use of ancillary testing methods such as ultrasound, aspiration, and biopsy.

Malignant masses that were stable in size for up to 4.5 years have been reported. Although such a long period of stability is unusual, these reports emphasize the need for suspicious appearing lesions to undergo biopsy regardless of their apparent lack of change in size on serial films. Such lesions may have been overlooked or misinterpreted on a previous study.

Any new microcalcifications or increase in number of such calcifications deserve special consideration. Appropriate workup with magnification views will allow analysis of the form of such calcifications. Any calcifications that are not clearly benign deserve biopsy. It is extremely rare for malignant microcalcifications to remain stable over time.

THE RADIOLOGIC REPORT AND PLAN

The radiologic report should be clear and concise. It should contain a description of the findings, with the radiologist's assessment of the probability of malignancy, as well as a plan of subsequent action based on that probability.

Mammographic and sonographic findings can be divided into four categories.

1. **Benign** findings include lipomas, oil cysts, lucent galactoceles, intramammary lymph nodes, hamartomas, fibroadenomas with macrocalcifications, simple cysts, scattered round calcifications of adenosis, arterial calcifications, sedimented calcium within microcysts, secretory calcifications in duct ectasia, skin calcifications, and multiple bilateral, well-circumscribed masses representing cysts or fibroadenomas. Such findings do not require a specific follow-up plan. These patients should undergo mammography and clinical breast examination at routine screening intervals. Clinicians must be cautioned, however, that the decision for a palpable abnormality that does not have a specific benign mammographic correlate to undergo biopsy must be based on clinical suspicion. Mammography has a false-negative rate of 8–10%.

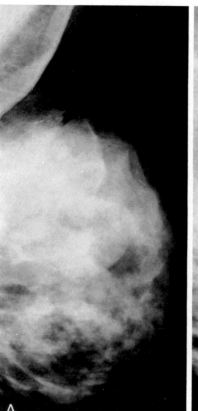
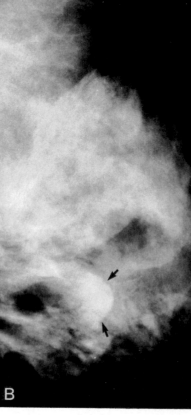
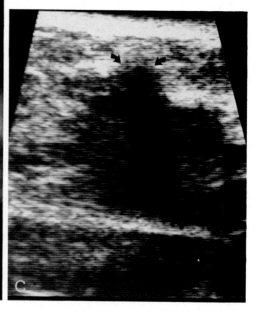

Figure 17.39.   Infiltrating Duct Carcinoma. A. Mediolateral oblique mammogram showing dense mammary parenchyma, but no evidence of malignancy. **B.** Mammogram 1 year later shows development of a subtle new mass (*arrows*). **C.** Ultrasound of the mass shows a shadowing, solid lesion (*arrows*). Biopsy demonstrated infiltrating duct carcinoma. (Courtesy of Patricia Bell, M.D., Auburn, California.)

2. **Probably benign** findings include small, well-circumscribed masses, clusters of smooth, round, similar-appearing microcalcifications, and asymmetric parenchymal densities that are not associated with palpable abnormalities. The probability that such abnormalities represent cancer is less than 1%; therefore, most mammographers recommend a plan of careful follow-up (25). The first follow-up mammogram of the affected breast should be performed 6 months following discovery of the abnormality. If the abnormality is stable, a bilateral study should be performed 6 months later, and then followup should occur at yearly intervals for a period of at least 3 years. Progression of a cancerous lesion depends upon tumor biology and doubling time; hence, the necessity of a lengthy follow-up period. Some cancers may grow slowly and others may change rapidly.

3. **Indeterminate** lesions which include lesions that are not classically malignant, but are suspicious enough to warrant fine-needle aspiration biopsy, core biopsy or surgical biopsy. The probability that such lesions will represent malignancy is approximately 25–35% in most practices in the United States.

4. **Probably malignant** lesions include classic spiculated masses and pleomorphic, clustered microcalcifications. These lesions have a very high probability of being malignant and should undergo biopsy.

INTERVENTIONAL PROCEDURES

Mammographically suspicious abnormalities require histologic or cytologic examination for definitive diagnosis. If the abnormality is clinically occult, an image-guided localization can be performed by the radiologist; this procedure is followed by an excisional biopsy. Although open surgical biopsy is the traditional method used for definitive diagnosis, percutaneous, image-directed aspiration or core biopsies performed in the radiology department are now an alternative.

Localization of Occult Breast Lesions

If an excisional biopsy of a mammographically suspicious, but nonpalpable, abnormality is to be performed, a localization will be required so that the surgeon is accurately directed to the lesion. Many methods for localization have been described. In choosing a technique, the radiologist should decide which method will allow sufficient accuracy so that the lesion can be removed without sacrificing large volumes of breast tissue. Malignancy will be found in only 25–35% of all biopsies performed for mammographically suspicious abnormalities. Since the majority of biopsies will be benign, it is extremely important to preserve as much breast tissue as possible.

Localizations can be performed using needle-wire systems or dye injection. There are several commercially available needle-wire systems. All allow placement of a wire through an introducing needle that has been positioned in the breast at the site of the abnormality. The wires differ mainly in the configuration of the anchoring end.

Injection of blue dye is a less frequently used method of localization. A needle is placed at the site of abnormality and dye is injected. If there is a delay between the time of injection and surgery, diffusion of the dye through the tumors can occur, resulting in a biopsy specimen that may be larger than necessary. Methylene blue, formerly in common usage for localizations, also interferes with estrogen receptor analysis.

Most mammographic units are equipped with a compression paddle that contains either one large hole marked on the edge with a grid, or a series of smaller holes marked with letters or numbers. The seated patient is placed in the mammographic unit so that the lesion to be localized is located under a hole in the compression plate. The breast is then filmed to determine the exact location of the abnormality. A needle is inserted parallel to the x-ray beam and through the abnormal area. The position of the needle with respect to the lesion is then checked by taking another film. If the needle position is satisfactory, the patient, with needle in place, is carefully removed from the mammography unit so that the tube can be rotated 90°. The patient is then positioned in the unit and compressed along an axis parallel to the needle. A film is taken to assess the depth of the needle tip with respect to the lesion. The needle must be in the lesion or deep to it in order to proceed. This assures a fixed relationship between the localizer and the lesion. Once the depth of the needle tip is satisfactory, the wire can be inserted through the needle and the needle withdrawn, leaving the wire in place (Fig. 17.40). Alternatively, dye can be injected through the needle and then the needle can be withdrawn. The patient is then sent to the operating room for surgical biopsy (26).

Once the biopsy has been performed the excised tissue should be sent for x-ray. This assures that the mammographic abnormality has been removed. In a small number of cases (1–5%), localization will fail and the lesion will not be removed. In most of these cases the localization will have to be repeated.

Most localizations are performed under mammographic guidance, but ultrasound can also be used to guide such procedures. The technique used is similar to that for ultrasound-guided percutaneous biopsy. A high-frequency transducer is placed over

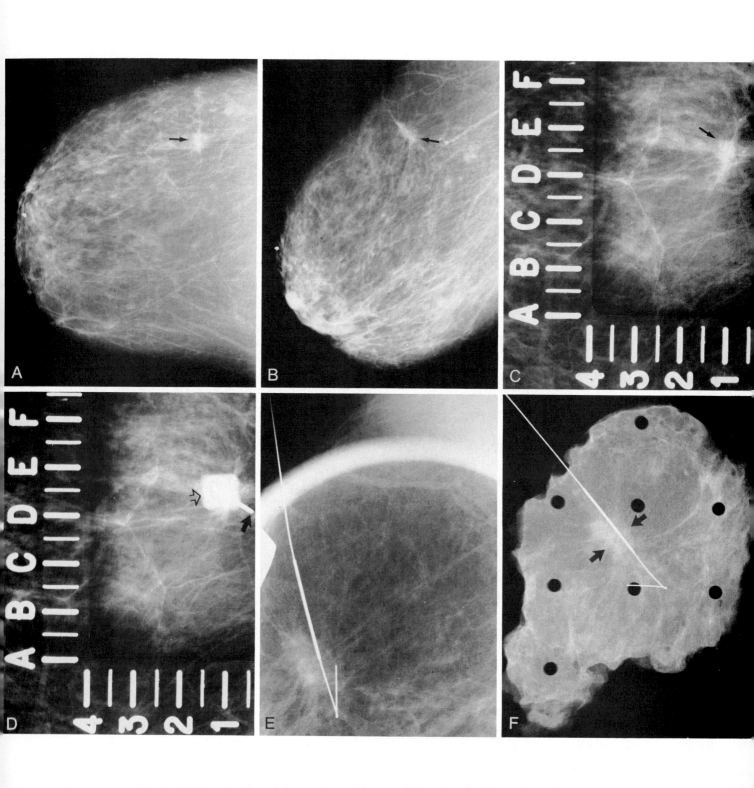

the lesion and the needle is introduced obliquely or vertically under real-time monitoring. When the tip is seen in the lesion, the wire can be inserted or the dye injected. Wire position should be confirmed by mammography.

Ultrasound is most useful in guiding a localization when the abnormality is seen well in one projection, but is obscured by dense tissue in the second. It may also be useful when lesions are located in areas of the breast that are difficult to position within the hole in the localized compression paddle. Ultrasound can only be used when the lesion can be visualized. Microcalcifications cannot be imaged, and only about half of all soft tissue masses are well delineated by ultrasound.

Percutaneous Aspiration and Biopsy of Occult Breast Lesions

Discovery of increasing numbers of potentially malignant occult breast masses has led to an increased number of excisional biopsies, the majority of which are benign. It has been estimated that the costs of surgical biopsies in a screening program can be greater than the costs of the screening mammograms themselves. Image-directed, FNAB and needle core biopsy of occult lesions can now be performed in the radiology department for about one-third the cost of an open surgical biopsy.

Fine-needle aspiration biopsy has been used to evaluate palpable breast masses for many years. Cells are withdrawn from the breast mass and examined under the microscope by a qualified cytologist. Diagnostic accuracy for FNAB ranges from 80 to 98%. In recent years there has been increasing interest in the use of both mammography and ultrasound to guide placement of needles for FNAB of clinically occult lesions (27).

Mammographic guidance of FNAB can be accomplished using a standard localization compression paddle or a dedicated stereotaxic device. If the localization paddle is used, the technique for placement of the needle is very similar to that used in performing a needle localization. The lesion is placed under the hole in the compression paddle and a 22-gauge aspirating needle is introduced (Fig. 17.41). Many times, the experienced operator can feel the lesion with the needle tip. The position of the needle in the lesion is then

confirmed by film. If the operator cannot feel the lesion, the patient can be removed from the unit, the tube rotated 90°, and a film taken so that the depth of the needle can be adjusted. The tip should be within the lesion. A syringe is then attached to the needle and suction is applied together with movement of the needle through the lesion in fanning planes so that all areas are sampled. If more than one specimen is required and the lesion is not easily felt with the needle tip, a coaxial system may be used. In so doing, an introducing needle can be placed at the superficial edge of the lesion and successive samples can be taken through it with thinner needles.

Dedicated stereotaxic devices can also be utilized to guide needle placement. These allow the x-ray tube to move independent of the compressed breast. The lesion is again placed deep to the hole in the compres-

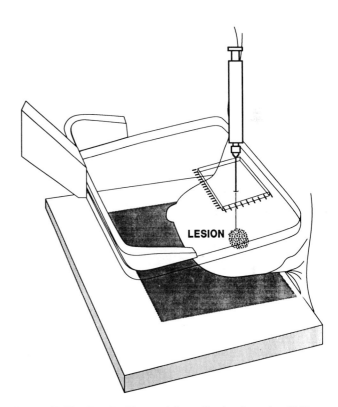

Figure 17.41. Needle Biopsy. Schematic drawing of a FNAB accomplished with mammographic guidance and a standard localizing paddle. The needle is placed into the lesion through the fenestration in the compression paddle. (From Kline TS, Kline IK. Guides to clinical aspiration, biopsy breast. New York: Igaku-Shoin, Medical Publishers, 1989:205.)

Figure 17.40. Needle Localization. Craniocaudal **(A)** and mediolateral **(B)** mammograms show a highly suspicious spiculated mass in the upper outer quadrant (*arrows*). **C.** Localization was performed by placing the fenestrated compression plate over the lesion (*arrow*) and then placing a needle parallel to the x-ray beam through the lesion. **D.** The hub of the needle (*open arrow*) is superimposed on the lesion; the tip (*solid arrow*) is at the posterior edge. A

film is then taken in the 90° orthogonal projection and, once the depth is adjusted, the hook wire is passed through the needle. **E.** A film in the same projection demonstrates the final depth of the wire. **F.** The excised tissue is sent for specimen x-ray to confirm that the abnormality (*arrows*) has been removed. Histologic examination in this case revealed invasive lobular carcinoma.

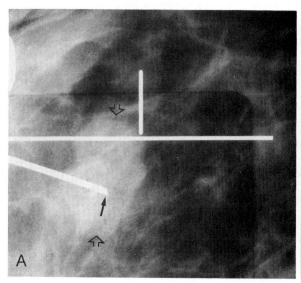
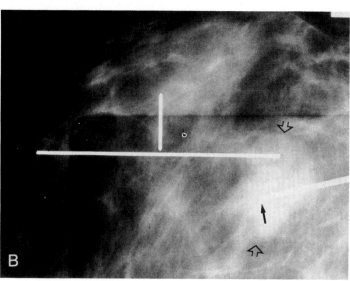

Figure 17.42. Stereotaxic Biopsy. A and **B.** Fine-needle aspiration biopsy performed with a stereotaxic device added on to a standard mammography unit. The two views are taken 30° apart to confirm that the needle tip (*black arrow*) is within the lesion (*open arrows*) on both views. Cytologic diagnosis was fibroadenoma.

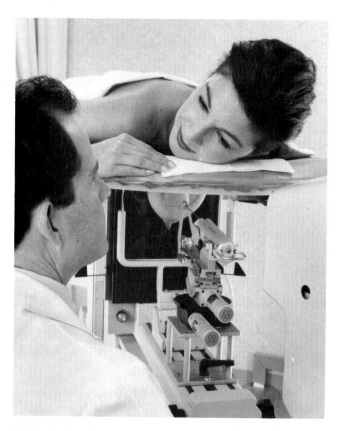

Figure 17.43. Dedicated Prone Stereotaxic Biopsy Unit. (Reproduced with permission from Fischer Imaging Corporation, Denver, Colorado.)

sion plate. Two views are taken 30–40° apart. Calculation of the amount of deviation of the lesion in these two views allows exact determination of the location of the lesion. The needle guide is adjusted in three di-

mensions and the needle is placed through the skin into the lesion. After confirmation that the needle lies within the lesion on both views, a sample can be aspirated (Fig. 17.42).

Currently there are two types of stereotaxic units available. One can be added on to a standard mammography machine, but has limited working space and requires a seated patient. The other is a prone dedicated unit that is more costly, but offers the advantages of having the patient in a prone position so as to minimize movement and vasovagal reactions (Fig. 17.43). Needle-core biopsies are more suited to performance on a prone unit.

Needle-core biopsies are performed using an automated push button biopsy gun with larger gauge trucut type needles, which obtain a thin core of tissue. Samples of breast tissue obtained in this way are processed in the pathology department exactly like surgically obtained biopsy samples; histologic diagnoses are obtained. Histologic interpretation of core biopsy samples does not require the specialized expertise of a cytologist, and therefore may become more widely accepted.

Ultrasound may also be used to guide placement of needles for either FNAB or core biopsy (Fig. 17.44). Aspiration of fluid cannot be performed if a core biopsy needle is used; many lesions chosen for ultrasound-guided biopsy will be atypical cysts from which fluid can be easily aspirated using a 22-gauge needle. If the lesion is clearly solid, a core biopsy needle can be advanced to the proximal edge of the mass and then fired under real time visualization.

Only those lesions that are suspicious enough to warrant biopsy should be investigated by FNAB or

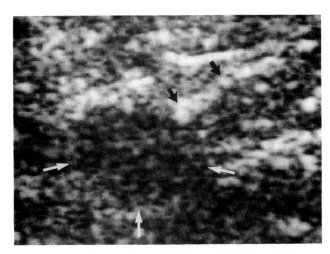

Figure 17.44. Ultrasound-guided Biopsy. Ultrasound shows the needle (*black arrows*) at the edge of a solid, hypoechoic mass (*white arrows*), which was a ductal carcinoma.

core biopsy. These techniques should not replace short-interval mammographic follow-up of probably benign lesions as they are more expensive.

Both FNAB and core biopsy are techniques that have only recently come into use for sampling occult breast lesions. Reported sensitivities for these procedures range from about 70–95%; specificities vary from 85–100%. Specimens with insufficient material can be a problem if FNAB is utilized. Both FNAB and core biopsy are subject to sampling error. It is very important to correlate cytologic or histologic results with the mammographic degree of suspicion. If a highly suspicious lesion yields a benign diagnosis, the patient should undergo surgical biopsy. All patients undergoing FNAB or core biopsy with benign results should have mammograms at 6, 12, and 24 months after the procedure to ensure stability of the lesion sampled (28).

Acceptance of FNAB and core biopsy of occult breast lesions is varied. Guidelines for use of these procedures are still evolving.

Other Interventional Procedures

Aspiration of sonographically atypical cysts can be performed for confirmation of the diagnosis using either ultrasound or mammographic guidance. The majority of such lesions will be smooth-walled masses that are atypical either because they lack through transmission or because the fluid within them is not anechoic. In such cases a 22-gauge needle can be inserted using a technique similar to that used for FNAB. If fluid is withdrawn, the lesion should be totally aspirated. After aspiration, air can be insufflated into the cyst cavity. This may prevent recurrence. If fluid cannot be withdrawn, the lesion is presumably

solid, and FNAB or needle localization can be performed using the aspiration needle.

In cases where there is irregularity or nodularity of the cyst wall by sonography, some mammographers advocate pneumocystography for confirmation. Surgical biopsy should be undertaken in these cases even though intracystic carcinomas are rare. Cytologic evaluation of aspirated fluid is unreliable for diagnosis.

Galactography can be used to investigate the cause of a spontaneous nipple discharge. The procedure involves the injection of contrast material into a duct, after which films are taken to look for intraductal tumors. These are most frequently papillomas, and less commonly carcinomas. The utility of this study is controversial. If the patient has a bloody discharge, some surgeons prefer to inject the discharging duct with methylene blue in the operating room before dissecting along it. Others utilize preoperative galactography to evaluate bloody discharge, and feel that if the galactogram is negative the patient can be observed. The use of galactography in the evaluation of a unilateral, spontaneous serous discharge is similarly controversial, since both bloody and serous fluid can be associated with small cancers that may not be visible mammographically (28).

Conclusion

Breast cancer represents a significant public health problem. Over 175,000 new cases are diagnosed and nearly 50,000 women die of the disease each year in the United States. Early detection with screening mammography is the only proven way to lower mortality from breast cancer. Diagnostic accuracy can be increased with the use of special mammographic views, ultrasound, and percutaneous biopsy techniques. Other modalities, such as MR and positron-emission tomography, are under study to determine their potential utility in diagnosis of breast diseases.

Utilization of breast imaging has increased over the last decade, but there are still significant numbers of women who have never had a mammogram. It is estimated that up to one-third of all women over the age of 50 fall into this category. Our challenge, as radiologists, is to maintain the highest standards of quality in performance and interpretation of breast imaging studies; it is also to encourage more women to take regular advantage of these life-saving techniques.

References

1. Shapiro S. Evidence on screening for breast cancer from a randomized trial. Cancer 1977;39:2772–2782.
2. Tábar L, Fagerberg CJG, Gad A, et al. Reduction in mortality from breast cancer after mass screening with mammography. Lancet 1985;i:829–832.
3. Verbeek ALM, Hendricks JHCL, Holland R, et al. Reduction of breast cancer mortality through mass screening with

modern mammography. First results of the Nijmegen Project, 1975–1981. Lancet 1984;i:1222–1224.

4. Collette HJA, Day NE, Rombach JJ, de Waard F. Evaluation of screening for breast cancer in a non-randomized study (the DOM Project) by means of a case-control study. Lancet 1984;i:1224–1226.

5. Andersson I, Aspegren R, Janzon L, et al. Mammographic screening and mortality from breast cancer: the Malmö mammographic screening trial. British Medical Journal 1988;297:943–948.

6. Chu KC, Smart CR, Tarone RE. Analysis of breast cancer mortality and stage distribution by age for the Health Insurance Plan clinical trial. J Natl Cancer Inst 1988;80:1125–1132.

7. Tábar L, Fagerberg G, Day NE, Holmberg L. What is the optimum interval between mammographic screening examinations?—An analysis based on the latest results of the Swedish two-county breast cancer screening trial. Br J Cancer 1987;55:547–551.

8. Baines CJ, Miller AB, Kopans DB, et al. Canadian National Breast Screening Study: assessment of technical quality by external review. AJR 1990;155:743–747.

9. Baines CJ, McFarlane DV, Miller AB. The role of the reference radiologist. Estimates of inter-observer agreement and potential delay in cancer detection in the National Breast Screening Study. Invest Radiol 1990;25:971–976.

10. Feig SA, Ehrlich SM. Estimation of radiation risk from screening mammography: recent trends and comparison with expected benefits. Radiology 1990;174:638–647.

11. Baker LH. Breast cancer detection demonstration project: five-year summary report. CA 1982;32:4:194–225.

12. Dodd GD. American Cancer Society guidelines on screening for breast cancer: an overview. CA 1992;42:3:177–180.

13. Tábar L, Fagerberg G, Duffy SW, et al. Update of the Swedish two-county program of mammographic screening for breast cancer. Radiol Clin North Am 1992;30:187–210.

14. Sickles EA, Filly RA, Callen PW. Breast cancer detection with sonography and mammography: comparison using state-of-the-art equipment. AJR 1983;140:843–845.

15. Kopans DB, Meyer JE, Lindfors KK. Whole-breast US imaging: four-year follow-up. Radiology 1985;157:505–507.

16. de Paredes ES, Marsteller LP, Eden BV. Breast cancers in women 35 years of age and younger: mammographic findings. Radiology 1990;177:117–119.

17. Sickles EA. Mammographic features of 300 consecutive nonpalpable breast cancers. AJR 1986;146:661–663.

18. Kopans DB, Swann CA, White G, et al. Asymmetric breast tissue. Radiology 1989;171:639–643.

19. Marsteller LP, de Paredes ES. Well defined masses in the breast. Radiographics 1989;9:13–37.

20. Sickles EA. Breast masses: mammographic evaluation. Radiology 1989;173:297–303.

21. Bassett LW. Mammographic analysis of calcifications. Radiol Clin North Am 1992;30:93–105.

22. Harris JR, Lippman ME, Veronesi U, Willet W. Breast cancer (second of three parts). N Engl J Med 1992;327:390–398.

23. Eklund GW, Busby RC, Miller SH, Job JS. Improved imaging of the augmented breast. AJR 1988;151:469–473.

24. Gorczyca DP, Sinha S, Ahn CY, et al. Silicone breast implants in vivo: MR imaging. Radiology, 1992; 185:407–410.

25. Sickles EA. Periodic mammographic follow-up of probably benign lesions: results in 3,184 consecutive cases. Radiology 1991;179:463–468.

26. Kopans DB, Lindfors K, McCarthy KA, Meyer JE. Spring hookwire breast lesion localizer: Use with rigid-compression mammographic systems. Radiology 1985;157:537–538.

27. Jackson V. The status of mammographically guided fine needle aspiration biopsy of nonpalpable breast lesions. Radiol Clin North Am 1992;30:155–166.

28. Fajardo LI, Jackson VP, Hunter TB. Interventional procedures in diseases of the breast: needle biopsy, pneumocystography and galactography. AJR 1992;158:1231–1238.

Section V **CARDIOVASCULAR RADIOLOGY**

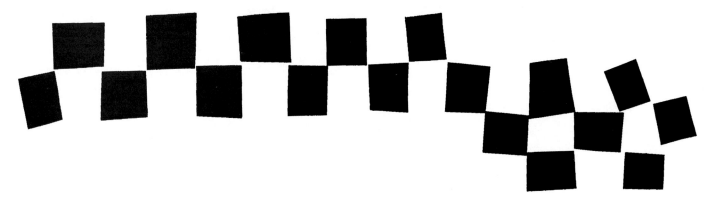

18

Cardiac Anatomy, Physiology, and Imaging Modalities

David K. Shelton, Jr.

IMAGING METHODS

Thorough knowledge of cardiac anatomy and physiology is important as a basis for cardiac imaging. Comprehensive knowledge of cardiac imaging also requires consideration of virtually all of the available imaging modalities. Chest radiography provides the initial evaluation of most cardiac patients. A barium esophagogram can be added for the additional information provided by the close esophageal relationship to cardiac structures. Fluoroscopy increases the detectability of coronary and valvular calcification as well as providing dynamic and positional information. Echocardiography, including pulse and color flow Doppler, and transesophageal technique provides additional detailed imaging of internal cardiac anatomy. Nuclear cardiology, positron emission tomography and pharmacologic testing provide key functional,

perfusion and physiologic information. Cardiac and coronary angiography, although invasive, provide detailed anatomic information that can lead directly to interventional or surgical therapy. Computed tomography (CT) and ultrafast CT with the use of intravenous iodinated contrast material are capable of providing critical information, particularly for pericardial or intracardiac disease. Magnetic resonance imaging (MR) adds three-dimensional tomographic and motion studies of the myocardium, valves, and chambers without utilizing ionizing radiation or intravascular contrast. In summary, cardiac imaging requires familiarity with all imaging techniques and their associated physics, three-dimensional cardiac anatomy, cardiac physiology, and cardiac disease processes.

ANATOMY

The four-chambered human heart lies primarily in the anterior left hemithorax with the left ventricle lying on the left hemidiaphragm (Figs. 18.1 and 18.2). The right atrium extends to the right of midline as it receives systemic blood from the superior vena cava (SVC), inferior vena cava (IVC), and coronary sinus. The right atrium and right ventricle lie primarily anterior to the planes of the left atrium and left ventricle. The right ventricle is the most anterior chamber and abuts the sternum (Fig. 18.3). The left atrium is subcarinal and midline in the thorax, being supplied by the right and left superior and inferior pulmonary veins.

Frontal Projection. The right border of the cardiac silhouette is formed primarily by the right atrium with the SVC entering superiorly and the IVC often seen at its lower margin (Figs. 18.1 and 18.3). The left border of the heart is created primarily by the left ventricle and left atrial appendage. The pulmonary artery, aortopulmonary window, and aortic knob extend superiorly.

Lateral Projection. The right ventricle is border-forming anteriorly adjacent to the sternum with its outflow tract extending superiorly and posteriorly (Fig. 18.2). The left atrium is border-forming in the

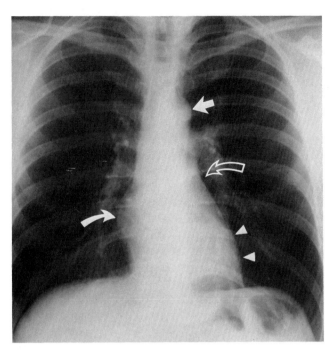

Figure 18.1. Normal PA Chest Radiograph. Frontal view of the chest demonstrates normal heart size, contours and chamber size. The hila and pulmonary vascularity are normal. The left ventricle (*arrowheads*) is border-forming on the left. The right atrium (*curved arrow*) is border-forming on the right. The aortic knob (*arrow*) is of normal contour and the pulmonary artery (*open arrow*) is concave.

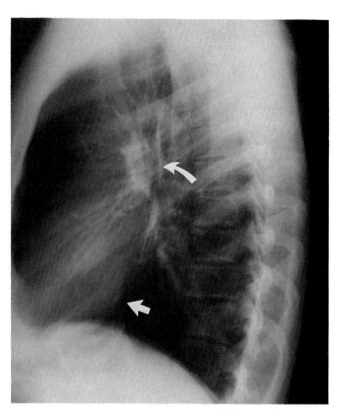

Figure 18.2. Normal Lateral Chest Radiograph. This well-positioned left lateral chest radiograph demonstrates the right ribs projected posterior to the left ribs because of divergence of the xray beam. The right and left bronchi are overlapped and the sternum is seen in the lateral view. The true lateral projection allows evaluation of the IVC intersection (*arrow*) with the left ventricle. There is no evidence of posterior displacement of the left bronchus (*curved arrow*) to indicate left atrial enlargement. There is no evidence of right ventricular encroachment into the retrosternal clear space.

high posterior, subcarinal region. The left ventricle is border-forming inferiorly and posteriorly.

Right Atrium. The right atrium is divided into two portions. The smooth posterior wall develops from the sinus venosus with the attached SVC and IVC in continuity posteriorly (Fig. 18.4). The trabeculated anterior wall is derived from the embryonic right atrium. The *right atrial appendage* extends superiorly and medially from the SVC opening. The *crista terminalis* is a muscular ridge that runs from the mouth of the SVC and fades inferiorly to the mouth of the IVC. It divides the two portions of the atrium and corresponds to an external *sulcus terminalis*. The medial wall of the right atrium is the interatrial septum, which contains a smooth, central dimpled area called the *fossa ovalis*. Inflow from the SVC, IVC and coronary sinus enters the smooth posterior portion of the right atrium. The SVC has a free opening, whereas the IVC is partially guarded by a thin *eustachian valve*, which is occasionally absent or perforated (network of Chiari). The large draining coronary vein or *coronary sinus* enters the right atrium anterior and medial to the IVC. Its opening is guarded by the *thebesian valve* between the orifice of the IVC and the tricuspid valve.

Right Ventricle. The right ventricle (Figs. 18.4 and 18.5) lies anterior to the left ventricular outflow tract and wraps around it and to the left. The right ventricular outflow is directed superiorly, posteriorly,

and to the left. The right ventricle is divided into a posterior/inferior portion (inflow or *sinus portion*), which is heavily trabeculated and a less trabeculated anterior/superior portion (outflow tract or *pulmonary conus*). The two portions of the right ventricle are divided by the *crista supraventricularis*, which is a muscular ridge with a septal band called the *moderator band*. This band is present in more than 40% of patients, connects the interventricular septum to the anterior papillary muscle, and contains the right bundle of His. The *infundibulum (conus arteriosus)* is the smooth cephalic portion of the right ventricle that leads to the pulmonary trunk.

Pulmonary Arteries. The muscular pulmonary conus extends to the semilunar, tricuspid pulmonary valve with the pulmonary trunk extending superiorly and to the left. The left pulmonary artery extends posteriorly as a continuation of the main pulmonary artery coursing over the top of the left main stem bronchus, then descending posteriorly. The right pulmonary artery extends horizontally to the right, bifurcates within the pericardial sac, and exits the right hilum as the truncus anterior and interlobar arteries. The right upper lobe bronchus is *eparterial*, meaning it lies above the right pulmonary artery. The left main stem bronchus is *hyparterial*, meaning it lies below the pulmonary artery.

The *ligamentum arteriosum* arises from the superior, proximal left pulmonary artery and crosses through the aorticopulmonary window to the floor of the aorta. The ligamentum arteriosum is the remnant of the ductus arteriosus, which closes functionally in the first 24 hours and closes anatomically by 10 days. Desaturated blood from the right heart circulates through the lungs and returns as oxygenated blood through the right and left superior and inferior pulmonary veins into the left atrium.

Left Atrium. The left atrium is the highest and most posterior chamber (Fig. 18.6). Its smooth walls are nestled between the right and left bronchi, and its posterior wall abuts the anterior wall of the esophagus. The *left atrial appendage* is a small pouch that projects superiorly and to the left and is smoother and

longer than the right atrial appendage. The left atrial appendage extends anterior to the left superior pulmonary veins and is commonly seen on MR and CT scans. The foramen ovale within the interatrial septum remains nominally patent in up to 25% of adults. Its inferior margin is a remnant of the septum primum and may be somewhat scalloped. The mitral valve is located anterior and inferior to the body of the left atrium with the mitral valve leaflets extending into the left ventricle.

Left Ventricle. The mitral valve is the conduit for blood flow from the left atrium to the left ventricle and is in the high posterior "valve plane" of the left ventricle (Figs. 18.5 and 18.6). The anterior or septal leaflet of the mitral valve lies near the interventricular septum and extends to the posterior (noncoronary) cusp of the aortic valve. The smaller posterior mitral leaflet lies posteriorly and to the left. The *chordae tendineae* are strong fibrous cords that extend from the mitral leaflets to the papillary muscles of the left ventricle. The inflow portion of the left ventricle is

Figure 18.3. Cardiothoracic Anatomy: Frontal View of the Heart after Cutaway of the Chest Wall, Pleural Surfaces, and Pericardial Surface. Note the relationship of the right atrium, right ventricle, left atrial appendage and left ventricle to the great vessels. (Reproduced with permission. Drawing by Frank H. Netter, M.D., from *Atlas of human anatomy*, the CIBA Collection of Medical Illustrations, Clinical Symposia. West Caldwell, NJ: CIBA-Geigy Corp, 1989.)

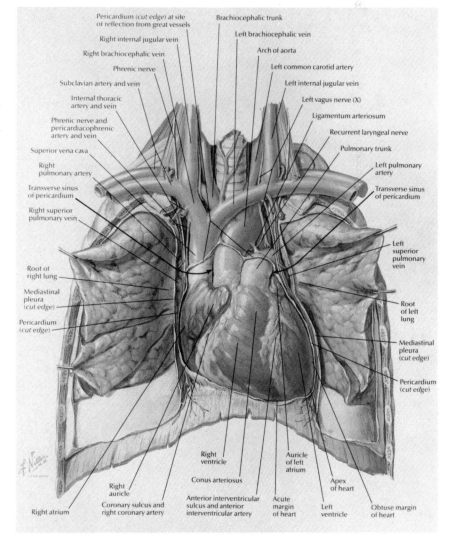

Figure 18.4. Cutaway Views of the Right Atrium and Right Ventricle. (Reproduced with permission. Drawing by Frank H. Netter, M.D., from *Atlas of human anatomy*, the CIBA Collection of Medical Illustrations, Clinical Symposia, 1989.

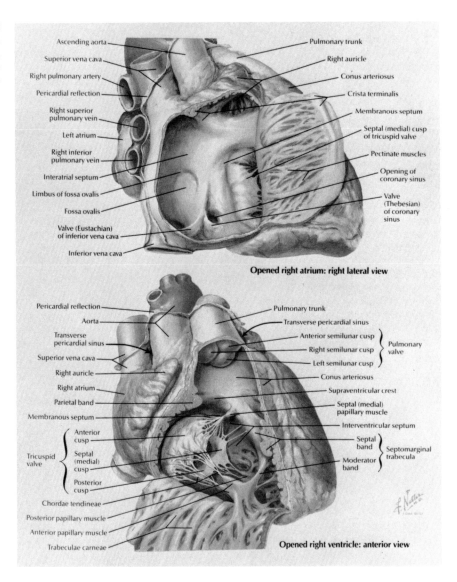

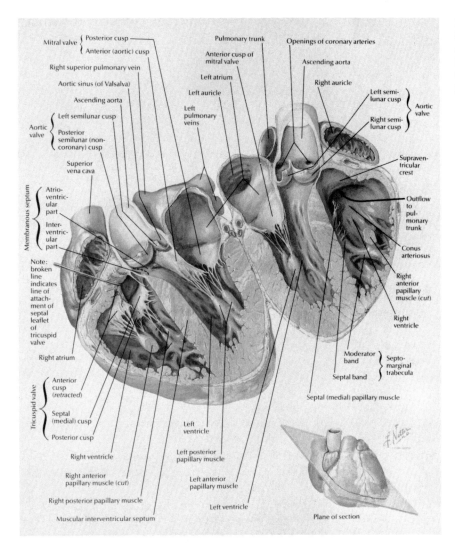

Figure 18.5. Bisection through the Heart Simulating a Four-Chamber View. (Reproduced with permission. Drawing by Frank H. Netter, M.D., from *Atlas of human anatomy*, the CIBA Collection of Medical Illustrations, Clinical Symposia, 1989.)

Figure 18.6. Cutaway Views of the Left Ventricle and Left Atrium. (Reproduced with permission. Drawing by Frank H. Netter, M.D., from *Atlas of human anatomy*, the CIBA Collection of Medical Illustrations, Clinical Symposia, 1989.)

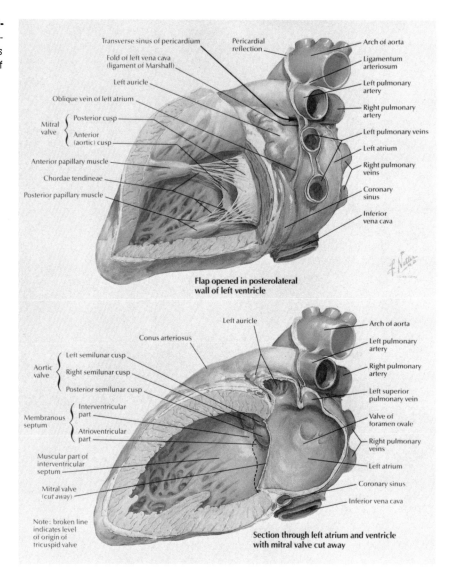

posterior to the anterior leaflet of the mitral valve. The outflow portion of the left ventricle is anterior and superior to the anterior mitral leaflet. The interventricular septum has a high membranous portion that is contiguous with the aortic root. The more muscular inferior portion of the septum extends to the left ventricular apex. The esophagus passes immediately posterior and is in contact with the muscular wall of the left ventricle.

Aorta. The outflow tract of the left ventricle leads into the aortic root which contains the aortic valve composed of right, left, and posterior (noncoronary) cusps. The *sinuses of Valsalva* are the reservoirs created by the closure of the aortic valve and from which the right and left coronary arteries arise. The posterior wall of the aorta is continuous with the anterior leaflet of the mitral valve and more superiorly abuts the anterior wall of the left atrium. The anterior wall of the aorta is continuous with the interventricular septum. After coursing superiorly and then to the left,

the aorta gives off the right innominate artery, left common carotid artery, and left subclavian artery. The aortic arch is the transverse portion of the aorta that abuts the left wall of the trachea causing a characteristic indentation.

Conduction System. The *sinoatrial node* is specialized neuromuscular tissue that measures approximately 5 × 20 mm and is located on the anterior endocardial surface of the right atrium just above the SVC and right atrial appendage junction, near the crista terminalis. Electrical propagation spreads to both atria via Purkinje-like fibers and is recorded as the P wave on an electrocardiogram. The *atrioventricular node* is a 2 × 5 mm neuromuscular tissue on the endocardial surface, along the right side of the interatrial septum, just inferior to the ostium of the coronary sinus. The impulse is collected and delayed approximately 0.7 seconds in the atrioventricular node before passing into the *bundle of His.* The bundle of His is a 20-mm long tract extending down the right

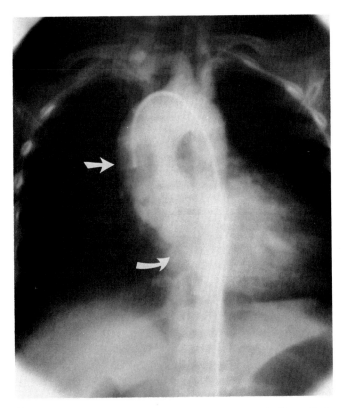

Figure 18.7. Aortogram via Transfemoral Approach. The catheter is placed in the mildly dilated ascending aorta (*straight arrow*). Notice the reflux of contrast from the aortic valve into the left ventricle (*curved arrow*) in this patient with aortic insufficiency.

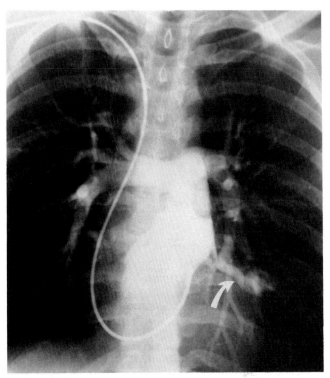

Figure 18.8. Right Heart Catheterization via the Right Subclavian Vein. The catheter is positioned in the pulmonary conus. Contrast fills the main, right, and left pulmonary arteries. Note the arteriovenous malformation with a large feeding artery (*arrow*).

Table 18.1. Normal Values for Cardiac Catheterization

Site	Pressures (mm Hg)	Saturation (%)
Vena cava	5	60–65
Right atrium	2–5	65–75
Right ventricle	25/0	70
Pulmonary artery	25/10	73
Left atrium	2–8	94–98
Left ventricle	120/0–5	94–98
Aorta	120/80	94–98

side of the membranous interventricular septum. The bundle of His bifurcates into a right and left bundle before arborizing through the two ventricles via the Purkinje system. The interventricular septum activates from superior to inferior with the anterior/septal right ventricle being the first to activate and the posterior/basal left ventricle being the last to activate. This information is particularly useful when evaluating phase analysis or phase propagation in gated cardiac scintigraphy.

CARDIAC CATHETERIZATION

Left-sided catheterization is normally accomplished via arterial puncture in the femoral or brachial artery (Fig. 18.7). It is typically utilized for aortography, coronary angiography, ventriculography, and evaluation for patent ductus arteriosus. Right-sided catheterization is typically accomplished by venous puncture in the femoral or brachycephalic vein (Fig. 18.8). It is utilized for pulmonary angiography, catheterization of the right atrium and ventricle, or for evaluation of shunt lesions such as an atrioseptal defect.

Important considerations include determination of the catheter course to help diagnose atrioseptal defects, ventriculoseptal defects, patent ductus arteriosus or persistent left SVC. During catheterization,

saturation percentages are commonly determined, along with pressure measurements and pressure gradients (Table 18.1). Contrast is injected to demonstrate additional details of anatomy, as well as to evaluate for valvular lesions, chamber size, ventricular function, and wall motion.

Right Atrial pressures are normally 2–5 mm Hg and oxygen saturation is 65–75%. Elevated right atrial pressures are seen with right heart failure, decreased compliance, and tricuspid valve disease. An 8% or larger increase in saturation from the IVC to the right atrium is considered evidence of a left-to-right shunt (ASD).

Right Ventricular pressures are typically 25 systolic/0–5 diastolic mm Hg. Elevated systolic pressures are seen with pulmonary hypertension, pulmonary stenosis and congenital heart lesions such as transpo-

Table 18.2. Average Physiologic Data for Cardiac Chambers

Parameter	Left Chambers	Right Chambers
Atrial end diastolic volume	50 ml	57 ml
Ventricular end diastolic volume	125–150 ml	165 ml
Ejection fraction	50–75%	45–55%
Stroke volume	70 ml	70 ml
Cardiac output	4–5 liters/min	4–5 liter/min
Cardiac index	2.8–4 liters/min/m²	2.8–4 liters/min/m²

sition and truncus arteriosus. Diastolic pressures increase with right heart failure. Saturations should be nearly the same as right atrial saturations. A 5% increase in saturation from right atrium to right ventricle suggests a ventriculoseptal defect.

Pulmonary Arterial pressures are normally 25 systolic/10 diastolic mm Hg with a mean pulmonary artery pressure of 15 mm Hg. A significant pressure gradient (>10 mm Hg) across the valve implies pulmonary stenosis. Increased pressures are seen with shunt lesions, pulmonary vascular disease and pulmonary venous obstruction. Pulmonary saturation should be approximately the same as right ventricular saturation, with a 3% difference considered significant for a shunt lesion.

Pulmonary Wedge pressure is typically 2–8 mm Hg and approximates the left atrial pressure unless there is evidence of pulmonary venous obstruction. Elevations in the left atrial or wedge pressure are usually seen with mitral stenosis and left-sided congestive heart failure. Normal left atrial saturation is approximately 94%, and a decrease greater than 5% implies a right-to-left shunt.

Left Ventricular pressures are 120 systolic/0–5 diastolic mm Hg. Decreased systolic pressures are seen with shock and congestive heart failure. Elevated systolic pressures imply systemic hypertension or outlet obstruction. Increased diastolic pressure is seen with congestive heart failure. Decreased saturation at the left ventricular level would imply a right-to-left shunt. Aortic pressure is normally 120/80 with a mean pressure of 70–100 mm Hg.

With each systolic contraction the average stroke volume of each ventricle is approximately 70 ml of blood (Table 18.2). End diastolic volume is normally 125–150 ml for the left ventricle and 165 ml for the right ventricle. A normal cardiac output is 4–5 liters/min with a normal cardiac index of 2.8–4.0 liters/min/m² of body surface area. The normal ejection fraction is 50–75% for the left ventricle and 45–55% for the right ventricle. Typical end diastolic volumes are 57 ml for the right atrium and 50 ml for the left atrium. Coronary blood flow averages 224 ml/min and increases up to six-fold during exercise.

Aortic Valve. The normal aortic valve orifice is 3 cm². Symptoms result from aortic stenosis when the orifice is less than 0.7 cm², or less than 1.5 cm² if there is aortic stenosis and insufficiency. Mild stenosis is indicated by a pressure gradient across the aortic valve greater than 25 mm Hg, moderate stenosis by a gradient greater than 40–50 mm Hg, and severe stenosis by a gradient exceeding 80 mm Hg.

Mitral Valve. The mitral valve orifice usually measures 4–6 cm². Mild mitral stenosis occurs with an orifice less than 1.5 cm², moderate mitral stenosis at less than 1.0 cm², and marked mitral stenosis at less than 0.5 cm².

Pulmonary Stenosis is significant if the right ventricular systolic pressures exceed 70 mm Hg.

Pulmonary Artery Hypertension is defined as a mean pulmonary artery pressure of more than 25 mm Hg.

CHEST RADIOGRAPHY

The chest radiograph remains the mainstay for imaging of the heart and lungs. There are many approaches to reading the radiograph. Although most radiologists initiate the process with "global perception," it is important to develop a checklist scan technique. This discussion concerns adult posteroanterior (PA) and lateral radiographs.

Cardiac Silhouette

Size. The cardiothoracic ratio should not exceed 0.5 on a 72-inch erect PA radiograph, or 0.6 on a portable or anteroposterior (AP) examination. Realize that other factors should be considered, such as fat pads and pectus deformity.

Shape. Various contour effects can be clues to underlying disease. "Water bottle" configuration occurs with pericardial effusion or generalized cardiomyopathy. Left ventricular or "Shmoo" configuration (after Al Capp's Shmoo) describes lengthening and rounding of the left heart border with a downward extension of the apex due to left ventricular enlargement. "Hypertrophy" configuration describes increased convexity of the left heart border and apex. Right ventricular hypertrophy and enlargement tends to lift the apex and create a more horizontal vector to the cardiac axis. Hypertrophy of either ventricle usually causes little enlargement of the silhouette unless dilation is also present. Hypertrophy typically results from increased afterload, whereas dilation occurs with failure or diastolic overload. "Straightening" of the left heart border is seen with rheumatic heart disease and mitral stenosis.

"Moguls of the Heart." Skiing the moguls of the heart refers to the left mediastinal outline beginning at the aortic knob. A prominent knob is a clue to ectasia, aneurysm, or hypertension. Notching or "figure three" sign of the aorta suggests coarctation (Fig.

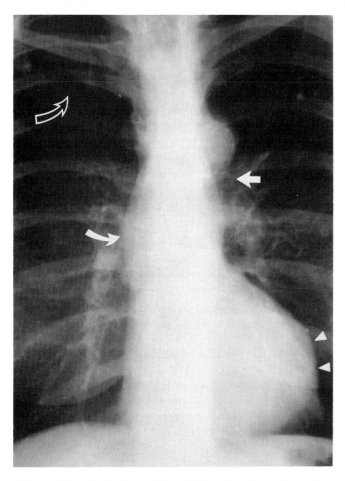

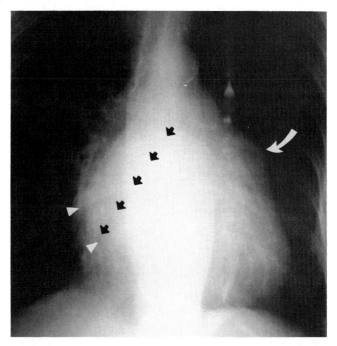

Figure 18.10. Rheumatic Heart Disease. The left atrial append-age is strikingly prominent (*curved arrow*). Splaying of the carina and a double density along the right heart border indicates left atrial enlargement (*arrowheads*). When the distance from the lateral margin of the left atrium to the midpoint on the under surface of the left bronchus exceeds 7 cm, left atrial enlargement is likely (*black arrows*).

Figure 18.9. Aortic Coarctation. Notice the "figure 3 sign" or notching of the aorta near the aortic knob (*straight arrow*). The ascending aorta (*curved arrow*) is prominent and the left ventricle is excessively rounded (*arrowheads*). Rib notching is noted along the right fifth rib margin inferiorly (*curved open arrow*).

18.9). The second mogul is the main pulmonary artery segment. Excessive convexity is seen with post-stenotic dilation, chronic obstructive pulmonary disease, pulmonary artery hypertension, left-to-right shunts, and pericardial defects. Severe concavity suggests right-to-left shunts. The third mogul is a prominent left atrial appendage that in 90% of cases, indicates prior rheumatic carditis (Fig. 18.10). It rarely is seen with other causes of left atrial enlargement. The fourth mogul is a bulge just above the cardiophrenic angle, seen with infarction or ventricular aneurysm. A fifth bulge at the cardiophrenic angle is caused by pericardial cysts, prominent fat pads, or adenopathy.

Chamber Enlargement

Left Atrial Enlargement is best confirmed by measuring the distance from the midinferior border of the left main stem bronchus to the right lateral border of the left atrial density (Fig. 18.10). This distance is less than 7 cm in 90% of normal patients and is greater than 7 cm in 90% of left atrial enlargement pa-

tients, as proven by echocardiography. This measurement can be approximated by placing one's right fifth finger under the left bronchus, and while keeping the fingers closed, if the left atrium is seen beyond one's four fingertips, the left atrium is enlarged. Less sensitive signs of left atrial enlargement include splaying of the carinal angle, uplifting of the left main stem bronchus, and prominence of the left atrial appendage. On occasion, the enlarged left atrium will displace the descending aorta to the left. Massive left atrial enlargement can result in the left atrium becoming border-forming on the right side, so called "atrial escape." On lateral views an enlarged left atrium will displace the left bronchus posteriorly with the bronchi creating right and left legs for the "walking man sign." An enlarged left atrium also impresses against the esophagus.

Right Atrial Enlargement is more difficult to define on chest radiographs than left atrial enlargement, but is fortunately less common. Clues include a prominent atrial bulge too far to the right of the spine (more than 5.5 cm from the midline on a well-positioned PA radiograph). Another sign is elongation of the right atrial convexity to exceed 50% of the mediastinal/cardiovascular shadow. Right atrial enlargement usually accompanies right ventricular enlargement.

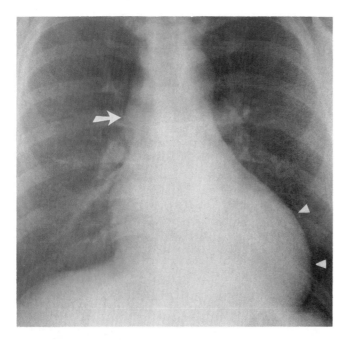

Figure 18.11.   Left Ventricular Enlargement. Prominence of the left ventricle with rounding along the inferior heart border and an apex that is pointing downwards (*arrowheads*) is indicative of "left ventricular configuration." The ascending aorta (*arrow*) is dilated because of aortic stenosis and insufficiency.

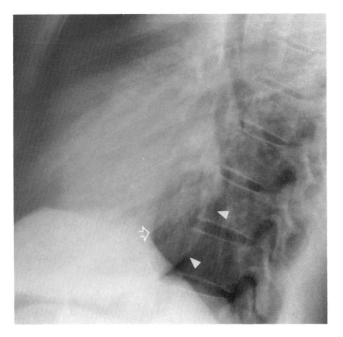

Figure 18.12.   Left Ventricular Enlargement. The posterior margin of the left ventricle (*arrowheads*) projects prominently behind the IVC (*open arrow*) and overlaps the thoracic spine. The Hoffman-Rigler sign is positive.

Left Ventricular Enlargement. On the PA view, an enlarged left ventricle creates an elongated left heart border with the apex pointing downward. Prominent rounding of the inferior left heart border is also seen (Fig. 18.11). The lateral view shows an en-

larged left ventricle extending behind the esophagus. The Hoffman-Rigler sign for left ventricular enlargement exists when the left ventricle extends more than 1.8 cm posterior to the posterior border of the IVC at a level 2 cm cephalad to the intersection of the left ventricle and IVC (Fig. 18.12). This sign requires a true lateral radiograph and can be false-positive if the lateral view is obliqued or there is volume loss in either lower lobe. This sign can be quickly applied by using one of the "2-cm fingertips" for a quick check without a ruler.

Right Ventricular Enlargement is not as easily detected as left-sided enlargement. If the heart is enlarged and Rigler's sign does not show left ventricular enlargement, then consider right-sided enlargement. If the right ventricle fills too much of the retrosternal clear space or "climbs" more than one-third of the sternal length, then right ventricular enlargement is likely. Indirect signs such as enlargement of the pulmonary outflow tract or hilar arteries add confidence.

Abnormal Mediastinal Contours

Aorta. Dilation of the ascending aorta due to poststenotic dilation is seen in approximately 80% of patients with aortic stenosis (Fig. 18.11). It can also be seen in patients older than 50 when there is tortuosity of the entire aorta or systemic hypertension. Ascending aortic aneurysm (calcific with syphilis, not calcified with Marfan's syndrome) is another possibility (Fig. 18.13). A ductus bump adjacent to the aortic knob is an indication of patent ductus arteriosus.

Azygos Vein dilation (greater than 6 mm on upright PA or 1 cm on supine radiograph) is seen with intravascular volume expansion, elevated central venous pressure, and right heart failure (Fig. 19.16). Additional causes include the Valsalva maneuver, pregnancy, renal failure, vena cava obstruction or azygos continuation of the IVC. Dilation of the SVC often accompanies volume expansion or elevated central venous pressure but is more difficult to detect with certainty.

Cardiac Calcifications

Coronary Calcification. Radiographs can commonly demonstrate coronary artery calcification in a 3 cm triangle along the upper left heart border, called the "CAC" (coronary artery calcification) triangle (Figs. 18.14 and 19.1). If chest pain and coronary calcification are present, there is a 94% chance the patient will have occlusive coronary artery disease at angiography. Fluoroscopic detection of coronary calcification actually has higher sensitivity and specificity in screening asymptomatic individuals than exercise tolerance testing. In symptomatic patients the detection of coronary calcification approaches exercise tol-

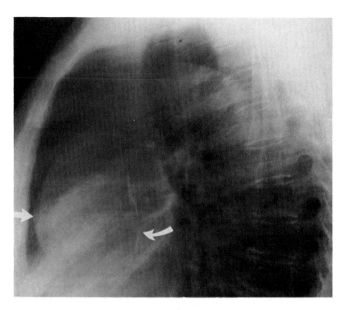

Figure 18.13. Calcified Aortic Aneurysm. The ascending aorta is enlarged in this patient with a syphilitic calcified aortic aneurysm. The anterior margin is identified by soft-tissue prominence (*straight arrow*) overlapping the retrosternal clear space. The posterior margin is identified by calcification in the wall (*curved arrow*).

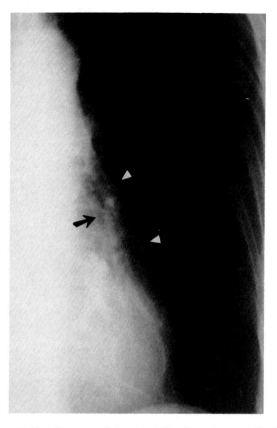

Figure 18.14. Coronary Artery Calcification. The calcification (*arrow*) is most commonly detected in the coronary artery calcification triangle along the upper left heart margin (*arrowheads*). The presence of coronary artery calcification may be indicative of coronary stenosis and ischemic heart disease.

erance testing in sensitivity and exceeds exercise tolerance testing in specificity. More than 82% of the patients with fluoroscopically demonstrated coronary artery calcification and positive exercise tolerance testing have significant coronary artery disease at angiography. Calcifications have more significance when seen in patients under 60 years of age. Heavier and more extensive calcification correlates with more severe coronary disease. Detection of coronary calcification helps to differentiate patients with ischemic from those with nonischemic cardiomyopathy.

Valvular Calcification is seen in 85% of patients with acquired valvular disease but is rarely detected in patients under 20 years of age. Aortic valve calcification is highly specific for valve disease. Calcific aortic stenosis is most often degenerative in origin and is usually seen in elderly males. Extensive aortic annulus calcification is atherosclerotic in nature and has been associated with conduction blocks.

Mitral valve calcification is highly suggestive of rheumatic valvular disease and is seen on chest x-ray in approximately 40% of patients with mitral stenosis. It is even more common in patients with stenosis and regurgitation. Atherosclerotic calcification of the mitral annulus occurs in approximately 10% of the elderly population (Fig. 18.15). It appears as circular, ovoid, or C- or J-shaped calcification in the mitral annulus and can lead to mitral valve incompetence.

Sinus of Valsalva Aneurysm calcification is seen as a curvilinear density anterior and lateral to the ascending aorta.

Calcified Ligamentum Arteriosum is seen as a linear calcification in the aortopulmonary window connecting the top of the left pulmonary artery to the floor of the aortic arch.

Calcified Left Atrium. Thin curvilinear calcification in the wall of the left atrium is usually associated with mitral stenosis, left atrial enlargement, atrial fibrillation, and left atrial thrombus.

Calcified Pericardium is typically anterior and inferior in location. It can be single- or double-layered and is associated with a high incidence of constrictive pericardial hemodynamics. Causes include viral, hemorrhagic, and tuberculous pericarditis.

Calcified Infarct. Dystrophic calcification may occur in the myocardial wall from prior myocardial infarction.

Calcified Ventricular Aneurysm. Thin curvilinear calcification anterolaterally near the apex is most often seen with true aneurysms. Posterior curvilinear calcification is usually seen in pseudoaneurysms (Fig. 18.16).

Calcified Thrombus is seen as clumpy calcification in the left atrium or, less commonly, in the left ventricle.

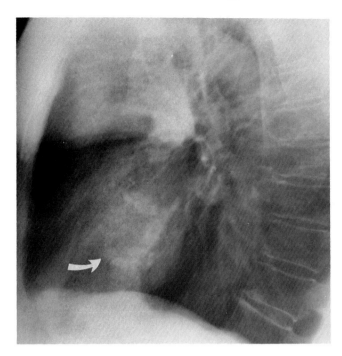

Figure 18.15. Mitral Annulus Calcification. Ovoid calcification of the mitral annulus (*arrow*) is secondary to atherosclerosis and is commonly associated with mitral insufficiency. Mitral calcification is best seen on a lateral radiograph.

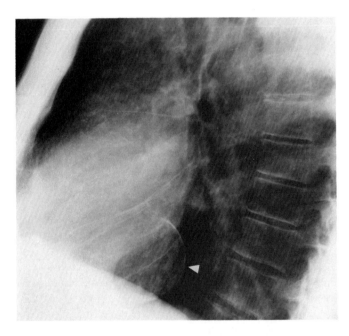

Figure 18.16. Calcified Ventricular Pseudoaneurysm. Thin, curvilinear calcification along the left ventricle (*arrowhead*) is indicative of a pseudoaneurysm.

Calcified Pulmonary Arteries. Thin eggshell-like calcification in the walls of the pulmonary arteries is virtually diagnostic of long-standing pulmonary arterial hypertension (Figs. 19.14 and 19.15).

Tumors. Rounded or stippled calcifications are seen occasionally in atrial myxomas and rarely in other cardiac neoplasms (Fig. 19.27).

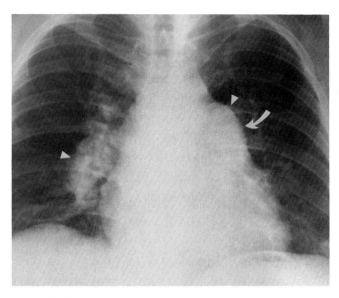

Figure 18.17. Idiopathic Pulmonary Hypertension. The main (*curved arrow*), right, and left (*arrowheads*) pulmonary arteries are dilated. The pulmonary arteries taper rapidly and peripheral pulmonary vascularity is decreased.

Pulmonary Vascularity

The lungs have dual blood supply with pulmonary arteries and systemic bronchial arteries.

Pulmonary Arteries. Increased circulation from left-to-right shunts results in enlargement of the main and hilar pulmonary arteries with increased blood flow to the upper and lower lobes. Asymmetrical blood flow can be seen with pulmonary hypoplasia, Swyer-James syndrome, and congenital lesions such as pulmonary stenosis (increased to the left lung) or tetralogy of Fallot (increased to the right lung).

Bronchial Arteries arise from the aorta and penetrate into the lungs, traveling with the bronchi. Tetralogy of Fallot and pseudotruncus arteriosus result in a shift to bronchial circulation. Bronchial arteries are also important in Rasmussen's aneurysms from tuberculosis and systemic hypervascularity of any chronic infection.

Pulmonary Arterial Hypertension (Fig. 18.17) results in (*a*) dilated main pulmonary artery, (*b*) right-sided cardiac enlargement, (*c*) central enlargement of left and right pulmonary arteries, (*d*) rapid pruning of the peripheral pulmonary arteries, (*e*) decreased peripheral pulmonary circulation, (*f*) calcification of the central pulmonary arteries, and, (*g*) secondary enlargement of the azygos vein.

Pulmonary Aneurysms and peripheral pulmonary coarctation can also cause unusual enlargements of the pulmonary arteries and may be seen in Williams' syndrome, Marfan's syndrome, and collagen disorders.

Pulmonary Venous Hypertension (Fig. 18.18) results from mitral stenosis, mitral regurgitation, or elevated left ventricular pressure (aortic stenosis or congestive heart failure). The normal vessel caliber in the lower lobes is greater than that in the upper lobes by a 3:2 ratio, due to hydrostatic pressure and the high compliance of the venous system. Elevated ve-nous pressure causes progressive, edematous perivas-cular cuffing, which occurs first in the lower vessels which have higher hydrostatic pressures. Perivascu-lar edema in the lower lobes results in decreased com-pliance and progressive cephalization of blood flow. The chest radiograph shows decreased caliber of lower lobe vessels and increased caliber of upper lobe ves-sels. Cephalization of blood flow is the earliest radio-graphic sign of congestive heart failure and pulmo-nary venous hypertension. Cephalization begins at 10–13 mm Hg wedge pressure. Equalization of upper to lower pulmonary blood flow occurs at 14–16 mm Hg. Reversal of the normal distribution with the up-per lobe vessels distended and the lower lobe vessels constricted occurs at 17–20 mm Hg. Hilar fullness, "Viking helmet sign" in the hila, and filling out of the right hilar angle commonly accompany reversed flow distribution.

Pulmonary Edema. Interstitial edema with Kerley A, B, and C lines and thickened pulmonary fis-sures occurs at 20–25 mm Hg wedge pressure (Fig. 18.19). Kerley lines represent thickened interlobular septa: A-lines are long straight lines radiating toward the hila, B-lines are horizontal lines connecting to the pleural surface near the costophrenic angle, and C-lines are random reticular lines seen throughout the lungs. Alveolar edema begins at 25–30 mm Hg wedge pressure (Fig. 18.20). Chronic failure "toughens" the interstitium (often resulting in hemosiderosis and pulmonary ossification) and can add an additional 5 mm Hg protective zone prior to developing interstitial or alveolar edema. These progressive signs of failure have been classified as stages 1–4 (Table 18.3).

Congestive Heart Failure. Radiographic find-ings include: (*a*) cardiomegaly, (*b*) left ventricular and left atrial enlargement, (*c*) cephalization of blood flow,

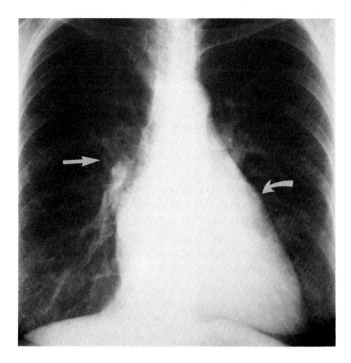

Figure 18.18. Pulmonary Venous Hypertension. Cephalization of blood flow is evident in this patient with mitral stenosis and enlarged left atrial appendage (*curved arrow*). The lower lobe vessels are constricted and the upper lobe vessels are distended. Fullness in the hilar angle (*straight arrow*) is due to enlargement of the superior pulmonary veins crossing between the interlobar artery and the up-per lobe artery.

Figure 18.19. Interstitial Edema. The edema is indicated by prominent Kerley lines. Thickening of the fissures (*arrow*) is also present, along with prominence of the left ventricle, left atrium, and cephalization of blood flow.

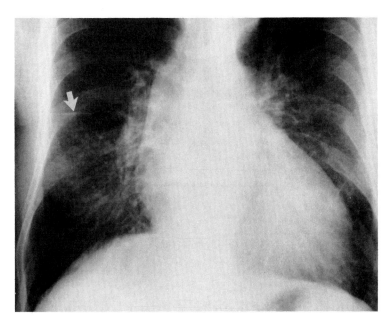

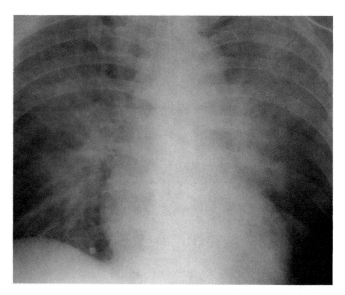

Figure 18.20. Alveolar Pulmonary Edema. Classical bat wing or butterfly perihilar alveolar infiltrates are present in a symmetrical cloud-like pattern.

Table 18.3. Signs of Progressive Cardiac Failure

Stage	Sign	Wedge Pressure (mm Hg)
1	Progressive cephalization	10–20
2	Interstitial edema and septal lines	20–25
3	Alveolar edema, often in bat wing perihilar distribution	>25–30
4	Chronic or severe pulmonary venous hypertension resulting in hemosiderosis, pulmonary ossification, and chronic interstitial disease such as from long-standing mitral stenosis	>30–35

(*d*) azygos vein and SVC distension, (*e*) perivascular cuffing with haziness and unsharpness of the pulmonary vessels, (*f*) peribronchial cuffing with thickening of the bronchial walls seen as small "Cheerios" when viewed end on, (*g*) Kerley lines, (*h*) thickening of the pulmonary fissures, (*i*) subpleural edema, (*j*) pleural effusions, usually larger in the right hemithorax, and (*k*) alveolar edema in a "bat wing" or "butterfly" distribution, also often more pronounced on the right.

Right Heart Failure. The most common cause of right heart failure is left heart failure. Elevated left-sided pressures manifest in the pulmonary circuit and then the right side of the heart. Long-standing venous hypertension leads to pulmonary arterial hypertension. Elevated right-sided pressures cause right ventricular hypertrophy and dilation, as well as systemic venous dilation involving azygos vein, SVC, and jugular veins. Dilation of the right heart can also cause tricuspid valve incompetence. Right heart failure protects the pulmonary circuit by accumulating edema and fluid outside the lungs, similar to the old therapeutic maneuver of rotating tourniquets.

Right heart failure may also occur with the dilated cardiomyopathies, including viral and alcoholic cardiomyopathy. When right heart failure is due to pulmonary disease such as chronic obstructive pulmonary disease, destructive lung disease, or primary pulmonary hypertension, the term *cor pulmonale* is utilized.

The Pericardium

The pericardium is composed of one continuous fibrous membrane that is folded back on itself, creating two layers. The inner layer of visceral pericardium or epicardium is closely attached to the myocardium and subepicardial fat. The outer layer or parietal pericardium is thicker and is often referred to simply as the pericardium.

Pericardial Effusion. Between the visceral and parietal layers is the pericardial space, which usually contains 20 ml of serous fluid. More than 50 ml of fluid is clearly abnormal, but 200 ml is required for detection by plain film radiography. Mediastinal and epicardial fat allow the pericardium to be visualized as a thin arcuate line paralleling the anterior heart border in the retrosternal region. A pericardial stripe exceeding 2–3 mm is indicative of pericardial thickening or effusion. Unfortunately, the thickened pericardial stripe can be seen on the lateral radiograph in only about 15% of patients with pericardial effusion. The *differential density sign* refers to a lucent margin along the left heart border on the PA radiograph, or along the posterior cardiac border on the lateral radiograph. It is seen in up to 63% of patients with pericardial effusion but is less specific than the thickened pericardial stripe. Large pericardial effusions cause the heart to appear on frontal radiographs in the shape of a sac of water sitting on a tabletop (Fig. 18.21).

Pneumopericardium appears on plain films as radiolucency surrounding the heart and separated from the lung by a thin white line of pericardium (Fig. 18.22). Air may also be seen outlining the pulmonary arteries or the undersurface of the heart. Pneumopericardium can be caused by trauma, infection, or pneumomediastinum. Firm attachment of the pericardium to the ascending aorta just above the main pulmonary artery serves to delimit the air.

Other Signs of Cardiac Disease

Situs Anomalies. Careful attention should be directed at the location of the aortic arch, gastric fundus, heart, pulmonary fissures and the branching pattern of the bronchi. Normal anatomic positioning is termed *situs solitus*. *Situs inversus* means that the patient's entire anatomic arrangement is reversed in a right-to-left direction as a "mirror image." Situs inver-

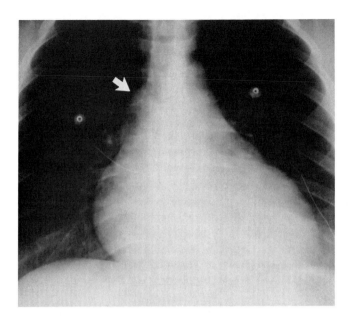

Figure 18.21. Pericardial Effusion. Water-bottle configuration of the cardiac silhouette is indicative of pericardial effusion or dilated cardiomyopathy. This patient with systemic lupus erythematosus has an enlarged azygos vein (*arrow*), decreased pulmonary vasculature, and clear lung parenchyma.

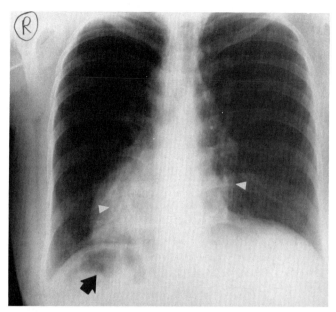

Figure 18.23. Kartagener's Syndrome. Situs inversus is evident with dextrocardia and the gastric air bubble (*black arrow*) on the patient's right. Evidence of bronchiectasis is present behind the heart and in the left lower lobe (*arrowheads*).

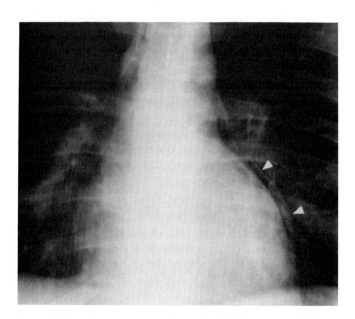

Figure 18.22. Pneumopericardium. Air within the pericardial sac allows visualization of the pericardium (*arrowheads*) seen as a thin white line parelleling the left heart border.

sus is associated with a 5–10% incidence of congenital heart disease, compared with less than 1% incidence for situs solitus. *Dextrocardia* indicates that the heart is in the right hemithorax. The apex of the heart lies to the right with the long axis of the heart directed from left to right. *Kartagener's syndrome* is a combination of situs inversus with dextrocardia, bronchiectasis and sinusitis (Fig. 18.23). The latter findings are because of the abnormal mucosal cilia.

Dextroposition means the heart is shifted toward the right hemithorax. It is associated with hypoplastic right lung and an increased incidence of congenital heart disease, particularly left-to-right shunts. *Dextroversion* means the cardiac apex is to the right, but the stomach and aortic knob remain on the left. The left ventricle remains on the left but lies anterior to the right ventricle.

Dextrocardia with situs ambiguous and polysplenia is also called "bilateral left-sidedness." Each lung contains only two lobes and hyparterial bronchi. Bilateral SVCs are also common. The incidence of congenital heart disease is increased, most commonly atrial septal defect or anomalous pulmonary venous return. Dextrocardia with asplenia is referred to as "bilateral right-sidedness" because of bilateral minor fissures and three lobes in each lung. The cardiac anomalies are usually more complex and severe than in polysplenia.

Bony Abnormalities

Postoperative changes of sternotomy suggest prior cardiac surgery and the presence of cardiac disease. Sternal fractures from motor vehicle accidents are associated with a 50% incidence of cardiac contusion. Hypersegmentation of the sternum (more than four to five segments) is present in 90% of Down's syndrome patients and offers a clue to the presence of endocardial cushion defect or complete atrioventricular canal. Wavy retrosternal linear opacities suggest dilated internal mammary arteries associated with coarctation of the aorta. Pectus excavatum is associated with an increased incidence of mitral valve prolapse and Marfan's syndrome. A barrel-shaped chest with pectus carinatum is associated with ventricular septal defects and complete atrioventricular canal. Scoliosis with a "shield chest" is seen with Marfan's syndrome, aortic valve disease, coarctation, and aortic dissection.

The presence of 11 or fewer ribs is highly associated with Down's syndrome and atrioventricular canal. "Ribbon ribs" or bifurcated ribs and an overcirculation pattern suggests truncus arteriosus whereas their association with an undercirculation pattern suggests tetralogy of Fallot. Rib notching and inferior rib sclerosis indicates collateral circulation through intercostal arteries and occurs with coarctation of the aorta and Blalock-Taussig operations. The third through the eighth ribs are most commonly involved. Fractures of the first and second ribs indicate high-velocity blunt trauma has occurred and there is an increased risk of aortic injury.

The spine offers clues to the presence of aortic valve disease when changes of ankylosing spondylitis, neurofibromatosis, or rheumatoid arthritis are present. Scoliosis is associated with an increased incidence of congenital heart disease.

NUCLEAR CARDIOLOGY

Cardiac nuclear medicine is a central modality in cardiac imaging and is covered in detail in Chapter 50. Perfusion scans with thallium or new technetium agents are useful for diagnosing coronary ischemia and myocardial infarcts. Normal perfusion scans appear in the shape of a horseshoe in the vertical and long axes, and of a doughnut in the short axis (Fig. 50.1). The scans are accomplished during rest, with controlled exercise or with pharmacologic stress with intravenous dipyridamole. The stress and redistribution or rest images appear identical in normal patients. Hypoperfused segments on stress images, which fill in on rest, are indicative of ischemia (Fig. 50.3). Hypoperfused segments on both rest and stress images are usually infarcts or scars. Myocardial infarction scanning can be accomplished utilizing rest perfusion agents for "cold spot" imaging or technetium pyrophosphate for "hot spot" imaging (Figs 19.7 and 19.8). The new antimyosin antibodies have also shown great promise for diagnosing and sizing myocardial infarction.

Electrocardiogram-gated myocardial blood pool studies examine wall motion and allow left ventricular ejection fraction calculations. Ventricular function, aneurysms, and valvular disease may be studied with volume curves and functional images (Figs. 50.4 and 50.5). Right ventricular ejection fraction calculations require first-pass examinations because of anatomic overlap of the right ventricle with the atria in the left

anterior oblique projection. First-pass cardiac studies can also diagnose SVC obstruction and left-to-right cardiac shunts. Right-to-left cardiac shunts can be evaluated and quantified with technetium macroaggregated albumin or microspheres.

Single Photon Emission Computed Tomography (SPECT) imaging greatly improves the diagnostic capabilities of perfusion imaging and infarct scans. Positron Emission Tomography (PET) is a new technology with increased resolution compared with single photon emission computed tomography imaging. Positron emission tomography can assess cardiac metabolism as well as perfusion, enhancing its ability to evaluate cardiomyopathies, ischemia, infarction, and "hibernating" or viable myocardium.

ECHOCARDIOGRAPHY

Echocardiography includes M-mode, real-time two-dimensional ultrasound, range-gated and color flow Doppler and transesophageal ultrasound. *Transesophageal echocardiography* utilizes a nasogastric probe with a steerable ultrasound beam that views the heart and aorta from the close posterior position provided by the esophagus (Fig. 18.24). *M-mode echocardiograms* are produced by a narrow ultrasonic beam that is directed at cardiac structures and observed over time or is swept across an area of anatomy (Figs. 18.25–18.27). The returning echoes produce a time-motion study of cardiac structures. With a transthoracic technique, anterior structures are usually displayed at the top of the image. The thickness and motion of the myocardium can be evaluated throughout the cardiac cycle. Pericardial effusions are shown as an echo-free space adjacent to the myocardium (Fig. 18.25). Large pleural effusions create an echolucent space posterior to the left ventricle and pericardium. The right atrium and atrial septum are not well seen by M-mode echocardiography.

The interventricular septum appears as a band of echoes near the midplane. It normally thickens and moves toward the posterior wall of the left ventricle during systole (Fig. 18.25). Paradoxic septal motion may be seen with pericardial effusion, tamponade, chronic obstructive pulmonary disease, asthma, atrial septal defects and septal ischemia. The interventricular septum measures less than 10–11 mm at end diastole and is compared with the thickness of the posterior wall of the left ventricle for asymmetric or concentric hypertrophy.

The aortic root lies immediately posterior to the right ventricle and measures 8–12 mm in neonates and 20–40 mm in adults (Fig. 18.26). The thin parallel aortic walls move anteriorly during systole. The aortic root is dilated with aortic stenosis, aortic insufficiency, tetralogy of Fallot, and aortic aneurysm. The thin aortic cusps seen within the aortic root should open widely during systole and should not reverberate.

The left atrium is seen posterior to the aortic root (Fig. 18.26). The normal size is no larger than 40 mm during diastole in adults. The left atrium is free of internal echoes and has a thin posterior wall that merges with the thicker left ventricular wall.

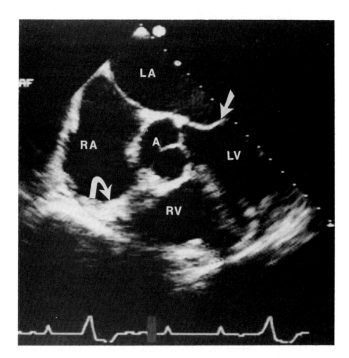

Figure 18.24. Transesophageal Echocardiogram. A five-chamber view of the heart is provided by an ultrasound probe within the esophagus. The probe is behind the left atrium and is depicted at the top of the image. All four chambers and the aortic valve are seen in one plane, the "five-chamber view." The left atrium (LA) and right atrium (RA) are separated by the interatrial septum. The aortic valve (A) is readily identified in the midplane. The right ventricle (RV) and left ventricle (LV) are separated by the interventricular septum. The tricuspid valve (curved arrow) is seen between the right atrium and right ventricle, and the mitral valve (straight arrow) is seen between the left atrium and left ventricle.

The left ventricle lies inferior and lateral to the left atrium and is an echo-free space except for the thin chordae tendineae and the echogenic projections of the papillary muscles. The left ventricular posterior wall thickens during systole and contracts anteriorly. The transverse diameter of the left ventricle does not normally exceed 5.7 cm during diastole. The wall measures approximately the same as the ventricular septum (10–11 mm).

The mitral valve produces a saw-toothed or M-shaped pattern posterior to the interventricular septum (Fig. 18.27). The anterior leaflet is the dominant echo and is continuous with the posterior wall of the aortic root. Immediately posterior to the anterior leaflet is the W-shaped pattern of the posterior leaflet. The two leaflets close during systole. The echo pattern of the anterior leaflet should be carefully scrutinized for evidence of thickening, delay in closure (seen with mitral stenosis), vegetations, prolapse, myxoma, or high-frequency vibration secondary to aortic regurgitation (Austin Flint phenomena). The specific points of the mitral waveform are (Fig. 18.27):

A point: **A**trial contraction with peak anterior opening motion.

B point: notch **B**etween the A and C points representing rapid rise in systolic pressure.

C point: **C**losure of the mitral valve occurs with contraction of the left ventricle during systole.

D point: early **D**iastole when mitral valve begins to open.

E point: maximal **E**xcursion of the valve opening. This is the peak of early diastolic opening and the most anterior position of the valve during diastole.

F point: most posterior point of early diastolic **F**illing prior to atrial contraction.

The E-F slope is a function of left atrial emptying rate and should be steep. With mitral stenosis, the

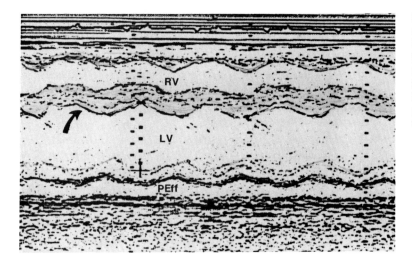

Figure 18.25. Pericardial Effusion. An M-mode echocardiogram with the ultrasonic probe at the top of the image demonstrates the right ventricle (RV), interventricular septum (curved arrow), and left ventricle (LV). Note the normal myocardial contractility with the interventricular septum contracting toward the posterior left ventricular wall during systole. A pericardial effusion (PEff) is seen as an echolucent space posterior to the left ventricular wall.

Figure 18.26. Aortic Root. An M-mode echocardiogram demonstrates anterior movement of the anterior (*curved arrow*) and posterior (*straight arrow*) walls of the aortic root during systole. The right ventricle (*RV*) is seen anterior to the aortic root and the left atrium (*LA*) is seen posterior to the aortic root. Aortic valve motion can be seen within the aortic root.

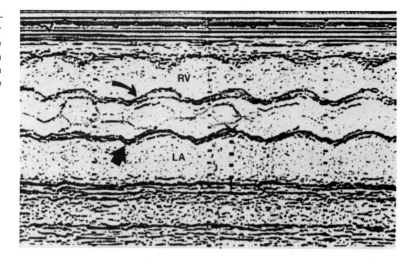

Figure 18.27. Normal Mitral Valve. An M-mode echocardiogram demonstrates the right ventricular cavity and left ventricular cavity separated by a band of echoes representing the interventricular septum (*arrow*). The moving mitral valve can be seen within the left ventricular cavity. Because of plane of section, the full systolic motion of the myocardium is not well visualized. The points of the mitral waveform are labelled with letters.

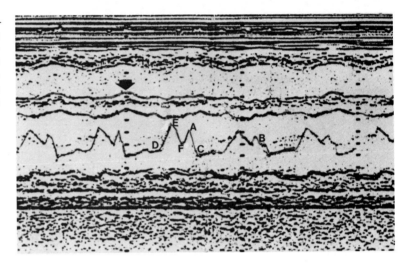

slope will be flattened and look more squared off than M-shaped. With valve thickening and calcification, the squared off part appears thickened.

The tricuspid valve is identified by locating the mitral valve and rotating the transducer medially. It has an M-shaped echo pattern similar to that of the mitral valve. The E-F slope is decreased with tricuspid stenosis and is increased with Ebstein's anomaly, tricuspid regurgitation, and atrial septal defect.

The pulmonic valve is rather difficult to evaluate by M-mode echocardiography. The diameter of the pulmonary trunk is similar to the aortic root. Pulmonary valve motion is similar to aortic valve motion, except that only the posterior leaflet is well seen and there may be a small "A wave" because of atrial contraction.

CORONARY ANGIOGRAPHY

Selective catheterization of the coronary arteries was first accomplished in 1959 by Sones using a flexible, tapered tip catheter utilizing a cut-down procedure on the brachial artery. In 1966 Amplatz utilized J-shaped, preformed catheters with better torque control from a transfemoral approach. In 1968 Judkins used separate preformed catheters for the right and left coronary arteries. After selective catheterization of the coronary artery, hand injections of contrast verify the size and flow of the artery. The left coronary artery generally requires 7–9 ml of contrast at 4–6 ml/sec whereas 6–8 ml at 3–5 ml/sec is sufficient for the smaller right coronary artery. Pressure limits for power injectors should be set at less than 150 psi. The catheter tip should not be left wedged in the coronary ostium, as this might occlude blood flow.

Complications of coronary angiography include hematoma, pseudoaneurysm, and fistula formation at the puncture site, arrhythmias including premature ventricular contractions, heart block and asystole, myocardial infarction, stroke, emboli, and death. Indications for coronary arteriography include (*a*) confirmation of an anatomic cause for angina, (*b*) identification of high-risk lesions, (*c*) evaluation of asymptomatic patients with abnormal exercise tolerance test or occupational risk, (*d*) preoperative evaluation for cardiac surgery, (*e*) evaluation of patients with coronary artery bypass grafts for stenosis or oc-

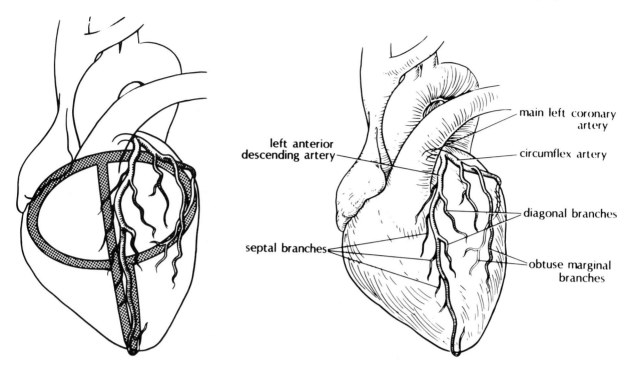

Figure 18.28. Left Coronary Artery in the Left Anterior Oblique Projection. The LCA divides into the circumflex artery that makes up the left side of the circle, and the left anterior descending artery that makes up the anterior portion of the loop. Obtuse marginal branches extend from the circumflex artery; diagonal and septal branches extend from the left anterior descending artery. (From Kubicka RA, Smith C. How to interpret coronary arteriograms. *Radiographics* 1986;6:661–701.

clusion, and (f) after myocardial infarction, for evaluation of interventional therapy.

Coronary Anatomy

The *right coronary artery* (RCA) arises from the right coronary cusp and the *left coronary artery* (LCA) arises from the left coronary cusp. Approximately 85% of patients are right dominant, meaning that the RCA supplies the posterior descending artery and the posterior and inferior surface of the myocardium. In 10–12% of patients the LCA is dominant and supplies the inferior and posterior surface. Approximately 4–5% of patients are co-dominant. The LCA measures 0.5–1.5 cm in length before it divides beneath the left atrial appendage (Figs. 18.28 and 18.29). The *left anterior descending artery* (LAD) extends anteriorly in the interventricular groove. The *circumflex artery* extends laterally and posteriorly under the left atrial appendage to the atrioventricular groove. An occasional third branch is the *ramus intermedius*, which extends as a first diagonal branch (d1) or a first marginal branch (m1).

The *LAD* gives off several *septal branches* that penetrate into the septum. One or more *diagonal branches* extend toward the anterolateral wall. Occasionally a conus branch comes off after the first septal branch and extends to the right ventricular infundibulum. The *circumflex artery* gives off one or more *ob-tuse marginal* branches that supply the lateral wall of the left ventricle.

The *RCA* passes anterior and to the right between the pulmonary artery and the right atrium (Figs 18.30 and 18.31). Its first branch is a *conus branch* to the pulmonary outflow tract. The second branch is the *sinus node branch* with a smaller branch to the right atrium. *Muscular branches* extend into the right ventricular myocardium. At the posterior turn a large *acute marginal* branch is given off anteriorly toward the diaphragmatic surface of the right ventricle. The RCA then extends posteriorly in the atrioventricular sulcus and makes a 90° turn toward the apex in right dominant systems. As the *posterior descending artery* it supplies branches to the diaphragmatic myocardium and the posterior one-third of the interventricular septum.

The coronary arteries can be visualized as a circle and loop with the atrioventricular groove being the circle and the interventricular septum being the attached loop (Figs. 18.28–18.31). In the right anterior oblique projection, the circle is superimposed on itself and the loop is in profile. In the left anterior projection, the circle is more open and the loop is foreshortened. In the left anterior craniad view there is a better, elongated view of the left main coronary artery, LAD, circumflex, and ramus intermedius. For additional details on the circle and loop concept, please refer to

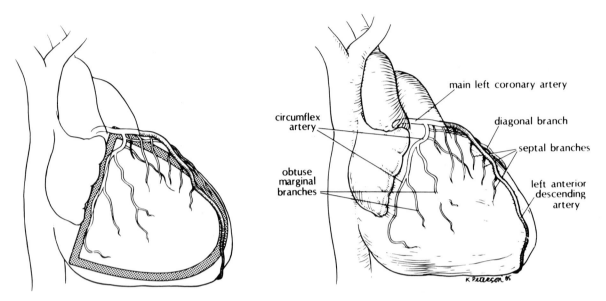

Figure 18.29.   Left Coronary Artery in the Right Anterior Oblique. The loop is more open in this projection, whereas the circle is superimposed. The left anterior descending artery makes up the anterior portion of the loop. The circumflex artery and its obtuse marginal branches make up the left side of the circle. (From Kubicka RA, Smith C. How to interpret coronary arteriograms. *Radiographics* 1986;6: 661–701.

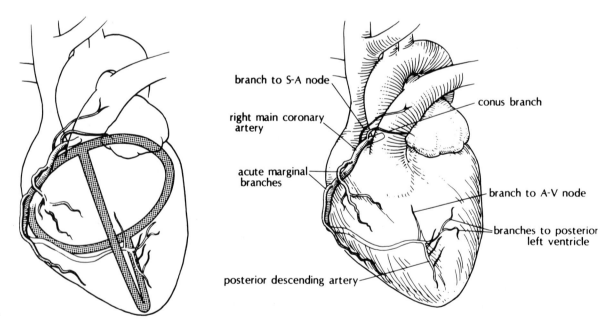

Figure 18.30.   Right Coronary Artery in the Left Anterior Oblique Projection. The right portion of the circle represents the RCA and the posterior portion of the loop represents the posterior descending artery. *S-A,* sinoatrial; *A-V,* atrioventricular. (From Kubicka RA, Smith C. How to interpret coronary arteriograms. *Radiographics* 1986;6:661–701.)

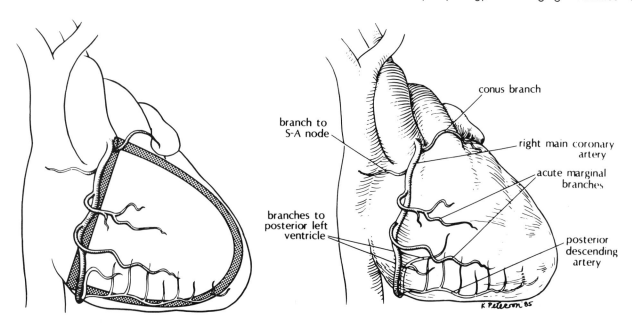

Figure 18.31. Right Coronary Artery in the Right Anterior Oblique Projection. The RCA forms the atrioventricular circle. The loop is more opened in this projection with the posterior descending artery making up its inferior margin. *S-A*, sinoatrial. (From Kubicka RA, Smith C. How to interpret coronary arteriograms. *Radiographics* 1986;6: 661–701.)

the excellent primer on this subject by Kubicka and Smith.

Coronary Pathology

Fixed Coronary Stenosis. A 75% reduction in cross-sectional area is required to cause a significant reduction in blood flow (Fig. 19.3). A 50% reduction in diameter corresponds to a 75% reduction in cross-sectional area. Other significant findings include coronary calcification, ulcerative plaques, and aneurysm formation. Collateral flow typically develops when there is greater than 85% stenosis.

Catheter Spasm is most often seen in the RCA as a smooth transient narrowing, 1–2 mm distal to the catheter tip. The patient usually remains asymptomatic.

Prinzmetal Variant Angina is angina secondary to prolonged coronary spasm. Intravenous ergonovine may be used in a provocative test to incite coronary spasm and typical symptoms and electrocardiographic changes. Prinzmetal angina is usually treated medically.

Kawasaki's Syndrome is an inflammatory condition of the coronary arteries, probably due to prior viral syndrome, that results in coronary stenosis and aneurysms.

Myocardial Bridging describes a normal variant in which the coronary arteries penetrate and then emerge from the myocardium rather than running along the surface of the epicardium. This causes arterial constriction during systole, which reverts to normal flow during diastole.

Anomalies of the coronary arteries include multiple coronary ostia with more than one coronary artery arising directly from one coronary cusp, a single coronary artery, and origination of the LCA from the pulmonary artery (Fig. 18.32).

Therapeutic Considerations

The primary modes of therapy for coronary artery disease include many efficacious medical regimens, percutaneous coronary angioplasty, and coronary artery bypass graft. Coronary artery bypass grafting utilizes native internal mammary arteries or saphenous vein grafts. Surgical bypass has been shown to prolong life in left main coronary artery disease and three-vessel disease. Percutaneous coronary angioplasty (Fig. 19.4) is considered the therapy of choice for single-vessel disease and has an 85–90% success rate. Angioplasty is typically accomplished by balloon dilation of the stenotic lesion over the guidewire. Angioplasty is considered successful when the stenosis is reduced to less than 50% of diameter narrowing, although long-term prognosis is better when there is less than 30% remaining stenosis. Percutaneous atherectomy, laser angioplasty, and coronary stents are additional percutaneous techniques that are currently being evaluated.

CARDIAC ANGIOGRAPHY

Angiography of the heart in adults most often involves left-sided catheterization via arterial puncture with retrograde examination of the aorta, left ventricle, and left atrium. Selective catheterization of the

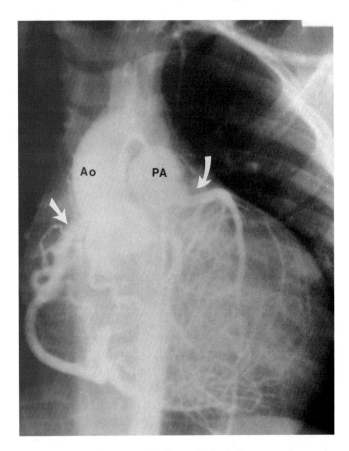

Figure 18.32. Aberrant LCA. The catheter in the ascending aorta (*Ao*) opacifies a dilated RCA (*straight arrow*). The LCA (*curved arrow*) arises from the pulmonary artery (*PA*) and is filled in a retrograde fashion via collateral flow from the RCA.

coronary arteries is also accomplished from the arterial side. Right heart angiography utilizes puncture of the femoral vein with catheter placement in the right atrium, right ventricle, pulmonary outflow tract, or pulmonary artery. Additionally the left atrium or left ventricle may be seen on delayed or "levo-phase" views from a right-sided injection. It is also possible to access the left side during right heart catheterization by puncturing the atrial septum. End-hole catheters are used for pressure measurements and pigtail or multiple side-hole catheters are used for intracardiac injections to avoid contrast injection into the myocardium itself. Blood flow is estimated with standard oximetry and indicator dilution techniques.

Wall motion is evaluated globally and regionally. *Hypokinesia* describes diminished contractility or less systolic motion than normal. *Akinesia* means no systolic wall motion. *Dyskinesia* means there is paradoxic wall motion during systolic contraction. *Asynchrony* refers to cardiac motion that is out of phase with the remainder of the myocardium.

Ventricular aneurysms appear as a bulge in the wall that moves paradoxically compared with other areas of the left ventricle (Fig. 18.33). True aneurysms are lined by thinned, scarred myocardium and are typically located near the apex or anterolateral wall. Pseudoaneurysms are focal, contained ruptures that are often larger but have narrower ostia, and are most commonly located at the inferior and posterior aspect of the left ventricle. Intramural thrombi may be seen in up to 50% of ventricular aneurysms.

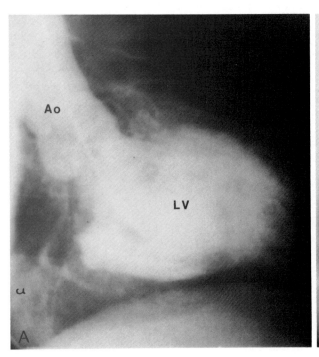

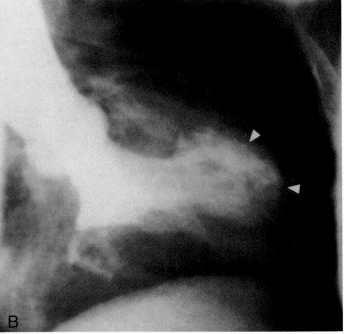

Figure 18.33. Left Ventricular Aneurysm. Diastole (**A**) and end systole (**B**). The left ventriculogram (*LV*) is accomplished with the pigtail catheter entering the left ventricle from the aortic root (*Ao*). A paradoxic bulge near the apex (*arrowheads*) indicates a left ventricular aneurysm.

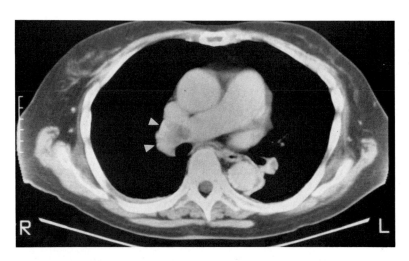

Figure 18.34. Pulmonary Artery Embolus. Contrast-enhanced CT examination shows a filling defect within the right pulmonary artery (*arrowheads*). Disappearance with time confirms an embolus. Primary neoplasms or metastatic emboli may cause a similar filling defect.

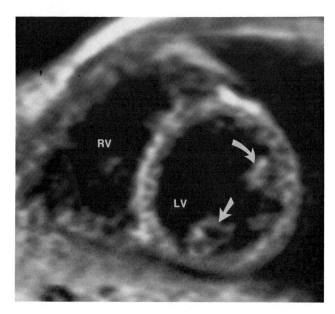

Figure 18.35. Spin-Echo MR. A tomographic slice in the short axis projection demonstrates the right ventricle (*RV*), interventricular septum, and left ventricle (*LV*). The anterior (*straight arrow*) and posterior (*curved arrow*) papillary muscles are seen within the left ventricular cavity. The spin-echo technique creates a black blood appearance because of the signal void of moving blood.

COMPUTED TOMOGRAPHY AND ULTRAFAST CT

Computed tomography is useful in evaluating aortic aneurysms, aortic dissections, central pulmonary thrombosis (Fig. 18.34), intracardiac masses and thrombi, pericardial thickening, fluid collections and pericardial calcifications. Optimal contrast enhancement is required for most studies. Ultrafast CT offers the advantage of high-speed scanning to stop action and eliminate motion artifact. Angled couch views supplement standard axial imaging. With cardiac gating, cine-CT can provide wall motion studies and valve evaluation. Ultrafast CT has also been used to screen for coronary artery calcification and to document patency of coronary bypass grafts.

CARDIAC MAGNETIC RESONANCE IMAGING

Cardiac MR combines many of the capabilities of the other imaging modalities into one examination. These include excellent static anatomic images and dynamic motion studies for function. Cardiac MR applications include congenital heart disease, aortic and pulmonary artery disease, pericardial disease, ventricular function, valvular function, cardiomyopathies, and cardiac masses. Cardiac pacemakers are considered contraindications, but most prosthetic valves can be safely studied.

The best anatomic depiction is accomplished on spin-echo T1-weighted images where the moving blood produces a signal void or "black blood" appearance (Fig 18.35). Gradient-echo or fast-field echo images impart bright signal to coherently flowing blood, creating a "white blood" appearance similar to contrast studies (Fig. 18.36). Electrocardiographic gating can be used similar to gated cardiac blood pool scintigraphy. Slice-specific information is acquired with reference to specific phases within the cardiac cycle. With gradient recalled echo technique applied, motion studies can show flowing blood as well as myocardial contractility.

Magnetic resonance images are acquired as tomographic slices through any selected plane. The planes may be angled to match cardiac or vascular anatomy. Tissue characterization of the myocardium is accomplished using T1- and T2-weighted images, contrast enhancement, and spectroscopy. This may be useful for neoplastic, infiltrative, or inflammatory conditions of the myocardium.

Cardiac MR motion studies provide functional information including wall motion analysis, systolic wall thickening, chamber volumes, stroke volumes, right and left ventricular ejection fractions and valve evaluation (Fig. 18.37). Flowing blood becomes turbulent and loses its coherence when it passes through stenotic or regurgitant valves. The high-velocity stenotic

Figure 18.36. Fast-Field Echo MR. The fast-field echo technique creates a white blood depiction that shows flowing blood and turbulence during motion studies. The end diastole image (*straight arrow*) has the largest ventricular size. The end systole image (*curved arrow*) has the smallest ventricular cavity and the thickest wall.

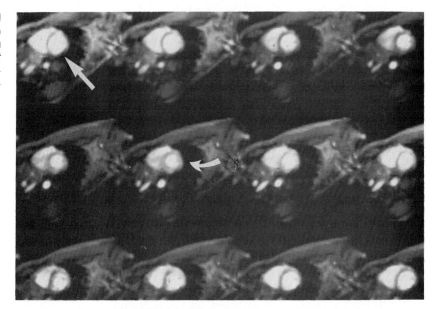

Figure 18.37. Magnetic Resonance Imaging Ejection Fraction Technique. Regions of interest are drawn on the diastolic image (*straight arrow*) and the end systolic image (*curved arrow*) of each slice. An area ejection fraction (*EF*) is then calculated for each slice. Volume ejection fraction calculations are calculated using sequential slices that include the entire ventricular volume. *EDV*, end diastolic volume; *ESV*, end systolic volume; *SV*, stroke volume; *CO*, cardiac output; *ED*, end diastole; *ES*, end systole.

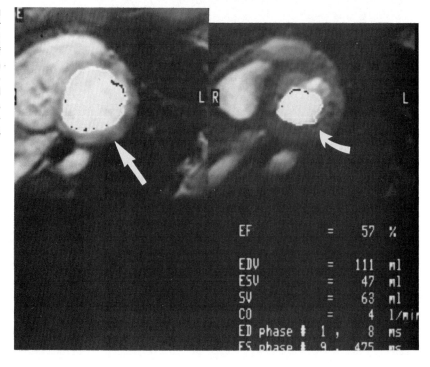

jet or regurgitant flow is displayed as a wedge-shaped puff of dark turbulent flow readily identified on the white blood background with the gradient-echo technique (Figs. 19.21 and 19.22). Visual and region of interest grading can be accomplished for stenotic or regurgitant flow based on distance, area, or regurgitant volume (see Chapter 19). The regurgitant fraction is calculated by comparing the right and left stroke volumes. Velocity encoded cine-MR techniques, utilizing phase analysis, can calculate flow velocities and flow volumes in addition to the regurgitant volumes. These techniques can be employed in lieu of angiography for many cases. Understanding MR signal characteristics

and details of three-dimensional cardiac anatomy displayed in different tomographic planes is critical to the accurate utilization of cardiac MR.

Suggested Readings

Brundage BH. Comparative cardiac imaging. Rockville, MD: Aspen Publications, Inc, 1990.

Chapman S, Nakielny R. Aids to radiological diagnosis. 2nd ed. London: WB Saunders, 1990.

Chen CE, Cooper C. Review of radiology. Philadelphia: WB Saunders, 1990.

Cooley RN, Schreiber MH. Radiology of the heart and great vessels. 3rd ed. Baltimore: Williams & Wilkins, 1978.

Dahnert W. Radiology review manual. Baltimore: Williams & Wilkins, 1991.

Feigenbaum H. Doppler echocardiography. Philadelphia: Lea & Febiger, 1986.

Gedgaudas E, Moffer JH, Castaneda-Zuniga WR, Amplatz K. Cardiovascular radiology. Philadelphia: WB Saunders, 1985.

Higgins CB. Essentials of cardiac radiology and imaging. Philadelphia: JB Lippincott, 1992.

Kelley MJ. Chest radiography for the cardiologist. Cardiology clinics. Philadelphia: WB Saunders, 1983.

Kubicka RA, Smith C. How to interpret coronary arteriograms. Radiographics 1986;6:661–701.

Marcus ML, Schelbert HR, Skorton DJ, Wolf GL. Cardiac Imaging—a companion to Braunwald's heart disease. Philadelphia: WB Saunders, 1991.

Miller DD, Burns RG, Gill JB, Ruddy TD. Clinical cardiac imaging. New York: McGraw-Hill, 1988.

Miller SW, ed. Symposium on advances in cardiac imaging. Radiol Clin North Am 1985;23:587–793.

Miller SW, ed. Cardiopulmonary imaging. Radiol Clin North Am 1989;27:1059–1266.

Netter FH, Atlas of human anatomy. The CIBA collection of medical illustrations. West Caldwell, NJ: CIBA-GIEGY Corporation, 1989.

Putnam CE. Cardiopulmonary imaging. Radiol Clin of North Am. Philadelphia: WB Saunders, 1983.

Ravin CE, Cooper C. Review of radiology. Philadelphia: WB Saunders, 1990.

Taveras JM, Ferrucci JT. Radiology. Philadelphia: WB Saunders, 1991.

Wolfe CL. Cardiac imaging. Cardiology clinics. Philadelphia: WB Saunders, 1989.

Cardiac Imaging in Acquired Disease

David K. Shelton, Jr.

Cardiac disease remains among the most common problems affecting patient morbidity and mortality today, despite many important dietary, pharmaceutical, interventional, and surgical advances. Most acquired cardiac diseases can be classified under six general categories: ischemic heart disease, cardiomyopathies, pulmonary vascular disease, acquired valvular disease, cardiac masses, and pericardial disease. Utilization of plain film, fluoroscopy, ultrasound, computerized tomography (CT), magnetic resonance imaging (MR), nuclear imaging, and angiocardiography must be integrated with knowledge of specific disease processes.

ISCHEMIC HEART DISEASE
Coronary Artery Disease

Coronary artery disease is the most common cause of mortality in the United States, with approximately one American dying every minute. Six to seven million Americans have active symptoms related to ischemic heart disease. Approximately 300,000 coronary artery bypass grafts (CABG) are accomplished per year in the United States with a similar number of percutaneous transluminal coronary angioplasties (PTCA).

Clinical presentations include (*a*) stable angina, (*b*) unstable angina (often preinfarction), (*c*) acute myocardial infarction, (*d*) congestive heart fail-

ure secondary to chronic ischemia or prior infarction sequelae, (*e*) arrhythmias, and (*f*) sudden death. Clinical symptoms are due to luminal abnormalities of the coronary arteries including (*a*) atheromatous disease, (*b*) coronary thrombosis, (*c*) intraluminal ulceration and hemorrhage, (*d*) vasoconstriction, and (*e*) coronary ectasia and aneurysm.

Risk factors for development of atherosclerotic coronary artery disease include elevated serum cholesterol, high cholesterol intake, tobacco smoking, diabetes, hypertension, ventricular hypertrophy, hyperlipidemia, gout, inactivity, age, male sex, and heredity. Aggravating conditions include aortic stenosis, ventricular hypertrophy, cardiomyopathy, coronary embolism, congenital anomalies, Kawasaki's disease, and anemia. Noninvasive imaging is often utilized as a screening test. However, selective coronary angiography with ventriculography is usually required to determine coronary anatomy and to direct the specific therapy.

A typical imaging workup would include chest radiography, nuclear medicine perfusion scans, and consideration for coronary angiography. Indications for coronary angiography include angina refractory to medical therapy, unstable angina, high-risk occupations such as pilots, and abnormal electrocardiograms or stress perfusion tests. Coronary angiography is considered following myocardial infarction when PTCA or intracoronary thrombolysis are being considered. Additional indications include development of mechanical dysfunction, progressive congestive failure, refractory ventricular arrhythmias, and follow-up of intravenous thrombolytic agents.

Coronary artery calcification occurs in the intima and is directly related to advanced atheromatous disease and coronary narrowing (Figs. 18.14 and 19.1). Coronary calcification is detected at angiography in 75% of patients with 50% diameter stenosis. Only 11% of men without significant coronary artery disease have coronary calcification. In the asymptomatic population, the detection of coronary calcification has a predictive accuracy of 86%. In symptomatic patients, coronary calcification is seen in 50% of patients with single-vessel disease, 77% of those with two-vessel disease, and 86% of those with three-vessel disease. Fluoroscopically detected coronary calcification in the presence of angina-like chest pain is associated with coronary stenosis 94% of the time. Overall, fluoroscopic detection of coronary artery calcification has a 73% sensitivity and 84% specificity for symptomatic patients. Exercise tolerance testing has sensitivity of 76–88%, and specificity of 43–77%. Exercise testing with planar thallium imaging has a sensitivity of 85% and specificity of 85%.

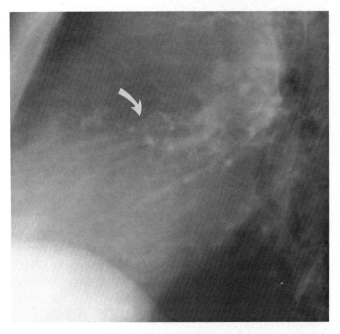

Figure 19.1. Coronary Artery Calcification. Lateral chest radiograph demonstrates coronary artery calcification (*arrow*).

Myocardial perfusion scanning, utilizing thallium, ^{99m}Tc-sestamibi or ^{99m}Tc-teboroxime, is the primary imaging modality for detecting myocardial ischemia. Stress images are obtained with exercise or pharmacologic agents such as dipyridamole. Single photon emission computed tomography (SPECT) has increased the sensitivity to 90–94%, and the specificity to 90–95%. The hallmark for segmental ischemia is a perfusion defect on stress testing that fills in during rest examination (Fig. 19.2). A defect that appears stable during both stress and rest examinations is usually an infarction. "Hibernating" regions of viable myocardium associated with tight coronary stenosis may appear as fixed defects on sestamibi/teboroxime images or redistribution thallium images obtained 4 hours after stress.

Gated blood pool scintigraphy will demonstrate exercise-induced wall motion abnormalities in 63% of patients with significant coronary artery disease. With exercise, the ejection fractions normally increase by at least 5%. Failure of ejection fraction to increase with exercise is an indication of myocardial dysfunction. Utilizing these two findings, exercise gated blood pool scintigraphy has a sensitivity of 87–95% and a specificity of 92% for coronary artery disease.

Coronary angiograms should be evaluated for the percent of stenosis, the number of vessels involved, focal versus diffuse disease, coronary anatomy, ectasia or aneurysm, coronary calcification and collateral flow (Fig. 19.3). Collaterals may include epicardial, myocardial, atrioventricular, inter-coronary or intracoronary vessels. The angiographer must count the number of major epicardial vessels with

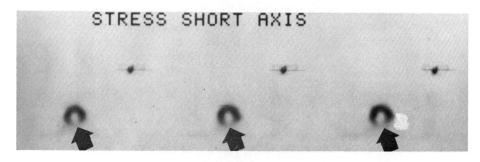

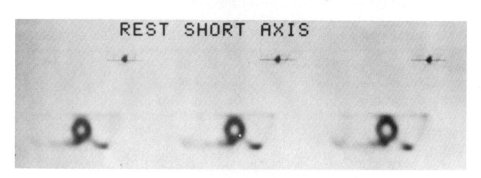

Figure 19.2. Myocardial Perfusion Scan. Single photon emission CT images of the left ventricle in short axis projection demonstrate a defect (*arrows*) in the inferior wall of the left ventricle during stress, which is well perfused on the rest images. This is strong evidence of ischemic heart disease utilizing ^{99m}Tc sestamibi as the radionuclide and pharmacologic stress testing with dipyridamole.

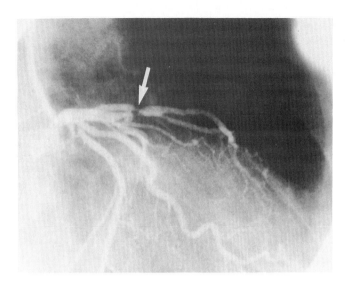

Figure 19.3.   Coronary Stenosis. An 80% stenotic lesion (*arrow*) is identified in the left anterior descending artery. This patient was experiencing classic angina.

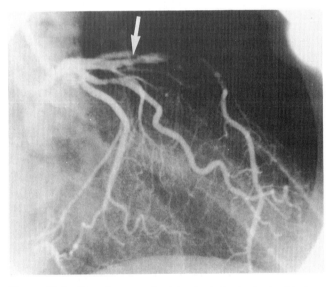

Figure 19.4.   Percutaneous Transluminal Angioplasty. Marked improvement in the LAD lesion (*arrow*) seen in Figure 19.3 is evident following PTCA. The angina symptoms resolved.

greater than 50% diameter narrowing. Patients are divided into one-, two-, or three-vessel disease based upon involvement of the right or left main coronary artery, left anterior descending artery and left circumflex artery. A 50% diameter narrowing results in a 75% cross-sectional area reduction, which is the physiologic point at which flow is restricted. Reliability for estimating the percent diameter narrowing depends upon the observer, projection, resolution, and presence of coronary calcification or ectasia. The degree of coronary disease may be assessed utilizing percent stenosis of each individual coronary artery or based on 5-mm segments of the coronary arteries. The right coronary artery is 10 cm long, the left main coro-

nary artery is 1 cm long, the left anterior descending (LAD) is 10 cm long, and the left circumflex is 6 cm long, for a total of 27 cm. These may be divided into 54 5-mm segments. This scoring system allows the interpreter to quantify the number of 5-mm segments with stenoses in the 0–25%, 25–50%, 50–75%, and 75–100% ranges. The significance of 30–70% lesions is often clarified by correlation with stress-induced perfusion scintigraphy.

Percutaneous transluminal angioplasty is usually accomplished for localized lesions in one- or two-vessel disease (Fig. 19.4). Coronary artery bypass grafting, utilizing saphenous veins grafts or the internal mammary artery, is usually reserved for more complex or longer segment disease. The CABG markers are often placed at the anastomotic site to help the angiographer during future selective angiography. Utilization of the internal mammary artery has better long-term results than saphenous vein grafts. Recurrence of symptoms after CABG may be due to occlusion, graft stenosis, or progression of native vessel disease. Graft stenoses and acute occlusions may be amenable to percutaneous interventional techniques.

Echocardiography is useful in detecting some of the long-term complications of ischemic disease, including ventricular aneurysm, thinning of myocardium, akinesia, or dyskinesia. Aneurysms are best seen at the apex and septum. Mural thrombi may also be diagnosed, but are difficult to visualize at the apex.

Computed tomography is capable of establishing the patency of coronary artery bypass grafts. Ultrafast CT has a 93% sensitivity, 89% specificity, and 92% accuracy for establishing patency of the CABG grafts. Ultrafast CT with contrast can evaluate wall motion, thrombi, old infarcts, aneurysm, and pericardial abnormalities.

Magnetic resonance can be utilized to (*a*) define the location and size of previous myocardial infarctions, (*b*) demonstrate complications of previous infarctions, (*c*) establish the presence of viable myocardium for possible revascularization, (*d*) differentiate acute versus chronic myocardial infarction, (*e*) evaluate regional myocardial wall motion and systolic wall thickening (Fig. 19.5), (*f*) demonstrate global myocardial function with right ventricular and left ventricular ejection fractions, (*g*) demonstrate regional myocardial perfusion, and (*h*) evaluate papillary muscle and valvular abnormalities. Gadolinium-enhanced T1-weighted images demonstrate areas of ischemia and reperfusion after myocardial infarction. Magnetic resonance imaging spectroscopy targeting myocardial phosphate metabolism can separate acute from chronic ischemia and reperfused, infarcted myocardium from reperfused, viable myocardium. With spin-echo imaging, MR has a 78% accuracy for establishing patency of CABGs. Cine MR with gradient echo

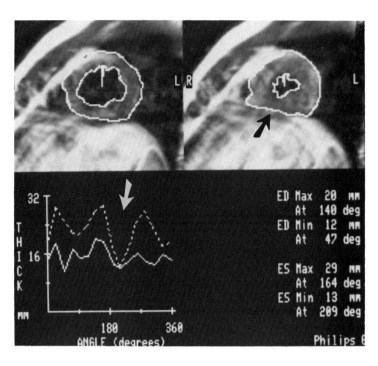

Figure 19.5. Wall Motion MR Evaluation. Short axis tomographic views of the left ventricle are utilized for evaluation of systolic wall thickening. Regions of interest are drawn around the myocardium in diastole (*left*) and systole (*right*). The inferior wall (*black arrow*) demonstrates hypokinesia and poor systolic wall thickening. The functional graph (*below*) confirms the findings (*white arrow*). The patient had a previous inferior wall myocardial infarction.

has a sensitivity of 88–93%, specificity of 86–100%, and overall accuracy of 89–91% for patency of CABGs.

Myocardial Infarction

After acute infarction, the chest radiograph will initially show a normal heart size in 90% of cases. Cardiomegaly and congestive failure will eventually develop in 60–70%, more frequently with anterior wall infarction, multivessel disease, or left ventricular aneurysm. Increasing stages of pulmonary venous hypertension, particularly alveolar edema, are associated with worsened prognosis.

Complications of myocardial infarcion include the following.

Cardiogenic shock implies that systolic pressure is less than 90 mm Hg and is typically associated with acute pulmonary edema and worsened prognosis.

Atrioventricular block is common after inferior wall infarcts due to injury to the atrioventricular nodal branch of the right coronary artery. Complete heart block occurs with larger infarcts and has a worse prognosis.

Right ventricular infarction occurs with 33% of inferior wall infarctions. Symptoms are caused by the reduction in right ventricular ejection infraction, which returns to normal within 10 days in approximately 50% of cases. The diagnosis may be established using technetium pyrophosphate (PYP) radionuclide scans. Complications include cardiac shock, elevated right atrial pressure, and decreased pulmonary artery pressure.

Myocardial rupture (3.3% of infarcts) may occur 3–14 days after infarction. The mortality rate approaches 100% and accounts for 13% of myocardial

infarction deaths. The chest radiograph shows acute cardiac enlargement secondary to leakage of blood into the pericardium. *Rupture of the interventricular septum* (1%) occurs day 4 to 21 as a complication of anterior myocardial infarction and LAD disease. Mortality is 24% within 24 hours, and 90% within 1 year. Swan-Ganz catheter measurements show an acute increase in saturation in the right ventricle, although the wedge pressures may be normal. Chest radiographs show acute pulmonary vascular engorgement and right-sided cardiac enlargement because of left-to-right shunt. Pulmonary edema is not a typical feature. Echocardiography readily demonstrates the septal defect.

Papillary muscle rupture (1%) is suggested by abrupt onset of mitral regurgitation with acute pulmonary edema on the radiograph. Typically, the left ventricle is only minimally enlarged, whereas the left atrium enlarges quickly. Inferior infarcts are associated with posteromedial papillary rupture. Anterior infarcts less commonly affect the anterolateral papillary muscle. Mortality is 70% within 24 hours and 90% within 1 year. Echocardiography confirms the diagnosis.

Ventricular aneurysm develops in approximately 12% of survivors from myocardial infarction. Ventricular aneurysms may also be caused by Chagas' disease or trauma and are rarely congenital, usually in young black males. Aneurysms present with congestive failure, arrhythmias and systemic emboli. *True aneurysms* are broad-mouthed, localized outpouchings that do not contract during systole (Fig. 18.33). They are typically anterior or apical and result from LAD disease. The chest radiograph shows a localized

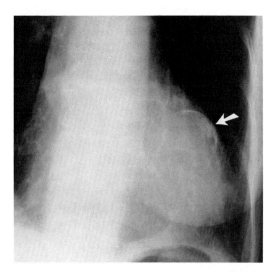

Figure 19.6. Left Ventricular Aneurysm. A localized calcified bulge (*arrow*) is seen along the left heart border, secondary to prior myocardial infarction complicated by left ventricular aneurysm.

bulge along the left cardiac border and may show rim-like calcification in the wall (Fig. 19.6). Fluoroscopy detects up to 50%, while 96% are detected by radionuclide ventriculography or myocardial perfusion scan. Echocardiography, contrast-enhanced CT, and MR are also very accurate at detecting true aneurysms.

Pseudoaneurysms are contained myocardial ruptures consisting of a localized hematoma surrounded by adherent pericardium. Etiologies include infarction and trauma. Patients are at high risk for delayed rupture. Pseudoaneurysms are typically posterolateral or retrocardiac in location and have smaller mouths than true aneurysms. Magnetic resonance imaging is the most accurate at detecting pseudoaneurysms. Their appearance can be confusing on echocardiography.

Dressler's syndrome (4%) is also known as the postmyocardial infarction syndrome and is similar to the postpericardiotomy syndrome complicating cardiac surgery. Onset is typically 1 week to 3 months postinjury (peak at 2–3 weeks), but relapses occur up to 2 years later. Presentation includes fever, chest pain, pericarditis, pericardial effusion, and pleuritis with pleural effusion usually more prominent on the left. Dressler's syndrome responds well to antiinflammatory medications.

Infarct Imaging

The indications for myocardial infarct imaging include late admission, equivocal enzymes, equivocal electrocardiogram, recent cardiac surgery or trauma, and suspicion of right ventricular infarction.

Radionuclide Imaging. "Cold spot" imaging is accomplished with thallium or technetium perfusion agents (Fig. 19.7). Sensitivity is 96% within 6 to 12

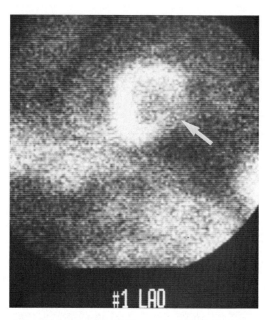

Figure 19.7. Myocardial Infarction. Resting, planar thallium image in the left anterior oblique projection demonstrates a defect in the inferoposterior wall (*arrow*), consistent with a myocardial infarction. Cold spot imaging can be accomplished within 6 hours of the acute event.

hours but only 59% for remote infarction. Acute infarction cannot be distinguished from remote infarction. "Hot spot" infarct imaging utilizes technetium PYP, technetium tetracycline, technetium glucoheptonate, indium-111 antimyosin antibodies, or F-18 sodium fluorine (Fig. 19.8). Pyrophosphate uptake occurs in myocardial necrosis due to PYP complexing with calcium deposits. The PYP scans turn positive at 12 hours, have peak sensitivity at 48–72 hours, and revert to normal by 14 days. Persistent abnormal uptake implies a poor prognosis or developing aneurysm. Cardiomyopathies and diffuse myocarditis show diffuse increased uptake. Contusions and radiation myocarditis show increased regional uptake.

Ultrafast CT with contrast demonstrates poor perfusion of the infarcted segment immediately after administration of contrast. After a delay of 10–15 minutes, the normal myocardium washes out, leaving a contrast enhanced periphery of the infarcted zone.

Magnetic resonance imaging demonstrates prolongation of T1 and T2 times secondary to edema of the acutely infarcted segment. Edema occurs within 1 hour after infarct and may be associated with myocardial hemorrhage. Magnetic resonance imaging has a 93% sensitivity, 80% specificity and 87% accuracy for acute myocardial infarction. The infarcted region is best delineated by high signal on T2-weighted images; however, surrounding edema tends to overestimate the size of the infarct. T1-weighted images with gadolinium demonstrate the acutely is-

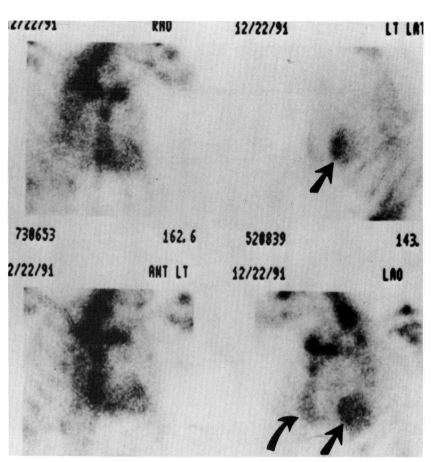

Figure 19.8. Myocardial Infarct Scan. Hot spot imaging was accomplished using PYP. Notice the uptake in the anterolateral wall of the myocardium (*arrows*) which is almost as "hot" as the sternum (*curved arrow*). Images are obtained in right anterior oblique (*RAO*), left lateral (*LT LAT*), anterior (*ANT LT*),and left anterior oblique (*LAO*) projections.

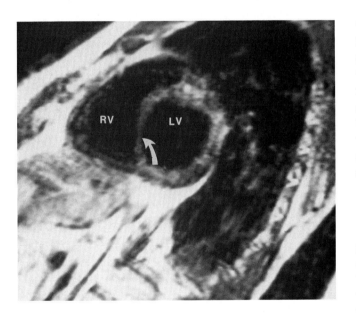

Figure 19.9. Old Septal Infarction. Spin-echo MR demonstrates fixed thinning of the myocardial wall (*arrow*) due to prior myocardial infarction. *RV*, right ventricle; *LV*, left ventricle.

chemic region and will help to differentiate reperfusion from occlusive myocardial infarction. Regional wall thinning and lack of systolic thickening are the best evidence of the size of the infarcted segment (Figs. 19.5 and 19.9). Scar tissue will not contract,

whereas viable myocardium will contract and thicken by at least 2 mm. Very high-grade stenotic lesions may result in chronically ischemic myocardium with altered metabolism. This "hibernating myocardium" may act like postinfarction scar but remains viable and may improve in function with revascularization. Unfortunately, it also remains at risk for acute infarction. "Stunned myocardium" describes postischemic, dysfunctional myocardium without complete necrosis, and which is potentially salvageable.

CARDIOMYOPATHIES

The prevalence of cardiomyopathies is approximately eight cases per 100,000 population in developed countries. One percent of cardiac deaths in the United States are due to cardiomyopathy. The mortality rate in males is twice that in females, and in blacks is twice that of Caucasians. In developing countries and in the tropics, the prevalence and mortality rates are much higher, probably because of nutritional deficiency, genetic factors, physical stress, untreated hypertension, and infection, especially Chagas' disease.

The cardiomyopathies are a group of anomalies with three basic features: (*a*) failure of the heart to maintain its architecture, (*b*) failure of the heart to maintain normal electrical activity, and (*c*) failure of the heart to maintain cardiac output. General features of cardiomyopathies include cardiomegaly, congestive heart failure, often with relatively clear lungs, dilated left and right ventricles with elevated end-diastolic pressures, decreased contractility, and decreased ejection fractions. Causes of congestive heart failure are listed in Table 19.1.

The cardiomyopathies may also be divided into dilated, hypertrophic, restrictive, and right ventricular forms (Table 19.2).

Dilated Cardiomyopathy

In the western world, dilated cardiomyopathy accounts for 90% of all cardiomyopathies (Fig. 19.10). The term "congestive cardiomyopathy" should be reserved for a subgroup of the dilated cardiomyopathies, where the etiology is unknown. Specific causes for dilated cardiomyopathies should be pursued as the specific therapy may vary: (*a*) ischemic cardiomyopathy (the most common cause) due to chronic is-

chemia, prior infarction or anomalous coronary arteries, (*b*) long-term sequelae of myocarditis (Coxsackie virus most common), (*c*) toxins (ethanol and adriamycin), (*d*) metabolic (mucolipidosis, mucopolysaccharidosis, glycogen storage disease), (*e*) nutritional deficiencies (thiamin and selenium), (*f*) infants of diabetic mothers, and (*g*) muscular dystrophies.

Clinical presentation is related to congestive heart failure, although the initial presentation may include cardiac arrhythmias, conduction disturbances, thromboembolic phenomena, or sudden death. Presentation may also differ, depending on left-sided dominance, right-sided dominance, or biventricular involvement.

Chest x-ray commonly demonstrates global cardiomegaly. Larger heart sizes are associated with worse prognosis. Coronary artery calcification may be a clue to ischemic cardiomyopathy. Gated myocardial scintigraphy shows decreased left ventricular ejection fraction, prolonged preejection period, shortened left ventricular ejection time, and a decreased rate of ejec-

Table 19.1. Causes of Congestive Heart Failure

Myocardial
  Cardiomyopathy (dilated, restrictive, hypertrophic)
  Myocarditis
  Postpartum cardiomyopathy
Coronary
  Transient ischemia
  Chronic ischemic cardiomyopathy
  Prior infarct or aneurysm
Endocardial
  Fibrosis
  Löffler syndrome
Valvular
  Stenosis
  Regurgitation
Pericardial
  Effusion
  Constrictive
Vascular
  Hypertension
  Pulmonary Emboli
  Arteriovenous fistula
  Vasculitis
Extracardiac
  Endocrinopathy (thyroid, adrenal)
  Toxic
  Anemic
  Metabolic

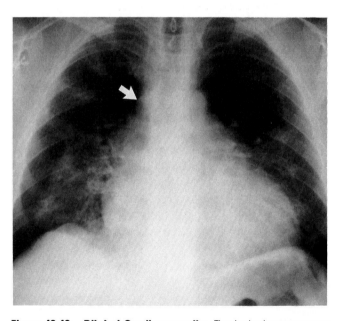

Figure 19.10. Dilated Cardiomyopathy. The typical appearance of a dilated cardiomyopathy is demonstrated with a water-bottle configuration and dilation of the azygos vein (*arrow*). Pulmonary infiltrates are due to pulmonary edema and capillary leak in this patient with viral myocarditis.

Table 19.2. Types of Cardiomyopathies

Type	Ventricular Wall[a]	Ventricular Cavity[a]	Contractility	Compliance
Dilated	LV thin	LV dilated	Decreased	Normal to decreased
Hypertrophic	LV thick	LV normal to decreased	Increased	Decreased
Restrictive	Normal	Normal	Normal to decreased	Severely decreased
Uhl's anomaly	RV thin	RV dilated	Decreased	Normal to decreased

[a]LV, left ventricular; RV, right ventricular.

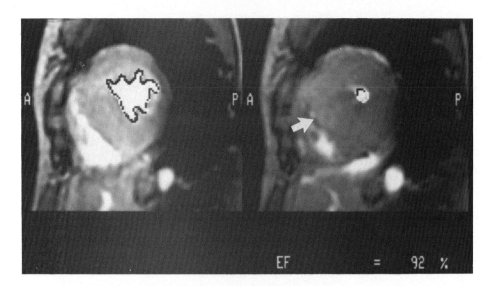

Figure 19.11. Hypertrophic Cardiomyopathy. Gradient-echo MR demonstrates marked left ventricular hypertrophy on these short axis views of the left ventricle. Note the asymmetric thickening of the septum (*arrow*) compared with the remainder of the left ventricular myocardium. Diastole is on the left and systole is on the right.

tion. Echocardiography shows a dilated left ventricle with hypokinesia, thinning of the left ventricular posterior wall and interventricular septum, decreased cardiac contractility, left atrial enlargement, and hypokinetic right ventricle. Magnetic resonance imaging shows dilation of the specific chambers, thickness of the myocardium with nonuniformity seen in prior infarctions, pericardial effusions, right and left ventricular ejection fractions, stroke volumes, wall-stress physiology and quality of systolic wall thickening.

Hypertrophic Cardiomyopathy

Hypertrophic Cardiomyopathy may be familial (60%), autosomal dominant with variable penetrance, associated with neurofibromatosis and Noonan's syndrome, or be secondary to pressure overload. The hypertrophic cardiomyopathies are divided into two basic types: (*a*) *concentric hypertrophy,* which may be diffuse, midventricular, or apical in distribution, and (*b*) *asymmetrical septal hypertrophy,* which includes *idiopathic hypertrophic subaortic stenosis* (Fig. 19.11). Either form may cause some degree of muscular outflow obstruction with a systolic pressure gradient. Systemic hypertension may cause left ventricular hypertrophy followed by dilation, pulmonary venous hypertension, and increased risk of coronary artery disease.

The clinical presentation includes angina, syncope, arrhythmias, and congestive heart failure. Sudden death occurs in 50% of patients. The overall mortality rate is 2–3% per year.

On chest radiography, 50% of patients with hypertrophic cardiomyopathy will have a normal chest radiograph and 30% have left atrial enlargement, commonly due to mitral regurgitation. Echocardiographic features include (*a*) hypertrophy of the interventricular septum (>12–13 mm), (*b*) abnormal ratio of thickness of the interventricular septum to left ventricular posterior wall (>1.3:1), (*c*) systolic anterior motion of the mitral valve with mitral regurgitation, (*d*) narrowing of the left ventricular outflow tract during systole, (*e*) high velocity across the left ventricular outflow tract with delayed systolic peaks on Doppler examination, and (*f*) midsystolic closure of the aortic valve.

Restrictive Cardiomyopathy

Restrictive Cardiomyopathy is the least frequent form of cardiomyopathy. Etiologies include infiltrative disorders such as amyloid, glycogen storage disease, mucopolysaccharidosis, hemochromatosis, sarcoidosis and myocardial tumor infiltration. In the tropics, endomyocardial fibrosis is highly prevalent. A rare form of endomyocardial fibrosis associated with eosinophilia is called *Löffler's endocardial fibrosis.* Restrictive cardiomyopathy should be considered when patients present with symptoms of congestive failure without radiographic evidence of cardiomegaly or ventricular hypertrophy (Fig. 19.12). The primary differential diagnosis is constrictive pericardial disease that can be differentiated by CT or MR.

Signs and symptoms are related to congestive failure, arrhythmias, and heart block. In late stages, the electrocardiogram shows low voltage. Pathophysiology includes impaired diastolic function with decreased ventricular compliance, poor diastolic filling, normal or near-normal systolic function, and elevation of right and left ventricular filling pressures.

The chest radiograph often shows a normal-sized heart with pulmonary congestion. Left atrial enlargement and pulmonary venous hypertension may be present. The PYP nuclear scans demonstrate hot spots in abnormal areas of myocardium in 50–90% of patients. Echocardiography shows decreased systolic and diastolic function with normal to decreased ejection fractions. Mild left ventricular wall thickening is often present with a granular appearance to

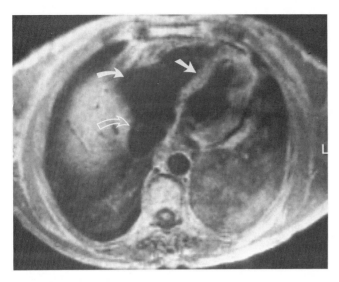

Figure 19.12. Restrictive Cardiomyopathy. Spin-echo MR demonstrates a variable high density signal within the myocardium, a dilated right atrium (*closed curved arrow*), and an enlarged inferior vena cava (*open curved arrow*). The interventricular septum has an abnormal contour (*straight arrow*) due to high right ventricular pressures in this biopsy-proven case of amyloid cardiomyopathy.

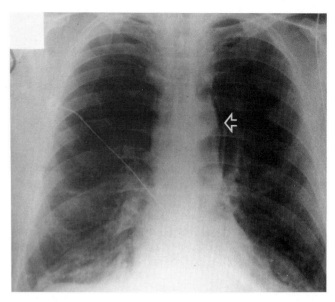

Figure 19.13. Cor Pulmonale. A posteroanterior chest radiograph demonstrates marked hyperinflation caused by chronic obstructive pulmonary disease. The anterior junction line (*arrow*) is herniated to the left of the aortic knob because of marked emphysema in the anterior segment of the right upper lobe.

the myocardium. Magnetic resonance imaging shows high signal in the myocardium on T2-weighted images in patients with amyloidosis and sarcoidosis. The atria are enlarged because of elevated diastolic pressures, but ventricular volumes are often normal. Mitral regurgitation and tricuspid regurgitation are readily depicted with gradient-echo cine MR. The inferior vena cava and superior vena cava may be greatly dilated.

Right Ventricular Cardiomyopathies

Cor pulmonale is defined as right ventricular failure secondary to pulmonary parenchymal or pulmonary arterial disease. It may be considered a secondary form of right ventricular cardiomyopathy. Etiologies include (*a*) destructive pulmonary disease such as pulmonary fibrosis and chronic obstructive pulmonary disease, (*b*) hypoxic pulmonary vasoconstriction due to chronic bronchitis, asthma, central nervous system hypoxia, and upper airway obstruction, (*c*) acute and chronic pulmonary embolism, (*d*) idiopathic pulmonary hypertension, and (*e*) extrapulmonary diseases affecting pulmonary mechanics such as chest deformities, morbid obesity (*Pickwickian syndrome*), and neuromuscular diseases.

The end result is alveolar hypoxia leading to hypoxemia, pulmonary hypertension, elevated right ventricular pressures, right ventricular hypertrophy, right ventricular dilation and right ventricular failure. Symptoms include marked dyspnea and decreased exercise endurance out of proportion to pulmonary

function tests. Blood gasses demonstrate hypoxemia and hypercapnia.

The chest radiograph shows a normal-sized heart or mild cardiomegaly (Fig. 19.13). Right ventricular and right atrial enlargement may be present. The main and central pulmonary arteries are prominent and the periphery is oligemic. The interlobar artery typically measures more than 16 mm. The lungs show signs of chronic obstructive pulmonary disease, emphysema, or pulmonary fibrosis. Nuclear scintigraphy shows right ventricular enlargement with decrease in the right ventricular ejection fraction on first pass examination. Echocardiography and MR show right ventricular and right atrial enlargement with thickening of the anterior right ventricular wall. M-mode echocardiography of the tricuspid valve shows a diminished A-wave and flat E-to-F slope. Therapy is aimed at the underlying pulmonary disorder.

Uhl's anomaly was initially described as a congenital disorder with "parchment-like thinning" of the right ventricle. More recently it has been described as an acquired disorder in infants or adults and is called "arrhythmogenic right ventricular dysplasia." This rare form of cardiomyopathy is limited to dilation of the right ventricle with marked thinning of the anterior right ventricular wall. Clinical presentation includes syncope, recurrent ventricular tachycardia, and premature death from early congestive failure or arrhythmias. Familial occurrence has been reported, and males outnumber females by 3:1. Right ventricular ejection fractions are commonly reduced to less

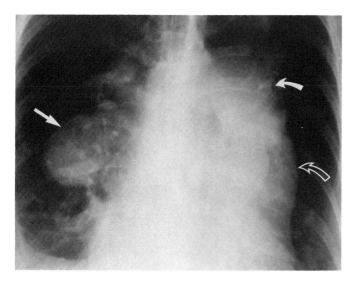

Figure 19.14. Pulmonary Arterial Hypertension. The main pulmonary artery (*open arrow*), left pulmonary artery (*curved arrow*), and right pulmonary artery (*straight arrow*) are extremely enlarged. Faint calcification is seen in the right pulmonary artery. The patient had schistosomiasis with resultant vasculitis and pulmonary arterial hypertension.

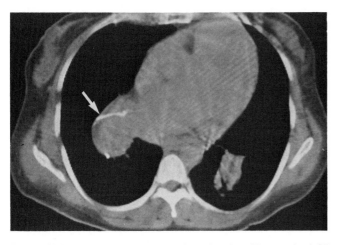

Figure 19.15. Pulmonary Arterial Hypertension. Non-contrast CT scan demonstrates calcification in the wall of the right pulmonary artery (*arrow*).

than half of normal, with mild reductions in the left ventricular ejection fraction.

PULMONARY VASCULAR DISEASE

Enlargement of the pulmonary outflow tract is seen in congenital heart disease with left-to-right shunts. Outflow tract prominence without evidence of a shunt lesion is usually due to poststenotic dilation of pulmonary stenosis, pulmonary arterial hypertension, Marfan's syndrome, Takayasu's arteritis, or idiopathic dilation of the pulmonary artery. Idiopathic dilation of the pulmonary artery demonstrates a dilated main pulmonary artery, normal peripheral pulmonary arteries, and normal, balanced circulation. This entity

is much more common in females and is often associated with a mild systolic ejection murmur, but without evidence of pulmonary stenosis.

Pulmonary arterial hypertension should be considered whenever the main pulmonary artery and left and right pulmonary arteries are enlarged (Fig. 19.14). Signs of right atrial and ventricular enlargement or hypertrophy are often present. Systolic right ventricular and pulmonary artery pressures exceed 30 mm Hg. Other findings include rapid tapering and tortuosity of the pulmonary arteries. The peripheral lung zones appear clear. Calcification within the pulmonary arterial walls is virtually diagnostic of pulmonary arterial hypertension (Fig. 19.15).

The differential diagnosis for pulmonary arterial hypertension includes long-standing pulmonary venous hypertension (mitral stenosis), Eisenmenger's physiology (from long-standing left-to-right shunts), pulmonary emboli, vasculitides (such as rheumatoid arthritis or polyarteritis nodosa), and primary pulmonary hypertension. Polyarteritis nodosa is a necrotizing vasculitis involving the medium-sized pulmonary arteries. Radiographic findings include small pulmonary arterial aneurysms, focal stenoses, small infarctions and signs of pulmonary hypertension. Primary pulmonary hypertension is most common in females in their 3rd and 4th decades. Histologic examination reveals plexiform and angiomatoid lesions with no evidence of emboli or venous abnormalities. Symptoms include dyspnea, fatigue, hyperventilation, chest pain, and hemoptysis.

Increased pulmonary blood flow is caused by high output states and left-to-right shunts. High output states include volume loading, pregnancy, peripheral shunt lesions (arteriovenous malformations), hyperthyroidism, anemia, and leukemia (Fig. 19.16). The main and central pulmonary arteries are enlarged with increased circulation to the lower lobes, upper lobes, and peripheral lung zones. Bronchovascular pairs show enlargement of the vascular component. The most common shunts in the adult are the acyanotic lesions including atrial septal defect, ventriculoseptal defect, patent ductus arteriosus, and partial anomalous pulmonary venous return. Cyanotic lesions with increased blood flow to the lungs include transposition of the great vessels, truncus arteriosus, total anomalous pulmonary venous return, and endocardial cushion defects. Ventriculoseptal defects may occur acutely following myocardial infarction.

Decreased pulmonary blood flow with a small heart is caused by chronic obstructive pulmonary disease, hypovolemia, malnourishment, and Addison's disease. When the cardiac silhouette is enlarged, the differential diagnosis includes cardiomyopathy, pericardial tamponade, Ebstein's anomaly, and right-to-left shunts from congenital heart disease.

Asymmetrical pulmonary blood flow may be evident on chest radiography, angiography or nuclear medicine pulmonary perfusion scans (Fig. 19.17 and see Fig. 19.24). This may result from either decreased or increased blood flow to one lung. Pulmonary valvular stenosis often results in increased blood flow to the left lung. Tetralogy of Fallot may cause increased blood flow to the right lung. Surgical shunts, such as the Blalock-Taussig procedure, increase blood flow to one lung. Decreased blood flow to one lung occurs in peripheral pulmonary stenosis (see Fig. 19.24), interruption of the pulmonary artery, scimitar syndrome, pulmonary hypoplasia, Swyer-James syndrome, pulmonary emphysema, pulmonary embolism, fibrosing mediastinitis, or carcinoma affecting one artery. One must be careful to exclude technical artifacts such as lateral decentering and soft-tissue asymmetry such as mastectomy. The balance of circulation and size of the central pulmonary arteries should be compared as well as the size of the bronchovascular pairs.

Pulmonary venous hypertension may be identified on radiographs, pulmonary angiogram or nuclear medicine perfusion scan (Figs. 18.18 and 19.18). Pulmonary venous hypertension is considered mild with wedge pressures of 10–13 mm Hg, moderate with equalization of upper and lower lobe blood flow and wedge pressures of 14–16 mm Hg, or severe with the upper lobe vessels being distended more than the lower lobe vessels and wedge pressure 17–20 mm Hg. Progressive cephalization is accompanied by progressive secondary enlargement of the pulmonary arteries and filling out of the hilar angles. The most common cause of pulmonary venous hypertension is elevation of left atrial pressures secondary to left ventricular failure (Table 19.3).

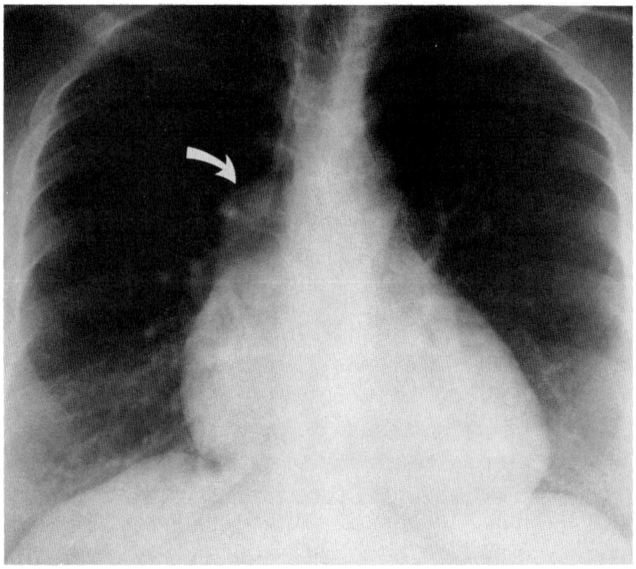

Figure 19.16. High Output Failure. Chest radiograph demonstrates cardiomegaly, vascular engorgement, and distension of the azygos vein in this pregnant patient with severe anemia. The azygos vein (*arrow*) is a good marker of intravascular volume expansion or elevated central venous pressures.

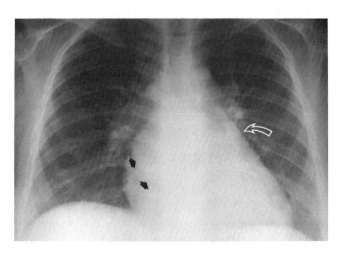

Figure 19.18. Moderate Mitral Stenosis. A chest radiograph demonstrates mild cardiomegaly with straightening of the left heart border, prominence of the left atrial appendage (*open arrow*), and evidence of left atrial enlargement (*arrows*). Cephalization of blood flow and enlargement of the pulmonary arteries indicate pulmonary venous and pulmonary arterial hypertension.

Figure 19.17. Asymmetrical Pulmonary Blood Flow. [99mTc] macroaggregated albumin pulmonary perfusion lung scan demonstrates marked reduction in the pulmonary blood flow to the left lung (*arrow*) in comparison with the right lung. A subtle left hilar mass was causing compression of the left pulmonary artery. *POST*, posterior; *RPO*, right posterior oblique; *RLAT*, right lateral; *ANT*, anterior; *LLAT*, left lateral; *LPO*, left posterior oblique.

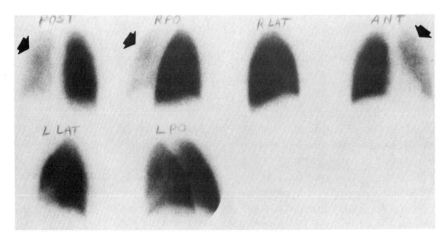

Table 19.3. Causes of Pulmonary Venous Hypertension

Left ventricular failure
Mitral stenosis
Mitral regurgitation
Aortic stenosis
Aortic regurgitation
Pulmonary venoocclusive disease
Congenital heart disease

Table 19.4. Causes of Mitral Regurgitation

Rheumatic heart disease
Congenital heart disease
Mitral valve prolapse
Ruptured chordae tendineae
Infectious endocarditis
Papillary muscle rupture
Mitral annulus calcification

ACQUIRED VALVULAR HEART DISEASE

Mitral stenosis in the adult is usually caused by rheumatic heart disease, with 50% of patients giving a history of rheumatic fever. Rarely, an atrial myxoma may mimic mitral stenosis. The incidence of mitral stenosis is higher in females by a ratio of 8:1. *Lutembacher syndrome* is a combination of mitral stenosis with a preexisting atrial septal defect, resulting in marked right-sided enlargement.

The normal mitral valve area is 4–6 cm². With mild mitral stenosis (mitral valve area <1.5 cm²), the chest x-ray may be normal and left atrial pressures are elevated only during exercise. Moderate mitral stenosis (valve area <1.0 cm²) produces signs of left atrial enlargement and pulmonary venous hypertension (Fig. 19.18). Dyspnea on exertion is common. Severe mitral stenosis (valve area <0.5 cm²) has marked left atrial enlargement, right ventricular enlargement, Kerley's lines, pulmonary edema, and, occasionally, calcification in the left atrial wall. Patients are often dyspneic at rest, with resting left atrial pressure exceeding 35 mm Hg. Palpitations and atrial fibrillation with risk of atrial thrombi and systemic emboli are also common. Long-standing pulmonary venous hypertension leads to pulmonary arterial hypertension. Stages of progression of mitral stenosis are (*a*) stage 1: pulmonary venous hypertension with hilar angle loss, (*b*) stage 2: interstitial edema with Kerley's lines, (*c*) stage 3: alveolar edema, (*d*) stage 4: chronic, recurrent congestive failure, hemosiderin deposits, and ossification or calcifications in the lung.

The chest x-ray is often characteristic with a long, straight, left heart border, left atrial enlargement, prominence of the left atrial appendage, cephalization of blood flow indicating pulmonary venous hypertension, pulmonary arterial hypertension, left atrial calcification, mitral valve calcification, prominent main pulmonary artery, right ventricular enlargement with filling of the retrosternal clear space, and dilation of the inferior vena cava. Echocardiography shows a decreased E-F slope on M-mode, slow left ventricular filling, left atrial enlargement, thickened mitral valve, decreased excursion of the mitral valve with a narrow mitral orifice, parallel movement of the anterior and posterior leaflets, and atrial fibrillation. Gated nuclear

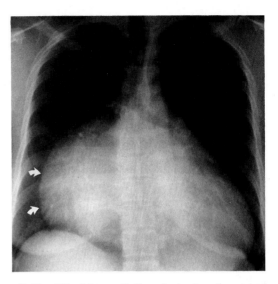

Figure 19.19. Mitral Regurgitation. A chest radiograph demonstrates marked left atrial enlargement with "atrial escape" where the left atrium (*arrows*) becomes border-forming along the right cardiac silhouette. Note the marked carinal splaying due to this massive left atrial enlargement.

angiograms are useful for following the left ventricular ejection fraction. Magnetic resonance imaging grades the valvular disease and determines chamber volumes and ejection fractions. Velocity-encoded cine MR quantifies peak velocity and instantaneous blood flow. The peak gradient across the stenotic valve can be calculated when the echo times (TE) are less than 7 μsec, allowing measurements of velocities up to 6 m/sec. Mitral commissurotomy may be performed if the leaflets are pliable. Mitral valve replacement should be considered before left ventricular failure occurs.

Mitral regurgitation associated with mitral stenosis of rheumatic heart disease is the most common hemodynamically significant form of mitral regurgitation in adults (Table 19.4).

The radiograph shows left atrial enlargement that is greater than that seen with pure mitral stenosis (Fig. 19.19). Left ventricular enlargement is also present. Pulmonary venous hypertension is less prominent than in mitral stenosis. The radiograph is near normal with mild mitral regurgitation, shows atrial enlargement and pulmonary venous hypertension with moderate disease, and shows progressive left atrial enlargement, left ventricular enlargement, pul-

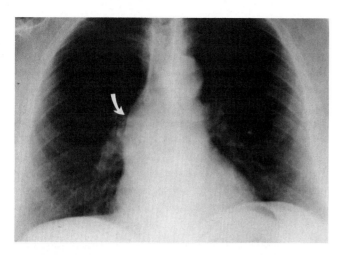

Figure 19.20. Aortic Stenosis. Note the enlarged ascending aorta (*arrow*), highly suggestive of poststenotic dilation in this patient with normal heart size.

monary venous hypertension, and pulmonary edema with severe mitral regurgitation.

Echocardiography shows left atrial enlargement, left ventricular enlargement and bulging of the atrial septum to the right. Nuclear angiogram shows a dilated left ventricle with an elevated left ventricular ejection fraction because of the hyperdynamic status. Magnetic resonance imaging using gradient echo and gated cine mode shows the regurgitant jet projecting from the left ventricle into the left atrium during systole. The regurgitant jet may be graded visually as mild, moderate or severe based upon its distance to the back wall. Grade 1 regurgitation is defined as turbulent flow extending less than one-third the distance to the back wall, grade 2 is less than two-thirds the distance to the back wall, and grade 3 is more than two-thirds of the distance to the back wall. The regurgitant fraction can be calculated by comparing the right and left ventricular stroke volumes, which are normally equal. The regurgitant fraction is equal to the right ventricular stroke volume minus the left ventricular stroke volume, divided by right ventricular stroke volume. Gated blood pool scintigraphy is used to follow the ejection fraction to optimize the timing of valve replacement.

Mitral valve prolapse is an interesting entity that has also been called "floppy mitral valve" or Barlow's syndrome. It is seen in 2–6% of the general population and is more common in young women. It has an autosomal dominant transmission and is more common in patients with straight backs, pectus excavatum and narrow anteroposterior diameters of the chest. Patients may be asymptomatic or have symptoms due to arrhythmias. A "honking" type of murmur or a murmur with midsystolic click is characteristic. The chest x-ray is usually normal, although occasionally patients will develop mitral regurgitation,

left atrial enlargement, and pulmonary venous hypertension. Echocardiography demonstrates a characteristic bulging of the anterior or posterior leaflets during midsystole when the valve should remain closed. This may also take the appearance of a pansystolic "hammock" type of leaflet bowing. Some patients develop myxomatous thickening of the mitral valve leaflets.

Aortic stenosis is caused by partial fusion of the commissures between the aortic valve cusps. Bicuspid aortic valve is found in 1–2% of the population and is present in 95% of congenital aortic stenosis. *Bicuspid aortic valve* is most common in males and is present 25–50% of patients with aortic coarctation. Sixty percent of patients older than 24 years of age have calcification within the bicuspid valve. *Calcific or degenerative aortic stenosis*, on the other hand, is usually seen in older patients with systemic hypertension. Aortic valve calcification is best seen on the lateral or right anterior oblique chest radiographs and implies an aortic gradient greater than 50 mm Hg. Noncalcific stenosis is usually due to rheumatic heart disease and coexists with mitral valve disease. The radiograph typically shows left ventricular hypertrophy with poststenotic dilation of the aorta (Fig. 19.20). Remember that the ascending aorta is not normally seen on frontal chest radiographs in patients less than 40 years of age. The echocardiogram shows dense aortic valve echoes, dilated aortic root, hyperdynamic function, and left ventricular hypertrophy. A bicuspid valve may be directly visualized. The aortic valve area is normally 2.5–3.5 cm². Symptoms occur when the valve area is less than 0.7 cm², or less than 1.5 cm² if there is combined aortic stenosis and aortic insufficiency. Mild aortic stenosis is associated with a 13–14 mm orifice and greater than 25 mm Hg gradient. Moderate aortic stenosis has an 8–12 mm orifice and greater than 40–50 mm Hg gradient. Severe stenosis occurs at less than 8 mm orifice with a gradient greater than 150 mm Hg. Cardiac MR and echocardiography show increased ventricular muscle mass with hypertrophy (Fig. 19.21). Magnetic resonance imaging and blood pool scintigraphy show decreased left ventricular ejection fraction, increased left ventricular emptying time, decreased rate of ejection, and a normal left ventricular filling rate.

Symptoms progress from angina to syncopal episodes to congestive failure with the possibility of sudden death with severe stenosis. Therapy is usually valve replacement, although some cases are amenable to valvulotomy.

Aortic insufficiency is primary when it is due to aortic valve disease or is secondary when due to aortic root disease (Table 19.5). Physical examination reveals a water-hammer pulse and Austin Flint mur-

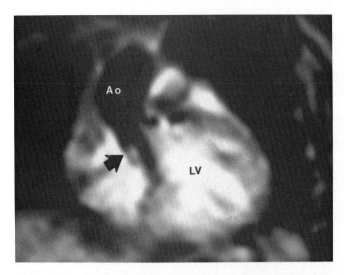

Figure 19.21. Aortic Stenosis. Gradient-echo MR coronal plane image of the ascending aorta (*AO*), aortic valve (*arrow*) and left ventricle (*LV*). Note the signal void in the entire ascending aorta due to marked turbulence caused by severe aortic stenosis.

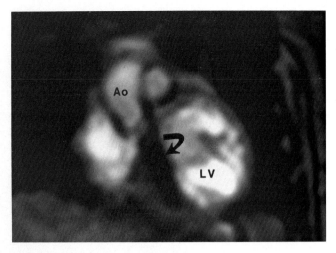

Figure 19.22. Aortic Regurgitation. Gradient-echo MR coronal plane image through the ascending aorta (*AO*) and left ventricle (*LV*) demonstrates regurgitant flow from the aortic valve into the left ventricle (*arrow*).

Table 19.5. Causes of Aortic Insufficiency

Valvular
  Congenital
  Rheumatic
  Infectious endocarditis
  Trauma
Aortic Root
  Syphilis
  Dissecting aneurysm
  Marfan's syndrome
  Rheumatoid arthritis
  Reiter's syndrome
  Relapsing polychondritis
  Giant cell arteritis
Subvalvular
  Aneurysm of sinus of Valsalva
  Subaortic stenosis
  High ventricular septal defect

mur due to vibrations of the mitral valve by regurgitant flow.

Chest x-ray shows a dilated, calcified aortic root with a normal heart size in mild disease. With moderate disease, the left ventricle and cardiac silhouette enlarge. With severe disease, left atrial enlargement and congestive heart failure develop. Symptoms include dyspnea on exertion, fatigue and symptoms of congestive failure.

Echocardiography and MR show the dilated aortic root, regurgitant aortic flow, diastolic flutter of the interventricular septum or anterior mitral leaflet (Austin Flint phenomena), left ventricular dilation, increased wall motion, increased ejection fraction and early mitral valve closure (Fig. 19.22). The ratio of the regurgitant flow width to the aortic root is helpful for grading the severity. Ventricular function may be fol-

lowed by MR, echocardiogram or nuclear scintigraphy.

Supravalvular aortic stenosis is due to a localized hourglass-type narrowing above the valve, a discrete fibrous-type membrane, or a diffuse hypoplastic tubular configuration of the ascending aorta. Supravalvular aortic stenosis is often associated with peripheral pulmonary stenosis and valvular or subvalvular aortic stenosis. This combination of findings are found with Marfan's syndrome or William's syndrome. The coronary arteries are dilated because of the elevated systolic pressure and narrowing of the aortic root (<20 mm). The aortic cusps themselves are normal.

Subvalvular/subaortic stenosis may be a fixed anatomic defect or a dynamic functional obstruction. Fixed subaortic stenosis is associated with congenital heart disease, especially ventricular septal defect, in approximately 50% of cases. Type 1 subaortic stenosis is a thin membrane located less than 2 cm below the valve. Type 2 is a thick, collar type constriction. Type 3 subaortic stenosis is an irregular, fibromuscular type of narrowing. Type 4 is a funnel-like constriction of the left ventricular outflow tract. The mitral valve is normal.

The functional type of subaortic stenosis has also been called asymmetrical septal hypertrophy, idiopathic hypertrophic subaortic stenosis, or hypertrophic obstructive cardiomyopathy. The appearances vary slightly. Findings may be evident with nuclear scintigraphy, but are more obvious on echocardiography and MR. The interventricular septum is significantly thicker than the left ventricular free wall in 95% of patients. The left and right ventricular cavities are normal or small in 95% of patients. Systolic anterior motion of the mitral valve is best seen on echo-

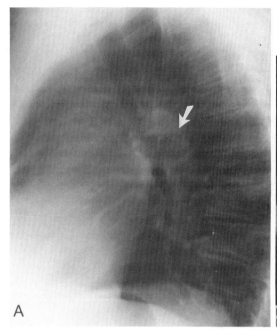
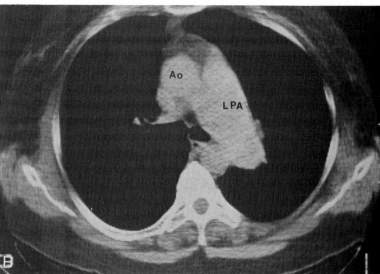

Figure 19.23. Pulmonary Stenosis. A., Lateral chest radiograph demonstrates marked post-stenotic dilation of the left pulmonary ar-tery (*arrow*). **B**, A CT scan through the ascending aorta (*Ao*) demon-strates marked dilation of the left pulmonary artery (*LPA*)

cardiography, but may also be identified with MR. Asymmetric septal hypertrophy may partially obstruct outflow in systole. The aortic cusp may flutter or par-tially close during systole. Mitral regurgitation is a common secondary finding due to abnormal mitral valve position or papillary muscle attachment.

Pulmonary stenosis is seen in approximately 8% of congenital heart disease and is uncommon as an acquired disease in adults. Symptoms may be second-ary to cyanosis or heart failure. A systolic ejection murmur is heard over the sternal border. The chest radiograph often shows dilation of the main left pul-monary arteries with increased flow into the left lung (Fig. 19.23). Right ventricular hypertrophy or enlarge-ment are seen on chest radiographs, MR, and echo-cardiography. Systolic doming of the pulmonic valve is secondary to incomplete opening and is best seen on echocardiography. Rarely, calcification may be identified in the pulmonary valve.

Valvular pulmonary stenosis is due to partial com-missural fusion in 95% of cases. Symptoms typically start in childhood and progress into adulthood. A pul-monic click is common and the electrocardiogram of-ten shows right ventricular hypertrophy. On angiog-raphy, a jet of contrast may be seen extending well into the left pulmonary artery. In dysplastic pulmo-nary stenosis (5% of cases) the cusps are immobile, thick, and redundant. There is no click and typically no poststenotic dilation.

Infundibular or subvalvular stenosis is common with tetralogy of Fallot and often occurs with ventricu-

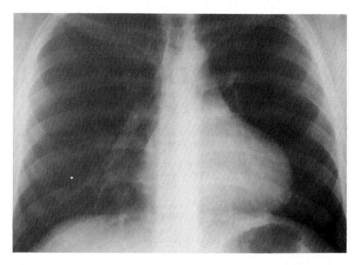

Figure 19.24. Peripheral Pulmonary Stenosis. A chest radiograph demonstrates classic right ventricular configuration indicative of right ventricle hypertrophy. Asymmetric blood flow is noted with de-creased markings in the left lung because of peripheral stenosis.

lar septal defects. Because of the location of the steno-sis, preferential flow goes to the right lung.

Peripheral pulmonary stenosis or supravalvular stenosis commonly (up to 60%) accompanies pulmo-nary valvular stenosis. Sites of narrowing include the main pulmonary artery, bifurcation, lobar, and seg-mental arteries (Fig. 19.24). Associated syndromes in-clude William's syndrome, tetralogy of Fallot, Ehlers-Danlos syndrome, and postrubella syndrome. Post-rubella syndrome is associated with intrauterine growth retardation, deafness, cataracts, mental retardation and patent ductus arteriosus. Williams' syndrome is associated with hypercalcemia, elfin facies, mental retardation, and supravalvular aortic stenosis. Ehlers-Danlos syndrome is a defect in collagen formation associated with joint laxity, skin stretchability, aneurysms, and mitral regurgitation.

Pulmonary insufficiency is very uncommon in adults and is usually due to subacute bacterial endocarditis. Pulmonary insufficiency demonstrates regurgitant flow into the right ventricle.

Bacterial Endocarditis. Patients predisposed to subacute bacterial endocarditis (SBE) include those with rheumatic heart disease, mitral valve prolapse, aortic stenosis, aortic regurgitation, bicuspid aortic valves (50% of aortic SBE), mitral stenosis, mitral regurgitation, congenital heart disease (especially ventricular septal defect and tetralogy of Fallot), prosthetic valves (4% of SBE), and drug addicts. Intravenous drug abusers are particularly at risk for tricuspid valve involvement. Tricuspid valve disease is suspected when multiple septic pulmonary emboli are seen on chest radiography. *Streptococcus viridans* was previously reported as the most common bacteria, however, *Staphylococcus aureus* has now become the most common bacterial agent. *Serratia* and *Pseudomonas* organisms are also common offenders, particularly in certain geographic locations. *Candida* is the most common fungal agent, followed by Aspergillus.

Valve vegetations can be detected in 50–90% of patients with known bacterial endocarditis. The vegetations cause excessive vibration of the valves during systole and the leaflets may appear slightly thickened or fuzzy. The actual vegetations may be seen to prolapse when the valve is closed. The vegetations may cause valvular incompetence or acute valvular destruction. The vegetations, or chronic areas of thickening, may remain even after successful antibiotic therapy. It is therefore difficult to discern acute infective vegetations from chronic changes. Infections of prosthetic valves result in exaggerated valve motion, partial valvular obstruction, loosening of the sutures, and perisutural leak or frank dehiscence. Magnetic resonance imaging is quite good at detecting perivalvular or perisutural leaks. Noninfectious vegetations and focal valve thickenings may be seen with carcinoid syndrome (right heart valves), *Libman-Sack's vegetations* of systemic lupus erythematosus, *Lambl's excrescences* (focal benign thickening), and myxomatous degeneration.

Other forms of endocarditis include *Chagas' disease*, which is common in South America and Africa. Chagas' disease is a late sequelae of acute myocarditis involving the parasite *Trypanosoma cruzi*. This may result in cardiomyopathy or ventricular aneurysm. Patients with acquired immunodeficiency syndrome may also develop an endocarditis and cardiomyopathy, possibly due to viral infections. Indium-labeled white cell scans or gallium scans may prove useful in patients where echocardiography is inconclusive or where secondary endocardial or aortic abscess is suspected (Fig. 19.25).

CARDIAC MASSES

Cardiac masses include thrombi, primary benign tumors, primary malignant tumors, and metastatic tumors. Lipomatous hypertrophy, moderator bands, and papillary muscles may simulate cardiac masses. Since most cardiac masses do not deform the outer contours of the heart, chest radiography is typically not useful, except for the occasional calcific mass. Nuclear scintigraphy, CT, and cardiac angiography identify intracardiac masses. However, echocardiography is usually the initial mode of evaluation and MR may be helpful when there is uncertainty.

Thrombi are the most frequent cause of an intracardiac mass and are most common in the left atrium and left ventricle where they present a risk of systemic emboli. Intraatrial thrombi are usually associated with atrial fibrillation, often secondary to rheumatic heart disease. Thrombosis commonly occurs along the posterior wall of the left atrium. Clots within the left atrial appendage are difficult to detect on echocardiography, but are readily identified with MR. Left ventricular thrombi are usually secondary to recent infarction or ventricular aneurysm (Fig. 19.26). The differentiation of tumor versus clot is best done with MR using gradient-echo techniques. Clots typically have low signal while tumors have intermediate signal. Neoplasms appear as nonenhancing masses on CT or MR. Cine-mode gradient-echo MR is useful for determining the morphology of the lesion. Intracardiac lipomas or lipomatous hypertrophy have characteristic bright signal on T1-weighted images and remain relatively bright on T2-weighted images. Fat saturation sequences help to make the specific diagnosis of lipoma, which is the second most common benign tumor.

Benign Tumors. Atrial myxoma makes up 50% of primary cardiac tumors and is the most common primary benign tumor. It occurs most frequently in patients in the 30–60 year age range and is often accompanied by fever, anemia, weight loss, embolic symptoms (27%), or syncope. Most (75–80%) myxomas are in the left atrium and may mimic rheumatic valvular disease (Fig. 19.27). Cardiomegaly, left atrial enlargement, pulmonary venous hypertension, and ossific pulmonary nodules may be seen. Enlargement of the left atrial appendage is uncommon. Echocardiogram and MR show the atrial filling defect that may prolapse into the left ventricle during diastole. Left atrial myxomas may be pedunculated and are usually

Figure 19.25. Subacute Bacterial Endocarditis. Indium-labeled white cell scan shows migration of indium-labeled white cells to the area of severe aortic endocarditis. Note the marked increased activity (*arrows*) to the left and posterior to the sternum (*curved arrow*) on these anterior (*ANT*) and left anterior oblique (*LAO*) views of the chest. *L*, liver. *S*, spleen.

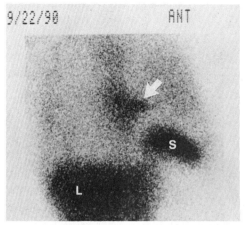

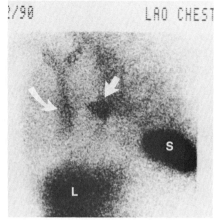

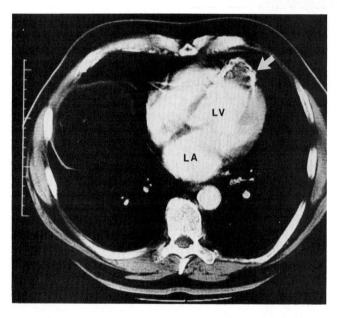

Figure 19.26. Left Ventricular Thrombus. Contrast enhanced CT scan through the left ventricle (LV) demonstrates calcification in an apical, left ventricular aneurysm (arrow). Note the nonenhancing low density thrombus within the aneurysm. LA = left atrium.

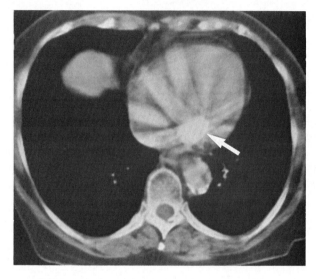

Figure 19.27. Left Atrial Myxoma. A CT scan demonstrates a densely calcified mass (*arrow*) within the left atrium, indicative of left atrial myxoma.

lobulated. On M-mode echo, the E-F slope is typically decreased with numerous echos seen behind the mitral valve.

Other benign tumors include lipoma, rhabdomyoma (Fig. 19.28) (found in 50–85% of tuberous sclerosis patients), fibromas (12% of which may calcify), and the rare teratoma. Hydatid cysts typically show a bulge along the left heart border with associated curvilinear calcification and are at risk for rupture into the pericardium or myocardium.

Malignant Tumors. Metastatic cardiac tumors are 10 to 20 times more common than primary cardiac tumors. Breast, lung, melanoma and lymphoma are the most common neoplasms to metastasize to the heart. Magnetic resonance imaging is excellent for detecting direct extension, intracardiac metastases and

pericardial involvement. Angiosarcoma is the most common primary malignant cardiac tumor, followed by rhabdosarcoma, liposarcoma, and other sarcomas.

PERICARDIAL DISEASE

Pericardial effusion is the most common abnormality of the pericardium. The normal pericardial stripe is 2–3 mm on chest x-ray and CT, and less than 4 mm on MR. Plain films show thickening of the pericardial stripe or differential density sign in up to 63% of patients with pericardial effusions. The water-bottle configuration is seen in chronic effusions. Fluoroscopy shows decreased cardiac pulsations. The normal pericardium contains approximately 20 ml of fluid, whereas it takes approximately 200 ml to be detectable by plain film. Echocardiography detects very small quantities (<50 ml) of pericardial fluid as a posterior sonolucent collection (Fig. 19.29). Small effusions (<100 ml) will appear as anterior and posterior so-

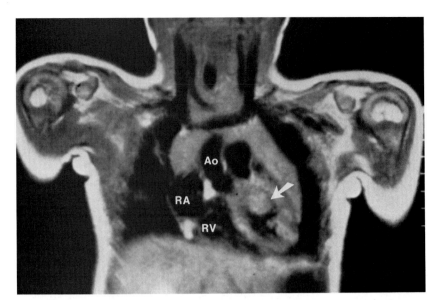

Figure 19.28. Left Ventricular Rhabdomyoma. Coronal spin-echo MR scan through the aorta (*Ao*) and left ventricle demonstrates a large polypoid mass near the outflow tract of the left ventricle (*arrow*). This patient had tuberous sclerosis and a presumptive diagnosis of ventricular rhabdomyoma was made. Note the good delineation of the right atrium (*RA*) and right ventricle (*RV*).

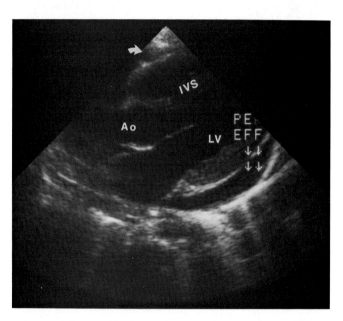

Figure 19.29. Pericardial Effusion. Longitudinal echocardiogram through the interventricular septum (*IVS*), aortic root (*Ao*), and left ventricle (*LV*) demonstrates a pericardial effusion (*PE EFF*). A smaller anterior effusion is also noted (*arrow*).

Table 19.6. Causes of Pericardial Effusion

Idiopathic
Infectious
  Viral (Coxsackie, echovirus, adenovirus)
  Bacterial (*Staphyloccocus, Streptococcus, Haemophilus influenza*)
  Fungal (*Candida, Aspergillus, Nocardia*)
  Mycobacterial
Autoimmune
  Systemic lupus erythematosus
  Rheumatoid arthritis
  Scleroderma
  Dressler's and postpericardiotomy syndromes
  Radiation-induced
Neoplastic
  Lymphoma, lung, breast metastases
Drug Induced
  Procainamide, hydralazine, phenytoin
Metabolic
  Uremia
  Myxedema
  Cholesterol
Miscellaneous
  Congestive heart failure
  Aortic dissection
  Sarcoidosis
  Pancreatitis
  Trauma

nolucent regions. Moderate-sized effusions (100–500 ml) demonstrate a sonolucent zone around the entire ventricle. Very large effusions (>500 ml) extend beyond the field of view and may be associated with the "swinging heart" inside the pericardium. Computed tomography is useful in detecting loculated pericardial effusions. Magnetic resonance imaging may characterize the fluid. Simple serous fluid appears dark on T1-weighed images (probably because of fluid motion), and bright on gradient-echo images. Complicated or hemorrhagic effusions appear bright on T1-weighted images, and dark on gradient-echo imaging (probably because of susceptibility artifact). The dif-

ferential diagnosis for pericardial effusions is listed in Table 19.6.

Cardiac tamponade refers to cardiac chamber compression by pericardial effusion under tension, compromising diastolic filling. Pulsus paradoxus describes an exaggeration of the normal pulse with a drop in systolic pressure greater than 10 mm Hg during inspiration. This occurs as a result of septal shift and paradoxic septal motion during right ventricular filling. Clinical examination shows marked jugular venous distension, distant heart sounds, and pericardial rub. The chest radiograph shows rapid enlargement of the cardiac silhouette with relatively normal-appearing vascularity. Echocardiography typically shows the septal shift, paradoxic septal motion, diastolic collapse of the right ventricle, and cyclical collapse of the atria.

Constrictive pericardial disease is due to fibrous or calcific thickening of the pericardium, which chronically compromises ventricular filling through restriction of cardiac motion. Age of onset is usually 30–50 years, and males exceed females by 3:1. The most common cause is postpericardiotomy. Other etiologies include virus (Coxsackie-B), tuberculosis, chronic renal failure, rheumatoid arthritis, neoplastic involvement, and radiation pericarditis. Calcification

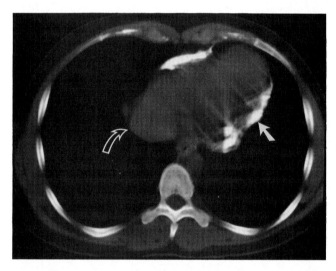

Figure 19.30. Constrictive Pericarditis. Nonenhanced CT demonstrates pericardial calcification (*closed arrow*) and a dilated inferior vena cava (*open arrow*). Note the distortion of the ventricles.

is seen on radiographs in up to 50% of patients. Pleural effusions and ascites are common and there may be an associated protein-losing enteropathy. Clinical findings include ankle edema, neck vein distension, pulsus paradoxus, pericardial diastolic knock and ascites. Chest radiographs show normal to mildly enlarged cardiac silhouette with small atria, dilated superior and inferior vena cava and azygos vein, and a flat or straightened right heart border. Echocardiography shows thickened pericardium, abnormal septal motion, and increased left ventricular ejection fraction with small end-diastolic volume. Small effusions may be seen with "effusive constrictive pericarditis," which has both thickening and effusion.

Computed tomography is particularly good at demonstrating pericardial thickening (>3 mm) in difficult cases (Fig. 19.30). Reflux of contrast into the coronary sinus, a bowed interventricular septum, flattening of the right ventricle, ascites, pleural effusions, and pericardial calcifications may also be seen. Magnetic resonance imaging shows pericardial thickening (>4 mm), dilation of the right atrium, inferior vena cava and hepatic veins, sigmoid septal shift, and narrowing of the right ventricle. Abnormal flow mechanics may also be seen in the vena cava and atria. The finding of an abnormally thick pericardium is important in differentiating constrictive pericardial disease from restrictive cardiomyopathy.

Pericardial cysts are most common in the cardiophrenic angles, right more common than left (Fig. 19.31). They are usually asymptomatic and are more frequent in males. The cysts are attached to the parietal pericardium, are lined with epithelial or mesothelial cells, contain clear fluid, and range in size from 3–8 cm.. They occasionally communicate with the pericardial space. Computed tomography attenuation

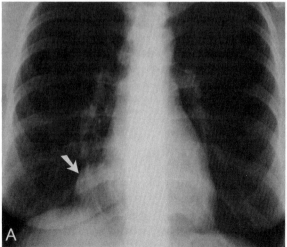

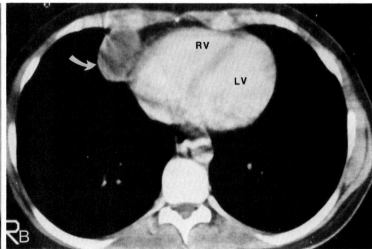

Figure 19.31. Pericardial Cyst. A. A chest radiograph demonstrates a soft-tissue mass in the right cardiophrenic angle (*arrow*). **B.** Contrast-enhanced CT scan demonstrates water density within the nonenhancing mass in the cardiophrenic angle, consistent with pericardial cyst. *RV*, right ventricle; *LV*, left ventricle.

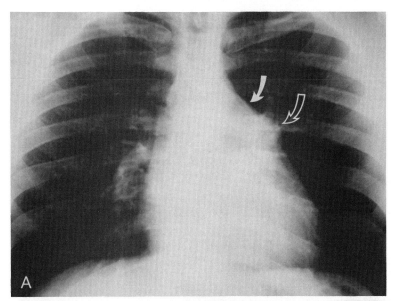

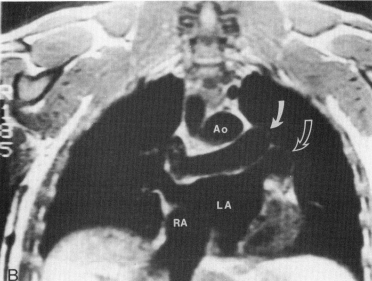

Figure 19.32. Partial Absence of the Pericardium. A. A chest radiograph demonstrates a prominence of the main pulmonary artery (*closed arrow*) and an unusual bulge along the left heart border (*open arrow*). **B.** Coronal spin-echo MR scan confirms enlargement of the main pulmonary artery (*closed arrow*) and shows herniation of the left atrial appendage (*open arrow*). *Ao,* ascending aorta; *LA,* left atrium; *RA,* right atrium.

numbers are 20–40 HU (Fig. 19.31). Magnetic resonance imaging demonstrates characteristic low signal on T1-weighted images and bright signal on T2-weighted images. The differential diagnosis for a cardiophrenic angle mass includes pericardial cyst, fat pad, lipoma, enlarged lymph nodes, diaphragmatic hernia, and ventricular aneurysm.

Congenital absence of the pericardium (Fig. 19.32) is more common in males than females by 3:1. The age at diagnosis is infancy through age 81. Complete left-sided absence (55%) is more common than foraminal defects (35%) or total absence (10%). Associated conditions include bronchogenic cysts, ventricular septal defects, diaphragmatic hernias, and sequestrations. With complete absence, the heart is shifted toward the left with a prominent bulge of the right ventricular outflow tract, main pulmonary artery and left atrial appendage. Insinuation of the lung into the anteroposterior window and beneath the heart is

characteristic. Decubitus views show a widely swinging cardiac silhouette. Partial absence of the pericardium risks strangulation of cardiac structures, with the possibility of sudden death. Surgical closure of partial defects is usually recommended.

Suggested Readings

Brundage BH. Comparative cardiac imaging. Rockville, MD: Aspen Publications, 1990.

Chapman S, Nakielny R. Aids to radiological diagnosis. 2nd ed. London: WB Saunders, 1990.

Chen CE, Cooper C. Review of radiology. Philadelphia: WB Saunders, 1990.

Cooley RN, Schreiber MH. Radiology of the heart and great vessels. 3rd ed. Baltimore: Williams & Wilkins, 1978.

Dahnert W. Radiology review manual. Baltimore: Williams & Wilkins, 1991.

Eisenberg RL. Chest and cardiac imaging. New York: Raven Press, 1993.

Feigenbaum H. Doppler echocardiography. Philadelphia: Lea & Febiger, 1986.

Gedgaudas E, Moffer JH, Castaneda-Zuniga WR, Amplatz K. Cardiovascular radiology. Philadelphia: WB Saunders, 1985.

Higgins CB. Essentials of cardiac radiology and imaging. Philadelphia: JB Lippincott, 1992.

Kelley MJ. Chest radiography for the cardiologist. Cardiology clinics. Philadelphia: WB Saunders, 1983.

Kubicka RA, Smith C. How to interpret coronary arteriograms. *Radiographics* 1986;6:661–701.

Marcus ML, Schelbert HR, Skorton DJ, Wolf GL. Cardiac imaging—a companion to Braunwald's heart disease. Philadelphia: WB Saunders, 1991.

Miller DD, Burns RG, Gill JB, Ruddy TD. Clinical cardiac imaging. New York: McGraw-Hill, 1988.

Miller SW, ed. Advances in cardiac imaging. Radiology clinics of North America. Philadelphia: WB Saunders, 1985.

Miller SW, ed. Cardiopulmonary imaging. Radiology clinics of North America. Philadelphia: WB Saunders, 1989.

Putnam CE. Cardiopulmonary imaging. Radiology clinics of North America. Philadelphia: WB Saunders, 1983.

Ravin CE, Cooper C. Review of radiology. Philadelphia: WB Saunders, 1990.

Taveras JM, Ferrucci JT. Radiology. Philadelphia: WB Saunders, 1991.

Wolfe CL. Cardiac imaging. Cardiology clinics. Philadelphia: WB Saunders, 1989.

Zaret BL, Beller GA. Nuclear cardiology. St. Louis: Mosby, 1993.

20

The Great Vessels

John E. Williams
Arnold B. Honick

IMAGING METHODS

Imaging of the vascular system is unique in that for many years it was largely limited to the relatively invasive modality of conventional angiography (CA). With the advent of both intravenous and intraarterial digital subtraction angiography (DSA), significant improvements were made in decreasing overall patient risk; however these new modalities continued to be relatively invasive. Over the last two decades, computed tomography (CT), ultrasound, and now magnetic resonance imaging (MR) have demonstrated remarkable abilities in vascular imaging and satisfy the need for noninvasive screening techniques.

Computed tomography and MR provide excellent visualization of both the vessel and its relationship to surrounding structures. Both mediastinal fat and aerated lung within the thoracic cavity serve as excellent contrast to optimally display the vascular structures being investigated. Although the MR characteristics of flowing blood depend on velocity, turbulence, and direction of flow, in general MR demonstrates the vessel lumen as "black blood" or flow void on routine cardiac-gated spin-echo imaging and "bright blood" with gradient refocused MR imaging techniques. Computed tomography depicts the vessel lumen optimally only when contrast enhancement is utilized.

Conventional angiography employs film-screen imaging in combination with rapid film changers and thus has the advantage of superb spatial resolution (six line pairs per mm versus 2 line pairs per mm for DSA). Digital subtraction angiography utilizes digital images acquired both immediately prior to and following the injection of contrast with subsequent electronic subtraction of the noncontrast (mask) images from those containing contrast. Its advantage is in better contrast resolution when compared with CA, along with decreased exam time and lower contrast dose. It is severely limited by motion artifact that may occur between the precontrast and subsequent contrast images. Digital subtraction angiography and CA are limited to imaging of the vessel lumen. They provide little detailed information concerning extraluminal pathology and are best utilized in addressing specific questions for pretreatment planning purposes, during percutaneous intravascular intervention, and when noninvasive imaging is equivocal or fails to provide adequate information.

THORACIC AORTA

Anatomy

Arteries are composed of three layers: a thin lining known as the intima, a relatively thick muscular layer called the media, and an outer layer termed the adventitia. These are not typically differentiated by the imaging modalities mentioned and are only of pathologic significance.

The thoracic aorta extends from the level of the aortic valve to the diaphragmatic hiatus and is divided into three main sections: ascending, arch, and descending aorta. The ascending portion terminates at the origin of the innominate artery and is further subdivided into the sinus and tubular regions and lies predominantly within the pericardial sac. The three

Figure 20.1. Normal Aortic Arch and Variants. A. Aortogram with "classic" origin pattern of the great vessels right brachiocephalic artery (*straight black arrow*), left common carotid artery (*open black arrow*), and left subclavian artery (*curved black arrow*). **B.** Normal variant aortic arch anatomy with common origin of the right brachiocephalic artery and left common carotid artery (*curved open black arrow*) and the origin of the left vertebral artery from the aortic arch (*white arrow*).

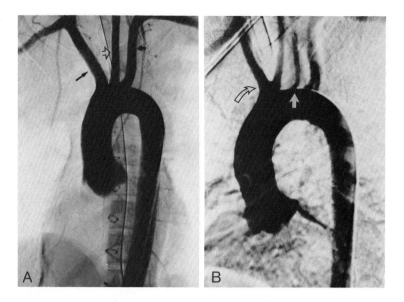

aortic valve leaflets have corresponding dilations within the sinus region of the aorta known as the sinuses of Valsalva. Two of the sinuses give rise to the right and left coronary arteries and are termed "right and left coronary sinuses." The remaining sinus is termed the "noncoronary sinus" and is located posteriorly. At the junction of the sinus and tubular portions, the aorta has a diameter of approximately 3–4 cm in the adult and tapers gradually to 1.5–2 cm at the aortic bifurcation within the abdomen. At no point is the descending aorta larger than the ascending aorta (1).

The aortic arch extends from the innominate artery origin to the insertion of the ligamentum arteriosum, coursing from right anterolaterally to left posterolaterally, in front of the trachea at approximately the level of T-4. It gives rise to the innominate, left common carotid, and left subclavian arteries. This is termed the classic origin pattern and is seen in approximately 70% of the population, (Fig. 20.1**A**). The most common variant pattern is a common trunk for the innominate and left common carotid arteries occurring in 22% of cases (2). The second most common pattern is an arch origin of the left vertebral artery that arises between the left common carotid and left subclavian arteries, present in approximately 5% of cases (Fig. 20.1**B**) The innominate, or brachiocephalic, artery then divides into the right subclavian and common carotid. The remainder of the arch distal to the left subclavian ending at the ligamentum attachment is termed the "isthmus" and may narrow slightly within this short segment.

The descending portion comprises the remainder of the thoracic aorta. A normal variant fusiform dilation along the ventromedial aspect of the proximal descending aorta adjacent to the ligamentum, known as a *ductus diverticulum*, is seen in approximately 10% of cases (2). Usually nine pairs of intercostal arteries

arise from the posterior descending aorta at intercostal spaces 3–11. The superior two intercostal arteries arise from the superior intercostal artery, which is a branch of the costocervical trunk. The bronchial arteries have an extremely variable anatomy and arise from the posterolateral descending aorta, usually from the level of T4 through T7. The most common patterns are three arteries (usually one right and two left) seen in approximately 40% of cases, single arteries bilaterally in 30%, and four arteries seen in approximately 25% of cases.

Basic Angiographic Techniques

There are several routes of access that can be utilized to study the thoracic aorta and its branches. The most common and safest route is the common femoral artery, with others including the axillary and brachial arteries. If the femoral approach is not feasible, the right axillary is the most useful for studying the ascending and arch regions, while the left axillary allows easier access to the descending thoracic and abdominal aorta because of their relative anatomic positions on the arch. An additional access route to the abdominal aorta is the translumbar approach, which employs a direct puncture of the abdominal aorta with the patient in the prone position.

The common femoral artery is palpated below the inguinal ligament with the skin puncture site located near the inferior margin of the femoral head. The artery lies along the junction of the medial and middle thirds of the femoral head. After sterile preparation and drape and following local anesthesia, a small skin incision is made. While palpating the artery, the opposite hand is used to puncture the artery by passing the needle at approximately 45° to the skin surface. The doublewall technique involves passing the needle through both walls of the artery. The stylet is then

Table 20.1. Angiographic Techniques

Procedure	Catheter	Injection Rate (ml/sec/total volume contrast)	Filming Rate (films/sec/total secs)
Thoracic aorta	Pigtail	30 / 60 (CA)	3/3; 1/6[b]
		20 / 40 (DSA)[a]	three frames / sec
Superior venacavagram	Pigtail	15 / 30 (CA)	2/3; 1/3[c]
		10 / 20 (DSA)[a]	two frames / sec
	Multiple side-hole straight catheters	Manual injection[d]	2/3; 1/8
		50 ml total volume (CA)	two frames / sec
		40 ml total volume (DSA)[a]	
Inferior venacavagram	Pigtail	20 / 40 (CA)	2/3; 1/3[b]
		15 / 30 (DSA)[a]	two frames / sec
Pulmonary	Pigtail, Grollman, balloon catheter	20 / 40 (CA)	3/3; 1/6[b]
		15 / 30 (DSA)[a]	three frames / sec

[a]May use either reduced rates / amounts of "full-strength" (76%) contrast as presented here, or same rates / amounts as CA using "half-strength" (30%) contrast.
[b]These techniques are for single-plane imaging; for biplane imaging these values may need to be doubled, depending on the type of equipment being used (e.g., 6/3; 2/6).
[c]Biplane SVC study performed for evaluation of mediastinal tumor involvement.
[d]Simultaneous injection of bilateral antecubital approach with catheters in axillary veins. This technique used for suspected SVC obstruction.

removed and the cannula withdrawn until pulsatile blood return is obtained. This is termed the "Seldinger technique" for percutaneous arterial access. The singlewall technique involves puncturing the artery with a hollow needle through the anterior wall only. After brisk, pulsatile flow is seen using either techique, a guidewire is then carefully passed through the needle and used to pass dilators and eventually the catheter into the artery of interest. The guidewire is advanced within the artery under fluroscopic control to prevent passing the wires and catheters subintimally. A test hand injection of contrast through a newly positioned catheter is always performed to assure intraluminal position and confirm placment within the desired vessel. Careful flushing of the catheter with heparinized saline is done throughout the procedure to prevent thrombus formation within the catheter. Following the procedure, the catheter is removed and hemostasis obtained at the puncture site using manual compression.

For imaging of the thoracic aorta, a pigtail catheter is placed approximately 1–2 cm above the valve. If only the great vessel origins need to be visualized, the catheter may be placed just proximal to the innominate artery, or within the descending aorta if this is the area of interest. The 45° left anterior oblique projection best displays the arch and great vessel origins, but as with all other radiographic imaging, orthogonal views are usually required. If machine capabilities for biplane imaging are available, this can be used initially and supplemented by various oblique projections to best demonstrate the anatomy of interest. When using DSA, either the contrast volume or the concentration can be reduced (Table 20.1).

General Risks and Contraindications. The overall complication rate for the three most commonly used sites for arterial access are femoral (1.7%), trans-

lumbar (2.9%), and axillary (3.3%). Problems related to arteriography can be categorized in to those related to direct vascular trauma and those secondary to contrast media. The most comon problem encountered in arteriography is puncture site bleeding/hematoma, which is of special concern in hypertensive patients. Other less common direct vascular injuries include subintimal dissection caused by guidewire or catheter trauma, either locally at the puncture site or distally within the vessel, and thrombus formation within or around the catheter. Both can lead to vessel occlusion either locally or distally because of embolization. These complications then necessitate further percutaneous intervention or surgery and may, in the extreme, lead to limb loss (3).

Complications related to iodinated contrast administration include renal toxicity and idiosyncratic reactions. Factors predisposing to contrast related acute renal dysfunction include dehydration, diabetes mellitus, preexisting renal insufficiency, multiple myeloma, and hyperuricemia. Most cases of renal toxicity are self-limiting and resolve completely. The best preventive measure is adequate patient hydration, either orally or intravenously. Idiosyncratic, or anaphylactoid-like, reactions are classified as mild, moderate, and severe and appear to be less prevalent with low-osmolality contrast agents as well as intraarterial versus intravenous use. Most reactions are mild to moderate (approximately 5% of contrast administrations), with manifestations ranging from nausea and vomiting to hives, urticaria, and mild bronchospasm, and require little or no treatment. More severe reactions (0.1% of contrast administrations) are manifested by marked bronchospasm and cardiovascular collapse and require immediate lifesaving intervention. Death attributable to iodinated contrast occurs in approximately 0.001% of cases. Risk factors that predispose

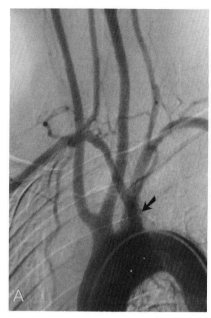

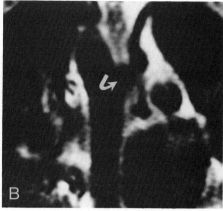

Figure 20.2. Congenital Anomalies of the Aortic Arch. A. Left Arch/Aberrant Right Subclavian Artery: Aortogram shows origin of the right subclavian artery distal to the left subclavian artery (*arrow*). Note the normal variant common origin of the right brachiocephalic artery and left common carotid artery. **B**. *Right Arch/Aberrant Left Subclavian Artery*: Coronal MR demonstrates a diverticulum of Kommerell at the origin of the aberrant left subclavian artery (*arrow*)

to an increased incidence of these types of reactions include prior contrast reaction, atopic history, patient anxiety, and age less than 1 year or greater than 60 years. Prophylaxis with corticosteroids and diphenhydramine has been shown to decrease the chances of idiosyncratic reaction by approximately 50% in those high-risk patients (4).

Congenital Anomalies

Left Arch/Aberrant Right Subclavian Artery. This is the most common arch anomaly, being found in 1% of otherwise normal individuals, and is rarely symptomatic. The right subclavian artery arises as the fourth branch of the arch ascending obliquely toward the right upper extremity and crossing behind the esophagus in 80% of cases, between the trachea and esophagus in 15%, and anterior to the trachea in 5% of cases (Fig. 20.2**A**) (2). A dilation at the origin of the anomalous vessel is commonly seen and is termed an "*aortic divertivulum*," or *diverticulum of Kommerell* (Fig. 20.2**B**) (5). This dilation represents the residua of the right arch of the embryonic arch system and, if large enough, may cause significant posterior impression on the esophagus resulting in *dysphagia lusoria* (6). There is a 10% association with congenital heart disease with coarctation and tetrology of Fallot being the most common. Plain film findings may be normal but not infrequently demonstrate widening of the superior mediastinum and anterior deviation of the trachea. Magnetic resonance imaging and CT demonstrate a higher than normal arch with a more

directly anteroposterior orientation, in addition to the aberrant vessel and its course through the mediastinum (6). Arteriography is rarely needed.

Right Arch/Aberrant Left Subclavian Artery (Fig. 20.2**B**) is much less common, occurring in approximately 0.1% of cases. The posterior arch may lie directly posterior to the esophagus; thus, the retroesophageal component may be due to the aberrant vessel or the arch itself. There is a 12% association with congenital heart disease, with tetrology of Fallot, atrial septal defect, and coarctation being the most common in descending order of frequency (2).

Right Arch with Mirror Image Branching is, as its name implies, a mirror image of the normal left arch branching system and thus has no retroesophageal component. There is a 98% association with congenital heart disease, with 90% of those being tetrology of Fallot (6).

Coarctation. This represents a primary abnormality of the media with a resultant eccentric narrowing of the aortic lumen due to infolding of the aortic wall. It occurs more commonly in males, in a ratio of 4:1, and is extremely rare in blacks. The more common localized (adult or postductal) type is characterized by focal, short-segment narrowing near the ligamentum arteriosum with almost all occurring distal to the left subclavian artery. The aortic isthmus may be narrowed proximal to the coarctation. Approximately 70% of cases are associated with congenital cardiac anomalies, the most common being bicuspid aortic valve. Other associated congenital defects include patent ductus arteriosus, ventricular septal de-

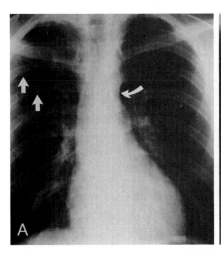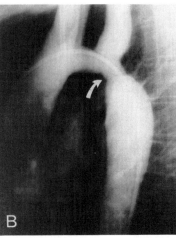

Figure 20.3.   Coarctation of the Aorta. A. Frontal chest radiograph shows inferior rib notching (*straight arrows*) and "3" sign (*curved arrow*). **B.** Aortic arch injection shows "diffuse" type of coarctation, distal to the left subclavian artery (*curved arrow*).

fect, and Berry aneurysms involving the circle of Willis. Coarctation is also often seen in patients with Turners syndrome (5).

Plain film findings include the characteristic "3" sign, formed by an indentation in the contour of the descending aorta just below the knob in the anteroposterior projection which represents the area of the coarctation and resultant poststenotic dilation. Rib notching along the inferior aspect of ribs three through nine represents defects in the ribs due to dilation and tortuosity of the intercostal arteries, which act as collateral pathways transmitting flow to the poststenotic descending aorta (Fig. 20.3**A**) (5). The first two intercostal arteries are not involved because of their origin from the thyrocervical trunk proximal to the coarctation. This implies longstanding obstruction and may not be seen in young children. This is most commonly bilateral; however it may be unilateral if the coarctation occurs proximal to the left subclavian artery, which would produce unilateral right rib notching. If an aberrant right subclavian artery arises distal to a coarctation, collateral flow would be provided via the left internal mammary/intercostal system, resulting in unilateral *left* rib notching (5, 6). Other findings that may be seen on the chest radiograph are dilation of the prestenotic aorta and brachiocephalic vessels, left ventricular hypertrophy, and linear retrosternal soft tissue densities caused by dilated internal mammary providing collateral flow.

The *diffuse* (infantile or preductal) type of coarctation is defined as long-segment hypoplastic narrowing distal to the origin of the innominate artery (Fig. 20.3**B**). This is typically identified early in infancy or early childhood depending on the severity of the stenosis, and has a higher association with other cardiac anomalies (bicuspid aortic valve in 85% of cases) (5). The prognosis tends to be worse than the local type.

The abdominal aorta is involved in coarctation in approximately 2% of cases. The *congenital* form rep-resents a developmental fusion anomaly of the paired primitive dorsal aorta, while the *acquired form* has a number of different etiologies including idiopathic inflammatory conditions, postradiation vasculitis, rubella syndrome, and neurofibromatosis. Imaging will demonstrate smooth diffuse or segmental narrowing and may even present as diffuse hypoplasia of the abdominal aorta.

Magnetic resonance imaging is currently the initial imaging modality of choice for aortic coarctation. Parasaggital imaging in the 30–40° left anterior oblique plane with cardiac gating will demonstrate both the ascending and descending aorta. This accurately defines the site and extent of the stenosis as well as defining collateral vessels. Cine MR enhances routine spin-echo imaging and GRE imaging and provides hemodynamic information as well. Thus, MR may preclude the need for angiography in selected cases and provides an excellent method for postsurgical evaluation. Two-dimensional echocardiography is also useful for diagnosis and follow-up of thoracic coarctations, especially in infants. In addition, it accurately evaluates the congenital cardiac defects associated with coarctation. Transabdominal ultrasound employing both gray scale and color duplex imaging is also useful in evaluating abdominal coarctation.

Angiography provides excellent visualization of the extent of aortic involvement and remains the most accurate technique in defining collateral vessel anatomy, which can be extremely valuable at the time of surgery. In addition, accurate pressure gradient measurements can be acquired.

Pseudocoarctation (aortic kink) of the thoracic aorta is a misnomer, and essentially represents a mild form of coarctation. The infolding occurs near the ligamentum arteriosum, similar to the localized form of more severe coarctation. Patients are asymptomatic because of the lack of a hemodynamically significant stenosis with <10 mmHg pressure gradient across kink. The ascending aorta is elongated with a high, transverse arch and redundant descending portion distal to the kink. The plain film findings are similar to true coarctation, with the exception that no rib notching or other evidence of collateral vessel formation is present. In adults, as the aorta becomes more elongated and tortuous, the segment distal to the kink may resemble an enlarging left upper mediastinal mass. There is a similar incidence of associated bicuspid aortic valve.

Aortic Trauma

Pathology. Aortic transection generally results from a sudden deceleration injury as in high-speed motor vehicle accidents or falls. The laceration may involve all three layers of the aortic wall (40% of cases) or only the intima; most often in the transverse orientation (2). Chronic pseudoaneurysms are formed when a periaortic hematoma is contained by the adventitia or the mediastinal connective tissues. The mechanism of injury is most likely a combination of both shearing and torsional forces at points of relative fixation or immobility along the course of the aorta. Thus, the most common site for injury is the aortic isthmus near the attachment of the ligamentum arteriosum (approximately 85% of cases), followed by the aortic root with fixation at the valve plane and ascending aorta (9%), and at the diaphragmatic hiatus (2%). The percentage of injuries occurring at the aortic root is actually higher, however, these are usually fatal and are more likely responsible for those fatalities occurring prior to reaching the hospital.

Prognosis. This is a highly lethal injury with an approximate 90% mortality rate before reaching the hospital (7). For patients that do survive and in whom the appropriate diagnosis and surgical intervention is not made, 80% die within 1 hour, 85% die within the first 24 hours, and 98% die within 3 months. Those that do survive without the diagnosis being made are at risk for developing chronic pseudoaneurysms, which occur in approximately 2% of cases (7).

Clinical. Asymmetric peripheral pulses, chest pain, and dyspnea are some of the clinical signs and symptoms seen with aortic injury, but these are largely nonspecific and may be masked by other injuries. Relative hypertension in the upper extremities following aortic laceration is known as *acute traumatic coarctation*, but is rarely seen.

Technical Considerations. The technique for catheterizing the thoracic aorta should be performed as already described, with extreme caution as the region of the isthmus adjacent to the ligamentum arteriosum is crossed. Any resistance to passing the J-wire or catheter should be suspect for aortic laceration, and gentle hand injection of contrast should be done. The cusps of the aortic valve must be opacified to ensure a complete examination, and biplane conven-

Table 20.2. Chest Radiograph Findings in Patients with Blunt Chest Trauma and Aortic Injury[c]

Chest Radiograph Findings	Sensitivity (%)	Specificity (%)
Mediastinal to chest width ratio >0.25	95	75[b]
Mediastinal widening >8 cm	75	26[b]
Indistinct aortic arch contour	75	5
Nasogastric tube displacement to right	67	68[a]
Tracheal displacement to right	61	77[c]
Inferior displacement left mainstem bronchus	53	74
Left apical pleural cap	37	58
Rib fractures, first and second ribs	17	70

[a]Adapted from Kadir S: Diagnostic angiography. Philadelphia: WB Saunders, 1986.
[b]Artifactual widening may resolve with upright positioning and optimal inspiration, although this may not be feasible in the setting of acute trauma.
[c]Combination of both nasogastric tube and tracheal displacement may have 96% sensitivity.

tional filming at a rapid rate should be used whenever possible. It is imperative that at least two views be obtained to exclude aortic injury. Digital subtraction angiography is not recommended because of the superior spatial resolution, large field of view, and decreased susceptibility to the motion artifact experienced in trauma situations that conventional filming offers. The examination should attempt to encompass the entire aorta, including the proximal arch vessels and celiac axis, to guarantee a comprehensive study.

RADIOGRAPHIC FINDINGS

Chest Radiograph. There are several well-described plain film findings that suggest aortic laceration (Table 20.2) (2,7). Any one of these alone carries little value in predicting vascular injury, although their presence suggests significant thoracic trauma (Fig. 20.4**A**). At the other extreme, a near-normal chest film may be seen in the presence of serious aortic injury. Because the consequences of a missed diagnosis are so ominous, a high clinical suspicion of aortic trauma based on mechanism of injury alone or any plain film abnormality should dictate the need for aortography! Other causes of mediastinal widening in the trauma patient include venous mediastinal bleeding, which is commonly seen in blunt chest trauma, and complications secondary to central venous catheter placement.

Arteriography. Computed tomography and MR are not presently indicated in the acute setting if aortic trauma is suspected. The findings on aortography may range from subtle intimal tears (seen in 10% of cases) (Fig. 20.4**B** and **C**) to complete transection. Others include traumatic aneurysms (common) (Fig. 20.4**D**), posttraumatic dissection (10% of cases), and posttraumatic coarctation. Multiple injuries are present in up to 20% of patients. A *ductus diverticulum* represents a normal variant bulging of the anter-

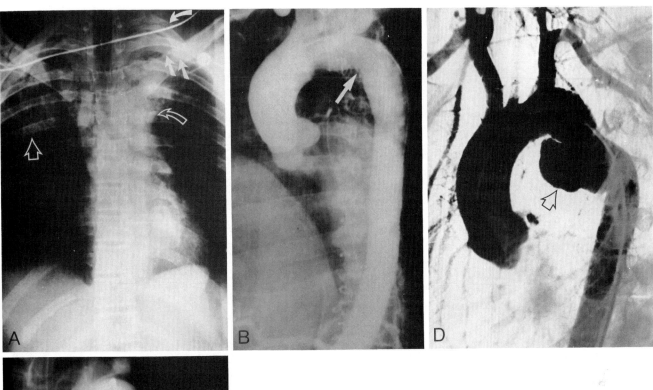

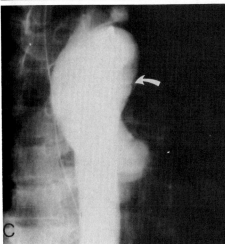

Figure 20.4. Acute Aortic Trauma. A. Manifestations of significant acute trauma and possible aortic laceration on this frontal chest radiograph include a widened mediastinum, ill definition to the aortic arch (*curved open arrow*), fracture of the left first rib (*curved closed arrow*), a left apical cap (*straight arrows*), and a right apical pulmonary contusion (*straight open arrow*). **B.** Left anterior oblique aortic arch injection demonstrates subtle irregularity of the intimal contour in the region of the ligamentum arteriosum attachment (*arrow*). **C.** Right anterior oblique projection of the aortagram in **B** helps confirm intimal injury manifested by a linear lucency (*curved arrow*). **D.** Another manifestation of acute aortic trauma is the formation of a contained rupture or *pseudoaneurysm* at the level of aortic laceration (*arrow*).

omedial aortic isthmus in the region of the ligamentum arteriosum and is seen in approximately 10% of the population. It may be differentiated from aortic injury by its smooth transition with the aorta, lack of intimal irregularity, and absence of delayed washout of contrast material.

Aneurysms

Aneurysms are localized dilations of the vessel wall and may be classified as *true* (all three layers intact) or *false* (disruption of all three layers with containment provided by surrounding connective tissue). The majority of thoracic aneurysms are asymptomatic (1). Symptoms are usually due to aneurysm size with secondary mass effect: stridor and dysphagia due to tracheobronchial and esophageal compression, superior vena cava (SVC) syndrome due to venous compression, and hoarseness due to recurrent laryngeal nerve compression. Substernal chest pain occurs in approximately 25% of cases.

IMAGING

Standard chest radiographs demonstrate contour abnormality and tortuosity of either the ascending and/or descending aorta as well as calcifications within the vessel wall (Fig. 20.5**A**). Differentiation from other mediastinal masses can be difficult and requires further evaluation by either CT or MR.

Computed tomography and MR are the best methods for initial assessment and follow-up of thoracic aortic aneurysms. Both techniques demonstrate vessel diameter, mural thrombus, calcifications, degree of luminal patency, and mass effect on adjacent mediastinal structure (1). Computed tomography is superior to MR in demonstrating calcifications within the wall. Both modalities are used to detect leaking or

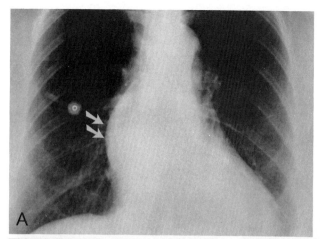

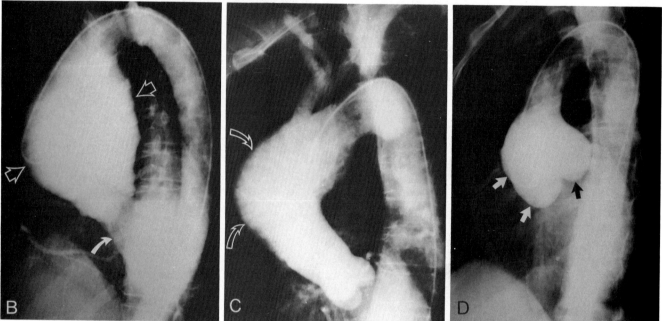

Figure 20.5.   Ascending Aortic Aneurysms. A. A posteroanterior chest radiograph with abnormal convexity to the right cardiac contour defined by a thin, curvilinear calcification (*arrows*) representing aneurysmal dilation of the ascending aorta. **B.** Same patient with marked dilation of the ascending aorta (*open arrow*) with associated aortic valvular regurgitation (*curved arrow*) is seen as a sequelae of *syphilis.* **C.** An *atherosclerotic* ascending aortic aneurysm (*arrows*). **D.** "Tulip bulb" aorta of Marfan's syndrome created by symmetric dilation of the sinuses of Valsalva (*arrows*).

ruptured aneurysms. Computed tomography shows increased soft-tissue density due to mediastinal hematoma and associated left pleural effusion, if present. A focus of direct extravasation is rarely seen. Magnetic resonance imaging will demonstrate signal intensities typical for acute or subacute blood products within the mediastinal soft tissues. Magnetic resonance imaging has the advantage of better demonstrating the relationship of the aneurysm with the arch vessels because of its ability to directly image in the sagittal plane.

Angiography may be reserved for preoperative planning when it is vital to know the relationship with the great vessels and coronary arteries, as well as the vascular supply to the spinal cord. Depending on the type of aneurysm being assessed, imaging of the abdominal aorta may also be needed. Because of the enlarged vascular space requiring opacification, a greater volume of contrast (70–80 ml) may be required. Angiography is unreliable in accurately assessing aneurysm size in the presence of mural thrombus because only the patent portion of the lumen is visualized.

TYPES OF ANEURYSMS

Atherosclerotic Aneurysms (Fig. 20.5**C**) are caused by impaired blood supply to the aortic wall via the vasa vasorum, with subsequent degeneration and loss of muscle fibers within the media. Most are fusiform with irregular walls due to mural thrombus and are most commonly seen in the distal arch and descending aorta (1). Calcifications, like those associated with nonaneurysmal atherosclerotic disease, are typically discontinuous, curvilinear, plaque-like formations. The risk of aneurysm rupture is related to size, with those measuring less than 5 cm in diameter rupturing very rarely, while those greater than 10 cm demonstrate a rate in excess of 40% of cases. The 1-year survival rate for aneurysms greater than 10 cm is 60%, with a 5-year survival rate of 19%. A rapidly expanding aneurysm of any size carries a poorer prognosis (1).

Syphilitic Aneurysms are a late sequelae of the disease and are seen in approximately 10–15% of untreated patient (1). They are caused by obliterative endarteritis of the vasa vasorum following obstruction of these vessels by the treponeme. This results in necrosis of the media, with weakening of the vessel wall and subsequent aneurysm formation. Scarring and contracture of the aortic wall produces wrinkling of the intima known as "tree-barking" (1). Involvement of the ascending aorta occurs in 36% of cases transverse arch 34%, descending arch 25%, and descending aorta in 5% of cases (1). Isolated abdominal aortic involvement is rare. Those involving the aortic root tend to be asymmetric, and are saccular in 75% of cases. Characteristic thin, "pencil-like" calcifications within the media are present in 15% of cases. Syphilis also causes aortic insufficiency (Fig. 20.5**B**) because of either aneurysm or valvulitis. Death results from aneurysm rupture in approximately 40% of cases.

Mycotic Aneurysms are similar to those seen with syphilis and are due to a bacterial infection in the vessel wall with resultant weakness and aneurysm formation. The bacteria can gain access to the wall of the aorta by several mechanisms, including seeding via the vasa vasorum in association with generalized septicemia, septicemia with secondary infection of a pre-existing atheromatous plaque, and direct invasion from an extravascular source. Predisposing factors include bacterial endocarditis, intravenous drug abuse, postoperative aortic surgery, and any immunocompromised state (1). They occur most commonly in the ascending aorta and sinuses of Valsalva, are almost always saccular, and rarely contain calcifications. Mycotic aneurysms account for approximately 3% of all abdominal aortic aneurysms

CONNECTIVE TISSUE DISORDERS

Marfan's Syndrome is an autosomal dominant connective tissue disorder that may have ocular, skeletal, and cardiovascular manifestations. These result from abnormal collagen production and in the aorta is termed "*cystic medial necrosis*," with eventual vascular elastic fiber fragmentation and weakening of vessel wall. Cardiovascular involvement (aorta, pulmonary artery, mitral valve, splanchnic vessels) is present in approximately 60% of cases and responsible for 93% of the deaths. Aortic involvement alone is responsible for 55% of the deaths. Manifestations within the aorta include aortic aneurysms (predominantly ascending), aortic dissection, dilation of the aortic sinuses, and coarctation. The characteristic symmetric dilation involving the sinuses of Valsalva is termed "sinotubular dilation" or "tulip bulb aorta" (Fig. 20.5**D**) This serves to differentiate Marfan's from atherosclerotic involve-

ment; however, other processes such as aortitis can have a similar appearance. Aortic dilation leads to aortic valvular insufficiency in all cases when the aortic root exceeds 6 cm.

Ehlers-Danlos Syndrome represents a group of heritable connective tissue disorders characterized by skin and joint hyperextensibility, soft-tissue calcifications, and vascular fragility. The ecchymotic or arterial type (type IV) is a rare form of Ehlers-Danlos Syndrome and is typified by fragile, thin skin, which in contrast to the other forms is not hyperextensible. The arterial manifestations include aortic aneurysms, aortic dissections, and pulmonary arterial ectasia and may be rarely complicated by spontaneous rupture. Because of the extreme vascular fragility that may be present, arteriography is *contraindicated* and other imaging modalities (CT, MR, possibly intravenous DSA) are utilized.

Congenital. As the name implies, these aneurysms represent a congenital discontinuity in the media and are similar pathologically to intracranial aneurysms. These comprise approximately 2% of thoracic aortic aneurysms and predominantly involve the sinuses of Valsalva, most commonly the right, followed by the noncoronary sinus (1). Congenital aneurysms usually are asymptomatic prior to rupture unless they produce valvular insufficiency due to valve leaflet distortion or there is encroachment on adjacent structures (i.e., the left coronary artery or the right ventricular outflow tract). The right sinus aneurysms typically rupture into the right ventricular outflow tract, while the noncoronary sinus aneurysms rupture into the right atrium. Both of these lesions result in left-to-right shunts. Other less common sites of rupture are the left atrium, left ventricle, or pericardial space. The plain chest radiograph findings are usually normal but occasionally may show enlargement of the aortic root or a contour abnormality along the right heart border if the aneurysm is large. Calcification is rare in a truly congenital sinus of Valsalva aneurysm, which serves to differentiate from one secondary to bacterial endocarditis.

Posttraumatic/Surgical. With the recent increase in aortocoronary bypass, postoperative aneurysms are increasing in frequency. In addition, blunt chest trauma, particularly deceleration injuries, may result in aneurysms. These are properly termed "chronic *pseudo*aneurysms" as the aneurysm wall does not contain all three layers. Posttraumatic pseudoaneurysms occur most commonly in the region of the ligamentum arteriosum and appear on plain film as left upper mediastinal mass (Fig. 20.6). They frequently demonstrate wall calcification but uncommonly contain mural thrombus. Because of low operative mortality and the tendency for rupture, these lesions are usually treated surgically. Postoperative

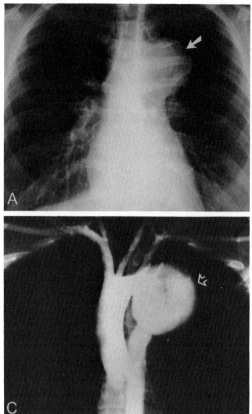

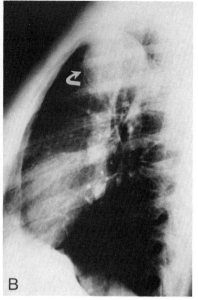

Figure 20.6. Chronic Pseudoaneurysm. A. A chest radiograph shows a double density to the aortic knob with abnormal convex contour (*arrow*). **B.** Lateral chest radiograph defines thin, curvilinear calcification about the enlarged aortic arch (*curved arrow*). Calcification helps define chronicity of the pseudoaneurysm. **C.** Aortic arch angiogram with definition of a large pseudoaneurysm (*arrow*).

aneurysms and dissections usually involve the ascending aorta, while postoperative aneurysms involving the abdominal aorta are located at the proximal or distal graft sites. Computed tomography and MR can be used to confirm the diagnosis; however, angiography is usually required for preoperative evaluation.

Aortic Dissection

Pathology. A dissection is defined as a separation of the layers of the vessel wall initiated either by a tear in the weakened intima or by rupture of a vasa vasorum and resultant subintimal hemorrhage into a diseased aortic media. This may also be termed a "*dissecting hematoma.*" A natural cleavage plane exists between the middle and outer thirds of the media. The defect in the media can either be present on a congenital (Marfan's syndrome) or an acquired basis. Predisposing factors include hypertension, bicuspid aortic valve, coarctation, pregnancy (accounting for 50% of dissections in women under 40 years of age), scoliosis, pectus excavatum, trauma (rare), and prior aortic surgery. Dissections originating in the abdominal aorta are rare and are usually the result of distal extension of a thoracic dissection.

Prognosis. Death from aortic dissection usually occurs secondary to retrograde dissection into the pericardium resulting in cardiac tamponade, massive aortic regurgitation, or rupture into the pleural space. If signs of rupture are present, the mortality rate is approximately 70%, and surgery is indicated, regardless of type. Dissections involving the ascending aorta usually require surgery (8). Those involving only the descending aorta exhibit a mortality rate of approximately 10% and may be managed medically.

Clinical Findings. Aortic dissection is more common between the ages of 30 and 85, and is more common in men in a ratio of 3:1 (2). A history of hypertension is obtained in 60% of cases. Dissection is often signaled by sudden, severe, tearing substernal chest pain with radiation to the back, which is present in 75% of patients. Neurologic symptoms resulting from involvement of the cranial or spinal vessels are present in 25% of cases, and aortic valvular murmurs are present in 65%. Asymmetric pulses in the upper extremities are often found if the arch is involved, and the femoral pulses are absent in 25% of cases.

CLASSIFICATION

There are currently two classification systems in wide use that describe the regions of the aorta in-

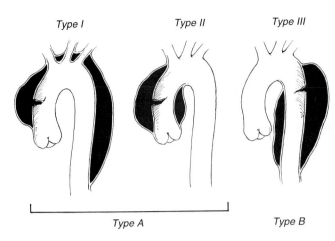

Figure 20.7. Classification Schemes of Aortic Dissection. DeBakey types I, II, and III, and Stanford types A and B. See text for details.

volved and have bearing on prognosis and patient management (Fig. 20.7) (8).

DeBakey: Type I (30% cases) involves the ascending aorta, arch, and variable portion of the descending aorta. Treatment: surgical.

Type II (20% cases) is limited to the ascending aorta and carries the worst prognosis. Treatment: surgical.

Type III (50% cases) originates near the isthmus distal to the left subclavian artery origin. This lesion carries the best prognosis. Treatment: medical or surgical.

Stanford: Type A (60% cases) involves the ascending aorta with variable involvement of the arch and descending aorta. Treatment: surgical.

Type B (40% cases) limited to the arch and descending aorta, similar to DeBakey III. Treatment: medical or surgical.

Technical Considerations. The femoral approach is used for arterial puncture if the pulse is normal or near normal. If not, then the axillary approach is used, again depending on strength of the pulse. Lead with a floppy tip straight or J-guidewire to avoid extending the dissection. *Do not force* the catheter or guidewire at any time. When in doubt, stop and perform a gentle hand injection. The false channel is recognized by inability to pass the guidewire beyond certain points within the aorta. When advancing the guidewire, it may imperceptibly go in and out of true lumen, or the false channel may be entered initially if the dissection extends to the groin. The position within the false lumen is confirmed with test injection, and if attempts to manipulate wire into the true lumen are unsuccessful, then judicious injection (amount and rate determined by observed flow) may be performed in order to identify the reentry point.

The pigtail catheter is then positioned above the aortic valve, and biplane imaging performed. Biplane imaging of the abdominal aorta may be necessary to image the distal extent of the dissection. Delayed imaging is necessary to allow for opacification of the false channel.

IMAGING

Chest Radiograph. Mediastinal widening is the most common plain film finding in dissection (80% of cases), followed by a double-aortic contour or "double-aortic knob sign" (40% of cases) (2,8). Other findings include diffuse enlargement of the aorta with ill definition or irregularity of the contour, inward displacement of intimal calcification >10 mm, tracheal displacement to the right, pleural effusion (more common on the left and suggestive of leakage), pericardial effusion, and cardiac enlargement. All findings are nonspecific but serve to support the diagnosis and prompt further workup in the appropriate clinical setting (Figs. 20.8**A** and 20.9**A**).

Computed Tomography is a valuable tool for evaluating dissection, with accuracy exceeding 90%. *Dynamic* scanning involves simultaneous injection of 2 ml/sec contrast for a total of 100 ml with approximately seven sequential rapid scans obtained at three separate levels in the aorta (mid-ascending, arch, and mid-descending). This method is useful in establishing the diagnosis as well as assessing flow characteristics between the true and false lumen. A second technique, *drip infusion*, uses a slower rate of contrast injection coupled with routine sequential scanning of the entire aorta to provide a prolonged period of opacification. This is best utilized for determining the full extent of the dissection, should it extend into the abdominal aorta. Noncontrast scanning is not recommended.

Findings in dissection include identification of an intimal flap seen as a linear filling defect within the aortic lumen along with the double-barrel aorta representing opacification of both the true and false lumen (Figs. 20.8**B** and **C** and 20.9**B**). The false lumen may exhibit delayed opacification, compression of the true lumen such that the false lumen may appear larger, and contain thrombus in 25% of cases. Other findings include an increase in aortic diameter (usually larger than 5 cm), hemopericardium, and hemothorax.

Magnetic Resonance Imaging is also an extremely accurate tool, with sensitivities and specificities exceeding 90% (8). This accuracy of both MR and CT may obviate the need for angiography in some cases at initial presentation. However, both are the primary imaging modalities of choice in the postoperative patient and in the evaluation of chronic dissection, which occurs in up to 10% of cases. Routine

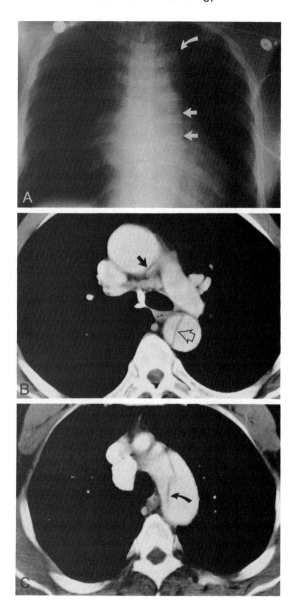

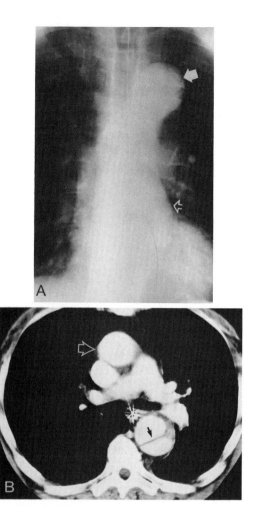

Figure 20.9. Type III (Stanford B) Aortic Dissection. A. A posteroanterior chest radiograph with prominent aortic knob (*open arrow*) and clinical history suspicious for a possible aortic dissection. **B.** Dynamic enhanced CT at the level of the main pulmonary artery with a well-defined intimal flap involving the descending aorta (*closed arrow*). No abnormality is noted in the ascending aorta (*open arrow*).

Figure 20.8. Type I (Stanford A) Aortic Dissection. A. A posteroanterior chest radiograph with widened superior mediastinal contour with double aortic knob sign (*curved arrow*). Irregularity of the descending aortic contour is also seen (*straight arrows*). **B.** Dynamic contrast-enhanced CT at the level of the left pulmonary artery shows the intimal flap within the ascending (*closed arrow*) and descending (*open arrow*) aorta. The larger false lumen compresses the true lumen. **C.** An image superior to **B** demonstrates the utility of CT in defining the two channels within the aortic arch, separated by the intimal flap (*arrow*).

spin-echo imaging will demonstrate findings similar to CT. The intimal flap will be outlined by "dark blood" (Fig. 20.10**A**), representing signal void in the true and false lumens, while GRE MR will delineate the flap surrounded by bright blood (8). This appearance will vary with the presence of thrombus or exceptionally slow flow within the false channel (Fig. 20.10**B**).

Aortography is the procedure of choice in the initial evaluation of acute dissection in order to limit contrast. It is important in preoperative planning in

order to demonstrate extent of the dissection, site of intimal tears, aortic valve regurgitation (30% of cases), coronary artery involvement, and filling of branch vessels (Figs. 20.10, **C** and **D**) (8). The classic finding with aortography is a double-barrel aorta, with an interposed intimal flap seen in 87% of cases. The intimal flap classically begins in the right anterolateral ascending aorta and spirals to the left posterolateral aspect of the descending aorta into the abdomen. Thus, the left renal artery is frequently supplied by the false lumen, and the left iliac is more commonly involved when the dissection extends this far distally. Flow within the false lumen may be slow or nonexistent, which can lead to late filling of branch vessels having their origin from this lumen. Nonexistent flow due to thrombus in the false channel, seen in up to 25% of patients, will appear as thickening of the aortic wall frequently up to 1 cm. The true lumen is com-

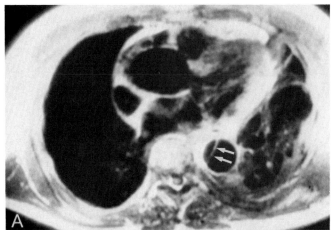

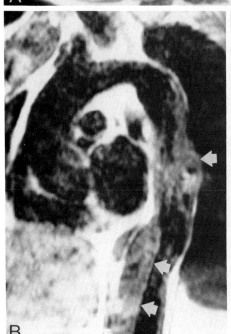

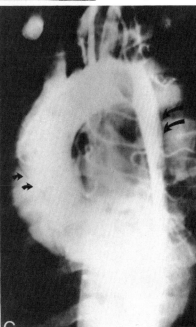

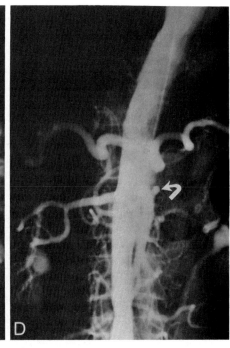

Figure 20.10. Aortic Dissection. A. Axial MR of a type III (Stanford B) dissection shows the intimal flap within the descending aorta (*arrows*). The flap is outlined by dark blood created by flow void on this sequence. **B.** An oblique sagittal MR of the aorta in the same patient depicts a spiraling false lumen (*arrows*) manifested as intermediate signal due to slow-flowing blood. **C.** Aortic arch injection in another patient with a type I (Stanford A) dissection shows the intimal flap beginning within the ascending aorta (*small curved arrows*) and extending into the descending aorta. The true lumen is flattened (*large curved arrows*) by this extension into the descending aorta. **D.** As the dissection extends into the abdominal aorta there is no identifiable filling of the left renal artery (*arrow*) (now supplied by blood within the false lumen).

pressed and narrowed by the false channel in 85% of cases, causing a deformity of the true lumen that may deviate the normal course of the catheter.

Aortitis

Aortitis is an inflammation of the aortic wall that can result from any number of etiologies including *inflammatory arthropathies* (rheumatoid arthritis, ankylosing spondylitis, scleroderma, systemic lupus erythematosus, Reiters disease, and Behçet's disease), *infection* (suppurative, syphilis, and tuberculosis), *radiation*, *rheumatic fever*, and *idiopathic aortitis*.

Takayasu's Disease ("pulseless disease") is an idiopathic, systemic, granulomatous vasculitis that principally affects the aorta and its major branches and, less commonly, the pulmonary arteries. Takayasu's disease is seen most commonly in young females (female:male = 9:1). The *acute* stage is manifested by nonspecific systemic symptoms such as

fever, myalgia, arthralgia, and malaise, with the diagnosis frequently being missed. The *fibrotic* stage is recognized by pulse deficits, claudication, bruits, renovascular hypertension, and other symptoms of vascular insufficiency (9).

Chest radiographic findings include calcification in the aortic wall, a hallmark in young women. On arteriography, long or short segment, smooth narrowing of the proximal branches of the aorta along with focal narrowing of the thoracic and abdominal aorta are seen (Fig. 20.11) Associated aneurysms may also be seen in approximately 10–15% of cases.

PULMONARY ARTERIES

Anatomy

The main pulmonary artery is confined within the pericardium, measuring approximately 3 cm in diameter and 5 cm in length, and extends from the pul-

Figure 20.11. Takayasu Arteritis. A. Aortic arch injection shows diffuse narrowing of the right brachiocephalic and right subclavian arteries (*open arrows*) and right common carotid arteries (*closed straight arrows*). An associated aneurysm is seen within the right common carotid artery (*curved arrow*). **B.** Abdominal aortogram with focal smoothly bordered narrowing of the proximal abdominal aorta (*curved arrow*) and a second segment just distal to the superior mesenteric artery origin (*straight arrows*).

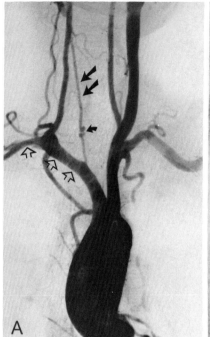

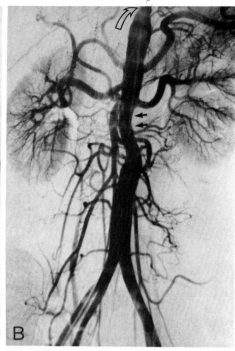

monic valve to its bifurcation into the right (RPA) and left (LPA) pulmonary arteries, which each measure approximately 2 cm in diameter. The RPA courses posterior to the ascending aorta and SVC to divide into an ascending branch (truncus anterior) supplying the upper lobe and descending branch (interlobar artery), which supplies the middle and lower lobe segments. The LPA, which is shorter than the right, essentially represents the continuation of the main pulmonary artery as it arcs over the left mainstem bronchus following the curve of the aortic arch to which it is connected by the ligamentum arteriosum. The LPA subsequently divides into an ascending branch, supplying the upper lobe, and descending branch supplying the lingula, superior and basilar segments of the lower lobe. Normal pulmonary artery pressures average approximately 25/8 mm Hg.

Imaging Methods

The decision for imaging of the pulmonary arteries will depend on the condition being evaluated. For the evaluation of embolic disease, plain film examination in concert with nuclear medicine ventilation-perfusion scanning (V/Q) is followed by angiography, if required. For the evaluation of vascular abnormalities, plain film examination supplemented by CT and MR may be all that is required. Angiography is utilized if there remains doubt as to diagnosis or if detailed anatomic information is needed, or if surgical or percutaneous intervention is planned.

Basic Angiographic Technique

The most common access site is the common femoral vein, although the right internal jugular vein or antecubital veins may also be used. The common femoral vein is located just medial to the artery and is entered by localizing the pulse as in arterial puncture and passing the needle just medial to it. Having the patient Valsalva during this maneuver distends the vein and improves the probability of access. The procedure is otherwise the same, with the exception that gentle aspiration is maintained on the needle as it is withdrawn until free return is encountered. Several catheters are available for pulmonary angiography, with most having a basic pigtail configuration in addition to a special curve allows easy maneuverability through the heart. Balloon occlusion catheters are used in selective cases when detailed visualization is required or standard LPA or RPA injections are contraindicated. Tip-deflecting wires may be necessary to provide further directionality for negotiation of large right heart chambers or congenital septal abnormalities. The catheter is passed via the tricuspid valve into the right ventricle and eventually through the pulmonic valve into the main pulmonary artery. As it is passed through the right ventricle, careful attention must be made of the cardiac monitor to observe for catheter-induced, life-threatening dysrhythmias. The catheter is then directed into either the LPA or RPA and imaging is performed in full inspiration using either CA or DSA (Table 20.1) Biplane CA is the preferred initial imaging modality supplemented by ipsilateral posterior oblique positioning.

Table 20.3. Relative Contraindications for Pulmonary Angiography

Pulmonary artery pressure >70mm Hg
Right ventricular end-diastolic pressure >20mm Hg
Left bundle branch block
Bleeding abnormalities
History of contrast reaction
Renal insufficiency

Precautions/Contraindications (Table 20.3). *Pulmonary artery hypertension* with systolic pressures >70 mm Hg represents a relative contraindication to angiography. Subselective hand injections may be necessary to prevent the complication of acute right heart failure or *cor pulmonale*. In the presence of *left bundle branch block*, catheter manipulation in the right ventricle may induce right bundle branch block, leading to life-threatening complete heart block. Such patients require placement of a temporary pacemaker prior to pulmonary angiography.

Congenital Anomalies

Unilateral Agensis or absence of the pulmonary artery is an uncommon anomaly associated with systemic arterial supply, small hemithorax, elevated hemidiaphragm, and shift of the mediastinum to the affected side. Ipsilateral rib notching may also be evident because of hypertrophy of the intercostal arteries to supply the lung. Ventilation-perfusion scanning demonstrates absence of perfusion with normal ventilation. Both CT and MR can be used to further document the absent pulmonary artery.

Aberrant Left Pulmonary Artery or *pulmonary sling* is caused by an abnormal origin of the LPA from either the distal main pulmonary artery or proximal RPA. The aberrant artery then courses over the right mainstem bronchus back across the mediastinum between the trachea and esophagus to the left hilum. Plain film findings include a small left hilum, right-sided mediastinal mass, indentation of the anterior barium-filled esophagus, and obstructive emphysema involving the right lung, if compression of the right mainstem bronchus is present. Computed tomography and MR are used for further documentation.

Pulmonary Embolism

The correct diagnosis of pulmonary embolism (PE) is essential because the mortality rate for untreated patients is 30%, versus 8% for treated PE. The clinical diagnosis is rarely straightforward, with patients presenting with a variety of nonspecific symptoms including dyspnea, pleuritic chest pain, cough, hemoptysis, and syncope. The classic triad of dyspnea, pleuritic chest pain, and hemoptysis is seen in only 20% of patients with pulmonary emboli. Similarly, electrocardiographic and arterial blood gas changes are unreliable (10).

The most common source for emboli is deep venous thrombosis (DVT) of the lower extremities. Thus, the risk factors for PE follow those for DVT (see Chapter 21). Other sites include internal iliac veins of the pelvis and the inferior vena cava (Fig. 20.12); upper extremities (increasing incidence because of greater use of long-term indwelling central venous catheters), mural thrombus within the right heart, renal veins, and tumor emboli (Fig. 20.13**B**). The risk of PE when a diagnosis of DVT is confirmed depends on the site of involvement. Untreated calf DVT carries less than a 10% incidence of PE, while clot present within the popliteal vein and above places the patient at approximately a 50% chance of PE (11). However, 30% of cases with confirmed PE have no evidence of lower extremity DVT. Death from PE is usually associated with obstruction of greater than 50% of the pulmonary arterial bed. This creates a sudden rise in pulmonary vascular resistance and pulmonary arterial pressure leading to acute strain on the right ventricle and then failure (10).

IMAGING

Chest radiograph. Although most patients with PE will have some abnormality on the chest radiograph, these findings are typically nonspecific and may be seen in a variety of diseases. The most common abnormalities seen are pulmonary infiltrates (indicating hemorrhage or infarction), pleural effusions (associated with infarction), and atelectasis (see Chapter 15). Other less common findings include elevation of the hemidiaphragm, cardiomegaly, congestive heart failure, and pulmonary hypertension. *Westermark's sign*, the most specific finding, is enlargement of the central vessels and segmental or lobar oligemia. A *Hampton's hump* is a pleural-based, wedge-shaped opacity that indicates pulmonary infarction, but is an uncommon finding. The utility of the chest radiograph is in excluding other conditions that can mimic PE clinically (e.g., pneumothorax, pneumonia, rib fracture) and in the interpretation of the V/Q scan (11).

Ventilation-perfusion scans are interpreted in degrees of probability of having PE: low probability (14%), intermediate (32%), and high probability (87%), using the PIOPED criteria (see Chapter 49). A normal V/Q scan essentially excludes PE. The V/Q scan can also be used to direct the pulmonary angiogram to the most likely affected area and determine the optimal projection for best demonstrating PE.

Angiography is performed when less invasive methods fail to provide adequate information or planned therapy requires definitive diagnosis (Table 20.4). It should *not* be performed in the presence of a normal V/Q scan. Angiography is best performed within

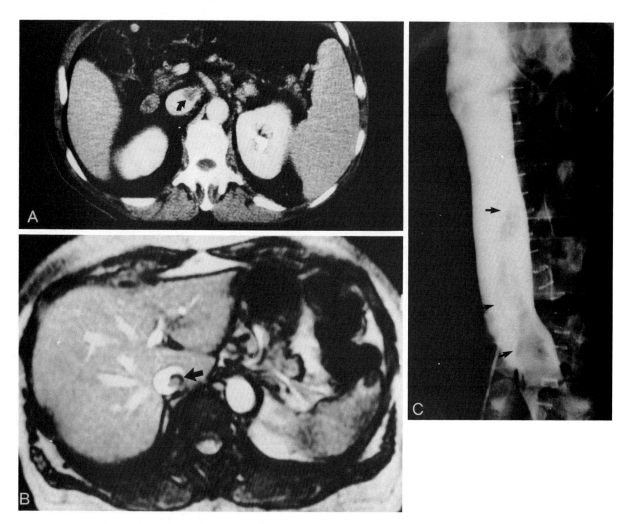

Figure 20.12. Inferior Vena Cava Thrombus. A. Transaxial contrast-enhanced CT of the abdomen with intraluminal clot within the IVC (*curved arrow*). **B.** Gradient recalled echo transaxial MR of the abdomen shows bright signal within blood vessels and intraluminal thrombus within the IVC manifested as an ovoid focus of intermediate signal surrounded by a crescent of dark signal (*arrow*). **C.** Inferior vena cavagram shows an extensive thrombus propagating from the left iliac vein (*arrows*).

24 hours of the onset of clinical symptoms to avoid larger clots from fragmenting and becoming less easily detectable. Most emboli are found in the lower lobes and more often involve the posterior segment (10).

The classic finding for PE is an intraluminal filling defect or vessel cutoff with thrombus extending into the contrast column (Fig. 20.13**A**). Magnification technique may be necessary to demonstrate small, distal emboli. Nonspecific signs include areas of decreased perfusion, prolonged arterial phase, delayed venous phase, and tortuous peripheral vessels. The diagnosis of PE should not be based on these findings alone as they may be seen in chronic obstructive pulmonary disease, bronchial asthma, mitral stenosis, and left ventricular failure. *Chronic PE* represents the residua of unresolved emboli, which occurs in approximately 1% of cases. It is manifested angiographically by stenoses, webs, and irregular tapering of the artery. These changes result in increased vascular resistance and pulmonary hypertension (10).

Magnetic Resonance Imaging and CT have successfully demonstrated large central emboli identified as filling defects using techniques applicable to these modalities. Both are limited by spatial resolution and thus are not currently useful for the initial evaluation of acute PE (10).

Nonembolic Pathology

Pulmonary Arteriovenous Malformation or *pulmonary arteriovenous fistula* represents an abnormal communication between the pulmonary artery and vein, creating a right-to-left shunt. While these fistulous communications may have an acquired etiology (trauma or infection), the majority are congenital. Most commonly, a single artery and vein are involved; however, more complex lesions may involve multiple vessels. One-third are multiple and most are located in the lower lobes. Nearly 60% of patients with multiple pulmonary arteriovenous

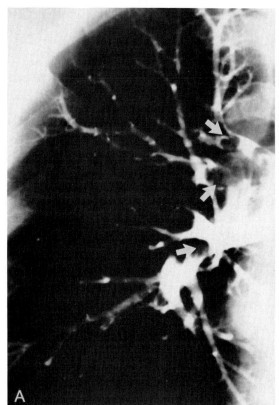

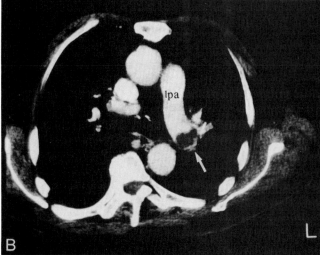

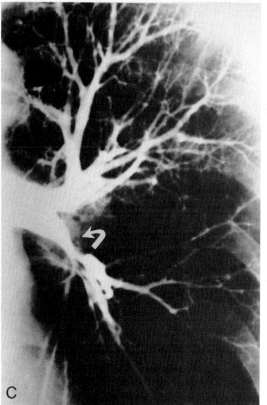

Figure 20.13. Pulmonary Embolism. A. Right pulmonary artery injection shows multiple intraluminal filling defects consistent with pulmonary emboli (*arrows*) . **B.** Contrast-enhanced CT at the level of the left pulmonary artery (*lpa*) with a large intraluminal tumor thrombus (*arrow*) from renal cell carcinoma. **C.** Other causes of pulmonary arterial obstruction include encasement by tumor, as seen in this primary bronchogenic squamous cell carcinoma (*arrow*).

malformations have associated extrathoracic hemangiomas or telangiectasias in a condition known as *hereditary hemorrhagic telangiectasia* or *Rendu-Osler-Weber syndrome*. On the other hand, approximately 15% of patients with the syndrome have pulmonary arteriovenous malformations. Complications of arteriovenous malformations include cyanosis, hemoptysis, thrombocytopenia, paradoxic embolus, and brain abscess.

Plain film findings include lobulated masses of variable size usually located within the inner third of the lung adjacent to the hila. The feeding artery and draining vein may also be detected. Computed tomog-

raphy and MR are useful for documenting multiple lesions and further defining the anatomy. Angiography is reserved for those cases that remain equivocal and for planned embolization or surgery.

Aneurysms. *Mycotic aneurysms* result from inflammatory processes such as chronic tuberculosis (*Rasmussen's aneurysm*), septic emboli, and necrotizing pneumonias. They may rupture into a bronchus, with resultant hemoptysis. *Connective tissue disorders* such as Marfan's syndrome characteristically involve the large central pulmonary arteries. Similar massive dilation may be seen with long standing *pulmonary hypertension* and atrial septal defect.

Table 20.4.   Indications for Pulmonary Angiography

Inadequate information from less invasive studies
    Intermediate probability V/Q scan
    Low probability V/Q scan with high clinical suspicion
    Underlying disease process that may cause false-positive V/Q
        scan
Possible adjustment of planned therapy
    Planned thrombolytic therapy
    Contraindication to anticoagulation with high probability V/Q
        scan
    Contemplate cava filter placement for recurrent PE

Occlusive Disorders. Other nonembolic etiologies that create narrowing or occlusion of the pulmonary arteries include arteritis (e.g., Takayasu's), primary or metastatic pulmonary neoplasms (Fig. 20. 13**C**), extrinsic compression from granulomatous or neoplastic hilar nodes, and fibrosing mediastinitis. *Coarctation* represents fibrous intimal proliferation and may be located either centrally or peripheral, depending on etiology. The congenital type usually presents centrally and may be associated with pulmonary valve stenosis and other congenital cardiac abnormalities. Acquired coarctations seen in the *postrubella syndrome* can be either central or peripheral.

CENTRAL VEINS
Anatomy

The SVC is formed by the junction of the short, vertically oriented right and longer obliquely oriented left bracheocephalic veins at approximately the level of T-1. The SVC contains no valves and measures approximately 7 cm in length and is usually less than 2 cm in diameter. It descends along the right side of the mediastinum and ends in the right atrium at the level of T-3. The trachea, right mainstem bronchus, right main pulmonary artery, and the innominate artery lie posterior and to the left of the SVC. Anteriorly and to right, the SVC is bordered by lung and mediastinal fat. The major tributary of the SVC is the azygos vein, which enters the dorsal aspect at its midpoint.

The inferior vena cava (IVC) is formed by the junction of the right and left (which crosses posterior to the aortic bifurcation) common iliac veins at approximately L-5. It ascends to the right of the abdominal aorta and anterior to the spine to enter the right atrium at about T-8. A rudimentary valve (*eustachian valve*) is present just prior to its entrance into the right atrium. The main tributaries of the IVC are the hepatic (T-10), renal (L-2), right adrenal and gonadal, and lumbar veins.

The azygos venous system is an asymmetrically paired paravertebral venous complex that provides an important collateral communication between the SVC and IVC. This system is divided into the *azygos* and *hemiazygos* veins, which lie to the right and the left of the spine, respectively. They are derived from their respective supracardinal vein. Both are continuations of the ascending lumbar and subcostal veins and begin at approximately L-1 level. The azygos follows the aorta through the diaphragm and into the chest to the T-6 level,where it arches anteriorly over the right mainstem bronchus to join the SVC. The hemiazygos vein ascends into the chest and traverses the midline to join the azygos vein at approximately T-8.

IMAGING

Computed tomography and MR are the best noninvasive methods for evaluating both congenital and pathologic entities involving the vena cava and azygos systems. Venography may be reserved for cases where more anatomic detail and functional characteristics are required, or as a precursor to intervention (Table 20.1).

Congenital Anomalies

Left SVC occurs in approximately 0.3% of the population and represents a persistence of the left anterior cardinal vein. The left SVC descends through the left mediastinum anterior to the aorta and left main pulmonary artery to join the coronary sinus, which subsequently drains into the right atrium. The coronary sinus is enlarged to accommodate the increased flow. A double SVC (left SVC with a normal right SVC) is the most common variation (85% of cases) and approximately one third of these will have a transverse anastamosis between the paired cavas; a single left SVC is rare. Approximately 75% of left SVC are asymptomatic, while the remainder are associated with a variety of congenital cardiac anomalies (12).

Azygos Continuation of the IVC represents absence of the intrahepatic portion of the IVC because of failure of the right subcardinal vein to anastomose with the hepatic veins. It occurs in approximately 0.6% of patients with congenital heart disease. The hepatic veins drain directly into the right atrium via the posthepatic segment of the IVC, and the renal and iliac veins drain via the azygos and hemiazygos systems. Findings due to the increased flow carried by the azygos include dilation of the azygos vein, azygos arch, and the SVC (Fig. 20.14). Hemiazygos continuation is much less common and may drain via the normal communication with the azygos vein, through a persistent left SVC, or by the accessory hemiazygos system (13).

Duplicated IVC is present in approximately 3% of the population and represents a persistence of the right and left supracardinal veins. The left IVC is a continuation of the left iliac vein and ascends to the left of the aorta before crossing over to join the right IVC, usually via the left renal vein (Fig. 20.15).

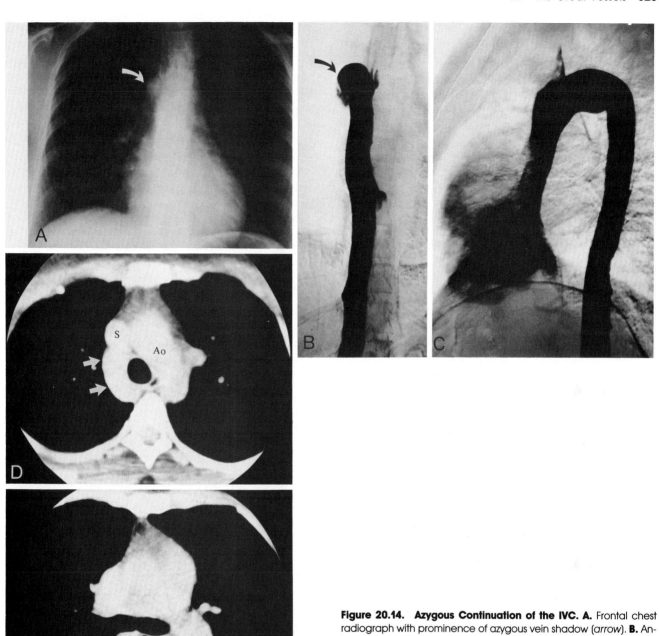

Figure 20.14. Azygous Continuation of the IVC. A. Frontal chest radiograph with prominence of azygous vein shadow (*arrow*). **B.** Anteroposterior view of contrast injection into the IVC show continuity with the enlarged azygous vein (*arrow*). **C.** Lateral view outlines the expected course of the azygous vein and its continuity with the SVC. **D.** Contrast-enhanced chest CT shows an enlarged azygous vein (*arrows*) joining SVC (S); *Ao,* aorta. **E.** Computed tomography inferior to **D.** demonstrates the enlarged but normally positioned azygous vein (*arrow*). *Ao,* aorta.

Left IVC without a normal right IVC occurs in approximately 0.2% of the population and, similar to the duplicated IVC, crosses the midline at the level of the renal veins and ascends normally into the intrahepatic segment.

Retroaortic/Circumaortic Left Renal Vein. The circumaortic left renal vein essentially represents a venous ring encircling the aorta to join the IVC. It is slightly more common (8% of cases) than the retroaortic left renal vein (2%), which crosses behind the aorta instead of its usual path anterior to the aorta.

Occlusive Disorders

Superior Vena Cava Obstruction results from either extrinsic compression or intraluminal thrombosis, which in turn leads to marked venous hypertension in the head and upper extremities known as *SVC syndrome.* This is manifested clinically as progressive dilation of the veins of the head and upper extremities; edema and plethora of the face, neck, and upper torso; cyanosis and conjunctival edema; dizziness, syncope, and headaches; and respiratory distress due to airway edema. If obstruction occurs slowly, a compensatory collateral network via the azygos, internal mammary, vertebral, and/or lateral thoracic veins will develop, and the clinical complex may not be readily apparent (Fig. 20.16**A**).

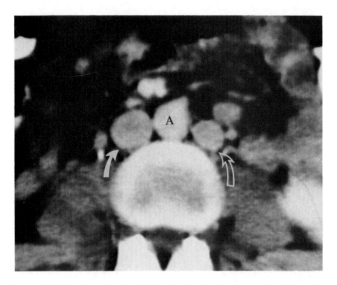

Figure 20.15. Duplicated IVC. Contrast-enhanced CT of the abdomen shows two vessels on either side of the aorta (A), consistent with duplication of the IVC (arrows). More inferior images defined the left IVC in continuity with the left common iliac vein.

Causes of SVC obstruction include malignancy, thrombosis from long term indwelling central venous catheters (Fig. 20.16**B**), mediastinal granulomatous disease, aortic aneurysm, and fibrosing mediastinitis. Malignancy is by far the most common cause (65–97% of cases) and may extrinsically compress or directly invade the lumen (Fig. 20.16**C**), or occlude the lumen by tumor thrombus. The majority of these are secondary to primary bronchogenic carcinoma, with the remainder caused by lymphoma and metastatic disease. Breast carcinoma is the most common metastatic process to cause SVC syndrome (14).

Inferior Vena Cava Obstruction, similar to SVC obstruction, is most commonly due to tumor. Renal cell carcinoma is the most common tumor to cause intraluminal obstruction by extension via the renal veins. Retroperitoneal lymphadenopathy is typically the cause for extrinsic compression in the adult, with renal and adrenal tumors predominating in children.

Nonneoplastic causes include thrombus extension from the lower extremities (Fig. 20.12), following placement of caval filters (Fig. 20.17) or surgical clip, coagulopathy, congestive heart failure, infection, and Budd-Chiari syndrome (which may be due to thrombotic occlusion or membranous obstruction of the suprahepatic IVC, or due to primary hepatic venous obstruction). Extrinsic nonneoplastic causes include

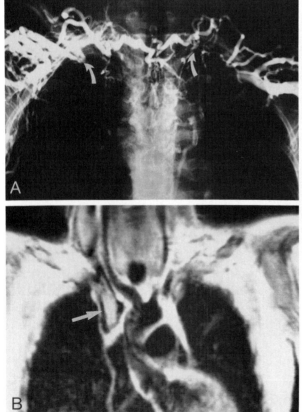

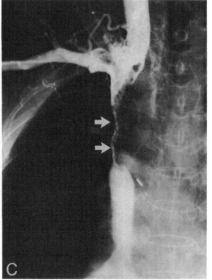

Figure 20.16. Superior Vena Cava Obstruction. A. Complete SVC obstruction recruits collateral veins (arrows) to permit venous return from the upper extremity. **B.** Coronal MR shows bright signal (arrow) within the SVC, consistent with thrombus. **C.** Contrast injection into the right subclavian vein displays a near-complete obstruction of the SVC created by tumor invasion (arrows).

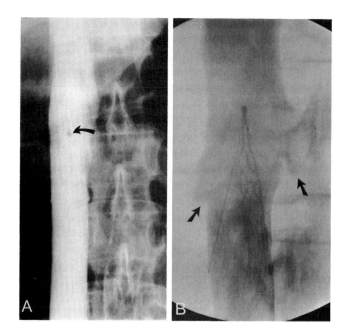

Figure 20.17. **Inferior Vena Cava Filter. A.** Inferior vena cavagram show a small thrombus within the filter (*arrow*). **B.** This subtraction image from a contrast injection into the IVC shows ideal placement of a Greenfield filter. Placement just inferior to the renal veins (*arrows*) limits potential dead space for thrombus formation.

hepatomegaly, massive ascites, retroperitoneal fibrosis, or inflammatory abdominal aortic aneurysm. Functional obstruction can result from compression by the gravid uterus or a large abdominal mass without primary involvement of the IVC.

Vena Cava Filters

Vena Cava Filters are devices placed percutaneously in the IVC with the goal of preventing pulmonary emboli by trapping clot fragments originating in the lower extremities or pelvis (Fig. 20.17**A**). The indications for filter placement include recurrent PE on adequate anticoagulation, patients in whom there is a contraindication to anticoagulation, and preoperative patients who are at an inordinate risk for PE. Prior to filter placement, an inferior vena cavogram is performed (Table 2.1) to assess the following: (*a*) presence of IVC thrombus, (*b*) caval size (if cava is too large a filter may not anchor properly, leading to filter migration), (*c*) level of the renal veins, and (*d*) presence of IVC and renal vein anomalies. Ideally, filters

are placed in the infrarenal IVC adjacent to the most inferior renal vein in order to provide flow across the filter to prevent clot propagation above the filter should it become filled with thrombus (Fig. 20.17**B**). Filters may be inserted from either a femoral or internal jugular vein approach, and placed above the renal veins if clot extends to the level of the renal veins. The recurrent PE rate for IVC filters ranges from 2 to 5% and a caval thrombosis rate of approximately 35%, depending on brand of filter (15). Complications include filter migration, tilting or malpositioning, caval perforation, and femoral and IVC thrombosis.

References:

1. Posniak HV, Demos TC, Marsan RE: Computed tomography of the normal aorta and thoracic aneurysms. Semin Roentgenol 1989;24:7–21.
2. Kadir S: Diagnostic angiography. Philadelphia: WB Saunders, 1986:124–171.
3. Hessel SJ, Adams DF: Complications of angiography. Radiology 1981;138:273–281.
4. Cohan RH, Dunnick NR. Intravascular contrast media: adverse reactions. AJR 1987; 149:665–670.
5. Jaffe RB: Radiographic manifestations of congenital anomalies of the aortic arch. Radio Clin North Am 1991;29:319–334.
6. Predy TA, McDonald V, Demos TC, Moncada R: CT of congenital anomalies of the aortic arch. Semin Roentgenol 1989;24:96-111.
7. Dee PM: The radiology of chest trauma. Radiol Clin North Am 1992;30:291–306.
8. Petsanick JP: Radiologic evaluation of aortic dissection. Radiology 1991;180:297–305
9. Stanson AW: Roentgenographic findings in major vasculitic syndromes. Rheum Dis Clin North Am 1990;16:293–308.
10. Dunnick NR, Newman GE, Perlmutt LM, Braun SD: Pulmonary embolism. Curr Prob Diagn Radiol 1988;17:203–27.
11. Ferris EJ: Deep venous thrombosis and pulmonary embolism: correlative evaluation and therapeutic implications. AJR 1992;159:1149–1155.
12. Cormier MG, Yedlicka JW, Gray RJ, Moncada R: Congenital anomalies of the superior vena cava: a CT study. Semin Roentgenol 1989;24:77–83.
13. Dudiak CM, Olson MC, Posniak HV: Abnormalities of the azygos system: CT evaluation. Semin Roentgenol, 1989;24:47–55
14. Yedlicka JW, Schultz K, Moncada R, Flisak M: CT findings in superior vena cava obstruction. Semin Roentgenol 1989;24:84–90.
15. Dorfman GS. Percutaneous inferior vena caval filters. Radiology 1990;174:987–992.

21

The Peripheral Vessels

John E. Williams
Arnold B. Honick

IMAGING METHODS

Imaging of the peripheral vasculature is done primarily by conventional angiography (CA) and intraarterial digital subtraction angiography (DSA). The principles of both these modalities, including their relative merits and disadvantages, have been discussed in Chapter 20. For lower extremity imaging, most angiographic equipment employs "step-table" capability using CA and DSA acquisition techniques. This involves synchronous contrast injection in the distal aorta with regular, sequential movements of the table. Rapid filming is done at each table stop, thus gaining maximal contrast utilization while imaging both lower extremities simultaneously. In addition, many modern angiographic suites utilize "C-arm" mounted image intensifier units coupled to both the digital imaging train and rapid film changer. This facilitates oblique imaging in order to optimally visualize the anatomy, thus obviating the need to move the patient, which may be difficult in certain clinical situations.

Computed tomography (CT) currently has limited use in the peripheral system but remains a mainstay in the evaluation of the abdominal aorta and the pelvic vessels. Magnetic resonance imaging (MR), with its inherent multiplanar imaging capability, is likewise well suited for evaluation of abdominal aorta. In addition, with the advent of flow-sensitive gradient-echo techniques and cine acquisition, MR angiography has demonstrated its applicability for noninvasive imaging of the peripheral vascular system.

Ultrasound is well suited for screening examinations of the abdominal aorta and proximal iliac arteries, usually for the detection of aneurysms. In addition, duplex ultrasound supplemented with color Doppler ultrasound is well established in noninvasive vascular evaluation of both the arterial and venous system of the neck and extermities. Thus, a basic understanding of Doppler physics is fundamental to the use and interpretation of vascular sonography.

Basic Doppler Physics

The Doppler equation is the foundation of interrogation and definition of blood flow in vascular structures (Fig. 21.1). The *Doppler effect* is a change in the frequency of sound due to motion of a reflector, which in this case is the red blood cell. The *Doppler shift* frequency is the difference between the frequency of the transmitted ultrasound beam from the transducer and the frequency of the reflected sound wave. Blood flow velocity, as defined by the Doppler equation, is proportional to the cosine of the angle (θ) between the ultrasound beam and the flowing blood pool, the speed of sound in body tissues (a constant: ~1540 m/sec), the frequency of the ultrasound transducer, and the frequency change between transmitted and received sound (1). Utilizing the Doppler equation, frequency shifts are converted to velocities; thus, velocity is now independent of the frequency of the transducer utilized and is easier to use for comparison studies. Ideally, the angle θ of 0° should be used. In practice,

$$\Delta F = \frac{2\,(V)\,(F_t)\,\cos\theta}{C}$$

ΔF = frequency shift

F_t = transducer frequency

C = velocity of sound in tissue (~1540 m/sec)

θ = angle between blood vessel and ultrasound beam

V = velocity of blood

Figure 21.1. Doppler Equation.

Table 21.1. High and Low Resistance Doppler Waveforms in Blood Vessels

High resistance waveforms
Sharp velocity upstroke in systole
Sharp fall following cardiac contraction
Possible postsystolic flow reversal
Limited or no diastolic forward flow

Examples: subclavian artery, ECA, arteries supplying muscular beds

Low resistance waveforms
Slow rise in systole
Gradual decrease after cardiac contraction
Flow never reaches baseline with continual forward flow in diastole
Flow never reaches zero baseline

Examples: umbilical artery, ICA, hepatic artery

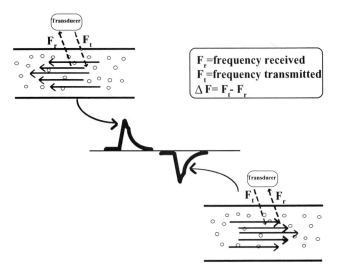

Figure 21.2. Doppler Ultrasound Spectral Display.

F_r = frequency received
F_t = frequency transmitted
$\Delta F = F_t - F_r$

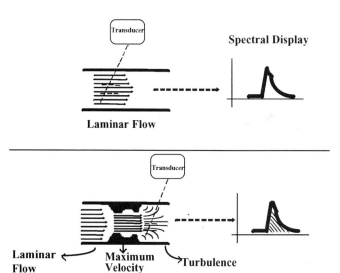

Figure 21.3. Laminar and Turbulent Flow on Duplex Ultrasound.

angles between 30 and 60° are utilized, with angles greater than 60° resulting in precipitous data loss.

Doppler signals returning to the transducer are analyzed and displayed as functions of time and velocity represented by a spectral display. In normal vessels the flow of blood is described as laminar. This means that in any well-defined portion of the blood vessel, there is a narrow range of velocities of the blood pool. The Doppler spectrum is thus displayed as a well-defined line, varying with systole and diastole (Fig. 21.2). Flow directed toward the Doppler beam is displayed as signal above the baseline, and flow away from the transducer as signal below the baseline (Fig. 21.2). Utilizing the characteristics of these waveforms, blood vessels are defined as being of low or high resistance (Table 21.1, see Fig. 21.5, **C** and **D**). This is determined by their function and the vascular beds they supply. Stenosis leads to turbulence of flow and loss of laminar characteristics, leading to varying velocities of individual red blood cells. This causes *spectral broadening*, depicted by "filling in" of the

spectral display, in a region of the vessel just distal to an area of stenosis (Fig. 21.3). This turbulence is maximal within 1 cm of the stenotic lesion. There is maximal elevation of blood flow velocity in the region of a stenotic lesion as well (Fig. 21.3, see Color Plate Fig. 21.3).

Duplex ultrasound combines B-mode gray scale imaging and Doppler scanning. This modality provides an accurate method to both quantify and characterize the significance of vascular pathology.

Color Doppler ultrasound is used as an adjunct to duplex sonography as it displays flowing blood in a color scheme on a real-time B-mode gray scale image (Color Plate Fig. 21.1). Mean velocity is assigned to picture elements (pixels) of the gray scale image. The typical color map displays flow toward the transducer as red and away from the transducer as blue, although any color spectrum can be used. Color Doppler ultrasound better depicts regions of turbulence and marked velocity elevation and can be used to more

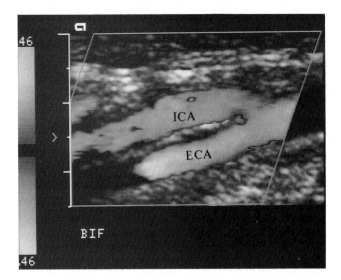

Color Plate Figure 21.1.   Normal Carotid Artery Color Doppler Ultrasound. Longitudinal color image of the carotid artery bifurcation. Note the homogeneous graduated color pattern within the common carotid, internal carotid (*ICA*), and external carotid (*ECA*), indicating laminar flow.

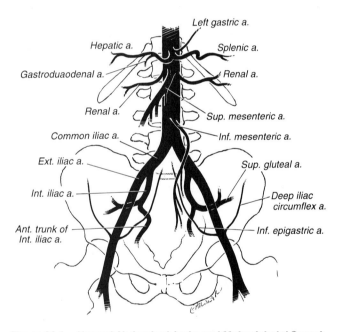

Figure 21.4.   Normal Abdominal Aorta and Major Arterial Branch Anatomy.

rapidly and efficiently perform pulsed Doppler interrogation of a blood vessel (2).

SYSTEMIC ARTERIES

Anatomy

Abdominal Aorta.   The abdominal aorta begins at the diaphragmatic hiatus and extends to its bifurcation into the right and left common iliac arteries at approximately L-4 (Fig. 21.4) It is positioned just slightly to the left of midline and measures less than

2.5 cm in diameter, tapering gradually to measure 1.5–2 cm at the bifurcation. Main branches and their approximate levels of origin include the celiac axis (T-12), superior mesenteric artery (T-12/L-1), inferior mesenteric artery (L-3), all of which arise from the ventral aorta, and the paired renal arteries (L-2), which arise laterally. A single renal artery to each kidney is present in approximately two-thirds of the population while multiple renal arteries occur in the remainder, with unilateral multiple more common than bilateral multiple. Other branch vessels include paired phrenic, adrenal, and gonadal arteries in addition to four pairs of lumbar arteries. All of these arise from the posterolateral aorta.

Neck.   The *right common carotid* artery arises from the bifurcation of the innominate artery. The *left common carotid* arises directly from the aortic arch, although it may have a common origin with the innominate artery in approximately 20% of individuals. Both common carotid arteries then bifurcate into the *internal* (ICA) and *external* (ECA) carotid arteries, with the division occurring anywhere from the C-1 to T-2 levels but most commonly at C3-4 level (Fig. 21.5). The ICA courses posterolateral to the ECA initially, then crosses to ascend slightly medial to the ECA. The *vertebral* arteries are the first branches of the subclavian arteries, with the left the same size or larger than the right in 75% of cases. They ascend within the transverse foramen of C-6 to C-2.

Upper Extremity.   The right subclavian artery arises from the innominate artery, while the left subclavian artery rises directly from the aortic arch. Both extend to the lateral aspect of the first rib and give rise to the following major branches, in order: *vertebral*, *internal mammary* (arises opposite the vertebral artery and descends to anastamose with the intercostal arteries and the superior epigastric artery), *thyrocervical trunk* (gives rise to inferior thyroid, superficial cervical, and suprascapular artery), *costocervical trunk*; and the *dorsal scapular* artery. The axillary artery then continues from the lateral aspect of the first rib, giving rise to the *anterior* and *posterior humeral circumflex* arteries. The brachial artery courses along the medial aspect of the arm with the median and ulnar nerves before branching into the *radial* and *ulnar arteries* near the elbow joint. Just distal to its origin, the ulnar artery gives rise to the *common interosseus* artery, which terminates in the distal forearm. If it continues into the hand, it is termed a *"persistent median"* artery, which is seen in approximately 4% of cases. The radial and ulnar arteries then form the *deep* and *superficial palmar arches* in the hand. The deep arch (complete in 95% of the population) is formed predominantly by the radial artery, while the chief contributor to the superficial arch (complete in 80%) is the ulnar artery (3).

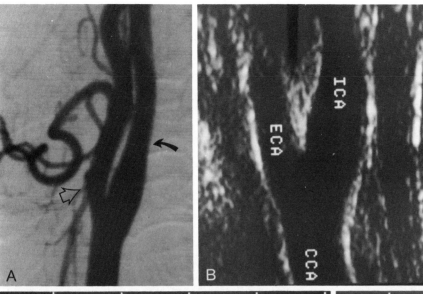

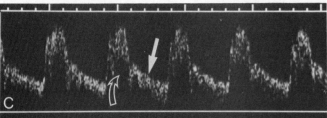

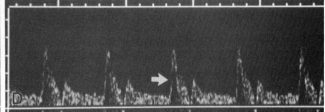

Figure 21.5. Normal Carotid Artery. A. Common carotid artery injection with normal internal carotid (*curved arrow*) and external carotid arteries (*open arrow*). **B.** Longitudinal ultrasound view from the posterolateral neck shows similar anatomy to that of the arteriogram: internal carotid artery (ICA), external carotid artery (ECA), and common carotid artery (CCA). Refer to Color Plate (Fig. 21.1) for color Doppler image of the normal carotid bifurcation. **C.** Internal carotid artery Doppler interrogation with low resistance waveform. Note the prominent diastolic flow (*straight arrow*) and clean envelope (*curved arrow*), typical of laminar flow in this low resistance vessel. **D.** Normal ECA Doppler waveform demonstrating high resistance waveform. Rapid systolic upstroke (*arrow*), seen in high resistance vessels.

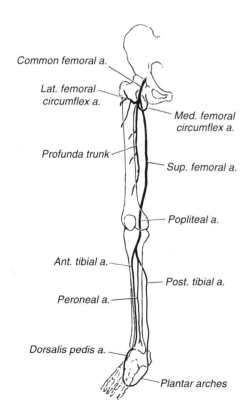

Figure 21.6. Normal Lower Extremity Arterial Anatomy

Lower Extremity. The *common iliac* artery originates at the aortic bifurcation and extends to its

bifurcation over the sacrum into the *external* and *internal iliac* arteries (Fig. 21.4). The internal iliac artery (*hypogastric*) divides into an anterior trunk (*superior and inferior vesicle, middle hemorrhoidal, internal pudendal, obturator, inferior gluteal, and uterine/prostatic* arteries) and a posterior trunk (*iliolumbar, lateral sacral, and superior gluteal* arteries). The external iliac artery courses to the inguinal ligament, giving off the *deep circumflex iliac* and the *inferior epigastric* arteries at that level. These branches represent the angiographic markers for the division between the external iliac and *common femoral* artery. The common femoral artery then bifurcates into the *profunda femoris* and *superficial femoral* arteries (SFA) near the inferior margin of the femoral head (Fig. 21.6). The SFA then continues in the anteromedial thigh to the adductor canal becoming the *popliteal* artery, giving off several small muscular branches along the way.

The popliteal artery travels in the popliteal fossa between the medial and lateral heads of the gastrocnemius muscle and terminates below the knee as the "trifurcation" vessels. In most cases, this does not represent a true trifucation but an initial branch, the *anterior tibial* artery and a short *tibioperoneal trunk*, which further divides into the *peroneal* and *posterior tibial* artery. The anterior tibial artery passes over the interosseous membrane below the knee to descend in the anterior compartment of the lower leg and then

Table 21.2. Angiographic Techniques

Procedure	Catheter	Injection Rate (m/sec/total volume contrast)	Filming Rate (film/sec/total secs)
Abdominal aorta	Pigtail	25/50 (CA)	2/4; 1/6[a]
		15/30 (DSA)[a]	two frames/sec
Bilateral lower extremity runoff	Pigtail	10/70 (CA)	2/3; 1/3
		8/42 (DSA)[b]	two frames/sec
Common carotid	Simmons	6/10 (CA)	2/4; 1/6[a]
	Headhunter	5/9 (DSA)[b]	three frames/sec
Internal carotid	Simmons	5/10 (CA)	2/4; 1/6†
	Headhunter	4/8 (DSA)[a]	three frames/sec
Subclavian	Simmons	6/18 (CA)	2/4; 1/8†
	Headhunter	4/16 (DSA)[a]	two frames/sec
Renal	Cobra	6/12 (CA)	2/4; 1/6
	Simmons	4/8 (DSA)[a]	two frames/sec
Celiac	Cobra/Simmons	10/50 (CA)	2/3; 1/4; 0.5/10[c]
SMA	Cobra/Simmons	8/48 (CA)	2/3; 1/4; 0.5/10[c]
SMA Portogram		8/60 (CA)	1/10; 0.5/10[c]
IMA	Cobra/Simmons	3/18 (CA)	2/3; 1/4; 0.5/10[c]

[a]These techniques are for singleplane imaging; for biplane imaging these values may need to be doubled, depending on the type of equipment being used (e.g., 6/3; 2/6).
[b]May use either reduced rates or amounts of "full-strength" (76%) contrast as presented here, or same rates/amounts as CA using "half-strength" (30%) contrast.
[c]The designation "0.5/10" denotes exposing one film every other second for a total of 10 seconds.

continues into the foot as the *dorsalis pedis* artery. The peroneal artery terminates above the ankle while the posterior tibial artery continues behind the medial malleolus and into the plantar aspect of the foot, giving off the *medial* and *lateral plantar* arteries. The *persistent sciatic* artery is a rare congenital variant representing failure in regression of embryologic anatomy. It is seen as an enlarged inferior branch from the internal iliac artery that exits the pelvis posteriorly and proceeds into the leg to join the distal SFA near the adductor canal. The proximal SFA may be absent or hypoplastic.

Angiographic Technique

The basic technique for accessing the arterial system is discussed in "Basic Angiographic Technique" in Chapter 20. Imaging of the abdominal aorta is best performed using a pigtail catheter placed at the T11-12 interspace using either DSA or biplane CA (Table 21.2). The lateral view is best suited for demonstrating the origins of the celiac axis, superior, and inferior mesenteric vessels. Visualizing the proximal renal arteries may require oblique imaging, usually right posterior oblique, with the pigtail catheter placed at the L1-2 interspace to optimally see the origins of the vessels. Selective injection of the renal artery is required for adequate evaluation of intrarenal branch disease.

The lower extremities are typically examined simultaneously with a pigtail catheter placed just proximal to the aortic bifurcation and step-table or full-length film changer imaging utilized. Accurate timing of step-table movements or exposure speed can be gauged using a small-contrast injection (5–10 ml) while either fluoroscopic visualization or 1 per sec digital imaging over the knee is performed. Once full opacification of the popliteal artery is seen, this time interval from bolus injection to arrival of the bolus at the knee is used to compute the optimum imaging rate. Individual evaluation of either lower extremity can be performed by passing a selective catheter over the bifurcation to examine the contralateral leg or by selective catheterization of the ipsilateral common femoral artery.

The upper extremities and neck vessels are usually examined from the femoral approach using selective catheters placed into each individual vessel. Direct access to the right common carotid or vertebral arteries is occasionally not feasible because of tortuosity or origin disease. The catheter may then be placed in the proximal subclavian or innominate artery and a blood pressure cuff placed on the ipsilateral arm. The cuff is then inflated to systemic arterial pressure just prior to the injection, thus diverting the majority of the flow into the vessel of interest.

Flow Enhancement. Several pharmacologic agents and manual maneuvers are available to enhance poor or sluggish flow in the distal extremities in order to optimally visualize vessel patency. *Tolazoline* is a powerful vasodilator with direct, local effect lasting approximately 15 minutes when injected intraarterially. The dose is typically 25–50 mg diluted in 5–10 ml normal saline and injected slowly through the catheter over 90 seconds prior to imaging. Adverse effects include hypotension, tachycardia, myocardial infarction, and arrhythmias. This is an excellent agent, and several runs in different projections may be performed per administration. *Nitroglycerin* is a vascular smooth muscle relaxant with direct, local effects when injected via the catheter. The dose is 100–

200 μg administered as a bolus. Caution must again be excercised to prevent inducing hypotension and its cardiac sequelae. (c) *Papaverine* is another direct acting, smooth muscle relaxant administered intraarterially into the vessel of interest and is useful in cases of spasm. The dose is 30 mg diluted in 10 ml of normal saline and administered slowly over 60–90 seconds. (d) *Reactive hyperemia* involves the application of a blood pressure cuff to the proximal extremity inflated to above systolic arterial pressure for approximately 5-7 minutes. Following release of the cuff, reactive vasodilation occurs, enhancing flow to the distal extremity. Similar results can be obtained through the application of warm moist towels to the foot or hand. Both are effective but are inconvenient, time-consuming, and uncomfortable for the patient and may not be appropriate in some cases.

Trauma

Abdominal aortic injury generally results from either blunt or penetrating trauma. As with the thoracic aorta, blunt abdominal aortic injury is most commonly associated with acute deceleration injuries in motor vehicle accidents. Clinical symptoms are often obscured by other intraabdominal or musculoskeletal injuries; however, loss of groin pulses or more peripheral embolic symptoms should raise the suspicion of significant injury to the abdominal aorta. Injuries to the abdominal aorta itself are much less common than are those that effect its major branch vessels such as the renal, lumbar, or mesenteric pedicles.

Angiographic findings of aortic trauma include intimal irregularity or flap, laceration with false aneurysm formation or retroperitoneal hematoma, post-traumatic dissection, or thrombosis. Penetrating trauma has the additional potential finding of arteriovenous fistula if adjacent arterial and venous structures were injured.

Peripheral vascular trauma on physical examination may range from normal to a cold, pulseless, ischemic extremity to frank, pulsatile bleeding. Only 40% of patients with documented arterial injury show any pulse abnormality on physical examination. The upper extremity is affected more frequently than the lower extremity. Penetrating trauma is the most common cause of peripheral vascular injury and is more commonly secondary to gunshot wounds (due to "proximity injury" damage) and less commonly from stab wounds. Approximately 10% of peripheral vascular injuries are secondary to nonpenetrating trauma. Most commonly, these are caused by long bone fractures or dislocations but may also be secondary to direct, blunt extremity injury. Piercing bone fragments associated with factures essentially represent "internal" penetrating trauma and thus may exhibit similar findings to those seen in gunshot and stab wounds. Dislocations classically cause stretch injuries, which can result in spasm, intimal flap, or complete vessel disruption.

The angiographic findings of peripheral vascular trauma (Fig. 21.7) are listed in Table 21.3. Diffuse vessel narrowing may be caused by hypotensive vasospasm and should not be mistaken for vascular injury. Similarly, if focal narrowing is seen (in the absence of contrast extravasation), the injection may be repeated following the intraarterial administration of one the vasodilating agents described. This will serve to (a) eliminate nontraumatic vasospasm unrelated to vessel injury, (b) reveal an underlying intimal tear or mural hematoma, or (c) exclude the possibility of extrinsic compression from hematoma if the spasm clears. In addition, this will allow improved opacification of more distal vessels and thus facilitate exclusion of more distal injury. Vessel occlusion may be secondary to occluding intimal flap, "recoil" spasm following complete transection of the vessel, extrinsic compression by bone or hematoma, or thromboembolization from a more proximal vascular injury. In cases of arterial extravasation in areas difficult access surgically such as the pelvis and segmental renal arteries, transcatheter embolization may be used (3).

Digital subtraction angiography is the imaging modality of choice in extremity trauma because of its superior contrast resolution, decreased contrast load, and real-time image projection. General anesthesia or adequate intravenous sedation may be necessary when a trauma patient is unable to cooperate fully during image acquisition to avoid motion artifacts that may obscure vessel injury. If an area of questionable intimal injury exists after DSA examination, CA may be used because of its superior spatial resolution. Because of the tachycardia and resultant high cardiac output inherent in trauma victims, greater contrast volume and injection rates as well as faster filming rates than normally used may be necessary.

Aneurysm

Abdominal aortic aneurysms are defined as dilation of the abdominal aorta greater than 3 cm. They are seen in approximately 2–6% of the population, occurring most commonly in white males (male:female = 8:1) over age 60. Most abdominal aortic aneurysms are asymptomatic and are detected incidentally on physical examination or plain film radiographs of the abdomen, or other imaging study (4). In those patients who are symptomatic, the most common manifestations are abdominal pain, abdominal mass, and distal embolization. Most abdominal aortic aneurysms are atherosclerotic in origin. Other much less common causes are syphilitic, mycotic, post-

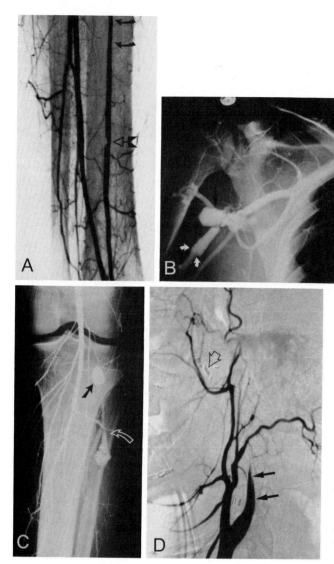

Figure 21.7. Manifestations of Peripheral Arterial Trauma. A. Intimal injury. Multiple stab wounds to lower leg shows eccentric defect in posterior tibial artery (*open arrow*). Note the area of spasm located more proximally (*curved arrows*). **B.** Traumatic pseudoaneurysm and arteriovenous fistula: Gunshot wound to the shoulder with a large pseudoaneurysm of the axillary artery (*straight arrow*) and formation of an arteriovenous fistula with opacification of vein (*curved arrows*) in early arterial phase. **C.** Gunshot wound to the left leg (*black arrow*) with fracture of the proximal fibula and pseudoaneurysm (*curved arrow*) formation. **D.** Carotid artery dissection. The smoothly bordered tapering of the ICA (*straight arrows*) is a typical configuration of traumatic dissection of the carotid artery created by gunshot wound (*open arrow*).

Table 21.3.   Manifestations of Peripheral Vascular Trauma

Intimal tear
Spasm
Extrinisc compression
Contrast extravasation
Occlusion
Pseudoaneurysm
Arteriovenous fistula

traumatic, and postsurgical complications (see "Types of Aneurysms" in Chapter 20).

TYPES OF ANEURYSMS

Atherosclerosis is responsible for most abdominal aortic aneurysms, with more than 90% involving the infrarenal aorta (6). As opposed to the thoracic and suprarenal aorta, there is insufficient vasa vasorum within the infrarenal aorta to provide adequate metabolic support. This creates a dependency on the process of diffusion to sustain the vessel wall.

As part of the atherosclerotic process, lipids and collagen are deposited in the media, which interfere with the diffusion process. This in turn results in a cycle of vessel wall ischemia, weakening, and progressive dilation. As the vessel diameter increases, flow within the aneurysm becomes slower and more turbulent, leading to deposition of mural thrombus. This can lead to occlusion of branch vessels within this region, notably the inferior mesenteric artery and lumbar arteries, seen in approximately 80% of cases (6).

Most abdominal aortic aneurysms are *fusiform* (concentric dilation) (Fig. 21.8) as opposed to *saccular* (asymmetric dilation) and will gradually enlarge at a rate of approximately 2–4 mm/year. Extension into the common iliac arteries occurs in 69% of cases, with extension into the external iliac being extremely uncommon (6). Isolated iliac artery aneurysms are rare, with the great majority being associated with abdominal aortic aneurysm. Complications of abdominal aortic aneurysm include rupture, peripheral embolization *(blue toe syndrome)*, thrombosis, and infection.

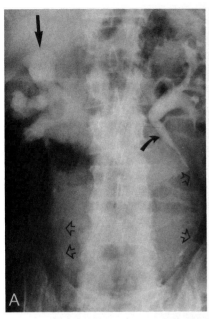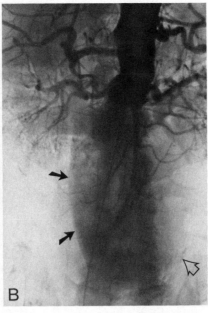

Figure 21.8. Abdominal Aortic Aneurysm. A. An intravenous pyelogram enhances some of the plain film findings of an aneurysm. Lateral displacement of the ureters (*curved arrow*) with lateral convexity to mural calcification (*open arrows*) are well seen. Also note the obstruction of the right renal collecting system (*straight arrow*). **B.** Aortogram shows smoothly bordered faint enhancement of this large aneurysm. The smooth borders (*straight arrows*) are commonly seen with thrombus lining the vessel lumen, as well as the mural calcification appearing displaced from the contrast-enhanced lumen (*open arrow*). Note also the lack of expected filling of lumbar arteries bilaterally.

The incidence of aneurysm rupture increases with increasing aneurysm size as follows: <4 cm = 10%, 4–7 cm = 25%, 7–10 cm = 45%, and >10 cm = 60% (7). Rupture usually occurs into the left retroperitoneal space, with rare instances of rupture into the adjacent gastrointestinal tract (*aortoenteric fistula*) and inferior vena cava (*aortovenous fistula*). Aortoenteric fistulas are usually related to prosthetic aortic grafts, with the duodenum the site of fistula formation in 80% (5).

Chronic Contained Rupture represents a break in the aneurysm wall with a focal rupture and leak restrained by the retroperitoneal soft tissues. Computed tomography demonstrates an extraluminal hematoma adjacent to the aneurysm; if flow into the hematoma is seen, this is termed a *false or pseudoaneurysm* (4).

Inflammatory Aneurysms constitute a subset of abdominal aortic aneurysms characterized by perianeurysmal fibrosis of unclear etiology occurring in 10% of cases. This fibrosis presents on CT as a thick, contrast-enhancing rind surrounding the aneurysm that may involve the ureters (25% of cases), left renal vein, inferior vena cava, duodenum, and adjacent small bowel and sigmoid colon, leading to obstruction (Fig. 21.9**D**). Ultrasound demonstrates a hypoechoic ring surrounding the aneurysm. There is evidence to suggest that this represents an autoimmune phenomenon and may respond to corticosteroids (5).

Infected (Mycotic) Aneurysms are rare and can result from primary infection of the aortic wall, secondary infection of a preexisting abdominal aortic aneurysm or contiguous spread from an adjacent abscess. The clinical presentation consists of sudden appearance of a pulsatile abdominal mass with fever. Computed tomography demonstrates a noncalcified, saccular aneurysm with associated periaortic fluid, gas, or vertebral osteomyelitis. *Staphylococcus* is the most common organism, followed by Gram-negative bacteria and *Salmonella*. Indium-labeled white cell radionuclide imaging is useful in differentiating mycotic from other types of abdominal aortic aneurysm (5).

Imaging

Although plain film examination of the abdomen can detect mural calcification in 50–86% of abdominal aortic aneurysm, ultrasound is the imaging modality of choice in the initial evaluation, screening, and follow-up of all asymptomatic abdominal aortic aneurysm, with accuracy rates exceeding 98% (6). Asymptomatic abdominal aortic aneurysms measuring less than 4–5 cm in diameter may be followed with serial ultrasound because of their low rupture rate, until size or symptoms dictate the need for surgery. Ultrasound is useful in detecting intraluminal thrombus (Fig. 21.9**A**), accurately sizing the aneurysm, and following extension into the proximal common iliac arteries. Ultrasound is limited by obesity and overlying bowel gas, and detection of renal artery involvement is difficult.

Computed tomography surpasses ultrasound in better defining the relationship of the aneurysm to the surrounding retroperitoneal structures. It is likewise extremely accurate in evaluating size, presence of intraluminal thrombus (Fig. 21.9**B**), and extension into the iliac arteries, although it may overestimate aneurysm size if the aorta is tortuous, thus imaging it obliquely. In addition, it is the imaging modality of choice for the evaluation of suspected rupture (Fig. 21.9**C**), *leaking aneurysm*, and perianeurysmal fibrosis (Fig. 21.9**D**) (5). Evaluation for these entities should include contrast enhancement with 10-mm

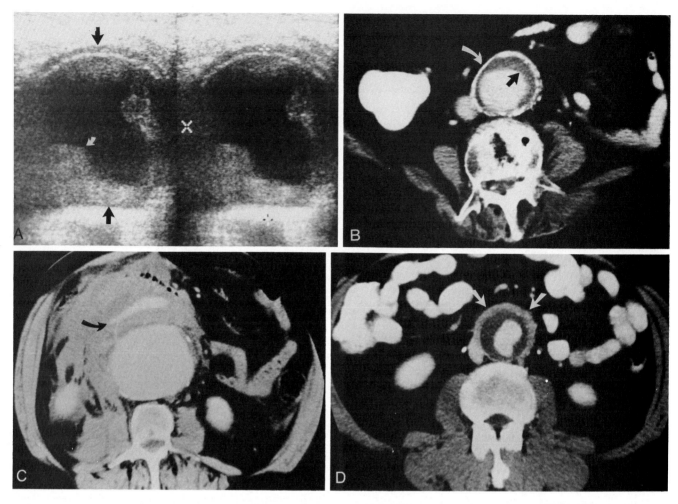

Figure 21.9. Abdominal Aortic Aneurysm. A. Transverse ultrasonographic images demonstrate an aneurysm with irregular intraluminal thrombus (*curved arrow*). **B.** Typical atherosclerotic aneurysm is seen in this contrast-enhanced CT with extensive mural calcification (*curved arrow*) and intraluminal thrombus (*straight arrow*). **C.** A ruptured aneurysm manifests as a crescentic collection of contrast (*arrow*) in the midst of extensive infiltration of the retroperitoneum and mesentery with intermediate density material consistent with thrombus. **D.** Enhanced CT image shows aneurysmal dilation of the aorta with enchancing irregular soft tissue surrounding the aorta (*arrows*), consistent with an inflammatory aneurysm.

contiguous slices with supplemental thin-slice imaging directed at areas of question. Magnetic resonance imaging is as accurate as CT in evaluating the described features of abdominal aortic aneurysm; however, it is currently limited by examination time and expense, and thus should be considered subordinate to CT. It may be useful when there is a contraindication to intravenous contrast (6).

Angiography is best utilized for the preoperative evaluation of abdominal aortic aneurysm in defining the number of renal arteries and their relationship to the aneurysm, the patency of the renal arteries and mesenteric vessels, and the patency of the external iliac and common femoral arteries. These factors may modify the surgical approach used and define additional procedures required in order to decrease postoperative morbidity. Angiography typically demonstrates a smooth, featureless aortic lumen that may or may not be widened. This is due to the deposition of mural thrombus that makes evaluation of lumen size inaccurate. This also accounts for nonvisualization of the lumbar and inferior mesenteric arteries, as described (6).

Arteriomegaly (*diffuse vascular ectasia, arteria magna, ectatic atherosclerosis*) is an unusual manifestation of aneurysmal disease that, as the name implies, represents diffuse, generalized dilation of the aortoiliac and femoral vessels (Fig. 21.10). It is associated with multiple aneurysms, predominantly abdominal aortic aneurysms, and characteristically produces severe tortuosity in the iliac arteries. Because of the capacious vascular system, increased amounts of contrast with prolonged imaging times are required.

Extremity Aneurysms are more often seen in the lower than the upper extremity. Atherosclerosis is the most common etiology for lower extremity aneurysms,

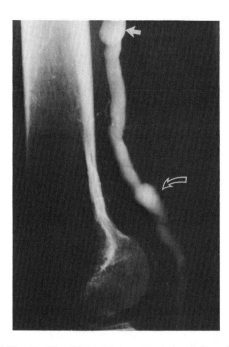

Figure 21.10. Popliteal Artery Aneurysm. Lateral view of the lower extremity arteriogram in a patient undergoing evaluation for an abdominal aortic aneurysm shows a proximal popliteal artery aneurysm (*curved arrow*). Note the associated distal SFA aneurysm (*straight arrow*) and arteriomegaly.

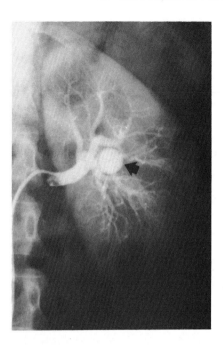

Figure 21.11. Renal Artery Aneurysm. This large segmental renal artery aneurysm (*arrow*) can be complicated by hypertension, hemorrhage, thrombosis, or arteriovenous fistula formation.

with the popliteal artery being the most prevalent site of involvement, followed by the femoral artery. Upper extremity aneurysms are more commonly secondary to trauma with atherosclerosis, arthritis, mycotic, and postsurgical aneurysms being secondary.

Popliteal aneurysms constitute two-thirds of all extremity aneurysms, and are associated with other aneurysms at other sites in 75% of cases (one-third are abdominal aortic aneurysms with approximately 60% being bilateral). Most are located in the proximal popliteal artery (Fig. 21.10), and usually contain thrombus. *Femoral* aneurysms are, likewise, bilateral in approximately 60% of cases, with 85% associated with abdominal aortic aneurysms and approximately 45% associated with popliteal aneurysms. Presenting symptoms include limb ischemia due to aneurysm thrombosis (more common with popliteal aneurysms), distal embolization, and gangrene. Other causes of lower extremity aneurysms include posttraumatic, mycotic, and postoperative complications.

Ultrasound is useful for initial evaluation and for accurately determining aneurysm size, with the exception of the subclavian aneurysms where CT or MR are better suited. Angiography is usually required for the final preoperative evaluation in order to determine the status of the peripheral vessels for planned bypass grafting and aneurysm repair.

Renal Artery aneurysms are uncommon and are usually detected incidentally. Approximately two-

thirds are located at the main renal artery bifurcation with the remainder arising from the segmental branches (Fig. 21.11). They are bilateral in 20% of cases and the majority are asymptomatic. Hypertension is present in approximately 15% of cases; the most common symptoms consist of pain and hematuria. Etiologies include atherosclerosis, fibromuscular dysplasia, polyarteritis nodosa (see later discussion), congenital, mycotic, and posttraumatic factors resulting in pseudoaneurysms. Calcification in the wall of the aneurysm may be seen on plain film but is better demonstrated on unenhanced CT and is associated with a low incidence of rupture. Noncalcified aneurysms demonstrate a 25% incidence of rupture.

Splenic Artery aneurysms are the second most common aneurysm found in the abdomen and are most commonly atherosclerotic in origin. Other causes include congenital, associated with pancreatitis, mycotic, associated with portal hypertension, and posttraumatic. They are more commonly seen in young women than are other aneurysms, and there is an increased rupture rate in pregnancy and in women of childbearing age. Patients are usually asymptomatic and most are discovered incidentally. Two-thirds of aneurysms contain calcification and thus have a lower propensity to rupture. However, almost 10% of aneurysms will rupture, with a mortality rate approaching 75%; thus, those exceeding 5 mm in diameter or those that present with symptoms are treated.

Arterial Occlusive Disease

Imaging

Imaging in arterial occlusive disease is done primarily with angiography. Ultrasound is utilized both for screening and follow-up with the examination directed to specific areas of interest. Angiography precedes planned surgical or percutaneous intervention, or is used to evaluate equivocal findings on other imaging studies. Magnetic resonance imaging angiography is steadily improving and may eventually become a valuable, noninvasive screening modality for the evaluation of the peripheral vascular system. It has shown greatest promise in the cervical carotid system (Fig. 21.12) and has demonstrated some usefulness in the lower extremity vessels (Fig. 21.13). However, signal degradation due to turbulence (which may simulate occlusion), insufficient spatial resolu-

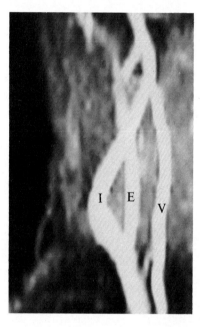

Figure 21.12. Cervical Carotid MR Angiography. A two-dimensional-time of flight MR angiography with normal anatomy of the right cervical carotid artery: ICA, *I*; ECA, *E*; vertebral artery, *V.*

tion in the periphery, and relative expense continue to plague MRA, currently relegating it to a subordinate role (8). Radionuclide imaging has special application in the evaluation of renovascular occlusive disease and is discussed in Chapter 50.

Duplex Ultrasound has proven its greatest utility in the evaluation of disease within the extracranial carotid system, although the principles discussed here will apply in general to other segments of the peripheral system.

The highest frequency transducer producing optimal images is utilized, most commonly linear 5–7.5 MHz. Complete evaluation of the visualized extracranial portions of the common, internal, and external carotid arteries utilizing gray scale, Doppler, and color flow Doppler techniques is performed.

Longitudinally, the common carotid artery (CCA), carotid bifurcation, and internal and external carotid arteries are imaged. Certain sonographic characteristics of the vessels aid in their identification (Table 21.4) (1). Transverse gray scale images follow the longitudinal evaluation when orientation of the vessels is confirmed as well as estimates of the type and degree of plaquing and stenosis obtained.

The ability to define plaque composition is controversial, with ulceration of plaque particularly difficult to assess. Gray scale images provide a more accurate definition of low-grade stenosis (<50% diameter). The use of real-time imaging to define the degree of stenosis becomes less accurate as the degree of stenosis increases. Diagnosing intraplaque hemorrhage is the most reliably predicted morphology detected by ultrasound. The importance of defining hemorrhagic plaque is its instability and the fact that it is prone to ulceration. Plaques that are homogeneous are rarely associated with ulceration or intraplaque hemorrhage (9).

Doppler interrogation of the carotid vessels allows identification of regions of altered flow dynamics. Analysis of the spectral waveform plays a key role in defining the degree and significance of stenotic lesions. The pulsatility of the components of the carotid arterial sys-

Figure 21.13. Iliac Arterial Occlusive Disease. Peripheral arterial MR angiography shows stenosis of the right common iliac artery (*arrow*) and complete occlusion of the left common iliac artery (*straight arrow*).

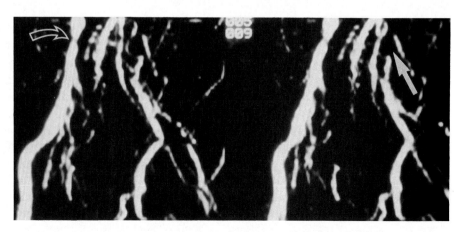

Table 21.4. Sonographic features of the External and Internal Carotid Arteries

Features	ECA	ICA
Size	Usually smaller	Usually larger
Branches	Yes	No
Doppler characteristics	High resistance	Low resistance
Orientation	Anteromedially toward face	Posterolateral toward mastoid

Table 21.5. Doppler Analysis[a]

Diameter Stenosis (%)	Degree Stenosis	Peak-Systolic Velocity (cm/sec)	End-Diastolic Velocity (cm/sec)	ICA/CCA Systolic Velocity Ratio	ICA/CCA Diastolic Velocity Ratio
0	None	<110	<40	<1.8	<2.6
1–39	Mild	<110	<40	<1.8	<2.6
40–59	Moderate	<130	<40	<1.8	<2.6
60–79	Severe	>130	>40	>1.8	>2.6
80–99	Critical	>250	>100	>3.7	>5.5

[a]Adapted from Bluth El, Wetzner SM, Stavros AT, et al. Carotid duplex sonography: a multicenter recommendation for standardized imaging and Doppler criteria. Radiographics 1988;8:487–506.

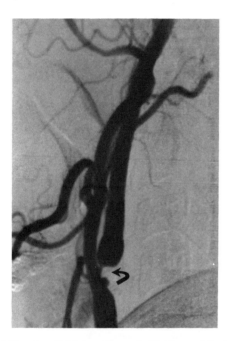

Figure 21.14. Carotid Artery Stenosis. Right carotid arterial injection demonstrates severe stenosis of the proximal ICA with associated ulceration (*arrow*). (Refer to Color Plates Figures 21.2 and 21.3 for corresponding duplex ultrasound evaluation, which also show critical stenosis in this region.)

tem differ. The ICA has a low resistance pattern, the external carotid artery a high resistance pattern, and the common carotid artery a mixture of the two, tending toward low resistance as 70% of this vessel's blood flow supplies the ICA. The degree of velocity elevation in systole and diastole, along with the degree of spectral broadening, are all used to determine the degree and significance of stenotic lesions (Table 21.5) (1). Areas of spectral broadening should alert one to possible stenotic lesions. Spectral broadening can also result from a sample volume that is too large, a Doppler sam-

ple gate that is too close to a vessel wall, and as a normal finding at the bifurcation of vessels. Peak systolic and diastolic velocities should be used to define the degree of stenosis. Flow-limiting stenosis is defined as that which is greater than 50% diameter. Velocity ratios are utilized in areas of suspected stenosis that do not display significant velocity elevations. End-diastolic, peak-systolic ICA-CCA ratios, and peak-diastolic ICA-CCA ratios are equal to peak systolic ratio in accuracy (10).

Color images allow a quick identification of abnormal areas of flow manifested as heterogeneous color patterns and luminal narrowing (Fig. 21.14, Color Plates Figs. 21.2 and 21.3). This is especially true in defining suspected occlusion and with stenosis encompassing less than 50% of the diameter of the vessel (9). In diagnosing complete occlusion, color duplex ultrasound appears to have value for detecting residual lumen patency, although it is still accepted practice to perform angiographic evaluation in patients suspected of having occlusion or preocclusive stenosis as defined by duplex sonography. Use of color duplex ultrasound shortens the examination time, helps resolve conflicts between gray scale and duplex images, and aids in defining the extent of stenosis (9).

Carotid duplex is a useful, accurate, and effective method of defining stenosis when compared with arteriography; it has sensitivities and specificities ranging from 84 to 99% and an accuracy rate of 90–95% (9).

Collateral Pathways

In the event of severe arterial stenosis or occlusion, collateral channels develop in an attempt to "bypass" the obstruction and provide flow to relatively ischemic distal territory. They represent small, preexistent arterial communications that enlarge in response to increased load requirements. The more chronic the occlusion and the more severe the stenosis, the larger and more numerous these accessory vessels tend to be. Knowledge of the anatomy of these pathways is important in planning catheter placement for optimal opacification of the vessels below the obstruction. For example, unilateral occlusion of the common and internal iliac artery may result in the ipsilateral intercostal arteries or even the internal mammary artery

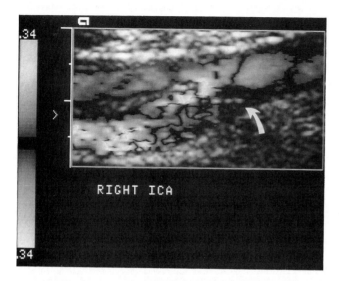

Color Plate Figure 21.2. Carotid Artery Stenosis. Longitudinal color image of the carotid artery bifurcation demonstrating an eccentric homogeneous atherosclerotic plaque (*arrow*) at the origin of the ICA. The marked heterogeneous color display distal to the plaque is suggestive of severe turbulence secondary to a significant stenosis. Refer to Figure 21.14 for angiographic correlation.

supplying the majority of flow to that leg. Therefore, placing the catheter at the aortic bifurcation for routine runoff imaging would not opacify that extremity. The catheter should be placed at a level sufficient to fill the lower intercostal arteries. Selective injection of the ipsilateral internal mammary artery may be necessary.

The major collateral pathways for occlusive disease involving the lower extremity are outlined in Tables 21.6 and 21.7 as these typically are the most complex. Other important collateral pathways in the lower extremity are (a) the *profunda femorus* artery, providing collateral flow around SFA or popliteal obstruction, and (b) the *peroneal* artery, supplying collateral flow for disease in the anterior or posterior tibial artery.

Collateral supply for disease in the renal artery may come from *periureteral* and *peripelvic* collaterals supplied by lumbar, subcostal, adrenal, and internal iliac arteries to anastamose with the distal renal artery and branches. These may be seen as multiple extraluminal impressions on the contrast-filled ureter during the angiogram or on intravenous pyelogram during workup for renal function abnormality. Renal *capsular* arteries anastamose to perforating branches of the lobar and interlobar arteries in the kidney, and *intrarenal anastamoses* provide the remainder of collateral pathways to the kidney.

Subclavian Steal Syndrome.   Upper extremity occlusive disease is usually confined to the subclavian artery; disease beyond this point is uncommon. If the obstruction is proximal to the origin of the vertebral

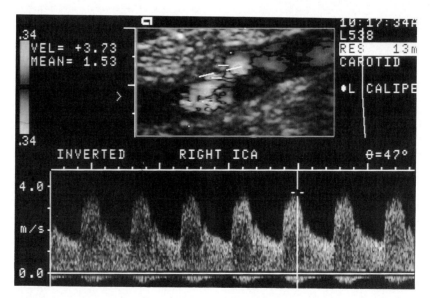

Color Plate Figure 21.3. Carotid Artery Stenosis. The same patient as in Color Plate Figure 21.2, demonstrating use of color flow to direct placement of Doppler cursor in the area of maximal flow velocity. Doppler waveform analysis shows measurement of peak systolic flow velocity (measuring cursor positioned at peak of systolic flow) with value of 3.73 m/sec (*upper left*), indicating critical stenosis (see Table 21.4). Note "filling in" of Doppler waveform, known as spectral broadening, indicative of turbulence. Refer to Figure 21.14 for angiographic correlation.

Table 21.6. Collateral Pathways for Aortic/Bilateral Common Iliac Occlusion[a]

Internal mammary	→	Superior epigastric	→	Inferior epigastric	→	External iliac
SMA to IMA	→	Superior to middle hemorrhoidal	→	Internal iliac	→	External iliac
Intercostals and lumbars	→	Superior gluteal and iliolumbar	→	Internal iliac	→	External iliac
Intercostals and lumbars	→	Deep circumflex iliac	→		→	External iliac

[a]Adapted from Kadir S: Diagnostic angiography. Philadelphia: WB Saunders, 1986. Arrows indicate direction of flow.

Table 21.7. Collateral Pathways for Unilateral Common Iliac Occlusion[a]

Intercostals and lumbars	→	Iliolumbar	→	Internal iliac	→	External iliac
Contralateral internal iliac	→	Lateral sacrals	→	Ipsilateral internal iliac	→	External iliac
Abdominal aorta	→	Testicular	→	Internal iliac	→	External iliac
Contralateral femoral	→	External pudendal	→	Ipsilateral external pudendal	→	Femoral
Intercostals and lumbars	→	Superficial circumflex iliac	→	Lateral femoral circumflex	→	Femoral
Reconstituted internal iliac	→	Superior/inferior gluteal, obturator	→	Medial femoral circumflex	→	Femoral

[a]Adapted from Kadir S: Diagnostic angiography. Philadelphia: WB Saunders, 1986. Arrows indicate direction of flow.

artery, reversal of flow in the ipsilateral vertebral artery may occur to provide collateral supply to the affected arm resulting in the *subclavian steal syndrome*. Flow is diverted from the intracranial circulation (*vertebrobasilar steal*) to the subclavian artery and may be manifested clinically as vertigo, syncope, paresthesias, dysarthria, and other neurologic symptoms in association with ipsilateral decreased radial pulse and upper extremity claudication. The left subclavian is more commonly affected (75% of cases), and it is more commonly seen in males (3:1). The most common cause is atherosclerosis, but it may be seen secondary to vasculitis, tumor compression, or on a congenital basis (e.g., coarctation associated with aberrant subclavian artery arising distal to the coarctation).

Angiography demonstrates the classic finding of delayed, retrograde flow in the ipsilateral vertebral artery and late opacification of the subclavian artery. Duplex ultrasound may suggest the diagnosis with reversal of flow in the vertebral artery.

Peripheral Occlusive Diseases

Atherosclerosis is the most frequent cause of chronic occlusive disease of the systemic arterial system. The arterial lesions, or *intimal plaques*, represent a combination of smooth muscle proliferation and extracellular lipid and collagen deposition that projects into the vessel lumen creating stenoses. *Complex plaques* result from calcification, ulceration, and intraplaque hemorrhage and thrombosis. The stenoses may be either *eccentric* or *concentric* in morphology and tend to occur at vessel bifurcations, at acute bends, and where vessels are deformed by overlying ligaments and around joints. The lesions appear angiographically as irregular areas of variable luminal narrowing. If the degree of stenosis is severe enough, *poststenotic dilation*, or fusiform dilation distal to a stenosis, may result. The stenoses may progress to complete vessel occlusion, at which time thrombosis occurs above the lesion with proximal propagation to the next largest branch.

The range of clinical manifestations in the extremities include intermittent *claudication* (pain or cramping) caused by exercise-induced muscle ischemia; *rest pain* consisting of severe pain, coolness, and numbness; and nonhealing ulcers and gangrene. The severity of the symptoms is closely related to the measurement of the ankle-to-arm systolic blood pressure ratio (*ankle-brachial index*). The level of claudication also correlates with the level of occlusive disease such that thigh and butt claudication indicates aortoiliac disease, while isolated calf claudication indicates SFA or popliteal involvement. Physical examination of the pulses will likewise indicate the level of disease and assist in choosing the best approach for performing the diagnostic study should percutaneous intervention be anticipated.

The disease is more common in males over 50 years of age, postmenopausal women, and diabetics. Diabetics typically have more severe distal calf vessel disease with an earlier age of onset. *Leriche's syndrome* is aortic or bilateral common iliac occlusion manifested by bilateral lower extremity claudication and impotence. In the carotid system, patients may present with transient ischemic attacks (*TIAs*) or transitory neurologic deficits localized to a particular vascular distribution, transient visual field deficits (*amaurosis fugax*) consistent with embolic phenomenon affecting the ophthalmic artery, or *stroke*, all of which are caused by slow flow or, more typically, emboli.

Atherosclerotic disease can occur anywhere in the arterial system, but is commonly found in the lower extremities and cervical carotid arteries. In the lower extremities, the most common location is the superficial femoral artery (Fig. 21.15) followed by the aortoiliac system (Fig. 21.16), trifurcation vessels, and popliteal arteries. Most carotid lesions classically

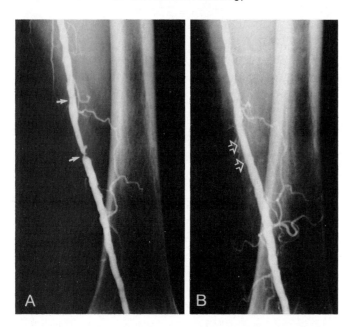

Figure 21.15. Superficial Femoral Artery Atherosclerotic Stenosis.
A. Atherosclerotic changes of the superficial femoral artery are seen with a focal dominant tight stenosis (*arrows*). **B.** Postangioplasty, there is marked improvement in the degree of stenosis (*arrows*).

involve the carotid bifurcation and proximal ICA adjacent to the bifurcation. Upper extremity involvement is less common than lower extremity involvement, and is usually confined to the subclavian artery.

Thromboembolic Occlusion is a common cause of extremity arterial occlusion. The heart is the most common source of emboli, with extracardiac aneurysms (abdominal aortic, iliac, popliteal, and subclavian) as the next most frequent site. The lower extremity vessels are more commonly affected, with branch points and preexisting stenoses as the most likely sites of involvement. The characteristic angiographic appearance is abrupt vessel occlusion with a superior convex meniscus (Fig. 21.17**A**).

Radiation-induced Injury to small and medium-sized arteries present with nonspecific symptoms typical of occlusive disease such as claudication, TIA, or stroke. The onset of symptoms correlate with three patterns of pathologic change: (*a*) intimal damage with resultant mural thrombosis usually occurring within 5 years postradiation, (*b*) fibrotic occlusion occurring within 10 years postradiation, and (*c*) acceleration of atherosclerotic changes in combination with periarterial fibrosis with latent onset of 20 years or more (11). Angiographic characteristics are smooth, long segment stenoses occurring in areas atypical for atherosclerotic disease, and confined within a radiation port (Fig. 21.18). Duplex ultrasound may demonstrate the unusual location, stenosis, as well as the periarterial fibrosis.

Fibromuscular Dysplasia (FMD) is found most often to involve the renal artery (Fig.21.19**A**). The next

most common sites of involvement are the carotid artery (3%) cases and the iliac artery (<1%) (Fig. 21.19, **B** and **C**). The usual location for carotid involvement is in the middle and distal third of the internal carotid artery (C-1 to C-2) (11, 12). The lesions are more common in middle-aged women and are frequently bilateral. Patients present with nonspecific symptoms of occlusive disease (TIA, amaurosis fugax, and stroke). The carotid lesions are associated with intracranial aneurysms in approximately 25% of cases (Fig. 21.19**B**) and there is a high association with FMD involving the renal artery (12). Iliac artery involvement likewise presents clinically with nonspecific symptoms of claudication similar to atherosclerotic disease. The external iliac artery is typically involved. (Fig. 21.19**C**). The pathology and angiographic appearance are identical to that seen in the renal artery and are discussed later.

Vasculitic Syndromes

Buerger's Disease (*thromboangiitis obliterans*) is an inflammatory vasculitis typically affecting young men under 40 years of age who almost invariably have a history of cigarette smoking. It is an obliterative process represented by intimal hyperplasia and thrombosis usually limited to the small and medium-sized arteries and veins, affecting the lower extremity more often than the upper extremity. The characteristic clinical symptoms consist of rest pain involving the feet and hands, which may progress to ulceration and gangrene. The angiographic findings include bilateral distal extremity occlusions, luminal irregularities, skip lesions, and abrupt segmental narrowings. Characteristic findings of "*corkscrew*" collateral vessels and the appearance of a normal-appearing major artery in the presence of occluded companion arteries are virtually diagnostic (Fig. 21.20) (13).

Temporal Arteritis (*giant cell arteritis*) is an uncommon granulomatous vasculitis typically affecting white females over 50 years old. The clinical presentation consists of a prodromal flu-like illness with eventual symptoms of jaw claudication, visual symptoms, myalgias, and tenderness of the superficial temporal artery. Laboratory values demonstrate a markedly elevated sedimentation rate; the diagnosis is usually confirmed on biopsy of the temporal artery. The most commonly affected arteries in decreasing order of frequency are the distal subclavian/axillary arteries, femoral arteries, and distal forearm and distal external carotid branches. Common carotid, proximal subclavian, and innominate artery involvement has not been seen (13). There is usually symmetric, bilateral involvement with the upper extremity more commonly involved. The lesions are typically long, smooth segments

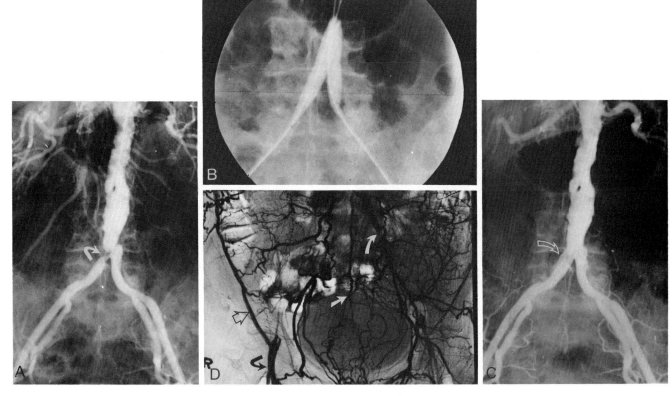

Figure 21.16. Common Iliac Artery Occlusive Disease and Angioplasty. A. Aortic injection preangioplasty shows a tight stenosis of the proximal right common iliac artery (*arrow*). **B.** To protect the contralateral common iliac artery, a "kissing" balloon technique is utilized for angioplasty. **C.** Postangioplasty result shows improved patency of the right iliac artery (*arrow*). Note the intimal cleft representing a normal intimal "crack" seen with angioplasty. **D.** Aortic injection with severe iliac occlusive disease demonstrates multiple collateral vessels. Complete occlusion of left common iliac artery (*curved white arrow*) and absence of definable right common iliac artery. There is reconstitution of the right femoral artery (*curved black arrow*) by the deep iliac circumflex artery (*open arrow*). Multiple collateral vessels are seen within the left pelvis. Median sacral artery (*straight arrow*).

of stenosis with tapering at both the proximal and distal extents and with abundant collateral vessels.

Takayasu's Arteritis is also a giant cell arteritis and has been discussed in Chapter 20. The lesions have similar appearance to temporal arteritis; however, their distribution remains the distinguishing feature. Takayasu's arteritis typically involves the proximal brachiocephalic and carotid arteries and rarely extends beyond the carotid bifurcation (Fig. 20.11). Aortic involvement seen in Takayasu's arteritis is not seen in temporal arteritis (13).

Collagen Vascular Diseases. Rheumatoid arthritis, systemic lupus erythematosus, and scleroderma all effect the small and medium-sized arteries of the distal upper extremities. It is typically bilateral and symmetric with poorly developed collateral vessels. There is progressive, concentric vessel narrowing leading to occlusion. The vasospastic disorder, *Raynaud's phenomenon*, is frequently associated.

Entrapment Syndromes

Thoracic Outlet Syndrome, more commonly seen in women, comprises a group of anatomic abnormalities in which the artery, vein, or nerve are compressed as they pass through three possible areas of constriction: (*a*) *interscalene triangle*, formed by the anterior and middle scalene muscles and the first rib inferiorly with the artery and nerve passing through and the vein in front, (*b*) *costoclavicular space*, formed by the clavicle above and the first rib below with all three components passing through it, and (*c*) *pectoralis minor tunnel*, formed by the pectoralis minor tendon anteriorly and the coracoid process involving all three structures. Compression can result from a number of *congenital* (cervical rib, abnormal first rib or muscle insertion) or *acquired* (muscular hypertrophy, aberrant healing of rib or clavicle fracture, tumor) etiologies. The most common is the *scalenus anterior syndrome* due to an abnormal insertion of the anterior scalene on the first rib.

Symptoms of the thoracic outlet syndrome include numbness, paresthesias, pain, sensory and motor deficits, and coolness that may be exacerbated with certain positioning. If the artery is involved, the radial pulse on the affected side may diminish or cease when the position (arm abduction, or neck extended and

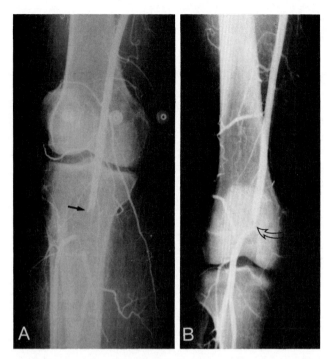

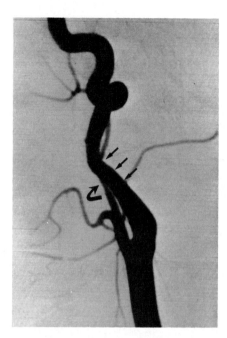

Figure 21.17 .**Popliteal Artery Occlusion. A.** Abrupt termination of flow is noted within the popliteal artery. Note the filling defect with subtle convex superior margin within the popliteal artery (*arrow*) and associated meniscus of contrast about this filling defect, typical for embolic occlusion. **B.** Smoothly bordered tapering (*arrow*) and near occlusion of the popliteal artery is typical of popliteal artery entrapment syndrome.

Figure 21.18.   Radiation Vasculitis. This carotid arteriogram in a 30-year-old patient who underwent radiation for rhabdomyosarcoma at age 5 shows the chronic sequelae of radiation with smooth tapering of the internal carotid artery (*straight arrows*) and ECA (*curved arrow*). A normal bifurcation helps differentiate this from atherosclerotic disease.

Figure 21.19.   Fibromuscular Dysplasia. A. Right renal artery injection shows the beaded appearance of medial fibromuscular dysplasia (*curved arrow*) with aneurysm formation (*straight arrow*). **B.** The cervical carotid artery (*curved black arrows*) shown with an associated intracranial aneurysm (*curved open arrow*) and Iliac arteries (**C.**) (*arrows*) are less commonly involved.

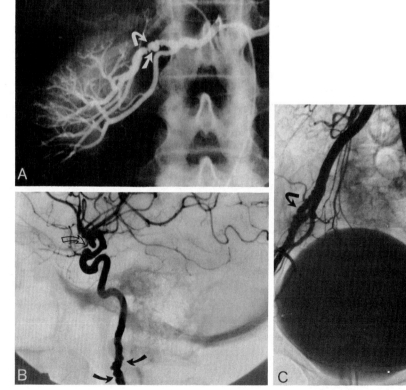

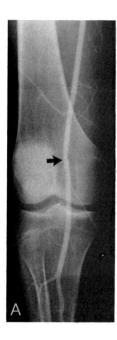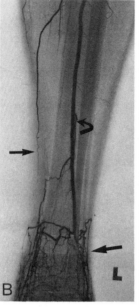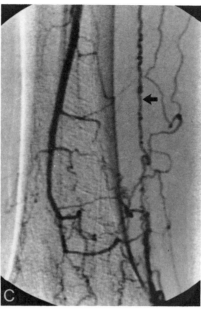

Figure 21.20. Buerger's Disease (Thromboangiitis Obliterans) . A. This arteritide typically is without atherosclerotic or other occlusive changes involving the proximal arteries. This 37-year-old male smoker has normal-appearing distal superficial femoral and popliteal arteries (*arrow*). **B.** Note the more distal arterial disease with corkscrew vessels (*straight arrows*) specific for this entity. Note the normal peroneal artery (*curved arrow*) associated with occlusion of the anterior and posterior tibial arteries. **C.** Opposite leg arteriogram, just above the ankle, with a typical corkscrew vessel (*arrow*).

head turned toward affected side) is assumed. However, this may also be seen in asymptomatic individuals and is thus an insensitive test. Venous involvement results in intermittent cyanosis, edema, and possible thrombosis.

Angiography is performed both in the neutral position with arms at the sides, and in the position that reproduces the patient's symptoms (Fig. 21.21). Both arteriography and venography may need to be performed if symptoms dictate. Most patients with arterial involvement will have fusiform aneurysmal dilation of the artery distal to the level of compression, representing poststenotic dilation. Other findings include focal stenosis, aneurysm, and distal embolization.

Popliteal Entrapment Syndrome represents compression of the popliteal artery either by abnormal medial course of the popliteal artery in relation to the medial head of the gastrocnemius muscle, an abnormal insertion of the muscle itself, or compression by the popliteus muscle. Bilateral disease is seen in 20% of cases, with males more commonly affected (8:1). Clinical presentation is unilateral calf claudication in a young male, which may be sudden in onset. Classic angiographic findings include medial deviation of the popliteal artery and stenosis (Fig. 21.17**B**). Stress views (active plantar flexion against resistance) may be necessary to evoke the findings. Other findings include popliteal artery thrombosis and aneurysm formation.

Vascular Grafts

Vascular grafts for the treatment of lower extremity occlusive disease and abdominal aortic aneurysms are commonplace procedures. The grafts frequently encountered in the abdomen and pelvis are the *aortobifemoral* (Fig. 21.22**A**) and *aortobiiliac* grafts which extend from the infrarenal aorta to the groins or proximal external iliac arteries, respectively, and are usually composed of GORETEX. *Extraanatomic* grafts are used in patients who require bypass for aortoiliac occlusive disease but are at high risk for a major abdominal procedure. The grafts extend from the axillary artery to the ipsilateral common femoral artery, with an accompanying graft extending to the contralateral femoral artery, and are known as "*ax-fem:fem-fem*" grafts. They too are composed of synthetic material. Puncturing grafts for access can be difficult and is usually performed using a singlewall technique. Because of the resistance of the graft material and the fibrosis present in the groin, overdilation may be required and a sheath should be placed. If no sheath is used, all catheters should be straightened over a guidewire prior to removal.

Femoropopliteal (fem-pop) grafts (Fig. 21.22 **B** and **C**) are used to bypass infrainguinal disease and extend from the common femoral artery to the popliteal artery either above or below the knee. A variant of this is the so called "*fem-distal*" graft, which bypasses to one of the trifurcation vessels at a variable distance into the calf. They are composed of either synthetic material or autologous vein graft, usually saphenous vein. If the vein is removed and reversed end for end, thus negating the function of the valves, it is termed *reverse saphenous vein*. If the vein is left in place and the proximal and distal ends anastomosed to the respective arteries (following valve excision using a valvulotome), it is termed *in situ vein graft*.

Graft complications include thrombosis, pseudoaneurysm formation (Fig. 21.22**D**), infection, postoperative hemorrhage, and graft-enteric fistula (14).

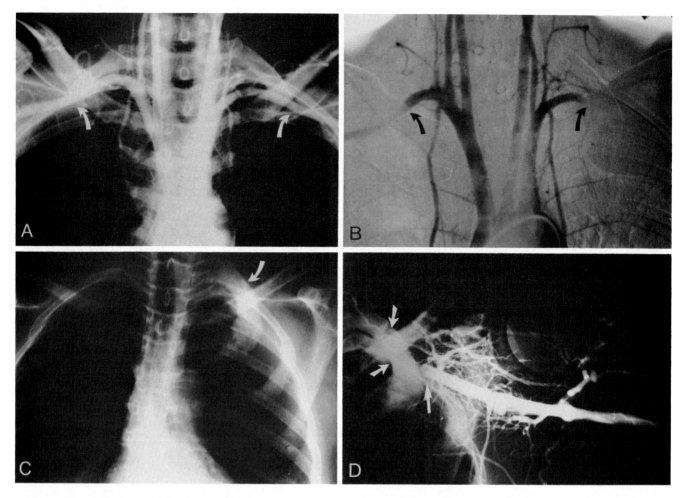

Figure 21.21.   Thoracic Outlet Syndrome. A. Aortic arch injection in a patient with thoracic outlet obstruction symptoms in the neutral position shows normal opacification of the subclavian arteries (*arrows*). **B.** With abduction of both arms there is occlusion of flow within the subclavian arteries bilaterally (*arrows*). **C.** Frontal projection of the upper ribs shows bony expansion and sclerosis of the left first rib, consistent with Paget's Disease (*arrow*). **D.** Upper extremity venogram demonstrates abrupt occlusion at the lateral margin of the enlarged first rib (*short arrows*) with the meniscoid filling defect representing thrombus (*long arrow*).

Duplex ultrasound is used to evaluate grafts below the inguinal ligament; angiography is reserved for cases in which a complication is suspected and intervention is planned. Grafts within the abdomen and pelvis are best evaluated for suspected complications by CT. Graft infections typically demonstrate perigraft fluid and gas. Pseudoaneurysms occur at the graft anastamoses, most commonly in the groin. Aortoenteric fistulas are discussed later.

Renal Occlusive Diseases

Atherosclerosis is the most common cause of renal artery stenosis (65% of cases) (Fig. 21.23) and is bilateral in approximately 40% of cases, occurring most frequently in patients over 50 years old. The stenoses are most commonly seen at the ostium and within the proximal third of the artery. Renal artery disease is nearly always associated with aortic disease, and osteal involvement reflects atherosclerotic plaque within the aorta extending across the renal artery orifice. Iso-

lated branch vessel disease is uncommon and is typically associated with main renal artery involvement. Atherosclerotic renal artery stenoses are responsible for approximately 65% of cases of renovascular hypertension. Angioplasty success rates depend on the location of the lesion—nonostial (80% of cases) versus ostial lesions (<40%).

Fibromuscular Dysplasia is the second most common cause of renal artery stenosis (30% of cases). The majority of lesions are seen in young females and more commonly affect the right renal artery, with bilateral involvement in 65% of cases. Fibromuscular dysplasia represents a heterogeneous group of lesions of unknown pathogenesis that affect the intima, media, or adventitia of the artery. Classification of the subgroups is made based upon the primary site of involvement in the arterial wall: *intimal hyperplasia, medial fibroplasia, fibromuscular hyperplasia,* and *subadventitial fibroplasia* (15). Medial fibroplasia is the most common of the subtypes, accounting for ap-

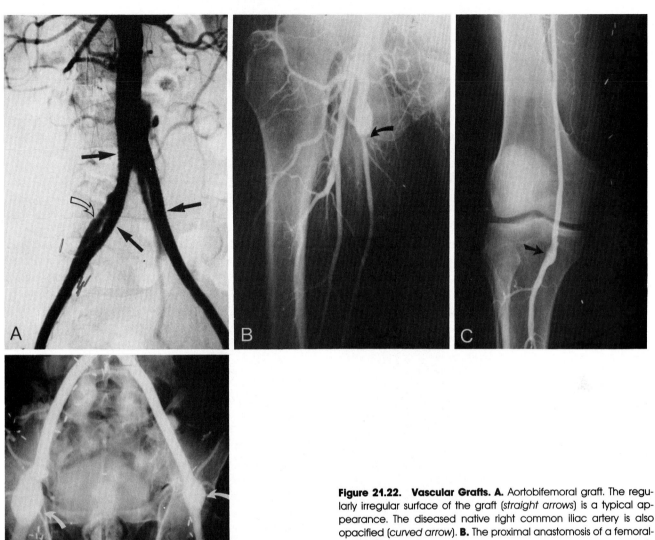

Figure 21.22. Vascular Grafts. A. Aortobifemoral graft. The regularly irregular surface of the graft (*straight arrows*) is a typical appearance. The diseased native right common iliac artery is also opacified (*curved arrow*). **B.** The proximal anastomosis of a femoral-popliteal graft using autologous reversed saphenous vein (*arrow*). **C.** The distal anastomosis of the femoral-popliteal graft in **B** is shown (*arrow*). **D.** One of the complications of grafts is pseudoaneurysm formation. Bilateral pseudoaneurysms, right greater than left, are shown (*arrows*) in this aortobifemoral graft.

proximately 75% of cases, and consists of the classic "string of beads" appearance on angiography, which represents alternating web-like stenoses and aneurysms (Fig. 21.19**A**). The middle and distal main renal artery is more frequently involved and is rarely seen involving the proximal renal artery alone. Fibromuscular dysplasia accounts for approximately one-third of the cases of renovascular hypertension and is the most common cause of hypertension in children. Angioplasty success rates approach 98%, thus making this the treatment of choice in FMD (14).

Neurofibromatosis can cause renal artery stenosis either by extrinsic compression of the renal artery by neurofibromata, or from disorganized intimal and medial proliferation, typically located at the renal artery orifice or proximal renal artery. Angiography demonstrates smooth or nodular-appearing stenoses with or without associated aneurysms. Hypertension secondary to neurofibromatosis is seen mainly in children.

Polyarteritis Nodosa is a rare necrotizing vasculitis that affects the small and medium-sized arteries. Multiple organs are typically involved with renal (85% of cases) and hepatic (65%) involvement being the most common. Characteristic subcutaneous nodules are seen in 15% of cases. The major angiographic findings include multiple, small, saccular "*microaneurysms*"; occlusions; and irregular stenoses throughout the abdominal viscera (Fig. 21.24) (13). The microaneurysms range in size from 1 to 12 mm and are typically located at branch points; they are seen in approximately 50% of patients. The differential diagnosis of the microaneurysms seen with polyarteritis nodosa include Wegener's granulomatosis, systemic lupus erythematosus, rheumatoid vasculitis, and drug abuse. (13)

Hemodialysis Access

Long-term hemodialysis access can be constructed by the use of internal arteriovenous fistulas or by the placement of synthetic graft material to bridge between artery and vein. The most common internal fistula is the *Brescia-Cimino fistula*, which is formed by anastamosing the radial artery to the cephalic vein at the wrist. The "arterialized" section of vein proximal to the anastamosis in the forearm is then punctured for access. *Arteriovenous bridge grafts* are composed of GORETEX and are usually placed within the subcutaneous tissues of the forearm. They may be in a loop configuration or straight, and bridge from brachial artery to antecubital vein or radial artery to antecubital vein (16). The graft material is then punctured for access.

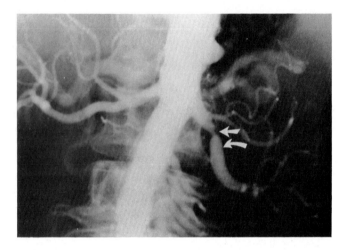

Figure 21.23.   Atherosclerotic Renal Artery Stenosis. Focal stenosis of the proximal left renal artery (*straight arrow*) with mild poststenotic arterial dilation (*curved arrow*) are typical of atherosclerotic stenosis.

Figure 21.24.   Polyarteritis Nodosa. Abdominal aorta injection with multiple microaneurysms involving the kidneys bilaterally (*curved arrows*). Although the kidneys are most commonly involved, other viscera can display similar vascular findings including the liver (*open arrow*) and spleen (*straight arrow*).

Complications include infection, bleeding, pseudoaneurysm formation (either at the graft anastamoses or from previous access puncture sites), thrombosis, stenosis, and vascular steal (flow through fistula "steals" blood from hand) (16). Stenoses can occur at either the arterial anastomosis or, more commonly, within the venous outflow limb. These are heralded by low arterial pressures and high venous pressures, respectively, at the time of dialysis.

Examination Technique involves puncturing the fistula in the venous limb with the needle directed toward the arterial inflow. Hand injections of contrast are made using either CA or DSA imaging. If visualization of the arterial anastomosis is indicated by the dialysis pressure abnormalities, a blood pressure cuff is applied to the upper arm and imaging performed once the cuff reaches systolic blood pressure. The cuff may then be released during the imaging sequence in order to visualize outflow through the venous limb. Duplex ultrasound is also useful for imaging and evaluation of graft complications.

Interventional Procedures

Percutaneous   Transluminal   Angioplasty (PTA) is indicated in the treatment of arterial occlusive disease that produces claudication interfering with life-style, rest pain, nonhealing ulcers, and gangrene; and is the treatment of choice for FMD. Percutaneous transluminal angioplasty is also used to treat the stenotic complications of hemodialysis access fistulas. Factors that predict technical success and long-term patency after angioplasty include (*a*) the artery involved—common iliac artery is better than SFA, which in turn is better than below-the-knee vessels; (*b*) the length of the disease—a short lesion better

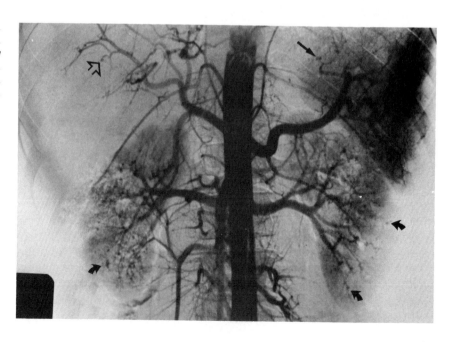

than a long one; (c) lesion morphology—concentric stenosis is better than eccentric; and (d) calcified lesion—which has a worse prognosis than noncalcified (Fig. 21.15). The PTA balloon creates controlled vessel injury by irreversibly stretching the vessel wall and "cracking" the plaque thus increasing the luminal diameter of the vessel. This produces a "cleft" in the lesion that extends through the intima and into the media, and is seen angiographically as a linear collection of contrast outside the main contrast column (Fig. 21.16C). Endothelium then grows into these clefts over a period of months and effectively heals the vessel open. Technical success at the time of PTA is defined as residual stenosis less than 30%, and less than 10 mm Hg pressure gradient across the lesion. Complications of PTA include intimal dissection, thrombosis, distal embolization, and vessel rupture (rare).

Basic technique of PTA is as follows: immediate preangioplasty heparin (5000 IU) and vascular antispasmodics (oral nifedipine, 10 mg, or intraarterial nitroglycerine, 100 μg); cross the lesion with guidewire and catheter; remove guidewire and inject contrast to confirm intraluminal position (not subintimal); replace guidewire, pass balloon across lesion, and dilate, watching for "waist" of balloon to resolve; and finally, inject contrast to check results, leaving a wire across PTA site *at all times* in case further dilation is required. The balloon size (in mm) is chosen by measuring the normal diameter artery near lesion, realizing that an inherent magnification factor of 20% will result in desired "overdilation" of the lesion.

Thrombolysis is most commonly utilized in acute native arterial or bypass graft thrombosis as well as in thrombosis of hemodialysis access shunts. The most commonly used agent is *urokinase*, which works by activating the body's endogenous enzyme plasmin with the end result being clot lysis, and has a half-life of approximately 17 minutes.

Contraindications to lytic therapy include active bleeding or recent gastrointestinal (GI) bleeding, central nervous system surgery in the past 2 months, intracranial tumor, recent stroke, and nonviable extremity. Lytic agents are administered locally into the clot through the arterial catheter at doses ranging from 800 U/min (low dose) to 4000 U/min (high dose). In general, the older the clot, the longer lysis will take for complete clot resolution. Complications of thrombolysis include bleeding, puncture site hematoma, pericatheter thrombus formation, and distal embolization.

SYSTEMIC VEINS
Normal Anatomy

Upper Extremity. As opposed to the lower extremity, the upper extremity is drained predominantly by the superficial venous system consisting of the *cephalic* and *basilic* veins in the upper arm. The basilic vein courses along the ulnar aspect of the forearm and medial forearm to continue as the axillary vein. The cephalic vein lies along the radial aspect of the forearm and ascends on the anterolateral upper arm to join the axillary vein below the clavicle. The deep system consists of small, paired veins that follow the artery (brachial in the upper arm) and empty into the basilic vein. The axillary vein becomes the subclavian vein at the lateral border of the first rib, which then receives the internal jugular vein to form the bracheocephalic vein.

Lower Extremity. The lower extremity is drained primarily by the deep venous system, which consists of paired veins in the calf that follow the arteries both in course and name (Fig. 21.25). Thus, there are paired *anterior tibial, posterior tibial*, and *peroneal* veins in the calf that join to form a single *popliteal* vein below the joint line of the knee. The deep veins from the *soleus* and *gastrocnemius* muscles drain into the tibioperoneal system and popliteal vein, respectively. The popliteal vein then continues into the thigh as the *superficial femoral* vein (SFV), which is then joined by the *profunda femorus* vein to form the *common femoral* vein (CFV) at the inferior margin of the femoral head. The popliteal and superficial femoral veins may be duplicated partially or completely in approximately 25% of patients.

The superficial system of the lower extremity is composed of the *greater* and *lesser saphenous* veins. The lesser vein begins at the lateral ankle and courses over the posterior calf to join the popliteal or greater saphenous veins. The greater saphenous vein originates near the medial malleolus and ascends the anteromedial leg to empty into the CFV at the inguinal ligament. Multiple small communicating veins between the superficial and deep system are present in the calf and lower thigh and are called *perforating* veins. These contain valves and are responsible for directing flow from the superficial to the deep system. The CFV then enters the pelvis medial to the common femoral artery to become the *external iliac* vein and eventually the *common iliac* vein at the sacrum, where it receives the *internal iliac* vein. The *ascending lumbar* vein empties into the common iliac vein directly, and is an important communication with the azygos system.

Imaging Methods

Imaging of the venous system of the lower extremities is performed in most cases for the exclusion of deep venous thrombosis, and relies predominantly on duplex ultrasound supplemented by contrast venography. Radionuclide venography is also utilized, typically in conjunction with ventilation-perfusion lung scanning, and can be used to examine both the upper

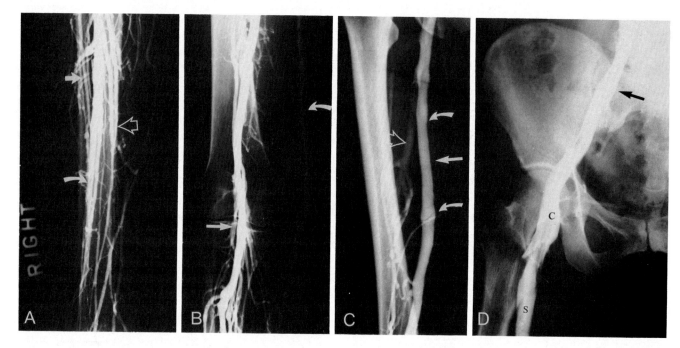

Figure 21.25.   Normal Lower Extremity Venogram. A. Following contrast injection into a vein of the dorsal aspect of the foot, there is homogeneous opacification of the calf veins. The anterior (*straight arrow*) and posterior (*open arrow*) tibial veins as well as the peroneal (*curved arrow*) veins are seen. **B.** The trifurcation vessels form the popliteal vein (*straight arrow*). Faint opacification of the greater saphenous vein (*curved arrow*) is also seen. **C.** The superficial femo-

ral vein (*straight arrow*) is well opacified without obstruction or filling defects. Note multiple, well-defined valves (*curved arrows*). Faint opacification of the profunda femoral vein is also seen (*open arrow*). **D.** A properly performed "dump" shot shows normal filling of the iliac vein (*arrow*). S, superficial femoral vein; *CFV*, common femoral vein.

and lower extremity veins. However, this technique suffers from poor spatial resolution and inability to detect nonocclusive thrombi in larger veins. Duplex ultrasound is limited in the upper extremity by overlying bony anatomy at the shoulder; thus, contrast venography remains a mainstay for evaluation of this region.

Basic Contrast Venogram Technique

Lower Extremity contrast venography may be performed using a variety of techniques. The nonweight bearing method is done by having the patient stand on a box placed under the unaffected extremity and tilting the table upright approximately 30–35°. A dorsal pedal vein along the lateral aspect of the foot is then cannulated (ideally directed toward the toes to facilitate filling of the deep system) and an intravenous infusion of heparinized saline begun. This not only flushes contrast out of the calf at the end of the procedure (contrast-induced thrombophlebitis occurs in <1% of cases), but also ensures flow without extravasation prior to the injection of contrast. A tourniquet is applied at the ankle to further assist in forcing the contrast into the deep system. Approximately 90–120 ml of 60% contrast is then injected over the course of the examination. Imaging may be performed using 14 × 17 inch film or fluoroscopic spot filming (with the former preferred because

of greater spatial resolution) over the calf, knee, thigh, and pelvis with the patient in the semiupright position. Filling of the iliac system and inferior vena cava is facilitated by having the patient Valsalva while the calf is gently massaged to push contrast into the SFV. The patient then relaxes, allowing the contrast to flow into the pelvis during the exposure.

Upper Extremity contrast venography is usually performed for the evaluation of axillary or subclavian vein obstruction. Thus, an antecubital vein is suitable for cannulation, and contrast is injected under fluoroscopic control with spot film or DSA imaging.

Venous Duplex Technique

The proximal deep veins of the lower extremity are examined from the inguinal ligament to the popliteal fossa. The examination of the common and superficial femoral veins is performed with the patient supine and with slight reverse Trendelenburg position. The leg is abducted and externally rotated. Utilizing linear 5 or 7.5 MHz transducers, the vessels are evaluated in the transverse plane. Compression and release of the venous structures is performed in the transverse plane every 1 cm to the level of the popliteal fossa. In the prone position with the knee bent approximately 15°, the popliteal vessels are examined. Compressibility of the veins and presence or absence of intraluminal thrombus is assessed (17). Longitudi-

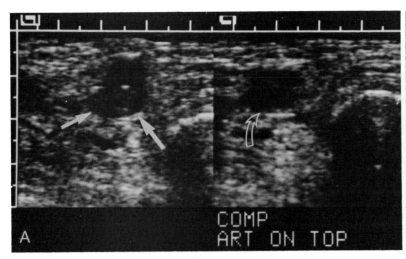

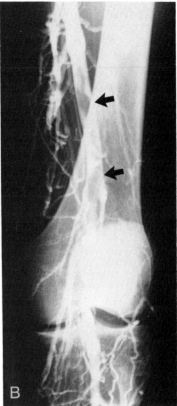

Figure 21.26. Lower Extremity DVT. A. Graded compression ultrasound demonstrates echogenic material with the superficial femoral vein (*straight arrows*). Compression image (*curved arrow*) shows distortion of the artery without coaptation of the vein, consistent with intraluminal venous thrombus. **B.** Left lower extremity venogram with serpentine intraluminal filling defect (*arrows*) consistent with thrombus within the popliteal vein.

nal views are utilized to determine the extent of thrombus. Calf veins can be examined for thrombosis as well, but this is a time-intensive examination and not routinely performed at most institutions.

Doppler interrogation of the veins provides a determination of spontaneous venous flow (that varying with normal respirations) and augmented flow created by squeezing the distal extremity. Color Doppler ultrasound is helpful in areas that are difficult to compress (distal SFV in Hunter's canal).

Deep Venous Thrombosis

Lower Extremity. The true prevalence of deep vein thrombosus (DVT) is unknown and DVT is a disease that remains asymptomatic in many patients. In patients who have symptomatic pulmonary emboli but who exhibit no signs of DVT, one-third will have lower extremity thrombus. In addition, the clinical diagnosis of DVT is unreliable such that when the signs and symptoms suggest DVT, the diagnosis is errant in 50% of cases (18). The most common symptoms associated with DVT are pain and swelling of the involved extremity, along with cyanosis, warmth, distension of the superficial veins and palpation of a tender, indurrated cord if a superficial vein developed thrombosis. Patients may be asymptomatic if the thrombus is incompletely obstructing the vein or one half of a duplication anomaly has thrombosed.

Risk Factors include prolonged immobilization, increasing age, pregnancy, oral contraceptive use, obesity, surgery (especially abdominal and orthopaedic), severe trauma, status postmyocardial infarction, congestive heart failure, malignancy, polycythemia, and previous acute DVT. In most patients, the thrombus originates in the calf; however, in patients who undergo hip surgery, DVT is more likely to develop in the iliofemoral system (18).

Upper Extremity. Deep venous thrombosis involving the upper extremities is much less common than that involving the lower extremity, but the incidence is increasing with the more frequent use of indwelling central venous catheters. Other causes include posttraumatic complications, secondary to thoracic outlet syndrome (see earlier discussion), central obstructing lesion such as rib abnormality (Fig. 21.21, **C** and **D**) or tumor, or postradiation. *Effort thrombosis* represents axillary vein thrombosis following vigorous exercise, with compression of the axillary vein during forced abduction. As with lower extremity DVT, thrombus within the upper extremity may be a source for pulmonary emboli (18).

Imaging

Duplex Ultrasound. The most reliable sign of thrombus within the deep veins is lack of compressibility (Fig. 21.26A) (17). Intraluminal thrombus will not allow normal coaptation to the venous walls. The amount of pressure to coapt the walls of the vein should not be enough to alter the contour to the adjacent artery. A less reliable sign is visualization of thrombus within the vein. The chronicity of thrombus is difficult to determine as acute and chronic clot can manifest as intraluminal echogenic material (16). If a vein is not visualized in its expected location, this may indicate thrombus that is isoechoic with muscle.

Doppler evaluation provides secondary information concerning the patency of the deep veins of the lower extremity. *Phasic flow* is that which varies with respiration, and if absent, bodes for a more proximal venous obstruction, either intrinsic or extrinsic. This is particularly helpful as a secondary sign of venous thrombosis involving the iliac veins. Detectable blood flow should also stop during the Valsalva maneuver in a patent venous system. *Augmented flow* is that which shows an increase in the proximal flow with compression of the distal vein.

For above-the-knee venous thrombosis, duplex compression sonography provides a sensitivity of 96% and specificity of 97% (17). Determination of acute versus chronic thrombus is problematic. Several sonographic signs are helpful in determining the chronicity of clot. As opposed to chronic thrombus, acute clot expands the normal caliber of the vein and tends to be more pliable. Older clot is firmer, tends to cause irregularity of the venous wall, and is associated with formation of collateral vessels (19).

Venography. The only conclusive finding of acute DVT on contrast venography is a persistent intraluminal filling defect within the vein lumen (Fig. 21.26**B**). Other findings highly suggestive of acute DVT include abrupt termination of the contrast column in the vein, inability to opacify a vein, and collateral formation. The more chronic the obstruction, the more collateral veins may be detected. This is especially true in the upper extremity. *Chronic DVT* represents the morphologic changes during clot organization and is manifested by persistent, eccentric mural filling defect, *recanalization* with establishment of an irregular, eccentric channel, loss of valves, persistent occlusion, and incompetent perforating veins and varicosities.

Post-Phlebitic Syndrome depicts the clinical manifestations of chronic DVT caused by valve destruction and inefficiency of the recanalized residual system to pump blood from the calf. This results in chronic venous stasis disease with the distinctive skin changes, pain, swelling, varicosities, and venous stasis ulcers typically seen at the ankles.

Phlegmasia Cerulea Dolens is a grave condition due to extensive DVT of the iliofemoral system leading to marked elevation of venous pressure in the extremity. This in turn leads to progressive swelling and compromise of the arterial circulation, with subsequent gangrene.

MESENTERIC VESSELS
Anatomy

Arterial. The *celiac axis, superior mesenteric (SMA),* and *inferior mesenteric (IMA)* arteries are the main arterial supply to the GI tract (Figs. 21.4**A** and 21.27). The celiac axis originates at the T-12 level, giving rise to the *splenic, common hepatic,* and *left gastric* arteries (Fig. 21.27**A**). The *common hepatic* artery becomes the *proper hepatic* artery after giving off the *gastroduodenal* artery, which then branches into the *superior pancreaticoduodenal* (anterior and posterior) and *right gastroepiploic* arteries. The *left gastroepiploic* artery and *short gastric* arteries are distal branches of the splenic artery. The *right gastric* artery is a small artery with variable origin, usually from the proper or left hepatic artery. The left gastric artery supplies the distal esophagus and the majority of the stomach (70%) running along the lesser curvature. The gastroepiploic arteries form an anastomosing arc along the greater curvature of the stomach, supplying the bulk of the remainder of gastric flow. A common normal variant is the *replaced right hepatic* artery, which originates from the SMA and is seen in 10% of individuals.

The SMA originates at the T-12/L-1 level and supplies the entire small intestine and the proximal two-thirds of the colon (Fig. 21.27**B**). The first branch is the *inferior pancreaticoduodenal* (anterior and posterior) artery, which freely anastomoses with the superior pancreaticoduodenal artery to supply the duodenum. The remaining branches in order of origin from the SMA are the *jejunal, ileal, middle colic, right colic,* and *terminal ileocolic* arteries. The middle colic artery divides into the left and right branches that freely anastomose with the respective right and left colic (IMA) arteries. The ileocolic artery supplies the terminal ileum and cecum; the right colic artery supplies the ascending colon and hepatic flexure, and the middle colic artery supplies the transverse colon.

The IMA originates at approximately the L-3 level and gives rise to the *left colic, sigmoid,* and *superior hemorrhoidal (rectal)* arteries (Fig. 21.27**C**). The superior hemorrhoidal artery branches freely anastomose with the hemorrhoidal artery branches of the internal iliac system.

Collateral Communications of the mesenteric vessels involve three arteries. (a) The *marginal artery of Drummond* represents the free anastomosis between the right colic, right and left branches of the

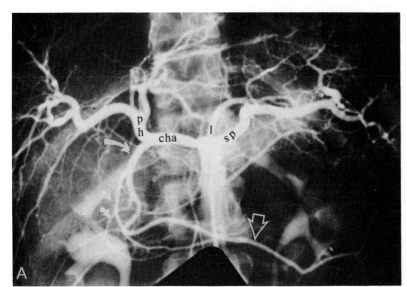

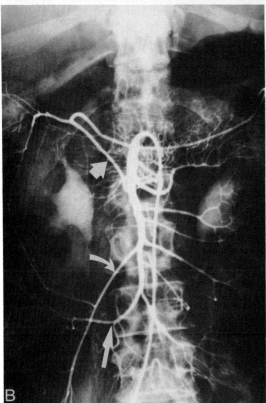

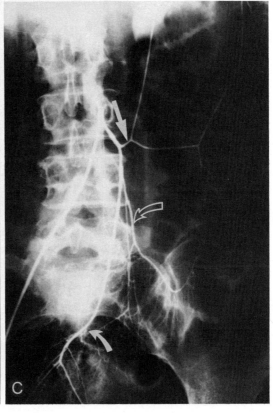

Figure 21.27. Normal Mesenteric Arteriogram. A. Celiac axis injection with the major branches: common hepatic artery *(cha)*, splenic artery *(sp)*, and left gastric artery *(l)*. The common hepatic artery continues as the proper hepatic artery *(ph)* after formation of the gastroduodenal artery *(large curved arrow)*. Major branches from the gastroduodenal artery include the pancreaticoduodenal arcade *(small curved arrows)* and continuation as the right gastroepiploic artery. **B.** Superior mesenteric artery injection: middle colic artery *(short straight arrow)*, right colic artery *(large straight arrow)*, and the ileocolic artery *(curved arrow)*. **C.** Inferior mesenteric artery (note attenuation of the vessel due to hypotension from GI bleeding at the time of the injection): left colic branches *(straight arrow)*, sigmoid branches *(curved open arrow)*, and superior hemorrhoidal *(curved arrow)*.

middle colic, and the left colic arteries. It is found along the mesenteric border of the colon and is an important collateral supply in IMA occlusions seen commonly with atherosclerosis and abdominal aortic aneurysm (Fig. 21.28); (*b*) the *Arc of Riolan* is a variable communication between the SMA and IMA and is located more centrally in the mesentery than the marginal artery, (*c*) the *Arc of Bühler* is a short, ventral artery between the main celiac and SMA representing a persistent fetal communication.

Portal Venous Anatomy (Fig. 21.29). The venous drainage of the GI tract generally follows the ar-

terial anatomy. The *inferior mesenteric* vein usually joins with the *splenic vein* near its junction with the *superior mesenteric* vein to give rise to the *main portal* vein. The *left* and *right gastric (coronary)* veins drain directly into the portal vein. The portal vein supplies approximately 70% of the blood supply of the liver. Normal antegrade flow in the portal venous system is termed "hepatopetal" flow." Reversal of flow is termed "hepatofugal" flow" and represents flow through portosystemic communications (e.g., coronary vein to azygos system, resulting in esophageal varices).

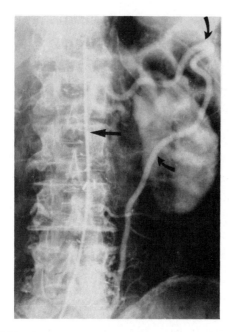

Figure 21.28. Marginal Artery of Drummond. In this patient undergoing an arteriogram for evaluation of an abdominal aortic aneurysm, there was notation of occlusion of the IMA. A catheter is seen within the aorta (*straight arrow*) with filling of the marginal artery of Drummond (*curved arrows*), providing collateral blood supply for the occluded mesenteric arterial segments.

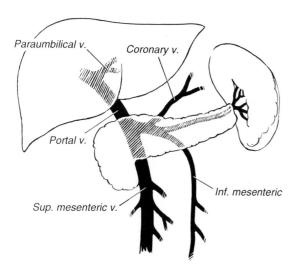

Figure 21.29. Portal Venous Anatomy.

Basic Angiographic Techniques

Selective injections of the individual vessels are required for accurate evaluation of the mesenteric arterial system (Table 21.2). Imaging of the portal venous system may be accomplished in one of two ways. The first involves selective celiac or SMA injections and late imaging to visualize the venous phase. Opacification may be enhanced with the direct arterial administration of tolazoline 25–50 mg into the SMA, which dilates end arterioles facilitating flow into the venous

system at the capillary level. Additionally, 15° left anterior oblique positioning projects the anatomy of interest off the spine and better profiles the main portal branches. The second method for portal venous imaging requires direct transhepatic puncture of the portal vein and is uncommonly used.

Gastrointestinal Hemorrhage

The evaluation of GI bleeding includes evaluation of the nasogastric tube (NG) aspirate, esophagogastric duodenoscopy, colonoscopy, radionuclide imaging (tagged-red blood cells and sulfur colloid), and angiography. The application of these modalities depends on the likely source of bleeding and the clinical status of the patient. Hemodynamically unstable patients may require emergency angiography and/or surgery, while the stable patient is able to undergo a more controlled, systematic evaluation and treatment. For suspected upper GI (UGI) bleeding (source proximal to the ligament of Treitz), the evaluation should begin with NG aspirate followed by endoscopy. For lower GI bleeding (essentially small bowel and colon source), the evaluation should consist of colonoscopy or radionuclide imaging to localize the site of bleeding and to guide the angiographic examination to the most likely vascular territory. Interventional procedures for the treatment of GI bleeding that can be provided by the radiologist consists of either vasopressin administration or transcatheter embolization (see "Interventional Procedures").

The most reliable angiographic sign of GI bleeding is contrast extravasation and this is seen as an amorphous contrast collection that persists through the venous phase. If the bleeding rate is rapid enough, the extravasated contrast may outline mucosal folds. One manifestation of this is the "*pseudovein*" sign, which represents a linear collection of contrast between mucosal folds, simulating an enlarged vein (Fig. 21.30). Other, less specific, signs include hyperemia and identification of a vascular malformation, aneurysm, or hypervascular mass. A bleeding rate of at least 0.5 ml per minute is necessary to be identified by angiography (20).

UPPER GI BLEEDING

Mallory-Weiss Tear is typically a single, longitudinal split in the mucosa located on the posterolateral aspect of the esophagogastric junction, usually on the gastric side. These account for approximately 14% of UGI bleeds and are usually associated with severe vomiting and retching as well as excessive alcohol consumption (20). Patients present with excruciating epigastric and left chest pain and may develop pneumothorax and pneumomediastinum if the injury is transmural. Arterial supply is left gastric, inferior

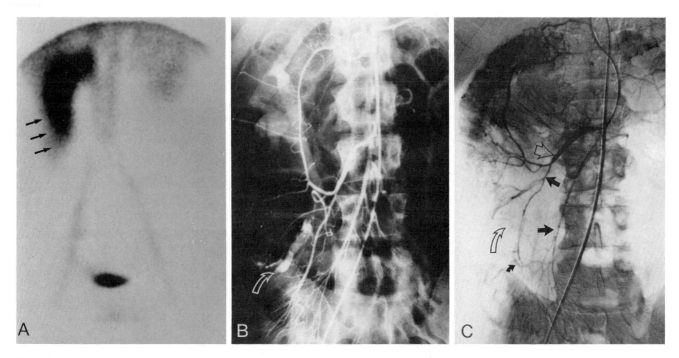

Figure 21.30. Lower GI Bleeding. A. A tagged red blood cell scan shows accumulation of radiotracer in the region of the hepatic flexure (*arrows*). The primary site of bleeding is not delineated. **B.** An SMA anteriogram demonstrates exstravasation of contrast in the right lower quadrant within a bleeding diverticulum with "pseudovein sign" (*arrow*). **C.** Following administration of intraarterial vaso-

pressin a repeat SMA injection shows no evidence of continued bleeding (*curved open arrow*). Note attenuation of vessels in response to the vasopressin infusion *(straight arrows)*, with a sudden decrease in caliber (*open arrow*). *Small curved arrow* show maintenance of venous return.

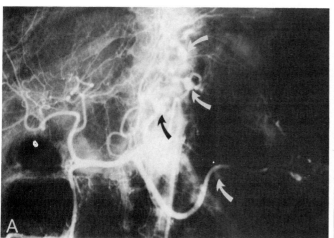

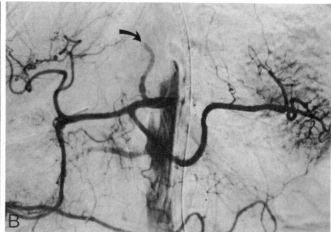

Figure 21.31. Bleeding Gastric Ulcers. A. Celiac artery injection shows multiple areas of extraluminal contrast within the stomach (*arrows*). These represent multiple foci of bleeding gastric ulceration. **B.**

The same patient, following embolization of the left gastric artery (*arrow*), fails to show evidence for continued gastric bleeding.

phrenic, or short gastrics. Treatment is (*a*) vasopressin, with 88% success, and (*b*) embolization (20).

Acute Hemorrhagic Gastritis accounts for approximately 27% of UGI bleeds and may occur without identifiable cause or may be seen in critically ill patients following surgery, burns, or trauma. It is also commonly seen in alcoholics. The angiographic appearance is a diffusely hyperemic mucosa with multiple punctate foci of contrast extravasation. Arterial

supply is left gastric, gastroepiploic. Treatment is (*a*) vasopressin, with 84% success, and (*b*) embolization (20).

Gastric Ulcers are responsible for approximately 10% of acute UGI bleeding (Fig. 21.31). The etiology may be idiopathic, seen in stress situations such as burns or major surgery, or associated with Zollinger-Ellison syndrome. It is usually seen as a single focus of contrast puddling or may demonstrate the "pseudovein" sign as contrast flows from the bleeding site between gastric rugae. Arterial supply is left gastric (most common), gastroepiploic. Treatment is (a) surgery, (b) embolization, which is used as temporary measure, and (c) vasopressin (20).

Duodenal Peptic Ulcer is the cause of UGI bleeding in approximately 25% of cases. The NG aspirate may be negative and in a small percent may present as lower GI bleeding. Other causes of duodenal bleeding include vascular malformations, visceral aneurysms, and neoplasm. Arterial supply is gastroduodenal, inferior pancreaticoduodenal. Thus, one may have to study both the celiac and SMA. Treatment is (a) surgery and (b) embolization (20).

Postsurgical Anastomoses following gastric bypass procedures (e.g., gastrojejunostomy) may be complicated by erosive ulceration, which is typically located on the jejunal side. Because of the distorted anatomy following surgery, several vessels may need to be studied. Arterial supply is usually SMA. Treatment is (a) vasopressin, and (b) embolization, with caution because of a surgically compromised vascular supply.

LOWER GI BLEEDING

Small Bowel

Aortoenteric Fistula accounts for approximately 10% of small bowel bleeding and usually represents a complication of abdominal aortic aneurysm surgery. It is located in the duodenum in 80% of cases, where it crosses over the aorta and can be seen as soon as 3 weeks postoperatively. Computed tomography findings suggestive of fistula formation is gas present in the retroperitoneal soft tissues in the region of the anastomosis. Others include loss of the normal fat plane between the duodenum and aorta, although this is nonspecific (14). Angiographically, it presents as an anterior nipple-like projection from the aortic graft anastomosis or rarely as contrast extravasation at the fistula site. Angiography is performed using an aortic injection, not selective injections of the SMA. Treatment is urgent surgery (20).

Tumor is the most common cause of bleeding from the small bowel. It is responsible for 20–50% of the cases of small bowel hemorrhage and is depicted angiographically as tumor neovascularity (enlarged, bizarre, irregular vessels with arteriovenous shunting) with or without contrast extravasation. Treatment is surgery.

Diverticula of the small bowel are an uncommon (6% of cases) cause of small bowel bleeding. They are located along the mesenteric border of the bowel; the jejunum is more common as a source for bleeding than the ileum. They typically bleed very slowly and

thus may be difficult to diagnose angiographically. Treatment is (a) vasopressin and (b) surgery.

Meckel's Diverticulum, or omphalomesenteric duct remnant, is found along the antimesenteric border in the distal ileum. Patients typically present with painless bleeding due to an ileal ulcer adjacent to heterotopic gastric mucosa contained in the diverticulum (Fig. 21.32). A radionuclide Meckel's scan is more sensitive than angiography as this demonstrates the gastric mucosa. Treatment is vasopressin, then surgery.

Inflammatory Bowel Disease is identified angiographically as diffuse hyperemia, arteriovascular shunting, and oozing. It has a similar appearance in the colon. Treatment is (a) vasopressin and (b) surgery.

Vascular Malformations are responsible for approximately 20% of small bowel bleeding. They may be solitary or multiple as seen in Osler-Weber-Rendu syndrome and usually present as chronic, recurrent bleeding.

Colorectal

Colonic Diverticula are the most common etiology of lower GI bleeding. Although diverticula are much more common in the left colon, a diverticulum that is bleeding is three times more likely to be found in the right colon (Fig. 21.31). Treatment is (a) vasopressin, with 90% success at controlling bleeding with a 20% rebleed rate, and (b) surgery or embolization (20).

Angiodysplasia is a vascular malformation or ectasia located more commonly in the right colon along the antimesenteric border. It is more common in patients over 55 years of age and is responsible for 50% of colonic bleeding in the older age group. However, angiodysplasia may be found in up to 15% of patients without a history of GI bleeding. Therefore, unless bleeding is detected, it becomes a diagnosis of exclusion after other possible causes (diverticula, ulcers, neoplasm, or colitis) have been ruled out. Classic angiographic features are (a) early opacification of an enlarged draining vein, (b) persistent dense opacification of the vein, and (c) vascular tufts located along the antimesenteric border of the cecum or ascending colon (Fig. 21.33). Treatment is surgery (20).

PORTAL HYPERTENSION

Bleeding from gastric and esophageal varices accounts for approximately 17% of acute, massive UGI hemorrhage (20). Varices represent normal venous channels that become massively dilated and tortuous in an attempt to circumvent flow around the diseased liver (Fig. 21.34). One of the more common routes is via the coronary veins that anastomose with the azygos system in the submucosa of the distal esophagus and gastric cardia. These abnormal vascular struc-

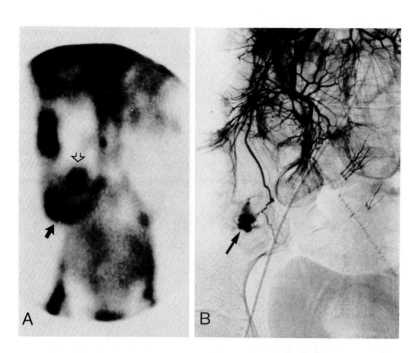

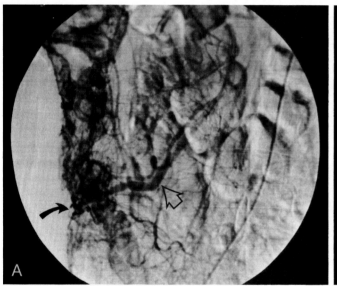

Figure 21.32. Bleeding Meckel's Diverticulum. A. In this young patient with suspected lower GI bleeding source, a tagged red blood cell study shows focal activity in the right lower quadrant of the abdomen (*open arrow*). Tracer activity is also seen in the distribution of the terminal ileum (*closed arrow*) and ascending colon. **B**. An SMA arteriogram shows a focal extraluminal pooling of contrast (*arrow*) in what was found at surgery to be a Meckel's diverticulum containing ectopic gastric mucosa.

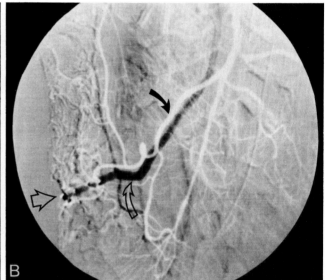

Figure 21.33. Colonic Angiodysplasia. A. In this patient with signs of lower GI bleeding, the typical angiographic findings of angiodysplasia are shown. A tangle of vessels is seen within the ascending colon (*curved arrow*) with an associated enlarged draining vein (*open arrow*). **B**. Subtraction technique demonstrates to better advantage the feeding artery (*curved closed arrow*) and draining vein (*curved open arrow*) with the associated tangle of vessels situated on the antimesenteric border of the colon (*open straight arrow*).

tures cause thinning of the overlying mucosa, project into the esophageal lumen, and are prone to erode and bleed. These are termed "uphill" varices as opposed to "downhill" varices seen with superior vena cava obstruction, in which the azygos system is the main collateral route carrying blood from the head and upper extremities. Other portosystemic communications can form in the presence of severe portal hypertension, such as spontaneous splenorenal shunts (Fig. 21.35).

In up to 60% of patients with documented varices, the source of bleeding may be due to something other than the varices, usually peptic ulcer disease or gastritis (20). Angiography is not performed for diagnosis but to plan surgical or percutaneous portosystemic shunt placement. This requires both celiac and SMA injections to fully evaluate the portal venous system, including splenic vein patency.

Mesenteric Ischemia

This entity comprises a group of disorders that all have a common end-point, bowel necrosis, with the current mortality rate approaching 70% (Table 21.8).

Figure 21.34. Esophageal Varices. A.
Transhepatic injection of the coronary vein shows typical configuration for "uphill" varices (*arrows*) in this patient with portal hypertension and variceal hemorrhage. **B.** Portal venous filling (*open straight arrow*) following SMA injection demonstrates esophageal and gastric fundal varices (*open curved arrows*) with a gastric occlusion balloon (*curved closed arrow*) expanded within the stomach in an attempt to temporarily stop variceal hemorrhage. The balloon also occludes the splenic vein (*small straight arrow*). The coronary vein is seen to good advantage (*large straight arrow*) supplying the large esophageal and gastric varices (*open curved arrows*).

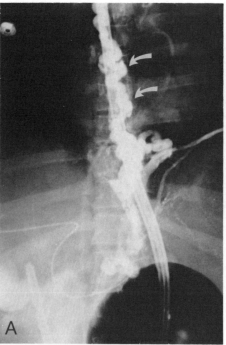

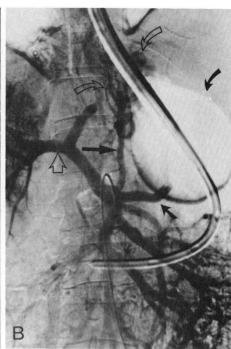

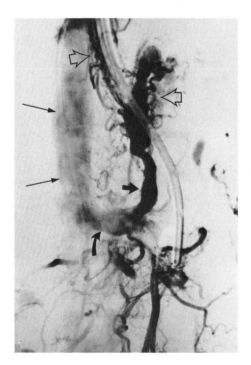

Figure 21.35. Portal Hypertension. A spontaneous splenorenal shunt (*short straight closed arrow*) is seen in this patient with portal hypertension. Multiple esophageal and gastric fundal varices are seen (*open straight arrows*) with filling of the left renal vein (*curved arrow*) and IVC (*long thin arrows*) by the spontaneous shunt.

Table 21.8.   Classification of Mesenteric Ischemia

Acute ischemia
   Arterial embolism
   Arterial thrombosis
   Venous thrombosis
   Nonocclusive ischemia
   Colonic ischemia
Chronic ischemia

bolus in the lumen of the SMA 4–6 cm from its origin. Arterial thrombosis usually occurs on a background of preexisting severe atherosclerotic occlusive disease involving the celiac and SMA. The symptoms of postprandial abdominal pain, weight loss, and altered bowel habits are typical.

Mesenteric venous occlusion generally affects the medium-sized veins of the middle small bowel and accounts for about 10% of cases. Nonocclusive ischemia is predominantly related to conditions that produce low flow states such as hypotension, dehydration, and low cardiac output. The bowel responds with disproportionate vasoconstriction, leading to ischemia. Angiography confirms diffuse vasoconstriction without evidence of underlying structural abnormality. Both mesenteric venous thrombosis and nonocclusive ischemia can present with GI bleeding. Chronic etiologies include atherosclerosis (Fig. 21.36), fibromuscular dysplasia, and various vasculitides (21).

Interventional Procedures

Embolization is indicated for the control of hemorrhage related to trauma and neoplasm, GI bleeding

Arterial embolism and thrombosis account for approximately 50% of cases, with nonocclusive ischemia accounting for an additional 25% (21). Emboli typically have a cardiac source, with angiography demonstrating a classic reverse meniscal sign typical of em-

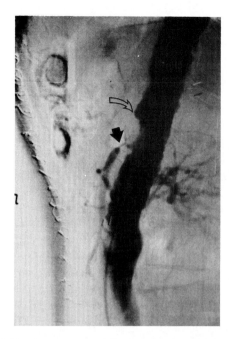

Figure 21.36. Mesenteric Ischemia. A lateral projection of an aortic injection shows severe atherosclerotic disease with occlusion of the celiac trunk (*curved arrow*) and severe stenosis to the origin of the superior mesenteric artery (*straight arrow*). The inferior mesenteric artery was also occluded.

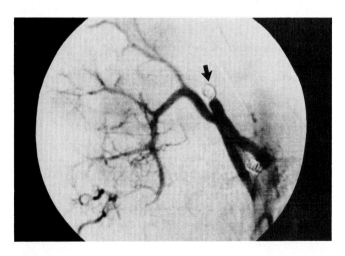

Figure 21.37. Therapeutic Embolization. Placement of an embolization coil (*arrow*) within the renal artery prior to surgery for a renal cell carcinoma is a permanent method of embolization used to limit potential surgical bleeding complications.

unresponsive to other therapies, preoperative tumor ablation (Fig. 21.37), gross hemoptysis, and vascular malformations, among others. Agents can be divided into two general categories: temporary and permanent. The most widely used temporary agent is Gelfoam gelatin sponge or powders that lasts for approximately 2 weeks before complete resorption. Permanent agents include polyvinyl alcohol (Ivalon), absolute ethanol, coils, and detachable balloons. *Postembolization syndrome* is characterized by pain, fe-

ver, nausea, and leukocytosis, and is typically seen with embolization of large tumors. This is usually a self-limiting situation and the symptoms resolve in 72 hours.

Vasopressin is the active hormone of the posterior pituitary gland and is used primarily for the control of acute GI bleeding. It results in splanchnic vasoconstriction and GI smooth muscle contraction, and demonstrates decreased complications when used locally and selectively by the intraarterial route. Complications include hypertension, myocardial infarction, arrhythmia, bowel infarct, and hyponatremia. The dose range is 0.2–0.6 U/min. When initiating therapy, patients are placed on lowest dose for a 20-minute infusion, at which time a repeat angiogram is performed to assess the following: (*a*) control of bleeding, (*b*) adequate vasospasm, and (*c*) venous return from the area being infused (Fig. 21.30). The latter is extremely important, for without venous return, adequate bowel perfusion could not be assured and bowel infarction may follow. The dose is incrementally increased until bleeding stops or the maximum dose is reached. The highest dose necessary to control bleeding is continued for 8–12 hours and tapered over 24–48 hours. *Postinfusion syndrome* occurs when the vasopressin is discontinued, and results in hypotension in the face of high urine output, which may be confused with rebleeding.

References

1. Taylor KJ, Holland S: Doppler ultrasound: part I. Basic principles, instrumentation, and pitfalls. Radiology 1990;174:297–307.
2. Mitchell DG: Color Doppler imaging: principles, limitations, and artifacts. Radiology 1990;177:1–10.
3. Kadir S. Diagnostic angiography. Philadelphia: WB Saunders, 1986.
4. Rose SC, Moore EE: Angiography in patients with arterial trauma: correlation between angiographic abnormalities, operative findings, and clinical outcome. AJR 1987;149:613–619.
5. Bower TC, Cherry KJ Jr, Pairolero PC: Unusual manifestations of abdominal aortic aneurysms. Surg Clin North Am 1989;69:745–754.
6. Bandyk DF: Preoperative imaging of aortic aneurysms. Surg Clin North Am 1989;69:721–735.
7. Darling RC, Messina CR, Brewster DC, et al: Autopsy study of unoperated abdominal aortic aneurysms. Circulation 1977;56(suppl 2):161–164.
8. Mulligan SA, Matsuda T, Lanzer P, et al: Peripheral arterial occlusive disease: prospective comparison of MR angiography and color duplex ultrasound with conventional angiography. Radiology 1991;178:695–700.
9. Carroll BA: Carotid sonography. Radiology 1991;178:303–313.
10. Zweibal W: Color duplex ultrasound of the carotid arteries: technique, normal features, and technical pitfalls. In: Rifkin M, ed. Syllabus special course: ultrasound 1991. Chicago: Radiological Society of North America Publications 1991:179–188.

11. Smullens SN: Surgically treatable lesions of the extracranial circulation, including the vertebral artery. Radiol Clin North Am 1986;24:453–460.
12. Wesen CA, Elliott BM: Fibromuscular dysplasia of the carotid arteries. Am J Sur 1986;151:448–451.
13. Stanson AW: Roentgenographic findings in major vasculitic syndromes. Rheum Dis Clin North Am 1990;16:293–308.
14. Vogelzang RL, Limpert JD, Yao JST: Detection of prosthetic vascular complications: comparison of CT and angiography. AJR 1987;148:819–823.
15. Tegtmeyer CJ, Selby JB, Hartwell GD, et al: Results and complications of angioplasty in fibromuscular disease. Circulation 1991;83:I-155–I-161.
16. Hunter DW, So SK: Dialysis access: radiographic evaluation and management. Radiol Clin North Am 1987;25:249–260.
17. Appleman PT, DeJong TE, Lampmann LE: Deep venous thrombosis of the leg: ultrasound findings. Radiology 1987;163:734–746.
18. Ferris EJ: Deep venous thrombosis and pulmonary embolism: correlative evaluation and therapeutic implications. AJR 1992;159:1149–1155.
19. Murphy TP, Cronan JJ: Evolution of deep venous thrombosis: a prospective evaluation with ultrasound. Radiology 1990;177:543–548.
20. Kadir S, Ernest CB: Current concepts in angiographic management of gastrointestinal bleeding. Curr Probl Surg 1983;20:281–343.
21. Hunter GC, Guernsey JM: Mesenteric ischemia. Med Clin North Am 1988;72:1091–1115.

Section VI

THE GASTROINTESTINAL TRACT

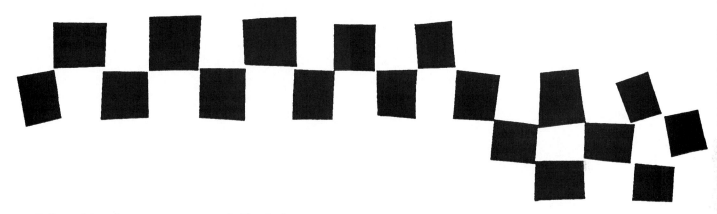

22

Abdomen and Pelvis

William E. Brant

Imaging Methods

Plain film radiographs of the abdomen are important for the assessment of the acute abdomen and to serve as "scout films" prior to contrast studies. Ultrasonography, computed tomography (CT), and magnetic resonances (MR) provide comprehensive evaluation of the abdomen, including the peritoneal cavity, retroperitoneal compartments, and major abdominal blood vessels and lymph nodes.

Compartmental Anatomy of the Abdomen and Pelvis

Knowledge of the complex compartmental anatomy of the abdomen is fundamental to understanding the effects of pathologic processes and to correctly interpret imaging studies of the abdomen. Understanding the shape and extent of anatomic compartments and their normal variations may clarify imaging findings that would otherwise be incomprehensible or lead to misdiagnosis. Fundamental considerations include constant anatomic landmarks, ligaments and fascia that define compartments, and normal variations in size and appearance of the various compartments and recesses. Identifying the precise compartment that an

abnormality determines to a great extent the nature of the abnormality (1).

The peritoneal cavity is divided into the greater peritoneal cavity and the lesser peritoneal cavity (the lesser sac) (Fig. 22.1). Within both portions of the peritoneal cavity are numerous recesses in which pathological processes tend to loculate (2, 3). The right subphrenic space communicates around the liver with the anterior subhepatic and posterior subhepatic space (Morison's pouch). The left subphrenic space communicates freely with the left subhepatic space. The right and left subphrenic spaces are separated by the falciform ligament and do not communicate directly. The right subphrenic and subhepatic spaces communicate freely with the pelvic peritoneal cavity via the right paracolic gutter. The phrenicocolic ligament prevents free communication of the left subphrenic and subhepatic spaces with the left paracolic gutter. Free fluid, blood, infection, and peritoneal metastases commonly settle in the pelvis because the pelvis is the most dependent portion of the peritoneal cavity and it communicates with both sides of the abdomen.

The falciform ligament consists of two closely applied layers of peritoneum extending from the umbilicus to the diaphragm in a parasagittal plane. The caudal free end of the falciform ligament contains the ligamentum teres, which is the obliterated umbilical vein remnant. The reflections of the falciform ligament separate over the posterior dome of the liver to form the coronary ligaments which define the "bare area" of the liver not covered by peritoneum (Fig. 22.2**A**). The coronary ligaments reflect between the liver and diaphragm and prevent access of ascites or other intraperitoneal processes from covering the bare area of the liver.

The lesser omentum, composed of the gastrohepatic and hepatoduodenal ligaments, suspends the stomach and duodenal bulb from the inferior surface of the liver. The lesser omentum separates the gastrohepatic recess of the left subphrenic space from the lesser sac (Figs. 22.1 and 22.2). The lesser sac is the isolated peritoneal compartment between the stomach and the pancreas. It communicates with the rest of the peritoneal cavity (the greater sac) through

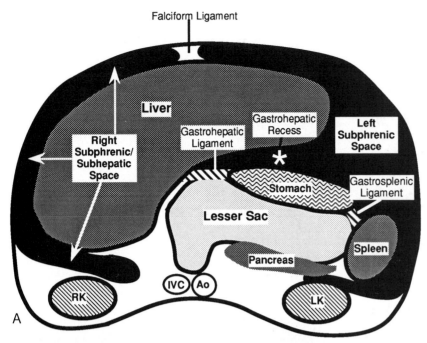

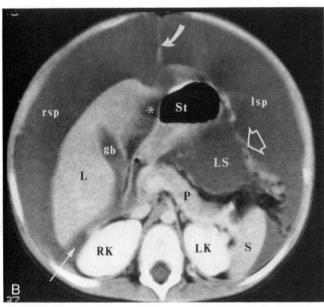

Figure 22.1.   Anatomy of the Peritoneal Cavity. A. Diagram of an axial cross-section of the abdomen illustrates the recesses of the greater peritoneal cavity and the lesser sac. **B.** CT scan of a patient with a large amount of ascites nicely demonstrates the greater peritoneal cavity and the lesser sac. The lesser sac (*LS*) is bounded by the stomach (*St*) anteriorly, the pancreas (*P*) posteriorly, and the gastrosplenic ligament (*open arrow*) laterally. The falciform ligament (*curved arrow*) separates the right (*rsp*) and left (*lsp*) subphrenic spaces. Fluid from the greater peritoneal cavity extends into Morison's pouch (*long arrow*) between the liver and the right kidney. Fluid in the gastrohepatic recess (***) separates the stomach from the liver (L). *S*, spleen; *gb*, gallbladder; *RK*, right kidney; *IVC*, inferior vena cava; *Ao*, aorta; *LK*, left kidney.

the foramen of Winslow. Pathologic processes in the lesser sac usually occur because of disease in adjacent organs rather than from spread from elsewhere in the abdominal cavity. The lesser sac is normally collapsed but can become huge when filled with fluid (Fig. 24.4).

The greater omentum is a double layer of peritoneum that hangs from the greater curvature of the stomach and descends in front of the abdominal viscera (Fig. 22.2). The greater omentum encloses fat and a few blood vessels. It serves as fertile ground for implantation of peritoneal metastases.

The retroperitoneal space between the diaphragm and the pelvic brim is divided into anterior pararenal, perirenal, and posterior pararenal compartments by

the anterior and posterior renal fascia (Fig. 22.3) (1, 4, 5). The anterior pararenal space extends between the posterior parietal peritoneum and the anterior renal fascia. It is bounded laterally by the lateroconal fascia. The pancreas, duodenal loop, and ascending and descending portions of the colon are within the anterior pararenal space.

The anterior and posterior renal fascia encompass the kidney, adrenal gland, and perirenal fat within the perirenal space. The anterior renal fascia is thin and consists of one layer of connective tissue. The posterior renal fascia is thicker, consisting of two layers of connective tissue (Fig. 22.3). The anterior layer of the posterior renal fascia is continuous with the anterior renal fascia. The posterior layer of the renal fascia is

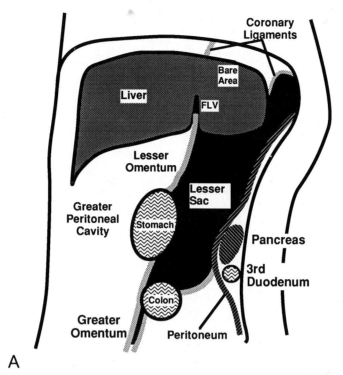

A

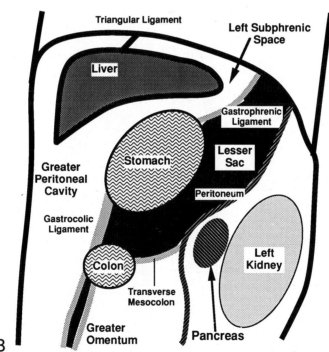

B

Figure 22.2.   The Lesser Sac. Sagittal plane diagrams of the medial **(A)** and lateral **(B)** aspects of the lesser sac illustrate its position
posterior to the stomach and anterior to the posterior parietal peritoneum covering the pancreas. Note that projections of the lesser
sac extend to the diaphragm, resulting in the potential for disease
processes in the lesser sac causing pleural effusions. The coronary
ligaments reflect between the liver and the diaphragm producing a
bare area of liver not covered by peritoneum.

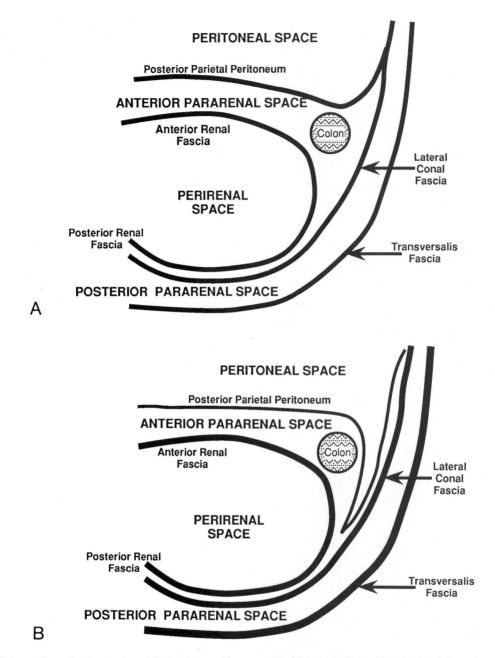

Figure 22.3. Retroperitoneal Compartmental Anatomy. Diagrams illustrate two normal variations of the reflections of the posterior parietal peritoneum around the descending colon. In A the colon is entirely retroperitoneal and in B the peritoneum forms a deep pocket lateral to the colon allowing intraperitoneal fluid to extend far posteriorly. Fluid or disease processes in the anterior pararenal space from the pancreas or colon may also extend posteriorly to the kidney by separating the two layers of the posterior renal fascia.

continuous with the lateroconal fascia, forming the lateral boundary of the anterior pararenal space. The anterior and posterior layers of the posterior renal fascia may be separated by inflammatory processes like pancreatitis extending from the anterior pararenal space. The perirenal space is discontinuous across the midline because of fusion of the renal fascial layers with connective tissue surrounding the aorta and vena cava.

The posterior pararenal space is a potential space, usually filled only with fat, extending from the posterior renal fascia to the transversalis fascia. The posterior pararenal fat continues into the flank as the properitoneal fat stripe seen on plain films of the abdomen. The compartment is limited medially by the lateral edges of the psoas and quadratus lumborum muscles.

The pelvis is divided into three major anatomic compartments (Fig. 22.4). The peritoneal cavity extends to the level of the vagina, forming the pouch of Douglas (cul-de-sac) in females (Fig. 22.5), or to the level of the seminal vesicles, forming the rectovesical pouch in males. The extraperitoneal space of the pelvis is continous with the retroperitoneal space of the

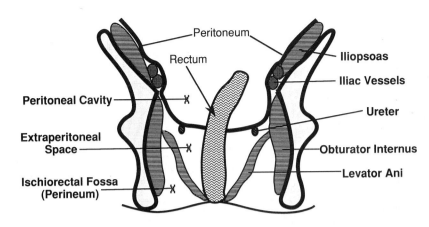

Figure 22.4. Compartmental Anatomy of the Pelvis. Diagram in the coronal plane illustrates the major anatomic compartments of the pelvis.

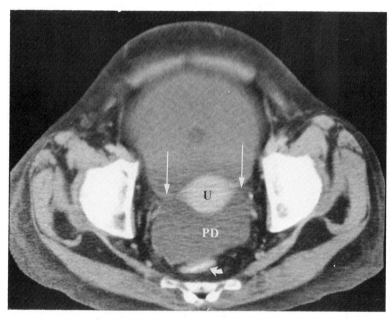

Figure 22.5. Pouch of Douglas. A CT of the pelvis in a woman with abundant ascites demonstrates fluid distension of the pouch of Douglas (*PD*) (cul-de-sac) posterior to the uterus (*U*) and anterior to the rectum (*curved arrow*). The broad ligament (*long arrows*) is outlined by fluid anteriorly and posteriorly.

abdomen, extends to the pelvic diaphragm, and includes the retropubic space (of Retzius). Pathologic processes from the pelvis spread preferentially into the retroperitoneal compartments of the abdomen. The perineum lies below the pelvic diaphragm and includes the ischiorectal fossa (Fig. 22.6).

Fluid in the Peritoneal Cavity

Fluid in the peritoneal cavity originates from many different sources and may vary greatly in composition. Ascites is serous fluid in the peritoneal cavity and commonly is caused by cirrhosis, hypoproteinemia, or congestive heart failure. Exudative ascites results from inflammatory processes such as abscess, pancreatitis, peritonitis, or bowel perforation. Hemoperitoneum may result from surgery or trauma. Neoplastic ascites is associated with intraperitoneal tumors. Urine, bile, and chyle may also spread freely within the peritoneal cavity.

Plain film findings associated with fluid in the peritoneal cavity include diffuse increase in density of the abdomen; indistinct margins of the liver, spleen, and psoas muscles; displacement of gas-filled colon away from the properitoneal flank stripe; bulging of the flanks; and increased separation of gas-filled small bowel loops.

Computed tomography demonstrates fluid density in the recesses of the peritoneal cavity (Fig 22.1**B**). The CT density of the fluid gives a clue as to its composition. Serous ascites has attenuation values near water (−10 to +10 H*U*). Exudative ascites is usually above +15 H*U*, while acute bleeding into the peritoneal cavity averages +45 H*U*.

Ultrasonography is sensitive to small amounts of fluid in the peritoneal recesses. Care must be taken to examine the most gravity-dependent portions of the peritoneal cavity, i.e., the pelvis in a supine patient. Simple ascites is sonolucent, while exudative, hemorrhagic, or neoplastic ascites often contains floating debris. Septations in ascites are usually associated with an inflammatory or malignant process.

Magnetic resonance shows limited specificity for defining the type of fluid present. Serous fluid is low

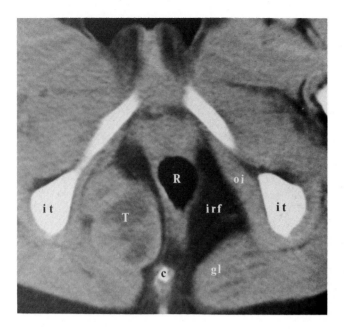

Figure 22.6.   Perineal Tumor. A CT scan of a 12-year-old girl with a history of a rhabdomyosarcoma of the right leg demonstrates a tumor metastasis (*T*) in the right ischiorectal fossa. The left ischiorectal fossa (*irf*) shows its normal appearance as a triangle of fat bordered by the rectum (*R*), obturator internus muscle (*oi*) and the gluteus muscles (*gl*). The ischiorectal fossa is entirely below the levator ani and is part of the perineum. *c*, tip of the coccyx. *it*, ischial tuberosities.

intensity on T1-weighted images and markedly increased in intensity on T2-weighted images. Hemorrhagic fluid shows high signal intensity on both T1- and T2- weighted images.

Pseudomyxoma Peritonei refers to gelatinous ascites and mucinous peritoneal implants that occur as a complication of rupture of appendiceal mucocele or intraperitoneal spread of mucinous adenocarcinoma of the ovary, colon, or rectum. Plain films may demonstrate ring-like calcification scattered throughout the peritoneal cavity. The CT demonstrates mottled densities, septations, and calcifications within the fluid (Fig. 22.7). The mucinous fluid is typically loculated and causes mass effect on the liver and bowel. Ultrasound demonstrates intraperitoneal nodules that range from hypoechoic to strongly echogenic.

Pneumoperitoneum

Free air within the peritoneal cavity is a valuable sign of bowel perforation, most commonly due to duodenal or gastric ulcer perforation. However, additional causes of pneumoperitoneum include trauma, recent laparotomy or laparoscopy, and infection of the peritoneal cavity with gas-producing organisms. Postoperative pneumoperitoneum usually resolves in 3 to 4 days. Serial films demonstrate a progressive decrease in the amount of air present. Failure of progressive

resolution or an increase in the amount of air present suggests a leak of bowel anastomosis or sepsis. Pneumoperitoneum in the absence of a ruptured viscus may occur with air introduced through the female genital tract by orogenital insufflation or associated with pulmonary emphysema, alveolar rupture, and dissection of air into the peritoneal cavity.

Plain film evidence of pneumoperitoneum is best seen on radiographs obtained with the patient in the standing or sitting position. Small amounts of air are clearly demonstrated beneath the domes of the diaphragm. Left lateral decubitus and cross-table lateral views may be used with very ill patients to demonstrate air outlining the liver. Signs of pneumoperitoneum on supine radiographs include gas on both sides of the bowel wall (Rigler's sign), gas outlining the falciform ligament, gas outlining the peritoneal cavity (the "football sign"), and triangluar or linear localized extraluminal gas in the right upper quadrant (Fig. 22.8) (6).

On CT, small amounts of extraluminal gas may be confused with gas within the bowel and be surprisingly difficult to recognize. Images should be examined at lung windows (window level (-)600 H*U*, window width 1000 H*U*) to detect free intraperitoneal air.

Acute Abdomen

The differential diagnosis of patients presenting with acute abdominal pain is extremely broad (Table 22.1). Accurate and efficient diagnosis requires cooperation between the referring physician and the radiologist to select the imaging method most likely to provide the correct diagnosis. Routine assessment of the acute abdomen commonly includes the "acute abdomen series," which consists of an erect posterior-anterior chest radiograph, and supine and erect radiographs of the abdomen. The chest radiograph provides optimal detection of pneumoperitoneum and intrathoracic diseases that may present with abdominal complaints. The supine abdominal film permits diagnosis of many acute abdominal conditions, while the erect abdominal film adds confidence to the diagnosis.

Mechanical bowel obstruction means stasis of bowel contents above a focal lesion. The obstruction may be due to obturation (occlusion by a mass in the lumen), stenosis due to intrinsic bowel disease, or compression of the lumen by extrinsic disease. Ileus means stasis of bowel contents due to an adynamic state. The goal of imaging is to confirm the presence of obstruction, identify its level, and demonstrate its cause. Radiographs can confirm the presence of bowel obstruction 6 to 12 hours before the diagnosis can usually be made clinically (7).

Normal Abdominal Gas Pattern. Interpretation of plain abdominal radiographs should routinely

Figure 22.7. Pseudomyxoma Peritonei. A CT scan of a 65-year-old male with a ruptured appendiceal mucocele demonstrates copious ascites (*A*) with prominent septations (*closed arrows*) and mass effect displacing bowel loops (*b*). Punctate calcifications (*open arrow*) are also present on peritoneal surfaces.

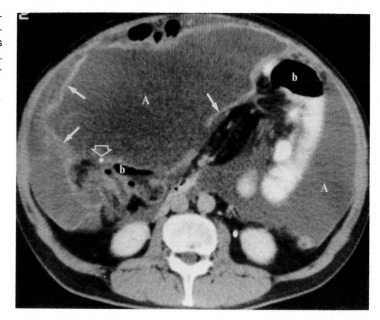

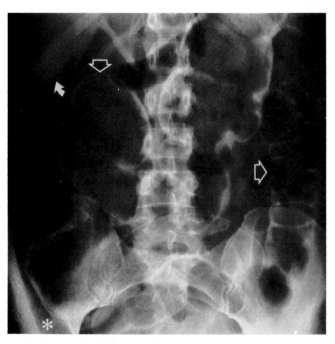

Figure 22.8. Pneumoperitoneum. Supine radiograph in a patient with a perforated gastric ulcer demonstrates visualization of both sides of the bowel wall (*open arrows*), free air outlining the edge of the liver (*curved arrow*), and free air outlining the pericolic gutter (***).

Table 22.1. Causes of Acute Abdomen

Appendicitis
Acute cholecystitis
Acute pancreatitis
Acute diverticulitis
Acute ulcerative colitis
Pseudomembranous colitis
Amebiasis
Acute intestinal ischemia
Peritonitis
Intraperitoneal abscess
Retroperitoneal abscess
Bowel obstruction
Urinary tract infection
Urinary tract obstruction
Pelvic inflammatory diseases

include assessment of gas, fluid, soft tissue, fat, and calcium densities. Normal gas in the abdomen is predominantly swallowed air. Air-fluid levels are seen in normal patients commonly in the stomach, often in the small bowel, and never in the colon distal to the hepatic flexure. Normal air-fluid levels in the small bowel should not exceed 2.5 cm in length. Small bowel air usually appears as multiple small, random gas collections scattered throughout the abdomen. Small bowel gas is increased in patients who chronically swallow air or drink carbonated beverages. Air-fluid levels longer than 2.5 cm suggest ileus or obstruction.

Dilated Bowel. In adults, dilated small bowel can usually be differentiated from dilated large bowel by assessment of location and anatomic features (7). Small bowel is more central in the abdomen and is characterized by valvulae conniventes, which cross the entire diameter of the lumen (Fig. 22.9). Dilated small bowel rarely exceeds 3 to 5 cm in diameter. Large bowel is more peripheral in the abdomen and is characterized by haustra that extend only part way across the lumen. Large bowel contains fecal material that has a characteristic mottled appearance. Large bowel usually exceeds 5 cm when dilated. The cecum, which has the largest normal diameter of the large bowel, always dilates to the greatest extent irrespective of the site of obstruction.

Ileus is a cause of stasis of bowel contents because of decreased or absent peristalsis. The common causes of ileus are listed in Table 22.2. Ileus typically

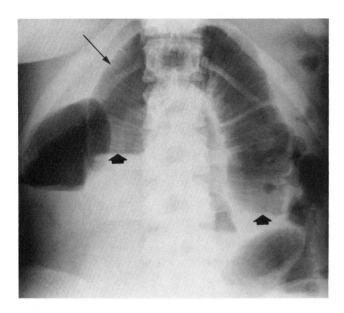

Figure 22.9. Small Bowel Obstruction. Plain, erect radiograph of the abdomen reveals dilated air-filled loops of small bowel containing air-fluid levels at different heights within the same loop (*arrowheads*). Note the valvulae conniventes (*long arrow*) that extend across the entire diameter of the bowel lumen. The small bowel obstruction was due to adhesions.

Table 22.2. Causes of Adynamic Ileus

Drugs
  Atropine, glucagon, morphine, barbiturates, phenothiazines
Metabolic causes
  Diabetes mellitus, hypothyroidism, hypokalemia, hypercalcemia
Inflammation
  Intraluminal: gastroenteritis
  Extraluminal: peritonitis, pancreatitis, appendicitis, cholecystitis, abscess
Postoperative: resolves in 4–7 days
Posttrauma
Postspinal injury

demonstrates diffuse symmetric, predominantly gaseous, distension of bowel. The small bowel, stomach, and colon are uniformly dilated without an abrupt termination. More loops are dilated than with obstruction. Occasionally ileus may result in a gasless abdomen with dilated loops of bowel that are filled only with fluid. Ultrasonography is useful in confirming decreased or absent peristalsis, although examination may be difficult if large amounts of gas are present.

Sentinel Loop refers to a segment of intestine that becomes paralyzed and dilated as it lies next to an inflamed intraabdominal organ. In essence, it is a short segment of adynamic ileus that appears as an isolated loop of distended intestine that remains in the same general position on serial films. A sentinel loop alerts one to the presence of an adjacent inflammatory process. A sentinel loop in the right upper quadrant suggests acute cholecystitis, hepatitis, or pyelonephritis. In the left upper quadrant, pancrea-

Table 22.3. Causes of Toxic Megacolon

Ulcerative colitis: 75% of cases
Pseudomembranous colitis
Crohn's colitis
Amebic colitis
Ischemic colitis
Bacterial colitis: cholera, typhoid

titis, pyelonephritis, or splenic injury may be suspected. In the lower quadrants, diverticulitis, appendicitis, salpingitis, cystitis, or Crohn's disease are causes of a sentinel loop.

Toxic Megacolon is a manifestation of fulminant colitis characterized by extreme dilation of all or a portion of the colon. In this state, peristalsis is absent and the large bowel loses all tone and contractility. The patient has progressive abdominal distension and is toxic, febrile, and obtunded. Bowel sounds and bowel movements are absent. The bowel wall becomes like "wet blotting paper," and the risk of perforation is extreme. Mortality approaches 20% in toxic megacolon. Acute ulcerative colitis is the most common cause of toxic megacolon (Table 22.3).

Plain films demonstrate distension of the colon with absent haustra. Dilation of the transverse colon is often the most striking observation. The diagnosis is suggested when the diameter of the colon exceeds 6.5 cm and the mucosa appears abnormal. Pseudopolyps due to islands of edematous mucosa surrounded by extensive ulceration appear as soft tissue nodules within the air-distended colon. Computed tomography demonstrates a distended colon filled with air and fluid. The wall of the colon is thin but has an irregular nodular contour; air may be seen within the colon wall. Barium enema is absolutely contraindicated because of risk of perforation.

Bowel Obstruction. When bowel obstruction occurs, the lumen of the bowel proximal to the obstruction progressively dilates because of continued secretions, swallowed fluid, air, and food, and eventual cessation of absorption. Stasis results in the overgrowth of bacteria and production of toxins that may injure the mucosa. Compromise of blood supply may occur because of distension of the bowel wall and increased intraluminal pressure. Simple obstruction refers to blockage of the luminal contents without interference with blood supply. Closed-loop obstruction means blockage of both the afferent and efferent segments of a bowel loop. This may occur with incarcerated hernias and volvulus. Strangulated obstruction means that the blood supply to the bowel wall is impaired.

Enteroclysis is recommended as the barium study of choice for evaluation of proximal or middle small bowel obstruction (7). Despite concern on the part of some surgeons, no risk of barium inspissation has

Table 22.4. Causes of Small Bowel Obstruction

Adhesions
  Postsurgical
  Postinflammatory
Incarcerated hernia
Malignancy, usually metastatic
Intussusception
Volvulus
Gallstone ileus
Parasites
  Bolus of ascaris
Foreign body

been shown in animal studies or many years of experience with human patients (7). For large bowel or distal small bowel obstruction, single-contrast barium enema is the usual study of choice. Water-soluble contrast is indicated when there is risk of perforation or evidence of peritonitis.

Strangulation obstruction refers to complete or partial bowel obstruction associated with impairment of blood supply. The obstruction is most commonly of the closed-loop type. Draining veins are usually obstructed first, resulting in extravasation of blood into the bowel lumen. Subsequent arterial obstruction may result in necrosis of the bowel wall. Radiographic diagnosis is difficult and early findings resemble simple obstruction with dilated gas-filled loops. A predominance of fluid-filled loops usually develops. A pseudotumor may be formed by completely fluid-filled obstructed loops that assume a coffee bean configuration. Mucosal folds are absent; ascites may develop. Air in the bowel wall indicates mural necrosis. Perforation of the small bowel uncommonly results in pneumoperitoneum because the small bowel usually contains little gas, and perforations are usually quickly walled off.

Small Bowel Obstruction

Small bowel obstruction accounts for 80% of all intestinal tract obstruction. The causes of small bowel obstruction are listed in Table 22.4. In the Western world, postsurgical adhesions account for 75% of small bowel obstruction, while in developing nations, 80% of small bowel obstruction may be due to incarcerated hernia, while only 10% are due to adhesions (7).

Plain film evidence of small bowel obstruction includes demonstration of dilated small bowel with air-fluid levels that exceed 2.5 cm in length (Fig. 22.9). The level of obstruction is determined by dilated loops above the obstruction and normal or empty loops below the obstruction. Stepladder or hairpin loops of small bowel are most characteristic. Air-fluid levels at differing heights within the same loop are strong evidence of obstruction. Small bubbles of gas trapped between folds in dilated, fluid- filled loops produce the "string of pearls" sign. Inguinal hernias, easily overlooked clinically in the obese, may be evident on radiographs.

Computed tomography can confirm small bowel obstruction and commonly reveal both its location and etiology, since both fluid-filled and gas-filled loops are clearly demonstrated. Thickening of the bowel walls suggests ischemia; ascites is commonly present. Body wall hernias are usually evident.

Ultrasonography is helpful when plain film findings are equivocal or the abdomen is gasless. Small bowel loops greater than 3 cm diameter suggest obstruction or ileus. The valvulae conniventes cause a "keyboard" pattern in fluid-filled loops (Fig. 22.10). Real-time examination confirms increased peristalsis with obstruction and decreased or absent peristalsis with ileus.

Adhesions are demonstrated on barium studies as abrupt, short segment narrowing of the dilated small bowel. The narrowed segment is compressed and the loop is fixated. The more distal small bowel is collapsed. Adhesions may be multiple and cause adherence of the small bowel to the anterior abdominal wall. Adhesions are not directly demonstrated by CT but may be evidenced by abrupt narrowing of small bowel without other causes evident. Adhesions may cause obstruction of the small bowel as soon as 2 weeks following intraabdominal surgery (7).

Incarcerated Hernias are associated with increased mortality if surgery is delayed for more than 24 hours. Most inguinal or femoral hernias (35% of the total) are apparent clinically, and barium studies are not needed. Incisional hernias are well demonstrated by CT but are usually wide-necked and do not cause obstruction. Internal hernias may be evidenced by compression of both afferent and efferent limbs of a small bowel loop.

Intussusception is a major cause of small bowel obstruction in children, but is less common in adults. In adults, intussusception is often chronic, intermittent, or subacute, and is usually caused by a polypoid tumor, such as lipoma. Additional causes of intussusception include malignant tumor, Meckel's diverticulum, lymphoma, mesenteric nodes, and foreign bodies. Enteroenteric intussusception occurs with small bowel tumors and sprue. Ileocolic intussuception is usually idiopathic in children, but is caused by a mass in adults. Colocolic intussusception is common in adults but rare in children. Plain films in intussusception demonstrate small bowel obstruction and a soft tissue mass. Barium studies demonstrate barium trapped between the intussusceptum and the receiving bowel forming a coiled spring appearance. Computed tomography is usually diagnostic, dem-

Figure 22.10. Small Bowel Obstruction. Ultrasonography demonstrates a fluid-filled, dilated loop of small bowel (*SB*) with the characteristic keyboard pattern (*arrows*) of the valvulae conniventes. Ultrasonography offers the advantage of demonstrating the size and peristaltic activity of fluid-filled bowel which are not apparent on plain radiographs.

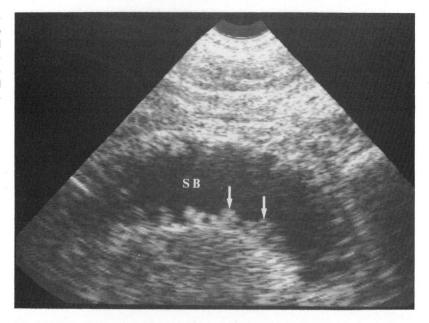

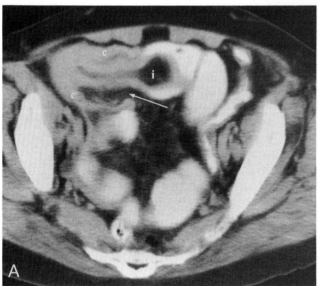

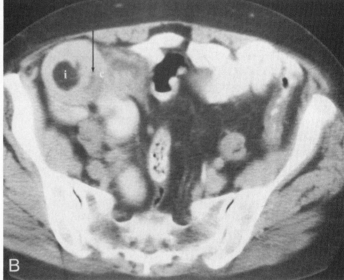

Figure 22.11. Intussusception. A. A CT scan demonstrates loop of ileum (*i*) invaginating into the cecum (*c*). Note the fat density (*arrow*) of the mesentery of the small bowel invaginating into the cecum adjacent to the ileal loop. **B.** A CT image at a higher level demonstrates a cross-section of the invaginating ileum (*i*) and the receiving cecum (*c*). Fat density (*arrow*) within the lumen of the cecum represents the invaginating ileal mesentery. (Case courtesy of Dr. Jim C. Chen, Roseville, CA.)

onstrating a characteristic target-like intestinal mass (8). On transverse section, the inner central density is the invaginating loop surrounded by fat density mesentery that is enveloped by the receiving loop (Fig. 22.11). Ultrasonography exhibits a similar "donut" configuration of alternating hyperechoic and hypoechoic rings representing alternating mucosa, muscular wall, and mesenteric fat tissues in cross-section.

Gallstone Ileus should be suspected in any elderly female with small bowell obstruction. It is the cause of 24% of small bowel obstruction in patients over age 70. Because it is a disease of the elderly, in-

sidious in onset, and difficult to diagnose, mortality is increased five times over that for small bowel obstruction due to adhesions. Bowel obstruction is caused by a large gallstone that erodes through the gallbladder wall and passes into the intestine, usually creating a cholecystoduodenal fistula. The gallstone most commonly lodges in the distal ileum. Specific radiographic signs are present in only about half the patients. Rigler's triad consists of dilated small bowel loops (80% of cases), air in the biliary tree or gallbladder (67%), and calcified gallstone in an ectopic location (50%). Barium studies should include instillation of contrast into the duodenum to demonstrate pas-

Table 22.5. Causes of Large Bowel Obstruction

Colon carcinoma (60%)
Metastatic disease, especially pelvic malignancies
Diverticulitis
Volvulus
Fecal impaction
Amebiasis
Ischemia
Adhesions

sage of barium into the biliary tree. Nonopaque obstructing gallstones are demonstrated as an intraluminal mass.

Large Bowel Obstruction

Large bowel obstruction is predominantly a condition of older adults, accounting for about 20% of all bowel obstruction. The cecum dilates to the greatest extent, irrespective of the site of large bowel obstruction. When the cecum exceeds 10 cm in diameter, it is at high risk for perforation with attendant risks of peritonitis and septic shock. The common causes of large bowel obstruction are listed in Table 22.5.

Plain films are commonly diagnostic in large bowel obstruction, demonstrating dilation of the colon from the cecum to the point of obstruction. The colon distal to the obstruction is devoid of gas. When the ileocecal valve is competent, the small bowel usually contains little gas; the colon is unable to decompress into the small bowel and gaseous distension of the cecum is progressive. When the ileocecal valve is incompetent, gaseous distension of the small bowel is often present; the colon can decompress into the ileum and jejunum, and risk of perforation of the cecum is reduced. Air-fluid levels distal to the hepatic flexure are strong evidence of obstruction unless the patient has had an enema. Barium enema confirms the presence of obstruction and demonstrates the site, and frequently the cause, of obstruction.

Sigmoid Volvulus is most common in the elderly, as well as in individuals on high-residue diets. The sigmoid colon twists around its mesentery, resulting in a closed-loop obstruction. The proximal colon dilates while the rectum empties. On plain films, the sigmoid colon appears as a large gas-filled loop without haustral markings, arising from the pelvis and extending high into the abdomen and often to the diaphragm (Fig. 22.12). The three white lines formed by the lateral walls of the loop and the summation of the two opposed medial walls of the loop converge inferiorly into the left iliac fossa. Barium enema demonstrates obstruction that tapers to a beak at the point of the twist. Mucosal folds spiral into the beak at the point of obstruction. Sigmoid volvulus causes 3–8%

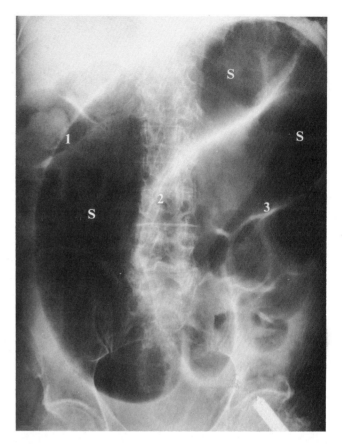

Figure 22.12. Sigmoid Volvulus. Plain radiograph demonstrates the characteristic massive dilation of the sigmoid colon (*S*) arising from the pelvis and extending to the left diaphragm. The three lines representing the walls of the twisted loop converging to the left lower quadrant are evident (*1, 2, 3*).

of large bowel obstruction in adults and has a reported mortality of 20–25%.

Cecal Volvulus. Twisting of the cecum usually occurs in the ascending colon above the ileocecal valve. Plain films demonstrate a massively dilated bowel loop projecting into the left middle or upper abdomen, usually with a single air-fluid level. The small bowel is distended while the distal colon is decompressed. The distal ileum encircles the cecum as it rotates. A contrast enema demonstrates a beak-like termination at the point of obstruction in the ascending colon. Cecal volvulus causes 1–3% of large bowel obstruction in adults and occurs most frequently in the elderly. Mortality rates of 20–40% are reported because of delays in diagnosis.

Fecal Impaction is the most common cause of large bowel obstruction in elderly and bedridden patients. Plain films demonstrate a large mass of stool having a characteristic mottled appearance in the distal colon. Following disimpaction, a barium enema should be performed to search for an obstructing carcinoma that may have caused the fecal impaction.

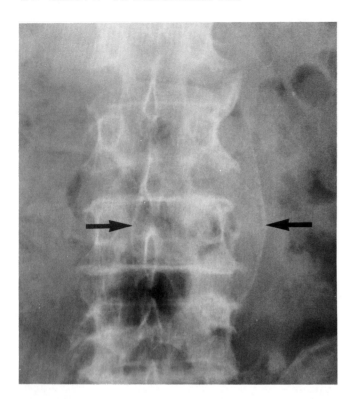

Figure 22.13. Abdominal Aortic Aneurysm. Plain radiograph demonstrates an aneurysm of the abdominal aorta evidenced by wide separation of calcifications in the aortic wall (*arrows*). Calcification in the wall overlying the spine may be difficult to visualize. A film taken with the patient in left posterior oblique position will project the aorta away from the spine and make visualization of wall calcifications easier.

Abdominal Calcifications

Intraabdominal calcifications may be an important sign of intrabddominal disease and should be searched for on every plain film examination of the abdomen.

Vascular Calcifications are common in the aorta (Fig. 22.13) and iliac vessels (Fig. 22.15) of older individuals. Plaque-like vascular calcifications overlie the lumbar spine and sacrum and commonly require detailed inspection to detect. Aneurysms of the aorta are manifest by luminal diameter exceeding 3 cm as measured between calcifications in the aortic wall (Fig. 22.13). Ring-like calcified aneurysms most commonly involve the splenic or renal arteries. *Phleboliths* are calcified thrombi in veins most commonly visualized in the lateral aspects of the pelvis. They are round or oval calcifications up to 5 mm size that commonly contain a central lucency.

Calcified Lymph Nodes result most commonly from granulomatous diseases such as tuberculosis or histoplasmosis. The calcification is usually mottled and 10–15 mm in size. Mesenteric nodes are the most commonly calcified.

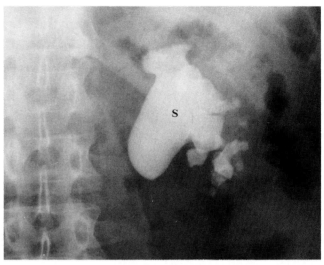

Figure 22.14. Staghorn Calculus. A plain radiograph reveals a large calculus occupying the collecting system of the left kidney and assuming its shape. Staghorn calculi (*S*) are usually composed of struvite and form in the presence of chronic urinary infection.

Gallstones and Gallbladder. Only about 15% of gallstones contain sufficient calcium to be identified on plain film. Most calcified gallstones contain calcium bilirubinate and have a laminated appearance with a dense outer rim and more radiolucent center. When there are multiple gallstones, they are commonly faceted. Calcifications in the gallbladder wall (porcelain gallbladder) are plaque-like and oval in configuration conforming to the size and shape of the gallbladder (Fig. 23.27). Milk of calcium bile is a suspension of radiopaque crystals within gallbladder bile. Layering of the suspension can be demonstrated on erect films.

Urinary Calculi. About 85% of urinary calculi are visible on plain film. They range in size from punctate up to several centimeters. Most characteristic are the staghorn calculi, which assume the shape of the renal collecting system (Fig. 22.14). Renal calculi are differentiated from gallstones by oblique projections that confirm their posterior position, as opposed to the more anterior positions of gallstones. Ureteral calculi may be seen anywhere along the course of the ureter, but are most common at the areas of narrowing: the ureteropelvic junction, the pelvic brim, and the vesicoureteral junction. Bladder calculi are single or multiple, commonly laminated, may be any size, and usually lie near the midline of the pelvis (Fig. 22.15). Calculi within bladder diverticula may be eccentric to the bladder.

Liver and Spleen Granulomas are usually multiple, small, and dense. They are healed foci of tuberculosis, histoplasmosis, or other granulomatous disease.

Appendicoliths and Enteroliths are concretions within the lumen of the bowel. Most are round or oval and have concentric laminations. Appendicoliths are strongly indicative of acute appendi-

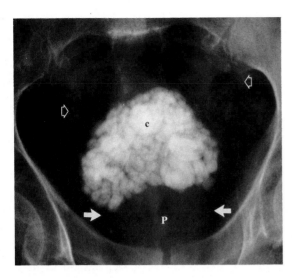

Figure 22.15. Bladder Calculi. Numerous calculi (*c*) in the bladder are evident on this plain radiograph of the pelvis. The large prostate (*P*, between *closed arrows*), responsible for urinary stasis leading to stone formation, makes a mass impression on the layering stones. Also evident are atherosclerotic calcifications in the iliac arteries (*open arrows*).

citis in patients with acute abdominal pain (Fig. 28.18). Enteroliths are most common in the colon and often due to calcium deposition on an undigestable material such as a fruit pit.

Calcified Adrenal Glands are associated with adrenal hemorrhage in the newborn, tuberculosis, and Addison's disease. The calcification is mottled and in the location of the adrenal glands on either side of the first lumbar vertebra (Fig. 29.6).

Pancreatic Calcification is associated with chronic alcohol-induced pancreatitis and hereditary pancreatitis. The calcifications are due to pancreatic calculi and are usually coarse and of varying size (Fig. 24.10).

Calcified Cysts may be found in the kidneys, spleen, liver, appendix, and peritoneal cavity. Calcification in the wall of a cyst is curvilinear or ring-shaped. *Echinococcus* cysts commonly calcify and may be found in any intraabdominal organ as well as within the peritoneal cavity.

Tumor Calcification. A wide variety of different tumors of abdominal organs may contain calcifications. The coarse "popcorn" calcification of uterine leiomyomas is most characteristic (Fig. 32.10). Benign cystic teratomas may form teeth or bone (Fig. 32.8). Calcified peritoneal metastases of ovarian or colon mucinous cystadenocarcinoma may outline the peritoneal cavity (Fig. 32.13**A**). Renal cell carcinoma calcifies in up to 25% of cases.

Soft-tissue Calcifications may be seen with hypercalcemic states, idiopathic calcinosis, and old hematomas. Calcified injection granuloma from quinine, bismuth, and calcium salts of penicillin are commonly

Table 22.6. Location of Abdominal Abscesses

Site	%
Pelvis	66
Subphrenic	18
Subhepatic	8
Infracolic	5
Lesser sac	3

evident in the buttocks. Cysticercosis causes characteristic "rice-grain" calcifications in muscles.

Tumors of the Peritoneal Surface

Peritoneal Mesothelioma is a primary tumor of the peritoneal membrane. Approximately 20–30% of mesotheliomas arise from the peritoneum, while most of the remainder arise from the pleura. All are closely related to asbestos exposure. Computed tomography demonstrates nodular, irregular thickening of the peritoneal surfaces. Ascites, when present, is often minimal. The tumor may involve the greater omentum and present as "omental cake," a layer of nodular soft tissue displacing the bowel away from the anterior abdominal wall. Adjacent bowel may be invaded and become fixed. Ultrasonography demonstrates the sheet-like superficial masses. Rare multilocular cystic forms of the tumor also occur.

Peritoneal Metastases are most commonly associated with ovarian carcinoma in females and colon, pancreas, or stomach carcinoma in males. The preferential sites for tumor implantation are the pelvic cul-de-sac, right paracolic gutter, and the greater omentum (Fig. 32.13). Computed tomography demonstrates tumor nodules on peritoneal surfaces, (Fig. 22.16) "omental cake", tumor nodules in the mesentery, thickening and nodularity of the bowel wall due to serosal implants, and ascites that is commonly loculated. Ultrasonography may directly visualize the peritoneal tumors, and demonstrates secondary signs of malignant ascites including echogenic debris in the fluid, septation, and matted bowel loops (9). Omental cake appears as diffuse nodular enlargement of the greater omentum (Fig. 32.14).

Abdominal Abscess

Abscesses occur within the peritoneal cavity because of spillage of contaminated material from perforated bowel or as a complication of surgery, trauma, pancreatitis, or acquired immunodeficiency syndrome (AIDS). Development of an abscess is commonly insidious, and the clinical presentation is often nonspecific and confusing. The pelvis is the most common site for abscess formation (Table 22.6).

Figure 22.16. Peritoneal Metastases. A CT scan demonstrates intraperitoneal spread of a rhabdomyosarcoma. The tumor is implanted on the omentum (o), causing the appearance of omental cake as the thickened omentum floats in ascites (A) between bowel loops and the abdominal wall. A calcified metastasis (arrow) is implanted on the peritoneal surface.

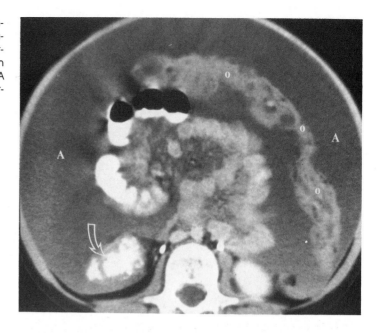

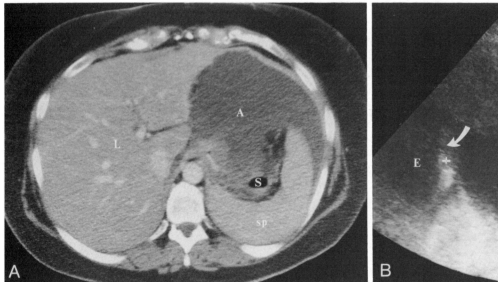

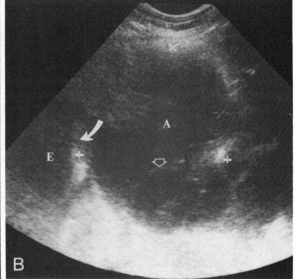

Figure 22.17. Left Subphrenic Abscess. A. A CT scan demonstrates a loculated fluid collection (A) in the left subphrenic space following gastric bypass surgery. The stomach (S) is displaced posteriorly. L, liver; sp, spleen. **B.** Ultrasonography in the same patient demon-strates internal septations (open arrow) within the fluid collection (A, between cursors) that are not apparent on the CT study. A pleural effusion (E) is seen above the diaphragm (curved arrow). The abscess contained Gram-negative organisms.

Plain film findings of abscess include soft tissue mass, collection of extraluminal gas, viscus displacement, localized or generalized ileus, elevation of the diaphragm, pleural effusion, and pulmonary basilar changes. A focal collection of extraluminal gas is the most specific sign of abscess but is unfortunately uncommon.

Computed tomography signs of abscess include a loculated fluid collection (Fig. 22.17A) often with internal debris and fluid-fluid levels. The walls of the fluid collection are often thick and irregular. Gas within the fluid collection is strong evidence of abscess. Fascia ad-jacent to the abscess is thickened, and fat surrounding the abscess may be increased in density and contain soft tissue strands due to inflammation.

Ultrasound demonstrates a focal fluid collection often containing echogenic fluid, floating debris, and septations (Fig. 22.17B). However, completely anechoic fluid collections may also be infected. A thickened wall is usually evident. Gas within the fluid collection is evidenced by echogenic foci producing comet-tail or reverberation artifacts. Computed tomography- or ultrasonography-directed aspiration confirms the diagnosis, provides material for culture,

Table 22.7. Lymphadenopathy—Upper Limits of Normal Node Size by Location

Node Location	Maximum Dimension (mm)	Comments
Retrocrural	6	May enlarge from disease above or below the diaphragm
Retroperitoneal	10	Multiple nodes 8-10 mm in size are usually abnormal
Gastrohepatic ligament	8	Must differentiate lymphadenopathy from coronary varices
Porta hepatis	6	May cause biliary obstruction
Celiac and Superior mesenteric artery	10	Also called preaortic nodes
Pancreaticoduodenal	10	Commonly involved by lymphoma and GI carcinoma
Perisplenic	10	Involved by lymphoma and GI carcinoma
Mesenteric	10	In the small bowel mesentery
Pelvic	15	Most commonly involved by pelvic tumors

and offers the opportunity for percutaneous catheter drainage (see Fig. 22.20).

Lymphadenopathy

A wide variety of neoplastic and inflammatory diseases result in abdominal lymphadenopathy (10–12). Computed tomography, ultrasonography, and MR can evaluate the entire abdominopelvic lymphatic system and have largely replaced lymphangiography in demonstrating lymphadenopathy. The abdomen and pelvis contain more than 230 lymph nodes, and lymphangiography fails to evaluate many lymph node groups including mesenteric, retrocrural, portal, and celiac nodes (10). Unfortunately, none of the cross-section imaging methods can demonstrate tumor involvement of a lymph node by alteration of internal architecture. Criteria for pathologic involvement is based primarily on alterations in node size (Table 22.7) (11).

Short axis measurements of lymph node size are preferred to determine abnormal enlargement. Morphologic patterns of pathologic lymphadenopathy include single enlarged nodes, multiple separate lobulated enlarged nodes, or bulky conglomerate masses of lymph nodes. Calcification in enlarged nodes may be seen with inflammatory adenopathy, mucinous carcinomas, sarcomas, and treated lymphoma. Patients who have had previous lymphangiograms may also show high density nodes on CT.

Computed tomography to detect adenopathy requires optimal contrast opacification of blood vessels and the gastrointestinal tract. Normal nodes are oblong in shape, homogeneous in configuration, and have short axis diameters below the limits listed in Table 22.7. Most pathologically enlarged nodes have CT densities slightly less than skeletal muscle. Low density nodal metastases are commonly seen with nonseminomatous testicular carcinoma, tuberculosis, and occasionally lymphoma.

Ultrasonography is almost equal to CT in accuracy for detection of lymphadenopathy, however, a skillful dedicated examination is required. Lymphoma typi-cally produces hypoechoic or even anechoic lymphadenopathy (Fig. 22.18). Masses of retroperitoneal nodes may silhouette segments of the normally echogenic wall of the aorta (the "sonographic silhouette sign"). The "sandwich sign" refers to entrapment of mesenteric vessels by masses of enlarged lymph nodes in the mesentery.

Magnetic resonance usually provides excellent differentiation of lymph nodes from blood vessels because of flow void within vessels. However, because of the current lack of an effective gastrointestinal contrast agent, loops of bowel are commonly confused with masses of nodes. On T1-weighted images, lymph nodes show low signal intensity compared to surrounding fat. On T2-weighted images, lymph nodes show high signal intensity compared to muscle. Fat saturation technique highlights pathologic adenopathy (Fig. 22.19).

Hodgkin's Lymphoma is responsible for 20–40% of all lymphoma and is characterized histologically by the presence of the Reed-Sternberg cell. Hodgkin's lymphoma has a bimodal age distribution most commonly affecting patients aged 25–30 and over 70 years. At presentation, abdominal adenopathy is present in about 25% of cases. The spleen is involved in about 40% of cases and the liver in about 8%. Involvement of the gastrointestinal tract and urinary tract is much less common with Hodgkin's than with non-Hodgkin's lymphoma. Lymphoma staging is shown in Table 22.8.

Non-Hodgkin's Lymphoma is responsible for 60–80% of all lymphoma. Non-Hodgkin's lymphoma is a heterogeneous group of disorders with a confusing array of constantly changing names and classifications (12). Non-Hodgkin's lymphoma are particularly common in patients with AIDS and other immunocompromised states. The Non-Hodgkin's lymphoma commonly involve extranodal sites including the gastrointestinal and urinary tract. At presentation, abdominal adenopathy is present in about 50% of cases. The spleen is involved in about 40% of cases (Fig. 24.20) and the liver in about 14%. The Ann Arbor staging classification developed for

Figure 22.18. Lymphoma. An axial plane ultrasonographic image demonstrates multiple enlarged hypoechoic lymph nodes (*n*) surrounding and displacing the aorta (*A*) and celiac axis (*open arrow*). The adenopathy extends into the hilum of the right kidney (*K*). *L*, liver.

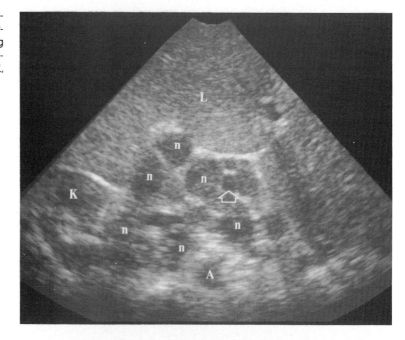

Figure 22.19. Lymphoma. Fat saturation MR image (TR = 2700, TE = 40, TI = 160) demonstrates a confluent mass of lymphoma nodes (*L*) with high signal intensity surrounded by low signal intensity fat and muscle. The iliac vessels (*arrow*) are encased by adenopathy.

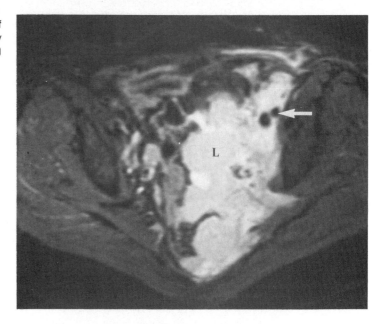

Hodgkin's lymphoma is also used for Non-Hodgkin's lymphoma (Table 22.8) (12).

Retroperitoneal Fibrosis

Retroperitoneal fibrosis is a rare condition manifest by formation of a fibrous plaque in the lower retroperitoneum that encases and compresses the aorta, inferior vena cava, and ureters (13). About two-thirds of cases are considered to be idiopathic. Methysergide, an ergot prescribed for migraine headache, is a cause of about 12% of cases. Small foci of metastatic malignancy that elicit a fibrotic reaction in the retroperitoneum account for another 8–10%. In-flammatory aneurysms, which induce a rind of peri-aneurysmal fibrosis, are responsible for 5–10% of cases. Other possible causes include tuberculosis, syphilis, actinomycosis, and fungi. About 15% of patients have additional fibrosing processes including mediastinal fibrosis, Riedel fibrosing thyroiditis, sclerosing cholangitis, and fibrotic orbital pseudotumors. The fibrotic plaque is usually located over the anterior surfaces of the fourth and fifth lumbar vertebrae. In the early stages the plaque is highly cellular and edematous; when mature, it consists of dense hyalinized collagen with few cells. Cases induced by malignancy have a few malignant cells scattered within the collagen.

Table 22.8. Staging of Lymphoma—Ann Arbor Staging Classification[a]

Stage	Description
I	Involves single lymph node region
Ie	Involves single extralymphatic organ or site
II	Involves two or more lymph node regions on the same side of the diaphragm
IIe	Involves a localized extralymphatic organ or site and one or more lymph node regions on the same side of the diaphragm
III	Involves lymph node regions on both sides of the diaphragm
IIIs	Also involves the spleen
IIIe	Also involves extralymphatic organ or site
IIIse	Also involves extralymphatic organ or site and the spleen
IV	Diffuse or disseminated involvement of one or more extralymphatic organs or tissues
Suffix A	Absence of fever, night sweats, unexplained weight loss of 10% or more of body weight in previous 6 months
Suffix B	Presence of above

[a]Modified from Castellino RA. The non-Hodgkin lymphomas: practical concepts for the diagnostic radiologist. Radiology 1991;178:315–321.

The hallmark of retroperitoneal fibrosis on excretory urography is smooth extrinsic narrowing of one or both ureters in the region of L4-5. Proximal hydronephrosis commonly results from impairment of ureteral peristalsis. The process may extend into the pelvis and cause a teardrop configuration to the bladder and narrowing of the sigmoid colon. Venography and aortography demonstrate smooth extrinsic narrowing of the vena cava and aorta.

Computed tomography demonstrates a fibrous plaque that envelops the cava, aorta, and often the ureters. The plaque may be midline or asymmetric, well-defined or poorly defined, localized or expansive.

On MR the plaque is typically of low signal intensity on both T1- and T2-weighted images. Plaque that shows high signal intensity on T2-weighted images should be considered supicious for malignancy as a cause, although early edematous plaques may have the same appearance.

On ultrasonograhphy, retroperitoneal fibrosis is easily confused with lymphoma in the retroperitoneum. Both show confluent hypoechoic masses encasing the cava and aorta. Typically, lymphoma extends behind the vessels and displaces them anteriorly while retroperitoneal fibrosis does not.

AIDS in the Abdomen

Acquired immunodeficiency syndrome in the abdomen is characterized by multiple coexisting diseases with multicentric involvement. Up to 90% of patients with AIDS develop complaints related to the gastrointestinal or hepatobiliary systems (14). Genitourinary tract disease affects 38–68% of AIDS patients (15). Manifestations of infectious and neoplastic processes in AIDS patients are effectively demonstrated by abdominal imaging techniques (Table 22.9) (14–18).

Acquired immunodeficiency syndrome is a disease of impaired cellular immunity caused by the retrovirus currently designated human immunodeficiency virus (HIV). The disease is characterized by multiple opportunistic infections and aggressive malignancies, most commonly Kaposi sarcoma and AIDS-related lymphoma. Infection by multiple organisms at multiple sites is the rule.

Opportunistic Infections are caused by organisms that are usually effectively controlled by normal cellular immunity (14–17). *Pneumocystis carinii* causes pneumonia in nearly 80% of AIDS patients. However, possibly because of prophylactic treatment with aerolized pentamidine, extrapulmonary *Pneumocystis* infections are increasingly common, affecting the liver, spleen, kidney, pancreas, and lymph nodes. *Mycobacterium avium-intracellulare* and *M. tuberculosis* are also frequent infections. *Mycobacterium avium-intracellulare* is a cause of bulky abdominal adenopathy, hepatosplenomegaly, and focal lesions in the liver and spleen. *Candida albicans* and cytomegalovirus are common causes of esophagitis as well as gastic antritis and duodenitis. *Cryptosporidium* and *Isospora belli* are protozoans, previously found only in animals, that infect the gastrointestinal tract and cause severe diarrhea. *Cryptosporidium* and cytomegalovirus are implicated as causes of AIDS-related cholangitis. Herpes virus, *Toxoplasma gondii*, *Entamoeba histolytica*, *Giardia lamblia*, and *Cryptococcus neoformans* are additional pathogens in AIDS patients.

Kaposi Sarcoma involves the abdomen as a multicentric neoplasm. *Kaposi Sarcoma* is more common in AIDS patients than all other neoplasms combined (14–17). Lymphadenopathy is frequent and can be distinguished from AIDS-related lymphoma and *M. avium-intracellulare* lymph node infection only by biopsy. Gastrointestinal involvement is manifest by wall thickening and multiple plaque-like nodules. *Kaposi sarcoma* may also cause focal lesions in the liver and spleen. Involvement of the skin is evidenced by subcutaneous nodules.

AIDS-related Lymphomas are extremely aggressive neoplasms that respond poorly to therapy (18). Most are non-Hodgkin's lymphoma, although Hodgkin's lymphoma is also increased in frequency. Ad-

Table 22.9. Abdominal Imaging Findings in AIDS

Persistent generalized lymphadenopathy (reactive lymphoid
    hyperplasia)
    Mild retroperitoneal adenopathy (<1 cm)
    Splenomegaly
    Perirectal infiltrate (90% of homosexual men)
Kaposi sarcoma
    Bulky adenopathy (>1.5 cm)
    Wall thickening gastrointestinal (GI) tract
    Rare focal lesions, liver + spleen
AIDS-related lymphoma
    Bulky adenopathy (>1.5 cm)—mesentery, paraortic, pelvic
    Hepatosplenomegaly
    Focal lesions in liver, spleen, kidney
    Focal masses/wall thickening GI tract
M. avium-intracellulare infection
    Bulky adenopathy (>1.5 cm)—retroperitoneal + mesenteric
    Hepatosplenomegaly
    Rare focal lesions, liver + spleen
P. carinii infection
    Tiny focal lesions in liver + spleen
    Diffuse or punctate calcification liver, spleen, kidney, adrenal
        glands, lymph nodes
AIDS-related cholangitis
    Irregular wall thickening of intrahepatic bile ducts
    Irregular dilation of intra- and extrahepatic bile ducts
    Inflammatory strictures of bile ducts
HIV nephropathy
    Global enlargement both kidneys
    Increased cortical echogenicity
Hemorrhagic cystitis due to cytomegalovirus (CMV), Candida,
    Salmonella, β-hemolytic streptococci
    Bladder wall thickening
Antritis/Duodenitis due to Cryptosporidium, CMV, Candida
    Wall thickening and ulceration gastric antrum and duodenum
AIDS enteritis due to Cryptosporidium, I. belli, M. avium-
    intracellulare
    Dilation of small bowel, especially jejunum
    Thickening of bowel wall
    Thickened or effaced mucosal folds
CMV colitis and ileitis
    Thickening of bowel wall with submucosal edema of entire
        colon, segment of colon, or cecum
    Toxic megacolon
    Colon perforation
Spinal osteomyelitis
    Lytic destruction of bone
    Paraspinal abscess

vanced disease with extensive extranodal involvement
is common at presentation. Multiple sites of involvement within the abdomen are usually evident. The diagnosis is confirmed by CT- or ultrasonography-directed biopsy.

More extensive descriptions of AIDS-related diseases affecting individual organs are provided in the
appropriate chapters.

Guided Percutaneous Biopsy

Over the past 15 years, guided percutaneous biopsy
has become a standard medical practice. In the abdomen, both CT and ultrasonography have proven effi-

cacious in providing safe precise guidance for percutaneous biopsy procedures (19-22). Guided biopsy
offers the advantages of accurate localization, avoid-
ance of vital structures, and markedly lowered morbidity and mortality compared to open surgical biopsy.

Indications. Percutaneous biopsy is performed
to (*a*) confirm suspected primary malignancy, (*b*) confirm metastases in a patient with known malignancy,
(*c*) establish the nature of an indeterminate lesion,
and (*d*) confirm the diagnosis of a likely benign lesion
(19–20).

Contraindications. Relative contraindications
to percutaneous biopsy include (*a*) uncorrectable
bleeding disorder, (*b*) lack of safe pathway to perform
a biopsy of the lesion, and (*c*) an uncontrolled patient
(19–21).

Complications from guided percutaneous needle
biopsy are infrequent and generally minor. The major
feared complication is uncontrolled hemorrhage. The
risk of hemorrhage is significantly increased by bleeding disorders, uncontrolled patient motion, and large
needle size. However, the overall mortality rate from
guided needle biopsy is 0.1% or less (20, 23). Additional complications include pneumothorax, localized
hematoma, vasovagal reactions, and infections. Hematuria may result from a biopsy performed in the urinary tract. Seeding of the needle tract with malignant
tumor is exceedingly rare and limited to isolated case
reports (20).

Choice of Guidance Method. The choice between CT and ultrasonography to guide biopsy procedures is largely one of equipment availability, as well
as personal preference and experience. Ultrasonography has the advantage of portability, continuous visualization of needle position, ability to guide
puncture in any direction, less expense, and generally
speedier performance of the procedure. However, ultrasound is limited by bone and bowel gas, as well as
surgical wounds and dressings. Ultrasound is optimal
for thin and average-sized patients and lesions located
superficially or at moderate depth. Transrectal and
transvaginal transducers improve access to sites traditionally difficult in biopsy by ultrasonography guidance. Most ultrasonography units have incorporated
optional biopsy guidance devices that attach to the
transducer and direct the needle to the visualized lesion. However, many experienced radiologists prefer
the freedom of the freehand technique: one hand is
used to hold the transducer, directing it at the lesion
and the intended biopsy path and the other hand is
used to pass the needle into the lesion. This technique frequently allows the transducer to be kept out
of the sterile field and optimizes flexibility for needle
direction (19–22).

Figure 22.20. Percutaneous Abscess Drainage. A. The patient is placed in an oblique right lateral decubitus position to optimize access to a fluid collection (*open arrow*) adjacent to the left psoas muscle (*p*). Metallic rods (*small arrow*) placed on the skin localize a puncture site directly above the fluid collection, allowing a direct vertical approach. The depth is measured from the skin surface to the center of the fluid collection (*1*). **B.** A needle is passed vertically into the fluid collection. The location of the needle tip (*long arrow*) is confirmed by identifying the black shadow (*short arrow*) cast from the needle tip. Aspiration of purulent fluid through the needle confirms the nature of the fluid collection and provides a specimen for laboratory analysis, Gram stain, and culture. **C.** A flexible guidewire (*arrow*) is passed through the needle and coiled within the fluid collection. **D.** The needle is removed leaving the guidewire in place. Dilators are passed over the guidewire to enlarge the tract extending to the abscess. A straightened pigtail catheter is guided into the abscess over the guidewire. The guidewire is removed and the pigtail loop is reformed at the end of the catheter to help maintain the catheter (*arrow*) in place. Aspiration is performed through the catheter until all fluid has been removed from the abscess. The catheter is sutured to the skin and attached to a drainage bag for continued drainage.

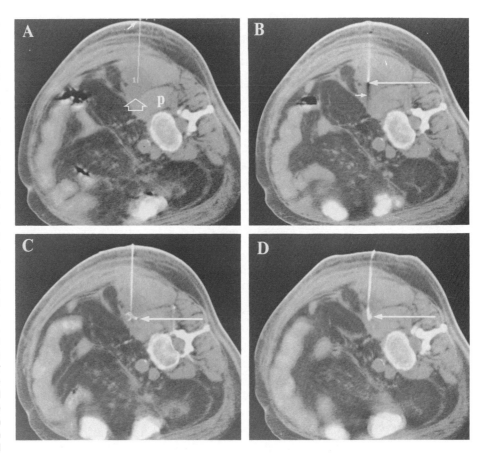

Computed tomography allows visualization of lesions without interference from wounds, dressings, bowel gas, or bone. Disadvantages of this method include needle placement without continuous visualization, higher cost, and often more lengthy procedure time. Biopsy of obese patients and very deep lesions is often best performed by CT guidance. Computed tomography also allows biopsy to be performed through bowel loops, allowing access to interloop abcesses and portions of the pancreas surrounded by bowel. Care must be taken to ensure that the true needle tip is visualized especially if the needle passes obliquely through the CT slice. The true needle tip has an abrupt termination, usually with a black streak due to beam hardening artifact extending from the needle tip (Fig. 22.20) (20). The needle shaft appears tapered due to volume averaging effect, and it lacks the black linear artifact.

Choice of Needle. The safest needles are the thin aspiration needles (20- to 22-gauge). These needles are most appropriate for fluid sampling and cell aspiration for cytologic analysis. Multiple passes can be made with thin needles with very low risk of significant hemorrhage. Larger needles (14- to 19-gauge)

provide tissue samples adequate for histologic analysis. Tissue recovery rates are increased, and most biopsies can be performed in one or two passes. Specially designed cutting-tip needles optimize recovery of tissue cores for histology. The disadvantage of larger needles is a greater risk of significant hemorrhage. Automated biopsy devices have recently been developed to reliably perform core biopsy for histology. The needle is aligned with the lesion, and biopsy is performed by activating a mechanical spring-driven biopsy motion. The exceedingly fast and precise motion improves recovery of histologic tissue specimens from solid lesions.

Patient Preparation includes assessment for coagulation disorders by obtaining prothrombin time, partial thromboplastin time, and platelet count. Known coagulation disorders should be corrected with vitamin K, fresh-frozen plasma, or platelets. The patient should be instructed as to the nature of the procedure and its potential risks and benefits. Informed patient consent must be obtained. Many biopsies can be performed on an outpatient basis, particularly when arrangements can be made to monitor the patient for a period of time following the procedure.

The skin is prepared with povidone-iodine solution. Local anesthesia is routinely used. Mild intravenous sedation is often helpful, especially when sampling deep lesions.

Biopsy Results. Biopsy of lesions can be performed in virtually every abdominal and pelvic organ, as well as in the intraperitoneal and extraperitoneal compartments. Overall accuracy rates vary from 82–100% for CT and 66–97% for ultrasound, depending on size and location of the lesion (20). Complication rates are reported at 0.3%–3.0% depending primarily on needle size (20).

Guided Percutaneous Drainage

Abscesses and fluid collections virtually anywhere within the abdomen or pelvis are routinely and preferentially drained percutaneously using radiographic guidance. Percutaneous nephrostomy and percutaneous biliary drainage are also routine procedures. All procedures are performed using the same general principles utilized for guided percutaneous biopsy.

Percutanous Abscess Drainage. Percutaneous catheter drainage is proven effective in treatment in a wide variety of fluid collections including unilocular and multilocular abscesses, pancreatic fluid collections, hematomas, lymphoceles, and amebic and echinococcal abscesses (24, 26). The abscess is localized and analyzed by CT or ultrasound (Fig. 22.20). Catheter placement can be performed using fluoroscopic, CT, or ultrasound guidance. A wide variety of specialized techniques and catheters have been developed and are continually being improved. Basic approaches utilize either the trocar method or the Seldinger technique. The trocar method utilizes a catheter loaded onto a stiff cannula with an internal, sharply pointed trocar. The catheter may be introduced by one-step puncture of the fluid collection with the complete assembly. The trocar is removed, fluid is aspirated to confirm location, then the catheter is advanced over the cannula and into the fluid collection. The Seldinger technique involves needle aspiration of a fluid collection, followed by passage of a guidewire through the needle into the collection (Fig. 22.20). The tract is enlarged using dilators passed over the guidewire, then the drainage catheter is placed into the fluid collection, and the guidewire is removed. The abscess is evacuated and may be irrigated with saline. The catheter is attached to a gravity drainage bag or to low suction. The abscess cavity and any potential communications to bowel, bladder, etc., can be studied by contrast injection into the cavity. Catheter care and termination of catheter drainage is provided by close and continuing communication between the radiologist and the patient's primary physician.

Percutaneous Nephrostomy. The urinary tract can be effectively drained by guided percutaneous passage of a catheter into the renal pelvis. Indications for urinary diversion include urinary tract obstruction, urosepsis, or urinary fistula. Percutaneous nephrostomies may also be performed preliminary to stone manipulation or removal, stricture dilation, or other urologic procedures. When renal function is normal, the procedure may be performed using fluoroscopic guidance following intravenous contrast injection to opacify the collecting system. Alternatively ultrasound or CT guidance is utilized. The renal collecting system is accessed by guided needle puncture through the renal parenchyma. Guidewires are placed, the tract dilated, and a pigtail nephrostomy drainage catheter is placed in the renal pelvis.

Percutaneous Biliary Drainage may be performed to relieve biliary obstruction, in the treatment of biliary sepsis, and preliminary to biliary interventional procedures such as stone extraction or stricture dilation. Ultrasonography or CT is used to guide needle puncture of intrahepatic bile ducts. Contrast is injected to opacify the biliary tree (percutaneous transhepatic cholangiography). Guidewires may then be advanced into the biliary tree and followed by placement of drainage catheters that may extend all the way through the ampulla of Vater, providing internal bile drainage.

References

1. Meyers MA. Dynamic radiology of the abdomen: normal and pathological anatomy. 3rd ed. New York: Springer-Verlag, 1988.
2. Dodds WJ, Foley WD, Lawson TL, et al. Anatomy and imaging of the lesser peritoneal sac. AJR 1985;141:567–575.
3. Rubenstein WA, Auh YH, Whalen JP, Kazam E. The perihepatic spaces: computed tomographic and ultrasound imaging. Radiology 1983;149:231–239.
4. Dodds WJ, Darweesh RMA, Lawson TL, et al. The retroperitoneal spaces revisited. AJR 1986;147:1155–1161.
5. Raptopoulus V, Kleinman PK, Marks S Jr, et al. Renal fascial pathway: posterior extension of pancreatic effusions within the anterior pararenal space. Radiology 1986;158:367–374.
6. Levine MS, Scheiner JD, Rubesin SE, et al. Diagnosis of pneumoperitoneum on supine abdominal radiographs. AJR 1991;156:731–735.
7. Herlinger H, Maglinte D, eds. Clinical radiology of the small intestine. Philadelphia: WB Saunders Company, 1989.
8. Balthazar E. CT of the gastrointestinal tract: principles and interpretation. AJR 1991;156:23–32.
9. Goerg C, Schwerk W-B. Peritoneal carcinomatosis with ascites. AJR 1991;156:1185–1187.
10. Einstein DM, Singer AA, Chilcote WA, Desai RK. Abdominal lymphadenopathy: spectrum of CT findings. RadioGraphics 1991;11:457–472.
11. Jackson FI, Lalani Z. Ultrasound in the diagnosis of lymphoma: a review. J Clin Ultrasound 1989;17:145–171.
12. Castellino RA. The non-Hodgkin's lymphomas: practical concepts for the diagnostic radiologist. Radiology 1991;178:315–321.
13. Amis ES Jr. Retroperitoneal fibrosis. AJR 1991;157:321–329.

14. Federle MP. A radiologist looks at AIDS: imaging evaluation based on symptoms complexes. Radiology 1988;166:553–562.

15. Kuhlman JE, Browne D, Shermak M, et al. Retroperitoneal and pelvic CT of patients with AIDS: primary and secondary involvement of the genitourinary tract. RadioGraphics 1991;11:473–483.

16. Jeffrey RB Jr, Nyberg DA, Bottles K, et al. Abdominal CT in acquired immunodeficiency syndrome. AJR 1986;146:7–13.

17. Kuhlman JE, Fishman EK. Acute abdomen in AIDS: CT diagnosis and triage. RadioGraphics 1990;10:621–634.

18. Townsend RR. CT of AIDS-related lymphoma. AJR 1991;156:969–974.

19. Gazelle GS, Haaga JR. Guided percutaneous biopsy of intraabdominal lesions. AJR 1989;153:929–935.

20. Charboneau JW, Reading CC, Welch TJ. CT and sonographically guided needle biopsy: current techniques and new innovations. AJR 1990;154:1–10.

21. Matalon TAS, Silver B. US guidance of interventional procedures. Radiology 1990;174:43–47.

22. McGahan JP, Brant WE. Principles, instrumentation, and guidance systems. In: McGahan JP, ed. Interventional ultrasound. Baltimore: Williams & Wilkins, 1990:1–20.

23. Smith EH. Complications of percutaneous abdominal fine-needle biopsy. Radiology 1991;178:253–258.

24. vanSonnenberg E, D'Agostino HB, Casola G, et al. Percutaneous abscess drainage: current concepts. Radiology 1991;181:617–626.

25. Peng-Qiu M, Zhi-Gang Y, QinFang L, et al. Peritoneal reflections of left perihepatic region: radiologic-anatomic study. Radiology 1992;182:553–557.

26. Lambiase RE, Deyoe L, Cronan JJ, Dorfman GS. Percutaneous drainage of 335 consecutive abscesses: results of primary drainage with 1-year follow-up. Radiology 1992;184:167–179.

23

Liver, Biliary Tree, Gallbladder

William E. Brant

LIVER

Imaging Methods

Ultrasound, computed tomography (CT), and magnetic resonance (MR) all produce high-quality images of the liver parenchyma. Ultrasound is an efficient screening method for patients who present with abdominal complaints. For focal liver metastases, its sensitivity is approximately equal to CT and MR (1); however, its images are difficult to reproduce for follow-up comparisons, and benign and malignant nodules cannot usually be distinguished (2). Color Doppler ultrasound is valuable in the assessment of liver vasculature and the diagnosis of portal and hepatic vein thrombosis and portal hypertension (3). Color Doppler ultrasound can effectively evaluate the vascularity of liver tumors, however, the utility of this information is not proven (1). Computed tomography and MR are generally preferred for liver tumor imaging because of their high sensitivity and specificity as well as their reproducibility for follow-up studies (1, 2, 4). Whether CT or MR is chosen as the imaging method of first choice currently depends mainly upon the availability of equipment, personal

choice, and experience. Both technologies continue to improve in their capacity for imaging the liver. Bolus dynamic CT, combining rapid scan acquisition with rapid high-dose contrast injection, is the currently favored CT technique (1). The accuracy of CT is increased by more invasive techniques including CT angiography and CT arterial portography. Both of these techniques involve CT following selective catheterization of the hepatic or superior mesenteric arteries (1). Magnetic resonance currently appears to be a bit more sensitive and specific in the diagnosis of focal lesions than is CT. However, CT is distinctly better than MR at demonstrating extrahepatic lesions as part of a comprehensive evaluation (1, 2, 4). Magnetic resonance is poor at demonstrating diffuse hepatic disease except for hepatic iron overload (4). T1-weighted images provide excellent depiction of anatomy; T2-weighted images demonstrate the most hepatic lesions. A wide variety of rapid scan acquisition techniques are being developed to overcome problems with motion.

Radionuclide scans utilizing technetium sulfur colloid demonstrate nonspecific defects in radionuclide activity where focal lesions are present. Lesions less than 2 cm in diameter are commonly missed by radionuclide scans, while CT and MR can demonstrate lesions a few millimeters in size. The sensitivity of radionuclide scanning in the liver is less than that of CT or MR. Radionuclide blood pool imaging is very useful for definitive diagnosis of cavernous hemangioma. Arteriography is used primarily for determining resectability of known liver tumors and demonstrating bleeding sites. It is currently rarely used in the diagnosis of liver masses.

Anatomy

The anatomy of the liver that is most relevant to liver imaging is the vascular anatomy that defines the surgical approach to lesion resection (5, 6). Hepatic vascular territories divide the liver into three lobes and four segments. The hepatic veins run in the *inter*lobar and *inter*segmental fissures, while the portal veins, hepatic arteries, and bile ducts run in the *intra*segmental parenchyma. Portal veins and hepatic arteries supply the parenchyma of the segments through which they course. Hepatic veins drain both segments bordering

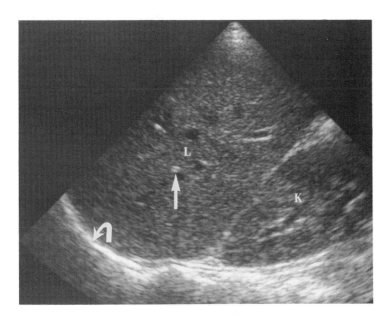

Figure 23.1. Normal Liver. Longitudinal ultrasound image demonstrates normal liver (*L*) and right kidney (*K*). The liver parenchyma is of uniform echogenicity, approximately equal to the parenchymal echogenicity of the kidney. The liver is well-visualized to the level of the diaphragm (*curved arrow*). Small portal triad structures (*straight arrow*) are seen throughout the liver parenchyma.

the fissures that the veins help define. The right and left lobes are separated by the major lobar fissure, defined by the middle hepatic vein. The right hepatic lobe is subdivided into anterior and posterior segments by the right intersegmental fissure, defined by the right hepatic vein. The left hepatic lobe is subdivided into medial and lateral segments by the left intersegmental fissure, defined by the left hepatic vein and by the fat-filled fissure of the ligamentum teres and falciform ligament. The caudate lobe lies between the fissure of the ligamentum venosum anteriorly and the inferior vena cava posteriorly. The caudate lobe is supplied by branches of both right and left hepatic arteries and portal veins. Hepatic venous drainage of the caudate lobe is by multiple small branches that enter the inferior vena cava directly.

The blood supply to the liver is approximately two-thirds via the portal vein and one-third via the hepatic artery. When intravenous contrast is administered as a bolus during rapid CT scanning, the maximum liver parenchymal enhancement will be delayed 1–2 minutes following initiation of injection. This delay reflects the transit time of contrast agent through the gastrointestinal tract before access to the liver through the portal vein. Tumors, which are supplied primarily by the hepatic artery, may maximally enhance during this time interval. The CT density of the normal liver is equal to or greater than the CT density of the normal spleen, both before and after intravenous contrast administration.

On ultrasound the normal liver is homogeneous with good visualization of small vascular structures within the parenchyma. The liver is isoechoic or slightly hyperechoic compared to the kidney, and is slightly hypoechoic compared to the spleen (Fig. 23.1).

On T1-weighted spin-echo MR sequences, the normal liver is of slightly higher signal intensity than the spleen, and most focal lesions appear as low density masses. With T2-weighted spin-echo sequences, the normal liver is less than or equal to the spleen in signal strength, and most focal lesions appear as high density masses (4, 7).

Diffuse Liver Disease

Hepatomegaly. Enlargement of the liver is usually judged subjectively on imaging studies. A liver length of greater than 15.5 cm measured in the midclavicular line has an 87% correlation with hepatomegaly. Causes of hepatomegaly include metabolic (fatty infiltration, glycogen storage disease), malignancy (lymphoma, diffuse metastases), inflammation (hepatitis), and vascular (passive congestion due to congestive heart failure).

Fatty Infiltration of the liver may be diffuse, focal, or diffuse with focal sparing. Fatty infiltration is a nonspecific response of hepatocytes to injury. Causes include alcoholism, obesity, malnutrition, hyperalimentation, steroid therapy, diabetes mellitus, pancreatitis, and chemotherapy. A characteristic feature of fatty infiltration is the lack of mass effect and lack of displacement of hepatic blood vessels.

Diffuse uniform fatty infiltration involving the entire liver is most common and is seen on ultrasound as a diffuse coarse increase in parenchymal echogenicity associated a loss of visualization of small vascular structures and with poor penetration of sound through the liver (Fig. 23.2). Computed tomography demonstrates diffuse low density of the liver parenchyma (lower density than spleen) (Fig. 23.3). Fatty changes can develop within 3 weeks of hepatocyte insult and may resolve within 6 days of removing the insult.

Focal fatty infiltration assumes a geographic or fan-shaped pattern with the same imaging features as diffuse infiltration. Vessels run their normal course through the area of involvement. Focal fatty infiltration may simulate a liver tumor, however, the area of involvement has a density characteristic of fat.

Diffuse infiltration with focal sparing may be the most confusing pattern because spared areas of normal parenchyma may simulate a liver tumor (Fig. 23.4). The fat-spared area is most commonly in the medial segment of the left lobe (quadrate lobe pseudotumor). The fat-spared area is hypoechoic relative to

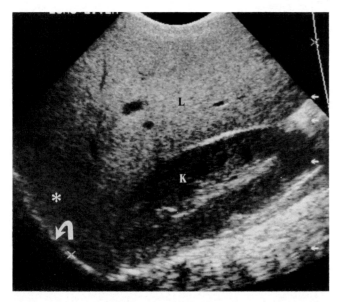

Figure 23.2. Diffuse Fatty Infiltration. Longitudinal ultrasound image demonstrates the liver parenchyma (*L*) to be coarsened and significantly more echogenic than the parenchyma of the right kidney (*K*). Decreased sound wave penetration is evidenced by decreased echo intensity (*) near the diaphragm (curved arrow). Visualization of small portal triad structures is lost.

Figure 23.3. Diffuse Fatty Infiltration. Computed tomography reveals the density of the enhanced liver parenchyma (*L*) to be significantly less than the density of the enhanced splenic parenchyma (*S*). Portal (*p*) and hepatic (*h*) veins run their normal courses without displacement or distortion. *V*, inferior vena cava; *Ao*, aorta.

the rest of the liver on ultrasound and is of higher density than the rest of the liver on CT. The remainder of the liver demonstrates features characteristic of diffuse fatty infiltration.

Cirrhosis is characterized pathologically by diffuse parenchymal destruction, fibrosis with alteration of hepatic architecture, and nodular regeneration as attempted repair. Causes of cirrhosis include hepatic toxins (alcohol, drugs), infection (viral hepatitis), biliary obstruction, and heredity (Wilson's disease). A variety of morphologic alterations are seen on imaging studies. These include hepatomegaly (early), hepatic atrophy (late), coarsening of hepatic parenchymal texture, irregularity (nodularity) of the liver surface, hypertrophy of the caudate lobe with shrinkage of the right lobe, and regenerating nodules. Extrahepatic signs of cirrhosis include evidence of portal hypertension, splenomegaly, and ascites.

Ultrasound demonstrates coarsening of and a heterogeneous increase in hepatic echotexture with decreased visualization of small portal triad structures. Regenerating nodules are usually isoechoic.

Computed tomograms may be normal or reveal parenchymal inhomogeneity with patchy areas of increased and decreased attenuation. The liver surface is often nodular (Fig. 23.5). Areas of fatty replacement may be evident. Regenerating nodules are usually isodense.

Magnetic resonance does not reflect a change in signal characteristics of the liver parenchyma with cirrhosis. However, the morphologic alterations in the liver are evident. Regenerating nodules may have increased signal intensity.

Radionuclide scans demonstrate a shift of colloid activity to the bone marrow and spleen. The gross

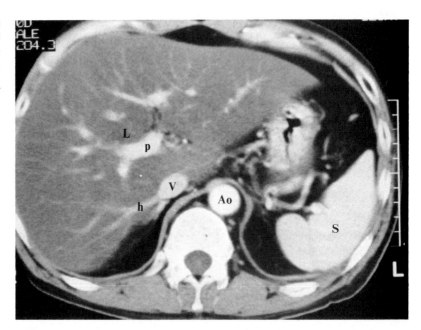

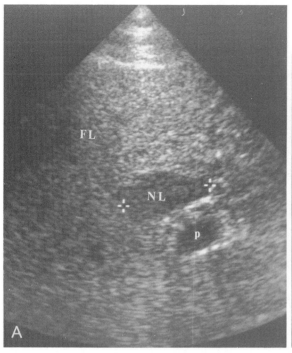

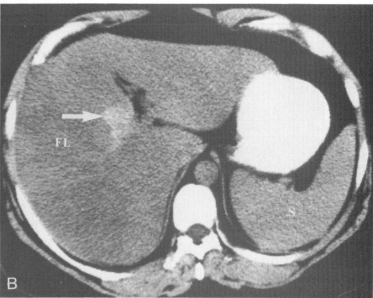

Figure 23.4. Fatty Infiltration with Focal Sparing. A, An ultrasound image demonstrates a focal hypoechoic area of normal liver (*NL*) near the portal vein (*p*) in a liver (*FL*) that is diffusely increased in echogenicity due to fatty infiltration. **B,** A CT image obtained without contrast enhancement demonstrates the spared area of normal liver (*arrow*) to be high density compared to the lower density of the fatty replaced liver (*FL*). *S*, spleen.

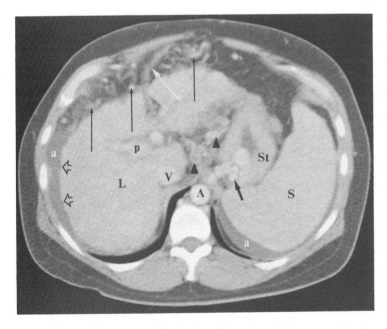

Figure 23.5. Cirrhosis and Portal Hypertension. A CT scan reveals atrophy of the liver (*L*) with diffuse nodularity of its surface (*open arrows*) and splenomegaly (*S*). Numerous enhancing portosystemic collateral vessels are evident including perihepatic (*long black arrows*), gastrohepatic (*arrowheads*), and gastric varices (*short arrow*). A dilated periumbilical vein (*white arrow*) is seen coursing out of the fissure of the ligamentum teres into the falciform ligament. Ascites (*a*) is also evident. *ST*, stomach; *V*, inferior vena cava; *A*, aorta.

morphologic changes in the liver are usually evident. Hepatic activity is inhomogeneous.

Portal Hypertension may result from a variety of causes including progressive vascular fibrosis associated with cirrhosis, portal vein obstruction, and congestive heart failure. As portal venous pressure increases, portosystemic collaterals develop and blood is shunted away from, instead of into, the liver. Portal hypertension carries the risk of hepatic encephalopathy and hemorrhage from varices. The signs of portal hypertension include portosystemic collaterals (coronary, gastroesophageal, splenorenal, hemorrhoidal, and retroperitoneal) (Fig. 23.5), increased portal vein diameter (>13 mm), increased superior mesenteric and splenic vein diameters (>10 mm), portal vein thrombosis, and splenomegaly due to vascular congestion (8).

Figure 23.6. Metastases. Computed tomography of the liver demonstrates multiple low density solid masses (*m*) of varying size representing metastases from adenocarcinoma of the colon. *st*, stomach. *sf*, splenic flexure of the colon.

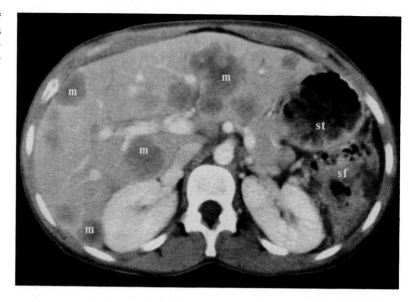

Hemochromatosis may be primary (hereditary) or secondary due to excessive iron intake from either parenteral or dietary sources. In severe cases, CT may demonstrate a diffuse increase in liver density to 75–130 HU. Magnetic resonance is more sensitive to hepatic iron overload and demonstrates marked diffuse loss of signal intensity on T2-weighted images, and moderate loss of signal intensity on T1-weighted images (4). Long-standing hemochromatosis places the patient at risk for cirrhosis and hepatocellular carcinoma.

Focal Liver Masses

A major challenge of liver imaging is to differentiate common and benign liver masses such as hepatic cysts and cavernous hemangioma from malignant masses such as metastases and hepatoma. Ultrasound can definitively characterize hepatic cysts; however, benign and malignant solid masses overlap in sonographic appearance. Computed tomography can characterize some cysts and cavernous hemangiomas but only with optimal technique and contrast administration. On MR, simple cysts and hemangiomas are hypointense on T1-weighted images and extremely hyperintense on T2-weighted spin echo images (7). These benign masses are typically homogeneous and have sharp outer margins. Malignant lesions on MR tend to be inhomogeneous with unsharp outer margins, peritumoral edema, and central necrosis.

Solid Liver Masses

Metastases are the most common malignant masses in the liver. Metastases are 20 times more common than primary liver malignancies. Hepatic metastases commonly originate from the gastrointes-

tinal tract, breast, and lung. A wide spectrum of appearance of metastatic disease is seen on all imaging studies (Fig. 23.6). Metastases may be uniformly solid, necrotic, cystic, or calicified; they may be avascular or hypervascular. Metastatic disease must be considered in the differential of virtually all hepatic masses.

Hepatocellular Carcinoma is the most common primary malignancy of the liver. Risk factors include cirrhosis, chronic hepatitis, and a variety of carcinogens. Hepatomas demonstrate three major growth patterns that affect their imaging appearance: diffuse infiltrative, solitary massive, and multinodular (Fig. 23.7). Invasion of tumor into the portal and hepatic veins and tumor necrosis are common (Fig. 23.8). The tumor metastasizes to lung, adrenal, lymph nodes, and bone. Detection of hepatoma on a background of cirrhosis and regenerative nodules is a major imaging challenge. Elevation in serum α-fetoprotein is found in 90% of patients and is strongly suggestive of hepatoma in patients with cirrhosis.

Fibrolamellar Hepatocellular Carcinoma is a subtype of hepatocellular carcinoma found in younger patients (mean age, 23 years). It is a very desmoplastic tumor with a characteristic stellate central scar (Fig. 23.9). Calcifications are common in these carcinomas.

Cavernous Hemangioma is second only to metastases as the most common cause of a liver mass. It is the most common benign liver neoplasm, found in up to 7% of the population. Up to 10% of patients have multiple lesions easily mistaken for metastases (Fig. 23.10). The tumor consists of large, thin-walled, blood-filled vascular spaces separated by fibrous septa. Blood flow through the maze of vascular spaces is extremely slow, resulting in characteristic imaging findings (9). Thrombosis within the vascular chan-

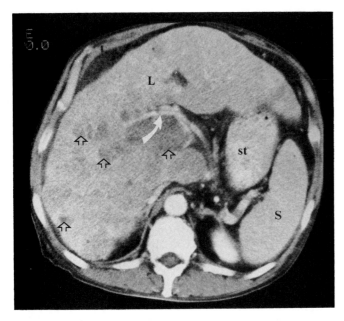

Figure 23.7. Hepatocellular Carcinoma. Contrast-enhanced CT demonstrates multiple hypodense nodules (*open arrows*) in the liver representing hepatocellular carcinoma. The portal vein (*curved arrow*) is compressed and distorted by tumor. *st*, stomach; *S*, spleen.

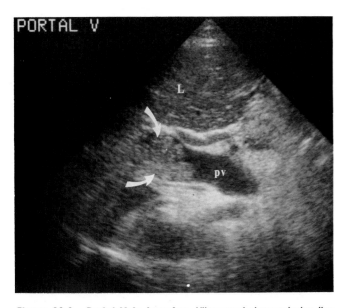

Figure 23.8. Portal Vein Invasion. Ultrasound demonstrates the portal vein (*pv*) to be enlarged and partially filled with tumor thrombus (*arrows*) from hepatocellular carcinoma. *L*, liver.

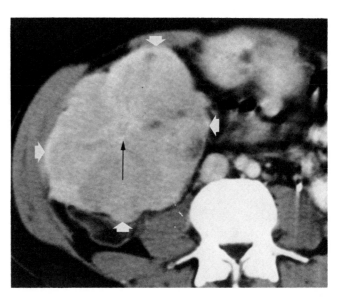

Figure 23.9. Fibrolamellar Hepatocellular Carcinoma. A CT scan demonstrates a large tumor (between *white arrows*) extending caudally from the right lobe of the liver. A characteristic stellate central scar (*black arrow*) is present.

No Doppler signal can be obtained from a cavernous hemangioma because the flow is too slow.

The CT generally shows a well-defined, hypodense mass on unenhanced scans. The characteristic pattern of enhancement with bolus intravenous contrast is nodular enhancement from the periphery with the lesion becoming isodense or hyperdense compared to the liver parenchyma. The contrast enhancement persists for 20–30 minutes following injection because of slow flow within the lesion.

Radionuclide scanning using technetium-labelled red blood cells as a blood pool agent is extremely accurate in the diagnosis of cavernous hemangioma (10). Hemangiomas are characterized by prolonged intense activity within the lesion on delayed images.

Magnetic resonance demonstrates a well-defined homogeneous mass that is hypointense or isotense on T1-weighted images and brightens markedly with increasing amounts of T2-weighting (Fig. 23.10).

Angiography has been the historical gold standard for hemangioma diagnosis. Normal-sized arteries feed an area of well-circumscribed vascular lakes with no neovascularity or arteriovenous shunting. Contrast remains pooled within the lesion late into the venous phase.

Biopsy may be required in atypical cases. Percutaneous biopsy can be safely performed using small needles (20-gauge and smaller). The characteristic finding is blood with normal epithelial cells and no malignant cells. Biopsy with large-bore needles has been associated with hemorrhage and death.

Focal Nodular Hyperplasia forms a nodule consisting of abnormally arranged hepatocytes, bile

nels may result in central fibrosis and calcification. Most lesions are less than 5 cm in size, cause no symptoms, and are considered incidental findings. Larger lesions occasionally cause symptoms by mass effect, hemorrhage, or arteriovenous shunting.

Ultrasound demonstrates a well-defined, uniformly hyperechoic mass in 80% of patients. In a patient with no history of malignant disease and normal liver chemistries, only follow-up is generally recommended.

Figure 23.10. Multiple Cavernous Hemangiomas. T2-weighted MR (TR = 2000, TE = 70) demonstrates multiple hyperintense cavernous hemangiomas (h) in the liver (L). These lesions were isointense with liver parenchyma on T1-weighted images. gb, gallbladder; rk, top of right kidney; lk, left kidney.

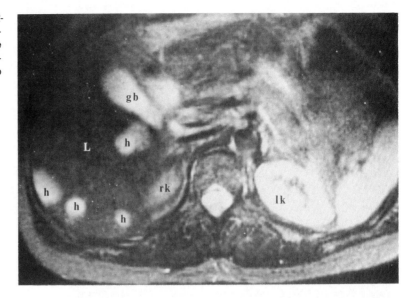

Figure 23.11. Multiple Hepatic Cysts. Unenhanced CT scan of a patient with adult polycystic disease shows multiple cysts (c) of varying size in the liver (L). Both right and left kidneys (rk, lk) are markedly enlarged, with parenchyma largely replaced by innumerable cysts.

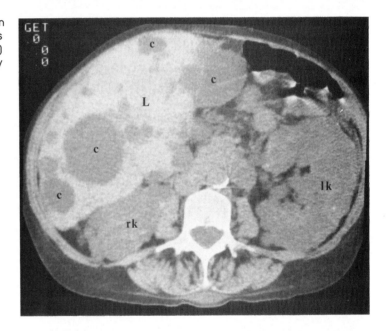

ducts, and Kupffer cells. Focal nodular hyperplasia is twice as common as hepatic adenoma. Because of the presence of Kupffer cells, most focal nodular hyperplasia nodules will show normal or increased radionuclide activity on technetium sulfur colloid liver-spleen scans. This finding is highly suggestive of the diagnosis. Focal nodular hyperplasia nodules are usually nonspecific in appearance on other imaging modalities. A central stellate scar, resembling the central scar of fibrolamellar carcinoma, is present in 15% of cases.

Hepatic Adenomas are rare, benign tumors that carry a risk of hemorrhage. They are found most commonly in women on long-term oral contraceptives. The imaging appearance on all modalities is nonspecific. Surgical resection is recommended because of

the risk of major hemorrhage and the question of malignant transformation.

Lymphoma involving the liver is usually diffusely infiltrative and undetectable by imaging methods. The focal nodular pattern found in 10% of cases resembles metastatic disease.

Cystic Liver Masses

Simple Hepatic Cyst is the second most common benign hepatic mass, found in up to 7% of the elderly population. Most are solitary, but they may be multiple, especially in patients with adult polycystic disease or tuberous sclerosis (Fig. 23.11). Cysts range in size from microscopic to 20 cm.

Ultrasound is the best imaging modality to characterize hepatic cysts (1). Typical cysts are anechoic

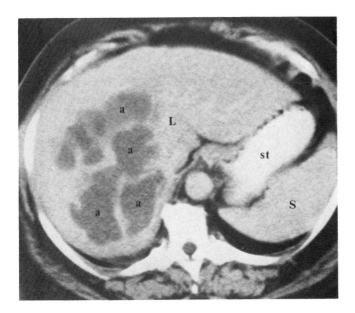

Figure 23.12. Pyogenic Abscess. A CT scan shows multiple low density areas (*a*) in the liver (*L*) representing a multiloculated pyogenic abcess. *st,* stomach; *S,* spleen.

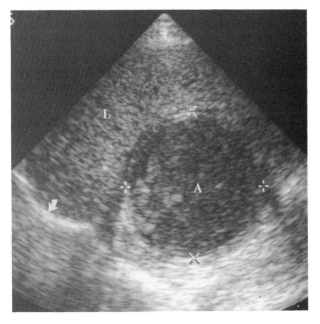

Figure 23.13. Amebic Abscess. Ultrasound demonstrates a well-defined hypodense mass (*A,* between calipers) in the right lobe of the liver (*L*). Note the proximity to the right hemidiaphragm (*arrow*).

with thin walls and posterior acoustic enhancement. Occasionally, hepatic cysts may have internal debris and septa, especially if they have been infected.

When a cystic mass does not meet criteria for a simple cyst, the following lesions must be considered (11).

Pyogenic Abscess is usually caused by *Escherichia coli, Staphylcoccus aureus, Streptococcus,* or anaerobic bacteria. Patients present with fever and pain. Lesions may be solitary or a tight group of individual microabscesses (Fig. 23.12). Gas is present

within the lesion in 20% of cases. Diagnosis is confirmed by percutaneous aspiration. Catheter or surgical drainage is indicated.

Amebic Abscess is usually solitary with thick nodular walls. The lesion may be indistinguishable from pyogenic abscess, however, the patient is usually not septic and has a history of travel to endemic areas. Amebic abscesses commonly occur in the right lobe of the liver (Fig. 23.13), often cause elevation of the right hemidiaphragm, and may rupture through the diaphragm into the pleural space. In the United States, the diagnosis is typically confirmed by serology and the patient is treated with metronidazole. In endemic areas, the diagnosis is confirmed by aspiration of "anchovy paste" material and the patient is treated by repeated aspiration or catheter drainage.

Echinococcus Cyst is due to infestation with *Echinococcus* tapeworm. Single or multiple cystic masses usually have well-defined walls that commonly calcify. Daughter cysts may be visualized within the parent cyst. Diagnostic aspiration carries a risk of anaphylactic reaction. Treatment is albendazole or surgical excision.

Cystic/Necrotic Tumor must always be considered for atypical cystic masses. Metastases may be necrotic or predominantly cystic. Biliary cystadenoma and cystadenocarcinomas are rare primary tumors that resemble mucinous cystic tumors of the pancreas.

Liver Trauma

Computed tomography is the imaging method of choice for blunt abdominal trauma. The extent of liver injury can be classified as contusion, laceration, or intrahepatic or subcapsular hematoma. Contusions are seen as low-density areas in the liver without associated hemoperitoneum. Lacerations are shown as jagged linear or stellate lucencies in the liver associated with intrahepatic hematoma and hemoperitoneum (Fig. 23.14). Subcapsular hematomas cause lenticular-shaped low-density areas beneath the liver capsule that compress the hepatic parenchyma. Computed tomography can accurately quantitate the severity of injury and the amount of hemoperitoneum, and help determine therapy.

BILIARY TREE
Imaging Methods

Imaging of the biliary tree utilizes diverse techniques with differing degrees of invasiveness. Ultrasound and CT are highly sensitive in the detection of dilation of the bile ducts, though they are somewhat less effective in identifying its cause. Ultrasound is the preferred screening method because of its low cost and convenience. Magnetic resonance can also dem-

Figure 23.14.   Liver Laceration. A CT scan of a patient involved in a motor vehicle accident demonstrates a jagged laceration (*arrows*) extending from posterior to the inferior vena cava (*V*) through the right lobe of the liver (*L*). Blood in the laceration is responsible for its low density. Hemoperitoneum was evident on lower CT slices (not shown). *S,* spleen.

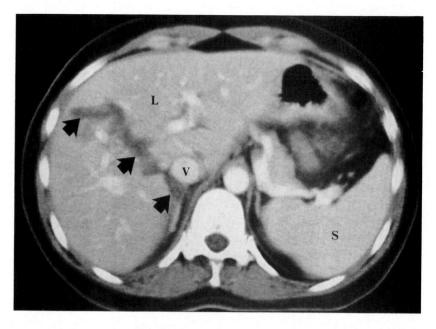

onstrate biliary dilation, and may be more effective than CT or ultrasound in demonstrating associated tumors. Endoscopic retrograde cholangiography (ERCP) and percutaneous transhepatic cholangiography supplement cross-sectional imaging methods by providing access to the biliary tree for contrast injection and subsequent catheter drainage. Operative cholangiography is used to visualize nonpalpable common duct stones at surgery, and T-tube cholangiography is used to visualize common duct stones following surgery. Radionuclide imaging, utilizing technetium-99m-iminodiacetic acid, is useful for showing the patency of biliary-enteric anastomoses and demonstrating bile leaks and fistulae. Scintigraphy has the greatest sensitivity for early obstruction (12). Intravenous cholangiography involved the use of highly toxic contrast agents and has been abandoned in favor of other techniques.

Anatomy

The bile ducts arise as bile capillaries between hepatocytes and join progressively larger branches until two main trunks are formed from the right and left lobes of the liver. The ducts of the left hepatic lobe are more anterior than those of the right hepatic lobe. This relationship must be kept in mind when cholangiography is performed. Contrast agents flow to the most dependent portions of the biliary tree and may not opacify nondependent ducts. Failure to fill ducts before gravitational positioning must not be interpreted as evidence of obstruction (12).

The right and left hepatic ducts combine to form the common hepatic duct that courses with the portal vein and hepatic artery in the porta hepatis. The cystic duct courses posteriorly and inferiorly from the gallbladder to join the common hepatic duct and form the common bile duct. The common bile duct runs ventral to the portal vein and to the right of the hepatic artery, descending from the porta hepatis along the free right margin of the hepatoduodenal ligament to the duodenal bulb. The distal third of the common duct turns caudally and descends in the groove between the descending duodenum and the head of the pancreas just anterior to the inferior vena cava. The duct tapers distally as it ends in the sphincter of Oddi, which protrudes into the duodenum as the ampulla of Vater. The common bile duct and the pancreatic duct share a common orifice in 60% of individuals and have separate orifices in the remainder. However, because of their close proximity, tumors of the ampulla region generally obstruct both ducts.

Normal intrahepatic ducts are not usually seen on ultrasound, CT, or MR. The extrahepatic common duct is routinely visualized and should not exceed 6 mm in internal diameter (12). Normal ducts are larger on cholangiography studies because of distension and magnification. Slightly larger common ducts are also normal in elderly patients because of elastic tissue degeneration with aging. Cholecystectomy is not proven to alter normal common duct size. Care must be taken to differentiate an enlarged common duct from an enlarged hepatic artery. Color Doppler is useful to make this differentiation on ultrasound. Contrast enhancement makes differentiation easy on CT. T2-weighted images demonstrate high signal intensity of static bile on MR.

Biliary Dilation

Biliary dilation demonstrated by ultrasound, CT, or MR is not to be considered equivalent to biliary obstruction (12–14). Biliary obstruction may be present intermittently or in the early stage, without biliary dilation being present. Biliary dilation may be present without obstruction following surgical decompression or bypass. Patients with clinical evidence of biliary obstruction (i.e., elevated alkaline phosphatase and direct hyperbilirubinemia) may not have biliary dilation. Hepatitis causes swelling of hepatocytes, which

blocks biliary capillaries and causes intrahepatic cholestasis without surgical obstruction.

Signs of biliary dilation include (a) multiple branching tubular, round, or oval structures that course toward the porta hepatis (Fig. 23.15), (b) dilation of the common duct greater than 6 mm (Fig. 23.16), and (c) gallbladder diameter greater than 5 cm, when obstruction is distal to the cystic duct. Benign disease is responsible for approximately 75% of cases of obstructinve jaundice in the adult, while malignant disease causes the other 25%. Gradual tapering of the common duct suggests benign stricture. Gallstones may be identified in the bile duct surrounded by a crescent of bile. Abrupt termination of the visualized common duct is characteristic of a malignant process.

Infected bile is present in up to 10% of cases of complete biliary obstruction and 60% of cases of partial or intermittent biliary obstruction. Intravenous antibiotic therapy is warranted prior to biliary interventional procedures in the obstructed patient.

Causes of biliary dilation and obstruction include the following.

Choledocholithiasis is responsible for approximately 20% of cases of obstructive jaundice in the adult (Fig. 23.17). Gallstones are present in the gallbladder in 10% of the population. Stones are present in the common duct in 8–20% of patients with gallbladder stones presenting at surgery (13). However, 1–3% of patients with choledocholithiasis will have no stones in the gallbladder. Operative cholangiography is a routine component of cholecystectomy for gallstones. T-tube cholangiography is routinely performed in the postoperative period to look for residual stones. Patients with prior cholecystectomy are at

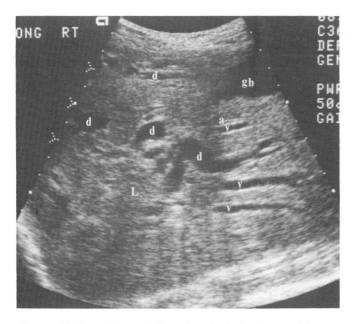

Figure 23.15. Biliary Dilation. Longitudinal ultrasound image demonstrates "too many tubes" in the liver (*L*). Dilated bile ducts (*d*), veins (*v*), and arteries (*a*) are most easily distinguished by use of spectral or color Doppler. Dilated bile ducts tend to be more tortuous and less uniform in diameter than arteries or veins. *gb*, gallbladder.

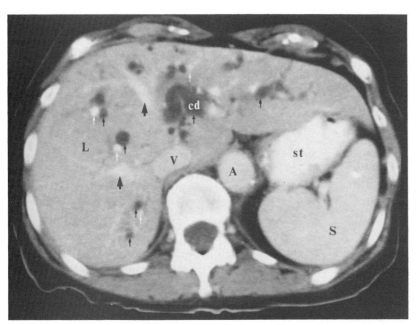

Figure 23.16. Biliary Dilation. A CT scan demonstrates dilated intrahepatic ducts (*small black arrows*) easily differentiated from portal veins (*small white arrows*) and hepatic veins (*black arrowheads*) by contrast enhancement of the blood vessels. The common hepatic duct (*cd*) is tortuous and dilated (12 mm diameter). Mild, diffuse, low density of the liver (*L*) compared to the spleen (*S*) indicates early diffuse fatty infiltration. *V*, inferior vena cava; *A*, aorta; *S*, stomach.

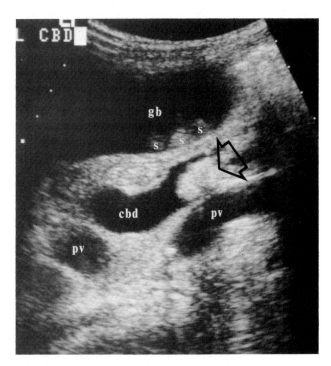

Figure 23.17. Choledocholithiasis. Ultrasound image of the porta hepatis demonstrates a large stone (*arrow*) obstructing the common bile duct (*cbd*) and resulting in its dilation (13 mm diameter). The gallbladder (*gb*) is dilated and contains several nonshadowing sludge balls (*s*) formed as a result of biliary stasis. *pv,* portal vein.

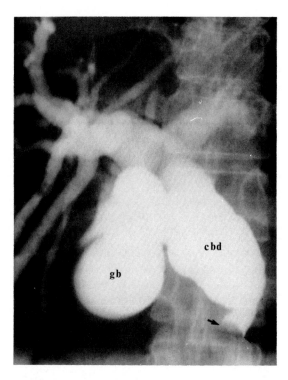

Figure 23.18. Choledocholithiasis. Percutaneous transhepatic cholangiogram demonstrates marked dilation of the common bile duct (*cbd*) and intrahepatic bile ducts. The gallbladder (*gb*) is also filled with contrast and distended. The cause of obstruction and dilation is a radiolucent stone (*arrows*) impacted in the distal common bile duct. The proximal aspect of the stone is well-outlined by contrast.

high risk for common duct stones when they present with jaundice, or evidence of cholangitis. Percutaneous transhepatic cholangiography and endoscopic retrograde cholangiography are the most efficacious examinations when common duct stones are highly suspected (Fig. 23.18).

Benign Stricture is the cause of 40–45% of obstructive jaundice in the adult. Causes of benign stricture include trauma, surgery, and prior biliary interventional procedures.

Pancreatitis is responsible for approximately 8% of cases of biliary obstruction.

Sclerosing Cholangitis is associated with a history of ulcerative colitis in 50% of cases (12). Sclerosing cholangitis is characterized by insidious onset of jaundice with progressive disease affecting both intrahepatic and extrahepatic bile ducts. Alternating dilation and stenosis producing a beaded pattern of intrahepatic ducts is characteristic. Small saccular outpouching (duct diverticula), demonstrated on cholangiography, are considered to be pathognomonic.

Acquired Immunodeficiency Syndrome (AIDS)-associated Cholangitis is characterized by thickening of the walls of the bile ducts as well as the gallbladder. Intrahepatic bile duct changes closely resemble sclerosing cholangitis. The presence of papillary stenosis is a clue to this diagnosis (12). Ulcers in the common duct, inflammatory changes in the duodenum, and evidence of infection with atypical mycobacterium, cytomegalovirus, and *Cryptosporidium* may be associated.

Oriental Cholangiohepatitis is an endemic disease in Southeast Asia characterized by recurrent attacks of jaundice, abdominal pain, fever, and chills (15). Intrahepatic and extrahepatic bile ducts are dilated and filled with soft pigmented stones and pus. The cause is unknown but it is associated with parasitic infestation and nutritional deficiency. Cholangiography demonstrates intraductal stones, severe extrahepatic biliary dilation, focal strictures, and straightening and rigidity of intrahepatic ducts.

Caroli's Disease is an uncommon congenital anomaly of the biliary tract characterized by saccular ectasia of the intrahepatic bile ducts. The cross-sectional imaging appearance is of diffusely scattered cysts that communicate with the bile ducts. The disease is associated with medullary sponge kidney and infantile polycystic kidney disease. Complications include pyogenic cholangitis, liver abscess, and biliary stones.

Choledochal Cysts are uncommon congenital anomalies of the biliary tree characterized by cystic dilation of the bile ducts (16). Cystic or fusiform dilation of the common bile duct accounts for 80–90% of cases (Fig. 23.19). Other types of choledochal cysts include

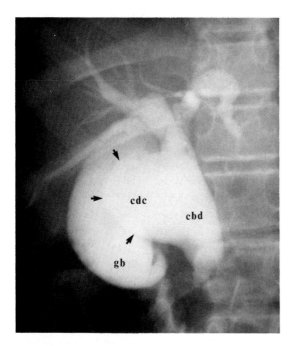

Figure 23.19. Choledochal Cyst. Endoscopic retrograde cholangiography demonstrates cystic dilation (*cdc, arrows*) of the common bile duct (*cbd*). The gallbladder (*gb*) and intrahepatic bile ducts are also opacified.

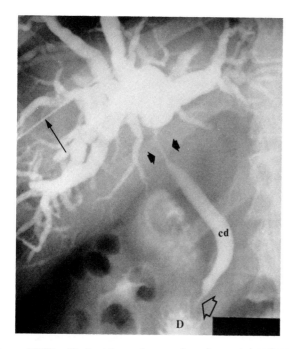

Figure 23.20. Cholangiocarcinoma. Percutaneous transhepatic cholangiogram demonstrates abrupt focal narrowing (*short arrows*) of the proximal common bile duct (*cd*) near the bifurcation. The intrahepatic bile ducts are diffusely dilated. The common bile duct shows normal narrowing at the ampulla of Vater (*open arrow*). The percutaneous transhepatic cholangiogram needle (*long arrow*) is evident. *D*, duodenum.

choledochal diverticulum, intraduodenal choledochocele, and multiple intrahepatic and extrahepatic

cysts. Caroli's disease is sometimes classified as a type of choledochal cyst.

Pancreatic and Ampullary Carcinomas are the cause of 20–25% of cases of biliary obstruction in the adult. Metastatic disease from lung, breast, gastrointestinal tumors, and lymphoma account for 2% of cases.

Cholangiocarcinoma is the second most common primary hepatic tumor. The histology is usually adenocarcinoma. Most cases involve the bifurcation or the common duct (Fig. 23.20). Predisposing conditions include choledochal cyst, ulcerative colitis, and primary sclerosing cholangitis. The tumor may be infiltrative, desmoplastic, and small, making imaging detection as well as needle biopsy difficult. Abrupt stricture with thickening of duct wall may be the only findings (12). Cross-sectional imaging is used to detect adenopathy and hepatic metastases. Prognosis is poor, with less than 20% of tumors resectable.

GALLBLADDER
Imaging Methods

Ultrasound is the imaging method of choice for the gallbladder. It offers high anatomic detail, convenience, and cost efficiency. Cholescintigraphy utilizing technetium-99m-iminodiacetic acid has sensitivity and specificity comparable to ultrasound for the diagnosis of acute cholecystitis (12). Oral cholecystograms remain useful in the diagnosis of cholelithiasis. Contrast agents taken orally are concentrated within the gallbladder and demonstrate gallstones as filling defects in the contrast pool. Plain films demonstrate calcified gallstones, porcelain gallbladder, and emphysematous cholecystitis. Gallstones and cholecystitis may be demonstrated by CT but the sensitivity is low. Computed tomography is useful in the diagnosis and staging of gallbladder carcinoma. Magnetic resonance has no significant role, at present, in gallbladder imaging.

Anatomy

The gallbladder lies on the underside of the liver in the fossa formed by the junction of the left and right lobes. While the position of the fundus is variable, the neck of the gallbladder is invariably positioned in the porta hepatis and major interlobar fissure (17). The gallbladder fundus frequently causes a mass impression on the top of the duodenal bulb. Kinking and folding of the gallbladder is common and generally easily recognized by careful image analysis (14, 17). The so-called phrygian cap, which is descriptive of folding of the gallbladder fundus, is a common normal variant. Septa within the gallbladder may be partial or complete. The spiral valves of Heister are small folds in the cystic duct.

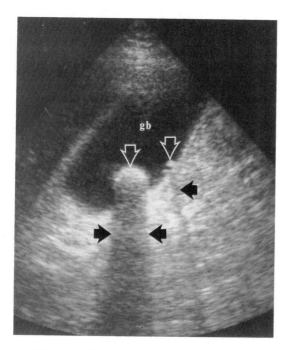

Figure 23.21. Gallstones. Ultrasound demonstrates focal echodensities of varying size (*open arrows*) within the gallbladder lumen (*gb*). Acoustic shadows (*closed arrows*) extend from the echodensities. Moving the patient into the upright position resulted in a change in position of the gallstones.

The normal gallbladder is well-distended with bile and is easily visualized following an 8–12 hour fast. A gallbladder greater than 5 cm in diameter is considered enlarged (hydropic), while a gallbladder less than 2 cm in diameter is considered contracted. The normal gallbladder wall does not exceed 3 mm in thickness, measured from gallbladder lumen to liver parenchyma, when the gallbladder is distended. The normal gallbladder lumen is free of particulate debris and is anechoic on ultrasound.

Gallstones

Gallstones are present in 8% of the general population and 15% of the population aged 40–60. Approximately 85% of gallstones are predominantly cholesterol, while 15% are predominantly bilirubin and are related to hemolytic anemia. Ten percent of stones are radiopaque, and are detectable by plain film as laminated or faceted calcifications. Fissures within gallstones may contain nitrogen gas, and are detectable on plain film as branching linear lucencies resembling a "crow's foot." An increased incidence of gallstones is found in women (female:male = 4:1), and patients with hemolytic anemia, diseases of the ileum, cirrhosis, and diabetes mellitus.

Ultrasound demonstrates gallstones as rounded echodensities in the gallbladder lumen that cast acoustic shadows and move with changes in patient position (i.e., "rolling stones") (Fig. 23.21). Ultra-

sound detects 95% of all gallstones. Small stones in the gallbladder neck are the most easily missed. Folds in the gallbladder can shadow and mimic gallstones. Air in adjacent bowel may also shadow and be mistaken for gallstones. When the gallbladder is contracted and completely filled with gallstones a "double arc shadow" may be seen. The first arc represents the gallbladder wall separated from the second arc of the gallstone surface by a thin rim of echolucent bile. The gallstone casts an acoustic shadow.

Computed tomography has a lower sensitivity for gallstone detection (80–85%) than does ultrasound. Gallstones vary in CT attenuation from fat density to calcium density. Some gallstones are not visible because they are isodense with bile; some gallstones are missed on CT because of their small size. Care must be taken to avoid interpreting contrast in adjacent bowel as cholelithiasis.

Oral cholecystogram demonstrates gallstones as filling defects within the contrast-filled gallbladder (Fig. 23.22). Mobile gallstones will move with changes in patient position. Oral cholecystogram has a 10% false-negative rate for gallstones because they are obscured by stool, contrast, or air in overlying bowel. Oral cholecystogram can reliably be performed only in patients on normal fat-containing diets who have bilirubin levels below 2 mg/100 ml. Obstruction of the cystic duct, associated with chronic cholecystitis and stones, causes nonvisualization of the gallbladder on oral cystogram. Additional causes of nonvisualization include poor intestinal absorption of contrast, prolonged fasting, and liver disease. Ultrasound may clarify the cause of gallbladder nonvisualization by confirming gallbladder disease.

Differential considerations for lesions in the gallbladder that may be mistaken for gallstones include the following (14).

Sludge Balls or tumefactive biliary sludge result from biliary stasis. The bile thickens and forms echogenic mobile masses that move with changes in patient position, but do not cast acoustic shadows (Fig. 23.17).

Cholesterol Polyps are common benign, polypoid masses that result from accumulation of triglycerides and cholesterol in macrophages in the gallbladder wall. They are of no clinical significance. All are 10 mm or less in size. They do not cast acoustic shadows (Fig. 23.23).

Adenomyomatosis may be focal and present as a polypoid mass fixed to the gallbladder wall.

Adenomatous Polyps are small, usually flat masses fixed to the gallbladder wall. They do not cast acoustic shadows.

Gallbladder Carcinoma may present as a polypoid mass. Most are 1 cm or more in size. Gallstones are usually present.

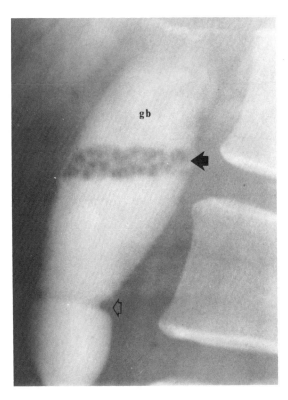

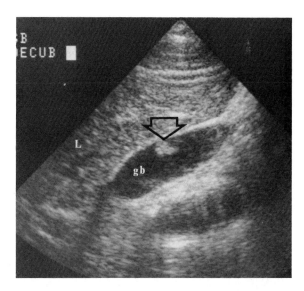

Figure 23.23. Cholesterol Polyp. Ultrasound demonstrates an echogenic nodule (*arrow*) extending from the nondependent wall of the gallbladder into the lumen (*gb*). The lesion does not cause acoustic shadowing. *L*, liver.

Figure 23.22. Gallstones. An upright film from an oral cholecystogram demonstrates multiple small gallstones (*closed arrow*) that float in contrast within the gallbladder lumen (*gb*). The high specific gravity of contrast causes some gallstones to float. A fold of mucosa (*open arrow*) produces partial septation of the gallbladder fundus. This is a normal variant.

Acute Cholecystitis

Acute inflammation of the gallbladder is caused 90% of the time by gallstones obstructing the cystic duct. About 5–10% occur in the absence of stones (acalculous cholecystitis). Cholescintigraphy and sonography have comparable sensitivities and specificities in the diagnosis of acute cholecystitis (12).

Scintigraphic diagnosis of acute cholecystitis is based upon obstruction of the cystic duct with nonvisualization of the gallbladder. The normal gallbladder demonstrates progressive accumulation of radionuclide activity over 30 minutes to 1 hour following injection of technetium-99m-iminodiacetic acid. Delayed visualization of the gallbladder may be seen in patients with biliary stasis due to fasting or hyperalimentation. Delayed images taken at 4 hours postradionuclide injection are needed to assess for this possibility. The test is considered positive if there is prompt tracer accumulation in the liver with excretion of tracer into the bowel and without gallbladder visualization at 4 hours. The test may be considered positive at 1 hour postradionuclide injection if the gallbladder does not visualize within 20 minutes of intravenous injection of morphine.

Confident ultrasound diagnosis of acute cholecystitis requires the presence of three findings: cholelithiasis, edema of the gallbladder wall seen as a band of echolucency in the wall, and a positive sonographic Murphy sign (Fig. 23.24). A sonographic Murphy sign is positive when transducer pressure over the gallbladder causes pain.

Although CT is not the imaging method of first choice for acute cholecystitis, findings that suggest the diagnosis include gallstones, distended gallbladder, thickened gallbladder wall, and pericholecystic fluid.

Acalculous Cholecystitis causes special problems in diagnosis because the cystic duct is not always obstructed. Inflammation may be due to ischemia or direct bacterial infection. Patients at risk for acalculous cholecystitis include those with biliary stasis due to lack of oral intake, posttrauma, postburn, postsurgery, or on total parenteral nutrition. Scintigraphy usually demonstrates lack of gallbladder visualization. Although this finding is 90–95% sensitive for acalculous cholecystitis, it is only 38% specific. False-positive conditions for nonvisualization include hyperalimentation and prolonged severe illness, which are predisposing conditions for acalculous cholecystitis. Ultrasound demonstrates a distended tender gallbladder with thickened wall but without stones (Fig. 23.25). Many patients are too ill to elicit a reliable sonographic Murphy sign.

Echogenic Bile. Sludge is a term used to describe the presence of echogenic particulate matter in the bile (Figs. 23.24 and 23.25). The particulate material is calcium bilirubinate and cholesterol crystals, which precipitate when biliary stasis is prolonged because of a lack of oral intake, hyperalimentation, or

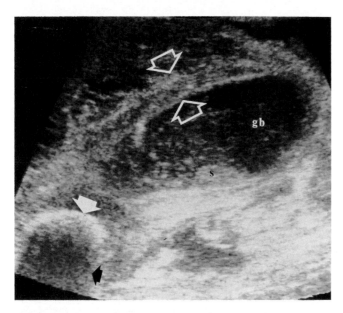

Figure 23.24.   Acute Cholecystitis. Ultrasound image through the long axis of the gallbladder (*gb*) demonstrates a large gallstone (*closed white arrow*) impacted in the neck of the gallbladder and casting an acoustic shadow (*black arrow*). The gallbladder wall is thickened (*open arrows*) and edematous. Echogenic sludge (*s*) is seen within the gallbladder lumen, giving evidence of bile stasis. A sonographic Murphy sign was present.

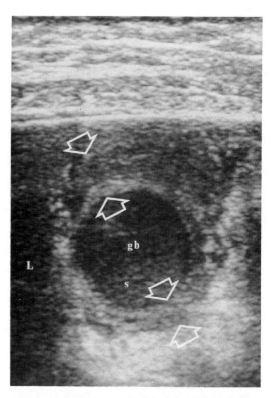

Figure 23.25.   Acalculous Cholecystitis. Transverse ultrasound image of the gallbladder (*gb*) demonstrates marked thickening and edema of the wall (*arrows*) and echogenic sludge (*s*) in the lumen. A sonographic Murphy sign was elicited. No gallstones were present. *L,* liver.

biliary obstruction. Since sludge may be found in a fasting, but otherwise normal patient, its presence is not definitive evidence of gallbladder disease. Pus, blood, and milk of calcium are additional causes of echogenic bile.

Complications of acute cholecystitis include the following.

Gangrenous Cholecystitis indicates the presence of necrosis of the gallbladder wall (Fig. 23.26). The patient is at risk for gallbladder perforation. Ultrasound findings include mucosal irregularity and asymmetric thickening of the gallbladder wall with multiple sonolucent layers, indicating mucosal ulceration and reactive edema.

Perforation of the Gallbladder is a life-threatening complication seen in 5–10% of cases. The perforation may occur adjacent to the liver resulting in pericholecystic abscess, into the peritoneal cavity resulting in generalized peritonitis, or into adjacent bowel resulting in biliary-enteric fistula. Overall mortality is as high as 24%. A focal pericholecystic fluid collection suggests pericholecystic abscess.

Emphysematous Cholecystitis results from infection of the gallbladder with gas-forming organisms, usually *E. coli* or *Clostridium perfringens*. About 40% of patients are diabetic. Gallstones may or may not be present. Gas is demonstrated within the wall or within the lumen of the gallbladder by plain film or CT. On ultrasound, intramural gas has an arc-like configuration difficult to differentiate from calcifica-

tion and porcelain gallbladder. Gas in the lumen characteristically appears as an echogenic focus with ring-down artifact.

Mirizzi's Syndrome refers to the condition of biliary obstruction resulting from a gallstone in the cystic duct eroding into the common duct and causing an inflammatory mass that obstructs the common duct. Visualization of a stone at the junction of the cystic duct and the common hepatic duct in a patient with biliary obstruction and gallbladder inflammation suggests the diagnosis.

Chronic Cholecystitis

Chronic cholecystitis includes a wide spectrum of pathology that shares the presence of gallstones and chronic gallbladder inflammation. Patients with chronic cholecystitis complain of recurrent attacks of right upper quadrant pain and biliary colic. Imaging findings include gallstones, thickening of the gallbladder wall, contraction of the gallbladder lumen, delayed visualization of the gallbladder on cholescintigraphy, and poor contractility. Variants of chronic cholecystitis include the following.

Porcelain Gallbladder describes the presence of dystrophic calcification in the wall of an obstructed and chronically inflamed gallbladder (Fig. 23.27). The

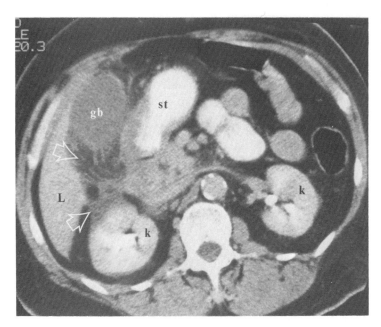

Figure 23.26. Gangrenous Cholecystitis. Computed tomography reveals a distended gallbladder (*gb*) with extensive pericholecystic inflammation manifest by globular and streaky soft tissue densities in the pericholecystic fat (*arrows*). *L*, liver; *k*, kidney; *s*, stomach.

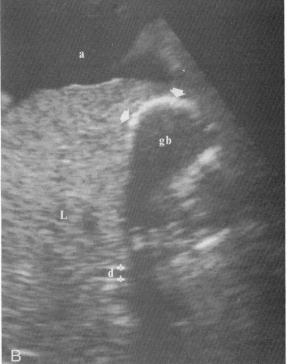

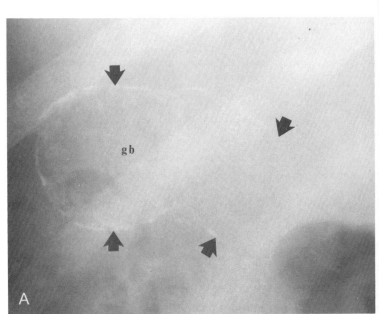

Figure 23.27. Porcelain Gallbladder. A, Plain radiograph of the right upper quadrant of the abdomen shows calcification (*arrows*) in the wall of the gallbladder (*gb*). **B**, An ultrasound image in the same patient demonstrates increased echogenicity of the gallbladder wall (*arrows*) producing shadowing of the gallbladder lumen (*gb*). Diligent analysis with multiple views is needed to differentiate calcification in the gallbladder wall from large stones filling the gallbladder lumen. This patient also has cirrhosis with a shrunken nodular liver (*L*) and ascites (*a*). *d*, common bile duct.

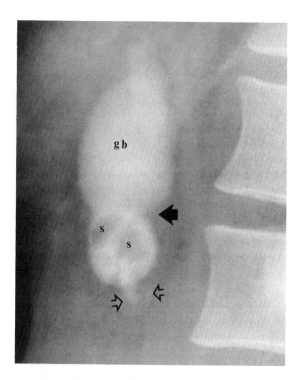

Figure 23.28.   Adenomyomatosis. An oral cholecystogram reveals compartmentalization of the gallbladder (*gb*) fundus by a thick septa (*closed arrow*). Contrast extends into the thickened wall at the fundus filling Rokitansky-Aschoff sinuses (*open arrows*). Stones (*s*) in the fundus are seen as lucent filling defects.

condition is associated with gallstones in 90% of cases. Porcelain gallbladder carries a 10–20% risk of gallbladder carcinoma. Cholecystectomy is usually indicated.

Milk of Calcium Bile, also called limy bile, is associated with an obstructed cystic duct, chronic cholecystitis, and gallstones. Particulate matter with a high concentration of calcium compounds is precipitated in the bile, making the bile radiopaque. Dependent layering of bile can be demonstrated on plain film radiographs. The bile is extremely echogenic on US and gallstones may be visualized within it.

Thickening of the Gallbladder Wall

Thickening of the gallbladder wall is present when the wall thickness measured on the hepatic aspect of the gallbladder exceeds 3 mm in patients who have fasted at least 8 hours. Conditions associated with wall thickening include the following (14).

Acute and Chronic Cholecystitis. Wall thickening is a usual feature of acute cholecystitis and is present in 50% of cases of chronic cholecystitis.

Hepatitis causes reduction in bile flow, which results in reduced gallbladder volume and thickening of the gallbladder wall in about half of the patients (12).

Portal Venous Hypertension and Congestive Heart Failure may cause wall thickening by passive venous congestion.

Acquired   Immunodeficiency   Syndrome causes thickening of the gallbladder wall for unknown reasons. Opportunistic organisms are sometimes present. Gallbladder wall thickening is also associated with AIDS cholangitis.

Hypoalbuminemia is associated with thickened gallbladder wall in 60% of patients.

Gallbladder Carcinoma usually presents as a focal mass but may cause only focal wall thickening.

Adenomyomatosis of the gallbladder is a benign condition of hyperplasia of the gallbladder mucosa with increased thickness of the muscular layer. It is usually focal in the fundus, but may be diffuse throughout the gallbladder. Outpouchings of mucosa into or through the muscularis form characteristic Rokitansky-Aschoff sinuses (Fig. 23.28).

Gallbladder Carcinoma

Carcinoma of the gallbladder is commonly misdiagnosed preoperatively. The presence of gallstones in 70–80% of cases commonly masks the findings of carcinoma, especially with ultrasound examination. Calcification of the gallbladder wall (porcelain gallbladder) is a risk factor. Imaging findings include (*a*) intraluminal soft tissue mass, (*b*) focal or diffuse thickening of the gallbladder wall, (*c*) soft tissue mass replacing the gallbladder, (*d*) gallstones, (*e*) extension of tumor into the liver, bile ducts, and adjacent bowel, and (*f*) metastases to regional lymph nodes (18).

References

1. Whalen E. Liver imaging–current trends in MRI, CT, and US: international symposium and course, June 1990. AJR 1990;155:1125–1132.
2. Ferruci JT. Liver tumor imaging: current concepts. AJR 1990;155:473–484.
3. Tessler FN, Gehring BJ, Gomes AS, et al. Diagnosis of portal vein thrombosis: value of color Doppler imaging. AJR 1991;157:293–296.
4. Thoeni RF. Clinical applications of magnetic resonance imaging of the liver. Invest Radiol 1991;3:266–273.
5. Mukai JK, Stack CM, Turner DA, et al. Imaging of surgically relevant hepatic vascular and segmental anatomy. Part 1. Normal anatomy. AJR 1987;149:287–292.
6. Mukai JK, Stack CM, Turner DA, et al. Imaging of surgically relevant hepatic vascular and segmental anatomy. Part 2. Extent and resectability of hepatic neoplasms. AJR 1987;149:293–297.
7. Rummeny E, Saini S, Wittenberg J, et al. MR imaging of liver neoplasms. AJR 1989;152:493–499.
8. Subramanyam BR, Balthazar EJ, Madamba MR, et al. Sonography of portosystemic venous collateral in portal hypertension. Radiology 1983;146:161–166.
9. Brant WE, Floyd JL, Jackson DE, Gilliland JD. The radiological evaluation of hepatic cavernous hemangioma. JAMA 1987;257:2471–2474.
10. Birnbaum BA, Weinreb JC, Megibow AJ, et al. Definitive diagnosis of hepatic hemangiomas: MR imaging versus Tc-99m-labeled red blood cell SPECT. Radiology 1990;176:95–101.

11. Murphy BJ, Casillas J, Ros PR, et al. The CT appearance of cystic masses of the liver. RadioGraphics 1989;9:307–322.

12. Burrell MI, Zeman RK, Simeone JF, et al. The biliary tract: imaging for the 1990s. AJR 1991;157:223–233.

13. Cronan JJ. The imaging of choledocholithiasis. Semin Ultrasound CT MR 1987;8:75–84.

14. Rosenthal SJ, Cox GG, Wetzel LH, Batnitzky S. Pitfalls and differential diagnosis in biliary sonography. RadioGraphics 1990;10:285–311.

15. Lim JH. Oriental cholangiohepatitis: pathologic, clinical, and radiologic features. AJR 1991;157:1–8.

16. Savader SJ, Benenati JF, Venbrux AC, et al. Choledochal cysts: classification and cholangiographic appearance. AJR 1991;156:327–331.

17. Meilstrup JW, Hopper KD, Thieme GA. Imaging of gallbladder varients. AJR 1991;157:1205–1208.

18. Lane J, Buck JL, Zeman RK. Primary carcinoma of the gallbladder: a pictorial essay. RadioGraphics 1989;9(2):209–228.

24

Pancreas and Spleen

William E. Brant

PANCREAS

Imaging Techniques

Ultrasound and computed tomography (CT) provide high-quality images of the pancreatic parenchyma and are used as primary imaging methods for detection of pancreatic masses and other abnormalities (1, 2). When CT or ultrasound is equivocal, endoscopic retrograde cholangiopancreatography (ERCP) usually provides excellent visualization of the lumen of the pancreatic duct, which is usually affected by any mass lesion of the pancreas (1–3). This procedure involves endoscopic cannulization of the bile and pancreatic ducts, followed by injection of a contrast agent and filming. The utilization of magnetic resonance (MR) for visualizing the pancreas is limited at present, because of respiratory motion artifacts and lack of a bowel contrast agent to allow differentiation of the bowel from the pancreas. Arteriography is used in selected cases to define tumor vascularity. Ultrasound and CT-directed biopsy and drainage procedures play a major role in the diagnosis and treatment of pancreatic diseases.

Anatomy

The pancreas is a tongue-shaped organ approximately 12–15 cm in length that lies within the anterior pararenal compartment of the retroperitoneal space (Fig. 24.1). The pancreas is posterior to the left lobe of the liver, the stomach, and the lesser sac. It is anterior to the spine, the inferior vena cava, and the aorta. Pancreatic tissue is best recognized by identification of the vessels around it. The neck, body, and tail of the pancreas lie ventral to the splenic vein, with the tail extending into the hilum of the spleen. The splenic vein and pancreas are anterior to the superior mesenteric artery. The head of the pancreas wraps around the junction of the superior mesenteric vein and the splenic vein, with the uncinate process of the pancreatic head extending under the superior mesenteric vein just anterior to the inferior vena cava. The splenic artery courses through the pancreatic bed in a tortuous course. Atherosclerotic splenic artery calicifications are easily mistaken for pancreatic calcifications. The lumen of the splenic artery may be mistaken for pancreatic cysts or a dilated pancreatic duct on US or CT without contrast.

Maximum dimensions for pancreatic size are 3.0 cm diameter for the head, 2.5 cm diameter for the body, and 2.0 cm diameter for the tail. The gland is somewhat larger in young patients and progressively decreases in size with age. Since the gland is not encapsulated, fatty infiltration between the lobules in older patients gives the pancreas a more delicate, less globular appearance on CT. The pancreatic duct is visualized with thin-slice (5 mm thick) CT and with ultrasound. It normally measures 3–4 mm in diameter in the head and tapers smoothly to the tail. The ERCP films show the normal duct to be a bit larger due to magnification effect and distension because of the contrast injection (Fig. 24.2). The duodenum cradles the pancreatic head in the C-loop. Many pancreatic abnormalities show secondary effects on the duodenum (Fig. 26.9), and occasionally on the stomach and colon.

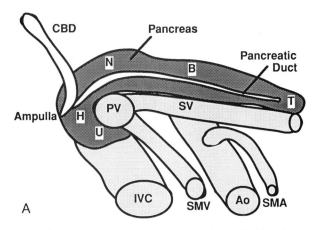

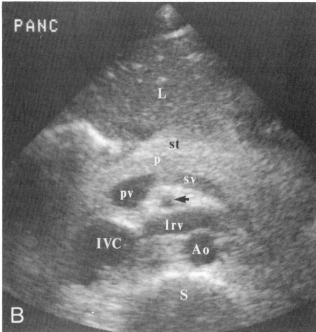

Figure 24.1. Normal Pancreas Anatomy. A diagram (**A**) and an ultrasound in transverse plane (**B**) demonstrate the normal anatomy of the pancreas. The majority of the pancreas lies anterior to the splenic vein (*sv*) and its junction with the superior mesenteric vein (*SMV*) forming the portal vein (*pv*). The head (*H*) and uncinate process (*U*) of the pancreas cradle the origin of the portal vein. The pancreatic neck (*N*) is anterior to the SV-SMV confluence, while the uncinate process and inferior vena cava (*IVC*) are posterior to the confluence. The superior mesenteric artery (*SMA, arrow*) arises from the aorta (*Ao*) dorsal to the splenic vein. The left renal vein (*lrv*) passes between the SMA and aorta to the inferior vena cava. The left lobe of the liver (*L*) offers a good sonographic window to the pancreas. The stomach (*st*) and lesser sac (collapsed) are anterior to the pancreas. *CBD*, common bile duct; *S*, spine; *B* body of the pancreas; *T*, tail of the pancreas; *p*, pancreas.

Acute Pancreatitis

The diagnosis of acute pancreatitis is generally made clinically. The role of imaging is to clarify the diagnosis when the clinical picture is unclear, to assess the severity of the condition, to determine prognosis, and to detect complications (1). Inflammation

of the pancreatic tissue leads to disruption of small pancreatic ducts, resulting in leakage of pancreatic secretions. Because the pancreas lacks a capsule, the pancreatic juices have ready access to surrounding tissues. Pancreatic enzymes digest fascial layers, spreading the inflammatory process to multiple anatomic compartments. Causes of acute pancreatitis include ethanol abuse, obstructing biliary stones, trauma, peptic ulcer, a variety of drugs, and hereditary predisposition.

Imaging studies of acute pancreatitis may be normal in mild cases. Computed tomography provides the most comprehensive initial assessment, while ultrasound is useful for follow-up of specific abnormalities, such as fluid collections. Abnormalities that may be seen in the pancreas include (*a*) focal or diffuse enlargement; (*b*) changes in density due to edema (Fig. 24.3); and (*c*) indistinctness of the margins of the gland due to inflammation. Abnormalities in the peripancreatic tissues include stranding densities in the fat with indistinctness of the fat planes and thickening of affected fascial planes. Complications demonstrated by imaging include (*a*) fluid collections in pancreatic and peripancreatic spaces and often widespread throughout the abdomen (Fig. 24.4); (*b*) liquefactive necrosis of portions of the pancreas, best demonstrated as lack of parenchymal enhancement during bolus contrast adminstration on CT (Fig. 24.5) (4); (*c*) phlegmon, pancreatic mass formation due to edema and inflammation; (*d*) abscess formation due to bacterial growth in necrotic tissues (Fig. 24.6); (*e*) hemorrhage due to erosion of blood vessels or bowel; (*f*) pancreatic ascites due to leakage of pancreatic secretions into the peritoneal cavity; and (*g*) pseudocyst formation resulting from encasement of a pancreatic fluid collection by a fibrous capsule. Barium studies may demonstrate mass effect or inflammatory changes affecting adjacent bowel. Ultrasound or CT-directed aspiration biopsy may be needed to confirm the presence of pancreatic abscess. Image-directed catheter placement is an alternative to surgical drainage of pancreatic fluid collections.

Chronic Pancreatitis

Chronic pancreatitis is caused by recurrent and prolonged bouts of acute pancreatitis that cause parenchymal atrophy and progressive fibrosis. Both the exocrine and endocrine function of the pancreas may be affected. The clinical diagnosis is often vague, so imaging is used both to confirm the diagnosis and to detect complications (3, 5). The morphologic changes of chronic pancreatitis include (*a*) dilation of the pancreatic duct, usually in a beaded pattern of alternating areas of dilation and constriction (Figs. 24.7 and 24.8); (*b*) decrease in visible pancreatic tissue due to atrophy (Fig. 24.9); (*c*) calcifications in the

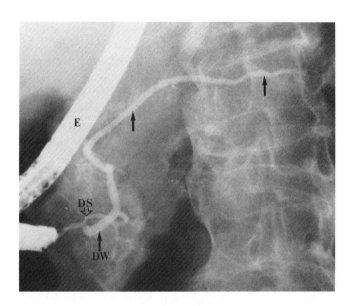

Figure 24.2.   Normal Pancreatic Ducts. Radiograph from an ERCP demonstrates the main duct of Wirsung (*DW, black arrows*) and the accessory duct of Santorini (*DS, open arrow*). In this patient the main duct drained separately into the major papilla (of Vater) with a different orifice for the common bile duct. The accessory duct drained into the minor papilla. Both ampullae were cannulated endoscopically and injected prior to this radiograph. A number of different variants of pancreatic duct anatomy exist. This variant is found in about 35% of individuals. Embryologically, the main duct is formed by the entire duct of the ventral pancreatic bud and the distal portion of the duct of the dorsal pancreatic bud. The main duct may join the common bile duct or have a separate orifice in the major papilla. The proximal portion of the duct of the dorsal pancreatic bud may be obliterated or persist as the accessory duct. *E,* endoscope.

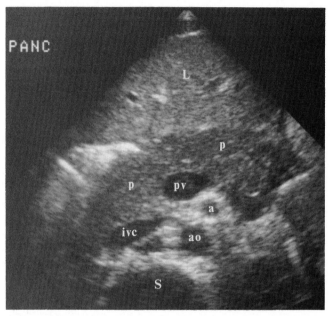

Figure 24.3.   Acute Pancreatitis. Ultrasound image in axial plane reveals a diffuse decrease in the echogenicity of the pancreatic parenchyma (*p*) compared to the liver (*L*) because of diffuse edema of acute inflammation. The normal pancreas is more echogenic than the normal liver (Fig. 24.1*B*). No discrete fluid collections were evident. *pv,* portal vein; *a,* superior mesenteric artery; *ivc,* inferior vena cava; *ao,* aorta; *S,* spine.

pancreatic parenchyma that vary from finely stippled to coarse, usually associated with alcoholic pancreatitis (Fig. 24.10); (d) fluid collections that are both intra- and extrapancreatic; (e) focal enlargement of the pancreas due to benign inflammation and fibrosis; (f) dilation of the biliary duct because of fibrosis or mass in the pancreatic head; and (g) fascial thickening and chronic inflammatory changes in surrounding tissues. Differentiation of an inflammatory mass due to chronic pancreatitis from pancreatic carcinoma frequently requires image-directed biopsy.

Pancreatic Carcinoma

Ductal adenocarcinoma of the pancreas is a highly lethal tumor that is usually unresectable at presentation. The average survival time of a patient with this disease is only 5–8 months (3, 6–9). It accounts for 3% of all cancers and is second only to colorectal cancer as the most common digestive tract malignancy

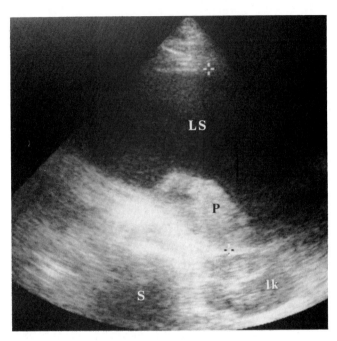

Figure 24.4. Pancreatic Fluid Collection in Lesser Sac. Ultrasound scan in axial plane shows a large collection of fluid anterior to the pancreas (P) in the lesser sac (LS). Ultrasound is excellent for following the evolution of pancreatic fluid collections. S, spine; lk, left kidney.

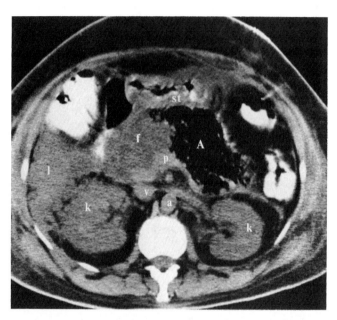

Figure 24.6. Pancreatic Abscess. Air (A) and fluid (f) extend from the bed of the pancreas (p) on this CT scan performed without intravenous contrast. Air in the pancreatic bed is indicative of abscess and/or fistulous communication with bowel. st, stomach; l, liver; v, inferior vena cava; a, aorta; k, kidney.

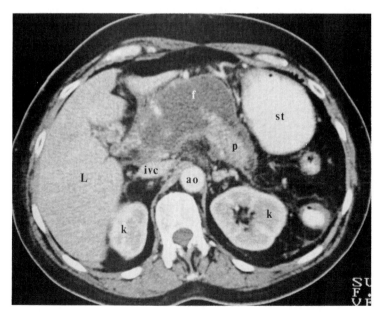

Figure 24.5. Acute Necrotizing Pancreatitis. A CT scan performed with rapid bolus adminstration of intravenous contrast demonstrates enhancement of only the distal body of the pancreas (p). The pancreatic head and neck did not enhance and are lost in the fluid (f) extending from the pancreatic bed. This CT finding is indicative of pancreatic necrosis. st, stomach; L, liver; ivc, inferior vena cava; ao, aorta; k, kidney.

Figure 24.7. Chronic Pancreatitis. Radiograph from an ERCP following contrast injection into the pancreatic duct (D) demonstrates irregular dilation of the duct with multiple filling defects (arrows) due to stones and debris. Contrast is also present in the lumen of the third portion of the duodenum (3). E, endoscope.

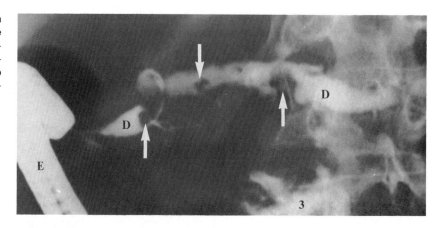

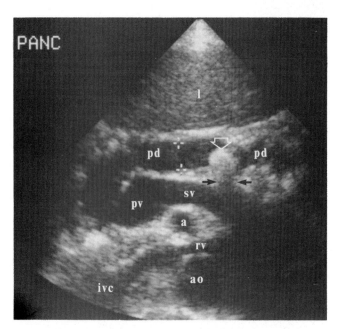

Figure 24.8. Dilated Pancreatic Duct with Calculus. Ultrasound in axial plane demonstrates a calculus (open arrow) in the markedly dilated pancreatic duct (pd). The calculus is seen as an echogenic focus with acoustic shadowing (black arrows). The pancreatic parenchyma is atrophic, consistent with chronic pancreatitis. The pancreatic duct measures 8.7 mm in diameter (calipers). A detailed knowledge of anatomy is needed to correctly identify all structures visualized. Doppler ultrasound is helpful in confirming vascular structures. ao, aorta; a, superior mesenteric artery; ivc, inferior vena cava; rv, left renal vein; sv, splenic vein; pv, portal vein; l, liver.

(6). Radiographic assessment of resectability is critical because surgical resection offers the only hope of cure, yet the surgery itself carries a high morbidity. Scanning by CT should include rapid bolus contrast injection and thin slices (5mm) (9). Pancreatic cancer appears as a hypodense mass distorting the contour of the gland. Associated findings include obstruction of the common bile duct (Fig. 24.11) and pancreatic duct, and atrophy of pancreatic tissue beyond the tumor. Metastases commonly go to regional nodes, liver, and the peritoneal cavity. Signs of potential resect-

ability include isolated pancreatic mass with or without dilation of the bile or pancreatic ducts or combined dilation of both the bile and pancreatic ducts without an identifiable pancreatic head mass. Signs of unresectabilty include (a) extension of the tumor beyond the margins of the pancreas (Fig. 24.12), (b) tumor involvement of adjacent organs, (c) enlarged regional lymph nodes (>15 mm), (d) encasement or obstruction of peripancreatic arteries or veins, (e) metastases in the liver, and (f) peritoneal carcinomatosis. Less than 10% of patients are potentially resectable using these criteria. Image-guided biopsy can confirm the diagnosis in patients who are deemed to be unresectable (Fig. 24.13).

Islet Cell Tumors

Functioning islet cell tumors, such as insulinomas or gastrinomas, produce distinct clinical syndromes and usually present while the tumors are small. Nonfunctioning islet cell tumors present with symptoms of a growing mass and are thus usually large when discovered. Functioning tumors vary in malignant potential from 10% for insulinoma to 60% for gastrinoma and to 80% for glucagonoma. Up to 80% of nonfunctioning tumors are malignant.

Functioning islet cell tumors vary in size from 0.4–4.0 cm and require strict attention to technique for accurate preoperative identification. Most small islet cell tumors cannot be identified on precontrast CT. Since the lesions tend to be hypervascular, bolus contrast administration during rapid thin-slice CT scanning through the pancreatic bed offers the best chance of lesion visualization. The tumor stands out as an enhancing nodule within the pancreas. Sonography has proven extremely valuable for tumor localization during surgery (3). Islet cell tumors appear as hypoechoic masses within the pancreas (10).

Nonfunctioning islet cell tumors tend to be much larger, 6–20 cm diameter. Many show contrast enhancement on CT. Coarse calcifications are common in these tumors.

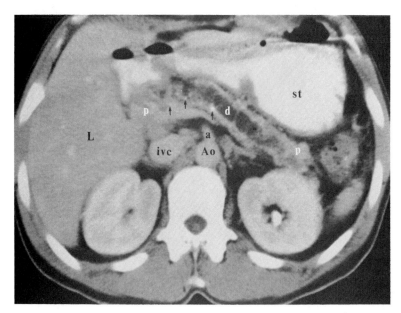

Figure 24.9. Chronic Pancreatitis. A CT scan with bolus intravenous contrast enhancement demonstrates marked dilation of the pancreatic duct (*d*) and atrophy of the pancreatic parenchyma (*p*). Punctate calcifications are also present (*arrows*). The aorta (*ao*) is seen at the origin of the superior mesenteric artery (*a*). *L*, liver; *st*, stomach; *ivc*, inferior vena cava.

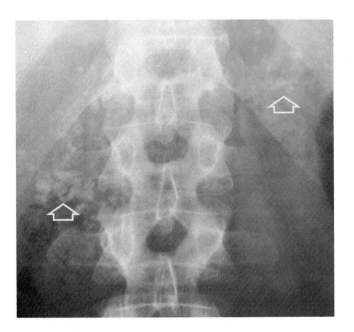

Figure 24.10. Pancreatic Calcifications. Plain radiograph of the upper abdomen demonstrates multiple calcifications (*arrows*) throughout the region of the pancreatic bed. Pancreatic calcifications of this type suggest chronic pancreatitis due to alcohol abuse or hereditary pancreatitis.

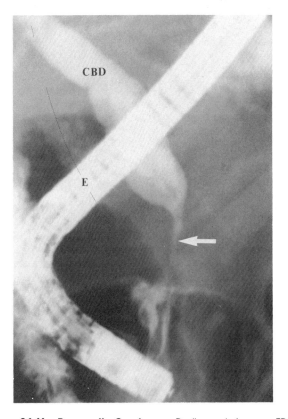

Figure 24.11. Pancreatic Carcinoma. Radiograph from an ERCP demonstrates a characteristic "rat-tail" appearance (*arrow*) of the dilated common bile duct (*CBD*) at the head of the pancreas due to pancreatic carcinoma. *E*, endoscope.

Figure 24.12. Unresectable Pancreatic Carcinoma. A CT with bolus intravenous contrast demonstrates an inhomogeneous necrotic tumor (T) in the head of the pancreas. The margins of the tumor are ill-defined (curved arrow), indicating invasion of peripancreatic tissues. The tumor extends (long arrow) to the superior mesenteric vein (v), but spares the superior mesenteric artery (a). Bile ducts (open arrow) in the liver (L) were dilated because of distal obstruction. ivc, inferior vena cava; rv, left renal vein; ao, aorta.

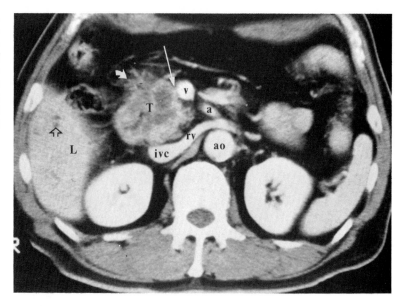

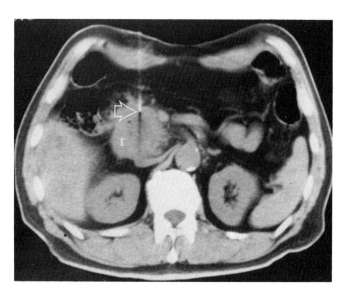

Figure 24.13. Percutaneous Pancreatic Biopsy. A CT is used to guide percutaneous biopsy of a pancreatic head tumor (T). A vertical needle course is selected to bring the needle tip (arrow) into the lesion. The black streak emanating from the needle indicates that the needle tip, not the needle shaft, is visualized. The biopsy confirmed pancreatic carcinoma.

Cystic Lesions

Pseudocysts resulting from pancreatitis are the most common pancreatic cystic lesions (11). They are of fluid density and generally have a definable fibrous wall that may be calcified. Internal septations are occasionally present.

Abscess must be considered in any patient with a cystic pancreatic lesion and a fever. Most abscesses have indistinct walls and contain fluid and debris. The presence of gas bubbles within the cystic mass is

good evidence for abscess (11). Image-directed aspiration confirms the diagnosis and may be followed by percutaneous catheter placement for treatment.

True Pancreatic Cysts are found in 10% of patients with adult polycystic disease, 30% of patients with von Hippel-Lindau syndrome, and some patients with cystic fibrosis (11). They appear as well-defined fluid-filled masses with walls of variable thickness.

Cystic Tumors of the pancreas are of two types: microcystic adenoma, which is always benign, and mucinous cystic tumor, which is usually malignant (3). Both tumor types are usually large (12–13 cm) at presentation (8, 11, 12). Microcystic adenomas are composed of innumerable small cysts 1 mm to 2 cm in size. The cysts may be so small that the tumor appears as a solid lesion on imaging studies. A characteristic feature is a central stellate fibrous scar that may be calcified. Approximately 80% of patients with this disease are age 60 or older. This tumor also occurs in patients with von Hippel-Lindau disease. Mucinous cystic tumors are all potentially malignant and require complete excision. They are composed of large cysts (>5 cm), which may be unilocular or multilocular (Figs. 24.14 and 24.15). The wall of the lesion is 1–2 mm thick and is commonly calcified. Metastases to the liver tend to be cystic.

Pancreatic Trauma

The spectrum of traumatic pancreatic injuries includes pancreatitis, laceration, and transection. Pancreatic injuries are best documented by CT. Pancreatic lacerations appear as irregular lucent clefts in the pancreatic parenchyma, most commonly at the junction of the body and tail just to the left of midline (Fig. 24.16). Complete transection is rare.

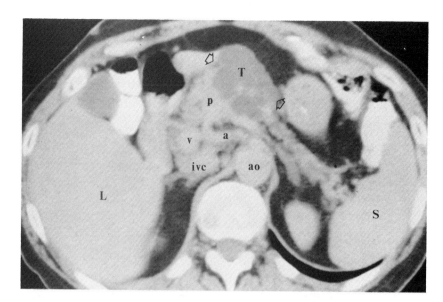

Figure 24.14. Mucinous Cystadenocarcinoma of the Pancreas. A CT demonstrates a multiloculated cystic tumor (*T*, between *arrows*) arising from the pancreas (*p*). No metastases in the liver (*L*) were evident. *v*, superior mesenteric vein; *a*, superior mesenteric artery; *ivc*, inferior vena cava; *ao*, aorta; *S*, spleen.

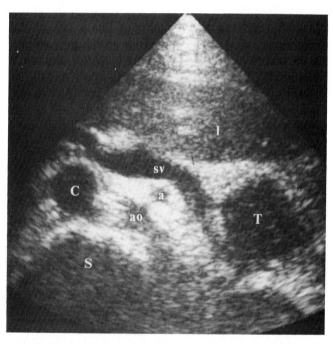

Figure 24.15. Mucinous Cystadenocarcinoma of the Pancreas. Axial plane ultrasound demonstrates a unilocular cystic tumor (*T*) arising from the tail of the pancreas. A cyst (*C*) was present on the right kidney. The inferior vena cava was not distended when this image was taken. *S*, spine; *ao*, aorta; *a*, superior mesenteric artery; *sv*, splenic vein; *l*, liver.

SPLEEN

Imaging Techniques

Ultrasound and CT remain the major techniques used to image the splenic parenchyma. Technetium sulfur colloid radionuclide images both the liver and the spleen. Magnetic resonance is disappointing in its ability to detect splenic abnormalities because the splenic parenchyma parallels pathologic lesions such as lymphoma and metastases in reaction to changes in pulse sequences, showing insufficient contrast differentiation to identify the lesions.

Anatomy

The spleen is intraperitoneal, occuping the left upper quadrant of the abdomen just below the diaphragm, and posterior and lateral to the stomach. Its diaphragmatic surface is smooth and convex, conforming to the shape of the diaphragm, while its visceral surface has concavities for the stomach, kidney, colon, and pancreas (13). The average spleen size in adults is 12 cm in length, 7 cm in breadth, and 3–4 cm in thickness. The spleen normally decreases in size with age. The splenic artery and vein maintain a close relationship to the pancreas as they course to the splenic hilum and divide into multiple branches entering the spleen.

Ultrasound demonstrates a very homogeneous midlevel echo pattern for the splenic parenchyma. The CT density of the normal spleen is always less than or equal to the CT density of the normal liver. The spleen enhances irregularly, following bolus administration of contrast agent. Transient pseudomasses are formed because of variable rates of blood flow through the splenic parenchyma. Images taken a few minutes later show homogeneous, enhanced parenchyma. Lobulations and clefts in the splenic contour are common and must not be mistaken for masses or splenic fractures (13).

Accessory spleens are found in about 10% of normal individuals (13). These appear as round or oval masses 1–3 cm in size and of the same texture as normal splenic parenchyma. They may be single or multiple and are usually located in the splenic hilum. Technetium sulphur colloid radionuclide scans can be

Figure 24.16.   Transected Pancreas. Contrast-enhanced CT scan in a 2-year-old boy struck by an automobile demonstrates a lucent fissure (*arrow*) in the pancreas (*p*) indicating disruption of the parenchyma. The portal vein (*pv*) and splenic vein (*sv*) enhance normally. Surgery confirmed complete transection of the pancreas with an intact splenic vein and artery. *L*, liver; *S*, spleen; *St*, stomach; *i*, inferior vena cava; *ao*, aorta; *k*, kidney.

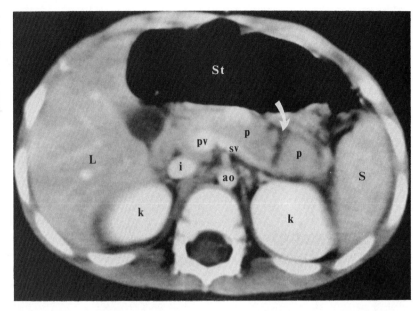

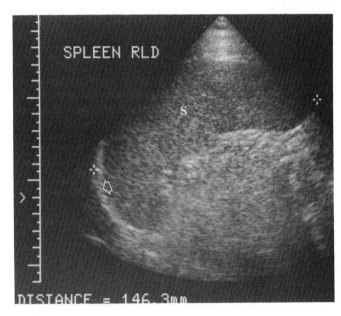

Figure 24.17.   Splenomegaly. Ultrasound image in coronal plane from the left side demonstrates enlargement of the spleen (*S*, between calipers). The spleen parenchyma is of homogeneous normal echogenicity. The diaphragmatic surface of the spleen conforms to the shape of the diaphragm (*arrow*).

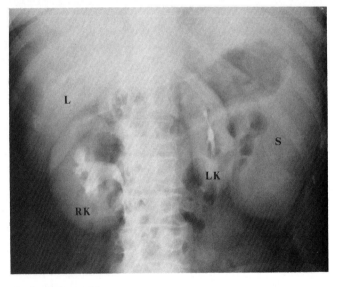

Figure 24.18.   Splenomegaly. Radiograph from an excretory urogram demonstrates a massively enlarged spleen (*S*) in a patient with rheumatoid arthritis and Felty's syndrome. The left kidney (*LK*) is compressed and rotated by the large spleen. The inferior margin of the spleen extends well below the inferior margin of the liver (*L*). *RK*, right kidney.

used to confirm suspected accessory spleens as functioning splenic tissue.

Splenomegaly

The diagnosis of splenic enlargement on imaging studies is usually made subjectively (Fig. 24.17) (13,14). Although quantitative methods have been attempted, none have proven popular. A few guidelines may be helpful. The measurements for normal spleen size listed above encompass 95% of the population. Larger measurements are indicative of splenomegaly (Fig. 24.17). On CT or MR the anterior margin of the normal spleen seldom projects ventral to the anterior axillary line (13), and the inferior spleen tip seldom extends more caudally than the inferior liver tip (Fig. 24.18). On ultrasound the spleen rarely extends to the lower pole of the left kidney.

The causes of splenomegaly are many. Most do not produce a change in spleen density so differentiation is based upon imaging findings elsewhere or clinical evaluation. Mild to moderate splenomegaly is seen with portal hypertension, acquired immunodeficiency syndrome (AIDS), storage diseases, collagen vascular disorders, and infection. More marked splenomegaly is usually associated with lymphoma, leukemia, infectious mononucleosis, hemolytic anemia, and myelofibrosis (14).

Cystic Lesions

Post-traumatic Cysts lack an epithelial wall. They generally have thick walls and septations that may be calcified. The internal fluid may be complex because of blood products, cholesterol crystals, and cellular debris.

Epidermoid Cysts are true epithelial-lined cysts that are probably developmental in origin. They have the same appearance as posttraumatic cysts, but less frequently have calcification in their walls.

Echinococcus Cysts generally have prominent calcifications in the wall and prominent internal septations and debris.

Pancreatic Psuedocysts extend beneath the splenic capsule by tracking along the pancreatic tail to the splenic hilum.

Abscesses generally occur in spleens that are already diseased. They present with vague symptoms and have a high mortality when left untreated. They appear as single or multiple low-density masses with ill-defined thick walls. They may contain gas or demonstrate air-fluid levels (Fig. 24.19). Image-guided aspiration confirms the diagnosis. Treatment is by catheter drainage or splenectomy.

Solid Lesions

Lymphoma is the most common malignant tumor involving the spleen (14). Lymphoma may cause diffuse splenomegaly, multiple masses of varying size (Fig. 24.20), or a large solitary mass (14,15). Hodgkin's lymphoma may involve the spleen without being detected by any imaging method. Adenopathy is frequently evident elsewhere in the abdomen when the spleen is involved with lymphoma.

Metastases are found in the spleen on autopsy series in 2–4% of patients who die of cancer. The most common primary tumors to affect the spleen are malignant melanoma, and lung, breast, gastrointestinal, and ovarian carcinoma. Metastases appear as single or multiple low-density masses.

Infarction classically appears as a wedge-shaped defect in the splenic parenchyma (Fig. 24.21). However, multiple infarcts may fuse and the wedge shape may be lost. The key finding is extension of a low-density area to an intact splenic capsule. Causes include emboli, and inflammatory or neoplastic involvement of local splenic vessels. Splenomegaly, especially due to lymphoma, is a predisposing condition.

Hemangiomas are the most common primary neoplasm of the spleen. Most are similar in appearance to liver hemangiomas on ultrasound and are seen as well-defined hyperechoic masses. The typical pattern of CT enhancement described for liver hemangiomas is not often seen with splenic hemangiomas. Multiloculated and cystic appearances of spleen hemangiomas have also been reported.

AIDS

Splenomegaly associated with generalized lymphoid hyperplasia is the most common finding in patients with AIDS. Focal lesions in the spleen are usually caused by opportunistic infections such as pneumocystis, atypical mycobacterium, or *Candida* (Fig. 24.22). *Pneumocystis carinii* infection may cause multiple splenic calcifications (Table 24.1). An AIDS-associated lymphoma and Kaposi sarcoma may also cause single or multiple solid-appearing lesions in the spleen.

Splenic Trauma

Contrast-enhanced CT is the modality of choice to demonstrate splenic injury. The spleen is the most commonly injured intraabdominal organ following blunt trauma. A splenic laceration is seen as an irregular cleft through the splenic parenchyma with associated perisplenic or intraabdominal blood (Fig. 24.23). Subcapsular hematomas are seen as peripheral low-density lenticular-shaped masses that displace the splenic parenchyma inward and may bow

Figure 24.19.   Splenic Abscess. Coronal plane ultrasound image demonstrates extensive destruction of the splenic parenchyma by a large abscess (*A*) containing air bubbles seen as mobile echogenic foci distributed through the fluid of the abscess (*small arrows*). Only a small remnant of normal splenic parenchyma (*S*) remains. The *open arrow* indicates the left hemidiaphragm.

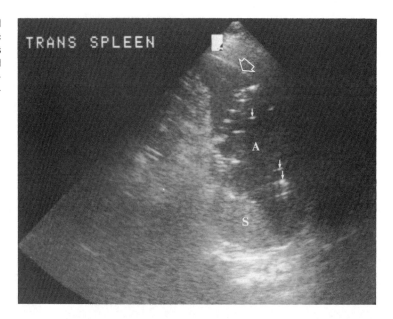

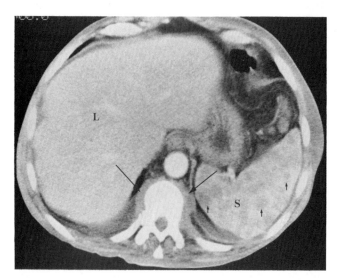

Figure 24.20.   Lymphoma. Contrast-enhanced CT demonstrates inhomogeneous splenic parenchyma (*S*) with multiple focal masses (*small arrows*) of varying size. Confluent retrocrural adenopathy (*long arrows*) is also present. The liver (*L*) appears normal.

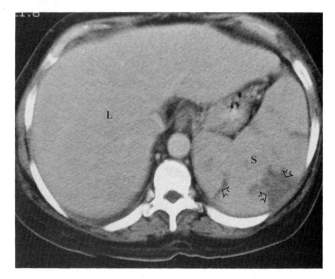

Figure 24.21.   Splenic Infarction. A CT scan demonstrates wedge-shaped and linear areas of infarction (*arrows*) in the spleen (*S*) in this patient with splenomegaly of an unknown cause. Note that the infarctions extend to the splenic capsule. The liver (*L*) has a normal appearance.

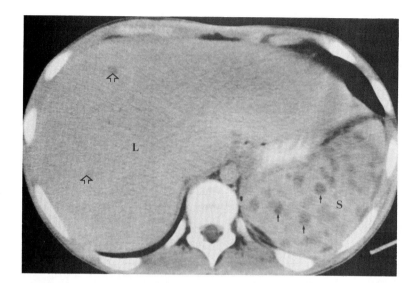

Figure 24.22. Candida Abscesses. Multiple Candida abscesses in the spleen (*S, small arrows*) and liver (*L open arrows*) are demonstrated by CT in this immunocompromised patient with *Candida* sepsis.

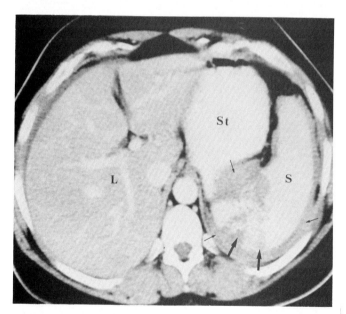

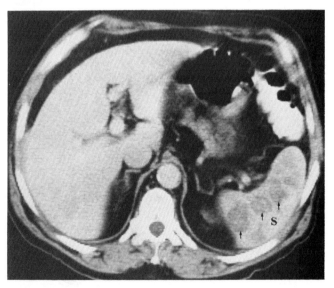

Figure 24.23. Ruptured Spleen. A CT scan obtained during bolus intravenous contrast administration demonstrates multiple ragged linear defects (*large arrows*) in the spleen (*S*) representing fractures of the splenic parenchyma. Blood is present in the peritoneal spaces (*small arrows*) around the spleen, indicating disruption of the splenic capsule. The liver (*L*) was not injured. This patient was involved in an auto accident. *St*, stomach filled with oral contrast.

Figure 24.24. Intrasplenic Hematomas. A CT scan demonstrates multiple low-density foci (*arrows*) in the spleen (*S*) representing intrasplenic hematomas in this patient with blunt trauma to the left flank.

Table 24.1.   Multiple Splenic Calcifications

Tuberculosis
Histoplasmosis
Pneumocystis (AIDS)
Phleboliths
Infarctions

the capsule outward. Intrasplenic hematomas appear as irregular low-density areas within the parenchyma (Fig. 24.24).

References

1. Freeny PC. Radiology of the pancreas: two decades of progress in imaging and intervention. AJR 1988;150:975–981.
2. Ormson MJ, Charboneau JW, Stephens DH. Sonography in patients with a possible pancreatic mass shown on CT. AJR 1987;148:551–555.
3. Gulliver DJ, Cotton PB, Baillie J. Anatomic varients and artifacts in ERCP interpretation. AJR 1991;156:975–980.
4. Balthazar EJ, Robinson DL, Megibow AJ, Ranson JH. Acute pancreatitis: value of CT in establishing prognosis. Radiology 1990;174:331–336.
5. Luetmer PH, Stephens DH, Ward EM. Chronic pancreatitis: reassessment with current CT. Radiololgy 1989;171:353–357.
6. Beazley RM, Cohn I Jr. Update on pancreatic cancer. CA 1988;38:310–319.
7. Shawker TH, Garra BS, Hill MC, Doppman JL, Sindelar WF. The spectrum of sonographic findings in pancreatic carcinoma. J Ultrasound Med 1986;5:169–177.
8. Friedman AC. Imaging pancreatic carcinoma. Appl Radiol Feb 1990;21–28.
9. Megibow AJ. Pancreatic adenocarcinoma: designing the examination to evaluate the clinical question. Radiology 1992;183:297–303.
10. Günther RW. Ultrasound and CT in the assessment of suspected islet cell tumors of the pancreas. Semin Ultrasound CT MR 1985;6:261–275.
11. Ros PR, Hamrick-Turner JE, Chiechi MV, et al. Cystic masses of the pancreas. Radiographics 1992;12:673–686.
12. Johnson CD, Stephens DH, Charboneau JW, et al. Cystic pancreatic tumors: CT and sonographic appearance. AJR 1988;151:1133–1138.
13. Dodds WJ, Taylor AJ, Erickson SJ, et al. Radiologic imaging of splenic anomalies. AJR 1990;155:805–810.
14. Taylor AJ, Dodds WJ, Erickson SJ, Stewart ET. CT of acquired abnormalities of the spleen. AJR 1991;157:1213–1219.
15. Goerg C, Schwerk WB, Goerg K. Sonography of focal lesions of the spleen. AJR 1991;156:949–953.

25

Pharynx and Esophagus

William E. Brant

Imaging Methods

The upper gastrointestinal series (UGI), also called a barium meal, is a barium examination of the alimentary tract from the pharynx to the ligament of Treitz. A barium swallow or esophagram is a study more dedicated to evaluation of swallowing disorders and suspected lesions of the pharynx and esophagus. Barium sulfate preparations are ingested orally and filming is performed during fluoroscopy. The fluoroscopic examination is commonly videotaped to allow for more detailed review of swallowing dynamics and motility (1–3). Double-contrast techniques utilizing mucosal coating with barium combined with luminal distension are preferred for mucosal detail. Distension of the pharynx is provided by having the patient phonate (4). Distension of the esophagus is attained by having the patient ingest gas-producing crystals. Full-column, or single-contrast, technique utilizes barium suspension alone to fill and distend the esophagus. Mucosal relief views are collapsed views of the barium-coated esophagus.

Computed tomography (CT) complements barium studies and endoscopy of the esophagus and its mucosa by demonstrating the esophageal wall and adjacent structures. The CT itself is poor at evaluating the mucosa. While CT is excellent for demonstrating the extent of disease, findings are seldom specific for the nature of the disease. Inflammatory and neoplastic abnormalities are commonly indistinguishable on CT.

Magnetic resonance (MR) offers an alternative to CT for demonstrating the extent of esophageal disease. The normal esophagus is usually clearly demonstrated throughout its length by MR. The clear depiction of blood vessels by MR is useful in confirming the presence of varices and evaluating mediastinal vascular anatomy.

The esophagus is generally not amenable to ultrasound examination except by an endoluminal approach. Endosonography currently shows much promise and is undergoing extensive clinical evaluation.

This chapter reviews the pharynx as studied as part of a barium examination and for assessment of swallowing disorders. Cross-sectional imaging of the neck and pharynx is reviewed in Chapter 9.

Anatomy

The pharynx extends from the nasal cavity to the larynx (5, 6). It is classically divided into three compartments (Fig. 25.1). The nasopharynx extends from the skull base to the soft palate. Its function is entirely respiratory, and it will not be considered further in this chapter. The oropharynx extends from the soft palate to the hyoid bone. The hypopharynx extends from the hyoid bone to the cricopharyngeus muscle. The base of the tongue forms the anterior boundary of the oropharynx (Fig. 25.1). The outline of the surface of the tongue is nodular because of the presence of lymphoid tissue forming the lingual tonsils and the circumvallate papillae, which contain taste buds. The lingual tonsils may hypertrophy and mimic a neoplasm. The epiglottis and aryepiglottic folds separate the larynx from the oropharynx and hypopharynx. The *valleculae* are two symmetric pouches formed in the recess between the base of the tongue and the epiglottis. They are divided medially by the median glossoepiglottic fold and bounded laterally by the lateral glossoepiglottic folds. The *pyriform sinuses* are deep, symmetric, lateral recesses formed by the protrusion of the larynx into the hypopharynx.

The esophagus extends from the cricopharyngeus muscle at the level of C5-6 to the gastroesophageal junction (GEJ). The esophagus is a muscular tube formed by an outer longitudinal muscle layer and an

Figure 25.1. Double-Contrast Pharyngogram.
Three radiographs of the pharynx coated with barium demonstrate normal anatomic structures: **A**, nondistended lateral view, **B**, distended lateral view, obtained by having the patient phonate "eee...", and, **C**, frontal (anteroposterior) view. The nasopharynx (*NP*) extends from the skull base to the soft palate (*sp*). The oropharynx (*OP*) spans from the soft palate to the hyoid bone (*HB*). The hypopharynx (*HP*) extends from the hyoid bone to the cricopharyngeus muscle (C5-6), which demarcates the pharynx and esophagus. The epiglottis (*e*) closes during swallowing to protect the larynx (*L*) from aspiration. The cricoid cartilage makes a prominent impression on the hypopharynx (*small white arrows*). The base of the tongue (*t*) has a normal lobulated appearance due to nodular lymphoid tissue. The valleculae (*v*) are recesses between the tongue and epiglottis, bordered by the median glossoepiglottic fold (*large black arrow*) and the lateral glossoepiglottic folds (*small black arrows*). The pyriform sinuses (*ps*) extend laterally and posterior to the larynx.

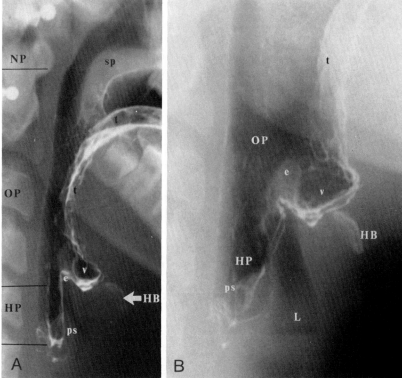

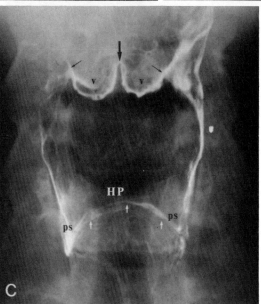

inner circular muscle layer lined by stratified squamous epithelium. The esophagus lacks a serosal layer, which allows for rapid spread of tumor into adjacent tissues. The proximal one-third of the esophagus is predominantly striated muscle, while the distal two-thirds is predominantly smooth muscle. Normal extrinsic impressions on the esophagus are made by the aortic arch, the left mainstem bronchus, and the left atrium.

On cross-sectional imaging, the esophagus appears as an oval of soft tissue density usually surrounded by fat. The esophagus may contain air or contrast lo-

cated centrally within its lumen. Eccentric contrast or air should be considered abnormal. The wall of the distended esophagus should not exceed 3 mm in thickness.

Anatomy of the esophagogastric region is complex and controversial (7). The length of the esophagus is tubular while its termination is saccular (Fig 25.2). The saccular termination is called the *esophageal vestibule*. The tubulovestibular junction is formed by a symmetrical muscular ring called the *A-ring*. The *B-ring* is an asymmetric mucosal ring or notch that occurs at the junction of esophageal squamous epithe-

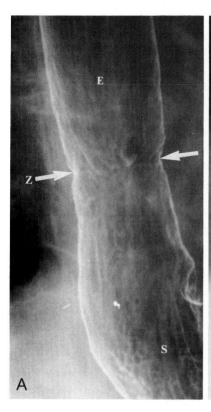
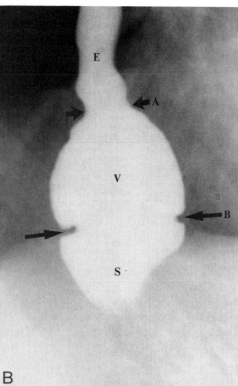

Figure 25.2. Anatomy of the Gastroesophageal Junction. Radiographs from a double-contrast barium study, **(A)** and a single-contrast barium study **(B)** demonstrate the physiologic and anatomic landmarks of the gastroesophageal junction. The Z-line (Z, *white arrows*), seen best on the double-contrast study, marks the junction of the squamous epithelium of the esophagus (*E*) and the columnar epithelium of the stomach (*S*). The single-contrast study demonstrates the esophageal vestibule (*V*) demarcated by the muscular A–ring (A, *short black arrows*) and the mucosal fold of the B-ring (B, *long black arrows*). The vestibule marks the location of the lower esophageal sphincter. The Z-line and the B-ring are markers of the gastroesophageal junction. Their location relative to the esophageal hiatus in the diaphragm varies with swallowing and other physiologic motions.

lium with gastric columnar epithelium. This squamo-columnar junction is also marked by the *Z-line*, a thin ragged line of demarcation seen on double-contrast views of the lower esophagus. The B-ring and the Z-line are considered to be radiographic markers of the GEJ.

The esophageal hiatus is an angled opening in the diaphragm formed by the edges of the diaphragmatic crura. On CT and MR, the crura often appear as prominent, teardrop-shaped structures of muscle density. With normal breathing, the proximal vestibule and A-ring lie in the thorax. The midvestibule is in the esophageal hiatus, and the distal vestibule and B-ring are in the abdomen. With swallowing, the vestibule opens and moves upward and the B-ring may be seen 1 cm above the diaphragm.

Normal Swallowing and Motility

The normal process of swallowing can be divided into oral, pharyngeal, and esophageal phases (1, 3, 5). The oral stage involves the voluntary transport of a bolus from the oral cavity into the pharynx. The soft palate elevates and the tongue depresses to accommodate the bolus and channel it into the oropharynx. The oropharynx and hypopharynx receive the bolus and conduct it to the esophagus. Breathing is halted while the larynx elevates, the laryngeal vestibule closes, and the epiglottis and aryepiglottic folds close over the opening into the larynx and deflect the bolus through the lateral piriform sinuses.

The functional upper esophageal sphincter (UES), formed by the cricopharyngeus and other pharyngeal muscles, opens to receive the bolus. Peristalsis conveys ingested material through the tubular esophagus to the stomach. *Primary peristalsis* is composed of a rapid wave of inhibition that opens the sphincters, followed by a slow wave of contraction that moves the bolus. Normal peristalsis will clear the esophagus completely with each swallow. Radiographically, primary peristalsis appears as a stripping wave that traverses the entire esophagus from top to bottom. *Secondary peristalsis* is initiated by distension of the esophageal lumen. The peristaltic wave starts in the midesophagus and spreads simultaneously up and down the esophagus to clear reflux or any part of a bolus left behind. Secondary waves have the same radiographic appearance as primary waves except that they start at the point of the retained barium bolus.

Tertiary waves are nonproductive contractions associated with motility disorders. Irregular contractions follow one another at close intervals from the top to the bottom of the esophagus. These nonperistaltic contractions cause a corkscrew or beaded appearance of the esophageal barium column. The functional lower esophageal sphincter (LES) at the level of the esophageal vestibule relaxes and opens in response to swallowing, primary peristalsis, and proximal esophageal dilatation.

Esophageal motility is best evaluated radiographically by observing fluoroscopically at least five sepa-

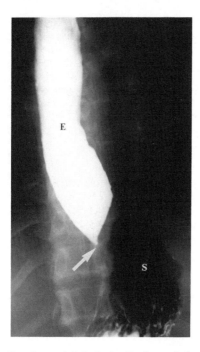

Figure 25.3.   Esophageal Achalasia. Radiograph from a UGI series reveals uniform dilation of the esophagus (*E*) to the level of the GEJ where a beak (*arrow*) is formed by the barium column. Repeated observation by fluoroscopy confirmed failure of relaxation of the LES and prolonged retention of barium in the esophagus even in the upright position. *S,* stomach.

rate swallows of barium with the patient in a prone position (8, 9). The patient must be instructed to swallow only once, as continuous swallowing distends the esophagus and makes impossible the evaluation of primary peristalsis.

Motility Disorders

Dysphagia is defined as the awareness of swallowing difficulty during the passage of solids or liquids from mouth to stomach (2). Patients complain of feeling a "lump in the throat," of food "sticking in the throat," of pain in the chest, or painful swallowing (odynophagia). These symptoms may be caused by anatomic abnormalities, tumors, or motility disorders of the pharynx or esophagus. Subjective assessment of the location of the abnormality is not reliable (1–3, 5). Detailed dynamic barium studies of the entire orophayngeal-esophageal pathway with videofluoroscopy are needed for complete evaluation (1–5). Motility disorders that may cause dysphagia or aspiration are reviewed below.

Cricopharyngeal Achalasia is due to failure of complete relaxation of the UES, resulting in dysphagia and aspiration. Barium swallow demonstrates a shelf-like impression on the barium column at the pharyngoesophageal junction at the level of C5-6. The pharynx is distended and barium may overflow into the larynx and trachea. Since some normal individu-

als have a prominent cricopharyngeal impression, controversy exists as to how prominent the impression must be to be considered significant. Narrowing of the lumen greater than 50% is generally accepted as a definite cause of dysphagia (3). Cricopharyngeal dysfunction is commonly associated with neuromuscular disorders of the pharynx.

Esophageal Achalasia is a disease of unknown etiology characterized by (*a*) absence of peristalsis in the body of the esophagus, (*b*) marked increase in resting pressure of the LES, and (*c*) failure of the LES to relax with swallowing. The abnormal peristalsis and LES spasm results in a failure of the esophagus to empty. Pathologically, cases show a deficiency of ganglion cells in the myenteric plexus (Auerbach's plexus) throughout the esophagus. The clinical presentation is insidious, usually at age 30–50, with dysphagia, regurgitation, foul breath, and aspiration. Radiographic signs include (*a*) uniform dilatation of the esophagus, usually with an air-fluid level present, (*b*) absence of peristalsis, with tertiary waves common in the early stages of the disease, (*c*) tapered "beak" deformity at the LES due to failure of relaxation (Fig. 25.3), and (*d*) increased incidence of epiphrenic diverticula and esophageal carcinoma.

Diseases that may mimic esophageal achalasia include the following.

Chagas Disease is caused by the destruction of ganglion cells of the esophagus due to a neurotoxin released by the protozoa, *Trypanosoma cruzi,* endemic to South America, especially eastern Brazil. The radiographic appearance of the esophagus is identical to achalasia. Associated abnormalities include cardiomyopathy, megaduodenum, megaureter, and megacolon.

Carcinoma of the GEJ may mimic achalasia, but tends to involve a longer segment of the distal esophagus, is rigid, and tends to show more irregular tapering of the distal esophagus and mass effect.

Diffuse Esophageal Spasm is a syndrome of unknown cause characterized by multiple tertiary esophageal contractions, thickened esophageal wall, and intermittent dysphagia and chest pain. Primary peristalsis is usually present but the contractions are infrequent. Most patients are middle-aged.

Neuromuscular Disorders are a common cause of abnormalities of the oral, pharyngeal, or esophageal phases of swallowing (1). The most common cause of neurologic dysfunction is cerebrovascular disease and stroke. Additional causes include Parkinsonism, Alzheimer's disease, multiple sclerosis, neoplasms of the central nervous system, and posttraumatic central nervous system injury. Diseases of striated muscle, such as muscular dystrophy, myasthenia gravis, and dermatomyositis, predominantly affect the pharynx and proximal third of the esophagus.

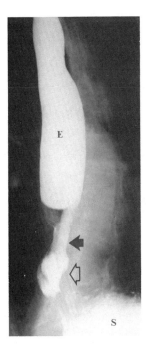

Figure 25.4 Scleroderma. Barium esophagram demonstrates the esophagus (*E*) to be dilated and lacking in peristaltic motion in its distal two-thirds on fluoroscopic observation. The GEJ (*open arrow*) is wide and is never observed to close. Reflux esophagitis causes stiffening and narrowing of the distal esophagus (*closed arrow*). *S*, stomach.

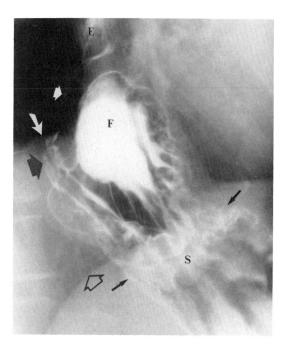

Figure 25.5. Hiatus Hernia. Left posterior oblique view from an UGI series demonstrates a large hiatus hernia. The fundus (*F*) of the stomach (*S*) extends well above the level of the left hemidiaphragm (*open arrow*). The widened (6 cm) esophageal hiatus makes an impression (*small black arrows*) on the body of the stomach. The GEJ (*fat black arrowhead*) is 5 cm above the left hemidiaphragm. The distal esophagus (*white arrowhead*) is bowed around the herniated stomach. The right hemidiaphragm (*white arrow*) projects well above the left hemidiaphragm on this view.

Scleroderma is a systemic disease of unknown etiology characterized by progressive atrophy of smooth muscle and progressive fibrosis of affected tissues. Females are most commonly affected, usually aged 20–40 at the onset of disease. The esophagus is affected in 75–80% of patients. Radiographic findings include (Fig. 25.4) (*a*) weak to absent peristalsis in the distal two-thirds (smooth muscle portion) of the esophagus, (*b*) delayed esophageal emptying, (*c*) a stiff dilated esophagus that does not collapse with emptying, and (*d*) wide gaping LES with free gastroesophageal reflux. Despite free reflux, tight strictures of the distal esophagus are uncommon.

Postoperative States, including surgery for malignancy of the tongue, larynx, and pharynx, commonly impair swallowing function as well as alter the morphology (1). Surgical resection is aimed at providing at least a 1-cm margin free of tumor, and often results in removing large blocks of tissue and functionally altering the structures which remain.

Esophagitis frequently results in abnormal esophageal motility and visualization of tertiary esophageal contractions.

Gastroesophageal Reflux (GER) occurs as a result of incompetence of the LES. The resting pressure of the LES is abnormally decreased, and fails to increase with raised intraabdominal pressure. As a result, increases in intraabdominal pressure exceed LES pressure, and gastric contents are allowed to re-

flux into the esophagus. Symptoms of GER include substernal burning pain ("heartburn"), postural regurgitation (in supine position), and development of reflux esophagitis, dysphagia and odynophagia. Complications of GER include reflux esophagitis, stricture, and development of Barrett's esophagus.

The radiographic diagnosis of pathologic GER may be difficult because 20% of normal individuals show spontaneous reflux on UGI examination, and patients with pathologic GER may not demonstrate reflux without provocative tests. Monitoring of esophageal pH for 24 hours in an ambulatory patient is the simplest and most sensitive means of diagnosing abnormal GER (8, 10).

Hiatus hernia has for years been considered synonymous with GER. However, there is poor correlation between the presence of hiatus hernia and GER or reflux esophagitis. One area of controversy is the definition of hiatus hernia and the criteria used for diagnosis. The simplest definition is protrusion of any portion of the stomach into the thorax. Two major types of hernia are described. The most common is the sliding hiatus hernia with the gastroesophageal junction displaced more than 1 cm above the hiatus (Fig. 25.5). The esophageal hiatus is often abnormally widened to 3–4 cm. The upper limit of normal hiatal width is 15 mm, most easily measured by CT. The

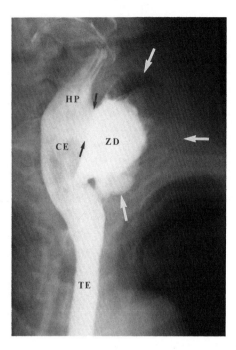

Figure 25.6. Zenker's Diverticulum. Barium swallow examination demonstrates a partially barium-filled outpouching (*ZD*) at the junction of the hypopharynx (*HP*) and cervical esophagus (*CE*). The full extent of the diverticulum is indicated by the *white arrows*. Note that the neck of the diverticulum (*black arrow*) is at a more cephalad location than its base, encouraging the trapping of food and liquid. *TE*, thoracic esophagus.

gastric fundus may be displaced above the diaphragm and present as a retrocardiac mass on a chest radiograph. The presence of an air-fluid level in the mass suggests the diagnosis.

Small, sliding hiatus hernias commonly reduce in the upright position. Much less common (1% of the total) is the paraesophageal hiatus hernia, in which the GEJ remains in normal location while a portion of the stomach, usually the fundus, herniates above the diaphragm. The mere presence of hiatus hernia is of limited clinical significance in most cases. The function of the LES and the presence of pathologic GER are the crucial factors in producing symptoms and causing complications. Large hiatus hernias, especially when the stomach is totally intrathoracic, are at risk for obstruction and volvulus.

Outpouchings

Zenker's Diverticulum arises in the hypopharynx just proximal to the UES. It is located in the posterior midline at the cleavage plane, known as Killian's dehiscence, between the circular and oblique fibers of the cricopharyngeus muscle (Fig. 25.6). The diverticulum has a small neck that is higher than the sac, resulting in food and liquid being trapped within the sac. The distended sac may compress the cervical esophagus. Symptoms include dysphagia, halitosis, and regurgitation of food.

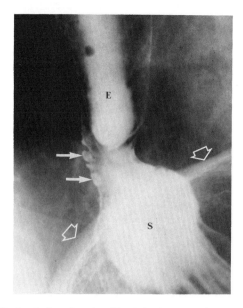

Figure 25.7. Reflux Esophagitis. A barium esophagram demonstrates stiffness and narrowing of the distal esophagus just above the level of the diaphragm (*open arrows*). Several prominent sacculations (*arrows*) are present, indicating long-standing and severe esophagitis. *E*, esophagus; *S*, stomach.

Midesophageal Diverticula may be pulsion or traction diverticula. Pulsion diverticula occur as a result of disordered esophageal peristalsis; traction diverticula occur because of fibrous inflammatory reactions of adjacent lymph nodes. Most midesophageal diverticula have large mouths, empty well, and are usually asymptomatic.

Epiphrenic Diverticula occur just above the LES, usually on the right side. They are rare and usually found in patients with esophageal motility disorders. Because of a small neck, higher than the sac, they may trap food and liquids and cause symptoms.

Sacculations are small outpouchings of the esophagus that usually occur as a sequela of severe esophagitis (see Fig. 25.7). They are thought to result from the healing and scarring of ulcerations. Sacculations tend to change in size and shape during fluoroscopic observation.

Esophagitis

Esophagitis is a common disease with many causes. Radiologic evaluation will detect most cases of moderate and severe esophagitis, but will demonstrate less than half the cases of mild esophagitis. Attention to excellent technique and use of double-contrast studies are essential (11). Radiographic signs of esophagitis include (*a*) thickened esophageal folds (>3 mm), (*b*) limited esophageal distensibility (asymmetric flattening), (*c*) abnormal motility, (*d*) mucosal plaques and nodules, (*e*) erosions and ulcerations, and (*f*) localized stricture.

Reflux esophagitis (RE) is the result of esophageal mucosal injury due to exposure to gastroduodenal secretions. The severity depends upon the concentration of caustic agents including acid, pepsin, bile salts, caffeine, alcohol, and aspirin, as well as the duration of contact with the esophageal mucosa. The findings of reflux esophagitis are always most prominent in the distal esophagus and gastroesophageal junction (Fig. 25.7). Early changes of reflux esophagitis include mucosal edema, which is manifest as a granular or nodular pattern of the distal esophagus (11). In contrast to the distinct borders of *Candida* plaques and nodules, reflux esophagitis nodules have poorly defined borders. Inflammatory exudates and pseudomembrane formation may mimic fulminant *Candida* esophagitis. However, the patient has symptoms of reflux rather than severe odynophagia.

Reflux esophagitis is the most common cause of esophageal ulcerations. The ulcers appear as discrete linear, punctate, or irregular collections of barium, usually surrounded by a radiolucent mound of edema. Distal prominence of the ulcerations is the key to differentiating RE ulcers from those of herpes esophagitis. Complications of reflux esophagitis include ulceration, bleeding, stricture, and Barrett's esophagus.

Barrett's esophagus is an acquired condition manifest by progressive columnar metaplasia of the distal esophagus caused by chronic gastroesophageal reflux (11, 12). The prevalence of Barrett's esophagus in patients with reflux esophagitis is about 10%, but may increase to 37% in patients with scleroderma. It is premalignant, with a 30–40 times increased risk of developing adenocarcinoma (see Fig. 25.11), resulting in a 15% prevalence of adenocarcinoma in patients with Barrett's esophagus. Clinical presentation is usually indistinguishable from reflux esophagitis. Adenocarcinoma may develop at any age. The characteristic radiographic appearance of Barrett's esophagus is a high (midesophageal) stricture or deep ulcer in a patient with GER. A reticular mucosal pattern of the esophageal mucosa, resembling areae gastricae of the stomach, is also suggestive. The diagnosis is confirmed by endoscopy and biopsy.

Infectious esophagitis is increasingly common because of the use of steroids and cytotoxic drugs, and the increasing incidence of acquired immunodeficiency syndrome (AIDS).

Candida is the most common cause of opportunistic esophagitis (8, 11). *Candida* of the oropharynx (thrush) is commonly present and is usually diagnosed clinically. Odynophagia is a prominent symptom. Discrete plaque-like lesions demonstrated by double-contrast esophagograms are most characteristic. The plaques appear as longitudinally oriented linear or irregular discrete filling defects with intervening normal-appearing mucosa. The lesions may be tiny and nodular, or giant and coalescent with pseudomembranes. The AIDS patients tend to have more fulminant disease with a diffuse "shaggy" esophagus.

Herpes simplex esophagitis begins as discrete vesicles that rupture to form discrete mucosal ulcers (8, 11). The ulcers may be linear, punctate, or ring-like and have a characteristic radiolucent halo. Discrete ulcers on a background of normal mucosa involving the midesophagus is most characteristic of herpes. Nodules and plaques are usually absent.

Cytomegalovirus is a cause of fulminant esophagitis in patients with AIDS. Cytomegalovirus esophagitis is characteristically manifest as one or more large, flat mucosal ulcers (8, 11). Endoscopic biopsy or culture confirms the diagnosis.

Tuberculosis. The esophagus is the least common portion of the gastrointestinal tract to be involved by tuberculosis. Manifestations include ulceration, stricture, and sinus tract formation.

Drug-induced esophagitis is due to intake of oral medications that produce a focal inflammation in areas of contact with the mucosa. Drugs that cause this condition include tetracycline, doxycycline, quinidine, aspirin, ascorbic acid, potassium chloride, alprenolol chloride, and emepronium bromide (11). The radiographic appearance may be identical to herpes esophagitis, with discrete ulcers separated by normal mucosa in the midesophagus. The diagnosis is suggested by a history of recent drug ingestion (8). Healing usually occurs within 7–10 days of discontinuing the offending medication.

Corrosive ingestion usually occurs as an accident in children or a suicide attempt in adults. Alkaline agents produce deep (full-thickness) coagulation necrosis. Acid agents tend to produce more superficial injury. Ulceration, esophageal perforation, and mediastinitis may complicate the acute injury. Late complications are fibrosis and long or multiple strictures.

Crohn's Disease may rarely be manifest as discrete aphthous ulcers in the esophagus. However, involvement of the small or large bowel by Crohn's disease is virtully always present. Crohn's disease of the esophagus should not be considered unless Crohn's disease of the bowel is already evident (8).

Radiation esophagitis obviously occurs in patients with a history of thoracic radiation therapy for malignant disease. Acute radiation may cause shallow or deep ulcers in the area of involvement. With the development of fibrosis, the peristaltic wave is interrupted and a long smooth stricture may develop within the radiotherapy field. Simultaneous radiotherapy and Adriamycin (doxorubicin hydrochloride) chemotherapy greatly accentuates esophageal inflammation.

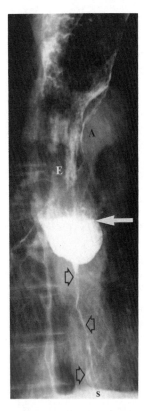

Figure 25.8. Stricture due to Reflux Esophagitis. A long segment stricture (*open arrows*) of the distal esophagus is apparent on this barium esophagram. The column of barium is abruptly narrowed to a thin irregular channel. Barium forms an air-fluid level (*white arrow*) on this upright view as it is retained in the esophagus before trickling through the stricture. Retained food particles and secretions cause a mottled appearance in the lumen of the proximal esophagus (*E*). The aorta (*A*) produces a normal impression on the left lateral aspect of the esophagus. *S*, stomach.

Esophageal Stricture

Strictures may be defined as any persistent intrinsic narrowing of the esophagus. The most common causes are fibrosis induced by inflammation and neoplasm. Since radiographic findings are not reliable in differentiating benign from malignant strictures, all should be evaluated endoscopically.

Esophagitis. Chronic inflammation induces progressive fibrosis that eventually narrows the esophageal lumen. Acute and chronic findings of esophagitis commonly overlap.

Reflux esophagitis is the most common cause of esophageal stricture. They are usually confined to the distal esophagus (Fig. 24-8), and may be smooth and circumferential, or asymmetric and irregular. Long segment stricture may be induced by long-term nasogastric intubation. A *Schatzki ring* is a pathologic ring-like stricture at the level of the B-ring due to reflux esophagitis.

Barrett's Esophagus strictures tend to be high in the midesophagus, and may be smooth and tapered,

or ring-like narrowings (12). The high position is because of a tendency to occur at the squamocolumnar junction, which has been displaced to a position well above the GEJ.

Corrosives strictures are long and symmetric. They commonly take years to develop.

Radiation strictures are confined to the radiotherapy field.

Neoplasm. An irregular, ulcerated, circumferential narrowing is most typical of malignant stricture. However, infiltrative tumors may cause smooth, rigid narrowing of the esophagus without a clear zone of transition. The mucosa may not be altered until tumor spread is substantial.

Webs are thin, delicate membranes that sweep partially across the lumen. They occur in both the pharynx and esophagus, and are commonly multiple. Pharyngeal webs arise most commonly from the anterior wall of the hypopharynx. Esophageal webs may occur anywhere, but are most common in the cervical esophagus just distal to the cricopharyngeus impression. Most are incidental findings; however, they occasionally cause sufficient obstruction to result in dysphagia.

Extrinsic Compression. Malignancy or inflammation in the mediastinum may encase the esophagus and narrow its lumen. Causes include lung carcinoma, lymphoma, metastasis to mediastinal nodes, tuberculosis, and histoplasmosis.

Enlarged Esophageal Folds

Esophagitis. Thick folds occur most commonly with reflux esophagitis. Additional findings associated with esophagitis, such as ulcerations and nodules, are commonly present.

Varices appear as serpiginous filling defects (Fig. 25.9) that change in size with changes in intrathoracic pressure, and collapse with esophageal peristalsis and distension. They are best demonstrated on UGI with mucosal relief views. Computed tomography with bolus contrast enhancement demonstrates varices as enhancing vascular structures within and adjacent to esophageal wall near the GEJ. Magnetic resonance is also effective in demonstrating varices as vascular spaces, with signal void because of flowing blood.

Uphill varices refer to the portosystemic collateral veins that enlarge because of portal hypertension. Coronary vein collaterals connect with gastroesophageal varices that drain into the inferior vena cava via the azygos system. Uphill varices are usually only present in the distal esophagus.

Downhill varices are formed as a result of obstruction of the superior vena cava with drainage from the azygous system through esophageal varices to the

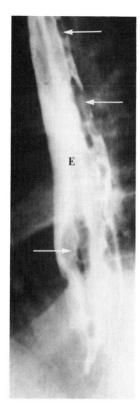

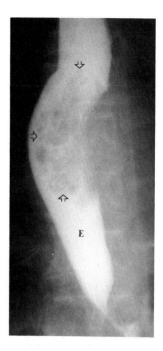

Figure 25.10. Squamous Cell Carcinoma appears as a polypoid mass (*arrows*) in the midesophagus (*E*) on this barium esophagram. Barium outlines the lobulations in the tumor.

Figure 25.9. Varices. A single-contrast barium esophagram demonstrates sinuous tubular and nodular filling defects (*arrows*) in the esophagus (*E*). This patient has cirrhosis, portal hypertension, and a history of upper gastrointestinal bleeding.

portal vein. Downhill varices usually predominate in the proximal esophagus.

Lymphoma may infiltrate the submucosa and thicken the folds. However, lymphoma rarely involves the esophagus directly and is virtually never primary in the esophagus.

Varicoid Carcinoma causes thick, tortuous, longitudinal folds that resemble varices but are rigid and persistent.

Mass Lesions/Filling Defects

Pharyngeal Carcinomas are well demonstrated by double-contrast pharyngography (8). Barium studies may detect tumors difficult to visualize endoscopically. Radiographic signs include (*a*) intraluminal mass seen as a filling defect, abnormal luminal contour, or focal increased density, (*b*) mucosal irregularity due to ulceration or mucosal elevations, and (*c*) asymmetric distensibility due to infiltrating tumor or extrinsic nodal mass. Most pharyngeal tumors are squamous cell carcinomas that may arise on the base of the tongue, palatine tonsil, posterior phayngeal wall, or the piriform sinus. Laryngeal tumors may impress upon the pharynx or extend into it. Staging is best performed by CT or MR.

Lymphoma of the pharynx is usually manifest as a large, bulky tumor of the lingual or palatine tonsils. Lymphoma constitutes 15% of oropharyngeal tumors.

Esophageal Carcinoma is squamous cell carcinoma (Fig. 25.10) in 90% of cases, while the remainder are adenocarcinoma arising in Barrett's esophagus (Fig. 25.11), undifferentiated, or miscellaneous cell types. The tumor assumes four basic radiographic patterns. An annular constricting lesion is most common. These appear as irregular ulcerated strictures. The polypoid pattern causes an intraluminal filling defect (Fig. 25.10). The infiltrative variety grows predominantly in the submucosa and may simulate a benign stricture. The least common pattern is that of a primary ulcerated mass. Predisposing conditions include cigarette and alcohol abuse, corrosive ingestion, and carcinoma of the head and neck. The typical patient is a 65-year-old male.

The tumor spreads quickly by direct invasion into adjacent tissues because of the lack of a serosal covering on the esophagus. Lymphatic spread may go to nodes in the neck, mediastinum, or below the diaphragm, depending on the location of the primary tumor in the esophagus. Hematogenous spread is to lung, liver, and adrenal gland.

Computed tomography and MR are used to define the extent of disease (Table 25.1 and Fig. 25.12) (13). Findings include irregular thickening of the esophageal wall, eccentric narrowing of the lumen, dilation of the esophagus above the area of narrowing, invasion of periesophageal tissues, and metastases to mediasti-

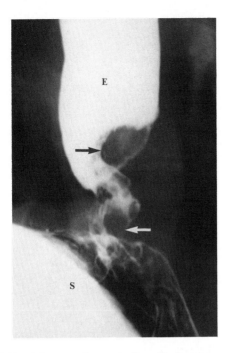

Figure 25.11. Adenocarcinoma in Barrett's Esophagus. A tumor in the distal esophagus (*E*) forms nodular (*arrows*) narrowing of the barium column. Endoscopy confirmed adenocarcinoma arising in Barrett's esophagus. *S*, stomach.

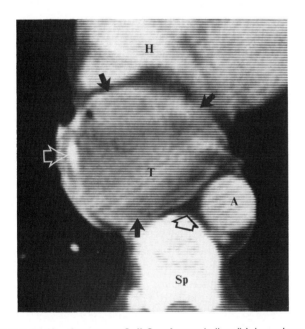

Figure 25.12. Squamous Cell Carcinoma in the distal esophagus causes a large tumor mass (*T, black arrows*) that nearly obliterates the esophageal lumen (*open white arrow*). Computed tomography is used to document the extraluminal extent of the tumor. The triangular fat space (*open black arrow*) between the esophagus, spine, and aorta is free of tumor. *H*, heart; *A*, aorta; *Sp*, spine.

nal lymph nodes and the liver. Obliteration of the fat space between the aorta, esophagus, and vertebral body is highly predictive of invasion of the aorta (14).

Gastric Adenocarcinoma spreads from the fundus and GEJ into the distal esophagus. Adenocarci-

Table 25.1. Staging of Esophageal Carcinoma

Stage	Description
0	Carcinoma in situ
I	Tumor invades lamina propria or submucosa
IIA	Tumor invades muscularis propria or adventitia
IIB	Tumor invades lamina propria, submucosa, or muscularis propria + regional node metastases
III	Tumor invades adventitia + regional node metastases or tumor invades adjacent structures
IV	Distant metastases

noma of the distal esophagus may be either primary gastric or primary esophageal arising in Barrett's esophagus.

Leiomyoma. Leiomyoma is the most common benign neoplasm of the esophagus. It is a firm, well-encapsulated tumor that arises in the wall. Ulceration is rare in the esophagus. Most are asymptomatic and discovered incidentally. Men aged 25–35 are affected most commonly (male:female = 2:1). On UGI, most appear as smooth, well-defined wall lesions, although rarely they may be pedunculated or polypoid. Coarse calcifications are occasionally present and strongly suggestive of leiomyoma. Evaluation by CT demonstrates a smooth, well-defined mass of uniform soft tissue density. The esophageal wall is eccentrically thickened.

Polyp. Fibroepithelial or fibrovascular polyps are a rare cause of esophageal filling defect. They appear as large ovoid or elongated intraluminal masses in the upper esophagus.

Extrinsic Lesions may invade the esophagus or simulate an esophageal mass or filling defect. Causes include mediastinal adenopathy, lung carcinoma, and vascular structures.

Aberrant right subclavian artery arises from the aorta distal to the left subclavian artery. To reach its destination it must cross the mediastinum behind the esophagus. It causes a characteristic upward-slanting linear filling defect on the posterior aspect of the esophagus.

Esophageal Perforation

Trauma. Endoscopy, esophageal dilation procedures, or any type of instrumentation may perforate the esophageal wall.

Boerhaave's Syndrome refers to rupture of the esophageal wall due to forceful vomiting. The tear is virtually always in the left posterior wall near the left crus of the diaphragm. Esophageal contents may escape into the left pleural space or into the potential space between the parietal pleura and left crus. Bleeding can be profuse and infection is a great risk. Radiographic findings include pneumomediastinum, left pleural effusion, and extravasation of contrast media into the mediastinum and/or pleura space.

Mallory Weiss tear involves only the mucosa and not the full thickness of the esophagus. While endoscopy usually identifies the lesion, it is commonly missed on UGI. It may be a cause of copious hematemesis.

References

1. Dodds WJ, Logemann JA, Stewart ET. Radiologic assessment of abnormal oral and pharyngeal phases of swallowing. AJR 1990;154:965–974.
2. Levine MS, Rubesin SE. Radiologic investigation of dysphagia. AJR 1990;154:1157–1163.
3. Jones B, Donner MW. Examination of the patient with dysphagia. Radiology 1988;167:319–326.
4. Rubesin SE, Jones B, Donner MW. Contrast pharyngography: the importance of phonation. AJR 1987;148:269–272.
5. Donner MW, Bosma JF, Robertson DL. Anatomy and physiology of the pharynx. Gastointest Radiol 1985;10:196–212.
6. Rubesin SE, Jessurun J, Robertson D, et al. Lines of the pharynx. Radiographics 1987;7:217–237.
7. Ott DJ, Gelfand DW, Wu WC, Castell DO. Esophagogastric region and its rings. AJR 1984;142:281–287.
8. Levine MS, Rubesin SE, Ott DJ. Update on esophageal radiology. AJR 1990;155:933–941.
9. Ott DJ, Chen YM, Hewson EG, et al. Esophageal motility: assessment with synchronous video tape fluoroscopy and manometry. Radiology 1989;173:419–422.
10. Wiener GJ, Morgan TM, Cooper JB, et al. Ambulatory 24-hour esophageal pH monitoring: reproducibility and variability of pH parameters. Dig Dis Sci 1988;33:1127–1133.
11. Levine MS. Radiology of esophagitis: a pattern approach. Radiology 1991;179:1–7.
12. Levine MS. Barrett's esophagus: a radiologic diagnosis? AJR 1988;151:433–438.
13. American Joint Committee on Cancer. Manual for staging of cancer. 4th ed. Philadelphia: JB Lippincott Company, 1992.
14. Takashima S, Takeuchi N, Shiozaki H, et al. Carcinoma of the esophagus: CT vs. MR imaging in determining resectability. AJR 1991;156:297–302.

26

Stomach and Duodenum

William E. Brant

Imaging Methods

The upper gastrointestinal (UGI) series is the standard radiographic method of examination of the stomach and duodenum. However, to attain a high sensitivity for the examination and to avoid missing significant pathology, multiple techniques must be utilized for the UGI (1). These include the single-contrast technique of filling and distending the stomach and duodenum with barium suspension. This technique is usually supplemented by compression procedures that are effective in demonstrating abnormalities of the distal stomach and duodenum. Mucosal relief technique, using small amounts of barium to coat the mucosa without distending the organ, is useful in demonstrating abnormalities such as varices. Double-contrast technique, using high-density barium suspensions to coat the mucosa and ingestible effervescent granules to distend the organ, is optimal for demonstration of subtle features of the mucosal surface. As with any radiographic examination, attention to detail and tailoring the examination for the clinical problem is essential in producing good results.

Computed tomography (CT) is used to assess abnormalities of the gastric and duodenal walls and to determine the extent of extraluminal disease. Optimal distension of the stomach and duodenum is mandatory for accurate CT interpretation. Nodular thicken-

ing of a nondistended but normal gastric wall, especially near the gastroesophageal junction (GEJ), may mimic a tumor (2). Gastric and duodenal distension may be attained by filling the organs with positive contrast agents or using effervescent granules to cause gaseous distension. The patient is positioned to optimize distension of the portion of the gastrointestinal tract of greatest interest.

Anatomy

The gastrointestinal tract is essentially a hollow tube consisting of four concentric layers (Fig. 26.1). The innermost layer exposed to the lumen is the mucosa. The mucosa consists of epithelium supported by loose connective tissue of the lamina propria and a thin band of smooth muscle called the muscularis mucosae. The submucosa provides the main connective tissue support for the mucosa. The submucosa contains the main vascular and lymphatic channels, lymphoid follicles, and autonomic nerve plexuses. The main muscular structure of the bowel wall is the muscularis propria, made up of inner circular and outer longitudinal layers. The serosa or adventitia is the outer covering of the bowel.

The appearance and position of the stomach and duodenum vary considerably from one individual to another. A number of terms have traditionally been used to describe the anatomic divisions of the stom-

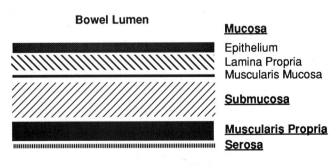

Figure 26.1. Layers of the Bowel Wall. The mucosa consists of three layers in close proximity to the bowel lumen. The submucosa consists of connective tissue, blood vessels, lymphatic channels and follicles, and autonomic nerve plexuses. The muscularis propria is the muscle layer responsible for peristalsis. The serosa is the outer covering layer.

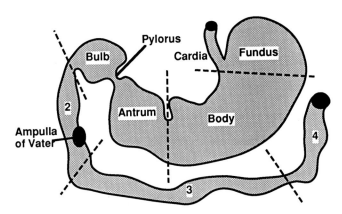

Figure 26.2. Anatomy of UGI Tract. The stomach is divided anatomically into fundus, body, and antrum. The pylorus serves as a valve that separates the stomach and duodenum. The duodenum is divided into bulb (or cap), descending (2), transverse (3), and ascending (4) portions.

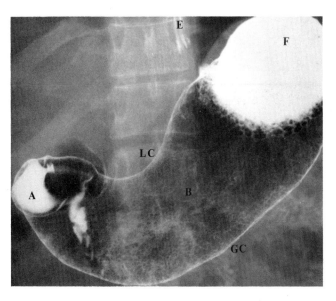

Figure 26.3. Normal Stomach. Double-contrast technique provides distension of the stomach with coating of its mucosa to demonstrate normal areae gastricae in the body (*B*) and antrum (*A*). *E*, esophagus. *F*, fundus. *LC*, lesser curvature. *GC*, greater curvature.

ach and duodenum (Fig. 26.2). Cardia refers to the region of the GEJ. The fundus is that portion of the stomach above the level of the GEJ. The body of the stomach is the central two-thirds portion from the cardia to the incisura angularis. The incisura angularis is an acute angle formed on the lesser curvature that marks the boundary between the body and the antrum. The parietal cells, which produce hydrochloric acid, and the chief cells, which produce pepsin precursors, are located in the fundus and body. The antrum is the distal one-third of the stomach, and contains gastrin-producing cells but no acid-secreting cells.

The pylorus is the junction of the stomach with the duodenum, and the pyloric canal is the channel through the pylorus. The duodenal bulb is the pyramidal first portion of the duodenum. The gallbladder frequently makes a prominant impression on the top of the bulb. The duodenum bulb, like the stomach, is covered on all surfaces by visceral peritoneum. The remainder of the duodenum is retroperitoneal and within the anterior pararenal compartment.

The second or descending portion of the duodenum is lateral to the head of the pancreas. The common bile duct and pancreatic duct pierce the medial aspect of the descending duodenum at the ampulla of Vater. The third or horizontal portion of the duodenum passes to the left between the superior mesenteric vessels and the inferior vena cava and aorta. The fourth or ascending portion of the duodenum ascends on the left side of the aorta to the level of L-2 and the ligament of Treitz, where its turns abruptly ventrally to form the duodenal-jejunal flexure.

The term areae gastricae refers to the detailed pattern of the gastric mucosa as demonstrated by double-contrast technique (Fig. 26.3). Normal areae gastricae varies from a fine reticular pattern to a course nodular pattern. The hallmark of normal is the regularity of

the pattern in all areas in which it is visualized. The term rugae refers to the gastric mucosal folds that produce distinct radiolucent ridges when the stomach is partially distended. Rugae are composed of mucosa, the lamina propria, the muscularis mucosae, and portions of the submucosa. Disease in any of these structures may cause thickening of the gastric folds.

The lesser curvature of the stomach is attached to the liver by the lesser omentum. The greater omentum attaches to the greater curvature of the stomach. The lesser sac is the intraperitoneal space posterior to the stomach and anterior to the pancreas.

On CT the normal gastric wall does not exceed 5 mm in thickness, while the normal duodenal wall is less than 3 mm thick. Both organs must be fully distended to accurately assess wall thickness. A prominent pseudotumor, caused by inadequate distension, is often seen on CT near the GEJ (2).

STOMACH

Gastric Filling Defects/Mass Lesions

Gastric Carcinoma is the third most common gastrointestinal malignancy, after colon and pancreatic carcinoma. Predisposing factors include pernicious anemia, atrophic gastritis, and gastrojejunostomy. Most (95%) are adenocarcinomas. The remainder are squamous cell carcinoma or rare cell types. The incidence of gastric carcinoma is higher in Japan, Finland, Chile, and Iceland than in the United States.

The tumor assumes four common morphologic growth patterns. Approximately one-third are polypoid masses that present as filling defects within the gastric lumen (Fig. 26.4). Many of these are broad-based and papillary in configuration. Another third are ulcerative masses presenting as malignant gastric ulcers. The remainder are infiltrating (Fig. 26.5), presenting as scirrhous carcinomas, or superficial spreading, producing plaque-like tumors or bizarre thickened folds. Scirrhous carcinoma is characterized by diffuse infiltration of the gastric wall by poorly differentiated or undifferentiated carcinomatous cells (3). The wall of the stomach is thickened and rigid. The terms linitis plastica or water-bottle stomach may be applied to describe the resulting stiff narrowed stomach (Fig. 26.6). Additional causes of narrowed stomach are listed in Table 26.1 (3).

Superficial spreading carcinoma spreads through the mucosa and submucosa producing nodular thick-ening or superficial mucosal ulceration. Intraluminal mass effect is minimal; however, the involved areas are thickened and rigid and involved rugae are thickened and distorted. Cancers are most common in the antrum, near the cardia, and along the lesser curvature.

The tumor may spread by direct invasion through the gastric wall to involve perigastric fat and adjacent organs, or may seed the peritoneal cavity. Lymphatic spread is to regional lymph nodes including perigastric nodes along the lesser curvature, celiac axis, and hepatoduodenal, retropancreatic, mesenteric, and paraaortic nodes. Hematogenous metastases involve the liver, adrenal glands, ovaries, and, rarely, bone and lung.

Computed tomography is used to determine the extent of tumor (4) (Fig. 25.5). Findings include (a) irregular thickening of the luminal surface, (b) asymmetric thickening of gastric folds, (c) intraluminal soft tissue mass, (d) extension of tumor into perigastric fat, (e) regional lymphadenopathy, and (f) metastases in the liver and adrenal. Staging of gastric cancer is shown in Table 26.2 (5).

Lymphoma accounts for 2% of gastric neoplasms. The stomach is the most common site of involvement for primary gastrointestinal lymphoma (6). Gastric lymphoma is 80% non-Hodgkin's, usually diffuse histiocytic lymphoma, and 20% Hodgkin's lymphoma. Lymphoma demonstrates three morphologic patterns: polypoid solitary mass, ulcerative mass, and diffuse infiltration. The UGI findings are strikingly similar to adenocarcinoma.

Computed tomography findings that are helpful in differentiating gastric lymphoma from carcinoma include (a) more marked thickening of the wall (may exceed 3 cm) (Fig. 26.7). (b) involvement of additional

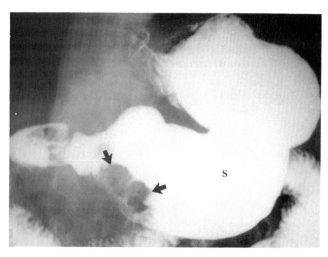

Figure 26.4. Polypoid Gastric Carcinoma. Single-contrast technique UGI series reveals a lobulated filling defect (arrows) in the antrum of the stomach (S).

Figure 26.5. Scirrhous Carcinoma. A CT scan demonstrates fixed nodular thickening (arrows) of the lateral wall of the stomach (S) caused by gastric adenocarcinoma. The outer margin of the stomach is well defined, giving evidence against extension of tumor through the wall. The CT also evaluates the liver (L) and regional lymph nodes for evidence of metastatic disease. C, splenic flexure of the colon.

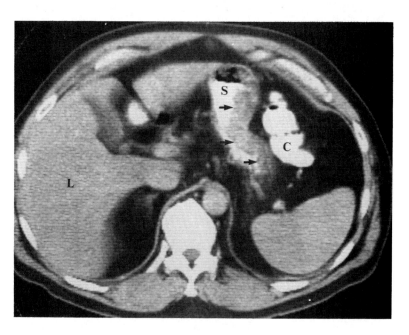

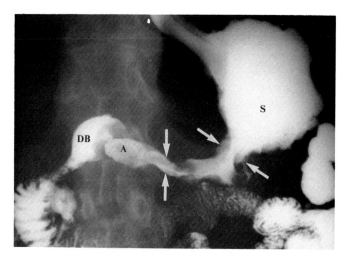

Figure 26.6.   Linitis Plastica. Scirrhous gastric carcinoma causes fixed nodular narrowing (*arrows*) of the body and antrum (*A*) of the stomach (*S*). No peristalsis through this portion of the stomach was observed at fluoroscopy. Biopsy yielded undifferentiated adenocarcinoma. *DB*, duodenal bulb.

Table 26.1.   Narrowed Stomach

Neoplastic
   Gastric adenocarcinoma (linitus plastica)
   Lymphoma (antral narrowing + extension into duodenum)
   Metastases (linitus plastica due to breast carcinoma)
Inflammatory
   Gastritis (usually antral narrowing)
   Peptic ulcer disease
   Corrosive ingestion (usually acid)
   Radiotherapy (after 4500 rads)
   AIDS[a] (*Cryptosporidium* infection) (narrowed antrum + small
      bowel involvement)
   Eosinophilic gastroenteritis (narrowing + wall thickening)
   Infection (tuberculosis + syphilis — both rare)
   Crohn's disease (rare)
   Sarcoidosis (usually asymptomatic)
Other
   Extrinsic compression (pancreatitis + pancreatic carcinoma)

[a]Acquired immunodeficiency syndrome.

Table 26.2.   Staging of Gastric Cancer

TMN Staging
Primary Tumor (T)

TX	Primary tumor cannot be assessed
T0	No evidence of primary tumor
Tis	Carcinoma in situ
T1	Tumor invades lamina propria or submucosa
T2	Tumor invades muscularis propria or subserosa
T3	Tumor penetrates serosa without invasion of adjacent structures
T4	Tumor invades adjacent structures

Regional Lymph Nodes (N)

NX	Regional lymph nodes cannot be assessed
N0	No regional lymph node metastasis
N1	Metastasis in perigastric lymph node(s) within 3 cm of the edge of the primary tumor
N2	Metastasis in perigastric lymph node(s) more than 3 cm from the edge of the primary tumor, or in lymph nodes along the left gastric, common hepatic, splenic, or celiac arteries

Distant Metastasis (M)

MX	Presence of distant metastasis cannot be assessed
M0	No distant metastasis
M1	Distant metastasis

Staging Grouping

Stage	T	N	M
Stage 0	Tis	N0	M0
Stage IA	T1	N0	M0
Stage IB	T1	N1	M0
	T2	N0	M0
Stage II	T1	N2	M0
	T2	N1	M0
	T3	N0	M0
Stage IIIA	T2	N2	M0
	T3	N1	M0
	T4	N0	M0
Stage IIIB	T3	N2	M0
	T4	N1	M0
Stage IV	T4	N2	M0
	Any T	Any N	M1

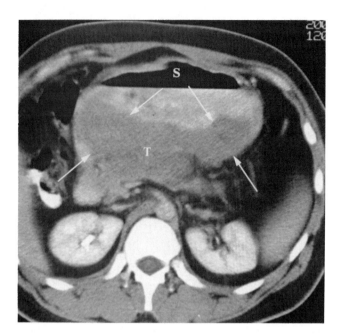

Figure 26.7.   Gastric Lymphoma. A CT scan demonstrates marked thickening (*arrows*) of the posterior gastric wall with a homogeneous tumor (*T*) extending into the lumen of the stomach (*S*). Endoscopic biopsy revealed large cell lymphoma.

areas of the gastrointestinal tract, (*c*) absence of invasion of the perigastric fat, and (*d*) more widespread and bulkier adenopathy.

Leiomyoma and Leiomyosarcoma arise from the smooth muscle of the gastric wall and grow as submucosal, subserosal, or exophytic tumors. Long-term silent growth to a large size is characteristic. The overlying mucosa is ulcerated in half the cases of leiomyoma and the majority of cases of leiomyosarcoma (Fig 26.8). Dystrophic calcification is relatively common in both benign and malignant tumors and helps to differentiate these lesions from other gastric tumors. Histologic differentiation of benign from malignant tumors is difficult; the differentiation is based upon size, gross appearance, and behavior of the tumor.

Computed tomography is useful in characterizing the tumors since they are predominantly extraluminal (7). Benign tumors are smaller (4–5 cm average size), homogeneous in density, and show uniform diffuse enhancement. Malignant tumors tend to be larger (12 cm, average size) with central zones of low density due to hemorrhage and necrosis (Fig. 26.8**B**), and show irregular patterns of enhancement.

Metastasis may present as submucosal nodules or ulcerated masses. They are commonly multiple. Common primary tumors are melanoma, and breast and lung carcinoma. Breast cancer metastases may simulate linitis plastica.

Kaposi Sarcoma, usually found in patients with acquired immunodeficiency syndrome, demonstrates a wide spectrum of appearances including polypoid

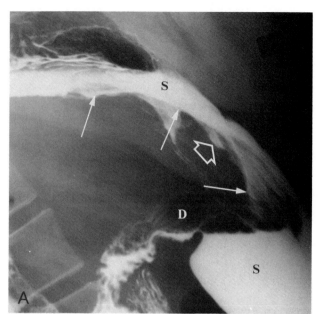

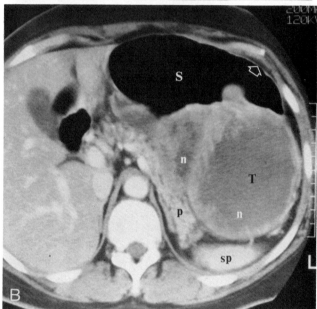

Figure 26.8.   Gastric Leiomyosarcoma. A. Radiograph in lateral upright position demonstrates a huge posterior mass distorting the lumen (*arrows*) of the stomach (*S*). A ulcer (*open arrow*) is evident. *D*, duodenal bulb. **B.** A CT scan of the same patient reveals the tumor (*T*) to be heterogeneous with large lucent areas representing necrosis (*n*). Note the thin, normal anterior wall (*open arrow*) of the stomach (*S*). The pancreas (*p*) is compressed against the spine by the mass. *sp*, spleen.

mass, thickened folds, and multiple submucosal masses.

Polyps are lesions that protrude into the lumen. Their appearance on double-contrast UGI series depends upon whether they are on the dependent or nondependent surface. A polyp on the dependent surface appears as a radiolucent filling defect in the barium pool; a polyp on the nondependant surface is covered with a thin coat of barium. The x-ray beam

Table 26.3. Multiple Gastric Filling Defects

Hyperplastic polyps
Adenomatous polyps (especially with polyposis syndromes)
Metastases
Lymphoma
Varices

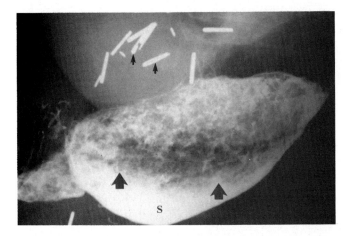

Figure 26.9. Bezoar. An UGI series reveals an irregular mottled mass (*large arrows*) floating in the lumen of the stomach (*S*). The mass is composed of retained food fibers in this patient with poor gastric emptying due to scleroderma and multiple gastric surgeries. Numerous surgical clips (*small arrows*) are evident.

catches its margin in tangent, resulting in a lesion whose margins are etched in white. The *bowler hat sign* (Fig. 28.5) is produced by the acute angle of attachment of the polyp to the mucosa. The *Mexican hat sign* consists of two concentric rings and is produced by visualizing a pedunculated polyp end-on.

Hyperplastic polyps account for 80% of gastric polyps. Most are less than 15 mm in diameter. They are not a neoplasm, but rather a hyperplastic response to mucosal injury, especially gastritis. They may be located anywhere in the stomach and are frequently multiple (Table 26.3). They have no malignant potential.

Adenomatous polyps account for 15% of gastric polyps and are true neoplasms with malignant potential. Most are solitary, located in the antrum, and are larger than 2 cm diameter.

Hamartomatous polyps occur in Peutz-Jeghers syndrome. They have no malignant potential.

Ectopic Pancreas is a common intramural lesion, usually found in the antrum. Lobules of heterotopic pancreatic tissue, up to 5 cm in size, are covered by gastric mucosa. Most are nipple- or cone-shaped with a small central orifice.

Bezoar/Foreign Body. The term bezoar refers to an intraluminal gastric mass consisting of accumulated ingested material (Fig. 26.9). Bezoars may be composed of a wide variety of substances: trichobe-

zoars are composed of hair; phytobezoars are composed of fruit or vegetable products. Any ingested foreign body may produce an intraluminal filling defect.

Extrinsic Impression. Masses adjacent to the stomach may produce filling defects. Extrinsic masses on the dependent surface produce ill-defined radiolucencies. The mucosa may be impressed upon by an extrinsic mass and be seen in profile as a white line. Pancreatic, splenic, hepatic and retroperitoneal masses may impress upon the stomach. Computed tomography is excellent for demonstrating the nature of an extrinsic mass impression.

Thickened Gastric Folds/Thickened Wall

Gastric folds are generally considered to be thickened if they exceed 1 cm in the fundus and 5 mm in the antrum.

Normal Variant. Gastric folds are normally most prominent in the fundus and upper third of the greater curvature. Thickened folds, even those larger than 1 cm, in this region are often normal, but require evaluation to exclude pathology.

Varices appear as smooth lobulated filling defects resembling thickened folds. They are most common in the fundus and usually accompany esophageal varices. Isolated gastric varices may occur with splenic vein occlusion.

Computed tomography with bolus contrast enhancement is an excellent method for confirming the presence of gastric varices, as well as demonstrating their cause.

Neoplasm. Lymphoma and superfical spreading gastric carcinoma may produce distorted rigid gastric folds that are commonly ulcerated and appear nodular. The distal stomach is the most common location for neoplasms.

Gastritis is a convenient label used to describe a wide variety of diseases affecting the gastric mucosa. Most, but not all, of these diseases are inflammatory. The hallmarks of gastritis are thickened folds and superficial mucosal ulcerations (erosions). The thickened folds are generally due to mucosal edema and superficial inflammatory infiltrate. Erosions are defined as defects in the mucosa that do not penetrate beyond the muscularis mucosae. Aphthous ulcers (also called varioliform erosions) are complete erosions that appear as tiny central flecks of barium surrounded by a radiolucent halo of edema (Fig. 26.10). Incomplete erosions appear as linear streaks and dots of barium. Erosions heal without scarring.

Acute erosive gastritis may be caused by peptic disease, alcohol, emotional stress, trauma, antiinflammatory medications (aspirin, steroids, indomethacin, phenylbutazone), corrosives (acids and alkalis), and infection with herpes simplex, cytomegalovirus, or *Candida*. Radiographic findings include erosions,

Figure 26.10. Aphthous Ulcers. Film from an air-contrast UGI series demonstrates multiple aphthous ulcers seen as spots of dense barium surrounded by a lucent halo (*arrows*). Aphthous ulcers are superficial mucosal erosions that do not penetrate the muscularis mucosae. (Case courtesy of C. John Rosenquist, M.D., University of California, Davis.)

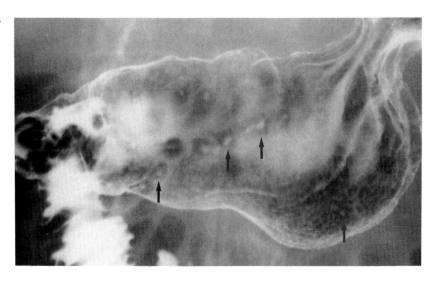

thickened nodular folds, limited distensibility, and poor peristalsis.

Crohn's gastritis appears identical to acute erosive gastritis. The disease characteristically involves the gastric antrum and proximal duodenum.

Phlegmonous gastritis is an acute, often fatal, bacterial infection of the stomach. α-Hemolytic streptococci are the most common cause, but a variety of other bacteria have also been identified. It may arise as a complication of septicemia, gastric surgery, or gastric ulcers. Multiple abscesses are formed in the gastric wall, which is markedly thickened. The rugae are swollen. Barium may penetrate into abscess crypts in the gastric wall. Peritonitis develops in 70% of cases. Healing usually results in a severely contracted stomach.

Emphysematous gastritis is a form of phlegmonous gastritis caused by gas-producing organisms, usually *Escherichia coli* or *Clostridium welchii*. Multiple gas bubbles are apparent within the wall of the stomach.

Eosinophilic gastroenteritis is a diffuse infiltration of the wall of the stomach and small bowel by eosinophils. Any or all layers of the wall may be involved. The condition is associated with a peripheral eosinophilia as high as 60%. Initially, the folds are markedly thickened and nodular, especially in the antrum. When chronic, the antrum is narrowed with a nodular "cobblestone" mucosal pattern.

Ménétrier's disease, also called giant hypertrophic gastritis, is a rare condition characterized by excessive mucus production, giant mucosal hypertrophy, hypoproteinemia, and hypochlorhydria. The UGI series demonstrate markedly enlarged and tortuous but pliable folds with hypersecretion (Fig. 26.11). Computed tomography exhibits wall thickening and nodular thick folds.

Gastric Ulcers

An ulcer is defined as a full-thickness defect in the mucosa. It frequently extends into the deeper layers of the stomach, including the submucosa and muscularis propria. About 95% of ulcerating gastric lesions are benign. All gastric ulcers should be examined endoscopically or be followed to complete radiographic healing.

Signs of an ulcer as demonstrated by a double-contrast UGI series include (*a*) a barium-filled crater on the dependent wall, (*b*) a ring shadow due to barium coating the edge of the crater on the nondependent wall, (*c*) a double ring shadow if the base of the ulcer is broader than the neck, and (*d*) a crescentic or semilunar line when the ulcer is seen on tangent oblique view. Some ulcers may be linear or rod-shaped.

Peptic Ulcer Disease. The pathogenesis of peptic disease is uncertain, despite extensive interest and investigation. Duodenal ulcers are usually associated with increased production of acid, while patients with gastric ulcers may have normal or even decreased acid levels. However, hydrochloric acid must be present for peptic ulceration to occur. Patients usually present with aching or burning pain within several hours after eating. Some patients with ulcers may be asymptomatic. The major complications of peptic ulcer disease are bleeding, obstruction, and perforation. Bleeding occurs in as many as 15–20% of patients. It is manifest by melena, hematemesis, or hematochezia. Gastric outlet obstruction complicates about 5% of cases. Ulcers may perforate into the free abdominal cavity or penetrate into adjacent organs. Free perforations generally present with an acute abdomen. Ulcer penetration into an adjacent organ is usually heralded by a marked increase in abdominal pain.

Benign Ulcers. The hallmark of benign ulcers and the basis for most radiographic signs of benignancy is mucosa that is intact to the very edge of an

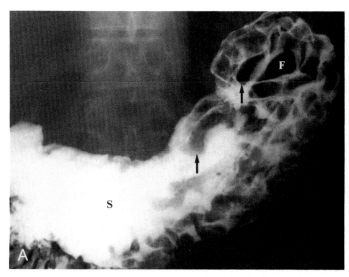

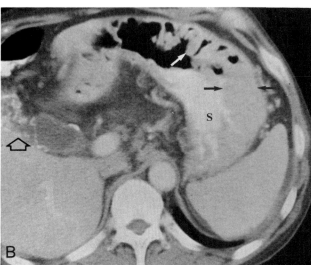

Figure 26.11. Ménétrièr's Disease. A. An UGI series reveals marked thickening of the mucosal folds (*arrows*) in the fundus (*F*) and proximal body of the stomach (*S*). **B.** A CT scan of the same patient confirms the marked thickening of the folds (*arrows*) of the stomach (*S*). This patient also had calcification of the wall of the gallbladder (*open arrow*).

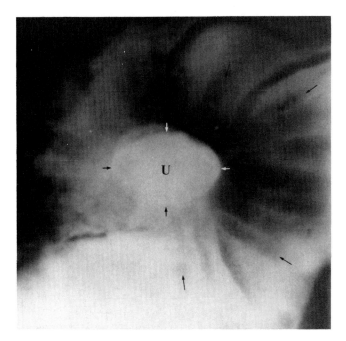

Figure 26.12. Benign Gastric Ulcer. Spot film from an UGI demonstrates a large benign gastric ulcer (*U, small arrows*). Prominent, well-defined folds (*larger arrows*) radiate to the ulcer crater.

undermining ulcer crater. However, it should be recognized that even if the ulcers are radiographically "benign," as many as 3% will actually be malignant. Demonstration of complete and sustained healing is considered the only reliable radiographic evidence of benign ulcer. Signs of benignancy include (*a*) a smooth ulcer mound with tapering edges, (*b*) an edematous ulcer collar with overhanging mucosal edge, (*c*) an ulcer projecting beyond the expected lumen, (*d*) radiating folds extending into the crater (Fig. 26.12), (*e*) depth of

ulcer greater than width, (*f*) sharply marginated contour, and (*g*) Hampton's line (a thin, sharp, lucent line that traverses the orifice of the ulcer). Hampton's line is caused by an overhanging gastric mucosa in an undermined ulcer. It is best demonstrated on spot films obtained with compression.

The size, depth, and location of the ulcer, and the contour of the ulcer base are of no diagnostic value in differentiating benign from malignant ulcers. The differential diagnosis of "benign ulcer" includes peptic disease, gastritis, hyperparathyroidism, radiotherapy, and Zollinger-Ellison syndrome.

Malignant Ulcers demonstrate signs that are the antithesis of benign ulcers. Evidence of irregular tumor mass or infiltration of the surrounding mucosa is evidence of malignancy. Signs of malignancy include (*a*) an ulcer within the lumen of the stomach, (*b*) an ulcer eccentrically located within the tumor mound, (*c*) a shallow ulcer with a width greater than its depth, (*d*) nodular, rolled, irregular, or shouldered edges, and (*e*) Carmen meniscus sign (describes a large flat-based ulcer with heaped-up edges that fold inward to trap a lens-shaped barium collection that is convex toward the lumen) (Fig. 26.13). The differential diagnosis of "malignant ulcer" includes gastric adenocarcinoma, lymphoma, leiomyoma, and leiomyosarcoma.

Computed tomography is useful in demonstrating the extent of the tumor mass and the degree of involvement of the gastric wall.

DUODENUM
Duodenal Filling Defects/Mass Lesions

In the duodenal bulb, 90% of tumors are benign. In the second and third portions of the duodenum, tu-

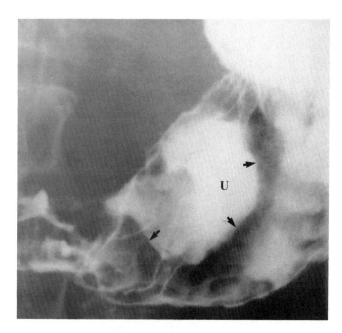

Figure 26.13.   Carmen Meniscus Sign. A large, flat malignant ulcer (*U*) traps barium within its rounded edges, seen as a band of lucency (*arrows*) surrounding the barium collection. The barium collection is convex toward the gastric lumen.

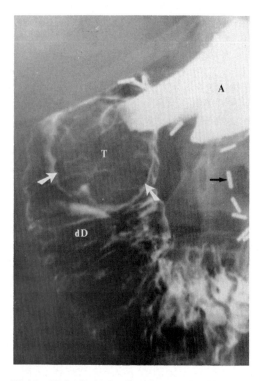

Figure 26.14.   Metastasis to Duodenum. Double-contrast view demonstrates a lobulated tumor (*T, white arrows*) within the lumen of the descending duodenum (*dD*). Surgical biopsy revealed renal cell carcinoma metastatic to the duodenum. The surgical clips (*black arrow*) are from a radical left nephrectomy. *A,* antrum of the stomach.

mors are 50% benign and 50% malignant. In the fourth portion of the duodenum, most tumors are ma-

lignant. Small, benign tumors of the duodenum usually present as smooth, polypoid filling defects. Except for larger lipomas which may be diagnosed by CT, precise diagnosis must be made by biopsy since these tumors are radiographically indistinguishable (8).

Duodenal Adenocarcinoma, while being the most frequent malignant tumor of the duodenum, is a rare lesion. Malignant tumors are most common in the periampullary region and are rare in the bulb. Morphologic patterns include polypoid mass, ulcerative mass, and annular constricting lesion. Metastases to regional lymph nodes are present in two-thirds of patients at presentation. Computed tomography demonstrates the local extent of the tumor, as well as nodal and liver metastases (8, 9).

Metastases to the duodenum may occur in the wall or subserosa of the duodenum. As the tumor grows it may extend into the lumen and present as an intraluminal mass (Fig. 26.14) that may ulcerate. The most common primaries are breast, lung, and other gastrointestinal malignancies.

Lymphoma in the duodenum usually presents as nodules with thickened folds (6). The nodules associated with lymphoma are distinctly larger than those seen with benign lymphoid hyperplasia.

Duodenal Adenoma usually presents as a polypoid lesion that may be pedunculated or sessile. Multiple adenomatous polyps are associated with polyposis syndromes. Villous adenomas have a high incidence of malignant degeneration and a characteristic "cauliflower" appearance on double-contrast UGI series.

Leiomyoma and Leiomyosarcoma present as an intramural, endoluminal, or exophytic mass. Ulceration is common. Leiomyosarcoma ranges up to 20 cm size and is most common in the more distal duodenum. Leiomyosarcoma is the second most common primary malignant tumor of the duodenum.

Lipoma of the duodenum is a soft tumor that may grow to large size. A definitive diagnosis can be made by CT demonstration of a uniform fat density mass (8, 9).

Lymphoid Hyperplasia presents as small (1–3 mm) polypoid nodules diffusely throughout the duodenum. The condition is usually benign, especially in children. It is associated with immunodeficiency states in some adults. There is no evidence that lymphoid hyperplasia is a precursor to lymphoma.

Gastric Mucosal Prolapse/Heterotopic Gastric Mucosa. Gastric mucosa may prolapse through the pylorus during peristalsis and cause a lobulated filling defect at the base of the duodenal bulb. The diagnosis is suggested by characteristic location and change in configuration with peristalsis.

Heterotopic gastric mucosa in the duodenal bulb is common histologically but less frequently evident radiographically. The lesion most commonly has the appearance of areae gastricae in the duodenal bulb. It may also appear as a solitary polyp that is indistinguishable from other polypoid lesions of the duodenum.

Brunner's Gland Hyperplasia/Adenoma. Brunner's glands are located in the submucosa of the proximal duodenum and secrete an alkaline substance into the lumen. Diffuse nodular gland hyperplasia is a common cause of multiple filling defects and is associated with hyperacidity. Brunner's gland adenoma presents as a solitary filling defect and is identical in appearance to other benign duodenal nodules.

Ectopic Pancreas may also occur in the duodenum, most commonly in the proximal descending portion. A solitary mass with a central dimple is most characteristic.

Extrinsic Mass impressions on the duodenum may be made by the gallbladder, masses in the liver, pancreas, adrenal gland, kidney, or colon, pancreatic fluid collections, adenopathy, or aneurysms.

Thickened Duodenal Folds

The valvulae conniventes, or Kerckring's folds, of the small bowel begin in the second portion of the duodenum and continue throughout the remainder of the small bowel. The valvulae conniventes are permanent circular folds of mucosa supported by a core of fibrovascular submucosa. They are normally several millimeters wide and remain visible even with full distension of the duodenum. Folds greater than 2–3 mm wide are usually considered thickened.

Normal Variant. Thickened folds are a nonspecific radiographic finding that may be found in normal individuals. The radiographic diagnosis of a pathologic condition is more confident when there are additional findings.

Duodenitis refers to nonspecific inflammation of the duodenum without discrete ulcer formation. Thickened folds may be the only radiographic manifestation. Severe cases (erosive duodenitis) show aphthous ulcers and erosions.

Pancreatitis and Cholecystitis thicken the duodenal folds by paraduodenal inflammation. Both may also cause mass impressions on the duodenal lumen. Computed tomography or ultrasound demonstrate the extent and nature of the paraduodenal process.

Crohn's Disease of the duodenum usually involves the first and second portions, and is almost always associated with contiguous involvement of the stomach. Duodenal involvement is manifest by thickened folds, aphthous ulcers, erosions, and single or multiple strictures.

Parasites. Giardiasis is due to an overgrowth of the parasite *Giardia lamblia* in the duodenum and jejunum. Many patients are asymptomatic carriers, but patients with invasion of the gut wall have abdominal pain, diarrhea, and malabsorption. Radiographic findings include spasm, distorted thickened folds, and hypersecretion.

Strongyloidiasis is caused by infection with the nematode, *Strongyloides stercoralis*, found in all areas of the world but most common in the warm, moist regions of the tropics. As with giardiasis, many patients are asymptomatic carriers. Invasion of the intestinal wall causes vomiting and malabsorption. The UGI findings include edematous folds, spasm, dilation of the proximal duodenum, and diffuse mucosal ulceration.

Lymphoma presents with nodular thickened folds (6).

Intramural Hemorrhage is caused by trauma, anticoagulation, and bleeding disorders. The regular pattern of thickened folds resembles a stack of coins. Partial or complete duodenal obstruction is usually present. The fixed retroperitoneal position of the third portion of the duodenum makes it susceptible to blunt abdominal trauma and compression against the lumbar spine.

Duodenal Ulcers and Diverticuli

Peptic Ulcer Disease clinically affects the duodenum three to four times as often as the stomach. Duodenal ulcers are associated with acid hypersecretion. Ninety- five percent are in the duodenal bulb with the anterior wall being most often involved. Radiographic diagnosis of a duodenal ulcer depends upon demonstration of the ulcer crater or niche. En face the crater appears as a persistent collection of barium or air. In profile, ulcers project beyond the normal lumen (Fig. 26.15). Thickened folds often radiate toward the ulcer crater which may be surrounded by a mound of edema. While the shape is usually round or oval, linear ulcers also occur. Giant ulcers larger than 2 cm may resemble diverticuli or a deformed bulb. Ulcer craters have no mucosal lining, so therefore have no mucosal relief pattern and do not contract with peristalsis. Ulcer scarring may cause a pattern of radiating folds with a central barium collection that is indistinguishable from an acute ulcer. Endoscopy may be required to make the differentiation. Postbulbar ulcers represent about 5% of the total. Most involve the second and third portions of the duodenum, which are frequently narrowed.

Complications of duodenal ulcer disease include obstruction, bleeding, and perforation. Bleeding from a duodenal ulcer is most efficiently diagnosed endoscopically. Perforation may be manifest by pneumoperitoneum or a localized abnormal gas collection. Peptic duodenal ulcer is not a premalignant condition.

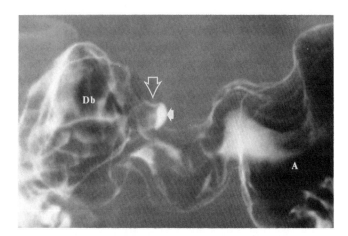

Figure 26.15. Peptic Ulcer. A UGI series demonstrates a persistent barium collection (*closed arrow*) that projects beyond the lumen of the base of the duodenal bulb (*Db*). A well-defined ulcer collar (*open arrow*) is present. *A*, gastric antrum.

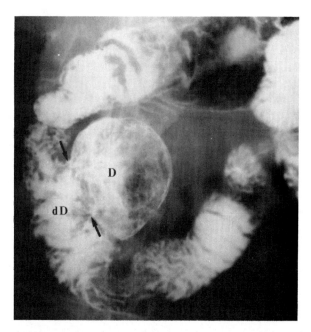

Figure 26.16. Duodenal Diverticulum. Radiograph from an UGI series demonstrates contrast and air filling a duodenal diverticulum (*D*) that originates from the medial aspect of the descending duodenum (*dD*). The neck of the duodenum is indicated by the *arrows*. (From Stone EE, Brant WE, Smith G. Computed tomography of duodenal diverticula. J Comput Assist Tomogr 1989;13:61–64.)

Figure 26.17. Duodenal Diverticulum. A CT scan demonstrates a diverticulum (*D*) of the descending duodenum (*dD*) that is completely fluid-filled and extends into the pancreatic bed, mimicking a pancreatic psuedocyst. *S*, stomach. *sv*, splenic vein. (From Stone EE, Brant WE, Smith G. Computed tomography of duodenal diverticula. J Comput Assist Tomogr 1989;13:61–64.)

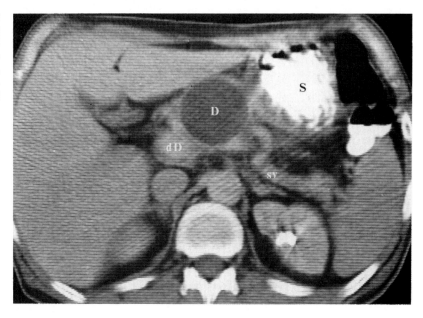

Zollinger-Ellison Syndrome is caused by a gastrin-secreting islet cell tumor of the pancreas. Continuous gastrin secretion results in marked hyperacidity and multiple peptic ulcers in the duodenum, stomach, and jejunum. Multiple recurrent or intractible postbulbar ulcers should suggest the diagnosis. Associated findings include thickened duodenal and gastric folds, Brunner's gland hyperplasia, prominent areae gastricae, and excessive gastric secretions. The islet cell tumor is malignant in 60% of cases.

Flexural Pseudotumors are a common cause of a duodenal filling defect with a central barium collection, mimicking an ulcerated lesions. They appear as rounded, swirled mucosal folds on the inner aspect of the flexure at the apex of the bulb. They are due to redundant mucosa and have a variable appearance on different projections.

Duodenal Diverticula are common (5% of UGI series) and usually incidental findings. They may be multiple and may form in any portion of the duodenum, but are most common along the inner aspect of the descending duodenum (Fig 26.16). Diverticula are differentiated from ulcers on a UGI series by demonstration of mucosal folds entering the neck of the diverticulum and change in appearance with peristalsis. On plain abdominal radiographs, duodenal diverticuli may be seen as abnormal air collections. On CT they may be filled with fluid and mimic a pancreatic pseudocyst (Fig. 26.17), or contain air and fluid and mimic a pancreatic abscess (10). Rare complications include perforation and hemorrhage. Diverticuli adjacent to the ampulla of Vater may rarely obstruct the common bile duct or pancreatic duct.

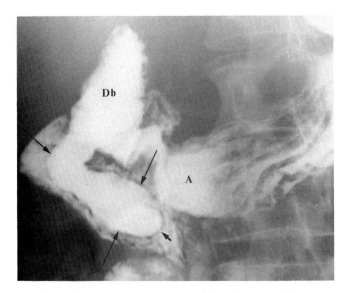

Figure 26.18.   Intraluminal Diverticulum. A UGI series demonstrates a barium-filled "sock" (*long arrows*) within the lumen of the descending duodenum. The radiolucent wall of the diverticulum (*short arrow*) is outlined by barium, both within the diverticulum and within the lumen of the duodenum. *Db,* duodenal bulb. *A,* gastric antrum.

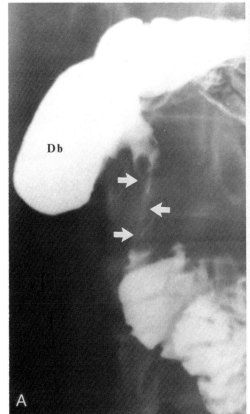

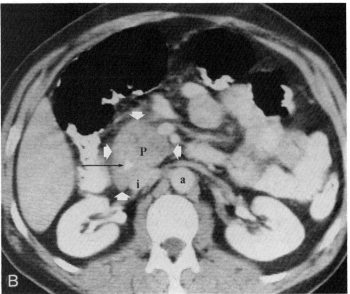

Figure 26.19.   Annular Pancreas. A. An UGI series demonstrates a 3-cm long circumferentially narrowed segment (*arrows*) of the descending duodenum. No ulceration was evident. *Db,* duodenal bulb. **B.** A CT scan reveals normal pancreatic tissue (*P, white arrows*) encircling the narrowed descending duodenum (*black arrow*) confirming the diagnosis of annular pancreas. *i,* inferior vena cava. *a,* aorta.

Intraluminal diverticula are caused by a thin, incomplete, congenital diaphragm that is stretched by moving intraluminal contents to form a "wind-sock" configuration within the duodenum (Fig. 26.18).

Duodenal Narrowing

Annular Pancreas is the most common congenital anomaly of the pancreas. Pancreatic tissue encircles the descending duodenum and narrows its lumen (Fig. 26.19). The abnormality occurs when the bilobed ventral component of the pancreas fuses with the dorsal pancreas on both sides of the duodenum (11). Although it often presents in childhood, especially in children with Down's syndrome, about half of the cases do not present until adulthood. Symptomatic adults present with nausea, vomiting, abdominal pain, and occasionally jaundice. The UGI series typically demonstrates eccentric or concentric narrowing of the descending duodenum. Annular pancreas is associated with a high incidence of postbulbar peptic ulceration in adults. Computed tomography confirms the diagnosis by demonstration of pancreatic tissue encircling the duodenum. Endoscopic retrograde cholangiopancreatography demonstrates an annular pancreatic duct encircling the duodenum.

Duodenal Adenocarcinoma can present as a circumferential constricting lesion with tumor shoulders giving evidence of mass effect. Ulceration is common. Computed tomography demonstrates the extent of the lesion.

Lymphoma causes marked wall thickening and bulky paraduodenal lymphadenopathy that may narrow the lumen.

Postbulbar Ulcer is commonly associated with narrowing of the lumen of the second and third portions of the duodenum.

Extrinsic Compression because of inflammation or tumor in adjacent organs, especially the pancreas, may constrict the duodenal lumen.

Upper Gastrointestinal Hemorrhage

Upper gastrointestinal hemorrhage refers to bleeding with the site of origin proximal to the ligament of Treitz. This hemorrhage has an average mortality of 8–10%. Causes in an approximate order of frequency are (a) duodenal ulcer, (b) esophageal varices, (c) gastric ulcer, (d) acute hemorrhagic gastritis, (e) esophagitis, (f) Mallory-Weiss tear, (g) neoplasm, (h) vascular malformation, and (i) vascular enteric fistula.

Barium studies should be avoided in the acute stages of UGI hemorrhage. Endoscopy is much more accurate than a UGI series in demonstrating the bleeding site (95% versus 45%). The UGI series may identify a lesion but does not indicate whether that lesion is responsible for the bleeding. Also, retained barium in the gastrointestinal tract following a UGI series will usually make performing angiography impossible. Angiography is useful to localize active bleeding sites and provide therapy by infusion of vasoconstrictors or performance of transcatheter embolization.

References

1. Gelfand DW. Correlative studies reveal efficacy of GI radiology. Diagnostic Imaging 1986;May:114–119.
2. Kaye MD, Young SW, Hayward R, Castellino RA. Gastric pseudotumor on CT scanning. AJR 1980;135:190–193.
3. Levine MS, Kong V, Rubesin SE, et al. Scirrhous carcinoma of the stomach: radiologic and endoscopic diagnosis. Radiology 1990;175:151–154.
4. Sussman SK, Halvorsen RA Jr, Illescas FF, et al. Gastric adenocarcinoma: CT versus surgical staging. Radiology 1988;167:335–340.
5. American Joint Committee on Cancer. Manual for staging of cancer. 4th ed. Philadelphia: JB Lippincott Company, 1992:63–66.
6. Smith C, Kubicka RA, Thomas CR Jr. Non-Hodgkin lymphoma of the gastrointestinal tract. Radiographics 1992;12:887–899.
7. Megibow AJ, Balthazar EJ, Hulnick DH, et al. CT evaluation of gastrointestinal leiomyomas and leiomyosarcomas. AJR 1985;144:727–731.
8. Kazerooni EA, Quint LE, Francis IR. Duodenal neoplasms: predictive value of CT for determining malignancy and tumor resectability. AJR 1992;159:303–309.
9. Farah MC, Jafri SZH, Schwab RE, et al. Duodenal neoplasms: role of CT. Radiology 1987;162:839–843.
10. Stone EE, Brant WE, Smith G. Computed tomography of duodenal diverticula. J Comput Assist Tomogr 1989;13:61–64.
11. Pantoja E, Nagy F, Thomas HA Jr, et al. Annular pancreas. Medical Radiography and Photography 1985;61(3):2–9.

27

Mesenteric Small Bowel

William E. Brant

Imaging Methods
Anatomy
Small Bowel Filling Defects/Mass Lesions
Mesenteric Masses
Diffuse Small Bowel Disease
Small Bowel Erosions and Ulcerations
Small Bowel Diverticula

Imaging Methods

Disease of the mesenteric small intestine is relatively rare. Detailed radiographic study of the small bowel is justified only when clinical suspicion of small bowel disease is high. Small bowel disease is usually manifest by four major symptoms: colic, diarrhea, malabsorption, and bleeding (1). Colic is defined as recurrent and spasmodic abdominal pain with periods of relief every 2–3 minutes. Diarrhea caused by small bowel disease is less urgent than that caused by colon disease. Malabsorption is manifest by steatorrhea, foul-smelling stools, and weight loss. Bleeding from small bowel disease is usually occult and manifest by anemia. Because the majority of the mesenteric small intestine is out of reach of the endoscopist, diagnostic radiology has the primary responsibility for its evaluation.

The traditional method for radiographic examination of the small bowel is the small bowel follow-through examination (Fig. 27.1) tacked onto a standard upper gastrointestinal series. The patient is asked to continue drinking barium while a series of supine abdominal films are obtained until the terminal ileum and cecum are filled with barium. Fluoroscopic examination of the small bowel is then attempted. This study is notoriously insensitive. It is limited by overlap of bowel loops, poor distension, flocculation of barium, intermittent barium filling, and unpredictable transit time.

Enteroclysis, or the small bowel enema, is the preferred method for detailed radiographic examination (Fig. 27.2) (1). This study provides more uniform distension of the bowel, even distribution of barium, su-

perior anatomic detail, and shorter overall examination time. The study is performed by passing a specially designed 12-14 French enteroclysis catheter through the mouth or nose and into the distal duodenum or proximal jejunum. A guidewire is used for directional control of the catheter during manipulation under fluoroscopy. The study may be performed single contrast using approximately 600 ml of barium or

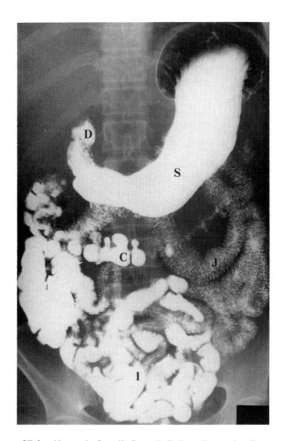

Figure 27.1. Normal Small Bowel Follow-through. The small bowel is demonstrated on an upper gastrointestinal series by having the patient ingest additional barium and by taking additional radiographs to document passage of barium through the small bowel into the colon. The loops of jejunum (*J*) have a delicate feathery appearance in the left upper abdomen, while the loops of ileum (*I*) are coarse and featureless in the right lower abdomen. Barium has filled portions of the ascending and transverse colon (*C*), identified by its haustral folds. Colonic haustral folds extend only partway across the bowel lumen, while small bowel folds extend completely across the bowel lumen. *S*, stomach. *D*, duodenum.

Table 27.1.   Diagnostic Findings of CT of the Gastrointestinal Tract

Benign Lesion	Neoplastic Lesion
Circumferential thickening	Eccentric thickening
Symmetrical thickening	Asymmetric thickening
Thickening <1 cm	Thickening >2 cm
Segmental or diffuse involvement	Focal soft tissue mass
Thickened mesenteric fat	Abrupt transition
Wall is homogeneous soft tissue density	Lobulated contour
"Double halo sign"—dark inner ring/bright outer ring	Spiculated outer contour
"Target sign"—bright inner-dark, middle-bright outer	Luminal narrowing
	Regional adenopathy
	Liver metastases

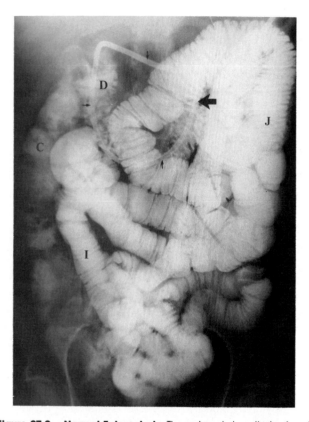

Figure 27.2.   Normal Enteroclysis. The enteroclysis catheter (*small arrows*) has been passed through the C-loop of the duodenum to the location of the ligament of Treitz (*large arrow*), using fluoroscopy to guide catheter manipulation. The enteroclysis technique provides uniform distension of the jejunum (*J*) and ileum (*I*). Barium fills portions of the ascending colon (*C*). Note the small bowel folds crossing the entire diameter of the small bowel lumen. *D,* duodenum.

double contrast using 200 ml of barium followed by 1000 ml of methylcellulose to advance the barium and distend the bowel.

The small bowel lumen and mucosal surface are best demonstrated by barium studies. Computed tomography complements the barium examination by demonstrating the extraluminal component of bowel disease (Table 27.1) (2, 3). In addition, CT evaluates

the mesentery, adjacent solid organs, the peritoneal cavity, and the retroperitoneum.

Ultrasound demonstrates the floating bowel loops in ascites and the dilated small bowel in ileus and small bowel obstruction (see Fig. 22.10). Real-time ultrasound may be used to evaluate peristalsis and help differentiate ileus and obstruction. Large small bowel masses and masses in the mesentery may be characterized by ultrasound.

Anatomy

The mesenteric small intestine is a tube approximately 7 m in length that lies totally within the greater peritoneal cavity. The jejunum is arbitrarily defined as the proximal two-fifths of the mesenteric intestine, while the ileum is the distal three-fifths (1). The jejunum and ileum are suspended from the posterior abdominal wall by the small bowel mesentery. The small bowel mesentery is composed of connective tissue, blood vessels, and lymphatic vessels, and is covered by peritoneum, which reflects from the posterior parietal peritoneum. The root of the small bowel mesentery extends obliquely from the ligament of Treitz, just left of the L-2 vertebra, to the cecum, near the right sacroiliac joint. On CT the mesentery is defined by its normal vascular structures outlined by fat between loops of bowel. Normal mesenteric lymph nodes may be seen as soft tissue density nodules 5 mm or less in size. The concave border of the small bowel loops is the mesenteric border where the mesentery attaches. The convex border, facing away from the mesentery, is called the antimesenteric border. Identification of the border involved by disease can be of diagnostic value.

On CT and barium studies, the jejunum has a feathery mucosal pattern, more prominent valvulae conniventes, a wider lumen, and a thicker wall. The ileum has a less featured mucosal pattern, thinner, less frequent folds, narrower lumen, and a thinner wall. The transition between jejunum and ileum is gradual, and all loops are freely mobile. The general structure of the layers of the small bowel wall is shown in Figure 26.1. The ileum has larger and more numerous lymphoid follicles in the submucosa. Villi are finger-like projections that extend from the entire mucosal surface of the small bowel. They are composed of loose connective tissue of the lamina propria. Tiny capillaries and lymphatic vessels (lacteals) extend to the submucosal vessels. The combination of valvulae conniventes and villi greatly expands the absorptive surface area of the small intestine. The caliber of the normal small bowel lumen is less than 3 cm with normal fold thickness of less than 3 mm and normal wall thickness of 2–3 mm (3).

Small Bowel Filling Defects/Mass Lesions

Neoplasms of the small intestine are rare accounting for only 2–3% of gastrointestinal tumors. Benign neoplasms are about equal to malignant neoplasms in overall frequency. However, when the patient presents with symptoms, malignancy is three times more common. Presenting afflictions include obstruction, pain, weight loss, bleeding, and palpable mass.

Carcinoid tumors are the most common neoplasm of the small intestine, accounting for about one-third of all small bowel tumors. They are considered a low-grade malignancy that may recur locally or metastasize to the lymph nodes, liver, or lung (1, 4). They arise from endocrine cells (enterochromaffin or Kulchitsky cells) deep in the mucosa. These cells produce vasoactive substances including serotonin and bradykinins. About 20% of all carcinoid tumors arise in the small bowel, most commonly in the ileum where 30% are multiple (4). Only 7%, those with liver metastases, present with carcinoid syndrome (cutaneous flushing, abdominal cramps and diarrhea) because the liver inactivates the vasoactive substances. The tumors grow slowly but are associated with a marked fibrotic response of the bowel wall and mesentery because the serotonin produced by the tumor induces an intense local desmoplastic reaction. Complications include stricture, obstruction, and bowel infarction induced by fibrosis of the mesenteric vessels. The tumors may be pedunculated and cause intussusception. Barium studies demonstrate mural nodules, usually smaller than 1.5 cm. Fixation of bowel loops and luminal narrowing may resemble Crohn's disease. Computed tomography findings may be virtually pathognomonic of carcinoid tumor (2). The primary lesion in the terminal ileum is seen as a small, lobulated soft tissue mass, occasionally with central calcification. A sunburst pattern of radiating soft tissue density is seen in the mesenteric fat. Adjacent loops of small bowel are fixed in position and distorted in appearance by the fibrosis in the mesentery.

Adenocarcinoma of the small bowel is about half as common as carcinoid tumor (1). It is most frequent in the duodenum and proximal jejunum, and is uncommon in the distal ileum, where carcinoid is most common. Most patients are symptomatic at presentation, and 30% have a palpable mass. Patients with adult celiac disease and Crohn's disease are at increased risk for small bowel carcinoma. Complications include bleeding, obstruction, and intussusception. Prognosis is poor, with a 5-year survival of 20%. Metastatic spread is by intraperitoneal seeding, lymphatic channels to regional nodes, and portal veins to the liver. Morphologically the tumor may be infiltrating, producing strictures; polypoid, producing filling defects; or ulcerating. The most common appearance on barium studies is an "apple core" stricture of the small bowel (1). Computed tomography demonstrates short segment asymmetric, irregular, circumferential thickening of the bowel wall, or an eccentric focal mass (Table 27.1).

Lymphoma is responsible for about 20% of all small bowel malignant tumors (5). The gastrointestinal tract is the most common site for extranodal origin of lymphoma, and the small bowel is most commonly involved. Most cases are non-Hodgkin's lymphoma. Non-Hodgkin's lymphoma clinically involves the gastrointestinal tract in 30% of cases overall. Lymphoma is most frequent in the terminal ileum where the concentration of lymphoid tissue is the greatest. Morphologic patterns of involvement include diffuse infiltration, exophytic mass, polypoid mass, and multiple nodules (1, 5). Barium studies most commonly reveal the infiltrative form with wall thickening, effacement of folds, and a wide lumen. Shallow ulceration is common, but strictures are rare. In fact, aneurysmal dilation of the lumen is a feature of lymphoma due to replacement of the muscularis and destruction of the autonomic plexus by tumor. Perforation is a danger, particularly along the unsupported antimesenteric border. Excavations in communication with the lumen are caused by ulceration and closed-off perforation into a lymphoid mass in the mesentery.

Polypoid masses of lymphoma may cause intussusception. The pattern of multiple nodules is uncommon. The nodules cause multiple filling defects that are larger than 4 mm, variable in size, and nonuniform in distribution. Computed tomography demonstrates nodular eccentric wall thickening, nodules, and polypoid masses (Fig. 27.3). Exophytic lymphoma is generally of uniform soft tissue density and enhances little, if any with intravenous contrast administration. This is a differentiating finding in comparison with leiomyosarcoma and adenocarcinoma, which usually enhance prominently. Computed tomography readily demonstrates associated findings of

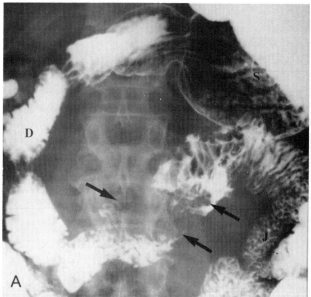 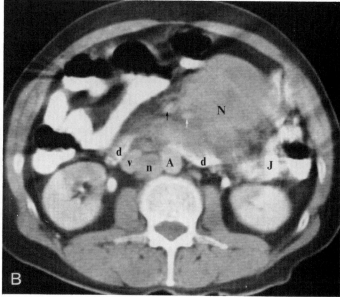

Figure 27.3. Non-Hodgkins Lymphoma. A. An UGI series demonstrates polypoid filling defects (*arrows*) in the third portion of the duodenum (*D*). The duodenal C-loop is widened and the jejunum (*J*) is displaced laterally. *S*, stomach. **B.** A CT scan of the same patient demonstrates the full extent of disease. A large mass of confluent enlarged lymph nodes (*N*) compresses and invades the duodenum (*d*), and displaces the jejunum (*J*). The adenopathy surrounds the superior mesenteric artery (*small white arrow*) and vein (*small black arrow*) creating a CT sandwich sign. An enlarged lymph node (*n*) is seen between the inferior vena cava (*v*) and the aorta (*A*).

lymphoma including mesenteric and retroperitoneal adenopathy and hepatosplenomegaly. The mesentery may show a large confluent mass encasing multiple bowel loops or enlarged individual nodes (Fig. 27.3**B**). The "sandwich sign," characteristic of lymphoma, refers to sparing of rind of fat surrounding mesenteric vessels encased by lymphoma.

Burkitt's lymphoma in North America usually presents with intestinal involvement, especially of the ileocecal area in children and young adults. The malignancy is aggressive, with rapid doubling time and poor prognosis. Imaging studies show bulky tumors.

Acquired immunodeficiency syndrome-related lymphoma is an aggressive high-grade non-Hodgkin's lymphoma with poor prognosis. Extranodal involvement, including small bowel lymphoma, is common. Adenopathy may be due to lymphoma, Kaposi's sarcoma, or *Mycobacterium avium-intracellulare* infection (see Table 22.9).

Mediterranean lymphoma, or immunoproliferative small intestinal disease, has been described in young adult Arabs and Jews of the Mediterranean area, Mexican Americans, and South African blacks (1). The disease progresses from plasma cell infiltrate of the proximal small bowel to immunoblastic NHL. It presents with malabsorption and diarrhea mimicking celiac disease. Involved segments of the bowel demonstrate features of lymphoma as described above.

Nodular Lymphoid Hyperplasia may involve the entire small bowel. The condition is differentiated from lymphoma by the uniform small size of the nod-

ules (2–4 mm) and even distribution through the area of involvement (see Fig. 28.7). Lymphoid hyperplasia confined to the terminal ileum and proximal colon is usually considered incidental and may be related to recent viral infection. Diffuse lymphoid hyperplasia is associated with hypogammaglobulinemia, especially low IgA.

Metastases to the small bowel are common. The two most frequent routes are by peritoneal seeding, usually involving the mesenteric border, and by hematogenous spread, which usually implants on the antimesenteric border. Intraperitoneal implantation of the small bowel serosa is most commonly due to ovarian carcinoma in women, and colon, gastric, and pancreatic carcinoma in men. The mesenteric border of the small bowel is favored by the flow of fluid along the small bowel mesentery from the left upper to the right lower abdomen. Implantation is most common along the terminal ileum, cecum, and ascending colon. Peritoneal implants on the parietal peritoneum, and omentum (omental cake), as well as in the pouch of Douglas, are demonstrated by CT. Barium studies demonstrate nodules and tethering of folds due to mesenteric fibrosis.

Hematogenous metastases are deposited along the antimesenteric border where the submucosal blood vessels arborize. Common primary malignancies are melanoma, lung, breast, and colon carcinoma, and embryonal cell carcinoma of the testes. Barium studies demonstrate mural nodules of uniform or varying

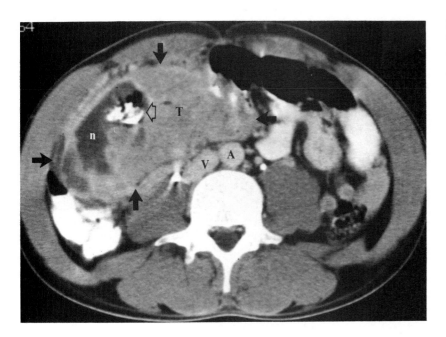

Figure 27.4. Leiomyosarcoma of the Ileum. Contrast-enhanced CT demonstrates a large tumor (*T*, between *closed arrows*) in the right abdomen encompassing a loop of ileum (*open arrow*). The tumor enhances with contrast (compare to muscle) and demonstrates low-density areas of necrosis (*n*). *V*, inferior vena cava. *A*, aorta.

size anywhere in the small bowel. They may appear as target lesions, or ulcerate or cavitate.

Kaposi's Sarcoma in AIDS patients commonly involves the small intestine. About half of the patients with skin lesions have intestinal lesions as well. Barium studies demonstrate multiple mural nodules, often centrally umbilicated. Computed tomography demonstrates mesenteric, retroperitoneal, and pelvic adenopathy.

Leiomyoma and Leiomyosarcoma. Leiomyoma is the most frequent benign neoplasm of the mesenteric small bowel. Eighty percent of small bowel leiomyomas occur in the jejunum and ileum and only 20% in the duodenum (1). They are circumscribed, round, or lobulated tumors of the bowel wall. They may project into the lumen, be pedunculated or exophytic. The overlying mucosa may ulcerate and be a source of intestinal bleeding. Computed tomography shows a focal, enhancing soft tissue mass. Angiography demonstrates a hypervascular mass.

Leiomyosarcoma represents about 8% of small bowel malignant tumors. The tumor is somewhat more common in the ileum than the jejunum. Most are exophytic and grow to large size, developing areas of necrosis and cystic changes. Ulceration and bleeding is common. They spread by direct extension to adjacent structures and by hematogenous routes to liver, lungs, and bone. Nodal metastases are uncommon. Like leiomyomatous tumors elsewhere, the malignant tumors are larger and more heterogeneous than benign tumors (Fig. 27.4). Computed tomography demonstrates the central tumor necrosis. Because the tumor is hypervascular, solid portions enhance avidly.

Adenoma accounts for about 20% of benign small bowel neoplasms. It is more common in the duode-

num than in the mesenteric small intestine. The tumor is a benign proliferation of glandular epithelium, and has the potential for malignant degeneration. Barium studies demonstate an intraluminal polyp with a finely lobulated surface.

Lipoma is most common in the ileum. The tumor arises from the fat of the submucosa. Lipomas account for about 17% of benign small bowel tumors. Most are asymptomatic incidental findings, although some cause bleeding or intussusception. Computed tomography demonstration of a fat density (−50 to −100 HU) tumor is diagnostic (2). Thin (5 mm) sections are recommended for the demonstration of fat density within small lesions.

Hemangioma is usually solitary and submucosal, projecting into the lumen as a polyp. These tumors are located predominantly in the jejunum. About two-thirds present with bleeding. Barium studies demonstrate a small polyp. The occasional presence of a calcified phlebolith suggests the diagnosis. They account for less than 10% of benign small bowel tumors.

Polyposis Syndromes cause multiple polypoid lesions of the small bowel. The differential diagnosis includes metastases, lymphoma, nodular lymphoid hyperplasia, Kaposi's sarcoma, and carcinoid tumors.

Peutz-Jeghers syndrome consists of multiple hamartomatous polyps in the small intestine associated with melanin pigmentation on the facial skin, palmar aspects of the fingers and toes, and mucous membranes (6). Most cases occur with autosomal dominant inheritance. Hamartomatous polyps are a nonneoplastic, abnormal proliferation of all three layers of the mucosa, epithelium, lamina propria, and muscularis mucosae. Hamartomatous polyps are most common in the jejunum, are usually pedunculated, and are variable in size up to 4 cm. Additional

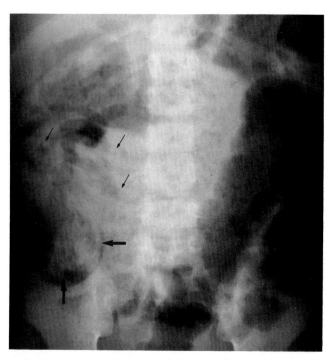

Figure 27.5. Ascaris Infestation. Plain radiograph demonstrates diffuse intestinal dilation. Roundworms in the ileum are seen as round and tubular soft tissue densities outlined by intestinal gas (*small arrows*). A large bolus of entangled worms (*large arrows*) plugged the distal ileum, causing small bowel obstruction.

polyps are often found in the stomach and colon. Some of these polyps are adenomatous and premalignant. Patients with Peutz-Jeghers syndrome also have a greatly increased risk of extraintestinal malignancy. Most patients present with colicky abdominal pain due to intermittent intussusception. Barium studies demonstrates myriad polyps in involved areas of small intestine, separated by normal bowel segments.

Gardner's syndrome of inherited adenomatous polyposis coli usually includes a few adenomatous polyps in the small bowel.

Juvenile gastrointestinal polyposis is most common in the colon but occasionally involves the small bowel. Inflammatory polyps containing cysts filled with mucin develop secondary to chronic irritation. Most are round, smooth, and pedunculated.

Cronkhite-Canada syndrome involves the small bowel in about half the cases with multiple inflammatory polyps. The colon and stomach are always involved.

Ascariasis is caused by infestation with the roundworm *Ascaris lumbricoides*. Ascariasis is found worldwide, but is most common in Asia and Africa. Endemic areas in the United States include rural southern Appalachia and the Gulf Coast states. Infestation is acquired by ingesting food or water contaminated with *Ascaris* eggs. The eggs hatch in the small

bowel. Larvae penetrate the wall and migrate through the vascular system to the lungs, where they molt and grow before migrating up the bronchi and trachea to the larynx where they are again swallowed. Worms mature in the small bowel, especially in the jejunum, and may reach 15–35 cm in size. New generations of infective ova are excreted in feces. A large bolus of worms may obstruct the small bowel, especially in children, or cause intussusception. Worms can be identified on plain abdominal radiographs in 70% of cases (Fig. 27.5). Barium studies demonstrate worms as long linear filling defects. Barium ingested by the worms may be seen in their intestinal tract as a long, string-like white line.

Mesenteric Masses

Masses arising in the small bowel mesentery frequently present as a palpable abdominal mass. They may be related to disorders of the small intestine or be primary to the mesentery itself (7). Computed tomography and ultrasound provide the most diagnostic information. Lymphoma, carcinoid tumors, metastases, leiomyoma, and leiomyosarcoma may all have a prominent component of disease in the mesentery, and must also be considered.

Mesenteric Desmoid tumors are solid mesenteric masses (7). Most are associated with Gardner's syndrome, however, they may occur as an isolated lesion. Both ultrasound and CT demonstrate a heterogeneous solid mass.

Mesenteric Cyst arises in the root of the small bowel mesentery. Some authors consider them to be cystic lymphangiomas. They are usually unilocular cysts, occasionally containing a few septa. The internal fluid may be serous, bloody, or chylous. Ultrasound demonstrates a well-defined cyst with occasional fluid-debris or fluid-fat levels. Computed tomography demonstrates a cystic mass, displacing loops of small bowel anteriorly and laterally.

Gastrointestinal Duplication Cyst is a congenital, partial, or complete replica of the small bowel. Most arise from the distal small bowel and may communicate with the normal intestinal lumen at one or both ends, or not at all. They are lined by intestinal epithelium. They closely resemble mesenteric cysts on CT and ultrasound.

Mesenteric Teratoma is heterogeneous in composition. Calcium components demonstrated by CT or ultrasound are a clue to radiographic diagnosis.

Diffuse Small Bowel Disease

The most useful radiographic features in the differential diagnosis of diffuse small bowel disease are the size and contour of the bowel lumen, the thickness, shape, and distribution of mucosal folds, the thick-

Table 27.2.   Dilated Small Bowel Lumen[a]

Normal Fold Thickness
    Mechanical obstruction
    Adynamic ileus
    Adult celiac disease
    Scleroderma
    Lactase deficiency
Thickened Folds
    Lymphoma
    Intestinal Ischemia
    Zollinger-Ellison syndrome
    Amyloidosis
    Abetalipoproteinemia

[a]Size >3 cm.

Table 27.3.   Thick, Straight Small Bowel Folds[a]

Diffuse
    Edema
        Hypoproteinemia
        Congestive heart failure
        Portal hypertension
Long Segment
    Intramural hemorrhage
        Trauma
        Ischemia
        Vasculitis
        Anticoagulant therapy
        Bleeding disorders
    Radiation enteropathy
    Abetalipoproteinemia
    Eosinophilic gastroenteritis
Short Segment
    Crohn's disease (early)
    Venous or lymphatic obstruction
        Metastases
        Surgery

[a]Size >3 mm.
Modified from Herlinger H, Maglinte DDT, Rubesin SE. Small bowel imaging—An overview of indications and a practical approach to the interpretation of abnormalities. In: Herlinger H, Maglinte DDT, eds. Clinical radiology of the small intestine. Philadelphia: WB Saunders Company, 1989:577.

Table 27.4.   Thick, Irregular Small Bowel Folds[a]

Diffuse
    Lymphangiectasia
    Amyloidosis
    Eosinophilic gastroenteritis
    Histoplasmosis
    Systemic mastocytosis
    Lymphoma
Proximal Bowel
    Giardiasis
    Whipple's disease
Distal Bowel
    With narrowing
        Crohn's disease
        Tuberculosis
        Behçet's disease
    Without narrowing
        Yersinia/Campylobacter
        Salmonella
        Lymphoma
With Gastric Involvement
    Crohn's disease
    Lymphoma
    Eosinophilic gastroenteritis
    Zollinger-Ellison syndrome
    Amyloidosis
With AIDS
    Cryptosporidiosis
    Toxoplasmosis
    Giardiasis
    Candidiasis
    Cytomegalovirus infection
    M. avium-intracellulare

[a]Size >3 mm.
Modified from Herlinger H, Maglinte DDT, Rubesin SE. Small bowel imaging—An overview of indications and a practical approach to the interpretation of abnormalities. In: Herlinger H, Maglinte DDT, eds. Clinical radiology of the small intestine. Philadelphia: WB Saunders Company, 1989:579.

ness of the bowel wall, associated mesenteric findings, and the location and extent of any abnormalities detected (Tables 27.2 through 27.4) (1, 8). A specific diagnosis can usually only be made by integrating clinical information with radiographic findings (8).

Obstruction and Ileus (Table 27.2). Mechanical small bowel obstruction and adynamic (paralytic) ileus are the most common causes of dilated small bowel with normal fold thickness (Fig. 27.6). Ileus is usually diagnosed by clinical and plain radiograph findings. Barium studies are used to demonstrate the site and cause of obstruction (see Table 22.4). The barium column terminates in a bulbous head at the site of obstruction when peristalsis is active. Peristalsis is hyperactive early in the course of obstruction, but diminishes as the bowel fatigues. These entities are discussed in greater detail in Chapter 22.

Adult Celiac Disease (nontropical sprue) presents with malabsorption, steatorrhea, and weight loss (8, 9). Gluten, an insoluble protein found in wheat, rye, oats, and barley, acts as a toxic agent to the small bowel mucosa. The mucosa becomes flattened and absorptive cells decrease in number; villi disappear. The submucosa, muscularis, and serosa remain normal. Patients with long-term sprue have an increased risk of lymphoma and gastrointestinal carcinoma. The classic radiographic appearance is dilated small bowel with normal or thinned folds predominantly involving the jejunum (Fig. 27.7). Visible folds show an increased amount of separation. Fluid excess is often evident in the ileum. Transient intussusceptions may be observed.

Tropical sprue has the same clinical and radiographic findings as nontropical sprue but is confined to India, the Far East, and Puerto Rico. The disease responds to administration of folate and antibiotics.

Scleroderma produces atrophy of the muscularis of the small bowel resulting in flaccid, atonic, dilated bowel. The valvulae conniventes are normal or thinned. A "hide-bound" appearance of thinned folds tethered together is produced by contraction of the longitudinal muscle layer to a greater extent than the

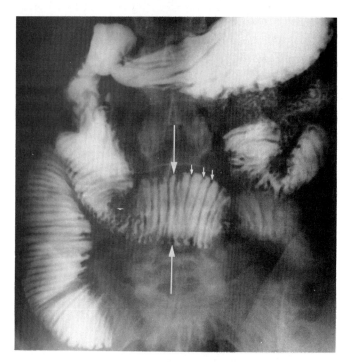

Figure 27.6. Small Bowel Obstruction. Small bowel follow-through examination reveals dilation of the small bowel lumen (>5 cm between *large arrows*) with normal thickness of well-defined folds (*small arrows*). The obstruction was due to adhesions.

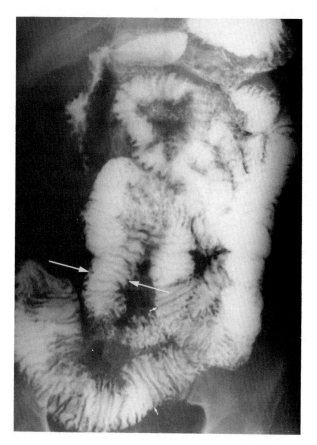

Figure 27.7. Adult Celiac Disease. Small bowel follow-through examination demonstrates dilation of the lumen of the small bowel (>4 cm between *long arrows*). The folds are of normal thickness (*small arrows*), less than 3 mm. Differential considerations are listed in Table 27.2. This patient with malabsorption became asymptomatic on a gluten-free diet.

circular muscle layer. Excessive contraction of the mesenteric border of the small bowel results in formations of mucosal sacculations along the antimesenteric border. The jejunum and duodenum are more severely involved than the ileum. The diagnosis is confirmed by skin changes and characteristic involvement of the esophagus (Chapter 25).

Lactase Deficiency. Lactase is required within the absorptive cells of the jejunum to properly digest disaccharides. Several population groups, including Chinese, Arabs, Bantu, and Eskimos, may become totally deficient in lactase during adult life. Secondary lactase deficiency may develop with alcoholism, Crohn's disease, and drugs such as neomycin. The nondigested lactose in the small bowel causes increased intraluminal fluid and dilated small bowel with normal folds.

Amyloidosis is a disease complex associated with infiltration of an amorphous protein material in body tissues (1). Most cases are associated with multiple myeloma or inflammatory disorders such as rheumatoid arthritis. Amyloid deposits are seen throughout the wall of the small bowel, especially within the walls of small blood vessels. Deposits in the muscularis impair motility. Diffuse, irregular thickened folds may be seen throughout the small bowel. Nodules are sometimes present.

Abetalipoproteinemia is a rare, autosomal recessive disease characterized by defective lipoprotein

synthesis by intestinal mucosa cells. Mucosal folds are uniformly thickened in the duodenum and jejunum and are normal in the ileum. The lumen of affected bowel may be normal or dilated.

Edema (Table 27.3) affects all layers of the bowel wall; however, interstitial fluid is concentrated in the submucosa with extension into the core of the folds. The bowel wall and mucosal folds are uniformly and diffusely thickened. Causes of small bowel edema include decreased oncotic pressure from hypoproteinemia (cirrhosis or renal failure), fluid overload, and increased venous pressure (congestive heart failure or portal hypertension).

Intramural Hemorrhage may involve any portion of the small intestine. Intramural bleeding due to trauma most commonly involves the third portion of the duodenum. Spontaneous mural hemorrhage may occur with bleeding disorders, anticoagulant therapy, or vasculitis. Patients may present with acute abdomen, vomiting, hematemesis, melena, fever, or palpable mass. Barium studies demonstrate a discrete hematoma as a focal intramural mass, while infiltrative hemorrhage is shown as uniform fold thickening as-

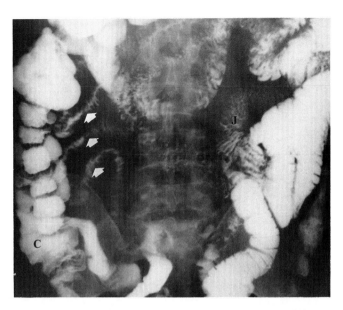

Figure 27.8. Intestinal Ischemia. Barium examination demonstrates a striking separation of multiple loops of ileum (*arrows*), indicating thickening of the bowel walls. The folds in involved loops are thickened and nodular due to edema and hemorrhage resulting from ischemia. A repeat study 1 month later documented complete resolution of all findings. *C*, colon. *J*, jejunum.

sociated with thickening of the bowel wall (Fig. 27.8). Parallel uniformly thickened folds give a "stack of coins" appearance. Computed tomography demonstrates the wall thickening of affected segments of bowel. Additional areas of spontaneous hemorrhage in the psoas muscle or rectus shealth may also be evident.

Intestinal Ischemia may result from embolism or thrombosis of the superior mesenteric artery or vein. Patients may present with an acute abdomen or vague symptoms. Arterial occlusion may be due to embolus, vasculitis, trauma, or adhesions. Venous thrombosis result from hypercoagulability states (neoplasms, oral contraceptives), inflammation (pancreatitis, peritonitis, abscess), or stasis (portal hypertension, congestive heart failure). Plain films demonstrate ileus, marked thickening of the bowel wall, and irregular thickened mucosal folds. Computed tomography is preferred to barium studies to demonstrate characteristic abnormalities. Thrombus within the mesenteric artery or vein is usually well demonstrated with contrast-enhanced studies.

Radiation Enteritis occurs when large doses of radiation are given to adjacent organs. The small bowel is the most radiosensitive organ in the abdomen. Long segments of bowel may be involved, with thickening of folds and bowel wall. Peristalsis is impaired. Progressive fibrosis leads to tapered strictures commonly involving long segments. The bowel may be kinked and obstructed by adhesions. Fistulas to the vagina or other organs may also result. Computed to-

mography demonstrates wall thickening and increased density of the mesentery, and fixation of bowel loops.

Eosinophilic Gastroenteritis virtually always affects the gastric antrum, as well as all or part of the small bowel. Intense infiltration of eosinophils in the lamina propria causes thickening of the bowel wall and mucosal folds, often with luminal narrowing. Barium studies show thickened and straightened folds. Thickening of the bowel wall is evidenced by wide separation between bowel loops and is demonstrated by CT.

Lymphangiectasia (Table 27.4) refers to gross dilation of the lymphatic vessels in the small bowel mucosa and submucosa. The primary form is a congenital lymphatic blockage, often associated with asymmetric edema of the extremities. Despite being congenital, symptoms often do not occur until young adulthood. Patients present with protein-losing enteropathy, diarrhea, steatorrhea, and recurrent infection. Secondary lymphangiectasia refers to lymphatic obstruction due to radiation, congestive heart failure, or mesenteric node involvement by malignancy or inflammation. The diagnosis is confirmed by jejunal biopsy. Barium study findings include diffuse fold thickening that is most pronounced in the jejunum, increased intraluminal fluid, and groups of tiny (1 mm) nodules due to distended villi. The pattern closely resembles Whipple's disease. Computed tomography helps the differentiation by revealing thickening of the bowel wall and mesenteric adenopathy in secondary lymphangiectasia.

Systemic Mastocytosis is a proliferation of mast cells in the skin, bones, lymph nodes, and gastrointestinal tract. Urticaria pigmentosa is the characteristic skin manifestation. Osteoblastic bone changes are found in 70% of cases. Lymphadenopathy and hepatosplenomegaly are often present. The bowel wall and mucosal folds are thickened, and mucosal nodules up to 5 mm size are often evident.

Whipple's Disease is an uncommon systemic disorder affecting the gastrointestinal tract, joints, central nervous system, and lymph nodes (1). The disease is caused by Whipple's bacilli, Gram-positive, rod-shaped bacteria that are found within macrophages in many organs and tissues. Patients may present with arthritis, neurologic symptoms, or steatorrhea. Generalized lymphadenopathy is usually present. Enteroclysis demonstrates irregularly thickened folds most prominent in the jejunum (Table 27.4). Demonstration of tiny (1 mm) sand-like nodules spread diffusely over the mucosa or in small groups is strong evidence of the disease. Increased luminal fluid is usual. Computed tomography reveals enlarged mesenteric lymph nodes that may have fat density (1).

AIDS Enteritis. In addition to lymphoma and Kaposi's sarcoma, AIDS patients are predisposed to multiple opportunistic infections of the gastrointestinal tract. Infective agents usually occur in combination and in multiple gastrointestinal sites.

Cryptosporidium and *Isospora belli* are protozoans that may infest the proximal intestine and cause a cholera-like diarrhea with life-threatening fluid loss. Barium studies show thickened folds and marked increased fluid (Table 27.4).

Cytomegalovirus causes disease in the small bowel and colon as well as the lungs, liver, and spleen. Mucosal ulceration with bleeding and perforation are the major intestinal manifestations. Barium studies may show thickened folds, loop separation, ulcers, and fistulae.

Mycobacterium avium-intracellulare is a common systemic infection in AIDS, involving lung, liver, spleen, bone marrow, lymph nodes, and intestinal tract. Barium studies show thickened, nodular folds with a sand-like mucosal pattern. Computed tomography demonstrates retroperitoneal and mesenteric adenopathy and focal lesions in the liver and spleen.

Candida, Amoeba histolytica, Giardia, Strongyloides, herpes simplex, and *Campylobacter* may also occur in AIDS patients.

Small Bowel Erosions and Ulcerations

Crohn's Disease is an inflammatory disease of uncertain etiology that may involve the gastrointestinal tract from the esophagus to the anus (1, 10). The disease is characterized by erosions, ulcerations, full-thickness bowel wall inflammation, and formation of noncaseating granulomas. Patients present, usually in their 20s and 30s, with diarrhea, abdominal pain, weight loss, and often fever. The typical course is one of remissions, relapse, and progression of disease. Patterns of gastrointestinal involvement include colon and terminal ileum (55%), small bowel alone (30%), colon alone (15%), and proximal small bowel without terminal ileum (3%) (1). Radiographic hallmarks of Crohn's disease include aphthous and confluent deep ulcerations, thickened and distorted folds, fibrosis with thickened walls, contractures and stenosis, involvement of the mesentery, asymmetric involvement both longitudinally and around the lumen, skip areas of normal intervening bowel between disease segments, and fistula and sinus tract formation. Aphthous ulcers are shallow, 1–2 mm depressions usually surrounded by a well-defined halo. Deep ulcerations are larger and often linear, forming fissures between nodules of elevated edematous mucosa ("cobblestone pattern"). Fibrosis and progressive thickening of the bowel wall narrows the lumen, particularly of the terminal ileum, producing the "string sign" (Fig. 27.9). Mesenteric involvement is best demonstrated by CT (1–3, 10). Ulceration along the mesenteric border may extend between the leaves of the mesentery. The mesenteric fat is infiltrated; the mesentery is thickened and retracted.

Complications of Crohn's disease are common and most are best demonstrated by CT (10) (Fig. 27.10). Obstruction is usually partial and due to strictures or areas of severe ulceration and spasm. Fistulae are formed in 19% of patients with small bowel disease (Fig. 27.9). Fistulae are abnormal communications between two epithelial-lined organs. Most frequent are

Figure 27.9. Crohn's Disease. A small bowel study in a patient with long-standing Crohn's disease demonstrates numerous sinus tracts and fistulas (*small arrows*) and extraluminal abscesses (*long arrows*). Fistulous connections extended between loops of small bowel as well as between ileum and the right ureter (not shown). The distal ileum (*i*) demonstrates irregular narrowing and separation from adjacent loops. Asymmetric involvement of a portion of the ileum has resulted in the formation of a sacculation (*large arrow*). The terminal ileum (*ti*) is narrowed and stiffened with a thick wall evidenced by separation from adjacent loops. C, cecum.

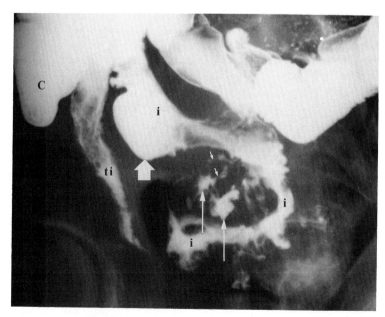

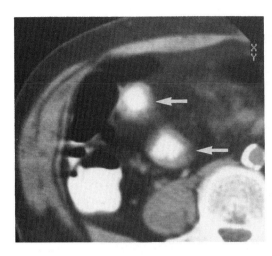

Figure 27.10. Crohn's Disease. A CT scan of the right midabdomen demonstrates thickening of the wall of two loops of ileum (*arrows*). Computed tomography is best for demonstrating the nature and extent of extraluminal disease.

ileocolonic and ileocecal, but enterocutaneous, enterovesical, and colovesical fistulae are also common. Sinus tracts extend into inflammatory extraluminal masses from the bowel lumen (Fig. 27.9). Abscess and phlegmon formation in the mesentery, peritoneal cavity, retroperitoneum, and abdominal wall are common. Free perforation occurs in 3% of cases. Most perforations are confined and form sinus tracts or fistulae. Carcinoma of the small and large bowel are increased in frequency with a prevalence of about 0.5% in Crohn's disease patients. Derangements of intestinal absorption cause megaloblastic anemia (vitamin B-12 deficiency) and an increased incidence of gallstones and renal stones. Up to 20% of patients have arthritis or spondylitis that mimics ankylosing spondylitis.

Yersinia Enterocolitis is caused by infection with the Gram-positive bacilli, *Yersinia enterocolitica* or *Y. pseudotuberculosis*. Infection causes an acute enteritis with abdominal pain, fever, and often bloody diarrhea that mimics acute appendicitis or acute Crohn's disease. Children and young adults are most often affected. The infection runs a self-limited course of 8–12 weeks. Diagnosis is confirmed by stool culture. Radiographic findings are most pronounced in the last 20 cm of the ileum. They include aphthous ulcers, nodules up to 1 cm size, wall thickening, and thickened folds that become effaced with increasing edema. Nodular lymphoid hyperplasia may appear during the resolution stage.

Campylobacter fetus subsp *jejuni* infection is clinically and radiographically similar to *Yersinia* enterocolitis. The disease usually lasts 1–2 weeks but relapses are common. Diagnosis is by stool culture.

Behçet's Syndrome is a multisystem disease due to a small vessel vasculitis that affects eyes, joints, skin, central nervous system, and occasionally the intestinal tract. Prominent clinical features include relapsing iridocyclitis, mucocutaneous ulcerations, vesicles, pustules, and mild arthritis. Intestinal disease most commonly involves the ileocecal region, where Crohn's disease is closely mimicked with ulceration, stenosis, and fistula formation.

Tuberculosis of the small intestine is uncommon in the United States and the Western world, but common in less developed areas. It typically involves the terminal ileum and cecum simultaneously and closely mimics Crohn's disease. Less than half of the patients have concurrent evidence of pulmonary tuberculosis. Barium studies demonstrate inflamed mucosa with transverse and stellate ulcers. The affected bowel becomes rigid and narrowed with nodular mucosa. Computed tomography demonstration of mesenteric adenopathy, high-density ascites, and peritoneal thickening suggests the diagnosis.

Small Bowel Diverticula

Small Bowel Diverticula are most common in the jejunum along the mesenteric border. They are outpouchings of mucosa through the bowel wall and between the leaves of the mesentery (1). They are commonly multiple and often asymptomatic. However, because of stasis of bowel contents within them, bacterial overgrowth may occur, resulting in deconjugation of bile salts and malabsorption. Vitamin B-12 absorption may also be impaired, resulting in megaloblastic anemia. Additional complications include obstruc-

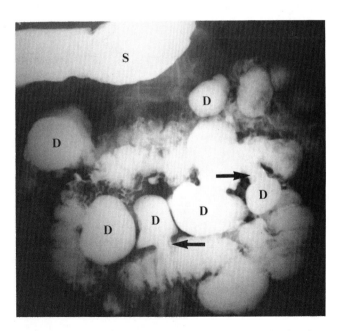

Figure 27.11. Small Bowel Diverticula. A small bowel series demonstrates numerous diverticula (*D*) extending from the duodenum and jejunum. The necks (*arrows*) of several diverticula are shown particularly well. *S*, stomach.

tion, acute diverticulitis, hemorrhage, and volvulus. Plain films may demonstrate featureless ovoid collections of air. Barium studies demonstrate the outpouchings, most with a neck smaller in diameter than the outpouching itself (Fig. 27.11). The diverticulum lacks mucosal folds and does not contract because of the lack of muscle within its wall.

Meckel's Diverticulum is the most common congenital anomaly of the gastrointestinal tract, present in 2–3% of the population. The diverticulum varies from 2 to 8 cm in length, and is located on the antimesenteric border of the ileum up to 2 m from the ileocecal valve. The tip of the diverticulum may be attached to the umbilicus by a remnant of the vitelline duct. Ectopic gastric mucosa is present in up to 62% of cases. Peptic secretions may cause ulceration and bleeding. Other complications include intussusception, volvulus, and perforation. Enteroclysis is the best method to demonstrate the diverticulum in an adult. The diverticulum appears as a blind sac attached to the antimesenteric border of the ileum. Radionuclide scanning for ectopic gastric mucosa is less reliable in adults than in children (1).

Pseudodiverticula or sacculations are outpouchings along the antimesenteric border of the small bowel that result from disease of the small bowel. They occur most commonly in association with Crohn's disease (Fig. 27.9) or scleroderma. With fibrosis and contraction of the mesenteric border of the bowel, the unsupported antimesenteric border becomes pleated and forms sacculations.

References

1. Herlinger H, Maglinte D, eds. Clinical radiology of the small intestine. Philadelphia: WB Saunders Company, 1989.
2. Balthazar EJ. CT of the gastrointestinal tract: principles and interpretation. AJR 1991;156:23–32.
3. Desai RK, Tagliabue JR, Wegryn SA, Einstein DM. CT evaluation of wall thickening in the alimentary tract. Radiographics 1991;11:771–783.
4. Buck JL, Sobin LH. Carcinoids of the gastrointestinal tract. Radiographics 1990;10:1081–1095.
5. Rubesin SE, Gilchrist AM, Bronner M, et al. Non-Hodgkin lymphoma of the small intestine. Radiographics 1990;10: 985–998.
6. Buck JL, Harned RK, Lichtenstein JE, Sobin LH. Peutz-Jeghers syndrome. Radiographics 1992;12:365–378.
7. Forte MD, Brant WE. Spontaneous isolated mesenteric fibromatosis. Diseases Colon Rectum 1988;31:315–317.
8. Rubesin SE, Rubin RA, Herlinger H. Small bowel malabsorption: clinical and radiologic perspectives—how we see it. Radiology 1992;184:297–305.
9. Rubesin SE, Grumbach K, Herlinger H, et al. Adult celiac disease and its complications. Radiographics 1989;9:1045–1066.
10. Javors BR, Wecksell A, Fagelman D. Crohn's disease: less common radiographic manifestations. Radiographics 1988;8:259–275.

28
Colon and Appendix

William E. Brant

COLON

Imaging Methods

The primary imaging methods for detection of colon abnormalities are the single-contrast and double-contrast barium enemas. The single-contrast is generally favored for the evaluation of colonic obstruction, fistulas, and in old, seriously ill or debilitated patients (1). The double-contrast is favored for detection of small lesions (<1 cm), for documentation of inflammatory bowel disease, and for detailed imaging evaluation of the rectum (1) (Fig. 28.1). Colonoscopy is a complementary procedure to barium studies that is limited by occasional failure to reach the right colon. Colonoscopy and proctoscopy are excellent for evaluating diagnostic problems posed by barium studies, and for biopsy of suspected neoplastic lesions (1).

As elsewhere in the gastrointestinal tract, computed tomography (CT) complements the barium examination by demonstrating intramural and extracolonic components of disease. It is excellent for demonstrating extrinsic inflammatory and neoplastic processes that affect the colon, abscesses, sinuses, and fistulas (1–3).

Computed tomography and magnetic resonance images (MR) have been utilized for initial staging of colorectal carcinoma. However, both methods are limited in their ability to determine the extent of bowel wall tumor infiltration and involvement of regional lymph nodes (1–5). Transrectal sonography is more accurate than CT or MR in determining local tumor extent of rectal carcinomas, but is inadequate for detection of regional lymph node involvement (5). For the initial staging of colorectal carcinoma, CT and MR should be reserved for patients with suspected widespread local or disseminated disease. Computed tomography is useful in screening for recurrence of

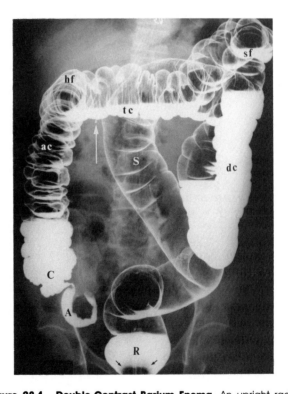

Figure 28.1. Double-Contrast Barium Enema. An upright radiograph from a double-contrast barium enema demonstrates normal colon anatomy. The appendix (A) extends from the cecum (C). The ascending colon (ac) extends to the hepatic flexure (hf), the coils of which must be examined by multiple oblique views. The transverse colon (tc) extends to the splenic flexure (sf), which continues as the descending colon (dc). This patient has a long sigmoid colon (S) that extends high into the abdomen. The transverse colon is relatively short. Patients with a short sigmoid colon usually have a long redundant transverse colon. The distended balloon at the tip of the enema catheter causes a lucent filling defect (small arrows) in the rectum (R). A tiny intramural diverticulum (long arrow) is seen in the proximal transverse colon.

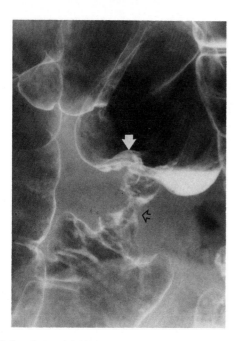

Figure 28.2.   Colon Carcinoma. Radiograph of the sigmoid colon from a double-contrast barium enema demonstrates a characteristic "apple core" constricting lesion of colon carcinoma. The lumen is markedly narrowed (*open arrow*) and shoulders of the tumor cause a mass impression on the adjacent distended lumen (*solid arrow*).

colorectal carcinoma because it can provide a comprehensive examination of the liver, abdominal cavity, and entire colon. Magnetic resonance imaging is sensitive but nonspecific in the detection of local recurrence of rectal carcinoma.

Anatomy

The large intestine consists of the cecum and appendix, colon, rectum, and anal canal. It is approximately 1.5 m in length from the ileum to the anus. The large intestine is characterized by the taenia coli, three longitudinal bands of muscle that traverse the colon shortening it to form haustra, sacculations created by puckering of the bowel wall. The major functions of the large intestine are the formation, transport, and evacuation of feces. These functions require mobility, absorption of water, and secretion of mucus. Infrequent peristalsis transports feces from the ascending and transverse colon to the sigmoid colon where fecal material is stored until defecation. The cecum and ascending colon absorb water from the highly liquid material received from the ileum. Mucus secreted by mucosal goblet cells protects the mucosa from injury, and is secreted in profuse amounts when the mucosa is irritated or injured.

The cecum is the large blind pouch that extends below the level of the ileocecal valve. The cecum generally lies in the right iliac fossa but may be quite mobile. It is usually covered on all sides by peritoneum (intraperitoneal), but may be fixed extraperitoneally, cov-

ered only on its ventral surface by peritoneum. The appendix is a long worm-like tube that hangs from near the apex of the cecum (Fig. 28.1). The ileocecal valve consists of two lips that project into the cecum forming a prominent mass. The ascending colon is extraperitoneal, lying in the anterior pararenal space, covered only on its ventral surface by peritoneum. The hepatic flexure forms two curves. The proximal, more posterior curve is closely related to the descending duodenum and right kidney. The more distal anterior curve is closely related to the gallbladder. The transverse colon is intraperitoneal and suspended from the transverse mesocolon that arises from the peritoneum covering the pancreas and sweeps transversely across the upper abdomen. The transverse mesocolon limits the superior extent of the small bowel loops. The splenic flexure is closely related to the tail of the pancreas and the caudal aspect of the spleen. The splenic flexure is anchored to the diaphragm by the phrenicocolic ligament, which serves as a boundary between disease processes of the left subphrenic space and the left paracolic gutter.

The descending colon, like the ascending colon, is extraperitoneal within the anterior pararenal space and is covered by peritoneum only on its ventral surface. The sigmoid colon forms a redundant loop of variable length from the distal descending colon in the left iliac fossa to the rectum. The sigmoid colon is completely intraperitoneal and is suspended by the sigmoid mesocolon that allows considerable mobility. The sigmoid colon penetrates the peritoneum at the level of vertebrae S-2 to S-4 to continue as the extraperitoneal rectum. The rectum extends for about 12 cm in close relationship with the sacrum. Peritoneum forming the pouch of Douglas covers the ventral and lateral aspects of the rectum. The anal canal is 3–4 cm long and is invested by the sphincter ani and levator ani muscles. A series of vertical folds form the rectal columns of Morgagni, beneath which are the veins that when dilated, are hemorrhoids.

The colon can be recognized on CT and MR by its course, haustral markings, and fecal content. The thickness of the wall of the normal colon does not exceed 5 mm (2, 3).

Colon Filling Defects/Mass Lesions

Colorectal Adenocarcinoma is the second most common malignant tumor in the United States and is the most common malignancy of the gastrointestinal tract (4–6). About 50% arise in the rectum and rectosigmoid area. Another 25% occur in the sigmoid colon, while the remaining 25% are evenly distributed throughout the remainder of the colon. Most tumors are annular constricting lesions, 2–6 cm in diameter, with raised everted edges and ulcerated mucosa (Fig. 28.2). Polypoid tumors are less common, some having

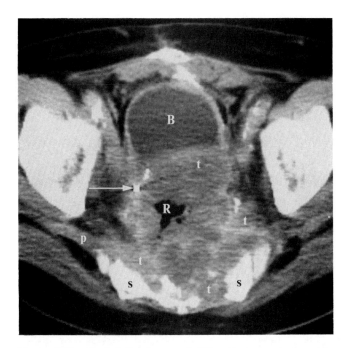

Figure 28.3. Rectal Carcinoma. A CT scan demonstrates widespread carcinoma of the rectum (*R*) with tumor extension (*t*) into the bladder (*B*), perirectal tissues, piriformis muscle (*p*), and sacrum (*s*). A stent (*arrow*) has been placed in the right ureter because of tumor obstruction at the ureteral vesical junction.

Table 28.1. Surgical-Pathologic Staging of Colorectal Carcinoma (Modified Dukes Classification)

Stage	Description
A	Limited to mucosa
B 1	Extension into, but not through, muscularis propria
B 2	Extension through muscularis propria; no nodes
C 1	Limited to bowel wall; positive nodes
C 2	Extension through bowel wall; positive nodes
D	Distant metastases

the frond-like appearance of villous carcinoma. Infiltrating scirrhous tumors, so common in gastric carcinoma, are rare in the large intestine, unless the patient has ulcerative colitis. The tumor spreads by direct invasion through the bowel wall (Fig. 28.3), lymphatic channels to regional nodes, and hematogenously through the portal veins to the liver and systemic circulation (Table 28.1). Intraperitoneal seeding from a tumor that penetrates the colon wall may also occur. Obstruction is the most frequent complication. Other complications are uncommon but include perforation, intussusception, abscess, and fistula formation. Up to 20% of patients have a second tumor of the large bowel at diagnosis, usually an adenoma or another carcinoma. Five percent of patients will have a second colorectal carcinoma either simultaneously or subsequently diagnosed. Patients with ulcerative colitis, Crohn's disease, familial polyposis, and Gardner's, Turcot's, and Peutz-Jeghers syndromes are at increased risk of colon carcinoma.

Table 28.2. Colorectal Carcinoma—CT and MR Staging[a]

Stage	Description
I	Intraluminal mass without thickening of wall
II	Thickened wall or pelvic mass; no invasion or extension to side walls
IIIa	Thickened wall or pelvic mass with invasion of adjacent structures but not to pelvic side walls or abdominal wall
IIIb	Thickened wall or pelvic mass with extension to pelvic side walls and/or abdominal wall without distant metastases
IV	Distant mestastases

[a]Adapted from Thoeni RF. Colorectal cancer: cross-sectional imaging for staging of primary tumor and detection of local recurrence. AJR 1991;156:910.

A scheme for CT staging of colorectal carcinoma is given in Table 28.2. This scheme may also be useful for staging by MR. The limitations of CT and MR staging are discussed above. Tumor recurrences are most common (a) at the operative site, near the bowel anastomosis, (b) in the peritoneal cavity, and (c) in the liver and distant organs. Because the entire abdominal cavity must be surveyed to detect tumor recurrence, CT is the current method of choice.

Polyps. A polyp is defined as a localized mass that projects from the mucosa into the lumen (6). Since the majority of colorectal cancers are believed to arise from preexisting polyps, the detection of colon polyps is a major indication for barium studies of the colon (6). The following "rules of thumb" can be applied. Polyps less than 5 mm are almost all hyperplastic, with a risk of malignancy less than 0.5%. Polyps 5–10 mm size are 90% adenomas, with a risk of malignancy of 1%. Polyps 10–20 mm size are usually adenomas, with a risk of malignancy of 10%. Polyps larger than 20 mm are 50% malignant.

On barium examinations, polyps may appear as flat plaques, lobulated filling defects, "bowler hats," (7) or pedunculated lesions (Fig. 28.4). The bowler hat sign refers to the appearance of intermediate-sized polyps on double-contrast examinations (Fig. 28.5). The differential diagnosis of polypoid lesions of the colon include bubbles, feces, mucus, and foreign objects.

Hyperplastic polyps are non-neoplastic mucosal proliferations. They are round and sessile. The great majority are less than 5 mm in size.

Adenomatous polyps are distinctly premalignant and a major risk for development of colorectal carcinoma. Up to 78% of early adenocarcinomas show histologic evidence of origin from adenoma. Adenomatous polyps are neoplasms with a core of connective tissue. Five to ten percent of the population older than 40 years have adenomatous polyps (6).

Hamartomatous polyps (juvenile polyps) represent about 1% of colon polyps. They are a common cause of rectal bleeding in children. The Peutz-Jeghers polyp is histologically similar (6).

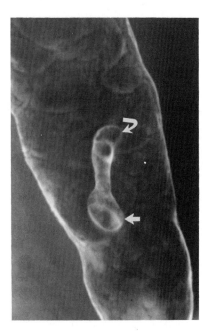

Figure 28.4. Pedunculated Polyp. Double-contrast barium enema demonstrates a long-stalked pedunculated polyp with a bulbous tip (*straight arrow*) arising (*curved arrow*) from the mucosa of the descending colon.

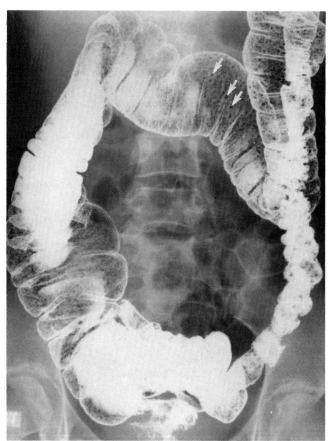

Figure 28.6. Familial Multiple Polyposis. Double-contrast barium enema reveals the entire colonic mucosa to be carpeted with innumerable small polyps seen as tiny filling defects (*arrows*).

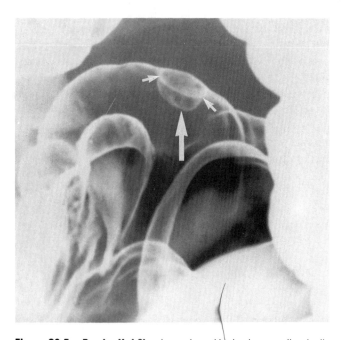

Figure 28.5. Bowler Hat Sign is produced by barium coating both the body of the polyp (*large arrow*) and the recesses (*small arrows*) between the base of the lesion and the normal colonic mucosa.

Inflammatory polyps are usually multiple and associated with inflammatory bowel disease (8). They account for less than 0.5% of colorectal polyps.

POLYPOSIS SYNDROMES

Familial Multiple Polyposis is an autosomal dominant condition of multiple adenomatous polyps

usually confined to the colon. Polyps, most under 5 mm in size, number in the thousands (Fig. 28.6). Multifocal origin of adenocarcinoma is part of the natural history of the disease. Colectomy and study of family members are recommended.

Gardner's Syndrome combines multiple adenomatous colon polyps with bone and skin abnormalities. This condition is also autosomal dominant. Associated bone abnormalities include cortical thickening of the ribs and long bones, osteomas of the skull, supernumerary teeth, and exostoses of the mandible. Fibromas, desmoids, and epidermal inclusion cysts are seen on the skin. Colon involvement is identical to familial multiple polyposis.

Turcot's Syndrome is autosomal recessive and rare. It consists of multiple adenomatous colon polyps and central nervous system tumors of various types, including malignant gliomas.

Cronkhite-Canada Syndrome is nonhereditary and consists of non-neoplastic inflammatory polyps, associated with ectodermal changes including nail atrophy, brownish skin pigmentation, and alopecia, as well as watery diarrhea and protein-losing enteropathy. The colon and stomach are always involved,

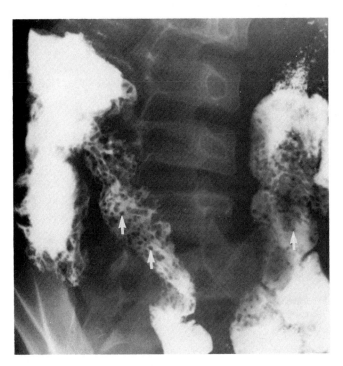

Figure 28.7. Lymphoid Hyperplasia. Single-contrast barium enema in a patient with hypogammaglobulinemia shows numerous small nodules (*arrows*) throughout the colon.

while the small bowel is involved in one-half of the cases. The mean age of onset is 60 years. The condition is usually rapidly fatal.

Peutz-Jeghers Syndrome of multiple hamartomatous polyps predominantly involves the small bowel, but most cases have gastric and colon polyps as well.

Lymphoid Hyperplasia may involve the colon with a diffuse pattern of tiny nodules 1–2 mm in diameter with characteristic umbilication (Fig. 28.7).

Lymphoma. The colon follows the stomach and small bowel as common sites for gastrointestinal lymphoma. Involvement of the cecum is most common; however, anal and rectal lymphoma are increasingly frequent in acquired immunodeficiency syndrome patients (9) (Fig. 28.8). Morphologic patterns include small to large nodules that may ulcerate, excavitate and perforate (Fig. 28.9), and diffuse infiltration of the bowel wall resulting in bulbous folds and thickened bowel wall. As in the small intestine, marked narrowing of the lumen is uncommon and aneurysmal dilation may occur when transmural disease destroys innervation. Non-Hodgkin's lymphoma is most common.

Leiomyoma and Leiomyosarcoma of the colon account for less than 1% of gastrointestinal tumors. They are more common in the stomach and small bowel than in the colon. As in the remainder of the gastrointestinal tract, they may appear as exophytic,

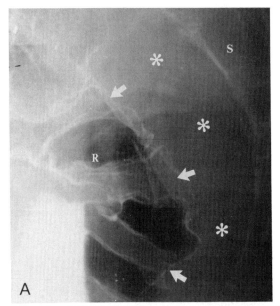

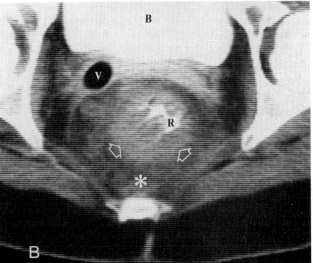

Figure 28.8. Rectal Lymphoma. A. Lateral view of the rectum from a double-contrast barium enema shows bizarre thickened folds (*arrows*) in the rectum (*R*) and marked widening of the presacral space (*). *S*, sacrum. **B.** A CT scan demonstrates irregular thickening of the wall (*arrows*) and distortion of the lumen of the rectum (*R*). The presacral space (*Q*) is infiltrated with soft tissue density. *B*, bladder; *V*, vagina containing a tampon.

mural, or intraluminal masses (Fig. 28.10). Most are 25 mm or larger. Ulceration is relatively frequent.

Lipoma is the most common submucosal tumor of the colon (10). It is most frequent in the cecum and ascending colon. Forty percent present with intussusception. Barium studies demonstrate a smooth, well-defined elliptical filling defect, usually 1–3 cm in diameter. The tumors are soft and change shape with compression. Computed tomography demonstration of a fat-density tumor is definitive.

Extrinsic Masses commonly cause mass effect on the colon that may simulate intrinsic disease.

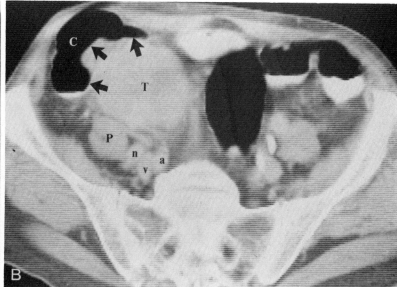

Figure 28.9.   Cecal Lymphoma. A. Radiograph of the cecum from a single-contrast barium enema shows mass impression (*arrows*) on both the cecum (C) and appendix (*open arrow*). **B.** A CT scan dem- onstrates the full extent of the tumor mass (*T*) impressing (*arrows*) on the cecum (*C*). An enlarged node (*n*) is also seen adjacent to the common iliac artery (*a*) and vein (*v*). *P*, psoas muscle.

Figure 28.10.   Leiomyosarcoma of the Rectum. A CT scan shows a large tumor (*T*) with an irregular low-den- sity area of central necrosis arising exophytically from the wall of the rectum (*r*), which is displaced laterally and anteriorly. The tumor obstructed the bladder out- let, necessitating placement of a suprapubic Foley catheter (*F*).

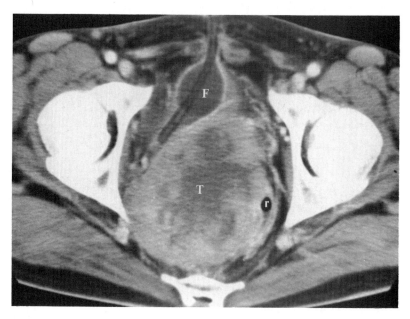

Endometriosis commonly implants on the sigmoid colon and rectum. Defects are frequently multiple and of variable size. Barium studies demonstrate sharply defined defects that compress but do not usually en- circle the lumen. Computed tomography demon- strates complex cystic pelvic masses with high-density fluid components. Multiple pelvic organs may be in- corporated into the mass. Magnetic resonance shows hyperintense lesions on all pulse sequences in about half of the cases and hypointense lesions on all pulse sequences in about one-third of the cases.

Metastases may involve the colon by contiguous spread, spread along mesenteric fascial planes, by in- traperitoneal seeding, through lymphatic channels, or by embolus through blood vessels. The involved colon demonstrates thickening of the wall, separation of folds, spiculation, angulations, narrowing, and sero- sal plaques (Fig. 28.11). Metastases often cannot be differentiated from primary tumors by imaging meth- ods. Crohn's disease and metastatic disease may also look exactly alike radiographically. Computed tomog- raphy or MR demonstrate contiguous involvement of the colon and rectum by pelvic tumors.

Extrinsic inflammatory processes, such as appen- dicitis, pelvic abscess, diverticular abscess, and pelvic inflammatory disease, may cause mass effect, asym- metric tethering, and spiculation.

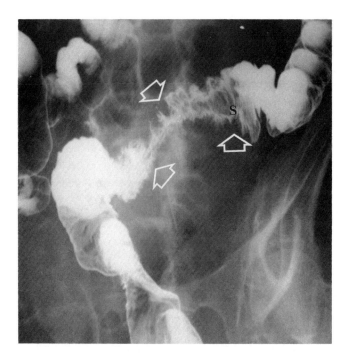

Figure 28.11. Serosal Metastases involving the Colon. Metastases from carcinosarcoma of the uterus implanted on the serosal surface of the sigmoid colon (*S*) cause narrowing and spiculation (*arrows*) of the lumen.

Colon Inflammatory Disease

Ulcerative Colitis is an uncommon idiopathic inflammatory disease involving primarily the mucosa and submucosa of the colon. The peak age for its appearance is 20–40 years, but onset of disease after age 50 is common. The disease consists of superficial ulcerations, edema, and hyperemia. The radiographic hallmarks of ulcerative colitis are granular mucosa, confluent shallow ulcerations, symmetry of disease around the lumen, and continuous confluent diffuse involvement (Table 28.3). An early fine, granular pattern is produced by mucosal hyperemia and edema that precedes ulceration. Superficial ulcers spread to cover the entire mucosal surface. The mucosa is stippled with barium adhering to the superficial ulcers. "Collar button ulcers" are deeper ulcerations of thickened edematous mucosa with crypt abscesses extending in the submucosa (Fig. 28.12). A coarse granular pattern is produced later by the replacement of diffusely ulcerated mucosa with granulation tissue. Late changes include a variety of polypoid lesions. Pseudopolyps are mucosal remnants in areas of extensive ulceration (8). Inflammatory polyps are small islands of inflammed mucosa. Postinflammatory polyps are mucosal tags that are seen in quiescent phases of the disease. Hyperplastic polyps may occur during healing after mucosal injury. Involvement typically extends from the rectum proximally in a symmetric and continuous pattern. The terminal ileum is nearly al-

ways normal. Rare "backwash ileitis" may produce an ulcerated but patulous terminal ileum.

Complications of ulcerative colitis include (a) strictures, usually 2–3 cm in length and commonly involving the transverse colon and rectum, (b) colorectal adenocarcinoma, with an approximate risk of 1% per year of disease, (c) toxic megacolon in 2–5% of cases (may be the initial manifestation), and (d) massive hemorrhage. Extraintestinal disease associations include sacroilitis mimicking ankylosing spondylitis in 20% of the cases, eye lesions including uveitis and iri-

Table 28.3. Ulcerative Colitis vs. Crohn's Colitis

Ulcerative Colitis	Crohn's Colitis
Circumferential disease	Eccentric disease
Regional (continuous disease)	Skip lesions (discontinuous disease)
Predominantly left-sided	Predominantly right-sided
Rectum usually involved	Rectum normal in 50%
Confluent shallow ulcers	Confluent deep ulcers
No aphthous ulcers	Aphthous ulcers early
Collar button ulcers	Transverse and longitudinal ulcers
Terminal ileum usually normal	Terminal ileum usually diseased
Terminal ileum patulous	Terminal ileum narrowed
No pseudodiverticula	Pseudodivertitula
No fistula	Fistula common
High risk of cancer	Low risk of cancer
Toxic megacolon	No toxic megacolon

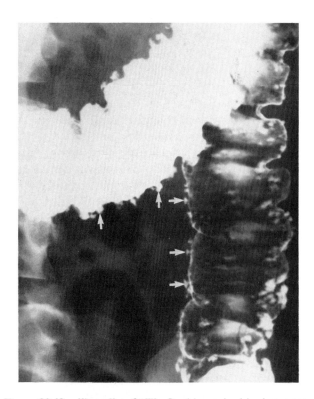

Figure 28.12. Ulcerative Colitis. Double-contrast barium enema shows a pattern of continuous involvement of the colon with innumerable submucosal collar button ulcers (*arrows*).

Figure 28.13. Crohn's Colitis. A. A CT scan through the transverse colon (*T*) demonstrates asymmetric thickening of the colon wall characteristic of Crohn's colitis. The anterior wall (*open arrows*) is normal, while the posterior wall (*closed arrows*) is thickened and nodular. **B.** A more caudal CT scan in the same patient demonstrates numerous air-containing perirectal cutaneous fistulas (*f*). *r*, rectum.

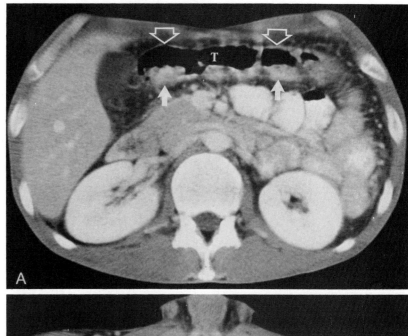

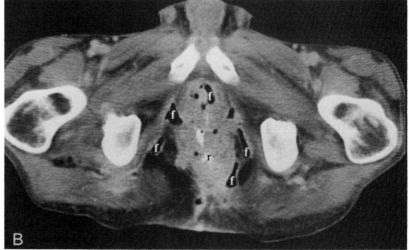

tis in 10% of the cases, cholangitis, and an increased incidence of thromboembolic disease.

Crohn's Disease involves the colon in two-thirds of all cases and is isolated to the colon in about one-third of all cases (11). Hallmarks of Crohn's colitis include early aphthous ulcers, later confluent deep ulcerations, predominant right colon disease, discontinuous involvement with intervening regions of normal bowel, asymmetric involvement of the bowel wall (Fig. 28.13**A**), strictures, fistulas, and sinus formation (Table 28.3). Pseudodiverticula of the colon are formed by asymmetric fibrosis on one side of the lumen, causing saccular outpouches on the other side. Involvement of the rectum is characterized by deep rectal ulcers and multiple fistulous tracts to the skin (Fig. 28.13**B**).

Pseudomembranous Colitis is an inflammatory disease of the colon, and occasionally the small bowel, characterized by the presence of a pseudomembrane of necrotic debris. There are many contributing causes including antibiotics (clindamycin, streptomy-

cin, lincomycin, any that change bowel flora), intestinal ischemia (especially following surgery), irradiation, long-term steroids, shock, and colonic obstruction. The disease presents as fulminant inflammatory bowel disease with diarrhea and foul stools. Plain radiographs reveal adynamic ileus with dilated large and small bowel. The colon may be greatly dilated, and toxic megacolon has been reported. Barium enema demonstrates an irregular lumen with thumbprint indentations similar to ischemic colitis. Superficial ulcers are common. Plaque-like defects on the mucosal surface are due to the pseudomembranes. The colitis is frequently patchy in distribution with sparing of the rectum.

Amebiasis is an infection by the protozoan parasite *Entamoeba histolytica*. The disease is worldwide but particularly common in South Africa, Central and South America, and Asia. At least 5% of the population of the United State harbor amebae. Encysted amebae are ingested with contaminated food and water. The cyst capsule is dissolved in the small

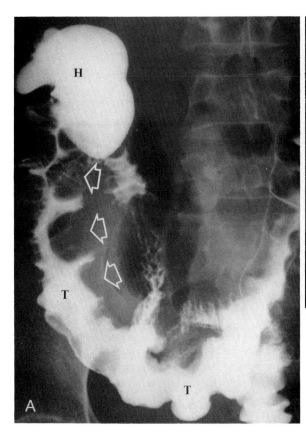

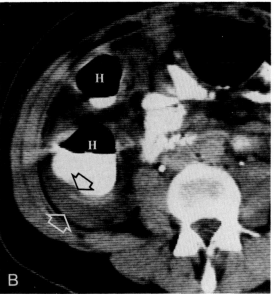

Figure 28.14.   Ischemic Colitis. A. Double-contrast barium enema shows thumbprinting pattern (*arrows*) involving the proximal portion of a redundant transverse colon (*T*). *H*, hepatic flexure. **B.** A CT scan in the same patient reveals marked thickening (*arrows*) of the walls of the hepatic flexure (*H*). The patient presented clinically with abdominal pain and bloody stools.

bowel, releasing trophozoites that migrate to the colon and burrow into the mucosa, forming small abscesses. The infection can spread throughout the body by hematogenous embolization or direct invasion. Amebic colitis produces dysentery with frequent bloody mucoid stools. Barium studies demonstrate a disease that closely mimics Crohn's colitis with aphthous ulcers, deep ulcers, asymmetric disease, and skip areas. The cecum and rectum are the primary sites of colonic disease. The terminal ileum is characteristically not involved. Complications include strictures, amebomas consisting of a hard fixed mass of granulation tissue that may simulate carcinoma, toxic megacolon, and fistulas, particularly following surgical intervention. Amebic liver abscess results from the spread of infection through the portal system and may be complicated by diaphragm perforation, pleural effusion, and thoracic disease.

Ischemic Colitis may mimic ulcerative colitis and Crohn's colitis both clinically and radiographically. The causes of ischemic colitis include arterial occlusion due to arteriosclerosis, vasculitis, or arterial emboli; venous thrombosis due to neoplasm, oral contraceptives and other hypercoagulation conditions; and low flow states such as hypotension, congestive heart failure, and cardiac arrhythmias. The pattern of involvement generally follows the distribution of a major artery and is the clue to diagnosis. The superior mesenteric artery supplies the right colon from the cecum to the splenic flexure. The inferior mesenteric artery supplies the left colon from the splenic flexure to the rectum. The splenic flexure region and descending colon are the most susceptible areas to ischemic colitis. Early changes include thickening of the colon wall, spasm, and spiculation. As blood and edema accumulate within the bowel wall, multiple nodular defects are produced in a pattern called "thumbprinting" (Fig. 28.14). Progression of the disease results in ulcerations, perforation, scarring, and stricture. Computed tomography demonstrates symmetrical or lobulated thickening of the bowel wall with an irregulary narrowed lumen. Submucosal edema may produce a low-density ring bordering on the lumen (2). Thrombus may occasionally be demonstrated within the superior mesenteric artery or vein.

Radiation Colitis may be indistinguishable radiographically from early ulcerative colitis. The diagnosis is made by confirmation of the involved colon being within an irradiation field. The rectosigmoid region is most commonly involved due to radiation of pelvic malignancy. Colitis is produced by a slowly progressive endarterits that causes ischemia and fibrosis. Radiographic findings include thickened folds, spiculation, ulceration, stricture, and occasionally fistula formation. Fibrosis results in a rigid, featureless bowel. Healing may include formation of pseudopolyps and postinflammatory polyps.

Figure 28.15. Diverticulosis. A CT scan demonstrates air-filled and contrast-filled outpouchings (arrows) representing diverticuli in the transverse (T) and descending (D) colon.

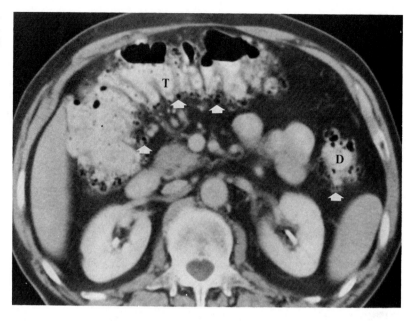

Cathartic Colon is due to chronic irritation of the mucosa by laxatives including castor oil, bisacodyl, and senna. The involved colon may be dilated and without haustra, or narrowed. The right colon is most commonly affected. Bizarre contractions are often observed. The diagnosis is made by clinical history.

Diverticular Disease

Colon Diverticulosis is an acquired condition in which the mucosa and muscularis muscosae herniate through the muscularis propria of the colon wall, producing a saccular outpouching (Fig. 28.15). Colon diverticula are classified as false diverticula because the sacs lack all of the elements of the normal colon wall. The condition is rare under age 25, but increases with age thereafter to affect 50% of the population over age 75. The major risk factor for diverticulosis is a low-residue diet. The condition is very uncommon in cultures where a high-residue diet is the norm, such as African native populations. The formation of diverticular sacs is usually associated with thickening of the muscularis propria, including both the circular muscle and the taenia coli. Severely affected portions of bowel are usually shortened in length, resulting in crowding of the thickened circular muscle bundles. Muscle dysfunction associated with diverticulosis may result in pain and tenderness without evidence of inflammation. Diverticulosis without diverticulitis is a cause of painless colonic bleeding that may be brisk and life-threatening.

Plain abdominal radiographs demonstrate diverticula as gas-filled sacs parallel to the lumen of the colon. Barium studies show diverticula as barium or gas-filled sacs outside the colon lumen. Sacs vary in size from tiny spikes to 2 cm diameter. Most are 5–10 mm

in diameter. They may occur anywhere in the colon but are most common and usually most numerous in the sigmoid colon. Some sacs are reducible and may disappear with complete filling of the lumen. Others may contain fecal residue. The associated muscle abnormality is seen as thickening and crowding of the circular muscle bands with spasm and spiked irregular outline of the lumen. Computed tomography demonstrates the muscle hypertrophy as a thickened colon wall and distorted luminal contour. The diverticula are shown as well-defined gas-filled or contrast-filled sacs outside the lumen (Fig. 28.15).

Diverticulitis is inflammation of diverticula, usually with perforation and intramural or localized pericolic abscess. Diverticulitis eventually complicates about 20% of the cases of diverticulosis. Clinical signs include painful mass, localized peritoneal inflammation, fever, and leukocytosis. Complications of diverticulitis include bowel obstruction, bleeding, peritonitis, and sinus tract and fistula formation. Diverticulitis is a less common cause of colon obstruction than is colon carcinoma. Obstruction due to diverticulitis is often temporarily relieved by smooth muscle relaxants such as glucagon. Colon bleeding is more often associated with diverticulosis than diverticulitis. Most diverticular abscesses are quickly walled off and confined, but free perforation with pus and air in the peritoneal cavity and diffuse peritonitis may also occur. Sinus tracts may lead to larger abscess cavities in the peritoneal or retroperitoneal compartments. Fistulas are most common to the bladder (Fig 28.16), vagina, or skin, but may develop to any lower abdominal organ including fallopian tubes, small bowel, and other parts of the colon. Diverticulitis is efficiently diagnosed radiographically by barium enema or CT. Barium enema examination is considered safe except when signs of free intraperitoneal perforation or sepsis are present.

Radiographic hallmarks of diverticulitis on barium enema include deformed diverticular sacs, demonstration of abscess, and extravasation of barium outside the colon lumen. The smooth outline of the involved sacs are deformed by inflammation and perforation. The resulting abscess causes extrinsic mass effect on the adjacent colon (Fig. 28.17**A**). The colon lumen is narrowed but tapers at the margins of narrowing in distinction with the abrupt narrowing of carcinoma. Barium leaks into the abscess cavities, or forms tracks paralleling the colon lumen and often connecting multiple perforated sacs (the "double track sign"). Computed tomography excels at demonstrating the paracolic inflammation and abscess associated with diverticulitis, as well as complications such as colovesical fistula. Pericolic fat is increased in density. The colon wall is thickened and the pericolic abscess appears as a soft tissue density or fluid density mass (Fig. 28.17B).

Lower Gastrointestinal Hemorrhage

While upper gastrointestinal hemorrhage is usually readily diagnosed by gastric aspirate and endoscopy, lower gastrointestinal hemorrhage is difficult to localize, even during surgery. The common causes of lower gastrointestinal hemorrhage are listed in Table 28.4. Radionuclide imaging studies are usually selected as the screening examination of choice for confirming the presence of, and often localizing, lower gastrointestinal bleeding (12). Technetium-99m-sulfur colloid or ^{99m}Tc-red blood cell studies are capable of detecting bleeding at rates below 0.1 ml/min. A negative scintigraphic study usually precludes the need for urgent angiography. Angiography requires bleeding rates of 0.5 ml/min or greater. However, angiography is more

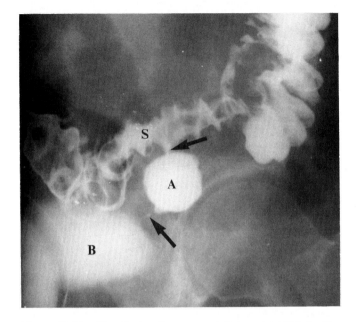

Figure 28.16.   Diverticular Abscess and Colovesical Fistula. Single-contrast barium enema demonstrates barium filling a diverticular abscess (A) and opacifying the bladder (B). Thin columns of barium (arrows) outline fistulous tracts extending from the bowel lumen to abscess and from abscess to the bladder. The lumen of the sigmoid colon (S) is irregularly narrowed by the inflammatory process.

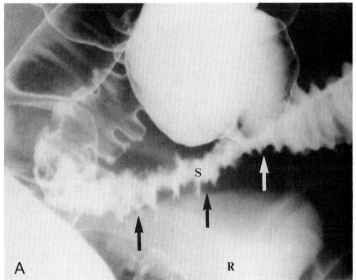

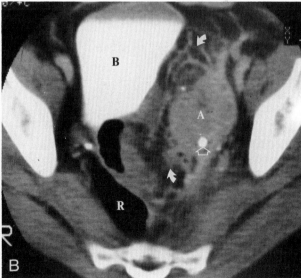

Figure 28.17.   Diverticulitis. A. Barium enema shows a narrowed spiculated lumen (arrows) of a segment of the sigmoid colon (S). R, rectum. **B.** A CT scan demonstrates the extraluminal component of the disease. A large inflammatory mass (A) is seen in the soft tissues of the pelvis. Inflammatory reaction causes rounded and streaky soft tissue densities (curved arrows) in the adjacent fat. A drop of barium (open arrow) is seen in a diverticulum, encompassed within the inflammatory mass. The loop of involved sigmoid colon shown in **A** is just cephalad to the CT slice shown. R, rectum. B, bladder.

Table 28.4.   Causes of Lower Gastrointestinal Hemorrhage

Cause	%
Colon diverticula	40
Angiodysplasia	17–30
Colon carcinoma	7–16
Polyps	8
Rectal trauma/fissure/hemorrhoids	7
Duodenal ulcer	Rare
Meckel's diverticulum	Rare
Bowel ischemia	Rare

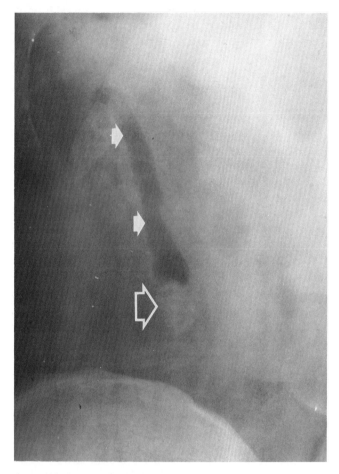

Figure 28.18.   Appendicolith. Plain radiograph of the abdomen demonstrates a faintly calcified appendicolith (*open arrow*) that obstructed the appendiceal orifice. The lumen of the appendix (*closed arrows*) is dilated and air-filled because of stasis and bacterial overgrowth. Surgery confirmed acute appendicitis with a retrocecal appendix.

specific than scintigraphy in demonstrating the anatomic cause of bleeding and offers the possibility of nonoperative treatment by embolization or infusion of Pitressin. Colonoscopy is usually unrewarding because of the large quantities of sticky, melanotic stool. Barium enema is not used to evaluate acute hemorrhage because it usually cannot locate the source of bleeding and it will interfere with any subsequently needed angiographic procedure.

Angiodysplasia refers to ectasia and kinking of mucosal and submucosal veins of the colon wall. The condition results from a chronic intermittent obstruction of the veins where they penetrate the circular muscle layer. A maze of distorted, dilated vascular channels replaces the normal mucosal structures and are separated from the bowel lumen only by a layer of epithelium. Angiodysplasia is acquired, and probably related to aging. The average age of affected patients is 65 years. Bleeding is usually chronic, resulting in anemia, but may be acute and massive. Angiography demonstrates a tangle of ectatic vessels without an associated mass.

APPENDIX

Imaging Methods

Filling of the appendix is attained most reliably by single contrast barium enema examination. The appendix is also frequently visualized on abdominal films obtained 6 to 48 hours following oral administration of barium. Failure to fill the appendix with barium on barium enema examination is not definitive evidence of appendiceal disease. The normal appendix is seldom recognized on CT, but may be demonstrated by graded compression ultrasound. Both CT and ultrasound have proven extremely useful in the diagnosis of appendiceal disease, especially acute appendicitis.

Anatomy

The appendix arises from the posteromedial aspect of the cecum at the junction of the taenia coli, about 1–2 cm below the ileocecal valve. The appendix is a blind-ended tube that is 5–10 mm in diameter (on barium studies) (Fig. 28.1) and approximately 8 cm in length, although it may be up to 30 cm long. Its mucosa is heavily infiltrated with lymphoid tissue. The appendix is quite variable in position: it may be pelvic, retrocecal, or retrocolic, and intraperitoneal or extraperitoneal in location. The appendix always arises from the cecum on the same side as the ileocecal valve. A posterior position of the ileocecal valve indicates a posterior position of the appendix.

Acute Appendicitis

Acute appendicitis is the most common cause of acute abdomen. Frequently the clinical diagnosis is straightforward. However, patients with atypical presentations cause diagnostic problems. The most difficult patients are women of childbearing age, in whom ruptured ovarian cysts and pelvic inflammatory disease may mimic acute appendicitis. Acute appendicitis results from obstruction of the appendiceal lumen. Continued mucosal secretions cause dilation and

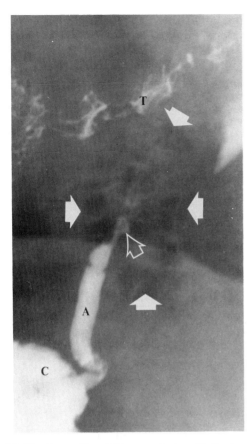

Figure 28.19. Appendiceal Abscess. Barium fills the lumen of the appendix (*A*) and extravasates from its tip (*open arrow*) into a large appendiceal abscess outlined by gas collections within it (*closed arrows*). *C*, cecum; *T*, transverse colon.

increased intraluminal pressure that impairs venous drainage and results in mucosal ulceration. Bacterial infection causes gangrene and perforation with abscess. Most periappendiceal abscesses are walled off, but free perforation and pneumoperitoneum occasionally occur.

Plain films will demonstrate an appendiceal calculus (appendicolith or fecalith) in about 14% of patients with acute appendicitis (Fig. 28.18). An appendicolith is formed by calcium deposition around a nidus of inspissated feces. The resultant calcification is usually laminated with a radiolucent center. Appendiceal abscess or periappendiceal inflammation may result in a visible soft tissue mass in the right lower quadrant (Fig 28.19). The lumen of the cecum, as outlined by gas, will be deformed; localized ileus may be evident.

Barium enema examination is frequently nonspecific. Complete filling of the appendix to its bulbous tip is strong evidence against appendicitis. However, nonfilling of the appendix, as would be expected with luminal obstruction, has no diagnostic value of its own. Mass impression on the cecum has many causes besides appendicitis.

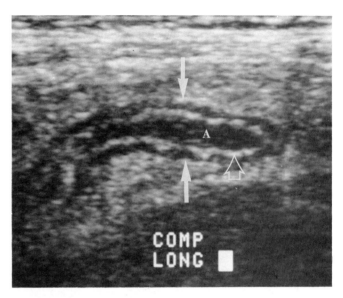

Figure 28.20. Acute Appendicitis. Graded compression ultrasound demonstrates a distended appendix (*A*) with a diameter (between *closed arrows*) of 10 mm. The mucosal interface produces a bright echogenic line (*open arrow*). Surgery confirmed an acutely inflamed and focally necrotic appendix. (Case courtesy of David A. Russell, M.D., Cedar Rapids, Iowa.)

Ultrasound, using the graded compression technique, is quite accurate in providing a definitive diagnosis (13, 14). Slow graded compression is applied with a near-focus transducer to the area of maximum tenderness. The normal appendix has a diameter of less than 6 mm when compressed. Visualization of an appendix larger than 6 mm diameter, or visualization of a shadowing appendicolith, is strong evidence of appendicitis (Fig. 28.20). With perforation, sonography may demonstrate a loculated pericecal fluid collection, a discontinuous wall of the appendix, and prominent pericecal fat. When the ultrasound examination is negative for appendicitis, an alternate diagnosis can frequently be suggested based upon visualized abnormalities.

Computed tomography is the imaging method of choice when periappendiceal abscess is suspected (Fig. 28.21). However, uncomplicated appendicitis cannot be excluded by CT. Appendicoliths are well demonstrated. A periappendiceal phlegmon is seen as an indurated soft tissue mass with a CT density greater than 20 HU. A liquified mass less than 20 HU in CT density is evidence of abscess. Abscesses larger than 3 cm generally require surgical or catheter drainage. Smaller abscesses or phlegmons commonly resolve on antibiotic treatment alone.

Mucocele of the Appendix

Mucocele refers to distension of all or a portion of the appendix with sterile mucus (15). The lumen is obstructed by appendicolith, foreign body, adhesions,

Figure 28.21. Periappendiceal Abscess. A CT scan demonstrates a dilated, fluid-filled cecum (C), an appendicolith (*open arrow*) obstructing the appendiceal orifice, and periappendiceal fluid and inflammation (*closed arrows*) resulting from appendiceal rupture.

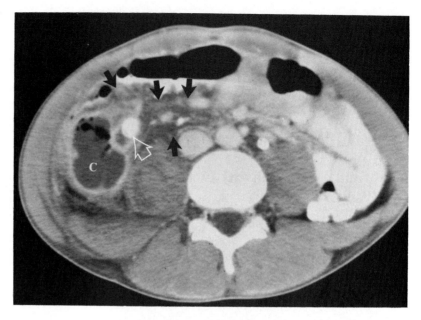

or tumor. Some cases are due to mucinous cystadenomas or cystadenocarcinomas of the appendix. Continued secretion of mucus produces a large (up to 15 cm), well-defined cystic mass in the right lower quadrant. Peripheral calcification may be present. Rupture of the mucocele may result in pseudomyxoma peritonei. Gelatinous implants spread throughout the peritoneal cavity, causing adhesions and mucinous ascites.

Appendiceal Tumors

Carcinoid is the most common tumor of the appendix, accounting for 85% of all tumors (16). The appendix is the most common location for carcinoid tumor, accounting for 60% of all carcinoids. Most occur near the tip and are round, nodular tumors up to 2.5 cm size. Most are solitary and have less tendency to metastasize than carcinoids elsewhere in the gastrointestinal tract. Carcinoid syndrome is rare and the mesenteric reaction seen with small bowel carcinoid is usually absent.

Adenomas occur in the appendix usually in association with familial multiple polyposis. Isolated adenomas are usually mucinous cystadenomas associated with mucocele of the appendix.

Adenocarcinoma of the appendix is rare.

References

1. Margulis AR, Thoeni RF. The present status of the radiologic examination of the colon. Radiology 1988;167:1–5.
2. Balthazar EJ. CT of the gastrointestinal tract: principles and interpretation. AJR 1991;156:23–32.
3. Desai RK, Tagliabue JR, Wegryn SA, Einstein DM. CT evaluation of wall thickening in the alimentary tract. Radiographics 1991;11:771–783.
4. Thoeni RF. Colorectal cancer: cross-sectional imaging for staging primary tumor and detection of local recurrence. AJR 1991;156:909–915.
5. Halvorsen RA Jr, Thompson WM. Gastrointestinal cancer: diagnosis, staging, and the follow-up role of imaging. Semin Ultrasound CT MR 1989;10:467–480.
6. Olmstead WW, Ros PR, Sobin LH, Dachman AH. The solitary colonic polyp: radiologic-histologic differentiation and significance. Radiology 1986;160:9–16.
7. Simms SM. Differential diagnosis of the bowler hat sign. AJR 1985;144:585–587.
8. Buck JL, Dachman AH, Sobin LH. Polypoid and pseudopolypoid manifestations of inflammatory bowel disease. Radiographics 1991;11:293–304.
9. Smith C, Kubicka RA, Thomas CR Jr. Non-Hodgkin lymphoma of the gastrointestinal tract. Radiographics 1992;12:887–899.
10. Taylor AJ, Stewart ET, Dodds WJ. Gastrointestinal lipomas: a radiologic and pathologic review. AJR 1990;155:1205–1210.
11. Javors BR, Wecksell A, Fagelman D. Crohn's disease: less common radiographic manifestations. Radiographics 1988;8:259–275.
12. Dorfman GS, Cronan JJ, Staudinger KM. Scintigraphic signs and pitfalls in lower gastrointestinal hemorrhage: the continued necessity of angiography. Radiographics 1987;7:543–562.
13. Jeffrey RB Jr, Laing FC, Townsend RR. Acute appendicitis: sonographic criteria based on 250 cases. Radiology 1988;67:327–329.
14. Rioux M. Sonographic detection of the normal and abnormal appendix. AJR 1992;158:773–778.
15. Madwed D, Mindelzun R, Jeffrey RB Jr. Mucocele of the appendix: imaging findings. AJR 1992;159:69–72.
16. Buck JL, Sobin LH. Carcinoids of the gastrointestinal tract. Radiographics 1990;10:1081–1095.

Section VII GENITOURINARY TRACT

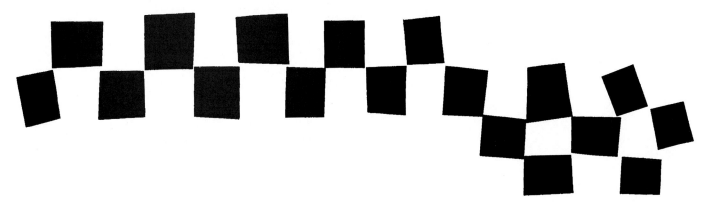

29

Adrenal Glands and Kidneys

William E. Brant

ARENAL GLANDS
Imaging Methods

Challenges in adrenal imaging occur in three major clinical settings. First, a patient is referred for adrenal imaging because a hormonally active adrenal tumor is suspected on a clinical basis. The role of imaging is to locate and characterize the lesion. Second, adrenal imaging is requested to evaluate for metastatic disease. Third, an adrenal mass is incidentally detected on imaging studies performed for other indications. The significance of the finding must be assessed both radiographically and clinically.

Computed tomography (CT) is usually the adrenal imaging modality of choice in adults (1–3). Ultrasound is excellent for screening the adrenal glands in infants and children, especially for detection of adrenal hemorrhage. Magnetic resonance (MR) can provide high-quality images of adrenal lesions and is useful in problem solving. Arteriography, venography, venous sampling, radionuclide imaging, and percutaneous biopsy are reserved for selected problem cases (4).

Anatomy

The adrenal glands are composed of an outer cortex and an inner medulla that are functionally independent and distinct. The cortex secretes steroid hormones including cortisol, aldosterone, androgens, and estrogens. The medulla produces catecholamines.

The adrenal glands lie within the perirenal space surrounded by fat. The right adrenal gland is located posterior to the inferior vena cava (IVC) at the level where the IVC enters the liver. The right adrenal gland is between the right lobe of the liver and the right crus of the diaphragm just above the upper pole of the right kidney. The left adrenal gland lies just medial and anterior to the upper pole of the left kidney, posterior to the pancreas and splenic vessels, and lateral to the left crus of the diaphragm. On cross-sectional imaging the adrenal glands appear triangular, linear, or inverted V- or Y-shaped." Each limb is smooth in outline and uniform in thickness with straight or concave borders. The limbs are up to 3 cm in length and 5–7 mm in thickness. The adrenal glands are of uniform soft tissue density on CT and ultrasound; MR may demonstrate corticomedullary differentiation in some normal patients and in most patients with adrenal hyperplasia. The cortex has higher signal intensity than the medulla.

Adjacent structures may cause major problems in adrenal imaging by mimicking adrenal masses. Tortuous splenic vessels, splenic lobulations, pancreatic projections, exophytic upper pole renal masses, portosystemic venous collaterals, retroperitoneal adenopathy, and portions of the stomach may all cause adrenal pseudotumors (1). Judicious use of oral and intravenous contrast on CT, or supplemental ultrasound or MR studies, will reveal the true nature of most of these conditions.

Figure 29.1. **Benign Adrenal Adenoma.** Longitudinal ultrasound demonstrates a homogeneous 3.5 cm mass (*A*, between *arrows*) arising from the right adrenal gland. The mass is outlined by echogenic fat. This is a nonhyperfunctioning adrenal adenoma that was discovered incidentally. *L*, liver; *RK*, right kidney.

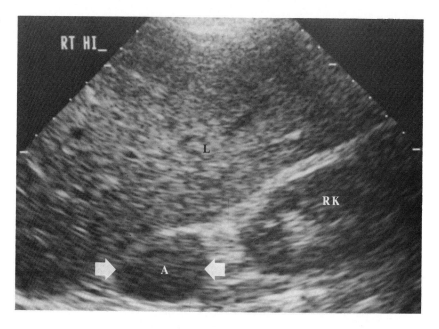

Adrenal Hyperplasia

Half of the cases of biochemically hyperplastic glands will appear normal on CT and MR. In the remainder of cases, both glands will be diffusely enlarged but maintain their normal adrenal shape. Uncommonly, hyperplasia may appear nodular and mimic solitary or multiple adenomas (4). In diffuse hyperplasia, the limbs of the adrenal glands are longer than 3 cm and exceed 10 mm thickness. Adrenal hyperplasia is present in 70% of the cases of Cushing's syndrome and 20% of the cases of Conn's syndrome. Adrenal hyperplasia is important to differentiate from adrenal adenoma as a cause of endocrine syndromes. The syndrome is usually treated medically when hyperplasia is causative, while surgical removal of hyperfunctioning adrenal adenomas is usually curative. Metastatic disease, tuberculosis, and histoplasmosis may also cause diffuse adrenal enlargement and mimic the appearance of adrenal hyperplasia.

Adrenal Adenoma

Adrenal adenomas may secrete excessive hormone and cause one of the endocrine syndromes or be nonhyperfunctional and present as an unsuspected adrenal mass. Function of the adenoma cannot be determined by imaging appearance, but is assessed clinically, or in problem cases, by venous sampling.

On CT, benign adenomas are typically small (<4 cm), well-defined, homogeneous, and nonenhancing (4). Malignant masses tend to be larger, irregular, inhomogeneous, and nonuniformly enhancing. The US appearance parallels that of CT, with benign adenomas being small (<4 cm), well-defined, and homogeneous in echogenicity (Fig. 29.1). Larger masses with heterogeneous echogenicity tend to be malignant.

On MR, T1-weighted images show adenomas to be hypointense or isointense relative to the liver. On T2-weighted images benign adenomas are slightly hyperintense to liver at high-field strength (Fig. 29.2) or hypointense to liver at low-field strength (4). Malignant lesions and pheochromocytoma tend to be hyperintense to liver at both high- and low-field strength. Gadolinium administration shows mild enhancement and rapid washout in benign lesions and strong early enhancement with slow washout in malignant lesions.

Adrenal Carcinoma

Adrenal carcinoma is an uncommon but lethal tumor. Most are large and invasive at presentation. About half the carcinomas are hyperfunctioning, causing endocrine syndromes, most commonly Cushing's syndrome, followed by virilization or feminization (1).

The typical CT appearance is a large mass (4–20 cm), with areas of central necrosis and hemorrhage, and a pattern of irregular enhancement. Adrenal tumors larger than 4–5 cm in size should be removed because of the significant risk of carcinoma. Calcification is present in 30% of the tumors (Fig. 29.3). Hepatic and lymph node metastases are common. Tumor thrombus in the renal vein or IVC may be evident. Large tumors may be difficult to differentiate from hepatic masses.

T1-weighted MR images demonstrate the inhomogeneous large mass. Signal intensity is increased on T2-weighted images. Gadolinium enhancement is useful to detect tumor thrombus.

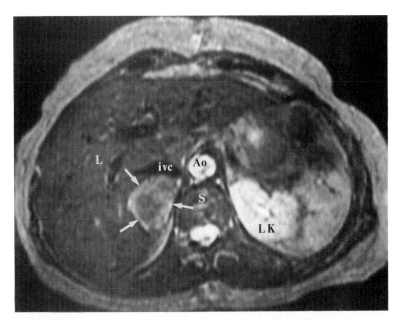

Figure 29.2. Benign Adrenal Adenoma. Axial plane T2-weighted (TR/1846; TE/80) 1.5 = tesla MR image demonstrates a right adrenal mass (arrows) that proved to be a benign hyperfunctioning adenoma causing Conn's syndrome in a 65-year-old woman. *Ao*, aorta; *ivc*, inferior vena cava; *L*, liver; *LK*, left kidney; *S*, spine.

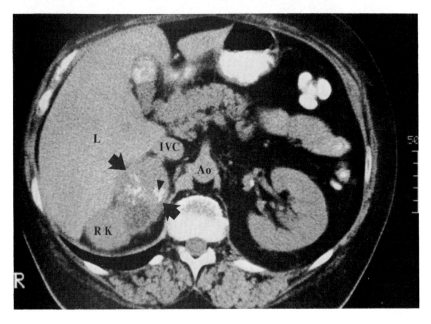

Figure 29.3. Adrenal Carcinoma. A CT scan in a 61-year-old woman with Cushing's syndrome demonstrates a 5-cm, irregularly marginated mass (arrows) with calcifications (arrowhead) replacing the right adrenal gland. *RK*, right kidney; *IVC*, inferior vena cava; *L*, liver; *Ao*, aorta.

Ultrasound with Doppler is also excellent for the evaluation of tumor thrombosis.

Adrenal Metastases

Adrenal metastases are exceedingly common, found in 27% of patients with malignant disease on autopsy series (1). The most common primary tumors are lung, breast, melanoma, gastrointestinal, and renal. Small lesions (<3–4 cm) tend to be homogeneous, well-defined, and indistinguishable from benign, nonhyperfunctioning adenomas. To complicate the issue, even in patients with known primary malignancy, up to 50% of small adrenal masses will be benign adenomas and not metastases. Percutaneous biopsy will be needed in many cases to determine the pathology (Fig. 29.4).

Larger lesions (>4 cm) generally show features of malignancy including inhomogeneous density, inhomogeneous enhancement, irregular outline, thick irregular rim, and invasion of adjacent structures. Magnetic resonance demonstrates metastases to be hyperintense relative to the liver on T2-weighted images. Gadolinium shows early enhancement and slow washout.

Adrenal Cysts

Adrenal cysts are rare and usually asymptomatic incidental findings. They may be seen at any age and are more common in females. Endothelial and epithelial cysts are the most common. Pseudocysts result from adrenal hemorrhage. Parasitic cysts are usually echinococcal in origin.

Figure 29.4. Adrenal Metastasis Biopsy. A CT-directed biopsy of a small right adrenal mass (*large arrow*) is performed using an approach through the right lobe of the liver (*L*). The needle tip is indicated by the *long white arrow*. Note the position of the right adrenal gland bounded by the inferior vena cava (*IVC*) anteriorly, the right lobe of the liver (*L*) laterally, and the right crus of the diaphragm (*black arrow*) medially. *Ao*, aorta.

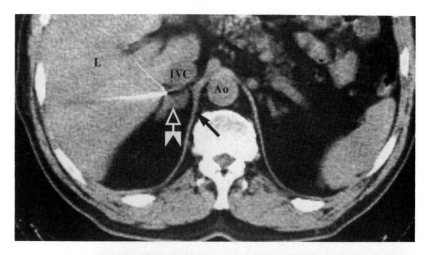

Ultrasound may define a classic, thin-walled, anechoic cyst. More often it demonstrates a cystic mass with thick walls, internal septations, and debris. Calcification is sometimes present in the wall. Differentiation from cystic degeneration of an adrenal malignancy is difficult in these cases and often requires percutaneous aspiration biopsy.

Computed tomography and MR are usually not helpful in providing further characterization of the mass.

Adrenal Myelolipoma

Myelolipomas are rare, nonfunctioning benign tumors arising from bone marrow elements. Identification of fat density within the tumor by CT or MR is definitive in making the diagnosis. They have no malignant potential. These tumors range in size up to 30 cm and are frequently internally inhomogeneous because of their mixed components. On ultrasound, they may be extremely echogenic and blend in with retroperitoneal fat.

Adrenal Hemorrhage

Adrenal hemorrhage is most common in newborn infants, usually induced by episodes of hypoxia or trauma. Most cases are bilateral. In adults, trauma and infection are the most common causes of adrenal hemorrhage. Unilateral hemorrhage is most common in adults, with the right adrenal most frequently affected.

Ultrasound initially demonstrates hyperechoic, mass-like enlargement of the adrenal gland (Fig. 29.5). With time, the adrenal mass becomes hypoechoic and progressively decreases in size. The gland may return entirely to normal or evolve into a thick-walled pseudocyst that commonly develops calcifications in its walls within 2–4 weeks of the hemorrhage. Eventual collapse of the pseudocyst results in coarsely calcified adrenal glands (Fig. 29.6).

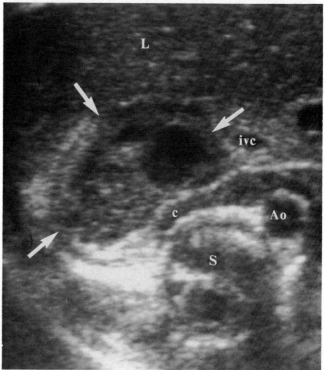

Figure 29.5. Adrenal Hemorrhage Enlarges the Right Adrenal Gland (*arrows*) in a 2-week-old Infant. The adrenal gland is identified by its location between liver (*L*), inferior vena cava (*ivc*), and right crus of the diaphragm (*c*). *Ao*, aorta; *S*, spine.

Magnetic resonance imaging demonstrates features of acute hemorrhage with short T1 and long T2 characteristics. T1-weighted images show areas of signal intensity brighter than liver, while T2-weighted images show bright signal intensity.

Adrenal Calcification

Adrenal calcifications, in both children and adults, most commonly result from adrenal hemorrhage (Fig. 29.6). Tuberculosis and histoplasmosis may cause diffuse adrenal calcification associated with Addison's disease. Adrenal tumors that calcify include neuro-

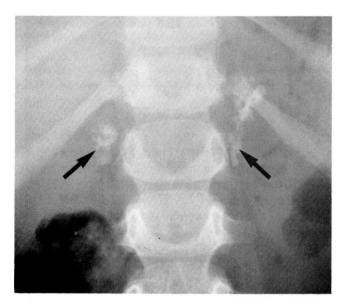

Figure 29.6. Adrenal Calcification. Plain radiograph of the abdomen in a 4-year-old girl demonstrates calcification of both adrenal glands (*arrows*) resulting from bilateral adrenal hemorrhage as an infant.

blastoma and ganglioneuroma in children, and carcinoma, pheochromocytoma, and ganglioneuroma in adults. Wolman's disease is a rare, autosomal recessive lipid disorder associated with enlarged calcified adrenal glands, hepatomegaly, and splenomegaly.

Endocrine Syndromes

Cushing's Syndrome is caused by excessive amounts of hydrocortisone and corticosterone released by the adrenal cortex. Clinical signs include truncal obesity, easy bruisability, generalized weakness, diabetes mellitus, and oligomenorrhea. Adrenal hyperplasia causes 70% of cases of noniatrogenic Cushing's syndrome. The hyperplasia is stimulated in 90% of cases by a pituitary microadenoma that produces adrenocorticotropic hormone (ACTH). In 10% of cases, the source of ACTH is ectopic, usually from lung malignancies. Benign adrenal adenomas cause 20% of cases of Cushing's syndrome, while adrenal carcinoma causes the remaining 10% (Fig. 29.2)(1).

Conn's Syndrome, produced by elevated levels of aldosterone, causes 1–2% of systemic hypertension. The clinical diagnosis is made by findings of persistent hypokalemia, increased serum and urine aldosterone, and decreased renin activity in the plasma. A solitary hyperfunctioning adrenal adenoma is the cause of 80% of cases (Fig. 29.2), while adrenal hyperplasia is the cause of the remaining 20%. Adenomas that produce Conn's syndrome tend to be small (<2 cm); therefore, strict attention to excellent CT technique using thin (5-mm) slices is necessary for accurate localization.

Adrenogenital Syndrome usually occurs in newborns and infants who have an enzyme deficiency (11β- or 22-hydroxylase) leading to deficient production of cortisol and aldosterone and an excess of precursors, especially androgens (4). These infants have adrenal hyperplasia, which is usually well-demonstrated by ultrasound. Both adrenal adenomas and carcinomas may be a cause of masculinizing or feminizing syndromes in older patients.

Pheochromocytoma is a rare tumor that causes hypertension, headaches, and tremors. Paroxysmal attacks of symptoms are characteristic, but not always present. Symptoms are produced by excessive secretion of catecholamines by the tumor. Pheochromocytoma is said to follow the "rule of tens": 10% are bilateral, 10% are extraadrenal, 10% are malignant, and 10% are familial. Pheochromocytoma is associated with multiple endocrine neoplasia (MEN II), von Hippel-Lindau syndrome, and neurofibromatosis. Since 90% of pheochromocytomas arise in the adrenal medulla, the adrenal glands are usually scanned first (Fig. 29.7). Most tumors are larger than 2 cm in diameter. Calcification is rare, but usually "eggshell" in configuration when present. If no lesion is found and clinical suspicion remains high, then scanning must be expanded to include the chest and remainder of the abdomen and pelvis. Extraadrenal sites for pheochromocytoma include the organ of Zuckerkandl near the bifurcation of the aorta, the bladder, and the paraaortic sympathetic chain. Magnetic resonance imaging may be the modality of choice to search for extraadrenal pheochromocytoma. The tumor demonstrates very bright signal intensity on T2-weighted images that makes it stand out from surrounding structures. Radionuclide scans utilizing I-131 or I-123 metaiodobenzylquanidine (MIBG) are also effective in localizing pheochromocytoma (Fig. 29.7); however, the agent is not widely available.

Addison's Disease refers to primary adrenal insufficiency, which occurs only after 90% of the adrenal cortex is destroyed. The most common cause (60–70%) in the United States is idiopathic atrophy, which is probably an autoimmune disorder (4). The adrenal glands shrink in size and may not be detectable with imaging methods. Additional causes include tuberculosis, histoplasmosis, infarction, disseminated fungal infection, lymphoma, and metastatic tumor (1). Adrenal calcification suggests prior tuberculosis or histoplasmosis. Bilateral enlargement is seen with active infection. Lymphoma and metastases replace the glands with tumor.

KIDNEYS
Imaging Methods

Excretory urography has been the traditional method of imaging the kidneys. However, US, CT, and

MR all provide better images of the renal parenchyma. Many renal masses will be detected initially by excre-

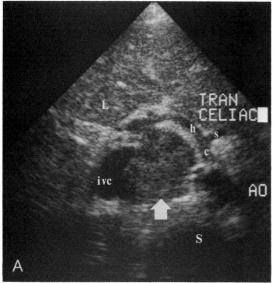

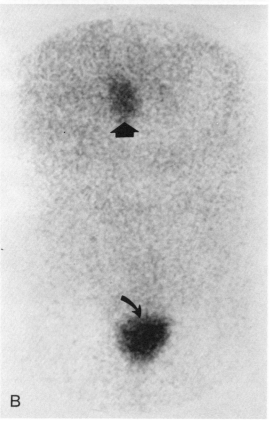

Figure 29.7. Pheochromocytoma in a 13-year-old male with hypertension. A. Axial plane ultrasound demonstrates the adrenal tumor extending between the inferior vena cava (*ivc*) and aorta (*AO*). The origin of the celiac axis (*c*) from the aorta and its branches, the common hepatic artery (*h*) and the splenic artery (*s*) are clearly seen. *L*, liver; *S*, spine. **B.** Radionuclide scan utilizing I-123 metaiodobenzylquanidine demonstrates focal radionuclide activity in the right adrenal tumor (*arrow*). Radionuclide activity is also seen in the bladder (*curved arrow*).

tory urography or ultrasound. Contrast-enhanced CT remains the most optimal imaging study to evaluate and stage suspected renal tumors (3, 5). Magnetic resonance imaging is a substitute for CT for patients in whom the use of intravenous iodinated contrast agents is contraindicated, or whenever the CT study is equivocal. Color Doppler ultrasound is valuable in the assessment of venous involvement by renal tumors. Venography remains useful whenever the question of venous involvement is not answered by CT, MR or color Doppler ultrasound. Arteriography is currently rarely used to diagnose or stage renal tumors, but may be required for embolization procedures (5). Percutaneous biopsy utilizing CT or ultrasound for guidance is used to provide histologic confirmation of tumors that have already metastasized.

Anatomy

The kidneys are located within the cone of renal fascia (Gerota's fascia), surrounded by the fat of the perirenal space. The kidney is made up of lobes that consist of a pyramid-shaped medulla surrounded by cortex except at the apex of the medullary pyramid. The cortex consists of all glomeruli, proximal and distal convoluted tubules, and accompanying blood vessels. The peripheral cortex is immediately beneath the renal capsule, while the septal cortex extends down between the pyramids as the columns of Bertin. Prominent columns of Bertin may simulate a renal mass. The medullary pyramids consist of the collecting tubules and the long, straight portions of the loops of Henle, as well as accompanying blood vessels. The apex of the pyramids is directed at the renal sinus and projects into the calyces. The term papilla refers to the innermost zone of the medulla, closest to the draining calyx. The kidneys gradually increase in size from birth to age 20. Renal length is relatively stable at 9–12 cm from ages 20–50, and gradually decreases thereafter.

Simple calyces are cupped-shaped structures that drain one renal lobe. Compound calyces drain several renal lobes and are more complex in shape. Compound calyces are more common at the poles of the kidney, and are more prone to intrarenal reflux. The shape of each calyx is determined by the shape of the papilla. Disease of the papilla is reflected in the appearance of the calyx. The minor calyces join to form major calyces (infundibula), which drain into the renal pelvis. The appearance of the calyces and pelvis varies widely from patient to patient, and often from one kidney to another, even in the same patient. About 10% of the renal collecting systems are bifid or completely duplicated.

The main renal arteries originate laterally from the aorta, just below the origin of the superior mesenteric artery. The right renal artery courses posterior to the

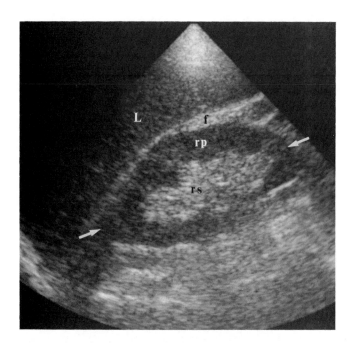

Figure 29.8. Normal Renal Ultrasound. A long axis ultrasound view of the right kidney (*between arrows*) obtained through the liver (*L*) demonstrates echogenicity of the normal renal parenchyma approximately equal to the echogenicity of the normal liver. The renal sinus (*rs*) containing vessels, the collecting system, and fat, is hyperechoic compared to the renal parenchyma (*rp*). The margins of the kidney are outlined by echogenic perirenal fat (*f*). Morison's pouch is a recess of the peritoneal cavity between the kidney and the liver that usually fills with fluid when ascites is present.

IVC, while the left renal artery courses posterior to the left renal vein. The main renal artery divides into ventral and dorsal branches as it enters the renal hilum. These branches divide into segmental arteries that supply separate portions of the kidney. Each is an end artery without anastomoses. Supplied segments of the kidney are therefore highly subject to infarction caused by emboli or occlusion. Interlobar arteries arise from segmental arteries and course in the columns of Bertin. Arcuate arteries are continuations of the interlobar arteries and course parallel to the renal capsule at the corticomedullary junction. Arcuate arteries give rise to intralobular arteries. Arterial divisions down to the level of the arcuate artery are demonstrable by color Doppler ultrasound.

The tight fibrous capsule that covers the kidney produces a sharp renal margin on CT. Perirenal fat continues into the renal sinus, outlining blood vessels and the collecting system. The renal fascia is commonly visualized on CT, especially when the fascia is thickened. Connective tissue septa extending between the renal capsule and the renal fascia subdivide the perirenal space into compartments and may be seen as linear strands in the perirenal fat.

T1-weighted MR images demonstrate a high-density cortex and a lower density medulla. With T2-weighted images, both the cortex and medulla

brighten, but corticomedullary differentiation is often lost. The collecting systems may be difficult to visualize unless filled with urine.

On ultrasound examination, the renal cortex of normal kidneys is isoechoic or slightly hypoechoic compared to adjacent liver or spleen (Fig. 29.8). Corticomedullary differentiation is best seen in infants. The medullary pyramids are lucent compared with the cortex. Lucent pyramids should not be mistaken for hydronephrosis. The central renal sinus is echogenic because of fat and multiple interfaces. Urine-filled collecting structures are easily visualized but blend with renal sinus echogenicity when collapsed. Care must be taken not to mistake prominent renal vessels for dilated collecting structures. Color Doppler ultrasound is useful in differentiating vessels from the collecting system.

Excretory urography will demonstrate corticomedullary differentiation when bolus contrast administration and rapid sequence filming are used. Since contrast agents are excreted by glomerular filtration, the cortex is opacified first, then the medulla is opacified as contrast passes into the collecting tubules. A tomogram late in the nephrogram phase will demonstrate uniform enhancement of the renal parenchyma. By 5 minutes postinjection, the collecting structures and ureters should be opacified (Fig. 29.9).

Since the kidneys actively concentrate contrast in the collecting tubules, renal masses seen on CT and excretory urography will be more lucent than the enhanced renal parenchyma.

Congenital Renal Anomalies

Renal Agenesis is associated with genital tract anomalies in the female. Ipsilateral adrenal agensis is found in 10% of cases. In the remainder, the adrenal gland may appear enlarged. Compensatory hypertrophy of the opposite kidney is usually evident.

Horseshoe Kidney is the most common renal fusion anomaly. The lower poles of the kidneys are joined across the midline by a fibrous or parenchymal band. As a result of fusion, the kidneys are malrotated, with the renal pelvices directed more anteriorly and the lower pole calyces directed medially (Fig. 29.10). The fused kidney is low in position in the abdomen because normal ascent is prevented by the fused parenchyma encountering the inferior mesenteric artery in the midline. Renal arteries are frequently multiple and ectopic in origin. Complications include increased susceptibility to trauma and urinary stasis leading to stones and infection.

Crossed-fused Renal Ectopia may present as an abdominal mass because both kidneys are on the same side of the abdomen (Fig. 29.11). Renal arteries

Figure 29.9. Normal Excretory Urogram. A radiograph of the kidneys taken 5 minutes after intravenous contrast injection demonstrates the enhanced renal parenchyma (between *arrowheads*) and the filled collecting system (*P*). The calyces (*long arrow*) are sharp and cup-shaped to accept the apex of the medullary pyramids. Upper pole calyces (*short arrow*) are usually compound because of drainage of multiple pyramids. Oblique views may be needed to confirm the normal appearance of calyces oriented anteriorly or posteriorly (*open arrow*). The normal kidney is equal in length to between three and four vertebral bodies.

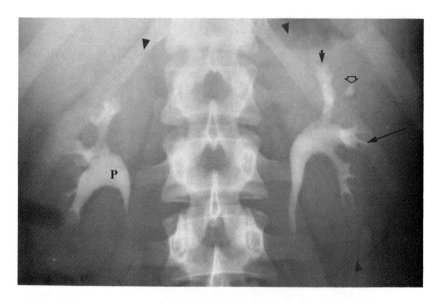

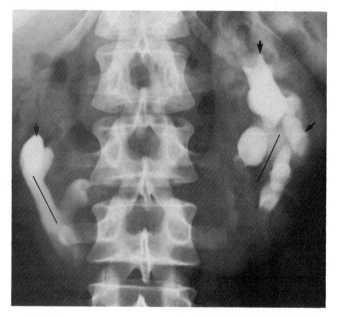

Figure 29.10. Horseshoe Kidney. Radiograph from an excretory urogram demonstrates the two kidneys extending across the spine and joined at their lower poles. Note the reversal of the long axis of each kidney (*black lines*) with the lower poles converging instead of diverging. The calyces (*arrows*) are blunted, reflecting urinary stasis created by the ureters having to cross anteriorly over the joined parenchyma.

are invariably aberrant. The ureters insert in their normal locations in the bladder trigone.

Solid Renal Masses

NEOPLASTIC

Renal Cell Carcinoma accounts for 85% of all renal neoplasms. It is most common in men (male:female = 3:1), at ages 50–70, and is bilateral in 2%. Since surgical resection provides the only chance for cure, early detection and accurate staging are critically important.

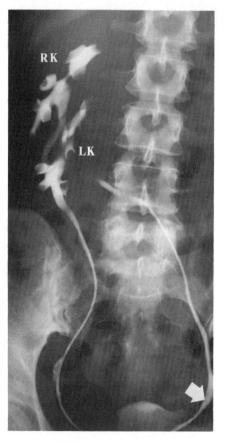

Figure 29.11. Crossed-fused Renal Ectopia. The left kidney (*LK*) is ectopic on the right side of the abdomen and its parenchyma is fused to the parenchyma of the right kidney (*RK*). Note that the left ureter (*arrow*) inserts normally into the bladder.

Any solid renal mass should be considered suspect for renal cell carcinoma (Figs 29.12 and 29.13). However, hemorrhage and necrosis are common, and cystic and multicystic forms are also seen (Fig. 29.14). Stippled central or peripheral calicifications are seen in 10% of cases. The tumors are commonly hypervas-

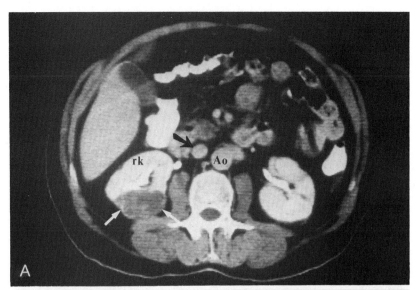

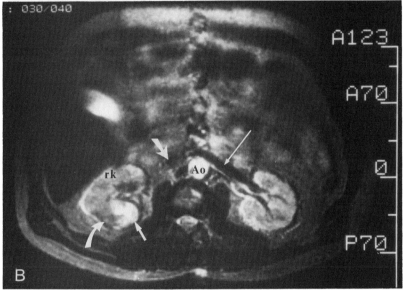

Figure 29.12. Renal Cell Carcinoma. A. Contrast-enhanced CT image demonstrates a heterogeneous low-density mass (*arrows*) in the right kidney (*rk*). **B.** T2-weighted (TR = 2000, TE = 60) MR image in the same patient demonstrates the cystic component of the tumor (*small arrow*) well, but the more solid portion (*curved arrow*) is isodense with the normal renal parenchyma. The IVC (*large arrow*) is free of evidence of tumor thrombus. The left renal vein (*long arrow*) is well demonstrated. *Ao*, aorta.

cular with numerous abnormal feeding vessels visualized. Tumor growth into the renal vein occurs in 30% of cases and extends into the IVC in 5–10%. Detection of venous invasion is critical to surgical planning.

Metastases are present at diagnosis in 40% of cases. The tumor metastasizes most commonly to lung, local lymph nodes, liver, bone, adrenal glands, and the opposite kidney. Chest CT and radionuclide bone scans are effective in demonstrating distant metastases.

Contrast-enhanced CT detects 96% of renal carcinomas (Fig. 29.12**A**) (5). However, when intravenous contrast is contraindicated, MR is preferred over noncontrast CT. Computed tomography is effective in staging renal cell carcinoma (Table 29.1). Venous invasion is seen as nodular, low-density tumor filling and expanding the vein.

Magnetic resonance imaging will commonly miss small, solid renal tumors (<3 cm) that do not distort the renal outline because the tumor demonstrates the same signal characteristics as normal renal parenchyma (Fig. 29.12**B**). Magnetic resonance imaging is effective in staging renal cell carcinoma and is more accurate than CT for advanced disease.

Ultrasound demonstrates solid renal cell carcinomas as a heterogeneous hypoechoic or mildly hyperechoic mass (Fig. 29.13). Areas of hemorrhage and necrosis appear cystic. Doppler ultrasound of the renal vein and IVC should be routine to assess for echogenic tumor thrombus diverting flow or occluding the vessel.

Angiomyolipoma is a benign mesenchymal tumor composed of abnormal blood vessels lacking elastic tissue, smooth muscle, and fat in varying amounts. Most (80%) are solitary unilateral tumors discovered most commonly in middle-aged women. The remaining 20% are found in patients with tuberous sclerosis. These tumors are commonly multicen-

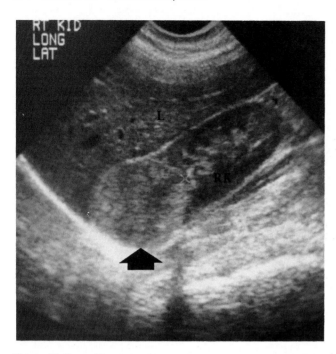

Figure 29.13. Renal Cell Carcinoma. An ultrasound image in the long axis of the right kidney *(RK)* reveals a solid, mildly hyperechoic mass *(arrow)* at the upper pole. *L,* liver.

tric and bilateral. Because of the abnormal thin-walled vessels, the tumors are prone to hemorrhage, which may be massive. Solitary lesions are usually surgically removed. Imaging studies reflect the tissue composition of the tumor.

Computed tomography demonstration of fat density within the tumor is considered diagnostic (Fig. 29.15). Smooth muscle and vascular components of the tumor are seen as nodules and strands of soft tissue density. Vascular areas of the tumor may show striking contrast enhancement.

Ultrasound characteristically demonstrates a strikingly hyperechoic solid mass (Fig. 29.16). Echogenicity of the tumor often exceeds renal sinus fat. Small tumors (<2 cm) are common incidental findings. Tumors may be as large as 20 cm and may be predominantly exophytic, mimicking nonrenal tumors.

T1-weighted MR images demonstrate the high-signal intensity of fat; however, differentiation from chronic hematoma may be difficult (3).

Angiography classically demonstrates a hypervascular mass with enlarged feeding arteries and tortuous, aneurysmally dilated vessels. Venous pooling is common, but there is no arteriovenous shunting.

Renal Adenoma. Controversy exists as to whether renal adenoma is a benign neoplasm or a small, well-differentiated renal cell carcinoma. By definition, adenomas are less than 3 cm in size, lack invasive features, and do not metastasize. Nevertheless, most are treated with total nephrectomy. They are in-

distinguishable from renal cell carcinoma by imaging methods.

Oncocytoma is a well-encapsulated, benign tumor composed of eosinophilic cells called oncocytes. Large tumors demonstrate a stellate central scar that is suggestive of the diagnosis. Angiography classically demonstrates a "spoke-wheel" configuration of radiating vessels. However, most oncocytomas are indistinguishable from renal cell carcinoma and must be surgically removed to confirm the diagnosis.

Lymphoma. While primary renal lymphoma is rare, the kidney is commonly involved by metastatic lymphoma, or by direct invasion. Most cases are non-Hodgkin's lymphoma. Patterns of renal involvement include diffuse disease enlarging the kidney, multiple bilateral solid renal masses, solitary bulky tumor, and tumor invasion into the renal sinus.

Metastases. The kidneys are a frequent site of hematogenous metastases; however, most are small and rarely symptomatic. Metastases usually appear as multiple, bilateral, small, irregular renal masses. Common primary tumors include lung, breast, and melanoma.

INFLAMMATORY

Xanthogranulomatous Pyelonephritis is a rare inflammatory lesion that may diffusely involve an obstructed kidney or present as a focal renal mass (6, 7). An obstructing stone, often a staghorn calculus, is usually present (Fig. 29.17). The kidney is chronically infected, most commonly with *Proteus mirabilis,* and does not function in the affected areas. Computed tomography and ultrasound demonstrate focal or diffuse hydronephrosis and a complex mass with areas of high and low density.

Cystic Renal Masses

Simple Renal Cyst is the most common renal mass. They are found in half the population over age 55. Small cysts are asymptomatic. Large cysts (>4 cm) occasionally cause obstruction, pain, hematuria, or hypertension. Cysts are commonly multiple and bilateral. Imaging by ultrasound, CT, and MR can all make a definitive diagnosis.

Ultrasound criteria for simple renal cyst are (a) round or oval anechoic mass, (b) increased through transmission, (c) sharply defined far wall, and (d) thin or imperceptible cyst wall.

Computed tomography signs include (a) sharp margination with the renal parenchyma, (b) no perceptible wall, (c) homogeneous attenuation near water density (−10 to +10 HU), and (d) absence of contrast enhancement (Fig. 29.18).

Magnetic resonance criteria include (a) homogeneous, sharply defined round or oval mass, (b) homogeneous low-signal intensity on T1-weighted images,

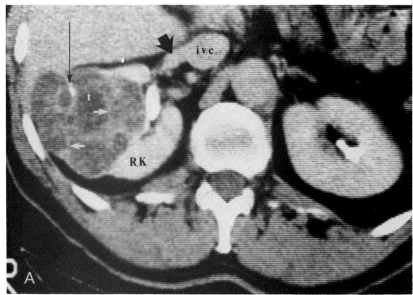

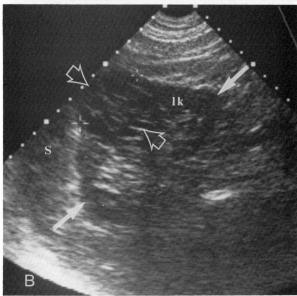

Figure 29.14. Renal Cell Carcinoma—multicystic appearance.
A. Contrast-enhanced CT scan reveals a lobulated tumor (*t*) in the right kidney (*RK*). Septations (*small arrows*) are evident between cystic areas. A focal calcification (*long black arrow*) is also present. The right renal vein (*black arrow*) and the inferior vena cava (*ivc*) are free of tumor thrombus. **B.** An ultrasound image in a different patient shows a multicystic mass (between *open arrows*) arising from the lateral aspect of the left kidney (*lk*, between *closed arrows*). The thin septations were lined by clear cells typical of renal carcinoma. *S*, spleen.

Table 29.1. Staging of Renal Cell Carcinoma

Stage		Description
I		Confined to the kidney (sharp renal margin on CT and MR)
II		Spread to perinephric fat but confined within Gerota's fascia (poorly defined margin on CT and MR)
III	A	Spread to renal vein or cava (intraluminal mass + enlarged vessel)
	B	Spread to local lymph nodes (nodes >15 mm diameter)
IV	A	Spread to adjacent organs
	B	Distant metastases

and (c) homogeneous high-signal intensity similar to urine on T2-weighted images.

Complicated Cyst. Simple renal cysts may be complicated by hemorrhage or infection. The resulting change in imaging characteristics may make differentiation from cystic renal tumors difficult.

Ultrasound usually demonstrates echoes within the fluid of complicated cysts. Cysts with thin septations and lobulated contours are still usually simple cysts. Cysts with thick septations, shaggy walls, or solid components are suspicious for neoplasm.

Computed tomography may demonstrate increased internal density in complicated cysts. Thick walls (Fig. 29.18), soft tissue components, or areas of enhancement are usually indications for percutaneous biopsy or excision.

Magnetic resonance signal intensity depends on the amount of blood or proteinaceous material present within the cyst. Cyst fluid with signal characteristics similar to urine suggests a simple cyst. Higher signal intensity on T1-weighted images suggests a complicated cyst, that may be indistinguishable from a solid mass.

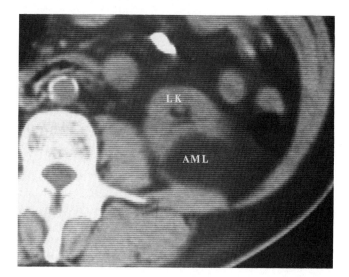

Figure 29.15. Angiomyolipoma. A CT image obtained without intravenous contrast demonstrates a fat-density tumor (*AML*) extending from the posterior aspect of the left kidney (*LK*) and blending imperceptibly with the perirenal fat.

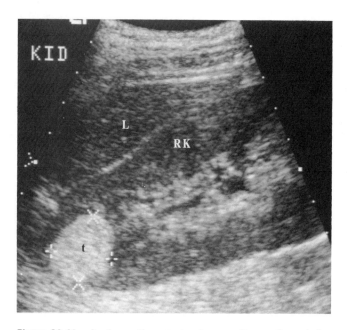

Figure 29.16. Angiomyolipoma. An ultrasound image through the long axis of the right kidney (*RK*) demonstrates a well-defined, uniformly hyperechoic tumor (*t*) in the upper pole. This appearance is strongly suggestive of angiomyolipoma. *L*, liver.

Renal Abscess usually results from pyelonephritis complicated by liquefactive necrosis. A focal renal mass with a thick wall is the most common appearance. Associated inflammatory changes include stranding densities in the perirenal space and thickening of the renal fascia. Renal abscesses may extend into the perirenal space and demonstrate an associated perirenal fluid collection (Fig. 29.19).

Renal Cell Carcinoma may appear as a predominantly cystic or multiloculated cystic mass (Fig.

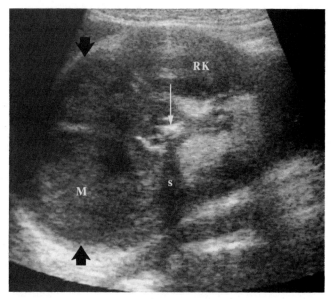

Figure 29.17. Xanthogranulomatous Pyelonephritis. Long axis ultrasound of the right kidney (*RK*) reveals a hypoechoic mass (*M*, between *arrows*) enlarging the upper pole. An obstructing stone (*long white arrow*) casting an acoustic shadow (*s*) is seen in the renal sinus. This kidney was chronically infected and was surgically removed, confirming xanthogranulomatous pyelonephritis.

29.14). Malignant tumor cells line the walls and septa. Thick walls, thick septations, and contrast enhancement are usually evident.

Multilocular Cystic Nephroma is an uncommon benign neoplasm consisting of a cluster of noncommunicating cysts of varying size separated by connective tissue septations. They are discovered most commonly in male infants and middle-aged women. Surgical excision is usually recommended in adults to exclude renal cell carcinoma.

Renal Cystic Disease

MULTIPLE BILATERAL RENAL CYSTS

Adult Polycystic Disease is transmitted by autosomal dominant inheritance (8, 9). Renal parenchyma is progressively replaced by multiple noncommunicating cysts of varying size (Fig. 29.20). Renal volume increases with the number and size of the renal cysts. The cysts are commonly complicated by internal hemorrhage. The condition can be detected in neonates and children, but most patients present clinically between ages 30 and 50 with hypertension and renal failure. Imaging diagnosis is confirmed by demonstration of cysts in the pancreas and liver, and occasionally in other organs. Aneurysms of the circle of Willis are present in 10–30% of cases.

Multiple Simple Cysts must be differentiated from adult polycystic disease. Patients with multiple simple cysts are usually older, have fewer number of cysts, usually no renal failure, and no family history of

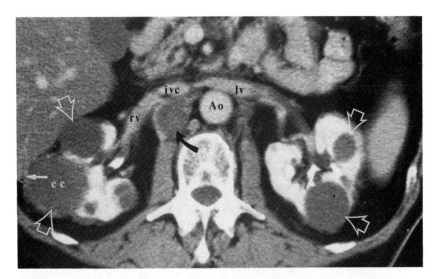

Figure 29.18. Multiple Renal Cysts. Contrast-enhanced CT demonstrates multiple cysts (*open arrows*) in both kidneys. The right kidney has one cyst (*cc*) that does not meet criteria for a simple cyst because of visible thickening of its wall (*closed arrow*). The thick wall was due to previous hemorrhage within the cyst. The renal veins (*rv, lv*) and inferior vena cava (*ivc*) are clearly seen. An enlarged retrocaval lymph node (*curved arrow*) is evident. *Ao*, aorta.

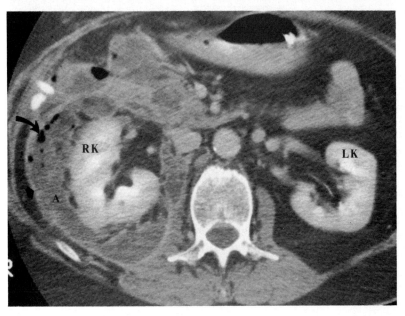

Figure 29.19. Perirenal Abscess. Contrast-enhanced CT scan discloses a low-density fluid collection (*A*) in the perirenal space between the right kidney (*RK*) and the thickened renal fascia (*arrowhead*). Gas bubbles (*curved arrow*) are seen within the perirenal abscess. *LK*, left kidney.

renal cystic disease (Fig. 29.18). Cysts are not found in other organs.

von Hippel-Lindau Syndrome is associated with multiple renal and pancreatic cysts, renal adenomas, and frequently multiple and bilateral renal cell carcinomas. Associated lesions include retinal angiomas and cerebellar hemangioblastomas. The disease is inherited with an autosomal dominant pattern.

Tuberous Sclerosis combines multiple renal cysts (Fig. 29.21) and multiple angiomyolipomas (10). Cutaneous, retinal, and cerebral hamartomas are associated. This condition also has an autosomal dominant inheritance pattern.

Acquired Cystic Kidney Disease is the term applied to the development of multiple cysts in the native kidneys of patients on long-term hemodialysis. Affected kidneys are usually small, reflecting the chronic renal disease. Cysts are predominantly cortical and rarely exceed 2 cm size. Solid adenomatous tumors

also develop and are prone to spontaneous hemorrhage.

MEDULLARY CYSTIC DISEASE

Medullary Sponge Kidney refers to dysplastic dilation of the collecting tubules in the papilla (8). The dilation is cylindrical or saccular in configuration. The condition is associated with urinary stasis, which may result in infection and stone formation (Fig. 29.22). Most patients are asymptomatic. There is no genetic predisposition and no risk of renal failure.

The kidneys remain normal in size. The condition is usually bilateral and symmetric, but may be focal, unilateral, or asymmetric. Striations or saccular contrast collections in the papilla on excretory urography are most characteristic. Stones in the papilla cause increased echogenicity in the medulla on ultrasounds.

Figure 29.20. Adult Polycystic Disease. Contrast-enhanced CT demonstrates massive enlargement of both right and left kidneys (*RK, LK*) and replacement of most of the renal parenchyma by multiple cysts (c). *p*, renal pelvis opacified with contrast.

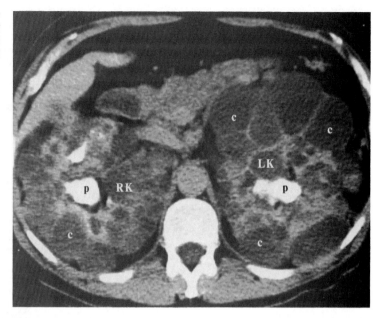

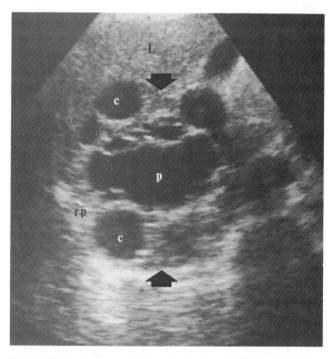

Figure 29.21. Tuberous Sclerosis. Transverse ultrasound view of the right kidney (between *arrowheads*) reveals multiple simple cysts (c) of varying size in the renal parenchyma (*rp*). The renal pelvis (*p*) is dilated because of mass effect and partial obstruction caused by the renal cysts. *L*, liver.

Uremic Medullary Cystic Disease presents with renal failure, anemia, and salt wasting. The basic defect is progressive tubular atrophy with glomerular sclerosis and medullary cyst formation. The medullary cysts are generally too small to be visualized by current imaging methods. Kidney size is normal or small. Renal parenchymal echogenicity is usually increased.

MULTICYSTIC RENAL DISEASE

Multicystic Dysplastic Kidney is usually diagnosed in utero or at birth. The classic multicystic dysplastic kidney appears as a mass of noncommunicating cysts of varying size (8). With time, the kidney progressively atrophies so that in the adult a nubbin of tissue, which is often calcified, is all that remains.

Renal Infections

Acute Pyelonephritis is usually due to ascending urinary tract infection caused by Gram-negative organisms, especially *Escherichia coli*. Uncomplicated infection requires no imaging, and often shows no imaging abnormalities. Imaging evaluation is indicated in patients who fail to respond to treatment or are severly ill. Computed tomography is more sensitive than ultrasound in demonstrating subtle changes in the renal parenchyma associated with uncomplicated pyelonephritis (6). Either CT or ultrasound can be used to detect complications such as renal or perirenal abscess.

Computed tomography demonstrates a swollen, edematous kidney usually with patchy areas of decreased density or a striated parenchymal nephrogram (6). Lobar nephronia refers to a preabscess state of focal bacterial infection seen as focal wedge-shaped or rounded area of decreased density. When liquefactive necrosis of the renal parenchyma occurs, an abscess is formed, seen as a thick-walled fluid collection within the kidney. Extension of fluid density into the perirenal space implies rupture of the renal capsule (Fig. 29.19).

Emphysematous Pyelonephritis is a form of acute pyelonephritis with air in the renal paren-

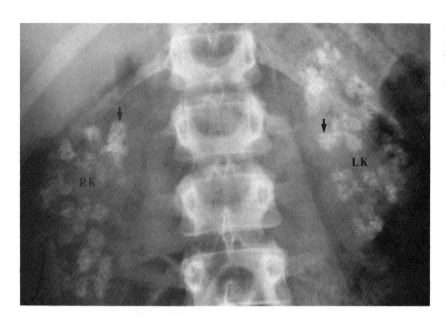

Figure 29.22. Medullary Sponge Kidney. Plain radiograph demonstrates innumerable calcifications (*arrows*) in the medullary regions of both right and left kidneys (*RK, LK*). The stones form in dilated collecting tubules in the medullary pyramids.

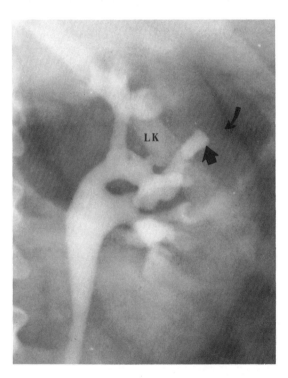

Figure 29.23. Reflux Nephropathy. Radiograph of the left kidney (*LK*) obtained as part of an excretory urogram demonstrates a blunted calyx (*arrow*) with an overlying cortical scar (*curved arrow*). These findings are indicative of reflux nephropathy.

chyma. The condition is rapidly progressive and often life-threatening (6). Mixed flora infection with Gram-negative organisms is most common. Computed tomography and plain films demonstrate gas collections within the renal parenchyma.

Chronic Pyelonephritis and Reflux Nephropathy.   Chronic pyelonephritis refers to chronic renal parenchymal infection (6, 7). In children, vesicoureteral reflux of infected urine is the most common

cause of chronic pyelonephritis. Intrarenal reflux, usually most prominent at the upper pole, damages the papilla, resulting in calyceal blunting with overlying cortical scarring. This process of progressive renal injury associated with reflux is referred to as *reflux nephropathy*. Adults may show stable residual findings of this childhood disease (Fig. 29.23). Chronic pyelonephritis in adults is most commonly associated with calculi and chronic obstruction (7). Neurogenic bladder, ileal conduits, and other causes of urinary stasis are predisposing conditions.

Both reflux nephropathy of childhood and chronic pyelonephritis in adults show similar imaging findings. The hallmark is a focal cortical scar that overlies a blunted calyx (Fig. 29.23). The disease is classically lobar, with normal lobes with normal calyces interposed between diseased lobes. These findings are demonstrated on excretory urography but may also be evident on ultrasound and CT.

Renal Tuberculosis may follow primary pulmonary tuberculosis by as much as 10–15 years (6, 7). Active pulmonary tuberculosis is present in only 10% of cases of renal tuberculosis. Only 30% show any chest radiograph evidence of prior tuberculosis. Patients present with asymptomatic hematuria or sterile pyuria. Since the disease is uncommon in the United States, imaging studies often initially suggest the diagnosis when it is unsuspected clinically. Computed tomography is generally preferred over ultrasound and excretory urography to demonstrate subtle findings (6, 7).

The hallmarks of renal tuberculosis include parenchymal destruction and cavity formation eventually leading to parenchymal scarring; parenchymal masses due to granuloma formation; fibrosis leading to strictures of the collecting system and ureters; and a wide variety of patterns of calcification. End-stage

Figure 29.24. Chronic Renal Failure. An ultrasound image of the right kidney (*RK*) demonstrates a diffuse increase in echogenicity of the renal parenchyma compared to the liver (*L*) in a patient with chronic renal failure. The kidney is of normal size.

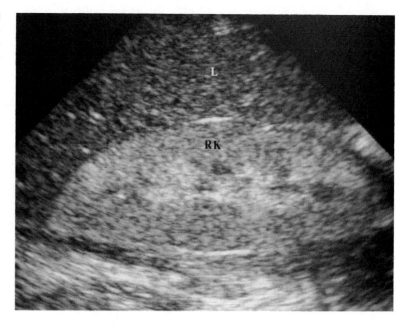

Table 29.2.   Medical Renal Diseases with Echogenic Renal Parenchyma in Adults

Acute glomerulonephritis
Chronic glomerulonephritis
Hypertensive nephrosclerosis
Diabetic glomerulosclerosis
Lupus nephritis
Lymphoma
AIDS
Amyloidosis

Table 29.3.   Causes of Bilateral Small Kidneys[a]

Arterial hypotension (acute contrast reaction)
Generalized arteriosclerosis
Nephrosclerosis due to systemic hypertension
Chronic glomerulonephritis
Uremic medullary cystic disease

[a]Adapted from Davidson AJ. Radiology of the kidney. Philadelphia: WB Saunders, 1985:179.

Table 29.4.   Causes of Bilateral Large Kidneys[a]

Proliferative disorders
    Acute glomerulonephritis
    Lupus nephritis
    Diabetic glomerulosclerosis
Parenchymal edema
    Acute tubular necrosis
    Acute cortical necrosis
    Acute bilateral pyelonephritis
Cell infiltration
    Lymphoma
    Leukemia
Protein deposition
    Multiple myeloma
    Amyloidosis
Urate deposition
    Urate nephropathy

[a]Adapted from Davidson AJ. Radiology of the kidney. Philadelphia: WB Saunders, 1985:221.

nonfunctional tuberculous kidneys may be hydronephrotic sacs, or appear as atrophic and calcified masses in the renal bed.

Renal Parenchymal Disease

Renal Failure. In patients with renal failure, ultrasound is usually requested to exclude hydronephrosis, assess renal size, and identify renal parenchymal disease. Bilateral hydronephrosis is a rare, but potentially reversible, cause of renal failure. Patients with acute renal failure and large (>12 cm) or normal-sized kidneys often require biopsy for definitive diagnosis of renal parenchymal disease. Patients with small (<9 cm) kidneys usually have irreversible end-stage renal disease and do not benefit from biopsy. Measurements of renal cortical thickness are unreliable in assessing residual renal function. Sonographic signs of renal parenchymal disease include a diffuse increase in parenchymal echogenicity often associated with loss of corticomedullary differentiation (Fig. 29.24) (11). Sonographic characterization of renal parenchymal changes correlated with renal size shortens the differential diagnosis of "medical renal disease" to a limited degree (Tables 29.2 through 29.4).

Acquired Immunodeficiency syndrome (AIDS). Renal disease in AIDS encompasses a broad spectrum of abnormalities (11). An AIDS-related nephropathy refers to focal and segmental glomerulosclerosis with associated tubular abnormalities. Diffuse renal infection with associated calcification due to *Pneumocystis carinii* and *Mycobacterium avium* and *M. intracellulare* have been reported. Patients with AIDS are exposed to nephrotoxic drugs such as pentamidine. Associated diseases such as

Table 29.5. Causes of Unilateral Small Kidney[a]

Renal artery stenosis
Global renal infarction
Radiation nephritis
Postobstructive atrophy
Postinflammatory atrophy
Congenital hypoplasia

[a]Adapted from Davidson AJ. Radiology of the kidney. Philadelphia: WB Saunders, 1985:151.

Table 29.6. Causes of Unilateral Large Kidney[a]

Acute renal vein thrombosis
Acute arterial infarction
Obstructive uropathy
Acute pyelonephritis
Duplicated collecting system
Compensatory hypertrophy

[a]Adapted from Davidson AJ. Radiology of the kidney. Philadelphia, WB Saunders, 1985:255.

Table 29.7. Causes of Medullary Nephrocalcinosis

Hyperparathyroidism
Medullary sponge kidney
Renal tubular acidosis (distal form)
Milk-alkali syndrome
Hypervitaminosis D
Hypercalcemic/hypercalciuric states

Table 29.8. Causes of Echogenic Renal Pyramids

Medullary nephrocalcinosis
Hyperuricemia
Papillary necrosis (dystrophic calcification)
Infection (*Candida*, cytomegalovirus)

lymphoma and dehydration due to diarrhea and vomiting may contribute to renal injury. Over 50% of patients with AIDS demonstrate increased renal parenchymal echogenicity.

Bilateral Small Kidneys (<9 cm) imply a systemic disease process that injures both kidneys and usually reduces their function (Table 29.3). The conditions listed are generally indistinguishable by imaging methods.

Bilateral Large Kidneys (>12 cm) imply a systemic process that adds to renal size by deposition of protein, cells, or fluid (Table 29.4). Acute tubular necrosis is the most common cause of acute renal failure (11). Acute tubular necrosis is most commonly precipitated by renal ischemia or exposure to nephrotoxic substances including radiographic contrast agents.

Unilateral Small Kidney suggests global injury to the renal parenchyma as a result of a local unilateral rather than a systemic process (Table 29.5). Renal artery stenosis causes chronic renal ischemia and is a cause of systemic hypertension. The involved kidney is small and demonstrates a delayed nephrogram and a delay in the collecting system opacification on XU. Global renal infarction occurs as a result of sudden occlusion of a main renal artery due to embolus, thrombus, or trauma. Radiation nephritis results from inclusion of the kidney in a field of therapeutic radiation. Postobstructive atrophy may follow relief of chronic obstruction. Postinflammatory atrophy follows chronic infection. Congenital hypoplasia is an underdeveloped kidney with a reduced number of lobes (<5 lobes); the opposite kidney usually shows compensatory hypertrophy.

Unilateral Large Kidney. With the exception of a duplicated collecting system and compensatory hypertrophy, unilateral large kidneys are due to acute local insults that affect only one kidney (Table 29.6). Renal vein thrombosis and renal artery infarction result in enlarged swollen kidneys in the acute state and small kidneys in the chronic state. Acute obstruction and acute pyelonephritis cause edematous swollen kidneys. Compensatory hypertrophy is usually associated with a small or poorly functioning opposite kidney. Duplication of the collecting system is proven by excretory urography.

Nephrocalcinosis

Nephrocalcinosis is a broad term that refers to pathologic deposition of calcium in the renal parenchyma. Nephrocalcinosis is usually bilateral and due to systemic disorders.

Cortical Nephrocalcinosis is unusual, representing less than 5% of nephrocalcinosis. Causes include acute cortical necrosis precipitated by severe ischemia, chronic glomerulonephritis, and primary hyperoxaluria.

Medullary Nephrocalcinosis is far more common and is usually related to hypercalcemic/hypercalciuric states (Table 29.7). Note that echogenic renal pyramids may result from medullary nephrocalcinosis as well as other causes (Fig. 29.25 and Table 29.8).

Renal Trauma

Contrast-enhanced CT provides the most comprehensive evaluation of renal trauma; however, excretory urography remains widely utilized. The types of renal injury include:

Renovascular Injury is evidenced by failure of the kidney to enhance following intravenous contrast injection. Occlusion of the renal artery because of an intimal tear resulting in thrombosis should be suspected (Fig. 29.26). Arteriography is required to identify the specific causative lesion. Immediate surgical repair is needed to preserve renal function.

Renal Contusion refers to extravasation of blood and urine into the renal parenchyma, but still con-

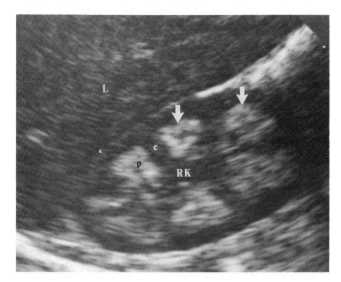

Figure 29.25. Medullary Nephrocalcinosis. Longitudinal ultrasound of the right kidney (*RK*) demonstrates abnormal increased echogencity of the medullary pyramids (*p, arrows*). Note the normal echogenicity of the intrarenal cortex (*c*) (columns of Bertin). *L,* liver.

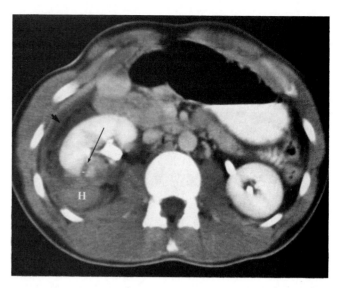

Figure 29.27. Renal Fracture. A CT scan of the kidneys following intravenous contrast administration demonstrates a linear defect (*long arrow*) in the parenchyma of the right kidney, indicating a renal fracture. Blood has escaped from the kidney resulting in a hematoma (*H*) in the perirenal space. The renal fascia (*short arrowhead*) is thickened.

Renal Fracture/Laceration. These are parenchymal injuries that extend to the periphery of the kidney, through the capsule and into the perirenal space (Fig. 29.27). Blood and urine spill into the perirenal space. Fragments of renal parenchyma may be deprived of their blood supply and do not enhance on CT following intravenous contrast administration.

References

1. Dunnick NR. Adrenal imaging: current status. AJR 1990;154:927–936.
2. Schultz CL. CT and MR of the adrenal glands. Semin Ultrasound CT MR 1986;7:219–233.
3. Baumgartner BR, Chezmar JL. Magnetic resonance imaging of the kidneys and adrenal glands. Semin Ultrasound CT MR 1989;10:43–62.
4. Francis IR, Gross MD, Shapiro B, et al. Integrated imaging of adrenal disease. Radiology 1992;184:1–13.
5. Singer J, McClennan BL. The diagnosis, staging, and follow-up of carcinomas of the kidney, bladder, and prostate: the role of cross-sectional imaging. Semin Ultrasound CT MR 1989;10:481–497.
6. Goldman SM, Fishman EK. Upper urinary tract infection: the current role of CT, ultrasound, and MRI. Semin Ultrasound CT MR 1991;12:335–360.
7. Kenney PJ. Imaging of chronic renal infections. AJR 1990;155:485–494.
8. Hayden CK Jr, Swischuk LE. Renal cystic disease. Semin Ultrasound CT MR 1991;12:361–373.
9. Mellins HZ. Cystic dilatations of the upper urinary tract: a radiologist's developmental model. Radiology 1984;153:291–301.
10. Bell DG, King BF, Hattery RR, et al. Imaging characteristics of tuberous sclerosis. AJR 1991;156:1081–1086.
11. Huntington DK, Hill SC, Hill MC. Sonographic manifestations of medical renal disease. Semin Ultrasound CT MR 1991;12:290–307.

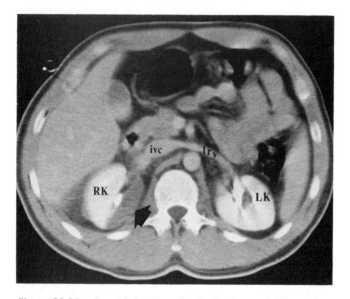

Figure 29.26. Renal Infarction. Contrast-enhanced CT reveals a lack of enhancement of the posterior-medial aspect (*arrow*) of the right kidney (*RK*) because of a trauma-induced intimal tear in the artery supplying this portion of the kidney. *LK,* left kidney; *ivc,* inferior vena cava; *lrv,* left renal vein.

tained within the renal capsule. Contused kidneys enhance poorly on excretory urography. Computed tomography demonstrates patchy areas of decreased enhancement.

Subcapsular Hematoma is the most frequent form of renal injury due to blunt trauma. The hematoma is confined next to the renal parenchyma by the tough renal capsule. Patients are at risk for developing fibrosis of the renal capsule and hypertension (Page kidney).

30

Pelvicalyceal System, Ureter, Bladder, and Urethra

William E. Brant

PELVICALICEAL SYSTEM AND URETER
Imaging Methods

Excretory urography is the usual method used to demonstrate the pelvicaliceal system and ureter. However, high-grade urinary tract obstruction may preclude adequate visualization because of delayed renal function or poor concentration of contrast. Retrograde pyelography, performed by cystoscopic catheterization of the ureteral orifice followed by injection of contrast, is independent of renal function and provides high-quality images of the ureter and the collecting system. Similiar images can be obtained by antegrade pyelography, performed via nephrostomy catheter; however, this procedure is more invasive. Computed tomography (CT) provides excellent images of the kidneys, collecting system, and ureter; it can demonstrate the extent of soft tissue lesions; and has

the capability of differentiating tumor from stones and blood clots. Ultrasound is the imaging method of choice for screening for hydronephrosis, but is limited in its ability to demonstrate small uroepithelial tumors. Magnetic resonance (MR) is seldom used in imaging the collecting system and ureters.

Anatomy

The collecting tubules of a medullary pyramid coalesce into a variable number of papillary ducts that pierce the tip of the papilla and drain into a receptacle of the collecting system called a *minor calyx*. The projection of a papilla into the calyx produces a cup shape. The sharp-edged portion of the minor calyx projecting around the sides of a papilla is called the *fornix* of the calyx (Fig. 29.9). Compound calyces, usually found at the poles of the kidney, are formed by the projection of two or more papilla into the calyx. *Infundibula* extend between minor calyces and the renal pelvis. The renal pelvis is triangular-shaped, with its base within the renal sinus. The apex of the pelvis extends downward to join the ureter. A so-called extrarenal pelvis is predominantly outside the renal sinus and is larger and more distensible than an intrarenal pelvis surrounded by renal sinus fat. An extrarenal pelvis should not be confused with hydronephrosis. There is endless variety in the size and arrangement of calyces, and in the shape and appearance of the renal pelvis.

The ureters have an outer fibrous adventitia that is continuous with the renal capsule and with the adventitia of the bladder (1). The muscularis, responsible for ureteral peristalsis, consists of outer circular and inner longitudinal muscle bundles. The mucosa lining the entire pelvicalyceal system, ureters, and bladder is transitional epithelium. The ureters enter the bladder at an oblique angle. When the bladder wall contracts, the ureteral orifices are closed. The ureters propel urine by active peristalsis, which can be visualized fluoroscopically and by ultrasound. Jets of urine opacified by contrast are frequently seen within the bladder on excretory urography and CT. Because of

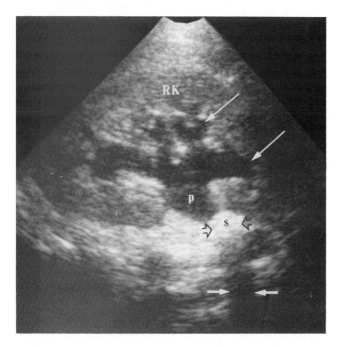

Figure 30.1. Hydronephrosis due to Ureteropelvic Junction Calculus. Coronal plane ultrasound of the right kidney (*RK*) reveals mild dilation of the calyces (*long white arrows*) and renal pelvis (*p*) due to an impacted stone (*s*, between *open arrows*) at the ureteropelvic junction. Note the dark acoustic shadow (between *short white arrows*) cast by the calculus.

peristalsis, the diameter of the ureter at any particular instant is highly variable. Three main points of ureteral narrowing, where calculi are likely to become impacted, are (a) the ureteropelvic junction, (b) the site at which the ureter crosses the pelvic brim, and (c) the ureterovesical junction.

Retrocaval Ureter is an anatomic variant in which the right ureter passes behind the inferior vena cava at the level of L3 or L4 vertebrae. The ureter exits anteriorly between the cava and the aorta to return to its normal position. The condition is associated with varying degrees of urinary stasis and proximal pyeloureterectasis. The anomaly is due to faulty embryogenesis of the inferior vena cava, with abnormal persistence of the right subcardinal vein anterior to the ureter instead of the right supracardinal vein posterior to the ureter.

Calculous Disease

Nephrolithiasis refers to the presence of calculi in the renal collecting system. Eighty percent of renal calculi are composed of sufficient calcium oxalate or calcium phosphate to be radiopaque on plain film. Struvite (magnesium ammonium phosphate) stones, formed in the presence of alkaline urine and infection, make up another 15% of renal calculi, and are also radiopaque. The remaining 5% of renal stones, primarily composed of urate or xanthines, are radiolucent. "Milk of calcium" refers to a fine sediment-con-

taining calcium that may be found in a calyceal diverticulum or hydrocalyx that lacks drainage. Complications of renal calculi include obstruction, ureteral stricture, chronic renal infection, and loss of renal function. High-quality plain films to detect calculi and calcification are mandatory prior to contrast studies of the urinary tract.

Renal Calculi. Most renal calculi are demonstrated on plain films. Excretory urography demonstrates stones within the collecting system as filling defects within contrast-opacified urine. Staghorn calculi form casts of the pelvicalyceal system (Fig. 22.14). Most are composed of struvite and are associated with chronic renal infection. Ultrasound demonstrates both radiopaque and nonradiopaque stones as echodensities with acoustic shadowing (Fig. 30.1). Large stones (>1.5 cm) are the easiest to identify with US. Small stones, which do not cast acoustic shadows, may blend in with renal sinus fat and are often not detected by ultrasound. However, ultrasound is more sensitive than plain film for subtle calcification in the renal parenchyma (Fig. 29.25). All calculi appear dense on CT. Computed tomographic attenuation values greater than 100 HU will differentiate a calculus from a tumor or blood clot. Computed tomography used to evaluate for calculi should be performed without intravenous contrast.

Ureteral Calculi are a major cause of acute urinary tract obstruction and renal colic. Stones that form in the kidney are prone to pass into and obstruct the ureter (Fig. 30.1). Stones less than 6 mm in size are likely to spontaneously pass through the ureter within 6 weeks. Stones larger than 6 mm are likely to become lodged in the ureter and require intervention for removal. Calculi are most likely to be found at the three points of ureteral narrowing mentioned previously (Fig. 30.2).

Hydronephrosis

Hydronephrosis is defined as dilation of the upper urinary tract. Hydronephrosis is not synonymous with obstruction, but has a number of causes that are listed below. The terms caliectasis, pyelectasis, and ureterectasis are more precise in describing dilation of portions of the urinary tract. Ultrasound is an excellent screening modality for determining the presence of urinary tract dilation.

Obstruction. The causes of obstruction include stone, stricture, tumor, and extrinsic compression. The degree of dilation produced by obstruction is variable. In general, the more proximal and the more chronic the obstruction, the greater is the degree of dilation. Acute obstruction produced by an impacted stone often produces minimal dilation.

Ultrasound demonstrates hydronephrosis as separation of normal sinus echogenicity by anechoic urine

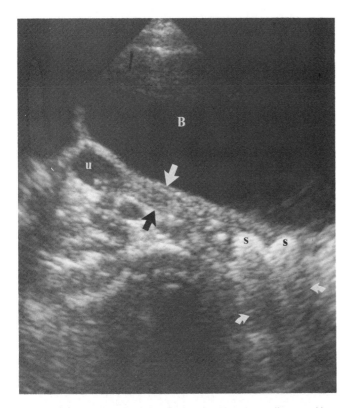

Figure 30.2. Calculi in Distal Ureter. Sagittal plane ultrasound image of the distal right ureter (*u*) demonstrates two stones (*s*) impacted at the ureterovesical junction. Faint acoustic shadows (*curved arrows*) are cast by the stones. Just proximal to the stones the ureter is filled with echogenic debris (*arrows*) due to infection developing as a result of urinary stasis. *B*, bladder.

in the collecting system (Fig. 30.1). The calyces become enlarged and blunted cystic structures that are seen to connect with the dilated renal pelvis. Medullary pyramids may be hypoechoic, especially in children, and must be differentiated from dilated calyces. Pyramids are more peripheral, surrounded by more echogenic cortex, and do not connect with the renal pelvis. A peripelvic cyst can easily be mistaken for hydronephrosis on ultrasound (Fig. 30.3).

Excretory urographic signs of obstruction include (a) increasingly dense nephrogram with time, (b) delay in appearance of contrast in the collecting system, and (c) dilated pelvicalyceal system and ureter to the point of obstruction (Fig. 30.4). *Pyelosinus reflux* may result from rupture of a fornix precipitated by contrast-induced diuresis superimposed on the increased hydrostatic pressure of an obstructed pelvicalyceal system. Urine and contrast extravasate into the renal sinus and perirenal space.

Computed tomography demonstrates dilation of the collecting system, either with or without use of intravenous contrast. Delay in opacification of the obstructed kidney and dependent layering of unopacified urine over heavier contrast media may also be evident. The location and cause of obstruction can frequently be identified

Pyonephrosis refers to infection in an obstructed kidney. Pyonephrosis can result in rapid destruction of the renal parenchyma and must be promply treated by relief of obstruction by ureteral stent or nephros-

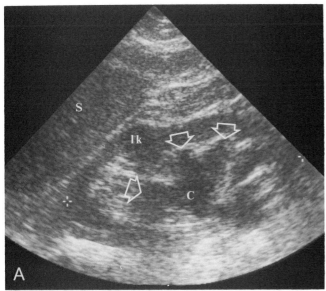

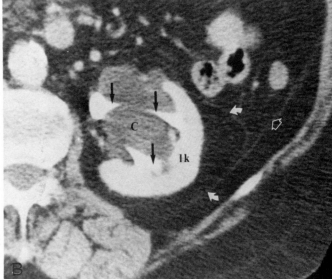

Figure 30.3. Peripelvic Cyst. A. Long axis ultrasound image of the left kidney (*lk*) reveals a fluid-filled structure (*C*) in the renal sinus. Lobulations (*arrows*) of the cystic mass resemble dilated calyces. *S*, spleen. **B.** A CT image of the left kidney (*lk*) reveals the calyces and pelvis (*black arrows*) to be stretched around the peripelvic cyst (*C*).

Cysts that arise in the renal sinus assume the shape of the sinus as they slowly enlarge, mimicking hydronephrosis. Note the visualization of the renal fascia (*curved arrows*) and lateroconal fascia (*open arrow*) in this patient.

Figure 30.4. Obstruction with Pyelosinus Reflux. A. Radiograph taken at 10 minutes following intravenous injection of contrast demonstrates a persisting dense nephogram in the left kidney (*LK*) with delay of contrast excretion into the collecting system. The patient had an obstructing stone at the ureterovesical junction. The right kidney (*RK*) is normal. **B.** Radiograph obtained 2 hours after contrast injection reveals leakage of contrast (*arrows*) out of the left collecting system and into the renal sinus and the perirenal and periureteric spaces. Overdistension of the obstructed collecting system due to the diuretic effect of the contrast agent resulted in rupture of a calyceal fornix. *u*, left ureter.

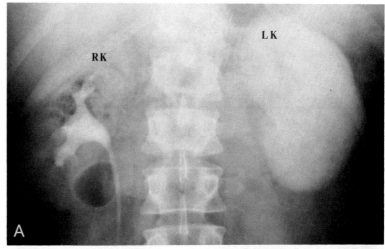

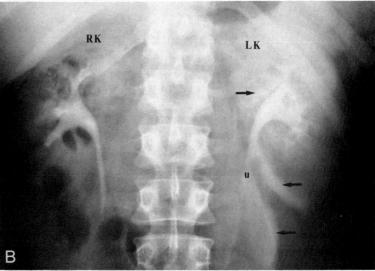

tomy tube placement and antibiotics. Ultrasound classically demonstrates a dilated collecting system filled with layering echogenic pus and debris [2]. Shadowing calculi may also be evident. Computed tomography may be better than ultrasound in demonstrating the site and cause of obstrution. Excretory urography is usually not useful because the affected kidney functions poorly or not at all.

Ureteropelvic Junction Obstruction is a common congenital anomaly that may go undiagnosed until adulthood. The amount of hydronephrosis and parenchymal atrophy present depends upon the severity of obstruction. The condition is bilateral in 30% of cases but is often not symmetric. Excretory urography and ultrasound demonstrate pelvicalyectasis with sharply defined narrowing at the ureteropelvic junction. The ureter is not dilated.

Vesicoureteral Reflux is a common cause of hydronephrosis in children. The basic defect is an abnormal ureteral tunnel at the ureterovesical junction and associated urinary tract infection. In adults, vesicoureteral reflux is usually associated with neurogenic bladder or bladder outlet obstruction. Chronic vesicoureteral reflux of infected urine causes reflux nephropathy. Vesicoureteral reflux is confirmed by demonstrating retrograde filling of the ureters on voiding cystourography or radionuclide cystography.

Congenital Megaureter is due to an aperistaltic segment of the lower ureter causing a functional obstruction and resulting in dilation of the proximal ureter. The aperistaltic segment of the ureter demonstrates smoothly tapered narrowing without evidence of mechanical obstruction.

Prune Belly Syndrome, also called Eagle-Barrett syndrome, is a congenital disorder manifest by absence of the abdominal wall musculature, urinary tract anomalies, and cryptorchidism. The ureters are markedly dilated and tortuous, the bladder is large and distended, and the posterior urethra is dilated.

Polyuria, associated with acute diuresis and diabetes insipidus may cause mild to moderate hydronephrosis.

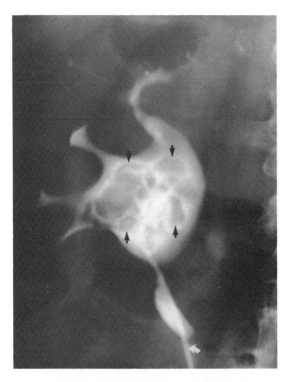

Figure 30.5. Multiple Calculi in the Renal Pelvis. A retrograde pyelogram demonstrates multiple filling defects (*arrows*) in the right renal pelvis which were proven to be radiolucent calculi. Contrast was injected into the renal pelvis via a catheter (*curved arrow*) in the right ureter that was inserted at cystoscopy.

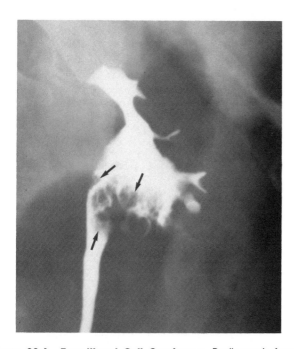

Figure 30.6. Transitional Cell Carcinoma. Radiograph from a retrograde pyelogram of the left kidney reveals a multilobulated filling defect (*arrows*) in the left renal pelvis. This was proven to be a TCC.

Filling Defect/Mass in Pelvicalyceal System or Ureter

Calculi are the most common cause of filling defects in the contrast-filled collecting system or ureter (Fig 30.5). Radiopaque calculi are evident on plain radiographs. Computed tomography demonstrates nonradiopaque calculi as high-density objects with a CT density of greater than 100 HU.

Blood Clots cause nonradiopaque filling defects that can be differentiated from soft tissue tumors by their change in appearance over time. Computed tomography demonstrates attenuation values of 50–65 HU (3).

Transitional Cell Carcinoma (TCC) accounts for 85–90% of all uroepithelial tumors [1, 3]. Most (85%) have a papillary growth pattern that is exophytic, polypoid, and attached to the mucosa by a stalk. These lesions cause a distinct filling defect in the collecting system or ureter (Figs. 30.6 and 30.7). A stippled pattern of contrast material within the interstices of the papillary lesion is characteristic. Tumors in the ureter may demonstrate a "champagne glass" sign of ureteral dilation distal to a filling defect (Fig. 30.7). This sign distinguishes tumor from calculus which impact in the ureter and cause distal spasm and narrowing. Nonpapillary tumors are nodular or flat, and tend to be infiltrating and aggressive. They cause strictures of the collecting system or ureter rather than filling defects.

Most TCC occur in males (male:female = 4:1) aged 60 and above. A variety of chemical agents used in the textile and plastic industries, drugs including cyclophosphamide and phenacetin, and chronic urinary stasis (horseshoe kidney) play a role in the etiology of these tumors. The tumor metastasizes most commonly to regional lymph nodes, liver, lung, and bone.

Transitional cell carcinoma exhibits a strong tendency toward multiplicity. Patients with upper tract TCC have multicentric tumors in 20–44% of cases, while those with TCC of the ureter develop bladder TCC in 20–37% of cases. Careful evaluation of the entire urinary tract is warranted both at initial diagnosis and for follow-up. Standard treatment of TCC is total nephroureterectomy and excision of a cuff of the bladder surrounding the ureteral orifice.

Computed tomography demonstrates a mass within the collecting system (Fig. 30.8). Computed tomography densities range from 8–30 HU unenhanced and 18-55 HU following contrast administration, allowing clear differentiation from calculi. Computed tomography demonstrates the extent of the tumor, including invasion of the kidney or surrounding structures, lymphadenopathy, and distant metastases (Table 30.1).

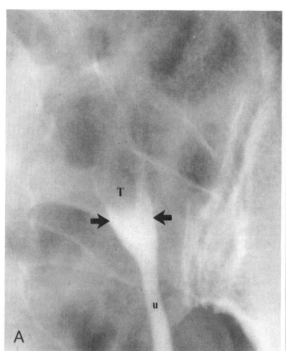

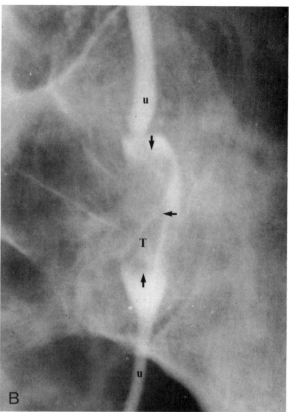

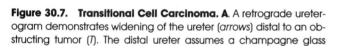

Figure 30.7. Transitional Cell Carcinoma. A. A retrograde ureterogram demonstrates widening of the ureter (*arrows*) distal to an obstructing tumor (*T*). The distal ureter assumes a champagne glass configuration because of the slow growth of the tumor. **B.** Additional contrast administration demonstrates the full extent of the tumor (*T*, between *arrows*). *u*, left ureter.

Ultrasound demonstrates renal TCC as a discrete hypoechoic mass within the renal sinus (Fig. 30.8). Small lesions may be subtle and easily missed. The absence of acoustic shadowing usually provides differentiation from calculi, although a few high-grade tumors have been reported to cast acoustic shadows [3].

Squamous Cell Carcinoma accounts for 10% of uroepithelial tumors. Chronic infection, calculi, and phenacetin abuse are major predisposing factors. Most tumors are infiltrating and superficially spreading, producing stricture or subtle filling defects.

Metastases are a rare cause of a filling defect. Common primary sites are the breast, melanoma, lung, stomach, and cervix.

Papillary Necrosis is ischemic necrosis of the tips of the medullary pyramids. Causes include infection, tuberculosis, sickle cell trait and disease, diabetes, and analgesic nephropathy. Necrotic papilla may remain in situ, slough into the collecting system causing a mobile filling defect, or disappear, resulting in a contrast collection in the papilla or a blunted calyx (see Fig. 30.14). Sloughed papilla may obstruct the ureter and cause renal colic.

Fibroepithelial Polyp is a benign fibrous polyp covered by transitional epithelium. It is most common

Table 30.1. Staging of TCC in the Renal Pelvis and Ureter[a]

Stage	Description
I	Tumor limited to uroepithelial mucosa and lamina propria
II	Tumor invades into, but not beyond, muscularis
III	Tumor invades beyond muscularis into periureteric or peripelvic fat or renal parenchyma
IV	Tumor invades adjacent organs or through the kidney into perinephric fat

[a]Adapted from American Joint Committee on Cancer. Manual for staging of cancer. 4th ed. Philadelphia: JB Lippincott Company, 1992:205–207.

in young adult men. The polyp is mobile and hangs from the mucosa by a long, thin stalk.

Pyeloureteritis Cystica is a benign process of submucosal cyst formation associated with chronic urinary tract infection. Multiple, small, smooth, round filling defects in the pelvis or ureter are characteristic (Fig. 30.9).

Stricture of Pelvicalyceal System or Ureter

A stricture is a fixed narrowing of the pelvicalyceal system or ureter. Strictures should be confirmed with multiple views taken in different projections. A diagnosis of ureteral stricture should never be made unless dilation of the ureter or pelvis above the point of

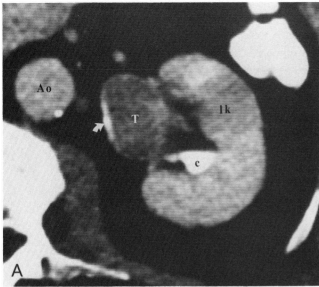

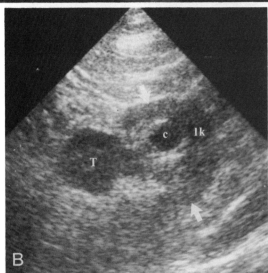

Figure 30.8. Transitional Cell Carcinoma. A. Contrast-enhanced CT of the left kidney (*lk*) demonstrates a tumor (*T*) in the enlarged left renal pelvis. A small amount of contrast (*arrow*) in the pelvis outlines the tumor. A calyx (*c*) proximal to the tumor is dilated. Note the CT density is slightly less than that of the enhanced renal parenchyma. *Ao,* aorta. **B.** An ultrasound image of the same kidney (*lk,* between *arrows*) in transverse plane shows the tumor (*T*) as a hypoechoic mass. The echogenicity of the mass is only slightly greater than that of a dilated calyx (*c*).

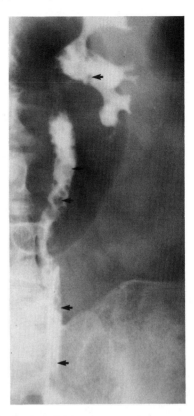

Figure 30.9. Pyeloureteritis Cystica. Retrograde pyeloureterogram demonstrates numerous well-defined, rounded filling defects (*arrows*) in the left renal pelvis and ureter, representing submucosal cysts. The patient had a history of recurrent urinary tract infection.

narrowing is present. Active peristalsis plus the numerous normal kinks and bends in the ureter mimic strictures but lack the combination of fixed narrowing with proximal dilatation.

Inflammation from Stone. An impacted calculus may cause inflammation, which results in scarring and fibrosis producing a stricture.

Posttraumatic strictures result from surgery and instrumentation.

Uroepithelial Tumor. The nonpapillary growth pattern of TCC characteristically causes strictures of the collecting system or ureters (Fig. 30.10). These account for 15% of TCC. Squamous cell carcinoma is usually manifest as a stricture of the pelvis or ureter.

Tuberculosis and Schistosomiasis are two chronic inflammatory processes that are characterized by fibrosis and strictures. Differentiation from TCC may be difficult (Figs. 30.11 and 30.12).

Extrinsic Encasement by tumor or inflammatory processes is a common cause of stricture. Causes include lymphoma, cervical carcinoma, colon carcinoma, endometriosis, Crohn's disease, diverticulitis, and pelvic inflammatory disease.

Papillary Cavities

Calyceal Diverticuli are uroepithelium-lined cavities in the renal parenchyma that communicate via a narrow channel with the fornix of a nearby calyx (Fig. 30.13). They may be congenital, developing from a ureteral bud remnant, or acquired because of rupture of a cyst, infection, or reflux.

Papillary Necrosis may result in cavities at the papillary tips that fill with contrast on both antegrade and retrograde studies (Fig. 30.14). Larger cavities cause blunting of the calyces.

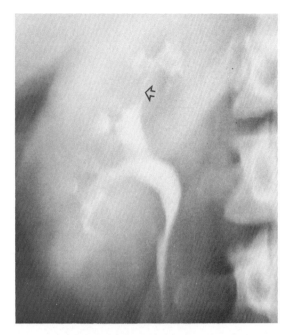

Figure 30.10.   Transitional Cell Carcinoma. Radiograph from an excretory urogram demonstrates fixed narrowing (*arrow*) of the upper pole infundibulum. Compare this view to Figure 30.11.

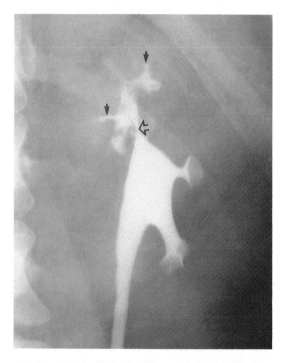

Figure 30.11.   Tuberculosis. Active renal tuberculosis causes narrowing (*open arrow*) of the upper pole infundibulum of the left kidney, very similar to that seen with TCC in Figure 30.10. Note the additional areas of narrowing and irregularity (*arrowheads*) affecting upper pole collecting structures. The study is a retrograde ureterogram.

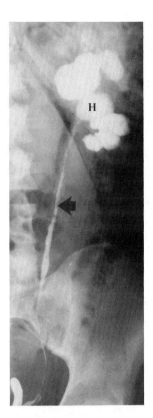

Figure 30.12.   Tuberculosis. Retrograde contrast injection shows numerous filling defects, areas of narrowing, and mucosal irregularity involving the left ureter (arrow). A high-grade stricture at the ureteropelvic junction causes marked hydronephrosis (*H*).

BLADDER

Imaging Methods

Evaluation of the bladder by standard excretory urography (XU) is usually sufficient to exclude most radiographically detectable bladder lesions. A cystogram, performed by instilling contrast agents directly into the bladder, provides a more detailed examination. Fluoroscopic examination is performed during bladder filling to detect reflux. Films are obtained in frontal, lateral, and oblique positions. Films obtained during voiding demonstrate the bladder outlet and urethra. Postvoid films document residual urine. While CT and MR play no significant role in bladder tumor detection, both are used to stage known bladder neoplasms [4, 5]. The urine-filled bladder is routinely used as a sonographic window to the pelvis. Intraluminal masses, calculi, bladder wall thickness, and bladder emptying can be reliably assessed by ultrasound [6].

Anatomy

The normal filled urinary bladder is oval in shape with the floor parallel to, and 5–10 mm above, the superior aspect of the symphysis pubis. The size and shape of the bladder varies with the degree of bladder

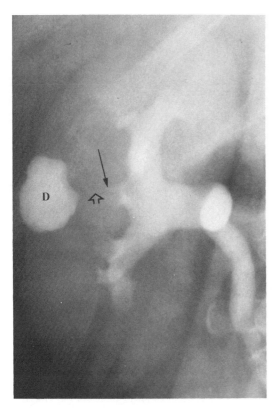

Figure 30.13. Calyceal Diverticulum. An excretory urogram reveals a contrast-filled diverticulum (*D*) in the renal parenchyma. A tiny stream of contrast (*open arrow*) fills the tract, providing communication between the diverticulum and the calyceal fornix (*arrow*).

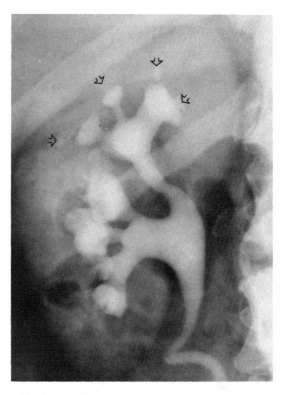

Figure 30.14. Papillary Necrosis. Multiple cavities (*arrows*) in the papilla fill with contrast during this excretory urogram in a patient with sickle cell trait. Most calyces are blunted. Low oxygen tension and high blood osmolality in the papillary tips predispose to sickling and ischemic injury.

filling. The superior surface is covered by peritoneum, which extends to the side walls of the pelvis. The sigmoid colon and loops of small bowel, as well as the uterus in females, lie on top of the bladder and may cause mass impressions on the bladder dome. The inferior surface is extraperitoneal. Anteriorly, the bladder is separated from the symphysis pubis by fat in the extraperitoneal space of Retzius. Posteriorly, the bladder is separated from the uterus by the uterovesical peritoneal recess in females, and from the rectum by the rectovesical peritoneal recess in males.

The lining mucosa of the bladder is loosely attached to the muscular coat so that when the bladder is contracted, the mucosa appears wrinkled. The *trigone* is a triangle at the bladder floor formed by the two ureteral orifices and the internal urethral orifice. With voiding, the trigone descends 1–2 cm and transforms from a flat surface into a cone with the urethra at the apex.

On MR T1-weighted images, the bladder wall is indistinguishable from low-intensity urine [4]. T2-weighted images demonstrate the low-intensity bladder wall, well outlined by high-intensity urine and perivesical fat. Chemical shift artifact at water-fat interfaces may interfere with assessment of tumor invasion of the bladder wall.

Thickened Bladder Wall/Small Bladder Capacity

The normal wall of a well-distended bladder should not exceed 5–6 mm in thickness as measured by ultrasound, CT, or MR. The following conditions are associated with abnormal thickening of the bladder wall and, usually, reduced bladder capacity.

Benign Prostatic Hypertrophy affects 50–75% of males over age 50. Prostate enlargement projects into the base of the bladder, uplifting the bladder trigone and causing "J-hooking" of the distal ureters (Fig. 31.24). Chronic bladder outlet obstruction results in thickening and trabeculation of the bladder wall. Prostate calcifications may be evident. Prostate carcinoma must also be considered as a cause of prostate enlargement, although imaging methods cannot reliably differentiate benign enlargement from malignancy.

Urethral Stricture and Posterior Urethral Valves cause chronic obstruction to the outflow of urine from the bladder. The bladder wall thickens reflecting muscle hypertrophy in an attempt to overcome the obstruction. Voiding or retrograde urethrography demonstrate the urethral abnormality.

Neurogenic Bladder may be spastic or atonic. Causes include meningomyelocele, spinal trauma, diabetes mellitus, poliomyelitis, central nervous system

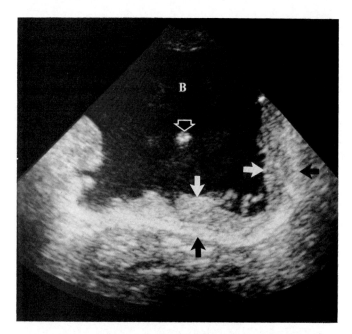

Figure 30.15. Neurogenic Bladder. Axial plane ultrasound of the bladder (*B*) demonstrates marked thickening (*arrows*) of the bladder wall with trabeculation. The patient had an indwelling foley catheter, the tip of which is evident (*open arrow*).

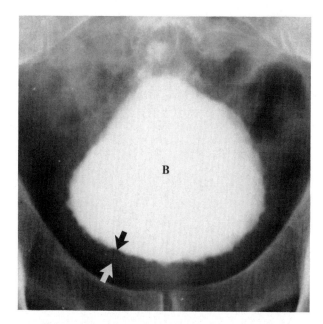

Figure 30.16. Bladder Wall Thickening. Radiograph from a cystogram in a patient with a neurogenic bladder and chronic urinary tract infections demonstrates a thickened bladder wall (between *arrows*) outlined by the contrast agent inside the bladder (*B*) and pelvic fat outside the bladder. Note the irregular contour of the bladder lumen caused by trabeculation of the muscle of the bladder wall.

tumor, and multiple sclerosis. Neurogenic bladders are prone to urinary stasis, chronic infection, and stone formation. Most neurogenic bladders eventually become trabeculated, thick-walled, and reduced in capacity (Figs. 30.15 and 30.16).

Cystitis. Inflammation of the bladder has many causes, including infection (bacteria, adenovirus, tuberculosis, schistosomiasis), drugs (cyclophosphamide), radiation, and autoimmune reaction.

Magnetic resonance demonstrates mucosal edema and inflammation as high-signal intensity on T2-weighted images, easily differentiated from normal low-signal bladder wall [4].

Cystitis Cystica is characterized by multiple fluid-filled submucosal cysts. Most cases are associated with bladder infection.

Cystitis Glandularis is a further progression of cystitis cystica with proliferation of mucous secreting glands in the lamina propria. The cysts vary in size and may obstruct the ureteral orifice. Cystitis glandularis may be a precursor of adenocarcinoma of the bladder.

Bullous Edema of the bladder wall is usually associated with chronic irritation from indwelling catheters. Grape-like cysts elevate the mucosa.

Interstitial Cystitis is a chronic, idiopathic inflammation of the bladder found most often in women. The bladder capacity is progressively diminished while the bladder wall thickens and becomes trabeculated.

Hemorrhagic Cystitis is characterized by hemorrhage into the mucosa and submucosa. It is caused by bacterial or adenovirus infection.

Eosinophilic Cystitis is an infiltration of the bladder wall by eosinophils. The cause is uncertain. The bladder wall is greatly thickened and frequently nodular.

Emphysematous Cystitis is a form of bladder inflammation with gas within the bladder wall or lumen (Fig. 30.17). It is associated with poorly controlled diabetes mellitus, bladder outlet obstruction, and infection with *Escherichia coli*, which ferment sugar in the urine to release carbon dioxide and hydrogen gasses. Additional causes of gas within the bladder lumen include instrumentation and vesicocolic fistula.

Calcified Bladder Wall

Schistosomiasis of the urinary tract is caused by infestation with *Schistosoma haematobium*. The larval cercariae of the blood fluke penetrate the skin of man in infected water, enter the lymphatic vessels, and circulate eventually to the portal system, where the organism matures into adulthood. Adult females migrate to the vesical venous plexus and lay their eggs in the wall of the urinary bladder and ureter. The eggs incite a fibrosing granulomatous reaction that results in beaded stenosis and irregular dilation of the ureters, and calcification of the walls of the distal ureters and bladder. The calcification is entirely due to calcification of the eggs embedded within the wall (Fig. 30.18). The ureters become aperistaltic; vesicoureteral reflux is common. Eventually, the bladder may become shrunken, fibrotic, and contracted. Renal dis-

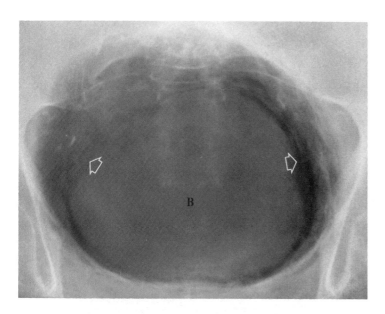

Figure 30.17. Emphysematous Cystitis. Air in the bladder wall is seen as a pattern of layering linear lucencies (*open arrows*) outlining the bladder (*B*) on this plain radiograph in a 67-year-old man with cystitis due to *E. coli.*

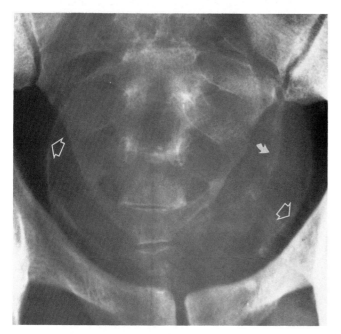

Figure 30.18. Schistosoma haematobium. Plain radiograph demonstrates calcification in the wall of the bladder (*open arrows*) and in the wall of the left ureter (*curved arrow*). The bladder is filled with urine. The patient is a 25-year-old Egyptian male.

ease develops slowly and secondary to functional obstruction and reflux.

Tuberculosis affects the kidneys primarily and the ureters and bladder secondarily. Calcification affects the ureters proximally and may eventually extend into the distal ureters and bladder. Tuberculous infection of the bladder causes wall thickening and reduced capacity. Calcification of the bladder wall is uncommon and patchy.

Cystitis. Postirradiation cystitis, chronic infection, and cyclophosphamide-induced cystitis have

been reported as causes of curvilinear or flocculent bladder wall calcification [7].

Neoplasm. Transitional cell and squamous cell carcinomas of the bladder may rarely calcify (1–7% incidence). Tumor calcification may be punctate or curvilinear, and is best demonstrated by CT.

Bladder Wall Mass/Filling Defect

Simple Ureterocele is a congenital prolapse of the dilated distal ureter and orifice into the bladder lumen at the normal insertion site of the ureter into the trigone. It is usually an incidental finding in adults, although larger, simple ureteroceles may be associated with ureter obstruction, infection, and stone formation.

Excretory urography demonstrates a rounded filling defect in the bladder at the ureteral insertion. A "cobra head" or "spring onion" appearance is characteristic. A radiolucent halo is produced by the wall of the ureter outlined both inside and outside by contrast (Fig. 30.19).

Ultrasound demonstrates a cystic mass at the ureteral oriface. Peristalsis of the ureter causes alternate filling and emptying of the ureterocele, as seen on real-time ultrasound.

Ectopic Ureterocele is usually associated with ureteral duplication. The Weigert-Meyer rule states that with complete ureteral duplication, the upper moiety ureter passes through the bladder wall to insert inferior and medial to the lower moiety ureter. The upper pole ureter usually ends as an ectopic ureterocele, and is usually obstructed because of its ectopic insertion. The lower pole ureter inserts in the normal location in the bladder trigone, but is subject to vesicoureteral reflux because of distortion of its passage through the bladder wall by the ectopic

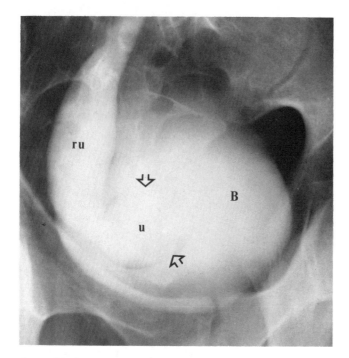

Figure 30.19. Simple Ureterocele. Oblique radiograph from an excretory urogram demonstrates dilation of the right ureter (*ru*) associated with a simple ureterocele (*u*) that protrudes into the lumen of the bladder (*B*). The radiolucent wall of the ureterocele (*arrows*) is outlined by contrast within the ureterocele and contrast within the bladder lumen. The wall of the ureterocele is made up of the wall of the ureter and the bladder mucosa.

ureterocele. Females with ectopic ureters are prone to urinary incontinence because the ureter may insert distal to the external sphincter into the vestibule, uterus, or vagina. In males, the ectopic ureter usually inserts proximal to the external sphincter; no incontinence results. Insertion sites include the lower bladder, posterior urethra, seminal vesicles, vas deferens, and ejaculatory duct. Large ectopic ureteroceles may obstruct the opposite ureter or cause bladder outlet obstruction because of their mass effect.

Excretory urography commonly demonstrates poor function or nonfunction of the obstructed upper pole system. The lower pole system is displaced inferiorly and commonly shows a "drooping lily" appearance. Reflux nephropathy of the lower pole system may be evident.

Ultrasound, CT, or MR demonstrates cystic dilation of the upper pole system, usually with marked parenchymal thinning. The upper pole ureter is commonly tortuous and dilated. The ectopic ureterocele (Fig. 30.20) and its associated dilated ureter may simulate a multiseptated cystic mass in the pelvis.

Transitional Cell Carcinoma of the bladder is the most common urinary tract neoplasm. Transitional cell carcinoma of the bladder is 50 times more common than TCC of the ureter [1]. While bladder tumors commonly develop in patients with primary TCC of the renal pelvis or ureter, only 2–4% of patients

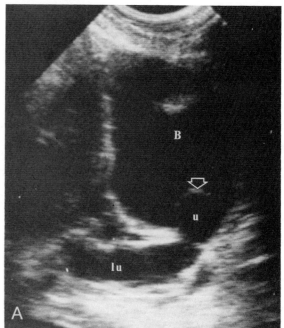

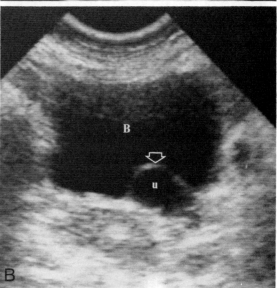

Figure 30.20. Ectopic Ureterocele. Ultrasound images in left sagittal **A**. and transverse **B**. planes demonstrate an ectopic ureterocele (*u*) of the left upper pole ureter (*lu*) protruding into the lumen of the bladder base. The upper pole collecting system was hydronephrotic, while the lower pole collecting system was normal. The wall of the ureterocele (*arrows*) is clearly seen. The ureterocele will change in size with peristalsis of the ureter. *B*, bladder.

with bladder carcinoma have TCC of the ureter [1]. Nonetheless, all patients with TCC deserve detailed screening of the entire uroepithelium.

Cross-sectional imaging is used to stage known bladder carcinoma (Table 30.2). Bladder carcinoma spreads by direct invasion through the bladder wall, by lymphatic spread to regional lymph nodes, and by hematogenous spread most commonly to bones, liver, and lung. Approximately 5% of patients have distant metastases at initial diagnosis.

Excretory urography plays a major role in screening the uroepithelium. Most bladder tumors appear as irregular filling defects (Fig. 30.21). Tumors larger than 1.5 cm are reliably detected by excretory urography, with inclusion of a postvoid film. Obstruction of an ureteral orifice may be associated. Cystoscopic biopsy is needed for histologic confirmation of the diagnosis.

Magnetic resonance T1-weighted images demonstrate tumor signal intensity as slightly higher than muscle but much lower than fat. With T2-weighted images, the tumor appears much brighter than bladder muscle. Magnetic resonance is better than CT in predicting the depth of bladder wall invasion, although it cannot differentiate stage II from stage III [5]. T2-weighted images demonstrate tumor invasion of the deep muscle layer as high-signal disruption of the normally low-signal bladder wall. Tumor extension into the perivesical fat is seen on T1-weighted images as low-signal tumor extending into high-signal fat. Pelvic lymph nodes larger than 1.5 cm are judged to be involved by MR. However, MR cannot detect tumor involvement of smaller lymph nodes.

Table 30.2.   Staging of TCC in the Bladder[a]

Stage	Description
0	Carcinoma in situ Papillary, noninvasive carcinoma
I	Tumor limited to uroepithelial mucosa and lamina propria
II	Tumor invades superficial muscle (inner half)
III	Tumor invades deep muscle (outer half) or tumor invades perivesical fat
IV	Tumor invades prostate, uterus, vagina, pelvic wall, abdominal wall or metastasis in lymph nodes or distant mets

[a]Adapted from: American Joint Committee on cancer. Manual for staging of cancer. 4th ed. Philadelphia: JB Lippincott Company 1992:195–197.

Computed tomography demonstrates TCC as a soft tissue mass projecting into the bladder lumen or as a focal thickening of the bladder wall (Fig. 30.22). Computed tomography is poor at differentiating superficial noninvasive tumors from those that invade the bladder muscle. Perivesical spread is seen as soft tissue density tumor in the perivesicial fat. Like MR, CT detects lymph node involvement only in nodes enlarged above 15 mm.

Ultrasound demonstrates exophytic tumors as polypoid masses extending from the bladder wall [6]. Infiltrating tumors may show as focal thickening of the bladder wall. Tumors may be difficult to recognize in the presence of diffuse bladder wall thickening and trabeculation (Fig. 30.15). Transrectal and transurethral sonography may play a role in the staging of bladder tumors [6].

Squamous cell carcinoma accounts for 4% of bladder malignancy. It tends to develop in bladders chronically irritated by stones and infection.

Adenocarcinoma is rare, accounting for less than 1% of bladder malignancy. Most cases are associated with bladder extrophy or urachal remnants.

Benign Bladder Tumors include leiomyoma, hemangioma, pheochromocytoma, and neurofibroma. Most produce smooth filling defects.

Blood Clots in the bladder are usually irregular in shape, move with changes in patient position, and change in size and appearance over time.

Bladder Stones may migrate from the kidney or form primarily within the bladder because of urinary stasis or a foreign body (Fig. 22.15). Solitary stones are most common. Stones must be removed to cure chronic bladder infection. Chronic bladder stones increase the risk of developing bladder carcinoma.

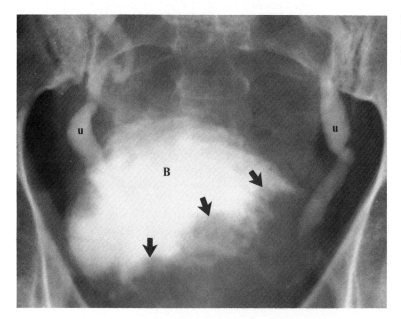

Figure 30.21. Transitional Cell Carcinoma. Radiograph from an excretory urogram reveals a lobulated mass (*arrows*) causing a large filling defect in the base of the bladder (*B*). Both ureters (*u*) are visualized.

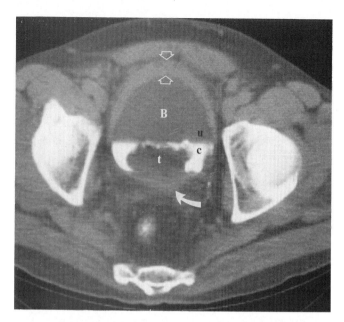

Figure 30.22.   Transitional Cell Carcinoma. A CT scan demonstrates a large tumor (*t*) arising from the posterior wall of the bladder (*B*) and extending through the bladder wall into the perivesical fat (*curved arrow*). This tumor is stage III. The bladder wall is thickened (*arrows*) because of benign prostatic hypertrophy. Note that contrast (*c*) layers posteriorly while unopacified urine (*u*) layers anteriorly in this supine patient. On an excretory urogram, routine films of the bladder may miss lesions of the anterior bladder wall if all films are taken in the supine position.

Pear-Shaped Bladder/Extrinsic Mass

Lymphadenopathy is a common cause of extrinsic mass impression on the bladder. Lymphoma and metastases from malignancy of pelvic organs are common causes.

Pelvic Hemorrhage indents the bladder and displaces it to the opposite side. Computed tomography and MR confirm the presence of hematoma.

Pelvic Lipomatosis refers to a condition of excessive perirectal and perivesical fat in the pelvis. The bladder is elongated and lifted up and out of the pelvis. Fat density is evident on CT and MR.

Iliac Artery Aneurysms tend to be clinically silent, but rupture is common and associated with high mortality. Calcification in the aneurysm may be apparent. Most are associated with aortic aneurysms.

Pelvic Tumors may be manifest on plain film or excretory urography by mass impression on the bladder.

Psoas Muscle Hypertrophy may also cause a pear-shaped bladder (Fig. 30.23).

Bladder Extravasation/Outpouchings

Bladder Diverticula are herniations of the bladder mucosa between interlacing muscle bundles. Most are located posterolaterally near the ureterovesical

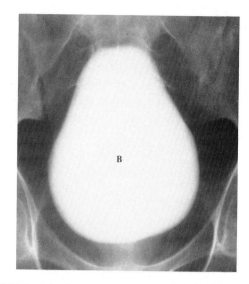

Figure 30.23.   Pear-Shaped Bladder. The bladder (*B*) on this excretory urogram is pear-shaped because of psoas muscle hypertrophy in this 16-year-old patient with muscular dystrophy.

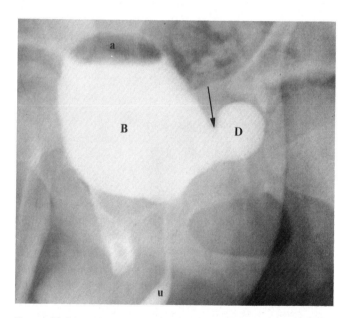

Figure 30.24.   Bladder Diverticulum. A smooth-walled diverticulum (*D*) extends from the posterolateral aspect of the bladder (*B*) on this oblique radiograph from a cystogram. The diverticulum fills with contrast through a wide neck (*arrow*) that connects with the bladder lumen. Diverticula that arise in this location near the ureteral orifice may cause vesicoureteral reflux. Air (*a*) was introduced into the bladder by the catheter placed to instill contrast. Contrast is seen in the urethra (*u*) on this film taken during voiding.

junction (Fig. 30.24). Diverticula may contain stones or tumor, and occasionally do not fill on cystograms.

Vesicocolonic Fistula most commonly occurs as a complication of diverticulitis (Fig. 28.16). Additional causes include colon or bladder carcinoma, ulcerative colitis, and Crohn's disease. The bladder is chronically infected, and the patient may complain of pneumaturia and fecaluria. The diagnosis is often made clinically. Barium enema and cystography detect only 35% of vesicocolonic fistulae. The fistulous tract is occasionally demonstrated by CT.

Vesicovaginal Fistula is usually a complication of gynecologic surgery, especially for cervical carcinoma. Obstetrical injury is an additional cause.

Vesicoenteric Fistula are almost always due to Crohn's disease.

Extraperitoneal Bladder Rupture (80% of bladder ruptures) results from puncture of the bladder by a spicule of bone from a pelvic fracture. Contrast extravasation is into extraperitoneal compartments, most commonly the retropubic space of Retzius (Fig. 30.25). Contrast extravasation may extend into the anterior abdominal wall, thigh, and scrotum. Excretory urography is not an adequate screening method. Cystography with distension of the bladder to at least 250 ml of contrast or CT is required to exclude bladder rupture.

Intraperitoneal Bladder Rupture (20% of bladder ruptures) results from blunt trauma applied to a distended bladder. The sudden rise in intravesical pressure results in rupture of the bladder dome and extravasation into the peritoneal space. Contrast material flows into the paracolic gutters and outlines the loops of the bowel (Fig. 30.26). Intraperitoneal bladder rupture may clinically mimic acute renal failure. Urine output is decreased or absent and serum creatinine is increased due to absorption of urine by the peritoneal surface.

URETHRA

Imaging Methods

The urethra is studied by retrograde and voiding urethrography. The retrograde urethrogram is a simple study of the anterior male urethra (Fig. 30.27). Contrast medium is injected into the anterior urethra by means of a syringe or catheter that occludes the meatal orifice. Films are exposed in the right posterior oblique projection. The anterior urethra normally distends fully because of resistance due to the external sphincter at the level of the urogenital diaphragm. Complete filling of the posterior urethra is not possible because contrast runs freely into the bladder. Voiding cystourethrography is performed by filling the bladder with contrast via a catheter. The catheter is removed, and films are obtained while the patient uri-

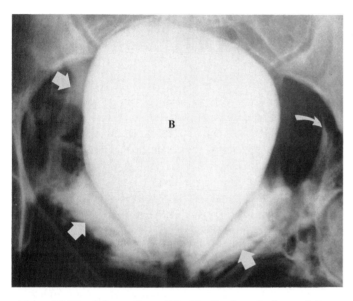

Figure 30.25. Extraperitoneal Bladder Rupture. Radiograph from a cystogram with the bladder (*B*) filled with contrast demonstrates extraperitoneal extravasation of contrast (*straight arrows*). A fracture of the acetabulum is evident (*curved arrow*).

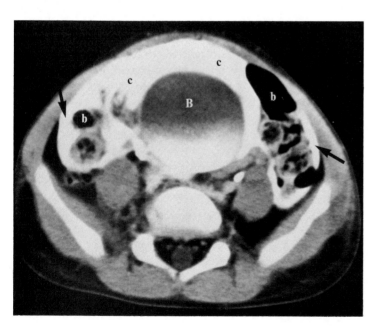

Figure 30.26. Intraperitoneal Bladder Rupture. A CT scan of a 5-year-old boy injured in a motor vehicle accident demonstrates contrast in the peritoneal cavity (*c, arrows*) surrounding loops of the bowel (*b*). The bladder (*B*) is distended with urine and layering contrast. The contrast agent in the peritoneal cavity strongly suggests bladder rupture. Perforated bowel would cause both air and oral contrast to be in the peritoneal cavity.

Figure 30.27. Retrograde Urethrogram. Contrast-injected retrograde through the penile meatus demonstrates the penile (*pu*) and bulbous (*bu*) urethra demarcated by the suspensory ligament of the penis at the penoscrotal junction (*curved arrow*). The urethra tapers to a point at the urogenital diaphragm (*straight arrow*), marking the location of the membranous urethra. The verumontanum (*open arrow*) marks the location of the prostatic urethra.

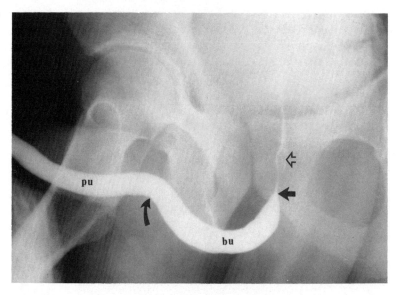

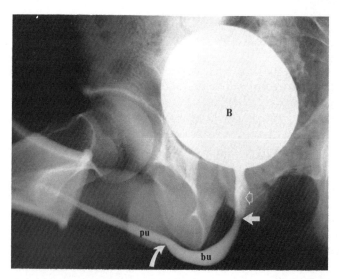

Figure 30.28. Voiding Cystourethrogram. Radiograph exposed while the patient is urinating demonstrates the entire urethra. The verumontanum (*open arrow*) is seen as an oval filling defect in the prostatic urethra. A slight constriction (*straight arrow*) at the lower edge of the verumontanum marks the location of the membranous urethra. The bulbous urethra (*bu*) extends to the penoscrotal junction (*curved arrow*). The penile urethra (*pu*) travels in the corpora spongiosum to the penile meatus. *B*, bladder.

nates into a basin on the fluoroscopy table. The voiding urethrogram demonstrates distension of both the posterior and anterior urethra (Fig. 30.28).

Radiographic study of the female urethra may be conducted with a voiding cysto- or retrograde urethrogram with a specially designed double-balloon catheter.

Anatomy

The male urethra is divided into posterior and anterior portions by the inferior aspect of the urogenital diaphragm [8]. The posterior urethra consists of the

prostatic urethra within the prostate gland, from the bladder neck to urogenital diaphragm, and the short *membranous urethra*, which is totally contained within the 1-cm thick urogenital diaphragm. The anterior urethra extends from the urogenital diaphragm to the external urethral meatus. It consists of the *bulbous urethra* extending from the urogenital diaphragm to the penoscrotal junction, and the *penile urethra* extending to the urethral meatus. The anterior urethra is entirely contained within the corpora-spongiosum penis except for the proximal 2 cm of the bulbous urethra, called the *pars nuda*.

The prostatic urethra runs vertically through the prostate over a length of 3–4 cm. An oval filling defect in the midportion of the posterior wall is the *verumontanum*. The ejaculatory ducts open into the urethra on either side of the verumontanum, while the prostatic glands empty into the urethra by multiple small openings that surround the verumontanum. The utricle, a müllerian remnant, is a small, saccular depression in the middle of the verumontanum.

The distal end of the verumontanum marks the beginning of the membranous urethra, which extends to the apex of the cone of the bulbous urethra (Fig. 30.28). The voluntary external urethral sphincter within the urogenital diaphragm entirely surrounds the membranous urethra. Cowper's glands are pea-sized accessory sex glands within the urogenital diaphragm on either side of the membranous urethra. Their ducts empty into the bulbous urethra 2 cm distally.

On retrograde urethrography, the bulbous urethra tapers to a cone shape as the urethra enters the external sphincter (Fig. 30.27). The apex of the cone marks the division between the membranous and bulbous urethra. The penoscrotal junction that divides the bulbous and penile urethra is marked by the suspensory ligament of the penis, which causes a normal

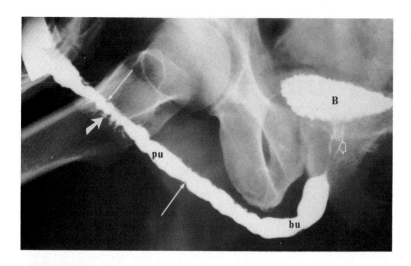

Figure 30.29. Urethral Strictures, Glands of Littre. Retrograde urethrogram demonstrates multiple strictures (*long arrows*) in the penile (*pu*) and bulbous (*bu*) urethra. Filling of the glands of Littre (*short arrow*) is evidence of urethritis. This patient had a history of multiple episodes of gonorrhea. The verumontanum (*open arrow*) marks the prostatic urethra. *B*, bladder.

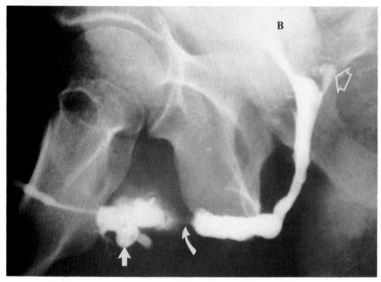

Figure 30.30. Periurethral Abscess and Fistula. Voiding cystourethrogram demonstrates a periurethral abscess (*arrow*) with a fistula into the scrotum. A stricture (*curved arrow*) is present, proximal to the abscess. Contrast is seen refluxing into the prostatic ducts (*open arrow*). *B*, bladder.

bend in the urethra. The entire anterior urethra is lined by the glands of Littre, whose secretions lubricate the urethra.

Cowper's ducts and the utricle occasionally fill with contrast during urethrography in a normal patient. However, filling of these structures with contrast occurs much more commonly in the presence of urethral strictures. Visualization of the glands of Littre is always abnormal and associated with chronic inflammation and urethral stricture (Fig. 30.29). Reflux of contrast into the prostatic ducts is also abnormal and is associated with prostatitis and distal urethral stricture (Fig. 30.30).

The female urethra varies in length from 2.5 to 4 cm. The urethra is embedded in the anterior wall of the vagina, and is lined throughout by periurethral glands.

Urethral Stricture

Urethral strictures are abnormal narrowings of the urethra due to fibrous scar tissue. They may involve the entire urethra or only a small portion. Abrupt, short-segment strictures are usually traumatic. Long-segment strictures may be either traumatic or inflammatory.

Causes of traumatic urethral strictures include instrumentation, indwelling catheters, prostatectomy procedures, chemical injury (podophyllin), saddle injuries (usually of the bulbous urethra), and pelvic fractures.

Most inflammatory strictures are due to gonorrhea. Additional etiologies include tuberculosis, schistosomiasis, and nonspecific urethritis.

Complications of urethral strictures include the following:

Periurethral Abscess is usually on the ventral surface, and may drain into the lumen or onto the skin, creating a periurethral fistula (Fig. 30.30).

False Passage is the most common complication of urethral stricture. It is usually iatrogenic because of attempted passage of catheters or instruments past the obstruction.

Figure 30.31. Urethral Diverticulum. Voiding cystourethrogram in a woman with recurrent urinary tract infections fills a urethral diverticulum (*D*). *B*, bladder; *U*, female urethra.

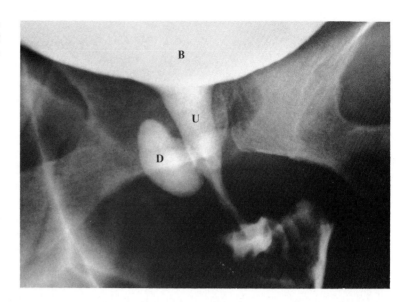

Stasis and Infection may cause disease of the upper urinary tracts including hydronephrosis, bladder hypertrophy, calculi, and chronic inflammation.

Carcinoma of the Urethra occurs as a complication of chronic urethritis and stricture. Carcinomas may appear as a filling defect in the urethra or as a change in appearance of the stricture. Most are squamous cell carcinoma and most involve the anterior urethra. Rare tumors of the posterior urethra are usually TCC that occur as part of multiple uroepithelial neoplasia.

Urethral Diverticulum

Urethral diverticuli are smooth, sac-like outpouchings of the urethra. They may be congenital or due to infection or trauma. Since they serve as a site of urinary stasis, stone formation and recurrent infection are common complications. A diverticulum of the female urethra is an uncommon cause of recurrent urinary tract infection. It may be demonstrated by a postvoid film of an excretory urogram, voiding cystourethrogram (Fig. 30.31), or by transabdominal or transperineal ultrasound.

Urethral Trauma

Traumatic injury to the posterior urethra occurs in about 10% of pelvic fractures. Straddle injuries, penile injury, and penetrating trauma also deserve urethrography to assess urethral injury. The classification of posterior urethral injury is as follows:

Type 1 is a stretch injury due to pelvic hematoma.

Type 2 is a rupture of the membranous urethra at the apex of the prostate with extravasation above the urogenital diaphragm.

Type 3 is a rupture of both the membranous and bulbous urethra with disruption of the urogenital diaphragm and contrast extravasation both above and below the diaphragm.

Complications of urethral injury are common and include stricture formation, incontinence, impotence, and pelvic and perineal sinus tracts and fistulas.

References

1. Winalski CS, Lipman JC, Tumeh SS. Ureteral neoplasms. Radiographics 1990;10:271–283.
2. Kenney PJ. Imaging of chronic renal infections. AJR 1990;155:485–494.
3. Leder RA, Dunnick NR. Transitional cell carcinoma of the pelvicalices and ureter. AJR 1990;155:713–722.
4. Lee JKT, Rholl KS. MRI of the bladder and prostate. AJR 1986;147:732–736.
5. Singer J, McClennan BL. The diagnosis, staging, and follow-up of carcinomas of the kidney, bladder, and prostate: the role of cross-sectional imaging. Semin Ultrasound CT MR 1989;10:481–497.
6. Abu-Yousef MM. Ultrasound of bladder tumors. Semin Ultrasound CT MR 1986;7:275–286.
7. Pollack HM, Banner MP, Martinez LO, Hodson CJ. Diagnostic considerations in urinary bladder wall calcification. AJR 1981;136:791–797.
8. Amis ES Jr, Newhouse JH, Cronan JJ. Radiology of male periurethral structures. AJR 1988;151:321–324.

31

Male Genital Tract

William E. Brant

SCROTUM AND TESTES
Imaging Methods

Ultrasound, supplemented by color Doppler, is the imaging method of choice to demonstrate the testes and scrotal contents (1–3). Magnetic resonance imaging (MR) using surface coils offers excellent spatial resolution, greater tissue contrast, and wider field of view, but has the disadvantages of greater cost and lesser availability (4). Radionuclide imaging provides useful information about perfusion, but with little anatomic detail. Computed tomography (CT) is useful in the staging of testicular tumors and in locating undescended testes that are not found by ultrasound (5, 6).

Normal Anatomy

The normal testis is ovoid and smooth, measuring approximately 3.5 cm in length and 2.0–3.0 cm in diameter (Fig. 31.1). It is covered by a dense fibrous capsule called the tunica albuginea. The testis consists of 250 lobules made up of seminiferous tubules that are the site of spermatozoa development. The seminiferous tubules unite to form the tubuli recti, rete testes, and finally efferent ductules, which exit the testis at the mediastinum. The mediastinum is an invagination of the tunica albuginea on the posterior surface of the testes that provides access for the efferent ductules and testicular vessels (Fig. 31.2). The efferent ductules carry seminal fluid to the epididymis. The epididymis is a highly convoluted tubule that is tightly applied to the posterior aspect of the testis. The head of the epididymis (globus major) is the enlarged (7–8 mm diameter) superior portion of the epididymis adjacent to the superior pole of the testes. The body of the epididymis is 1–2 mm in diameter and courses caudally along the posterior-lateral testis. The tail (globus minor) is the pointed lower extremity of the epididymis at the lower pole of the testis. The ductus deferens is the continuation of the epididymis that ascends along the posterior-medial aspect of the testis to become a component of the spermatic cord and traverse the inguinal canal. The appendix testis is a müllerian duct remnant seen as a small, oval structure just beneath the head of the epididymis. The appendix epididymis is a small, stalked appendage of the epididymal head. Torsion of the appendix testis or appendix epididymis may clinically mimic testicular torsion.

The scrotum consists of many layers of different tissue (Fig. 31.3). The thickness of the scrotal skin is usually 3–6 mm, with a maximum of 8 mm. The tunica vaginalis is a peritoneal membrane that forms a closed serous sac that covers the medial, anterior, and lateral aspects of the testis and the lateral aspect of the epididymis. This space normally contains 1–2 ml of fluid. Excessive fluid in this space is termed a hydrocele. The tunica vaginalis leaves a bare area posteriorly that anchors the testis to the scrotal wall. A midline septum divides the scrotum into two separate compartments (see Fig. 31.8).

The spermatic cord is formed at the internal inguinal ring, courses through the inguinal canal and abdominal wall, and suspends the testes in the scrotum (7). The spermatic cord consists of the ductus deferens; the testicular, deferential, and external spermatic arteries; the pampiniform plexus of veins; lymphatic vessels, and the covering cremaster muscle. Enlargement of the pampiniform plexus of veins is termed a varicocele. Doppler ultrasound can evaluate arterial flow in the spermatic cord (1, 2).

Ultrasound demonstrates the testes to be homogeneous in echogenicity with an echotexture similar to

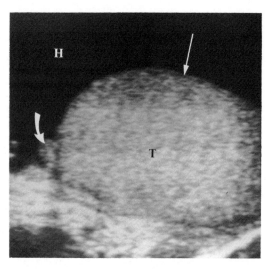

Figure 31.1.   Normal Testis, Large Hydrocele. An ultrasound image through the long axis of the testis (*T*) demonstrates its homogeneous midlevel echogencity. The head of the epididymis is seen as a small nodular structure (*curved arrow*) at the superior aspect of the testis. The tunica albuginea (*straight arrow*) is the tough fibrous capsule that covers the testis. The hydrocele (*H*) surrounds all portions of the testis except its posterior portion, where the testis is attached to the scrotal wall.

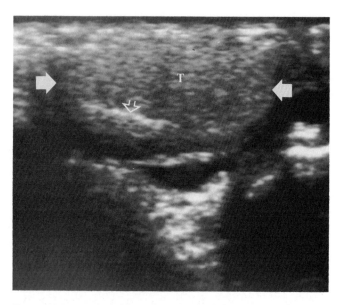

Figure 31.2.   Mediastinum of the Testis. The normal mediastinum testis is seen as an echogenic linear stucture (*open arrow*) paralleling the long axis of the testis (*T*, *between arrows*). Testicular vessels and ducts enter and exit the testis through the mediastinum.

the thyroid (3) (Fig. 31.1). The mediastinum is seen as a prominent echogenic line along the posterior aspect of the testis. Fluid in the space formed by the tunica vaginalis provides the best visualization of the components of the epididymis. The epididymis has a coarser, more heterogeneous appearance than the testis.

On MR the testis is of homogeneous signal intensity, well-demarcated by the dark signal of the tunica

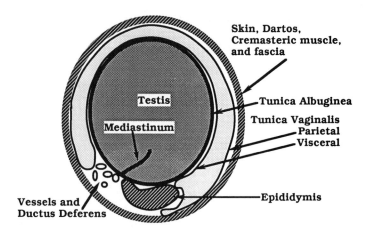

Figure 31.3.   Normal Scrotal Anatomy. Drawing of a cross-section of the scrotum demonstrates the testis encapsulated by the tunica albuginea and largely surrounded by the potential space lined by the tunica vaginalis. The testis is attached to the scrotal wall posteriorly, where the testicular blood vessels, ductus deferens, and epididymis reside.

albuginea. On T1-weighted images, the testis is slightly brighter than water and darker than fat (4). On T2 weighted images, the testis is approximately equal in signal strength to water and is brighter than fat. The epididymis is heterogenous and generally less intense than the testis.

Undescended Testis

About 3% of full-term newborns have an undescended testis. Most of these testes will spontaneously descend by 1 year of age, leaving 1% with cryptorchidism. Spontaneous descent after 1 year of age is unlikely. To preserve fertility, orchipexy is recommended by 2 years of age. Long-term retention of an undescended testis is associated with a dramatically increased risk of testicular neoplasm, especially seminoma. The undescended testis may be located anywhere along the course of descent, from the lower pole of the kidney to the superficial inguinal ring. Although they may be normal in size, most undescended testes are atrophic. They may be identified by ultrasound, CT, or MR as a soft tissue mass as small as 1 cm size (6) (Fig. 31.4). Many are identified in the inguinal canal, which runs an oblique, medially directed course through the flat muscles of the abdominal wall between the deep and superficial inguinal rings. The deep inguinal ring is located midway between the anterior superior iliac spine and the symphysis pubis. The superficial inguinal ring is located just above the pubic crest.

Scrotal Pathology

A major indication for diagnostic imaging of the scrotum is to differentiate intratesticular from extratesticular pathologic processes. Both ultrasound

Figure 31.4. Undescended Testis. A CT scan of a 25-year-old man demonstrates his right undescended testis (*arrow*) in the abdomen at the level of his right internal inguinal ring. The testis is similar to muscle in CT density. *B*, bladder; *iv*, external iliac vessels; *ra*, rectus abdominis muscle.

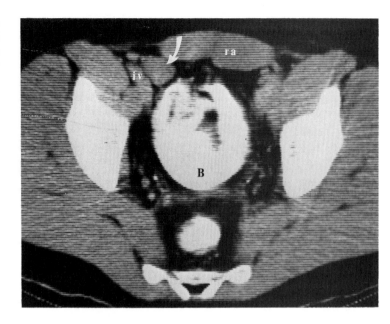

Table 31.1. Differential Diagnosis of Intratesticular Lesions

Malignant
 Primary germ cell tumor
  Seminoma
  Nonseminoma
   Embryonal cell carcinoma
   Teratoma
   Choriocarcinoma
   Mixed cell tumor
 Secondary malignancy
  Leukemia and lymphoma
  Metastasis
Benign
 Inflammatory
  Orchitis
   Epididymo-orchitis
   Mumps
  Abscess
 Torsion/infarction
 Gonadal stromal tumor
  Leydig cell tumor
  Sertoli cell tumor
 Cysts
  Cyst of the tunica albuginea
  Benign testicular cyst
 Trauma/hemorrhage

Table 31.2. Differential Diagnosis of Extratesticular Lesions

Extrinsic to epididymis
 Scrotal fluid collections
  Hydrocele
  Hematocele
  Pyocele
 Varicocele
 Scrotal hernia
Epididymal lesions
 Cystic
  Spermatocele
  Epididymal cyst
  Abscess
 Solid
  Sperm granuloma
  Epididymitis
  Sarcoidosis
  Adenomatoid tumor

and MR are 80–95% accurate in making this differentiation. The majority of intratesticular masses are malignant (Table 31-1). Every intratesticular lesion should be considered to be potentially malignant until it is proven to be benign. Most extratesticular lesions are benign and are caused by inflammation or trauma (Table 31.2).

Intratesticular Lesions

Primary Testicular Neoplasms constitute 4–6% of all male genitourinary tumors and 1% of all male malignancies. Ninety-five percent are germ cell tumors. They occur most commonly in the 25–35-year-old age group and present as a unilateral painless mass.

Seminomas constitute 50% of germ cell tumors. They are less aggressive and sensitive to radiation therapy. Seminomas are histologically monotonous, consisting of sheets of uniform cells intermixed with fibrous strands. Reflecting the histology, ultrasound demonstrates the tumor to be homogeneous and hypoechoic (Fig. 31.5), while MR demonstrates a well-demarcated tumor of uniform signal strength that is less than that of normal testis (3–5).

Non-Seminomatous Tumors. The remainder of germ cell malignancies can be grouped as non-seminomatous tumors. As a group they are more aggressive and resistant to radiation therapy. Cell types include embryonal cell carcinoma (20–25%), teratoma (5–10%), and choriocarcinoma (1–3%). The remainder are of mixed cell type. All tend to be heterogeneous

Figure 31.5. Seminoma. Longitudinal ultrasound demonstrates near-complete replacement of the testes (between *arrowheads*) by a homogeneous hypoechoic mass (*S*) that proved to be seminoma. Only a thin rim of normal testicular parenchyma remains (between *arrows*).

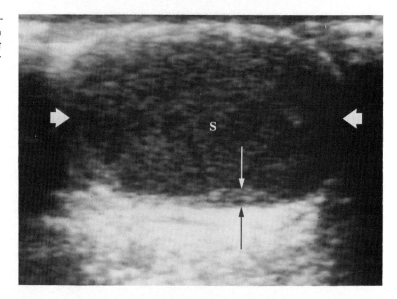

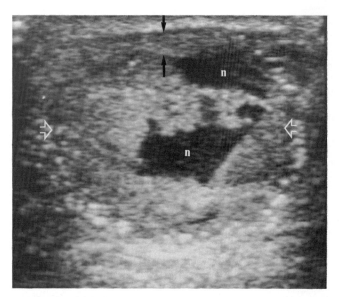

Figure 31.6. Choriocarcinoma. An ultrasound view of a testis in long axis demonstrates a large choriocarcinoma (between *open arrows*) replacing the testicular parenchyma. Note the marked inhomogeneity of the tumor with large areas of necrosis (*n*). The residual testicular parenchyma is indicated by the *black arrows*.

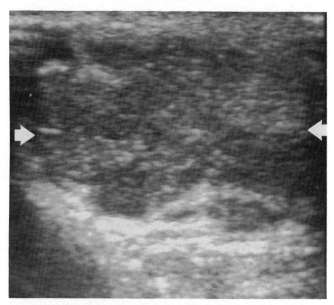

Figure 31.7. Malignant Melanoma Metastasis. Long axis view of the testis reveals complete replacement of parenchyma by an inhomogeneous, predominantly hypoechoic tumor (between *arrowheads*). No recognizable normal parenchyma remains.

because of mixed cellularity as well as the presence of hemorrhage and necrosis. Both ultrasound and MR demonstrate the heterogeneity and show irregular areas of high and low density, cystic areas, and calcification (Figure 31.6). A hydrocele is present in 15% of patients with germ cell tumors.

Lymphatic spread of tumor is most common, with a usual pattern of orderly ascending nodal involvement. Initial spread is along gonadal lymphatic vessels following the testicular veins to renal hilar nodes. Lymphatic metastases may also follow the external iliac chain to the paraaortic nodes. The internal iliac and inguinal nodes are rarely involved. Extensive metastatic involvement of the lymph nodes mimics lym-

phoma in young males. The primary tumor in the testis may be clinically occult, yet is effectively demonstrated by ultrasound. Hematogenous spread to the lungs usually follows lymphatic spread, except in choriocarcinoma, which spreads hematogenously early. Both CT and MR are excellent methods for initial tumor staging and follow-up.

Lymphoma, Leukemia, and Metastases from other primary tumors are more common than germ cell tumors in patients over age 50. The testis serves as a sanctuary for disease because of ineffective access of chemotherapy. Involvement of the testis may be diffuse or focal. Tumors are usually of lower density on imaging than normal parenchyma (Fig. 31.7). Careful

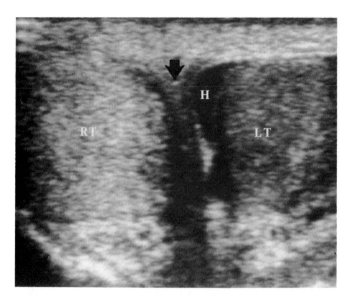

Figure 31.8. Acute Epididymo-orchitis. Transverse ultrasound view of the scrotum demonstrates the left testis (*LT*) to be diffusely hypoechoic compared to the right testis (*RT*). A small hydrocele (*H*) is seen in the left hemiscrotum. The midline septum (*arrow*) dividing the scrotum into two separate compartments is evident.

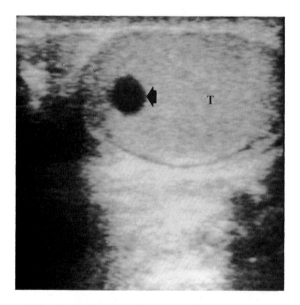

Figure 31.9. Testicular Cyst. A benign testicular cyst is viewed as a well-defined, spherical, uniformly anechoic mass (*arrow*) within the testis (*T*). Care must be taken to differentiate simple testicular cysts from cystic necrosis within testicular tumors.

comparison with the opposite testis may be necessary for detection of lesions. Renal cell and prostate carcinoma are the most common tumors to metastasize to the testis.

Orchitis and Abscess. Most inflammations of the testis are associated with epididymitis (8). Mumps is an additional cause of orchitis. The testis with orchitis is enlarged with edematous areas that may be irregular in outline (Fig. 31.8). A fluid-filled mass suggests abscess formation. Testicular abscess may rup-

ture through the tunica albuginea and result in a pyocele.

Infarction. Testis infarction may result from torsion or trauma. The infarct may appear as a focal low-density area or diffuse low density of the entire testis. With time, the testis shrinks and becomes fibrotic.

Gonadal Stromal Tumors. Leydig and Sertoli cell tumors account for 3–6% of all testicular tumors; 3% are bilateral; up to 15% are malignant. They appear as small, solid masses.

Cysts. Benign testicular cysts are incidental findings in 8–10% of males (9) (Fig. 31.9). Cysts of the tunica albuginea are well defined, small (2–5 mm in diameter), and peripheral. Both types are filled with serous fluid.

Trauma/Hemorrhage. In the setting of trauma, the role of imaging is to detect a ruptured testis. Ninety percent of ruptured testes can be salvaged by surgery performed in the first 72 hours following trauma. Intratesticular hematoma and hematocele are the major indicators of testis rupture. Discrete fractures are identified in a minority of cases. Color Doppler ultrasound is useful in detecting intratesticular vascular disruption and in avoiding mistaking a normal vascular cleft for a fracture.

Extratesticular Lesions

Scrotal Fluid Collections. A hydrocele is the accumulation of serous fluid between the visceral and parietal layers of the tunica vaginalis (Figs. 31.1 and 31.3). It is the most common cause of painless scrotal swelling. While many cases are idiopathic hydrocele may accompany malignant tumors, torsion, and inflammation. Hematoceles result from trauma or surgery. Pyoceles usually result from rupture of an abscess into the space between the layers of the tunica vaginalis. Internal septations and loculations are common with hematoceles and pyoceles.

Varicoceles are dilated serpiginous veins of the pampiniform plexus (Fig. 31.10). They occur in 15–20% of males and are the most common correctable cause of male infertility. Acute onset of a varicocele in an adult male aged 40 or older may be a sign of neoplastic obstruction of the ipsilateral gonadal or renal vein.

Scrotal Hernias may contain omentum, small bowel, or colon. The herniated mass extends through the inguinal canal to the scrotum (Fig. 31.11).

Cystic Epididymal Lesions. Spermatoceles are cysts of the epididymal head that contain sperm and cellular debris (Fig. 31.12). Epididymal cysts contain clear serous fluid and may occur anywhere along the course of the epididymis. Loculations and septations within the cysts are common. Spermatoceles range in size up to several centimeters.

Solid Epididymal Lesions. Sperm granuloma form when sperm extravasate into the soft tissues sur-

Figure 31.10.   Varicocele. Sagittal view of the scrotum demonstrates a network of curving tubular structures (*arrows*) at the superior pole of the testis (*T*). Doppler ultrasound confirmed slow venous flow within these dilated vessels.

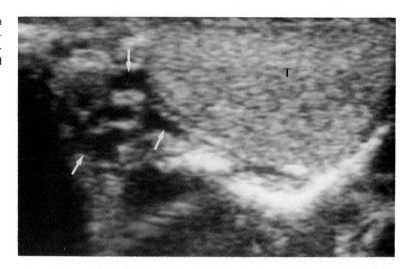

Figure 31.11.   Inguinal Hernia. Sagittal plane ultrasound reveals a moderately echogenic mass in the inguinal canal (*H*, between *arrowheads*). With straining, the mass approached the superior pole of the testis (*T*). With relaxation in the supine position the hernia was reduced. A small hydrocele (*h*) was also present. Surgery confirmed a small inguinal hernia with omentum extending through the inguinal canal into the superior aspect of the scrotum.

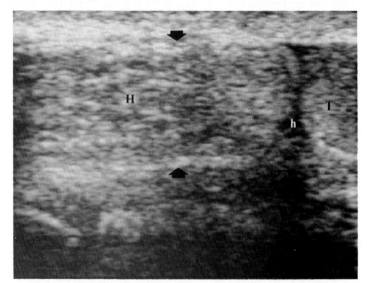

Figure 31.12.   Spermatocele. Long axis ultrasound image of the testis displays a well-defined extratesticular cyst (*S*) at the superior pole of the testicle (*T*). Debris within the spermatocele produces floating particles within the fluid. Acoustic enhancement (*arrows*) is evident deep to the spermatocele.

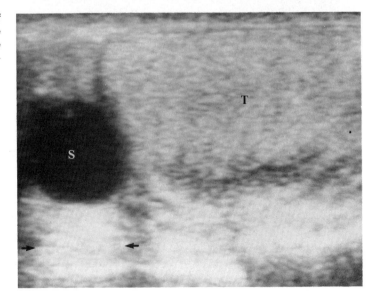

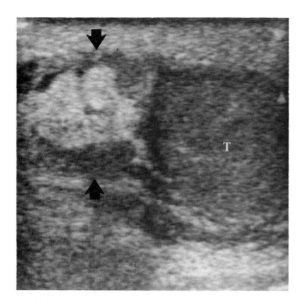

Figure 31.13. Chronic Epididymitis. The epididymis (*arrows*) is grossly enlarged and has a large central echogenic area, representing fibrosis and chronic inflammation. The testis (*T*) is diffusely hypoechoic because of diffuse orchitis.

rounding the epididymis. Chronic epididymitis, resulting from incompletely resolved acute epididymitis, causes an irregular, hard, tender mass (Fig. 31.13). Sarcoidosis may cause a painless, solid epididymal mass and involve the testis. Adenomatoid tumors are benign, slow-growing epididymal neoplasms.

Acute Painful Scrotum

Radionuclide flow studies have been the traditional methods of evaluating the acute painful scrotum, but more recently color Doppler ultrasound has been proven to be useful and accurate in differentiating torsion and epididymitis (Table 31.3).

Testicular Torsion results from anomalous suspension of the testis by a long spermatic cord with associated complete investment of the testis and epididymis by the tunica vaginalis resulting in the testis being not securely anchored to the scrotum. This has been termed the "bell and clapper" deformity. Surgical correction within 6 hours of torsion will usually preserve testicular function. Delay of surgery for 12 hours or more results in a salvage rate under 20%. The peak ages for testis torsion are the newborn period and ages 13–16 years.

Ultrasound findings of acute torsion include enlargement of the testis and epididymis with a diffuse but sometimes heterogeneous decrease in echogenicity. The spermatic cord is enlarged and the Doppler signal from the spermatic cord is decreased or lost (10). Demonstration of normal flow on one side and absent or decreased flow on the symptomatic side provide the most reliable evidence of torsion and testicular ischemia.

Table 31.3. Causes of Acute Painful Scrotum

Common
  Acute epididymitis
  Acute testicular torsion
Uncommon
  Torsion of appendix epididymis
  Torsion of appendix testis

Radionuclide perfusion studies utilizing technetium-99m pertechnetate demonstrate decreased vascular flow with a rounded cold area in the location of the affected testis. When torsion is present for more than 24 hours, the "doughnut sign" may appear. This is seen as a central cold area representing the underperfused testis surrounded by a rim of increased radionuclide activity due to dartos hyperemia.

Acute Epididymo-orchitis. While testicular torsion is most common in patients under 20 years, acute epididymitis is most common after age 20. The onset of pain and swelling is more gradual with epididymitis. Pyuria is commonly present. *Escherichia coli*, *Staphylcoccus aureus*, gonococcus, and tuberculosis are the most common causative organisms.

Ultrasound demonstrates thickening and enlargement of the epididymis (8). Color Doppler ultrasound demonstrates diffuse increased blood flow on the affected side as compared to the opposite side. Hydrocele is common. Inflammatory changes in the testis occur in 20% of cases.

Radionuclide perfusion imaging shows increased vascular flow in the spermatic cord on the affected side. Radionuclide activity in the affected hemiscrotum may also be increased because of reactive hyperemia.

PROSTATE AND SEMINAL VESICLES

Diseases of the prostate are a common cause of illness, particularly in elderly men. Prostate cancer is the third leading cause of cancer death in men. Ten percent of males over age 50 will develop clinical prostate carcinoma in their lifetime. Despite the high prevalence and importance of prostate disease, the diagnosis and treatment remain extremely controversial. The role of imaging in prostatic disease is also controversial. Computed tomography has traditionally been used to stage prostate cancer, but it has an accuracy of less than 60% (11). Magnetic resonance imaging using body coils offers promise of staging accuracy in the range of 90%. Transrectal ultrasound and MR using endorectal coils are being extensively investigated to determine their role in prostate cancer screening and local staging (12–15). The diagnosis of prostate cancer while it is localized to the prostate offers the best hope of improving survival.

Figure 31.14. Zonal Anatomy of the Prostate. The anatomy is illustrated in midsagittal plane (*left*) and axial plane (*right*) at the level of the vertical *dashed line* on the left.

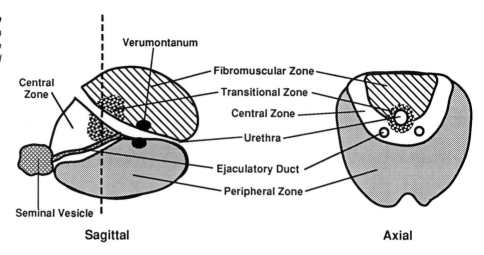

Sagittal   Axial

Normal Anatomy

High-resolution imaging of the prostate has revolutionized current concepts of prostate anatomy. Lobar anatomy, defined in most anatomy textbooks, has been abandoned in favor of zonal anatomy as demonstrated by ultrasound and MR (12–15). The prostate is divided into three glandular zones surrounding the urethra (Fig. 31.14). The *peripheral zone* contains approximately 70% of prostate tissue and is draped around the remainder of the gland like a glove holding a baseball. Most prostate cancers arise in the peripheral zone. The *transitional zone* consists of two small areas of periurethral glandular tissue. While it contains only 5% of prostatic tissue in the normal patient, it is the site of benign prostatic hypertrophy and may enlarge greatly. The *central zone* consists of the glandular tissue at the base of the prostate through which course the ducts of the vas deferens and seminal vesicles and the ejaculatory ducts. While the central zone makes up 25% of glandular tissue, only 5% of cancers arise there. The anterior portion of the prostate is occupied by nonglandular tissue called the anterior *fibromuscular stroma.*

The seminal vesicles are symmetrically sized, lobulated, teardrop-shaped masses that occupy the groove between the base of the bladder and the base of the prostate posteriorly (see Fig. 31.18). Prominent veins are frequently visualized in the periprostatic tissues. Lymphatic drainage of the prostate goes to regional pelvic lymph nodes with channels to paraaortic and inguinal nodes. Periprostatic venous connections to vertebral veins offer a route for the hematogenous spread of tumor to the axial skeleton

Computed tomography is poor at demonstrating intraprostatic architecture and cannot be used to differentiate tumor from benign hypertrophy (11). Computed tomography may, however, be used for demonstrating extraprostatic tumor extension and

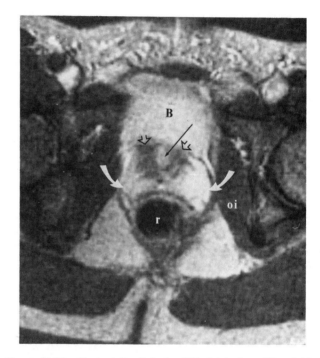

Figure 31.15. Normal Prostate by MR. Axial plane T2-weighted (TR/2000; TE/60) MR of a normal prostate obtained on a 1.5 tesla unit demonstrates the high-intensity peripheral zone (*curved arrows*), the urethra (*long arrow*), and the lower intensity transitional zone (*open arrows*). *B,* bladder; *r,* rectum; *oi,* obturator internus muscle.

metastatic spread. On MR the prostate is homogeneous and of uniform signal on T1-weighted images. The capsule margin may be demonstrated well by its interface with periprostatic fat. Zonal anatomy is demonstrated by T2-weighted images (Fig. 31.15). The peripheral zone is bright because of the high water content. The anterior fibromuscular zone is dark. The central and transitional zones are of low-signal intensity. While the central and transitional zones are difficult to differentiate from each other, they are easily separable from the peripheral zone on T2-weighted images. The seminal vesicles have an intermediate signal on T1-weighted images but tend to

Figure 31.16.   Normal Prostate by Ultrasound. Transrectal ultrasound image of a normal prostate in a sagittal plane just to the right of midline demonstrates a homogeneous inner gland (*IG*) surrounded by the peripheral zone (*arrow*). The fibromuscular zone (*FM*) is anterior. A, anterior; P, posterior; r, wall of the rectum.

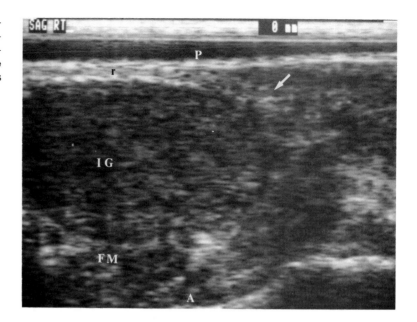

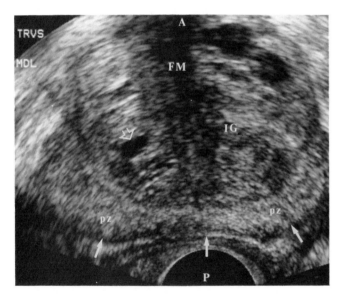

Figure 31.17.   Benign Prostatic Hypertrophy. Transrectal axial ultrasound view through the midprostate demonstrates excellent differentiation of a normal peripheral zone (*pz, solid arrows*). The inner gland (*IG*) demonstrates mild enlargement and heterogeneity that is characteristic of benign prostatic hypertrophy. A small prostatic cyst is evident (*open arrow*). The hypoechoic fibromuscular zone (*FM*) is anterior. A, anterior; P, posterior.

Table 31.4.   American Urological Association Staging of Prostate Cancer[a]

Stage	Description
A	No palpable lesion
A1	Focal
A2	Diffuse
B	Confined to prostate
B1	Small, discrete nodule
B2	Large or multiple nodules
C	Localized to periprostatic area
C1	No involvement of seminal vesicles, <70 g
C2	Involvement of seminal vesicles, >70 g
D	Metastatic disease
D1	Pelvic lymph node metastases or urethral obstruction
D2	Bone or distant lymph node or organ or soft tissue metastases

[a]Adapted from American Joint Committee on Cancer. Manual for staging of cancer. 4th ed. Philadelphia: JB Lippincott Company, 1992:181–183.

Prostate Carcinoma

One of the difficulties of dealing with prostate cancer is differentiating tumors with biological aggressiveness from those that are incidental findings. As many as 50% of men over age 75 will have prostate carcinoma on biopsy or autopsy. However, many of these cancers will not affect the patient's life span. The tumor is uncommon before age 50 and increases in incidence thereafter. The Gleason histologic grading system is used to assess the degree of differentiation of the tumor. A grade 1 is well differentiated, while a grade 5 is anaplastic. The Gleason score varies from 2 to 10 and adds the Gleason grade for the predominant and the secondary portions of the tumors. Tumor staging is by the American Urological Association system (Table 31.4). Ninety-five percent of tumors are adenocarcinoma.

brighten considerably on T2-weighted images. Any asymmetry in signal strength is abnormal. On transrectal US, the central and peripheral zones are equal in echogenicity and are usually distinguished only by position (Figs. 31.16 and 31.17). It is useful to describe the gland on ultrasound as having a peripheral zone and an inner gland comprising the central and transitional zones and their pathologic alterations. The anterior fibromuscular stroma is seen as a hypoechoic area at the anterior superior aspect of the gland.

Figure 31.18.   Seminal Vesicles. Transrectal axial plane ultrasound image of the seminal vesicles in a patient with prostate carcinoma demonstrates asymmetrical enlargement of the right seminal vesicle (*rsv*) compared to the left seminal vesicle (*lsv*) due to involvement by tumor. The normal seminal vesicles are symmetrical in size and shape. *A*, anterior; *P*, posterior.

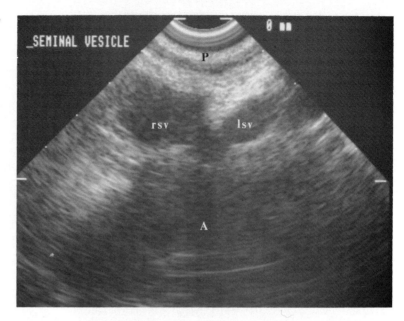

Table 31.5.   Differential Diagnosis of Peripheral Hypoechoic Nodule in the Prostate

Carcinoma
Benign prostatic hypertrophy
Prostatitis
Infarction
Fibromuscular hyperplasia

Prostate cancer spreads by local extension, lymphatic vessels to regional nodes, and by hematogenous dissemination. Penetration of tumor through the capsule or into the seminal vesicles greatly worsens the prognosis (Fig. 31.18). Both transrectal ultrasound and MR are used to assess local extension of known cancers. Computed tomography and MR are used to assess regional nodal involvement and distant metastases. Involvement of the axial skeleton by hematogenous metastases is common. Metastases to the lungs, liver, and kidneys occur in the terminal phases of the disease.

Detection of early tumors and the role of screening examinations is currently an area of great controversy. Both transrectal and endorectal MR have the ability to detect many tumors, but their exact sensitivity and specificity are debated (14–16). The sonographic appearance of prostate carcinoma is debated. Most authors currently agree that small cancers in the periphery are predominantly hypoechoic. Unfortunately, not all hypoechoic nodules in the peripheral zone are cancer (Table 31.5). In addition, up to 25% of cancers are isoechoic and indistinguishable from normal parenchyma. Detecting cancer in the midst of benign prostatic hypertrophy is a major challenge for any imaging modality.

Ultrasound signs of prostate cancer are (a) hypoechoic nodule, especially in the peripheral zone, (b) mass effect on surrounding tissues, (c) asymmetric enlargement of the prostate, (d) deformation of prostatic contour and, (e) heterogeneous area in the homogeneous gland (13, 14) (Fig. 31.19). Ultrasound is extremely useful in guiding prostate biopsy (Fig. 31.20). Both transrectal and transperineal routes are used for prostate biopsy. The transperineal route is more painful, while the transrectal route requires preprocedure antibiotics.

The MR appearance of malignant and benign prostate nodules overlap. On 1.5 tesla MR units, all cancer nodules had a low intensity compared to the high intensity of the peripheral zone on T2-weighted images (Fig 31.21). On medium field strength MR units, prostate carcinomas have been reported as showing heterogeneous, increased, or decreased intensity. The final diagnosis of any prostate nodule demonstrated by MR depends on biopsy and histology.

Benign Processes

Benign Prostatic Hypertropy is a nodular hypertrophy of the glandular tissue of the transitional zone, usually beginning in the 5th decade of life. The transitional zone becomes enlarged and heterogenous. Discrete nodules may be visualized (Fig. 31.22). The enlargement is often marginated circumferentially by a pseudocapsule. The prostatic urethra becomes elongated, tortuous, and compressed, causing bladder outlet obstruction. Stasis of urine may lead to the formation of bladder stones (Fig. 31.23). The bladder base is commonly elevated and the bladder wall may be thickened. (Figs. 31.22 and 31.24).

Acute Prostatitis is usually caused by *E. coli* infection. The gland is swollen and edematous. Streaky inflammatory changes may be seen in the periprostatic tissues. Prostatic abscess may be demonstrated

Figure 31.19. Prostate Carcinoma, Stage C1. Transrectal axial ultrasound reveals nodular hypoechoic carcinoma (*arrows*) extending irregularly into the periprostatic tissues on the left. The inner gland demonstrates the heterogeneous enlargement and nodularity of benign prostatic hypertrophy (*BPH*). *A*, anterior; *P*, posterior.

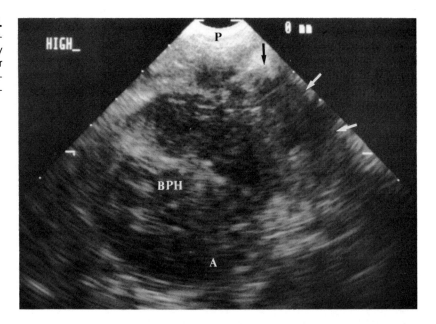

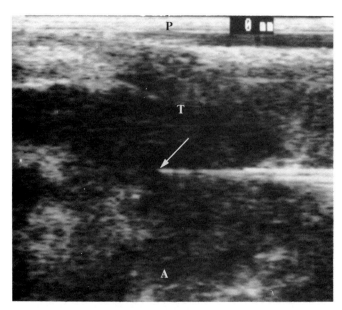

Figure 31.20. Transperineal Biopsy. Transrectal ultrasound image demonstrates transperineal biopsy of the tumor (*T*) that is also shown in Figure 31.19. This image is obtained in a sagittal plane well to the left of midline. The needle tip is indicated by the *arrow. A,* anterior; *P*, posterior.

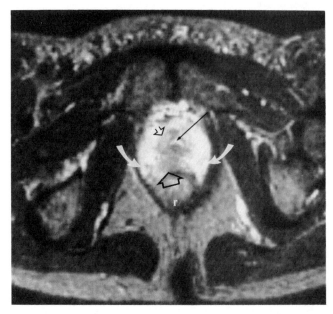

Figure 31.21. Prostate Carcinoma, Stage B2. Proton density-weighted axial plane 1.5 tesla MR image demonstates a low-intensity prostate carcinoma (*large open arrow*) in the peripheral zone (*curved arrows*). The tumor is confined to prostate gland and measures approximately 2 cm. The urethra (*long arrow*) and dark transitional zone (*small open arrow*) are evident. *r*, rectum.

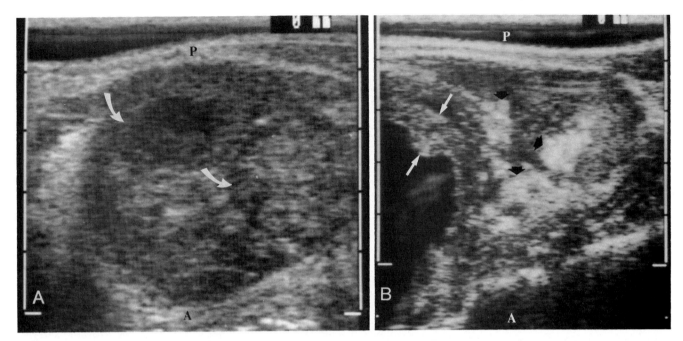

Figure 31.22.   Benign Prostatic Hypertrophy. A, Transrectal left sagittal ultrasound demonstrates nodular enlargement of the inner gland. Discrete hypoechoic and hyperechoic (*arrows*) nodules are defined. **B,** Transrectal left sagittal ultrasound image in a different patient demonstrates multiple calcifications (*black arrowheads*) in the inner gland. The bladder wall (between *white arrows*) is thickened and nodular because of chronic bladder outlet obstruction. *A,* anterior; *P,* posterior.

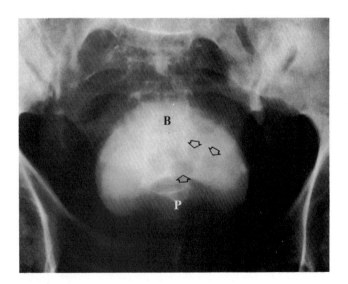

Figure 31.23.   Bladder Stones. A radiograph of the bladder (*B*) taken as part of an excretory urogram demonstrates a prominent prostate (*P*) impression on the base of the bladder. Multiple radiolucent bladder stones (*arrows*) are seen within the contrast-filled bladder.

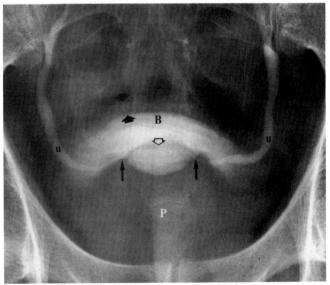

Figure 31.24.   Benign Prostatic Hypertrophy. A radiograph from an excretory urogram demonstrates marked uplifting of the bladder base due to massive enlargement of the prostate (*P*). The trigone (*open arrow*) and ureteral orifices (*black arrows*) are markedly elevated, resulting in a J-shaped appearance to the distal ureters (*u*). The bladder wall is thickened (between *black arrowheads*) and the bladder (*B*) mucosal pattern is prominent.

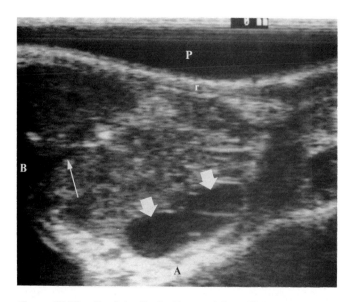

Figure 31.25. Prostate Cysts. Transrectal sagittal midline ultrasound image of the prostate demonstrates two prostatic cysts (*short arrows*). The urethral orifice (*long arrow*) is outlined by urine in the bladder (*B*). The wall of the rectum (*r*) is displaced anteriorly by fluid within the condom placed on the rectal transducer. *A*, anterior; *P*, posterior.

Table 31.6. Differential Diagnosis of Intraprostatic Cystic Lesions

Cystic degeneration of BPH[a] nodules
Prostatic retention cysts
Dilation of prostatic ducts
Cavitary prostatitis
Parasitic cysts

[a]Benign prostatic hypertrophy.

by ultrasound, CT, or MR as a focal fluid collection within the gland. Transrectal ultrasound may be used to direct needle aspiration of a suspected abscess.

Chronic Prostatitis results from incompletely resolved acute prostatitis. Large prostatic calculi are common and serve as a reservoir for persistent and relapsing infection.

Prostatic cysts are relatively common findings on prostate imaging examinations (Fig. 31.25). Cystic lesions of the prostate are listed in Table 31.6.

References

1. Horstman WG, Middleton WD, Melson GL, Siegel BA. Color Doppler US of the scrotum. Radiographics 1991;1:941–957.
2. Middleton WD, Thorne DA, Melson GL. Color Doppler ultrasound of the normal testis. AJR 1989;152:293–297.
3. Doherty FJ. Ultrasound of the nonacute scrotum. Semin Ultrasound CT MR 1991;12:131–156.
4. Mattrey RF. Magnetic resonance imaging of the scrotum. Semin Ultrasound CT MR 1991;12:95–108.
5. Steinfeld AD. Testicular germ cell tumors: review of contemporary evaluation and management. Radiology 1990;175:603–606.
6. Friedland GW, Chang P. The role of imaging in the management of the impalpable undescended testis. AJR 1988;151:1107–1111.
7. Gooding GA. Sonography of the spermatic cord. AJR 1988;151:721–724.
8. Tumeh SS, Benson CB, Richie JP. Acute diseases of the scrotum. Semin Ultrasound CT MR 1991;12:115–130.
9. Hamm B, Fobbe F, Loy V. Testicular cysts: differentiation with US and clinical findings. Radiology 1988;168:19–23.
10. Burks DD, Markey BJ, Burkhard TK, et al. Suspected testicular torsion and ischemia: evaluation with color Doppler sonography. Radiology 1990;175:815–821.
11. Demas BD. Computed tomography of the prostate gland. Semin Ultrasound CT MR 1988;9:339–342.
12. Fritzsche PJ, Wilbur MJ. The male pelvis. Semin Ultrasound CT MR 1989;10:11–28.
13. Hardt NS, Kaude JV, Li KC, Ros PR, Hackett RL. Sonography of the prostate: in vitro correlation of sonographic and anatomic findings in normal glands. AJR 1988;151:955–959.
14. Rifkin MD, Dähnert W, Kurtz AB. State of the art: endorectal sonography of the prostate gland. AJR 1990;154:691–700.
15. Chang Y, Hricak H. Magnetic resonance imaging of the prostate gland. Semin Ultrasound CT MR 1988;9:343–351.
16. Littrup PJ, Lee F, Mettlin C. Prostate cancer screening: current trends and future implications. CA 1992;42:198–211.

32

Female Genital Tract

William E. Brant

Imaging Methods
Anatomy
Congenital Anomalies
Cystic Pelvic Mass
Solid Pelvic Mass
Gynecologic Malignancy

Imaging Methods

Ultrasound is the primary imaging modality for evaluation of the female genital tract and pelvis. The utility and accuracy of ultrasound have been dramatically increased by the development of transvaginal tranducers and color flow Doppler imaging. Ultrasound is used as an adjunct to physical examination to confirm the presence or absence of a pelvic mass, and to evaluate its size, contour, and character, determine the organ of origin, evaluate for involvement of other organs, and detect the presence of ascites, hydronephrosis, and metastases. The transvaginal approach is used to improve visualization of small lesions and to overcome the limitations of limited bladder filling and obesity. Color Doppler ultrasound is used to identify pelvic blood vessels, identify vascular lesions of the pelvis, and detect neovascularity of tumors (1).

Magnetic resonance (MR) and computed tomography (CT) supplement ultrasound by providing additional characterization of lesions, and staging and follow-up of pelvic malignancies (2–5).

Hysterosalpingography is combined with ultrasound, CT, and MR to diagnose congenital anomalies of the female genital tract and mechanical causes of infertility (6–8). This study is performed by cannulating the cervix and injecting a contrast agent into the lumina of the uterus and fallopian tubes. Free communication of these lumina with the peritoneal cavity should be evident (Fig. 32.1).

Anatomy

The uterus is a thick-walled, muscular organ with a central cavity that opens to the peritoneum through the fallopian tubes and to the vagina through the cervix. In the adult woman, the uterus is 6–8 cm long, 4–6 cm in transverse diameter, and 3–4 cm in anteroposterior diameter. Following menopause, the uterus atrophies to infantile dimensions, 6 x 2 x 2 cm. The cervix makes up about two-thirds of the length of the uterus, until puberty, and about one-third the length of the uterus thereafter. Ultrasound and MR on T2-weighted images show zonal anatomy of the uterus (9–11). The endometrium is seen as a central bright stripe, separated from the thick intermediate density myometrium by a dark junctional zone representing the innermost layer of myometrium. The subendometrial halo of the junctional zone is important to evaluate for evidence of invasion by uterine malignancy. The thickness of the zones depends upon the stage of the menstrual cycle and exogenous hormone administration.

The parametrium is the fibrous tissue that separates the upper cervix from the bladder and extends laterally between the leaves of the broad ligament. The fundus and the body of the uterus are intraperitoneal and are well-demarcated by ascites. The peritoneum reflects over the anterior aspect of the uterus, forming a shallow vesicouterine pouch and over the posterior aspect of the uterus forming a deeper rectouterine pouch (of Douglas). The position of the uterus varies with the anatomy and size of the other pelvic organs, changing dramatically in position with filling of the bladder. The uterus is usually anteflexed over the bladder, but may normally be retropositioned toward the sacrum or directed laterally toward the pelvic side walls.

The fallopian tubes are approximately 12 cm in length and extend from the lateral angles of the uterus to the side of the pelvis in the free edge of the broad ligament. Hysterosalpingography is the principal method to image the tubes (Fig. 32.1).

The ovaries average 4 x 3 x 2 cm in size, with a maximum of 5 cm in any one dimension. In women of childbearing age, visualization of cystic follicles up to 2.5 cm in the periphery of the ovary is normal. The ovaries usually lie in a shallow ovarian fossa in the angle between the external iliac vessels anteriorly and the ureter posteriorly with the fallopian tubes draped

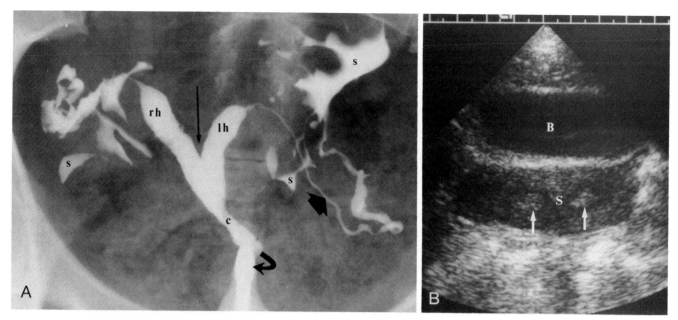

Figure 32.1. Septate Uterus. A. Hysterosalpingography demonstrates two horns of the uterine cavity (*rh, lh*) separated by a muscular septum (*long arrow*). The lumen of the left fallopian tube is well demonstrated (*arrowhead*), while the lumen of the right fallopian tube is obscured by the superimposed contrast. Free spill of contrast into the peritoneal cavity is evident (*s*), confirming the patency of both fallopian tubes. A contrast agent was injected into the uterus after placing a cannula (*curved arrow*) into the cervix (*c*). **B.** Axial plane ultrasound image of the uterus obtained through a filled bladder (*B*) demonstrates two separate uterine cavities (*arrows*) identified by their echogenic endometrium. The muscular septum (*S*) separating the uterine horns is evident.

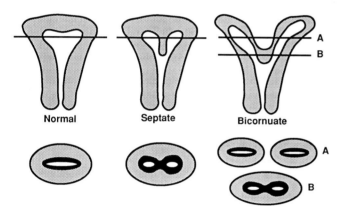

Figure 32.2. Uterine Anomalies. The normal uterus has a single oval endometrial cavity in axial plane images. The septate uterus has two endometrial cavities separated by a muscular septum. The fundus remains convex. The bicornuate uterus has two separate horns and a convex shape to the fundus. An axial plane image through the fundus (*A*) demonstrates no myometrial tissue between the two horns.

over and around them. Postmenopausal ovaries are atrophic, lack follicles, and are often difficult to visualize. Transvaginal ultrasound is the most effective way to evaluate postmenopausal ovaries.

The appearance of the uterus and ovaries varies dramatically with the physiologic changes of the woman being examined. To accurately interpret any imaging study of the female genital tract, the following information must be obtained: age of the patient, premenarchal or postmenopausal state, stage of the menstrual cycle, hormone therapy, and clinical presentation. Pregnancy must always be considered. Abnormalities of the first trimester of pregnancy are reviewed in Chapter 33.

Congenital Anomalies

Congenital anomalies of the female genital tract are a common cause of infertility, seen in up to 9% of women evaluated for infertility or repeated abortion. In addition, unrecognized anomalies may be mistaken for other types of pathology, such as leiomyoma.

Most anomalies result from arrested development or incomplete fusion of the paired müllerian duct that forms the uterus, cervix, and fallopian tubes (12, 13). Urinary tract abnormalities are associated in 20–50% of patients with uterine anomalies. Arrested müllerian duct development may result in uterine aplasia or unicornuate uterus with a single fallopian tube. Ipsilateral renal agenesis is found in 5–20% of patients with these anomalies. Failure of complete fusion of the müllerian duct results in varying degrees of duplication (Fig. 32.2), from uterus didelphys, with two uteri, two cervices, and two vaginas, to bicornuate uterus with two uterine horns, one (unicollis) or two (bicollis) cervices, and one vagina, to a septate uterus with a midline septum dividing the uterus into two cavities (Fig. 32.1). Uterine anomalies should be suspected when the uterus appears abnormal in size, contour, or position. The classification of the anomaly is made by a combination of physical examination, hysterosalpingography to demonstrate the uterine cavity and fallopian tubes, and MR or ultrasound to define the contour of the uterus (6, 7, 12).

Cystic Pelvic Mass

Cystic masses in the female pelvis are common imaging findings. However, it must be noted that the fluid contained within the cystic mass is frequently complex because of the presence of blood, pus, mucin, fat, or hair. Findings that suggest that a pelvic mass is cystic include visualization of a distinct wall, fluid-fluid layers, movement of internal contents with changes in patient position, and absence of visualization of blood vessels inside the mass (Fig. 32.3). Visualization of significant solid components in a cystic mass suggests the possibilty of malignancy.

Functional Ovarian Cysts are the most common ovarian masses. Small cysts, up to 2.5 cm, should generally be considered to be normal follicles. Pathologic follicular cysts up to 20 cm may result from excessive accumulation of fluid or internal hemorrhage (Fig. 32.4). Corpus luteal cysts result from hemorrhage into a physiologic corpus luteum. Functional cysts may rupture or undergo torsion. Diagnosis is made by the demonstration of a round, smooth, usually unilocular ovarian cyst that resolves on follow-up examination after one or two menstrual cycles.

Pelvic Inflammatory Disease and Endometriosis have a very similar appearance on all imaging studies and are considered together. Both cause masses which are predominantly cystic with complex internal fluid and adhesions that may encompass adjacent structures such as ovary or bowel into a complex mass. Differentiation is made primarily by clinical history.

Pelvic inflammatory disease is the term applied to acute or chronic inflammation of the tubes, ovaries, and pelvic peritoneum. Causes of the disease include gonococcus, chlamydia, anaerobic bacteria, and tuberculosis. The disease runs a spectrum from endometritis to salpingitis to hydrosalpinx (Fig. 32.5) and tubo-ovarian abscess. Patients are usually in their teens and 20s and present with pain, fever, and vaginal discharge.

Endometriosis is the occurrence of aberrant endometrial tissue outside the uterus. Most cases involve small implants on the peritoneum that are not visualized by any imaging method. Larger deposits may form cystic masses filled with old blood, a condition termed the "chocolate cyst" (Figs. 32.6 and 32.7). Patients are commonly in their 20s and 30s, and present with infertility, dysmenorrhea, and dyspareunia.

Ovarian Tumors, whether benign or malignant, are predominantly cystic. The tumors most commonly encountered are the epithelial tumors, serous and

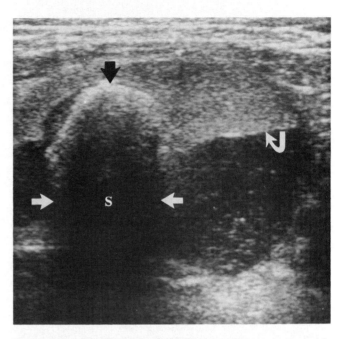

Figure 32.3. Benign Cystic Teratoma. An ultrasound of a pelvic mass demonstrates a fluid-fluid layer (*curved arrow*) and a large area of calcification (*black arrow*) with acoustic shadowing (S, between *white arrows*). Surgery confirmed a benign cystic teratoma containing teeth (the calcified portion), fat and hair (the fluid-fluid layer). (Case courtesy of Roy A. Kottal, M.D., Cedar Rapids, Iowa.)

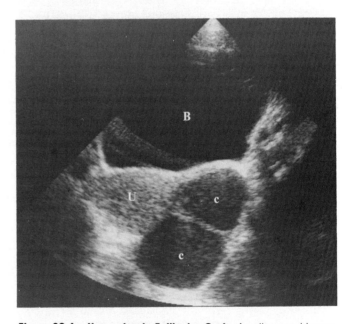

Figure 32.4. Hemorrhagic Follicular Cysts. An ultrasound image in a transverse plane through the full bladder (*B*) reveals two cystic masses (c) in the left adnexa. Note the low level internal echoes due to hemorrhage in these surgically confirmed follicular cysts. *U,* uterus.

mucinous cystadenoma and cystadenocarcinoma, and benign cystic teratoma. Epithelial tumors are discussed in the section on ovarian malignancy.

Benign cystic teratomas, also called dermoid cysts, are benign germ cell tumors usually discovered in patients aged 10–30. They are the most common ovar-

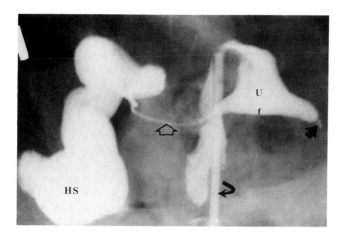

Figure 32.5. Hydrosalpinx. Hysterosalpingography demonstrates a retroflexed uterus (*U*) with the fundus (*f*) directed posteriorly and inferiorly. The left fallopian tube is occluded at the isthmus (*black arrow*). The right fallopian tube (*open arrow*) is massively dilated at its distal end, forming a hydrosalpinx (*HS*). Occlusion of the right fallopian tube is confirmed by the absence of peritoneal spill. The *curved arrow* indicates the cervical cannula.

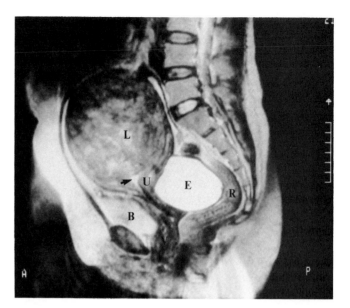

Figure 32.7. Endometrioma and Leiomyoma. A midsagittal plane, T2-weighted (TR = 1500, TE = 70) MR image of the pelvis demonstrates a large leiomyoma (*L*) arising from the anterior aspect of the uterus (*U*) and a large endometrioma (*E*) in the cul-de-sac between uterus and rectum (*R*). The high-signal intensity of the endometrioma on a T2-weighted image is nonspecific and compatible with any hemorrhagic cyst. The endometrial cavity of the uterus is indicated by the *arrowhead*. *B*, bladder; *V*, vagina. (Case courtesy of Roy A. Kottal, M.D., Cedar Rapids, Iowa.)

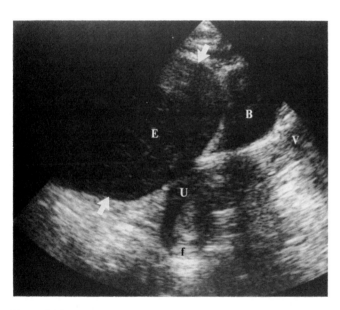

Figure 32.6. Endometrioma. A large endometrioma (*E*, between *arrows*) causes a mass impression on the bladder (*B*). The uterus (*U*) is retroflexed with the fundus (*f*) directed posteriorly. *V*, vagina.

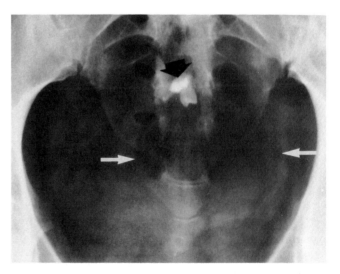

Figure 32.8. Benign Cystic Teratoma. A plain radiograph of the pelvis in a 22-year-old woman demonstrates several well-formed teeth (*black arrow*). A subtle, well-defined mass of fat density is also present (*white arrows*). These findings are diagnostic of cystic teratoma.

ian neoplasm. Fifteen to twenty-five percent of dermoid cysts are bilateral. Although predominantly cystic, the presence of mature ectodermal elements such as bone, teeth, and hair give them a complex and varied appearance (Fig. 32.3). The most characteristic appearance is a cystic mass with complex fluid and a mural nodule. Fluid-fluid levels are common. The diagnosis can often be confirmed by a plain film radiograph that demonstrates teeth or bone (Fig. 32.8).

Nongynecologic Cysts in the pelvis include abscess from appendicitis or diverticulitis, urachal cysts in the midline above the bladder, lymphocele in patients with prior pelvic node dissection, and paraovarian cysts in the mesosalpinx arising from wolffian duct remnants (14).

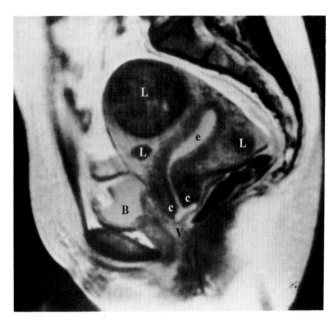

Figure 32.9. Multiple Leiomyomas. A midsagittal plane, T2-weighted MR image of the pelvis demonstrates multiple leiomyomas (L) which greatly enlarge and distort the uterus. The endometrial cavity (e) of the uterus and the cervix (c) are clearly demonstrated. B, bladder; V, vagina.

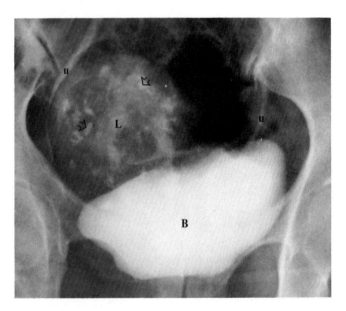

Figure 32.10. Leiomyoma Calcifications. A radiograph of the pelvis obtained as part of an excretory urogram demonstrates a leiomyoma (L) causing a mass impression on the bladder (B). Multiple characteristic "popcorn" calcifications (open arrows) are evident. u, ureters.

Solid Pelvic Mass

Leiomyoma is the most common tumor of the uterus. It is a benign tumor of smooth muscle origin arising in the myometrium (Fig. 32.7). Leiomyomas are virtually always multiple (Fig. 32.9). They may be completely within the myometrium, or subserosal or submucosal in location (13, 15, 16). Leiomyomas may

also be pedunculated and predominantly extrauterine, simulating an adnexal mass. Uncomplicated leiomyomas have the same imaging characteristics as the normal myometrium. They are suspected when the uterus is enlarged or altered in contour. Degenerative changes are common and dramatically affect imaging characteristics of the tumor. Leiomyomas may undergo atrophy, internal hemorrhage, cystic degeneration, fibrosis, and calcification. A "popcorn" pattern of calcification is characteristic, and definitive on plain film radiographs (Fig. 32.10). No imaging modality can reliably differentiate benign leiomyoma from the rare leiomyosarcoma. Retroposition of the uterus and uterine anomalies, such as a bicornuate uterus, must be differentiated from leiomyoma.

Solid Ovarian Tumors include benign fibroma, thecoma, Sertoli-Leydig tumors, and malignant germ cell tumors. Ovarian epithelial malignancies are occasionally predominantly solid. Metastatic disease to the ovary is usually solid. The most common malignancies to metastasize to the ovary are gastric carcinoma, lymphoma, and leukemia.

Nongynecologic Causes of a solid-appearing pelvic mass include adenopathy, pelvic kidney, and complex abscesses from appendicitis or diverticulitis.

Gynecologic Malignancy

Ovarian Cancer represents 3% of all malignancy in women, but accounts for 15% of all cancer deaths. There are more than 20 histologic types of ovarian malignancy, however, epithelial (70%) and germ cell (15%) tumors account for the majority. Epithelial tumors have a spectrum of histologic types from benign serous and mucinous cystadenoma to borderline malignancy to cystadenocarcinoma. Their appearance ranges from simple, thin-walled, unilocular cysts to multilocular cysts with thin septations (Fig. 32.11) to complex cysts with prominent solid elements (Fig. 32.12). The risk of malignancy increases with the amount of solid tissue visualized. Forty percent of ovarian tumors are malignant, two-thirds are cystic, and 25% are bilateral. The peak age of onset of ovarian cancer is 55–59. Ovarian malignancy has an insidious onset and a silent growth pattern that usually results in advanced disease at presentation. Transvaginal ultrasound utilizing color flow Doppler to detect neovascularity in the ovary offers promise for early detection of ovarian cancer.

Ovarian carcinoma spreads primarily by peritoneal seeding—with small tumor nodules implanting on the peritoneum, mesentery, and omentum—and malignant ascites (Figs. 32.13 and 32.14). Secondary patterns of spread include direct extension to adjacent structures, lymphatic metastases to pelvic and retroperitoneal nodes, and late hematogenous spread to lung, liver, and bones. Computed tomography is useful in the initial staging of advanced disease and in the follow-up of known ovarian cancer (Table 32.1). However, it is poor in the detection of peritoneal metastases. Only tumor implants 2–3 cm in size in the absence of ascites and 0.5–1 cm in the presence of ascites are reliably detected. At the present time, MR is inferior to CT for ovarian cancer staging because of the difficulty differentiating tumor from bowel (4). No imaging method can reliably differentiate benign from malignant ovarian masses. This is not surprising since many cases are borderline malignant, even histologically.

Cervical Cancer is the most common gynecologic malignancy. Squamous carcinoma accounts for 95% and adenocarcinoma for 5% of these cases. The peak age of onset is 45–55, but it is the second most common malignancy in women aged 15–34. Cervical cancer spreads predominantly by direct extension to involve the vagina, paracervical and parametrial tissues, and the bladder and rectum. Obstruction of the ureters is particularly common because of their proximity to the cervix. Lymphatic metastases to the pelvic, inguinal, and retroperitoneal nodes are common. Hematogenous metastases to the lung, bone, and brain occur only late in the course of the disease.

Computed tomography and MR are used to stage proven disease (2, 4, 17, 18) (Table 32.2); MR is generally preferred (Fig. 32.15). On T1-weighted images, cervical carcinoma is isointense with the myometrium. On T2-weighted images, the tumor is higher in signal compared with the lower signal in the normal tissue. Staging by CT requires excellent contrast enhancement to differentiate the tumor from normal tissue. Both MR and CT use node enlargement (>15 mm) as the primary criterion for involvement. This is inherently inaccurate since cervical cancer is known to involve nodes without enlarging them.

Endometrial Carcinoma is histologically 95% adenocarcinoma and 5% sarcoma. The peak age at onset is 62 years, with postmenopausal vaginal bleeding as the key symptom. The tumor spreads initially by invasion into the myometrium and cervix, followed by lymphatic spread to the pelvic and retroperitoneal nodes, then continued direct spread into the broad ligaments, parametrium, and ovaries. Peritoneal seeding will occur with penetration of the uterine serosa. Hematogenous spread to the lung, bone, liver, and brain occurs late in the course of the disease.

Both ultrasound and MR have been used to measure endometrial thickness in postmenopausal females to select patients suspected of having endometrial carcinoma for dilation and curettage. Endometrial thickness greater than 5–10 mm is used by many physicians as an indication for endometrial biopsy (16).

Magnetic resonance imaging is most often used to stage known endometrial carcinoma (4) (Table 32.3).

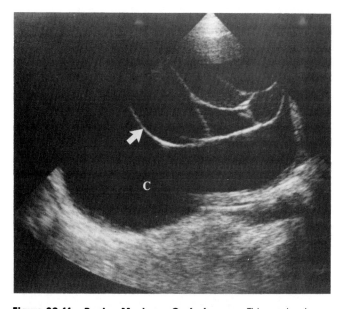

Figure 32.11. Benign Mucinous Cystadenoma. This ovarian tumor caused a huge mass, filling the pelvis and lower abdomen. An ultrasound confirmed a cystic mass (C) with a network of fine septations (*arrow*). The absence of detectable solid components suggested a benign tumor.

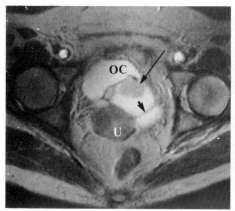
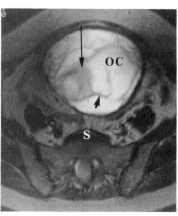

Figure 32.12. Ovarian Cystadenocarcinoma. Two axial plane, T2-weighted (TR = 2000, TE = 60) MR images demonstrated a complex pelvic mass (OC). The image on the left is at the level of the body of the uterus (U). The image on the right is 7 cm more superior, at the level of the sacral promontory (S). The fluid component of the mass was high intensity on both T1- and T2-weighted images, suggesting internal hemorrhage. Note the septations of varying thickness (*arrowheads*) and the solid nodular components (*arrows*).

Figure 32.13. Metastatic Ovarian Carcinoma. A. A plain film radiograph of the abdomen demonstrates calcified implants of ovarian carcinoma (C) throughout the peritoneal cavity. **B**. A technetium 99m MDP bone scan shows radionuclide uptake within the tumor nodules. Note the ghost of the liver (L) caused by tumor implantation on the peritoneal surface, rather than within, the liver. The pathologic diagnosis was metastatic papillary serous cystadenocarcinoma of the ovary.

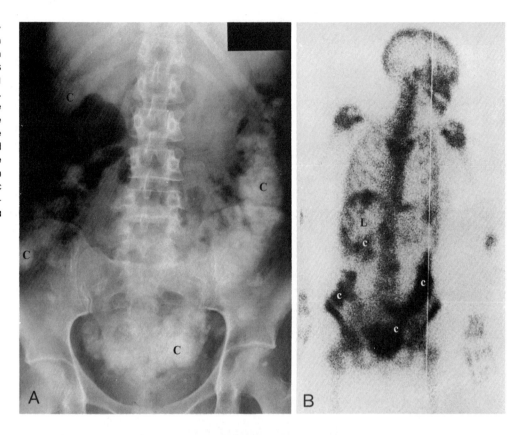

Figure 32.14. Metastatic Ovarian Carcinoma. A. An ultrasound image of the pelvis in a 68-year-old woman presenting with sudden onset of ascites confirmed ascites (A) with tumor implants (T) on the peritoneal surfaces. The uterus (U) is seen in transverse section, with the broad ligaments (arrows) outlined by fluid. **B**. A sagittal ultrasound image from the upper abdomen demonstrates tumor implantation (T) on the greater omentum outlined by fluid (A). This appearance has been called "omental cake."

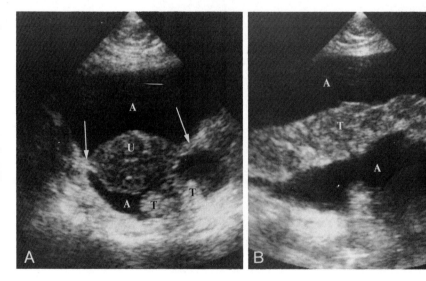

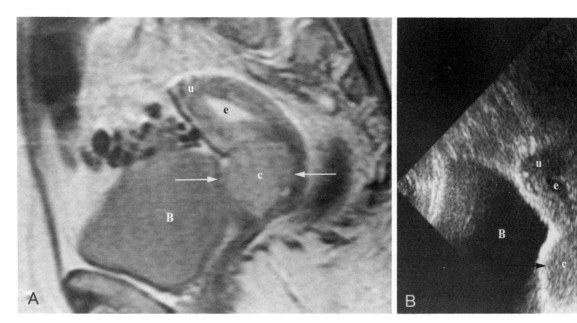

Figure 32.15. Cervical Carcinoma. Sagittal plane, proton density (TR = 2000, TE = 30) MR image (**A**), and sagittal ultrasound image (**B**), reoriented to match the MR, demonstrate a cervical carcinoma (c, between *arrows*) arising from the anterior lip of the cervix. The tumor invades the paracervical tissues anteriorly and the posterior lip of the cervix posteriorly. The tumor obstructs the endocervical canal, resulting in the accumulation of fluid in the endometrial cavity (e) of the uterus (u). This tumor was FIGO stage IIb. B, bladder. Magnetic resonance imaging is superior to US in revealing the extent of the tumor.

Table 32.1. Ovarian Cancer Staging (FIGO)[a]

Stage		Description
I		Tumor limited to ovaries
	Ia	Limited to one ovary
	Ib	Limited to both ovaries
	Ic	With malignant ascites
II		Tumor involves one or both ovaries with pelvic extension
	IIa	Involvement of uterus/fallopian tubes
	IIb	Extension to other pelvic tissues
	IIc	With malignant ascites
III		Tumor involves one or both ovaries with peritoneal extension outside the pelvis and/or regional lymph node metastasis
	IIIa	Microscopic peritoneal metastasis beyond pelvis
	IIIb	Macroscopic peritoneal metastasis beyond pelvis 2 cm or less in greatest dimension
	IIIc	Peritoneal metastasis beyond pelvis more than 2 cm in greatest dimension and/or regional lymph node metastasis
IV		Distant metastases

[a]Adapted from American Joint Committee on Cancer. Manual for staging of cancer. 4th ed. Philadelphia: JB Lippincott Company, 1992:167–169.

Table 32.2. Cervical Cancer Staging (FIGO)[a]

Stage		Description
0		Carcinoma in situ
I		Tumor confined to uterus
	Ia	Preclinical invasive carcinoma diagnosed by microscopy only
	Ib	Invasion confined to cervix
II		Tumor invades beyond uterus but not to pelvic wall or lower third vagina
	IIa	Without parametrial invasion
	IIb	With parametrial invasion
III		Tumor extends to pelvic wall and/or involves lower third vagina and/or causes hydronephrosis
	IIIa	Invasion of lower one-third of vagina
	IIIb	Extension to pelvic sidewall/hydronephrosis
IV	IVa	Tumor invades mucosa of bladder or rectum and/or extends to pelvic side walls
	IVb	Distant metastases

[a]Adapted from American Joint Committee on Cancer. Manual for staging of cancer. 4th ed. Philadelphia: JB Lippincott Company, 1992:155–157.

Table 32.3. Endometrial Cancer Staging (FIGO)[a]

Stage		Description
0		Carcinoma in situ
I		Tumor confined to uterine corpus
	Ia	Length of uterine cavity ≤8 cm
	Ib	Length of uterine cavity >8 cm
II		Tumor invades cervix but does not extend beyond uterus
III		Tumor extends beyond uterus but not outside true pelvix
IV	IVa	Tumor invades mucosa of bladder or rectum and/or extends beyond the true pelvis
	IVb	Distant metastases

[a]Adapted from American Joint Committee on Cancer. Manual for staging of cancer. 4th ed. Philadelphia: JB Lippincott Company, 1988:157–159.

Unfortunately the normal endometrium and endometrial cancer have similar signal characteristics. On T2-weighted images, carcinoma is brighter than the myometrium or cervix. Disruption of the junctional zone is evidence of myometrial invasion. Bright signal in the parametrial tissues is evidence of tumor spread. Lymph node metastases are judged by nodal enlargement (>15 mm). MR imaging and CT are equally accurate of the detection of lymph node metastases.

References

1. Kurjak A, Jurkovic D, Alfirevic Z, Zalud I. Transvaginal color Doppler imaging. J Clin Ultrasound 1990;18:227–234.
2. Sawyer RW, Walsh JW. CT in gynecologic pelvic diseases. Semin Ultrasound CT MR 1988;9:122–142.
3. Mitchell DG. Magnetic resonance imaging of the adnexa Semin Ultrasound CT MR 1988;9:143–157.
4. Chang YCF, Arrive L, Hricak H. Gynecologic tumor imaging. Semin Ultrasound CT MR 1988;9:29–42
5. Olson MC, Posniak HV, Tempany CM, Dudiak CM. MR imaging of the female pelvic region. Radiographics 1992;12:445–465.
6. Krysiewicz S. Infertility in women: diagnostic evaluation with hysterosalpingography and other imaging techniques. AJR 1992;159:253–261.
7. Pellerito JS, McCarthy SM, Doyle MB, et al. Diagnosis of uterine anomalies: relative accuracy of MR imaging, endovaginal sonography, and hysterosalpingography. Radiology 1992;183:795–800.
8. Yoder IC, Hall DA. Hysterosalpingography in the 1990s. AJR 1991;157:675–683.
9. Scoutt LM, Flynn SD, Luthringer DJ, et al. Junctional zone of the uterus: correlation of MR imaging and histologic examination of hysterectomy specimens. Radiology 1991;179:403–407.
10. Mitchell DG, Schonholz L, Hilpert PL, et al. Zones of the uterus: discrpancy between US and MR images. Radiology 1990;174:827–831.
11. Lin MC, Gosink BB, Wolf SI, et al. Endometrial thickness after menopause: effect of hormone replacement. Radiology 1991;180:427–432.
12. Mintz MC, Grumbach K. Imaging of congenital uterine anomalies. Semin Ultrasound CT MR 1988;9:167–174.
13. Baltarowich OH, Kurtz AB, Pennell RG, et al. Pitfalls in the sonographic diagnosis of uterine fibroids. AJR 1988;151:725–728.
14. Kier R. Nonovarian gynecological cysts: MR imaging findings. AJR 1992;158:1265–1269.
15. Karasick S, Lev-Toaff AS, Toaff ME. Imaging of uterine leiomyomas. AJR 1992;158:799–805.
16. Casillas J, Joseph RC, Guerra JJ Jr. CT appearance of uterine leiomyomas. Radiographics 1990;10:999–1007.
17. Waggenspack GA, Amparo EG, Hannigan EV, O'Neal MF. MRI of cervical carcinoma. Semin Ultrasound CT MR 1988;9:158–166.
18. Vick CW, Walsh JW, Wheelock JB, Brewer WH. CT of the normal and abnormal parametria in cervical cancer. AJR 1984;143:597–603.

33

Obstetric Imaging

William E. Brant

Imaging Methods

The development and continuing technological advancement of ultrasound has revolutionized the practice of obstetrics. An increasing percentage of all pregnancies is being evaluated by ultrasound. Modern ultrasound offers superb anatomic detail in real time, keeping up with the frequently vigorous motion of the fetus. Ultrasound is the imaging method of choice for evaluation of fetal anatomy and maternal pelvic organs, for dating the pregnancy, monitoring fetal growth, and assessing fetal well-being. Transvaginal sonography is particularly useful in the assessment of first trimester pregnancy and in demonstrating fetal anatomic structures deep in the pelvis. Magnetic resonance imaging is, at present, being used investigationally as a supplement to ultrasound imaging when the ultrasound examination is equivocal. Magnetic resonance imaging offers excellent detail of maternal pelvic organs unobscured by bone, gas, or fat (1). Demonstration of fetal anatomy is limited by fetal motion but may be overcome by fetal sedation and fast scan techniques (2). Computed tomography is the method of choice for pelvimetry. The use of plain radiographs in obstetrics has all but vanished.

Technique

An obstetric ultrasound examination consists of a survey of the uterus and maternal pelvic organs, measurements of the fetus to date the pregnancy and assess fetal growth, and a survey of fetal anatomy. Standards for the performance of obstetric ultrasound examinations have been published by the American Institute of Ultrasound in Medicine (3). In the first trimester the location and appearance of the gestational sac is documented. The embryo is identified, crown-rump length measured, and fetal cardiac activity confirmed. Fetal number is documented, and the uterus and adnexa are examined. Second and third trimester sonography includes assessment of fetal life and number, fetal position, amount of amniotic fluid, placental location and appearance, fetal measurements (biparietal diameter, head circumference, abdominal circumference, femur length), and evaluation of the uterus and adnexa. Assessment of fetal anatomy includes the cerebral ventricles, a four-chamber view of the heart, and images of the spine, stomach, bladder, umbilical cord insertion site, and renal regions. The literature refers to "Level I" obstetric ultrasounds as routine or standard examinations and "Level II" examinations as targeted to scrutinize fetal anatomy and detect anomalies (4).

FIRST TRIMESTER

The first trimester covers the period from conception to the end of the 13th menstrual week. This includes the entire embryonic period (0–10 weeks) and is a time of dynamic growth and the differentiation and development of most organ systems. The embryo and fetus have the greatest risk of maldevelopment, injury, and death during this period because of external factors or chromosome abnormalities. About 40% of implanted zygotes are menstrually aborted, while another 25–35% of surviving embryos will threaten to abort during the first trimester. Patients who present with vaginal bleeding and pelvic pain during the first trimester are commonly referred for ultrasound examination. The differential diagnosis includes anembryonic pregnancy, embryonic demise, ectopic pregnancy, subchorionic hemorrhage, and gestational trophoblastic disease.

Normal Gestation

The presence of a pregnancy is confirmed by a positive serum beta-human chorionic gonadotropin (β-hCG) test. Radioimmunoassay for βhCG allows pregnancy to be detected within 2 weeks of conception (as early as 23 menstrual days), and before a normal gestational sac can be detected by either transabdominal or transvaginal ultrasound. The early gestational sac can generally be seen by transvaginal sonography at 3.5–4.5 menstrual weeks as a tiny cystic structure within the echogenic decidua, the *intradecidual sign* (5) (Fig. 33.1). A normal gestational sac is often visualized by the transabdominal approach by 5 menstrual weeks. The normal gestational sac appears on US as a smoothly contoured, round or oval, fluid-containing structure positioned in the endometrial cavity near the fundus of the uterus (6). The normal sac has an echogenic border greater than 2 mm thick, which represents the choriodecidual reaction. A *double decidual sac sign* (Fig. 33.2) is evident in about 85% of normal pregnancies. The double sac sign is produced by visualization of three layers of decidual reaction early in pregnancy (7). The term decidua refers to the endometrium of the pregnant uterus. The decidua vera lines the endometrial cavity while the decidua capsularis covers the gestational sac. The decidua basalis contributes to the formation of the placenta at the site of implantation. A small amount of fluid in the endometrial cavity separates the decidua vera from the decidua capsularis allowing visualization of the "double sac." The double sac is not complete because of placental attachment to the uterine wall. A well-visualized double sac is excellent evidence of intrauterine pregnancy. However, a poorly visualized or absent double sac should be considered nondiagnostic. The normal gestational sac may be up to 25 mm mean sac diameter without visualization of an embryo by transabdominal sonography, or up to 16 mm mean sac diameter without visualization of an embryo by transvaginal sonography. (7, 8)

The yolk sac (Fig. 33.3) is a 2- to 6-mm diameter, spherical, cystic structure that is connected to the midgut of the embryo by a thin stalk, the vitelline duct. The yolk sac is the earliest site of blood cell formation in the embryo. It floats freely in fluid be-

tween the amniotic and chorionic membranes. It is generally the earliest structure visualized within the gestational sac and serves as definitive evidence of early pregnancy. The yolk sac should always be visualized in normal pregnancy in gestational sacs of 20

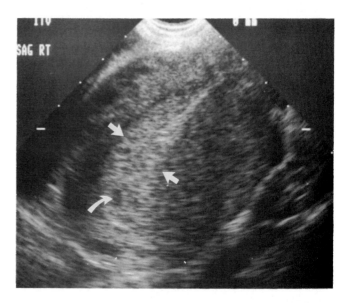

Figure 33.1. Intradecidual Sign. Transvaginal ultrasound image of the uterus in a sagittal plane demonstrates thickening of the endometrial stripe (*arrows*) due to decidual reaction. A tiny (6-mm) gestational sac (*curved arrow*) is implanted within the thickened decidua near the uterine fundus. The size of the sac corresponds to a pregnancy of approximately 4 weeks menstrual age.

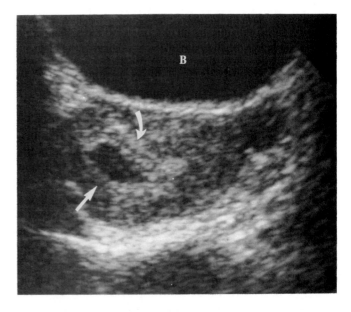

Figure 33.2. Double Decidual Sac Sign. A transverse image of the uterus obtained transabdominally through a filled bladder (*B*) demonstrates a gestational sac with two decidual layers in the endometrial cavity. The two echogenic lines (*curved arrow*) are formed by the decidua vera lining the endometrial cavity and the decidua capsularis covering the gestational sac. The placental implantation site on the posterior aspect of the uterus (*straight arrow*) has a single echogenic stripe due to the decidua basalis.

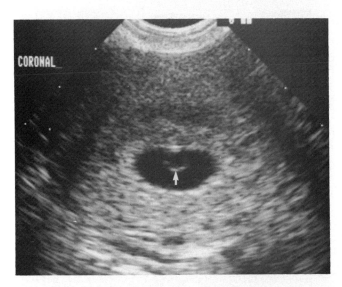

Figure 33.3.   Yolk Sac. The yolk sac (*arrow*) is demonstrated within the gestational sac by transvaginal ultrasound in a coronal plane. The normal yolk sac is less than 6 mm in diameter, spherical, and fluid-filled with a thin wall. Demonstration of the yolk sac within the uterus confirms intrauterine pregnancy.

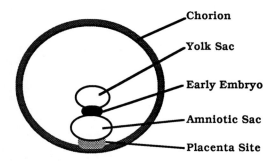

Figure 33.4.   Double Bleb Sign. The double bleb is formed by the yolk sac and the amniotic sac suspended in the fluid of the early chorionic sac. The embryo is seen as a tiny disc-like structure between the two blebs. Early cardiac activity can frequently be observed in the embryonic disc.

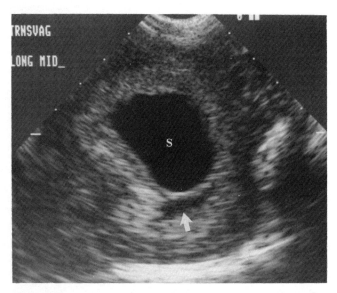

Figure 33.5.   Anembryonic Pregnancy. An empty gestational sac (*S*) measuring 28 mm in MSD is demonstated within the uterus by transvaginal US. Blood (*arrow*) is present in the endometrial cavity. In a normal intrauterine pregnancy, an embryo should always be demonstrable by transvaginal ultrasound when the MSD exceeds 16 mm.

mm mean sac diameter by transabdominal sonography or 8 mm mean sac diameter by transvaginal sonography (7, 8).

The earliest demonstration of the embryo is the *double bleb sign* (Fig. 33.4), produced by the amniotic sac and the yolk sac with the embryonic disc between them (9). Embryos as small as 2 mm long can be detected by transvaginal sonography. The earliest embryonic cardiac activity can be detected by careful inspection of the embryonic disc by real-time ultrasound. Transvaginal sonography may demonstrate tiny normal embryos in which cardiac activity cannot be confirmed. However, cardiac activity should always be seen transvaginally in embryos that can be visualized by transabdominal ultrasound.

Gestational age in the first trimester is estimated by measuring the mean diameter of the gestational sac (MSD, or mean sac diameter) or the crown-rump length of the embryo/fetus. A normal gestational sac grows at a rate of approximately 1 mm/day MSD.

Spontaneous Abortion

Abortion is the termination of pregnancy before 20 weeks, gestational age. *Spontaneous abortion* is the termination of pregnancy by natural causes. Approximately 10–15% of all known pregnancies end in spontaneous abortion. Up to 60% of spontaneous abortions have chromosomal abnormalities. A number of clinical terms are used to describe abortion. *Threatened abortion* refers to the appearance of vaginal bleeding and uterine cramping with a closed cervical os in early pregnancy. Threatened abortion complicates roughly 25% of all pregnancies (7). *Inevitable*

abortion presents with cervical dilation and fetal or placental tissues within the cervical os. With *complete abortion*, all uterine contents have been expelled. *Incomplete abortion* refers to the presence of residual products of conception within the uterus. In *missed abortion*, the fetus has died but remains within the uterus. *Habitual abortion* is defined as three or more successive spontaneous abortions. *Anembryonic pregnancy* or *blighted ovum* is a pregnancy in which the embryo has died and is no longer visible or never developed.

"Empty" Gestational Sac. A gestational sac without an embryo demonstrated by ultrasound is compatible with a very early intrauterine pregnancy, a nonviable intrauterine pregancy (blighted ovum) (Fig 33.5), or a pseudogestational sac associated with

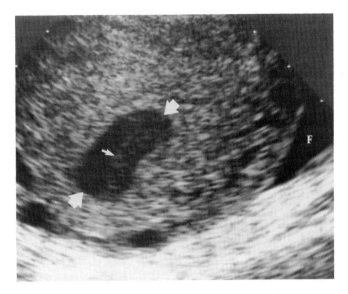

Figure 33.6. Pseudogestational Sac. Fluid within the endometrial cavity (*large arrows*) in a patient with an ectopic pregnancy mimics an intrauterine gestational sac. Echogenic material due to blood (*small arrow*) within the fluid cavity may mimic an embryo. The uterus is imaged in the sagittal plane with an intravaginal transducer. Fluid (*F*) is seen in the cul-de-sac.

Table 33.1. Ultrasound Criteria for Abnormal Gestational Sac[a]

Criteria	Transabdominal scan[b]	Transvaginal scan[a]
Major		
Sac size without yolk sac	≥20 mm MSD	≥8 mm MSD
Sac size without embryo	≥25 mm MSD	≥16 mm MSD
Distorted sac shape	Present	Present
Minor		
Irregular sac contour	Present	Present
Thin decidual reaction	≤2 mm	≤2 mm
Weak decidual echo amplitude	Present	Present
Absent double decidual sac	Present	Present
Low sac position in uterus	Present	Present

[a] The gestational sac diameter is measured in three orthogonal planes, and the measurements are averaged.
[b] Adapted from Nyberg DA, Laing FC, Filly RA, et al. Ultrasonographic differentiation of the gestational sac of early intrauterine pregnancy from the pseudogestational sac of ectopic pregnancy. Radiology 1983;146:755–759.
[c] Adapted from Levi CS, Lyons EA, Lindsay DJ. Early diagnosis of nonviable pregnancy with endovaginal US. Radiology 1988;167:383–385.

ectopic pregnancy (Fig. 33.6). A gestational sac is considered to be abnormal if it demonstrates the following features (Table 33.1): large size without an embryo or yolk sac, distorted shape, irregular contour, thin or weak choriodecidual reaction, absence of a double decidual sac, or abnormal position (7). Any one of the major criteria or three of the minor criteria are considered diagnostic. Large sac size and distorted contour have a reported 100% specificity and positive predictive value for identification of nonviable pregnancy. The original criteria reported by Nyberg et al. (7) have been refined by the use of transvaginal transducers, which improve visualization of anatomic detail (8). Most authors recommend allowing a 1–2 mm margin of error and repeating any equivocal scans in several days. Growth of the gestational sac by less than 1 mm/day MSD is additional evidence of abnormal sac development (10).

Embryonic or Fetal Demise is diagnosed by ultrasound confirmation of the absence of cardiac activity. Absence of cardiac activity in a fetus or an embryo large enough to be visualized by transabdominal ultrasound is definitive evidence of death. However, because of the increased sensitivity of transvaginal ultrasound in demonstrating cardiac activity, all cases of suspected demise of small embryos should be confirmed by transvaginal ultrasound, which may demonstrate cardiac activity even in embryos as small as 1.5 mm crown-ramp length (CRL) (11). However, transvaginal ultrasound may also visualize small, normal, living embryos (<5 mm CRL) without demonstrating cardiac activity (11). Absence of cardiac activity in embryos larger than 5 mm on transvaginal ultrasound is considered diagnostic of embryonic demise (missed abortion). Embryos smaller than 5 mm without cardiac activity should be rescanned in a few days to confirm demise.

Ectopic Pregnancy

Ectopic pregnancy occurs in only 1.4% of all pregnancies, but is the major cause of pregnancy-related deaths. Misdiagnosis of ectopic pregnancy remains one of the most common areas for medical malpractice litigation. Patients at high risk for ectopic pregnancy include those with a history of pelvic inflammatory disease, tubal surgery, endometriosis, ovulation induction, previous ectopic pregnancy, or use of intrauterine device for contraception. Ninety-five percent of ectopic pregnancies occur in the fallopian tube, most commonly in the isthmic portion. Interstitial ectopic pregnancies, developing in the portion of the tube passing through the uterine wall, may grow to large size before rupture, resulting in catastrophic hemorrhage. Additional sites for ectopic implantation include the abdominal cavity, ovary, and cervix. All patients with a positive pregnancy test (serum β-hCG), vaginal bleeding, pelvic pain, or adnexal mass must be considered at risk for ectopic pregnancy.

A completely confident diagnosis of ectopic pregnancy can be made sonographically only when a living embryo is positively demonstrated to be in a position outside of the uterus. However, this occurs in only 5–10% of ectopic pregnancies (12). Transvaginal sonography increases the possibility of demonstrating a live ectopic pregnancy (13). In any other circumstance, we are dealing with a situation of relative risk (Table 33.2). When an intrauterine pregnancy is documented by ultrasound, the risk of coexisting ectopic pregnancy is extremely low, estimated at 1 in 30,000. However, concurrent intrauterine and extrauterine

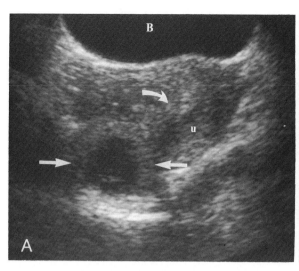
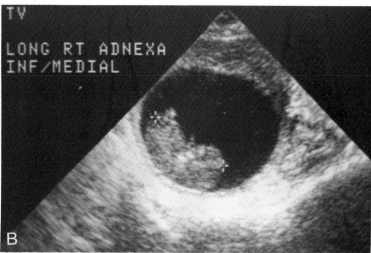

Figure 33.7. Ectopic Pregnancy. A. Transabdominal examination in a transverse plane through the bladder (*B*) demonstrates a cystic mass (*arrows*) with a thick echogenic wall in the right adnexa. The uterus (*u*) is empty but has a thickened endometrial stripe (*curved arrow*) due to decidual reaction. **B.** Transvaginal examination in the same patient demonstrates a 20-mm embryo (between caliper marks [+]) in the extrauterine sac. No cardiac activity was present.

Table 33.2. Risk Of Ectopic Pregnancy As Determined By Ultrasound Findings[a]

Ultrasound Finding	Approximate Risk
IUP Confirmed	
General population	1 in 30,000
Patient taking ovulation-inducing drugs	1 in 6–7,000
IUP Not Confirmed	43%
Living ectopic fetus	100%
Adnexal mass	83%
Moderate/large fluid	83%
Adnexal mass + pelvic fluid	94%
Normal pelvic sonogram	8%

[a]Adapted from Mahony BS, Filly RA, Nyberg DA, Callen PW. Sonographic evaluation of ectopic pregnancy. J Ultrasound Med 1985;4:221–228.

pregnancies do occur, especially in patients taking ovulation-inducing drugs (14). When an adnexal mass other than a simple corpus luteal cyst is demonstrated, or a moderate or large amount of fluid is present in the pelvis, the risk of ectopic pregnancy is high. Even when the ultrasound examination is entirely normal, a patient with a positive pregnancy test remains at risk for ectopic pregnancy. The role of ultrasound, then, is to demonstrate findings that determine relative risk. This assessment, in conjunction with clinical history and physical examination, determines the next step in the patient's evaluation.

Ultrasound findings in ectopic pregnancy include demonstration of an extrauterine gestational sac appearing as a fluid-containing structure with an echogenic ring (Fig. 33.7). A living or dead embryo may or may not be evident. The ectopic gestational sac must be differentiated from a corpus luteal cyst, which develops on the ovary at the site of ovulation. The corpus luteal cyst appears as a thin-walled cyst

projecting eccentrically from the ovary. Clotted blood from hemorrhage within a corpus luteal cyst may simulate an embryo. Hematosalpinx or ruptured ectopic pregnancy may appear as an amorphous solid or complex adnexal mass lacking an embryo or sac. Blood in the cul-de-sac usually appears as echogenic fluid, but may be entirely echolucent if liquid, or echogenic and solid-appearing if clotted. Stimulation of the endometrium by the hormones released by the ectopic pregnancy causes thickening of the central stripe of the uterus. Blood in the endometrial cavity causes a "pseudogestational sac" (Fig. 33.6) in up to 20% of ectopic pregnancies. A true gestational sac is differentiated from "pseudosac" by the presence of a yolk sac or embryo. A double decidual sac sign suggests a true gestational sac, but is not totally reliable since some pseudosacs may also show a double decidual sac sign. Doppler studies demonstrate absent or minimal peritrophoblastic flow with pseudosacs and high-velocity, low impedance flow with true gestational sacs (15).

Subchorionic Hemorrhage

Subchorionic hemorrhage (Fig. 33.8) is a common finding in the bleeding patient before 20 weeks gestational age. All cases are believed to develop because of venous bleeding from separation of the margin of the placenta. The hematoma collects preferentially beneath the chorion because the chorion is more easily separated from the myometrium than is the placenta. In the acute stage, the hemorrhage is hyperechoic or isoechoic relative to the placenta. By 1–2 weeks the hemorrhage becomes sonolucent. The prognosis can be related to the size of the hematoma in patients seen before 20 weeks. Hematomas larger than 60 ml have a

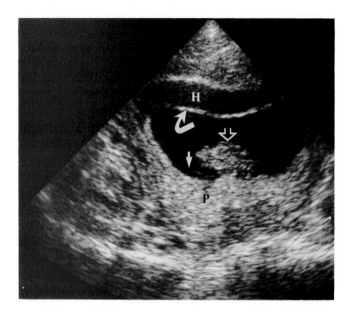

Figure 33.8.   Subchorionic Hemorrhage. Hemorrhage (*H*) extends beneath the chorion (*curved arrow*) from the edge of the placenta (*P*). A living 11-week fetus (*open arrow*) was present. Note the normal separation of the thin amniotic membrane (*straight arrow*) from the surface of the placenta.

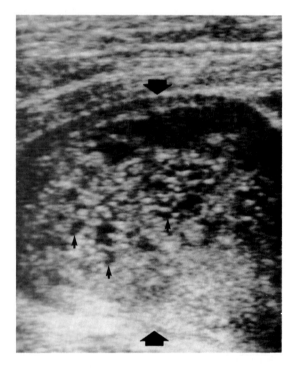

Figure 33.9.   Hydatidiform Mole. The uterus (between *large arrowheads*) is filled with echogenic material interspersed with numerous tiny cysts (*small arrows*), representing swollen chorionic villi.

greater than 80% chance of abortion or premature delivery (16).

Gestational Trophoblastic Disease

Gestational trophoblastic disease is a group of neoplasms that range from benign to highly malignant.

All are derived from abnormal placental tissues and occur as sequelae to pregnancy. Both benign and malignant tumors produce human chorionic gonadotropin. Serial measurement of β-hCG is a sensitive and reliable indicator of tumor activity. Gestational trophoblastic disease complicates about one in 1000–2000 pregnancies in the United States but has a much higher incidence in the Orient.

Hydatidiform Mole is the most benign form of the disease but maintains a potential for malignant sequelae. The placenta demonstrates edema and proliferation of trophoblasts. The villi become swollen and vesicular, resembling a "bunch of grapes." Patients present with hyperemesis, pregnancy-induced hypertension, or vaginal bleeding. The uterus may be enlarged (50%), normal (35%), or small (15%) for dates. Two types of hydatidiform mole exist. *Complete mole* (70%) involves the entire placenta, lacks a fetus, and is diploid in karyotype. *Partial mole* (30%) involves only a portion of the placenta, is usually associated with a fetus, and is triploid in karyotype.

Ultrasound in complete mole classically demonstrates the uterus to be filled with innumerable tiny cysts, often described as a "snowstorm" appearance because of the multiple interfaces (Fig. 33.9). Most vesicles are 1–2 mm in size but range up to 30 mm size. Partial mole demonstrates changes in only a portion of the placenta. The associated fetus usually has multiple anomalies. Early in the first trimester the classic appearance may not be evident; the mole may appear echogenic and solid (17). Transvaginal ultrasound helps to demonstrate the characteristic vesicles. Theca lutein cysts are seen as large, septated, bilateral cysts massively enlarging the ovaries in up to 50% of cases (Fig. 33.10).

Invasive Mole (chorioadenoma destruens) refers to invasion of molar tissue into, but usually not beyond, the myometrium.

Choriocarcinoma is a highly aggressive malignancy that forms only trophoblasts without any villous structure. Choriocarcinoma is locally invasive, spreads into the myometrium and parametrium, and hematogenously metastasizes to any site in the body. The hCG levels that rise or plateau in the 8–10 weeks following evacuation of molar pregnancy suggest invasive or metastatic gestational trophoblastic disease.

Ultrasound is relatively insensitive in demonstrating a locally invasive mole. Nodules in the myometrium are suggestive, but the sonographic appearance overlaps that of degenerating fibroids and ovarian dysgerminomas. Computed tomography and magnetic resonance demonstrate uterine enlargement, focal myometrial masses, dilated vessels, and areas of hemorrhage and necrosis within highly vascular tumor (18, 19). Metastases may be found in any organ.

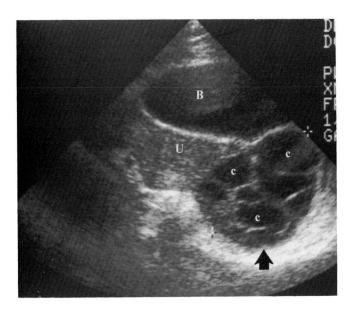

Figure 33.10. Theca Lutein Cysts. Transabdominal image in a transverse plane demonstrates the left ovary (*arrow*) to be greatly enlarged by numerous cysts (*c*) in this patient with persistent gestational trophoblastic disease. The uterus (*U*) is normal in size. *B,* bladder.

FETAL MEASUREMENTS AND GROWTH

Dating the pregnancy and determining the appropriateness of fetal growth is essential to obstetric care. Clinical dating is based upon maternal history of her last menstrual period and bimanual assessment of uterine size. Sonographic dating is based upon measurements of the gestational sac, embryo, or fetus. Serial measurements of fetal parameters are used to document growth. By convention, pregnancies are dated from the 1st day of the last menstrual period. The terms gestational age (GA), which is the clinical standard, and menstrual age are usually considered to be synonymous terms and are based on the average 28-day menstrual cycle. Conception is assumed to occur 14 days following the last menstrual period. Term is 40 weeks, with an acceptable range of 37–42 weeks.

Gestational Sac Size is used in the first trimester to estimate GA when no embryo is visualized. The gestational sac diameter is measured in three orthogonal planes and the results are averaged. The MSD is accurate to within approximately 1 week menstrual age.

Crown-Rump Length is measured from the top of the head to the bottom of the torso of the visualized embryo or fetus. The CRL is useful until about 10–12 weeks GA when other fetal measurements become more accurate. Charts provide GA estimations accurate to approximately 0.5 week menstrual age.

Biparietal Diameter is measured on an axial image of the fetal head at the level of the third ventricle and thalamus (Fig. 33.11). By convention, the mea-

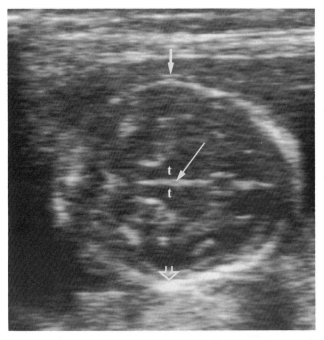

Figure 33.11. Transthalamic Plane. This axial image of the fetal cranium demonstrates the paired thalami (*t*) on either side of the midline third ventricle (*long arrow*). The biparietal diameter is measured in this plane from the outer surface of the near cranium (*closed arrow*) to the inner surface of the far cranium (*open arrow*). The head circumference is measured in this same plane.

surement is made from the outer table of the near cranium to the inner table of the far cranium. The measurement is affected by head shape and provides an inaccurate estimate of GA if significant dolichocephaly (elongated skull) or brachycephaly (round skull) is present.

Head Circumference is the outer perimeter of the fetal cranium measured in the same plane as the biparietal diameter. The head circumference measurement is relatively independent of head shape.

Abdominal Circumference is the outer perimeter of the fetal abdomen measured on an axial plane image at the level of the intrahepatic portion of the umbilical vein.

Femur Length is the measurement of the ossified portion of the femoral diaphysis. The entire femur must be imaged, and the femoral shaft must be centered in the beam so that it casts an acoustic shadow.

Gestational age estimates are most accurate in early pregnancy and become progressively less accurate as the pregnancy advances. The composite age, calculated by averaging the GA estimates of multiple parameters, is more accurate than any single parameter. Fetal anomalies may make individual parameters inaccurate for estimation of GA. Biparietal diameter, head circumference, abdominal circumference and femur length measurements predict GA accurate to about 1.2 weeks at 12–18 weeks, but are accurate to only about 3.1 weeks at 36–42 weeks. Gestational age is assigned at the time of the first ultrasound and is not changed thereafter. All subsequent ultrasound examinations are compared to the first examination to assess fetal growth.

Intrauterine Growth Retardation

Intrauterine growth retardation is defined as an estimated fetal weight below the 10th percentile for GA. This definition will include a number of normal fetuses. The challenge is to separate these normal fetuses from those who are pathologically affected. Estimated fetal weight is determined from established charts by measurement of abdominal circumference and biparietal diameter or abdominal circumference and femur length. *Symmetric IUGR* refers to fetuses in whom measurements of the head, abdomen, and femur are all proportionally small. Common causes of symmetric IUGR include chromosome abnormalities and intrauterine infections. In *asymmetric IUGR* the fetal abdomen is disproportionally small relative to the head and femur. The most common cause is placental insufficiency, which may be due to maternal hypertension, chronic illness, poor nutrition, smoking, drug or alcohol abuse. Infants with IUGR have up to 8 times the perinatal mortality of normal growth infants. Morbidity includes meconium aspiration and metabolic disorders. Additional parameters to assess by ultrasound in suspected IUGR cases include the thickness of fetal soft tissues and the volume of amniotic fluid. Severe IUGR is associated with oligohydramnios.

Fetal Macrosomia

Fetal macrosomia is variably defined as estimated fetal-weight above the 90th percentile for GA, or a fetal weight above 4000. Risk factors include maternal diabetes, maternal obesity, previous history of macrosomic infant, and excessive weight gain during pregnancy. Complications of macrosomia include traumatic delivery, fractures, brachial plexus injury, perinatal asphyxia, neonatal hypoglycemia, and meconium aspiration.

THE FETAL ENVIRONMENT
Uterus and Adnexa in Pregnancy

Uterine Leiomyomas are the most common solid pelvic masses encountered during pregnancy. Fibroids commonly enlarge and undergo cystic degeneration as the pregnancy advances. They are associated with bleeding, premature uterine contractions, malpresentation, and obstruction during labor. Leiomyomas must be differentiated from uterine contractions. Contractions are transient, although they may persist up to an hour. They typically appear homogeneous and isoechoic with the myometrium. They

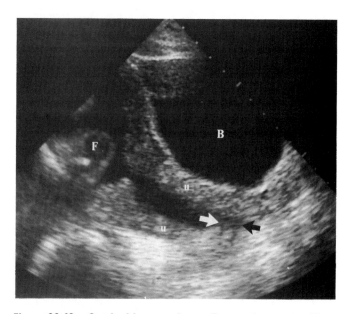

Figure 33.12.   Cervical Incompetence. The cervix, measured between the internal os (*white arrow*) and the external os (*black arrow*), is shortened to 9 mm in this patient with a history of multiple spontaneous abortions in the second trimester. An overdistended bladder (*B*) may compress the anterior and posterior walls of the lower uterine segment (*u*) together and mimic the cervix. The fetus (*F*) was 23 weeks GA.

bulge the inner, but generally not the outer, margin of the uterine wall. Leiomyomas are persistent, more heterogeneous, may have calcifications, and typically bulge the outer margin of the uterine wall.

Corpus Luteal Cysts are the most common cystic pelvic masses found in pregnancy. Internal hemorrhage causes enlargement up to 10–15 cm size, internal echoes, and septations. Most of these cysts regress by 16–18 weeks GA. Differential diagnosis includes benign cystic teratoma, cystadenoma, hydrosalpinx, and paraovarian cyst.

Theca Lutein Cysts form due to an exaggerated corpus luteum response to high levels of hCG. They appear as bilateral multicystic enlargement of the ovaries (Fig. 33.10). They occur most commonly with gestational trophoblastic disease, pregnancy with more than one fetus, and the use of ovulation-inducing drugs.

Cervical Incompetence may be congenital or result from cervical lacerations, excessive cervical dilation, or therapeutic abortion. The incompetent cervix is incapable of retaining a pregnancy to term. Preterm delivery is the single most common cause of a poor neonatal outcome. An obstetric history of recurrent loss of pregnancy in the second trimester establishes the diagnosis. Ultrasound is used to measure and follow cervical length and appearance (Fig. 33.12). Scans are performed through a partially filled bladder, transvaginally, or translabially from the introitus. The normal cervical length is 2.5–4 cm throughout gestation. Cervical length is measured between the internal and the external os. Cervical dilation is measured between the anterior and posterior surface of the cervical canal. Ultrasound criteria for cervical incompetence include cervical length <2.5 cm, cervical width >2 cm, dilation of the cervical canal >8 mm, and membranes bulging into the cervical canal. Sutures associated with cervical cerclage are seen on ultrasound as echogenic linear structures with acoustic shadowing.

Placenta and Membranes

Normal Placenta is first apparent on ultrasound at about 8 weeks as a focal thickening at the periphery of the gestational sac (20). The disc-like shape of the placenta becomes evident by 12 weeks, and by 18

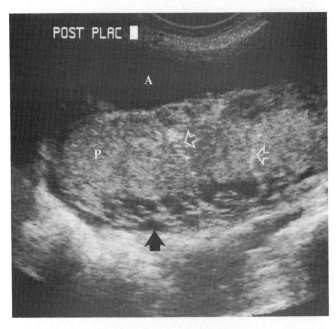

Figure 33.13. Normal Placenta. A transabdominal scan at 33 weeks GA demonstrates a normal placenta (*P*) with calcified septations (*open arrows*). The retroplacental complex of veins (*black arrow*) appears as a network of tubular lucencies beneath the placenta. *A*, amniotic cavity.

weeks the placenta is finely granular and homogeneous with a smooth covering chorionic membrane along its fetal surface. The retroplacental complex of decidual and myometrial veins forms a prominent sonographic landmark (Fig. 33.13). As the gestation advances the placenta becomes more heterogeneous, with focal echolucencies due to venous lakes and areas of fibrin deposition. Septations become prominent sonographic features throughout the placenta and cause undulations of the placental surface. Califications occur along the septations and are dispersed randomly throughout the placenta. These are normal changes of aging and should not be interpreted as indicators of disease. The normal placenta has a maximum thickness of 4 cm.

Placenta Previa is present when part or all of the placenta covers the internal cervical os (Fig. 33.14). Placenta previa is present at term in 0.3–0.6% of live births (20). However, placenta previa is suggested by ultrasound in as many as 45% of pregnancies examined in the first and second trimesters. These cases are due to low implantation. As the pregnancy progresses the lower uterine segment elongates and the placenta moves away from the cervical os. Risk factors for placenta previa include previous cesarean section, previous placenta previa, lower uterine surgical scars, and multiple previous pregnancies. Patients usually present with painless vaginal bleeding in the third trimester. Bleeding is initiated by the effacement of the cervix and dilation of the cervical os, which disrupts the vascular bed of the placenta. When the placenta covers the entire cervical os, the previa is complete. When an edge of the placenta covers a portion of the cervical os, the previa is partial or marginal.

Placental Abruption is defined as the premature separation of a normally positioned placenta from the myometrium. Separation is associated with hemorrhage from the maternal vessels at the base of the placenta. Abruption complicates 0.5–1.3% of pregnan-

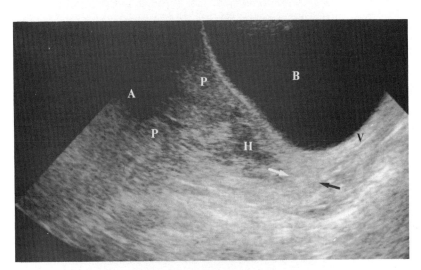

Figure 33.14. Placenta Previa. This patient, with a history of previous cesarean section, presented at 33 weeks GA with vaginal bleeding. The cervix (between *arrows*) is shortened to 18 mm. The placenta (*P*) covers the internal os (*white arrow*). A small hematoma (*H*) is seen between the placenta and the cervix. *A*, amniotic cavity; *B*, bladder; *V*, vagina.

Figure 33.15. **Placental Abruption.** The placenta (*P*) is displaced away from the wall of the uterus (*U*) by an echogenic hematoma (*H*). Note the absence of visualization of the retroplacental complex of veins. *A*, amniotic cavity.

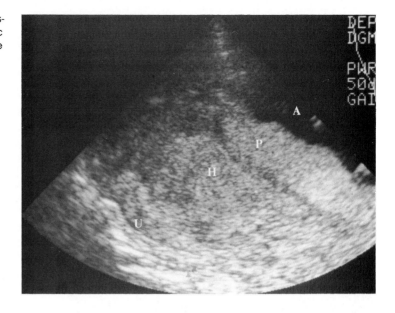

cies and is implicated in 15–25% of perinatal deaths. Risk factors include maternal hypertension, smoking, cocaine abuse, and previous history of abruption. *Subchorionic hemorrhage* occurs because of an abruption at the edge of the placenta (Fig. 33.8). Bleeding is usually venous and preferentially accumulates beneath the chorionic membrane adjacent to the placenta. *Retroplacental hemorrhage* occurs with more central abruption. Bleeding is usually arterial and accumulates beneath the placenta as an anechoic or mixed hypoechoic mass (Fig. 33.15). The hemorrhage may be isoechoic and difficult to differentiate from the placental tissue. The diagnosis is suggested by demonstrating disruption of the retroplacental complex of veins and thickening of the placenta (>4 cm).

Placenta Accreta is an abnormal adherence of the placenta to the uterine wall. Invasion of the uterine wall by the placenta is referred to as *placenta increta* and penetration of the uterine wall is *placenta percreta*. The decidua basalis and retroplacental complex of veins are completely or partially absent. The failure of the placenta to completely separate from the myometrium during labor results in hemorrhage. Risk factors include prior cesarean section, prior placenta accreta, and prior placenta previa. Scarring of the uterus results in the defective formation of decidua. Ultrasound findings include absence of vascular channels in the retroplacental region, increased echogenicity of tissues deep to the placenta, and visualization of retroplacental vessels within the bladder lumen. Placenta previa is usually also present.

Chorioangioma is a benign vascular placental mass supplied by the fetal circulation. It appears on ultrasound as a solid hypoechoic, sometimes septated, mass in the placenta usually close to the chorionic surface. Doppler demonstration of arterial waveforms at the fetal heart rate in vessels supplying the tumor is diagnostic. Vascular shunting may cause fetal high-output cardiac failure and fetal hydrops.

Umbilical Cord. The normal umbilical cord consists of two arteries and one vein surrounded by Wharton's jelly. It has a normal diameter of 1–2 cm. A single-artery umbilical cord is found in about 1% of pregnancies, and has a 10–20% association with congential malformations. Associated anomalies include cardiac, urinary tract, and central nervous system (CNS) malformations, omphalocele, trisomy 13, and trisomy 18. Masses in the umbilical cord include allantoic cysts, hematomas, hemangiomas, and teratomas.

Placental Membranes consist of an outer layer (*chorion*) and an inner layer (*amnion*). These membranes commonly remain separated by a layer of fluid (Fig. 33.16) until 14–16 weeks GA when the two membranes fuse. The amnion is visualized on ultrasound as a thin membrane floating in fluid. Occasional persistence of chorioamniotic separation into the third trimester is believed to be of no clinical significance.

Amniotic Band Syndrome is caused by the disruption of the amnion, allowing the fetus to enter the chorionic cavity (21). The fetus becomes entangled in fibrous bands that cross the chorionic cavity (Fig. 33.17). Entrapment of fetal parts results in amputation deformities that range from mild to incompatible with life. Typical abnormalities include asymmetric absence of the cranium resembling anencephaly, encephaloceles, gastroschisis and truncal defects, spinal deformities, and extremity amputations. The amniotic bands trapping the fetus may be visualized.

Amniotic Sheets (uterine synechia) are membranous structures that project into the uterine cavity (22). They demonstrate a characteristic appearance with a bulbous-free edge, thinner midportion, and a thickened base (Fig. 33.18). The fetus is able to move freely about the sheet of tissue. No fetal deformities are associated with this condition, which makes it distinct from the amniotic band syndrome. The amniotic sheets arise from folding of the chorioamniotic membranes over an intrauterine adhesion. Patients at

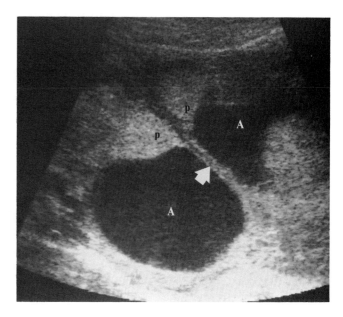

Figure 33.18. Amniotic Sheet. A fibrous band covered by chorioamniotic membranes (*arrow*) extends from the placenta (*p*) across the amniotic cavity (*A*). The uterine synechia forms a shelf-like structure that partially compartmentalizes the uterine cavity. The fetus has free access to both compartments.

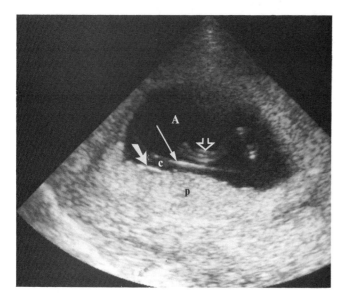

Figure 33.16. Normal Chorioamniotic Separation. The thin amniotic membrane (*long arrow*) is separated from the chorionic membrane (*short arrow*) covering the placenta (*p*) by fluid within the chorionic sac (*c*). The umbilical cord (*open arrow*) floats in the fluid of the amniotic sac (*A*).

increased risk for amniotic sheets include those with prior history of dilation and curettage or therapeutic abortion. An increased rate of cesarean section due to fetal malpresentation has been reported (23).

Amniotic Fluid

Normal Amniotic Fluid is essentially a dialysate of maternal serum in early pregnancy. As the pregnancy advances fetal urine becomes the major source of amniotic fluid. The composition of amniotic fluid is dynamic, with turnover of the entire volume every 3 hours. The fetus swallows amniotic fluid at a rate up to 450 ml per 24 hours. Transudate from the fetal lungs contribute a small volume. Water crosses placental membranes in response to osmotic gradients. Amniotic fluid is essential in promoting normal development and maturation of the fetal lungs. Suspended particles in amniotic fluid visualized by ultrasound may be due to normal vernix (desquamated fetal skin), blood, or meconium.

Polyhydramnios is an excessive amount of amniotic fluid, traditionally defined as greater than 2 liters of fluid at delivery. Ultrasound is used to confirm excessive fluid any time in pregnancy. Since amniotic fluid volume is difficult to measure, the diagnosis is usually made subjectively by visual inspection. The visual proportion of fluid relative to the size of the fetus is greatest early in the second trimester and decreases progressively to term. Polyhydramnios is suggested by large pockets of fluid relative to the age of the pregnancy. A fluid pocket greater than 8 cm deep

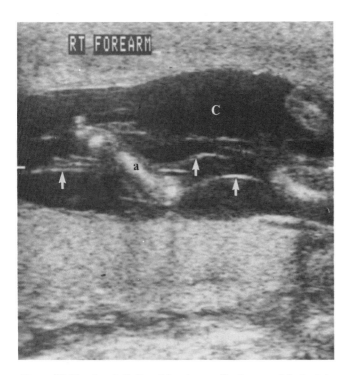

Figure 33.17. Amniotic Band Syndrome. The forearm (*a*) of a fetus at 15 weeks GA is entangled within fibrous bands (*arrows*) that extend across the chorionic cavity (*C*).

is strongly suggestive of polyhydramnios. Another clue is failure of the fetal abdomen to be in contact with both anterior and posterior uterine wall after 24 weeks GA. Excessive fluid is associated with preterm labor, premature rupture of membranes, and substantial maternal discomfort. About 60% of cases are idiopathic, 15–20% may be related to maternal disease (diabetes mellitus, preeclampsia, anemia, obesity), and 20–25% are associated with fetal anomalies. About half of all fetuses with anomalies will have polyhydramnios. Gross polyhydramnios has a higher association with fetal anomalies than mild polyhydramnios (24). Associated anomalies include anencephaly, encephalocele, gastrointestinal obstructions, abdominal wall defects, achondroplasia, and hydrops (isoimmunizaton).

Oligohydramnios refers to an abnormally low amniotic fluid volume. Like polyhydramnios, the ultrasound diagnosis is made by visual inspection. Fluid pockets are small, fetal parts are crowded, and fetal surface features like the face are difficult to visualize. Oligohydramnios is associated with premature rupture of membranes, intrauterine growth retardation, renal anomalies (lack of urine output), fetal death, eclampsia, and postdate pregnancies. A major complication of severe oligohydramnios is fetal lung immaturity.

Multiple Pregnancy

Twins occur in 1 of every 90 births (25). Morbidity and mortality are significantly increased in twin pregnancy compared to singleton pregnancy. Although twins represent less than 1% of all pregnancy, they account for 12–13% of all neonatal deaths. Twin morbidity includes prematurity, polyhydramnios, increased incidence of congenital anomalies, discordant growth, and cord accidents. Relative risk is increased if the fetuses share a placenta (monochorionic, 20%) as opposed to each fetus having its own placenta (dichorionic, 80%) (26). Twins that share a single amniotic cavity (monoamniotic) have the highest risk for morbidity, including conjoined twinning and intertwining of the umbilical cords. Visualization of two separate placentas, or determination that the twins are of different sex, is definitive proof of lower risk dichorionic twinning. Unfortunately, about half of dichorionic twins will have a fused placenta. Visualization of a membrane separating the twins confirms diamniotic twins. Monochorionic twins usually have vascular anastomoses at the placental level making them at risk for twin transfusion syndrome and twin embolization syndrome (26).

Twin Transfusion Syndrome results from shunting of blood from one twin to the other through vascular connections in the placenta. The abnormality ranges in severity from minor discordance in growth to severe intrauterine growth retardation in one twin with hydropic fluid overload in the other twin. Severe disparity in amniotic fluid volume may be present, with one twin experiencing polyhydramnios while the other twin is virtually anhydramniotic ("a stuck twin") (26). The mortality rate may be as high as 70%.

Twin Embolization Syndrome is an uncommon complication of the death of one twin in utero (26). Blood products from the dead twin are shunted through placental interconnections to the live twin, resulting in disseminated intravascular coagulopathy and multifocal tissue infarction.

FETAL ANOMALIES
General

Chromosome Abnormalities may be suspected when multiple or major fetal anomalies are detected by ultrasound. Advanced maternal age (>35 years at delivery) and a parent or previous child with aneuploidy or chromosomal translocation anomalies are risk factors for fetal chromosome abnormalities. Fetuses with structural anomalies detected on ultrasound have an 11–35% risk of associated chromosome abnormality. Fetal conditions with significant high risk of chromosome abnormality include holoprosencephaly, Dandy-Walker syndrome, cystic hygroma, cardiac malformations, omphalocele, duodenal atresia, facial anomalies, and early symmetric intrauterine growth retardation. Chromosome analysis is performed on samples obtained by amniocentesis or chorionic villous sampling.

Fetal Hydrops refers to the pathologic accumulation of fluid in body cavities and tissues. Ultrasound demonstrates ascites, pleural and pericardial effusions, and subcutaneous edema (Fig. 33.19). *Immune hydrops* is due to blood group incompatibility between mother and fetus. Modern treatment, including fetal transfusion, is highly successful. *Non-immune hydrops* is caused by a host of conditions including cardiac disorders, infections, chromosomal anomalies, twin pregnancy, urinary obstruction, and umbilical cord complications. The cause of many cases is not identified. The prognosis for nonimmune hydrops remains poor.

α-*Fetoprotein (AFP) Screening.* AFP is a protein produced by the fetal liver. Concentrations of AFP are highest in the fetal serum, with small amounts present in the amniotic fluid (AF-AFP), and minute amounts detectable in maternal serum (MS-AFP). Open neural tube and other skin defects allow AFP to leak into the amniotic fluid and maternal serum in abnormally large quantities. Routine MS-AFP screen-

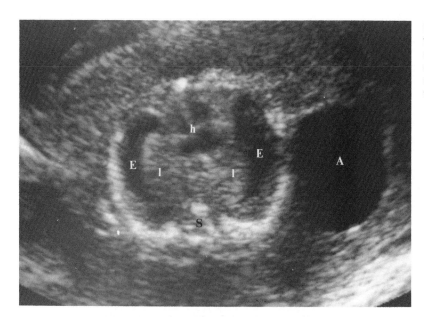

Figure 33.19. Fetal Hydrops. A transverse image through the fetal thorax at the level of the heart (*h*) demonstrates bilateral pleural effusions (*E*). The fetal chest is viewed from above, with the spine (*S*) posterior. This fetus also had ascites. A pocket of amniotic fluid (*A*) is seen adjacent to the right side of the fetus.

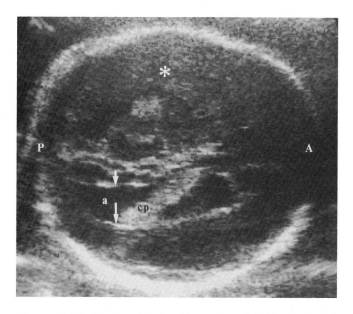

Figure 33.20. Transventricular Plane. The choroid plexus (*cp*) hangs dependently in the atria (*a*) of the lateral ventricle marking the lateral ventricular wall. The ventricular atrium is measured from its medial wall (*short arrow*) to its lateral wall (*long arrow*). The normal ventricular atrium does not exceed 10 mm in width at anytime during pregnancy. The near hemisphere (*) is obscured by reverberation artifact from the near skull. *A*, anterior; *P*, posterior.

ing is performed in Great Britain, California, and elsewhere to aid in detection of neural tube defects. The MS-AFP is measured at 16–18 weeks GA as determined by menstrual history. The normal values for MS-AFP vary with GA, reaching maximum values at 30–32 weeks gestation. Patients with abnormal MS-AFP are routinely referred for ultrasound evaluation and consideration of amniocentesis. The differential diagnosis for elevated AFP includes incorrect dates, multiple fetuses, fetal demise, anencephaly, encephalocele, myelomeningocele, gastroschisis, omphalocele, placental abruption, and cystic hygroma. Low AFP is associated with incorrect dating, fetal demise, normal fetuses, and Down's syndrome.

Central Nervous System, Face, Neck

Anomalies of the CNS occur in 1 of 1000 live births. Survivors are often severely handicapped and require long-term care. Effective ultrasound screening for CNS anomalies can be performed by examination of three crucial axial planes through the fetal brain (27). The *transthalamic plane* is used to measure the biparietal diameter and head circumference (Fig. 33.11). Abnormalities of head shape, microcephaly, macrocephaly, and major structural abnormalities are evident in this plane. The *transventricular plane* is an axial plane at the level of the ventricular atria (Fig. 33.20). The dominant landmark is the echogenic choroid plexus, which normally fills the atrium nearly completely. Measurements of atrial diameter made perpendicular to the walls do not normally exceed 10 mm. The *transcerebellar plane* is an axial scan in approximately 10–15° of inclination from the cantho-meatal line. The anatomic landmarks include the inferior portion of the third ventricle and the cerebellar hemispheres outlined by fluid in the cisterna magna (Fig. 33.21). The normal cisterna magna measures 2–11 mm in width. A small cisterna magna (<2 mm) suggests a Chiari II malformation, but may also be seen with massive ventriculomegaly. A large cisterna magna (>11 mm) may be a normal variant (mega-cisterna magna) or Dandy-Walker malformation, arachnoid cyst, or cerebellar hypoplasia. When these three planes are anatomically normal, the risk of CNS anomaly is approximately 0.005% (27). An algorithm for sorting out fetal CNS anomalies is given in Table 33.3 (28).

Table 33.3. Algorithm for Diagnosis of Congenital Brain Abnormalities^a

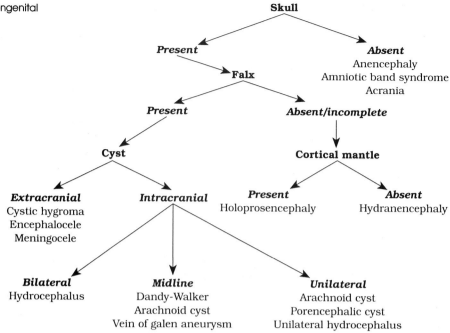

^aFrom Carrasco CR, Stierman ED, Hornsberger HR, Lee TG. An algorithm for prenatal ultrasound diagnosis of congenital CNS abnormalities. J Ultrasound Med 1985;4:163–168.

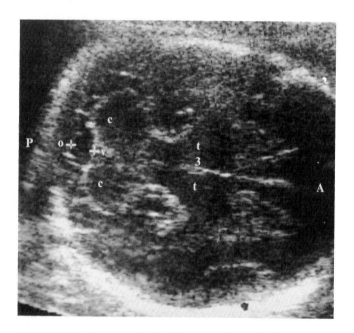

Figure 33.21.   Transcerebellar Plane. Landmarks for the transcerebellar plane include the thalami (*t*), third ventricle (*3*), and cerebellar hemispheres (*c*). The cisterna magna (between cursors [+]) is measured from the vermis (*v*) to the occiput (*o*). The normal cisterna magna measures 2–11 mm throughout pregnancy. *A*, anterior; *P*, posterior.

Ventriculomegaly is an anatomic finding with many causes that can be grouped into the categories of obstructive hydrocephalus (obstruction to flow of cerebrospinal fluid), cerebral atrophy (ex vacuo), and maldevelopment (such as agenesis of the corpus callosum). Ventriculomegaly detected in utero carries a poor prognosis. Up to 80% of fetuses with ventriculomegaly have associated anomalies. The US signs of ventriculomegaly include diameter of ventricular atrium >10 mm and a "dangling choroid." The choroid plexus hangs dependently in the ventricle and marks the position of the lateral ventricular wall (Fig. 33.22). The most common causes of ventriculomegaly seen in the fetus include Chiari II malformation and aqueductal stenosis.

Anencephaly is the most common neural tube defect. Ultrasound findings include absence of the cranial vault and cerebral hemispheres above the level of the orbits (Fig. 33.23). The cerebral hemispheres may be replaced by an amorphous neurovascular mass (area cerebrovasculosa) (29). The condition is inevitably fatal.

Cephaloceles are brain and/or fluid-filled sacs that protrude through a defect in the bony calvaria. They are found in the occipital (75%), frontoethmoid (13%), and parietal (12%) regions. Meningoceles contain only cerebrospinal fluid, while encephaloceles contain brain tissue (Fig. 33.24).

Spina Bifida refers to a spectrum of spinal abnormalities due to failure of the complete closure of the neural tube. The condition ranges from simple nonfusion of the vertebral arches with intact skin (spina bifida occulta), to protruding sacs containing cerebrospinal fluid, spinal cord, or nerve roots (myelomeningocele), to a totally open spinal defect (myeloschisis). Spina bifida may occur anywhere in the spine but most often occurs in the lumbosacral region. Ultrasound findings include outward splaying rather than inward convergence of the laminae, defect in the soft tissues overlying the bony abnormality, and a protruding sac containing fluid and often neural tissues (30) (Fig. 33.25). The associated functional neuromuscular defect often results in club foot deformities and dislocated hips. Associated cranial abnormalities of the Chiari II malformation provide clues to the presence of the spinal defect (31). Ventriculomegaly is present in 75% of cases. The "lemon sign" refers to bossing of the frontal bones causing a lemon-shaped appearance to the head in the axial plane (Fig. 33.26). The "banana sign" is produced by compression of the cerebellar hemispheres into a banana shape. The cisterna magna is small or obliterated (Fig. 33.26).

Chiari II Malformations are associated with 95% of myelomeningoceles (32). The cranial abnormality consists of caudal displacement of the cerebellar tonsils, pons, and medulla. The fourth ventricle is elongated, the posterior fossa is small, and the cisterna magna is obliterated.

Holoprosencephaly refers to a spectrum of disorders characterized by a failure of the prosencephalon to divide and form separate right and left hemispheres and thalami (32). Associated facial anomalies including hypotelorism, cyclopia, and proboscis are common (Fig. 33.27). Alobar holoprosencephaly is the most severe form and demonstrates absence of the falx and interhemispheric fissure with a single mid-line ventricle. The semilobar and lobar forms demonstrate greater degrees of midline separation.

Hydranencephaly refers to total destruction of the cerebral cortex, believed to be caused by the occlusion of the internal carotid arteries. The cranial vault contains fluid, but no cortical mantle is visible. The falx may be present but is usually incomplete. The brain stem and structures supplied by the vertebral arteries appear normal.

Dandy-Walker Malformation results from the maldevelopment of the roof of the fourth ventricle. The cisterna magna is enlarged and communicates directly with the fourth ventricle through its absent roof. The posterior fossa is enlarged and the tentorium is elevated (Fig. 33.28). The cerebellar hemispheres are usually hypoplastic. Hydrocephalus is usually present. The condition varies in severity across a broad spectrum. Less severe abnormalities are usually called Dandy-Walker variants. Arachnoid cysts and large cisterna magna are differentiated by their lack of communication with the fourth ventricle.

Cleft Palate and cleft lip account for 13% of all congenital anomalies found in the United States (33). Lateral clefting involves both lip and palate in 50% of cases, the lip alone in 25%, and the palate alone in 25%. The condition is bilateral in 20–25% of cases. Up to 60% of affected fetuses have additional anomalies including polydactyly, congenital heart disease, and trisomy 21. Ultrasound diagnosis is made on demonstration of a groove extending from one of the nostrils through the lip. Median cleft lip is a completely different entity associated with holoprosencephaly and accounting for less than 0.7% of all cases of cleft lip. A coronal plane sonogram of the face demonstrates a wide central defect in the upper lip and palate.

Cystic Hygroma is a fluid collection in the fetal neck due to failure of the lymphatic system to develop normal connections with the venous system in the neck. Ultrasound demonstrates a bilateral nuchal cystic mass with a prominent midline septum representing the nuchal ligament (Fig. 33.29). Up to 70% have an abnormal karyotype including Turner's syndrome and Down's syndrome. Generalized lymphangiectasia and fetal hydrops may occur and are always fatal when they do.

Chest and Heart

Congenital Diaphragmatic Hernia is a disorder in which abdominal contents protrude into the thorax through defects in the diaphragm. The most common type involves the foramen of Bochdalek at the posterolateral aspect of the diaphragm. The majority (75%) occur on the left side (Fig. 33.30). Anteromedial defects at the foramen of Morgagni also occur. Ultrasound findings include displacement of the

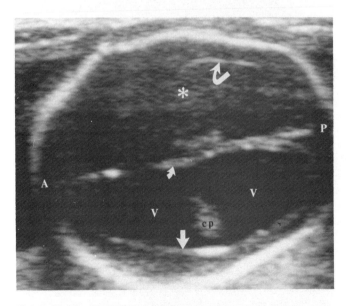

Figure 33.22. Ventriculomegaly. An axial image in the transventricular plane in a fetus with aqueduct stenosis demonstrates massive enlargement of the lateral ventricles (*V*). The choroid plexus (*cp*) dangles dependently from its medial attachment, marking the location of the lateral ventricular wall (*arrow*). The falx (*small curved arrow*) is seen as an echogenic stripe in the midline. The near hemisphere (*) is obscured by reverberation artifact from the near skull, but the lateral ventricular wall (*large curved arrow*) remains evident. *A*, anterior; *P*, posterior.

Figure 33.23. Anencephaly. A sagittal image through the head of a fetus with anencephaly demonstrates absence of the cranial vault (*) above the level of the eye (*e*). The mouth and lips are evident (*arrow*). *A*, fetal arm.

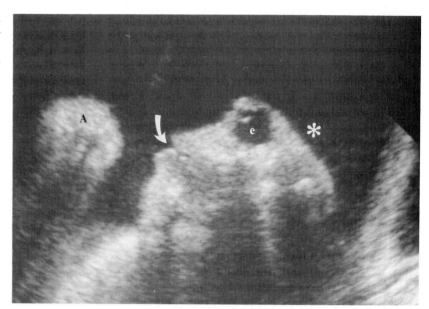

Figure 33.24. Encephalocele. Axial ultrasound image through the fetal skull demonstrates herniation of brain tissue (*B*) through a large defect in the skull (*black arrows*), forming an occipital encephalocele (*E*, between *open arrows*). The falx (*white arrow*) is seen as an echogenic midline stripe.

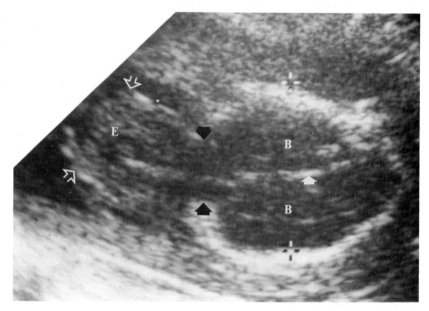

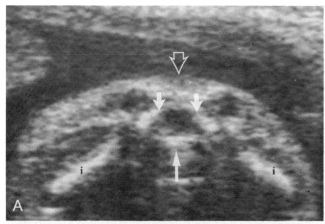

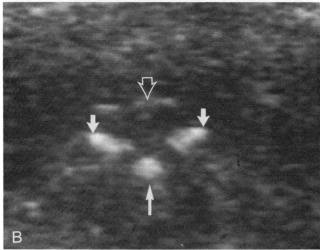

Figure 33.25. A. Normal Spine. Posterior transverse image through a normal fetal spine at the L4-5 level demonstrates the ossified portion of the vertebral body (*long arrow*) anteriorly and the converging ossified portions of the lamina (*short arrows*) posteriorly. The skin overlying the posterior aspect of the vertebra is intact (*open arrow*). *i*, iliac crest. **B. Meningomyelocele.** Posterior transverse image through a spina bifida defect demonstrates the ossified portion of the vertebral body (*long arrow*) anteriorly and the diverging ossified portions of the lamina (*short arrows*) posteriorly. A small fluid-containing sac (*open arrow*) protrudes through the defect.

heart and mediastinum, fluid-filled mass in the chest, absence of the stomach in the abdomen, and polyhydramnios. Associated defects, especially CNS, are common. Mortality is high (50–80%) because of pulmonary hypoplasia.

Cystic Adenomatoid Malformation is a congenital hamartomatous lesion of the lung usually affecting one lobe (34). The lesion consists of single or multiple cysts that vary in size from microscopic to larger than 2 cm size. Type I lesions appear on ultrasound as single or multiple cysts larger than 2 cm size. Type II lesions consist of multiple cysts of uniform size smaller than 2 cm. Type III lesions appear as echogenic solid masses because the cysts are microscopic. Polyhydramnios and fetal hydrops may occur.

Fetal Heart Anomalies. Congenital heart disease is a major cause of neonatal morbidity and mortality. Precise ultrasound diagnosis of fetal heart abnormalites often requires specialized equipment and a high level of expertise. However, the presence of many major structural abnormalities of the fetal heart can be recognized on the four-chamber heart view (35). The four-chamber view is obtained on an axial scan through the fetal chest just above the diaphragm (Fig. 33.31). The apex of the heart is directed at the left anterior chest wall at a 45 angle on the same side as the fetal stomach. Deviation from this position suggests a cardiac malformation or a thoracic mass (Fig. 33.30). Pericardial effusions appear as an anechoic band surrounding the myocardium. The ventricles are approximately equal in size and slightly smaller than their corresponding atria. Motion of the atrioventricular valves is observed in this plane. Papillary muscles in the ventricles may be echogenic and prominent. Discrepancies in chamber size or valve motion suggest cardiac malformations and the necessity to perform a more detailed examination.

Abdomen

Normal Fetal Abdomen. The normal fetal stomach should be visualized as a fluid-filled structure on the left side of the abdomen by 16 weeks GA. Failure to visualize the fetal stomach by 16 weeks suggests the possibility of esophageal atresia, diaphragmatic hernia, oligohydramnios, or recent gastric emptying. The colon is visualized after 20 weeks as a tubular structure around the periphery of the abdomen (36). The small bowel is more echogenic, centrally located, and blends with the liver. By the third trimester, peristalsis in small bowel loops can be observed. The visualized small bowel loops are normally <5 mm diameter and <15 mm in length. The colon progressively fills with meconium and approaches 2 cm in diameter near term. Normal fetal kidneys are seen as paired, slightly hypoechoic structures adjacent to the spine. The renal sinus appears as an echogenic stripe. Fetal lobulation causes an undulating contour of the kidneys. With advancing GA renal vasculature and the fluid-filled pelvis becomes evident. On axial section the normal renal pelvis anteroposterior (AP) diameter remains less than 50% of the AP diameter of the kidney.

Bowel Obstruction is suggested by dilation of the small bowel proximal to the obstructing lesion. Causes include atresia, stenosis, volvulus, enteric duplication, and Hirschsprung's disease. *Meconium ileus* is nearly always associated with cystic fibrosis. Thick meconium impacts in the distal ileum. Intraluminal meconium is quite echogenic. Perforation of a bowel segment results in *meconium peritonitis*. Ultrasound findings include calcifications in the peri-

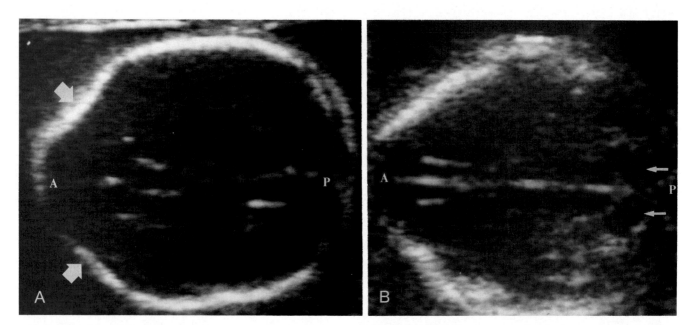

Figure 33.26. A. Lemon Sign. Concavity of the frontal bones (*arrows*) causes a "lemon" shape to the fetal skull in axial plane images. This appearance suggests a possible spina bifida defect. **B. Banana Sign.** Compression of the cerebellar hemispheres associated with downward herniation of the brain stem and the Chiari II malformation results in an hypoechoic "banana" (*arrows*) in the posterior aspect of the fetal skull in axial plane. *A,* anterior; *P,* posterior.

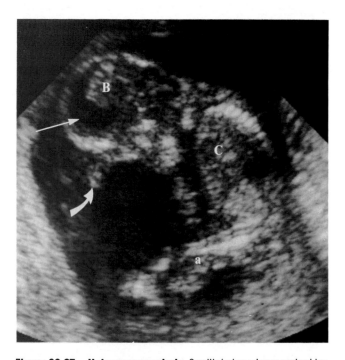

Figure 33.27. Holoprosencephaly. Sagittal plane transvaginal image of a 12-week fetus demonstrates a proboscis (*curved arrow*) protruding from the midface and the enlarged fused ventricles (*straight arrow*) of alobar holoprosencephaly. *B,* brain; *C,* chest; *a,* arm.

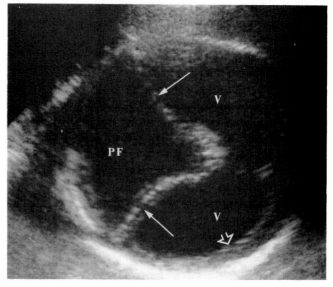

Figure 33.28. Dandy-Walker Malformation. Low axial plane image demonstrates cystic enlargement of the posterior fossa (*PF*) demarcated by the elevated tentorium (*arrows*). The lateral ventricles (*V*) are markedly enlarged and the cortical mantle (*open arrow*) is thinned.

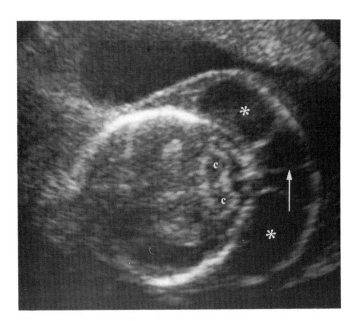

Figure 33.29. Cystic Hygroma. A multiseptated cystic mass (*) extends over the occipital region of the fetal skull. Cystic hygroma is differentiated from occipital cephalocele by demonstration of the midline septum (*arrow*) due to the nuchal ligament and absence of a bony defect in the skull.

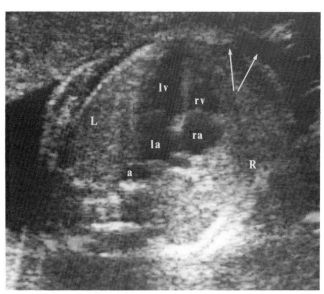

Figure 33.31. Four-Chamber View of the Heart. Axial plane image of the fetal thorax viewed from above demonstrates a normal four-chamber view of the heart. Note the orientation of the axis of the heart relative to the midline of the chest (*arrows*). *la*, left atrium; *lv*, left ventricle; *ra*, right atrium; *rv*, right ventricle; *a*, descending aorta; *L*, left thorax; *R*, right thorax.

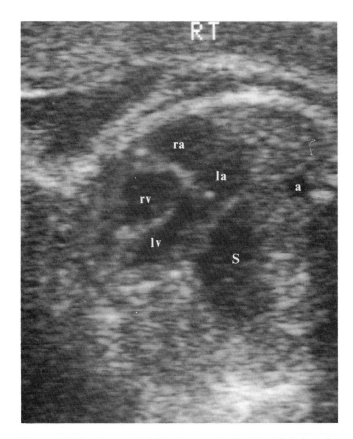

Figure 33.30. Congenital Diaphragmatic Hernia. Axial plane image of the fetal thorax viewed from above. Herniation of the stomach (*S*) into the left thorax displaces the heart into the right thorax. The heart is seen in four-chamber view. *ra*, right atrium; *rv*, right ventricle; *la*, left atrium; *lv*, left ventricle; *a*, descending aorta.

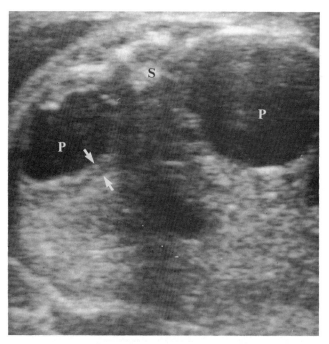

Figure 33.32. Hydronephrosis. Posterior axial plane ultrasound of the abdomen demonstrates marked bilateral enlargement of the renal pelves (*P*) in a male fetus with posterior urethral valves. The renal cortex is markedly thinned (*arrows*). *S*, spine.

Figure 33.33. Multicystic Dysplastic Kidney. The kidney (outlined by *arrows*) is largely replaced by multiple noncommunicating cysts (c).

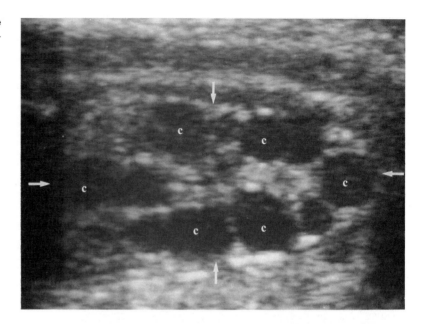

toneal cavity, meconium pseudocysts (hypoechoic mass with calcified wall), ascites, bowel dilation, and polyhydramnios.

Urinary Obstruction. Significant fetal hydronephrosis is usually defined as dilation of the renal pelvis >10 mm AP diameter, or >50% of the AP diameter of the kidney in axial section (37) (Fig. 33.32). Caliectasis is usually also evident. Assessment of bladder filling and amniotic fluid volume is necessary to determine the severity of obstruction. Renal pelvis measurements >4–6 mm before 24 weeks GA may progress to significant hydronephrosis in 41% of cases. Follow-up of these fetuses for evidence of progression of the collecting system dilation is recommended. Ureteropelvic junction obstruction is the most common cause of fetal hydronephrosis. Additional causes include ureterovesical junction obstruction, duplication and ectopic ureterocele, posterior urethral valves, and prune belly syndrome. Elective postnatal examinations of equivocal cases should be performed at 1–2 weeks of age to avoid underestimation of hydronephrosis due to early postnatal oliguria.

Renal Cystic Disease is commonly detected in utero. Multicystic dysplastic kidney appears as multiple noncommunicating cysts of varying size (Fig. 33.33). Since affected kidneys do not function, bilateral multicystic dysplastic kidney is associated with oligohydramnios and is not compatible with life. Infantile polycystic kidney disease (autosomal recessive) appears as massive enlargement of both kidneys. The kidneys are predominantly echogenic with a sonolucent rim. Discrete cysts are not evident. Adult polycystic kidney disease (autosomal dominant) is occasionally detectable in utero. The kidneys are enlarged but lack the sonolucent rim of infantile poly-

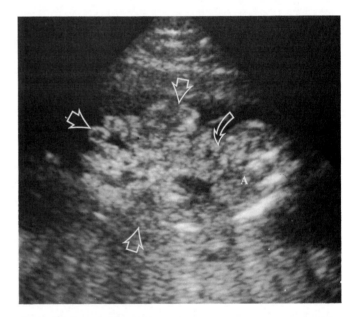

Figure 33.34. Gastroschisis. Transverse plane ultrasound through the fetal abdomen demonstrates herniation of multiple bowel loops (*arrows*) through a defect in the anterior abdominal wall (*curved arrow*). The bowel loops float freely in amniotic fluid and are not confined within a membrane. *A*, fetal abdomen.

cystic kidney disease. Occasional discrete cysts are visualized.

Gastroschisis results from a defect in the anterior abdominal wall on the right side of the umbilicus (38) (Fig. 33.34). The defect is usually 2–5 cm in size. The bowel herniates through the defect and floats freely in the amniotic fluid with no covering membrane. Small defects may be associated with bowel ischemia, resulting in thickening of the wall of the herniated bowel. The cord insertion site is normal. Gastroschisis is most commonly an isolated defect

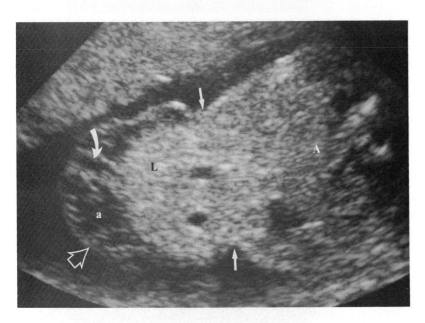

Figure 33.35. Omphalocele. The liver (*L*) herniates through a large defect (*small arrows*) in the anterior abdominal wall in this fetus with omphalocele. The umbilical vein (*curved arrow*) is included within the herniation. The herniated abdominal contents are confined within a membrane (*open arrow*). Ascites (*a*) is present within the omphalocele and within the fetal abdomen (*A*).

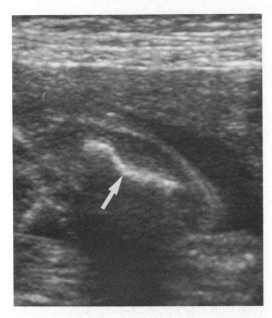

Figure 33.36. Osteogenesis Imperfecta. A longitudinal image of the femur demonstrates poor mineralization and central bowing due to a fracture (*arrow*).

without chromosomal anomaly or recurrence risk. Postnatal repair is usually successful so the prognosis is excellent.

Omphalocele is a more serious abdominal wall defect that is about equal in frequency to gastroschisis. The defect is midline at the umbilicus with herniation of abdominal contents into the base of the umbilical cord. Both liver and bowel are commonly present in the herniation. A membrane consisting of peritoneum and amnion always covers the omphalocele. The umbilical cord inserts through the membrane (Fig. 33.35). Associated anomalies are common (67–88%) including cardiac, CNS, urinary tract, and

gastrointesinal malformations. Chromosome anomalies are found in up to 40%. The ventral wall defect may include the heart (ectopia cordis).

Skeleton

Skeletal Dysplasias are a heterogeneous group of disorders of skeletal growth resulting in bones of abnormal size and shape (Fig 33.36). Thanatophoric dwarfism and achondrogenesis are the most common lethal skeletal dysplasias. Osteogenesis imperfecta and achondroplasia are common nonlethal dysplasias (Fig. 33.36). The presence of a skeletal dysplasia may be suggested by a short femur length measurement. This finding mandates measurements of foot length and of additional long bones, as well as assessment for structural skeletal abnormalities such as bowing, fractures, bone absence, and faulty mineralization. A ratio of femur length to foot length <0.9 suggests a skeletal dysplasia, while a ratio >0.9 is usually associated with a constitutionally small or growth-retarded fetus. Precise diagnosis of skeletal dysplasias may be difficult. An algorithmic approach is recommended (39).

References

1. Kier R, McCarthy SM, Scoutt LM, et al. Pelvic masses in pregnancy: MR imaging. Radiology 1990;176:709–713.
2. Benson RC, Colletti PM, Platt LD, Ralls PW. MR imaging of fetal anomalies. AJR 1991;156:1205–1207.
3. Guidelines for performance of the antepartum obstetrical ultrasound examination. Rockville: American Institute of Ultrasound in Medicine, 1991.
4. Sabbagha RE, Tamura RK. Some controversial issues. Clin Diagn Ultrasound 1987;20:319–325.
5. Yeh H-C, Goodman JD, Carr L, Rabinowitz JG. Intradecidual sign: a US criterion of early intrauterine pregnancy. Radiology 1986;161:463–467.

6. Nyberg DA, Laing FC, Filly RA. Threatened abortion: sonographic distinction of normal and abnormal gestation sacs. Radiology 1986;158:397–400.

7. Nyberg DA, Laing FC, Filly RA, et al. Ultrasonographic differentiation of the gestational sac of early intrauterine pregnancy from the pseudogestational sac of ectopic pregnancy. Radiology 1983;146:755–759.

8. Levi CS, Lyons EA, Lindsay DJ. Early diagnosis of nonviable pregnancy with endovaginal US. Radiology 1988;167:383–385.

9. Hsu-Chong Y, Rabinowitz JG. Amniotic sac development: ultrasound features of early pregnancy—the double bleb sign. Radiology 1988;166:97–103.

10. Nyberg DA, Mack LA, Laing FC, Patten RM. Distinguishing normal from abnormal gestational sac growth in early pregnancy. J Ultrasound Med 1987;6:23–27.

11. Levi CS, Lyons EA, Lindsay DJ. Ultrasound in the first trimester of pregnancy. Radiol Clin North Am 1990;28:19–38.

12. Mahony BS, Filly RA, Nyberg DA, Callen PW. Sonographic evaluation of ectopic pregnancy. J Ultrasound Med 1985;4:221–228.

13. Dashevsky SM, Lyons EA, Lyons CS, Lindsay DJ. Suspected ectopic pregnancy: endovaginal and transvesical US. Radiology 1988;169:181–184.

14. Hann LE, Bachman DB, McArdle CR. Coexistent intrauterine and ectopic pregnancy: a reevaluation. Radiology 1984;152:151–154

15. Dillon EH, Feyock AL, Taylor KJW. Pseudogestational sacs: Doppler US differentiation from normal or abnormal intrauterine pregnancy. Radiology 1990;176:359–364.

16. Nyberg DA, Mack LA, Benedetti TJ, et al: Placental abruption and placental hemorrhage: correlation of sonographic findings with fetal outcome. Radiology 1987;164:357–361.

17. Mendelson EB, Bohm-Velez M, Saker M. Transvaginal sonography in the abnormal first trimester. Semin Ultrasound CT MR 1990;11:34–43.

18. Sanders C, Rubin E. Malignant gestational trophoblastic disease: CT findings. AJR 1987;148:165–168.

19. Hricak H, Demas B, Braga CA, et al. Gestational trophoblastic neoplasm of the uterus: MR assessment. Radiology 1986;161:11–16.

20. Brant WE. Ultrasonography of the placenta. Perspectives in Radiology 1989;2:157–170.

21. Burton DJ, Filly RA. Sonographic diagnosis of the amniotic band syndrome. AJR 1991;156:555–558.

22. Randel SB, Filly RA, Callen PW, et al. Amniotic sheets. Radiology 1988;166:633–636.

23. Finberg HJ. Uterine synechiae in pregnancy: expanded criteria for recognition and clinical significance in 28 cases. J Ultrasound Med 1991;10:547–555.

24. Barkin SZ, Pretorius DH, Beckett MK, et al. Severe polyhydramnios: incidence of anomalies. AJR 1987;148:155–159.

25. Crane JP. Sonographic evaluation of multiple pregnancy. Semin Ultrasound CT MR 1984;5:144–156.

26. Filly RA, Goldstein RB, Callen PW. Monochorionic twinning: sonographc assessment. AJR 1990;154:459–469.

27. Filly RA, Cardoza JD, Goldstein RB, Barkovich AJ. Detection of fetal central nervous system anomalies: a practical level of effort for a routine sonogram. Radiology 1989;172:403–408.

28. Carrasco CR, Stierman ED, Harnsberger HR, Lee TG. An algorithm for prenatal ultrasound diagnosis of congenital CNS abnormalities. J Ultrasound Med 1985;4:163–168.

29. Goldstein RB, Filly RA, Callen PW. Sonography of anencephaly: pitfalls in early diagnosis. J Clin Ultrasound 1989;17:397–402.

30. Filly RA, Simpson GF, Linkowski G. Fetal spine morphology and maturation during the second trimester—sonographic evaluation. J Ultrasound Med 1987;6:631–636.

31. Campbell J, Gilbert WM, Nicolaides KH, Campbell S. Ultrasound screening for spina bifida: cranial and cerebellar signs in a high-risk population. Obstet Gynecol 1987;70:247–250.

32. Byrd SE, Osborn RE, Radkowski CB, et al. Disorders of midline structures: holoprosencephaly, absence of the corpus callosum, and Chiari malformations. Semin Ultrasound CT MR. 1988;9:201–215.

33. Hegge HN, Franklin RW, Watson PT, Calhoun BC. Fetal malformations commonly detectable on obstetric ultrasound. J Reproductive Med 1990;35:391–398.

34. Rosado-de-Christenson ML, Stocker JT. Congenital cystic adenomatoid malformation. Radiographics 1991;11:865–886.

35. McGahan JP. Sonography of the fetal heart: findings on the four-chamber view. AJR 1991;156:547–553.

36. Parulekar SG. Sonography of normal fetal bowel. J Ultrasound Med 1991;10:211–220.

37. Mandell J, Blyth BR, Peters CA, et al. Structural genitourinary defects detected in utero. Radiology 1991;178:193–196.

38. Hill LM. Sonographic detection of fetal gastrointestinal anomalies. Ultrasound Q 1988;6:35–67.

39. Spirt BA, Oliphant M, Gottlieb RH, Gordon LP. Prenatal sonographic evaluation of short-limbed dwarfism: an algorithmic approach. Radiographics 1990;10:217–236.

Section VIII   BONES AND JOINTS

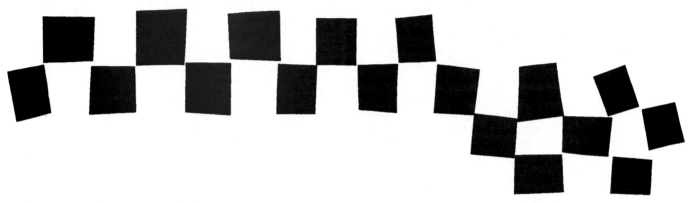

34

Benign Cystic Bone Lesions

Portions of this chapter were adapted from an earlier work by the author, *Fundamentals of Skeletal Radiology*, 1989, Philadelphia, W. B. Saunders Company. Reprinted by permission.

Clyde A. Helms

A benign, bubbly, cystic lesion of bone is one of the more common skeletal lesions a radiologist encounters. The differential diagnosis can be quite lengthy and is usually structured on how the lesion looks to the radiologist, using his or her experience as a guide. This method, called "pattern identification," certainly has merit, but it can lead to a very long differential diagnosis and many erroneous conclusions if not tempered with some logic.

In general, if a differential diagnosis will yield the correct diagnosis 95% of the time, most would consider it a useful differential list; however, it would not be appropriate to accept a 1-in-20 miss rate for fractures and dislocations. In general, the shorter the differential diagnosis list, the more helpful it is to clinicians, and the easier it is to remember. A shorter differential list will usually have a lower accuracy rate than a long list, however, many times the longer lists contain such rare entities that the accuracy does not really increase substantially. For most of the entities in bone radiology a 95% accurate differential is acceptable. If one wants to be more accurate than that, simply add more diagnoses to the list of differential possibilities.

When the differential diagnosis is long, as in the differential for bubbly, cystic lesions of bone, it can be difficult to recall all of the entities that should be mentioned. A mnemonic can be helpful in recalling long lists of information; therefore, a helpful mnemonic is recommended.

FEGNOMASHIC

FEGNOMASHIC is a mnemonic that serves as a nice starting point for discussing possibilities that appear as benign, cystic lesions in bone. This mnemonic has been in general use for many years. By itself it is merely a long list—14 entities—and needs to be coupled with other criteria to shorten the list into manageable form for each particular case. For instance, the age of the patient will help add or eliminate many of the possibilities. If multiple lesions are present, only half a dozen entities need to be discussed. Methods of narrowing the differential are discussed later in this chapter.

The first step in approaching a benign, cystic bone lesion is to be certain it is really benign. The criteria for differentiating benign from malignant are covered in Chapter 35. Once it is established that the lesion is truly a benign, cystic lesion, FEGNOMASHIC will allow a differential diagnosis that is at least 95% accurate. Merely memorizing the 14 entities in this differential is easily done (Table 34.1).

The next step after learning the names of all of the lesions is getting some idea of what each lesion looks like. This is where experience becomes a factor. For the medical student or 1st-year resident it is difficult to go beyond saying that they *all* look cystic, bubbly, and benign. However, the 3rd-year resident should have no trouble differentiating between a unicameral bone cyst and a giant cell tumor because he or she has seen examples of each many times before and knows what each looks like.

After getting a feel for what each lesion looks like radiographically, and overcoming the frustration that builds when one realizes that many of them look alike, try to learn ways to differentiate each lesion from the others. I have developed a number of keys that I call "discriminators," which will help to differentiate each lesion. These discriminators are 90–95% useful (I will

Table 34.1. Discriminators for Benign Lytic Bone Lesions—Mnemonic: FEGNOMASHIC

Letter	Represents	Characteristics
F	*Fibrous dysplasia*	No periosteal reaction.
E	*Enchondroma*	1. Must have calcification (except in phalanges).
		2. No periostitis.
	Eosinophilic granuloma	Must be under age 30
G	*Giant cell tumor*	1. Epiphyses must be closed.
		2. Must abut the articular surface.
		3. Must be well defined with a nonsclerotic margin.
		4. Must be eccentric.
N	*Nonossifying fibroma*	1. Must be under age 30.
		2. No periostitis.
		3. Cortically based
O	*Osteoblastoma*	Mentioned when ABC is mentioned (especially in the posterior elements of the spine).
M	*Metastatic diseases and myeloma*	Must be over age 40.
A	*Aneurysmal bone cyst*	1. Must be expansile.
		2. Must be under age 30.
S	*Solitary bone cyst*	1. Must be central.
		2. Must be under age 30.
H	*Hyperparathyroidism (brown tumor)*	Must have other evidence of HPT.
I	*Infection*	Must always mention.
C	*Chondroblastoma*	1. Must be under age 30.
		2. Must be epiphyseal.
	Chondromyxoid fibroma	No calcified matrix.

mention when they are more or less accurate, in my experience) and are by no means meant to be absolutes or dogma. They are guidelines, but have a high accuracy rate.

Textbooks rarely tell that a finding "always" or never occurs. They temper their descriptions with "virtually always," or "invariably," or "usually," or "characteristically." I have tried to pick out findings that come as close to "always" as I can, realizing that I will only be around 95% accurate. That is good enough for most radiologists.

The following will be only a brief description of each entity, as more complete descriptions are readily available in any skeletal radiology text. What will be emphasized, however, are the points that are unique for each entity, thereby enabling differentiation from the others. Table 34.1 is a synopsis of these discriminators.

FIBROUS DYSPLASIA

Fibrous dysplasia is a benign congenital process that can be seen in a patient of any age and can look like almost any pathologic process radiographically. It can be wild-looking, a discrete lucency, patchy, sclerotic, expansile, multiple, and many other descriptions. It is, therefore, difficult to look at a bubbly lytic lesion and unequivocally say it is or is not fibrous dysplasia. It would be better if the FEGNOMASHIC differential started on a positive note, say, with giant cell tumor or chondroblastoma, for which there are some definite criteria. However, since fibrous dysplasia is first on the list we might as well deal with it.

How do you know whether to include or exclude fibrous dysplasia if it can look like almost anything? Experience is the best guideline. In other words, look in a few texts and find as many different examples as possible; get a feeling for what fibrous dysplasia looks like.

Fibrous dysplasia will not have periostitis associated with it; therefore, if periostitis is present, one may safely exclude fibrous dysplasia. Fibrous dysplasia virtually never undergoes malignant degeneration and should not be a painful lesion unless there is a fracture. An occult fracture often occurs in long bones with fibrous dysplasia; therefore, it is not unusual to have it present with pain and no obvious fracture seen in a long bone. Pain in a flat bone, such as the ribs or pelvis (nonweight-bearing bones), should not occur with fibrous dysplasia.

Fibrous dysplasia can be either monostotic (most commonly) or polyostotic, and has a predilection for the pelvis, proximal femur, ribs, and skull. When it is present in the pelvis, it is invariably present in the ipsilateral proximal femur (Fig. 34.1). I have seen only one case in which the pelvis was involved with fibrous dysplasia and the proximal femur was spared. The proximal femur, however, may be affected alone, without involvement in the pelvis (Fig. 34.2).

Fibrous dysplasia often involves the ribs. It typically has an expansile, lytic appearance in the posterior ribs (Fig. 34.3), and a sclerotic appearance in the anterior ribs.

The classic description of fibrous dysplasia is that it has a ground-glass or smoky matrix. This description confuses people as often as it helps them, and I

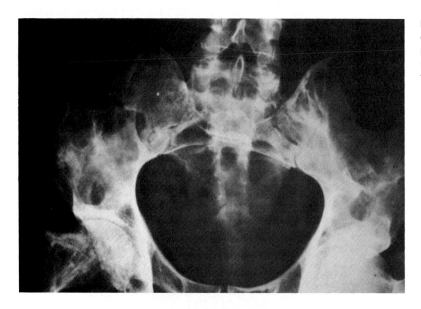

Figure 34.1. Fibrous Dysplasia. This patient has poly-ostotic fibrous dysplasia with diffuse involvement of the pelvis as well as the proximal right femur. When the pelvis is involved with fibrous dysplasia, the ipsilateral femur on the affected side is invariably also involved.

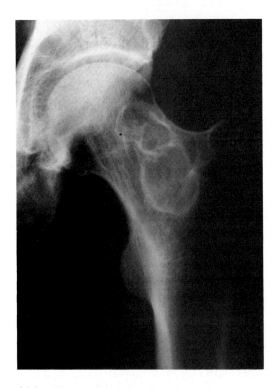

Figure 34.2. Fibrous Dysplasia. This patient has a well-defined lytic lesion with a hazy, ground-glass appearance in the neck of the left femur. The pelvis was uninvolved. It is not unusual for monostatic fibrous dysplasia to involve the proximal femur and spare the pelvis.

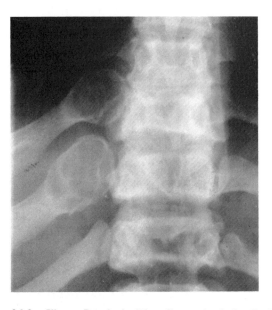

Figure 34.3. Fibrous Dysplasia. When fibrous dysplasia affects the ribs, the posterior ribs often demonstrate a lytic expansile appearance, as in this example. When the anterior ribs are involved, they are most often sclerotic in appearance. Note also the involvement of the thoracic spine.

do not recommend using ground-glass appearance as a buzz word for fibrous dysplasia. Fibrous dysplasia is often purely lytic and becomes hazy or takes on a ground-glass look as the matrix calcifies (Fig. 34.4). It can go on to calcify significantly, and then it presents as a sclerotic lesion (Fig. 34.5). Also, I often see lytic lesions with a pathologic diagnosis other than fibrous dysplasia that have a distinct ground-glass appear-

ance; therefore, the ground-glass quality can be misleading.

Adamantinoma. When a lesion is encountered in the tibia that resembles fibrous dysplasia, an adamantinoma should also be mentioned. An adamantinoma is a malignant tumor that radiographically and histologically resembles fibrous dysplasia (Fig. 34.6). It occurs almost exclusively in the tibia and the jaw (for unknown reasons), and is rare. Because it is rare, one may choose not to include it in the differential—a misdiagnosis will not occur more than once or twice in a lifetime.

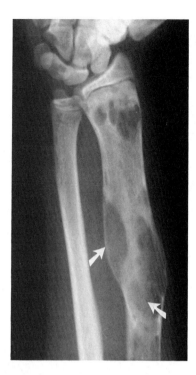

Figure 34.4. Fibrous Dysplasia. Polyostotic fibrous dysplasia is seen in the radius in this child. Parts of this lesion have a hazy, ground-glass appearance (*arrows*) while others are more lytic appearing. A hazy, ground- glass appearance is often present in fibrous dysplasia, but just as often, the appearance can be purely lytic, or even sclerotic.

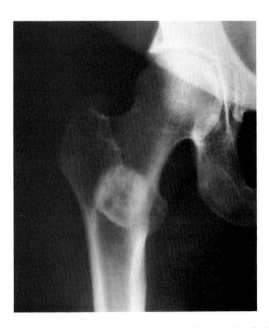

Figure 34.5. Fibrous Dysplasia. This predominantly sclerotic lesion in the intertrochanteric region of the right hip is a characteristic appearance for monostatic fibrous dysplasia in this location.

McCune-Albright Syndrome. Polyostotic fibrous dysplasia occasionally occurs in association with café au lait spots on the skin (dark-pigmented, freckle-like lesions) and precocious puberty. This

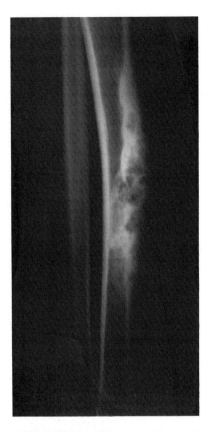

Figure 34.6. Adamantinoma. This expansile, mixed lytic and sclerotic process in the midshaft of the tibia is characteristic for fibrous dysplasia. However, an adamantinoma has an identical appearance and should be considered in any tibial lesion that resembles fibrous dysplasia. Biopsy showed this to be an adamantinoma.

complex is called McCune-Albright syndrome. The bony lesions in this syndrome, and even in the simple polyostotic form, often occur unilaterally, that is, throughout one-half of the body. This does not happen often enough to be of any diagnostic use in differentiating fibrous dysplasia from other lesions.

The presence of multiple lesions of fibrous dysplasia in the jaw has been termed "cherubism." This is from the physical appearance of the child with puffed-out cheeks having an angelic look. The jaw lesions in cherubism regress in adulthood.

Discriminator. No periosteal reaction.

ENCHONDROMA AND EOSINOPHILIC GRANULOMA

Enchondroma

Enchondromas occur in any bone formed from cartilage, and may be central, eccentric, expansile, or nonexpansile. They invariably contain calcified chondroid matrix except when in the phalanges. An enchondroma is the most common benign cystic lesion in the phalanges (Fig. 34.7). If a cystic lesion is present without calcified chondroid matrix anywhere ex-

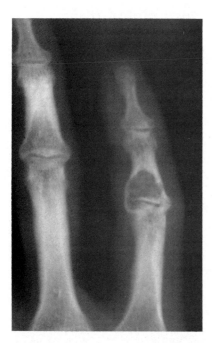

Figure 34.7.   Enchondroma. A lytic lesion in the phalanges is most commonly an enchondroma. This is the only location in the skeleton where an enchondroma does not contain calcified chondroid matrix. These most often present with pathologic fractures, as in this example.

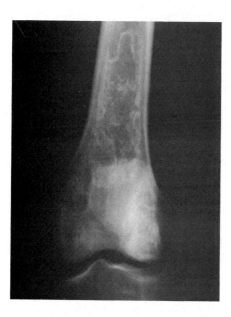

Figure 34.8.   Bone Infarct. This lytic lesion in the distal femur with a calcified, serpiginous border is typical for a bone infarct. Occasionally, the differential between a bone infarct and an enchondroma can be difficult on plain films; however, in this example an infarct is easily diagnosed.

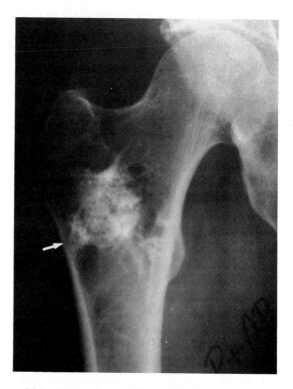

Figure 34.9.   Enchondroma. This mixed lytic, sclerotic lesion in the intertrochanteric region of the right femur shows the stippled punctate calcification typical for chondroid matrix seen in an enchondroma. Some endosteal scalloping is seen on the lateral cortex (*arrow*), but this is subtle.

cept in the phalanges, I will not include enchondroma in my differential.

Often it is difficult to differentiate between an enchondroma and a bone infarct. An infarct usually has a well-defined, densely sclerotic, serpiginous border (Fig. 34.8), whereas an enchondroma does not (Fig.

34.9). An enchondroma often causes endosteal scalloping, whereas a bone infarct will not. Although these criteria are helpful in separating an infarct from an enchondroma, they are not foolproof.

It is difficult, if not impossible, to differentiate an enchondroma from a chondrosarcoma. Clinical findings (primarily pain) serve as a better indicator than radiographic findings, and indeed pain in an apparent enchondroma should warrant surgical investigation. Periostitis should not be seen in an enchondroma either. Trying to histologically differentiate an enchondroma from a chondrosarcoma is also difficult, if not impossible, at times. Therefore, biopsy of an apparent enchondroma should not be performed routinely for histologic differentiation.

Multiple enchondromas occur on occasion; this condition has been termed "Ollier's disease" (Fig. 34.10). It is not hereditary and does not have an increased rate of malignant degeneration. The presence of multiple enchondromas associated with soft-tissue hemangiomas is known as Maffucci's syndrome (Fig. 34.11). This syndrome also is not hereditary; however, it does have an increased incidence of malignant degeneration of the enchondromas.

Discriminators.   1. Must have calcification (except in phalanges). 2. No periostitis or pain.

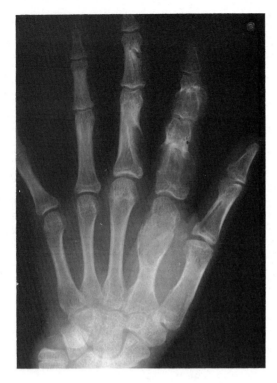

Figure 34.10. Ollier's Disease. Multiple enchondromas are present throughout the hand. This is a typical example of Ollier's disease.

Eosinophilic Granuloma

Eosinophilic granuloma (EG) is a form of histiocytosis X, the other forms being Letterer-Siwe disease and Hand-Schüller-Christian disease. Although these forms may be merely different phases of the same disease, most investigators categorize them separately. The bony manifestations of all three disorders are similar and are discussed in this review simply as EG.

Eosinophilic granuloma, unfortunately for radiologists, has many appearances (1). It can be lytic or sclerotic; it may be well defined or ill defined; it may or may not have a sclerotic border; and it may or may not elicit a periosteal response. The periostitis, when present, is typically benign in appearance (thick, uniform, wavy) but can be lamellated or amorphous. Eosinophilic granuloma can mimic Ewing's sarcoma and present as a permeative (multiple small holes) lesion.

How, then, can one distinguish EG from any of the other lytic lesions in this differential? Remember that it is difficult to exclude EG from almost any differential of a bony lesion, be it benign or malignant. Eosinophilic granuloma occurs almost exclusively in patients under the age of 30 (usually under the age of 20); therefore, the patient's age is the best criterion. I recommend mentioning EG as a differential possibility for *any* lesion in a patient under the age of 30. Therefore, since EG can look like anything, so long as the x-ray is not of an arthritide or trauma, EG can be mentioned without even looking at the film!

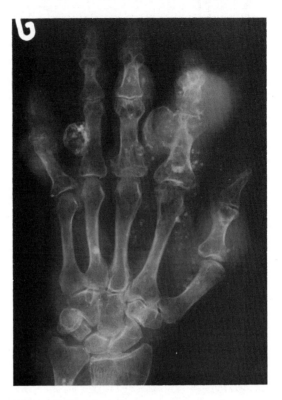

Figure 34.11. Maffucci's Syndrome. Multiple enchondromas associated with phleboliths are present in the phalanges. This combination of findings invariably represents hemangiomas and enchondromas in Maffucci's syndrome.

Eosinophilic granuloma is most often monostotic (Fig. 34.12), but it can be polyostotic (Fig. 34.13) and, thus, has to be included whenever multiple lesions are present in a patient under the age of 30.

Eosinophilic granuloma may or may not have a soft-tissue mass associated, so the presence or absence of a soft-tissue mass will not help in the differential diagnosis. In fact, I know of no entity in which presence or absence of an associated soft-tissue mass will warrant inclusion or exclusion of the process from a differential. It is important to note the presence of a soft-tissue mass (or its absence), but it will do little to narrow the differential diagnosis.

Most radiologists are inept at evaluating the soft tissues because they are difficult to see, and computed tomography (CT) and magnetic resonance imaging (MR) have made it unnecessary in most cases to rely on plain films for the soft tissues. Fortunately, in most cases, the presence or absence of a soft-tissue mass will not alter the differential diagnosis. The treating physician will undoubtedly want to know if the soft tissues are involved, and to what extent; this can be satisfactorily demonstrated with MR.

Eosinophilic granuloma occasionally has a bony sequestrum (Fig. 34.14). Only two other entities have been described that, on occasion, have bony sequestra: osteomyelitis and fibrosarcoma; therefore, when a

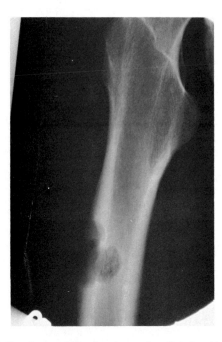

Figure 34.12. Eosinophilic Grauloma. A well-defined lytic lesion is seen involving the cortex of the proximal femur in this 20-year-old patient. Biopsy showed this to be EG.

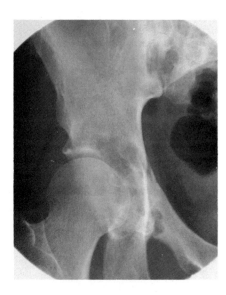

Figure 34.13. Eosinophilic Granuloma. Well-defined lytic lesions are present throughout the pelvis in this 24-year-old patient. In addition to the lesion around the right hip, a lesion is seen at the right sacroiliac joint. Biopsy showed this to be EG.

sequestrum is identified, EG, osteomyelitis, and fibrosarcoma should be considered. As will be discussed in Chapter 40, an osteoid osteoma will often give an appearance of a sequestration when the nidus is partially calcified.

Clinically, EG may or may not be associated with pain; therefore, clinical history is noncontributory for the most part.

Discriminator. Must be under age 30.

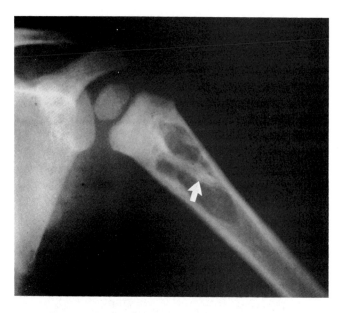

Figure 34.14. Eosinophilic Granuloma. This well-defined lytic lesion contains a bony sequestrum (*arrow*) which is typical for osteomyelitis or EG. Biopsy revealed this to be EG.

GIANT CELL TUMOR

Giant cell tumor is an uncommon, somewhat controversial lesion with several schools of thought as to its radiographic appearance. I subscribe to the most widely used approach, as do the majority of radiologists and pathologists (2).

First, it is important to realize that one is unable to tell if a giant cell tumor is benign or malignant, regardless of its radiographic appearance. In fact, histologically, a giant cell tumor cannot be divided into either a benign or a malignant category. Most surgeons curettage and pack the lesions and consider them benign unless they recur. Even then they can still be benign and recur a second or third time. About 15% of giant cell tumors are thought to be malignant, based on their recurrence rate. They can metastasize to the lungs, but do so late.

There are four classic radiographic criteria for diagnosing giant cell tumors. If any of these criteria are not met when looking at a lesion, giant cell tumor can be eliminated from the differential diagnosis.

Number one. Giant cell tumor occurs only in patients with closed epiphyses; this is valid at least 98–99% of the time and is extremely useful. I will not entertain the diagnosis of giant cell tumor in a patient with open epiphyses.

Number two. The lesion must be epiphyseal and abut the articular surface (Fig. 34.15). There is disagreement over whether giant cell tumors begin in the epiphyses, metaphyses, or from the physeal plate itself; however, except for rare cases, when radiologists see the lesions, they are epiphyseal and are flush against the articular surface. The metaphysis also has

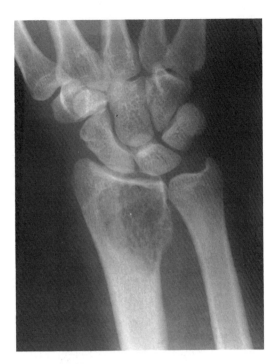

Figure 34.15. Giant Cell Tumor. A well-defined lytic lesion without a sclerotic margin is seen abutting the articular surface of the distal radius in a patient who has closed epiphyses. These are all characteristics of a giant cell tumor.

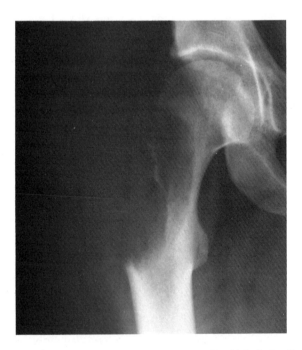

Figure 34.16. Giant Cell Tumor. This well-defined lytic lesion that does not have a sclerotic margin completely involves the greater tuberosity. The apophyses have the same differential diagnosis as lesions in the epiphyses, which makes giant cell tumor a strong possibility in this example. Biopsy showed this to be a giant cell tumor.

some of the tumor in it because the lesions are generally very large. When one sees a giant cell tumor, it will be epiphyseal. Perhaps more importantly, it should be

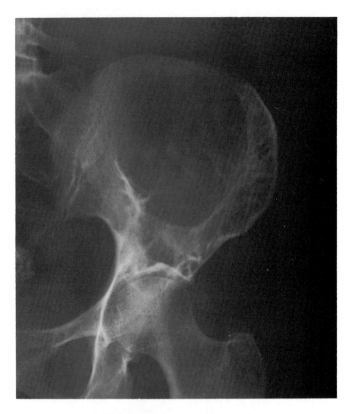

Figure 34.17. Giant Cell Tumor. A large, well-defined lytic lesion in the iliac wing is seen, which does contain a sclerotic margin and does not appear to abut any articular surface. The pelvis is a good location for giant cell tumor, which this proved to be at biopsy. The usual rules for giant cell tumors such as a nonsclerotic margin do not apply in flat bones.

flush against the articular surface of the joint. This occurs in 98–99% of giant cell tumors; therefore, if I have a lesion that is separated from the articular surface by a definite margin of bone, I will not include giant cell tumor in the diagnosis. This rule does not apply in flat bones, such as in the pelvis or in the apophyses, which have no articular surfaces (Fig. 34.16).

Number three. Giant cell tumors are said to be eccentrically located in the bone, as opposed to being centrally placed in the medullary cavity. When a bony lesion is quite large, it can be difficult to tell if it is central or eccentric. I do not find this to be a terribly useful description, but it is one of the classic "rules" of a giant cell tumor.

Number four. The lesion must have a sharply defined zone of transition (border) that is not sclerotic. This is a very helpful finding in giant cell tumor. The only places this does not apply is in flat bones, such as the pelvis (Fig. 34.17), and the calcaneus.

It is important to realize that the four criteria for a giant cell tumor apply only to giant cell tumors and not to any other lesion. For instance, I know of no other lesion that depends on whether the epiphyses are open or closed. No other lesion in any of my lists

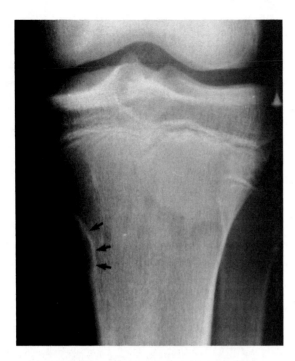

Figure 34.18. Fibrous Cortical Defect. A well-defined lytic lesion is seen in the medial metaphysis of this tibia (*arrows*), which is typical for a fibrous cortical defect.

use as a diagnostic factor whether the zone of transition is sclerotic or not (many lesions, such as nonossifying fibromas, will usually have a sclerotic margin, but it does not occur enough to include as a discriminator). No other lesion must always abut the articular surface, and no other lesion has the classic description of being eccentrically placed (although several lesions, including nonossifying fibroma and chondromyxoid fibroma, are in fact eccentric most of the time).

So, although these four criteria apply well for giant cell tumor, they do not apply at all for any other lesions. Residents have a tendency to apply these criteria to every lytic lesion encountered for the simple reason that they have learned the four criteria.

Once one of the criteria is violated, the remainder do not even have to be used to eliminate a giant cell tumor. For instance, if a lytic lesion is found in the middiaphysis of a bone, giant cell tumor can be excluded. There is no need to check further to see if it is eccentric, if it has a nonsclerotic margin, or if the epiphyses are closed.

Again, these rules will be greater than 95% effective and, in my experience, close to 99% effective. If one or two cases are found that do not fit the criteria, another pathologist should review the slides. Many pathologists refer to aneurysmal bone cysts as giant cell tumors; hence they have giant cell tumors that do not obey any of the criteria. These pathologists may be correct, but they are not in the mainstream of what

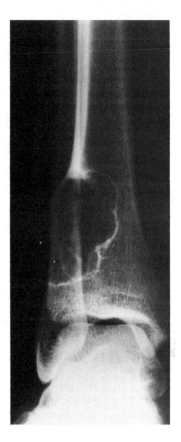

Figure 34.19. Nonossifying Fibroma. A large, well-defined lytic lesion, which is slightly expansile with scalloped sclerotic margins, is seen in the distal tibia in this young patient. This is a characteristic appearance of an NOF. The examination was obtained for a sprained ankle and not for this asymptomatic lesion.

most people use for giant cell tumor criteria, both radiographically and histologically.

Discriminators. 1. Epiphyses must be closed. 2. Must abut the articular surface. 3. Must be well defined with a nonsclerotic margin. 4. Must be eccentric.

NONOSSIFYING FIBROMA

A nonossifying fibroma (NOF) is probably the most common bone lesion encountered by radiologists. It reportedly occurs in up to 20% of children and usually spontaneously regresses so as to be seen only rarely after the age of 30. "Fibrous cortical defect" is a common synonym, although some people divide the two lesions on the basis of size, with a fibrous cortical defect being smaller than 2 cm in length (Fig. 34.18) and an NOF being larger than 2 cm (Fig. 34.19). Histologically, these lesions are identical; therefore, it seems appropriate to refer to them all as NOFs rather than to subdivide them by their size.

Nonossifying fibromas are benign, asymptomatic lesions that typically occur in the metaphysis of a long bone, emanating from the cortex. They classically have a thin, sclerotic border that is scalloped and

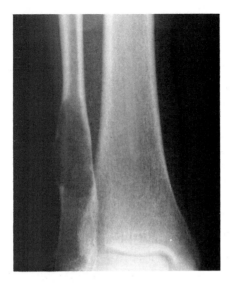

Figure 34.20. Nonossifying Fibroma. A well-defined, expansile lytic lesion in the distal fibula is noted in this asymptomatic patient, which is characteristic for an NOF.

slightly expansile (Fig. 34.20); however, this is a general description that probably applies to only 75% of the lesions, and could equally apply to most of the lesions in FEGNOMASHIC. They do not have to have expansion or a scalloped or sclerotic border, and are not limited to the metaphyses. Then how are they best recognized? The best way is to familiarize one's self with their general appearance is by looking at examples in textbooks. That can be done in 15 minutes. It is important to recognize these lesions because they are what I call "do not touch" lesions (see Chapter 39); that is, the radiologist's diagnosis should be the final word and thereby supplant a biopsy. These lesions are so characteristic that no differential diagnosis should be entertained, although a few entities can indeed occasionally simulate them.

If a CT or MR is obtained of an NOF, there will often appear to be interruption of the cortex, which can be misinterpreted as cortical destruction (Fig. 34.21). This merely represents cortical replacement by benign fibrous tissue and should not warrant further investigation.

If the patient is over 30 years of age, NOF should not be included in the differential diagnosis. Nonossifying fibromas must be asymptomatic and exhibit no periostitis, unless there is an antecedent history of trauma. They routinely "heal" with sclerosis and eventually disappear (Fig. 34.22), usually around the ages of 20–30. During this healing period they can appear hot on a radionuclide bone scan because there is osteoblastic activity. These lesions can occasionally get quite large (Fig. 34.23); therefore, growth or change in size will not alter the diagnosis. They are most commonly seen about the knee but can occur in any long

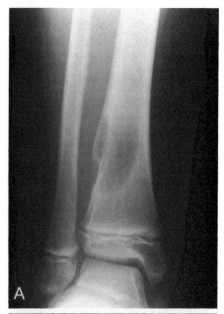

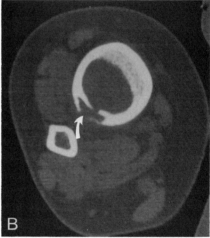

Figure 34.21. Nonossifying Fibroma. A. A well-defined, lytic lesion that is minimally expansile is seen in the distal tibia in this child who was examined for a sprained ankle. **B.** A CT examination showed apparent cortical destruction (*arrow*) which was felt to be suggestive of an aggressive lesion. Biopsy showed this to be a nonossifying fibroma. Both CT and MR will often show apparent cortical destruction, which is merely cortical replacement by benign fibrous tissue.

bone. Occasionally multiple NOFs are seen about the knee, each of which is characteristic in appearance.

Discriminators. 1. Must be under age 30. 2. No periostitis or pain. 3. Cortically based.

OSTEOBLASTOMA

Osteoblastomas are rare lesions that could justifiably be excluded from this differential without the fear of missing a diagnosis more than once in a lifetime. Why, then, include them? The mnemonic FEGNOMASHIC would not have nearly the same ring without the extra vowel, so osteoblastoma remains.

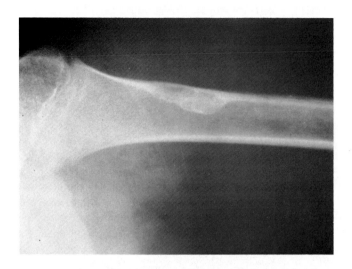

Figure 34.22. Healing Nonossifying Fibroma. A predominantly sclerotic lesion, which is minimally expansile and well defined, is seen in the proximal humerus in this child who is asymptomatic. This is a typical appearance of a disappearing or healing, NOF. With time, this lesion will melt into the normal bone and essentially disappear.

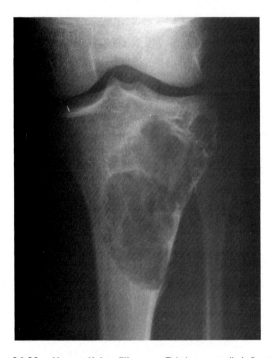

Figure 34.23. Nonossifying Fibroma. This large, well-defined lytic lesion with faint sclerotic margins is seen in the proximal tibia. It has a very typical appearance for a giant cell tumor; however, it has sclerotic margins and does not abut the articular surface. The lesion underwent biopsy and found to be an NOF. (Case courtesy of Larry Yeager, M.D., Redwood City, CA.)

Osteoblastomas have two appearances. (a) They look like large osteoid osteomas, and are often called giant osteoid osteomas. Because osteoid osteomas are sclerotic lesions and do not resemble bubbly lytic lesions, this is not the type of osteoblastoma we are concerned with in this differential. (b) They simulate an-

eurysmal bone cysts (ABCs). They are expansile, often having a soap bubble appearance. If an ABC is being considered, so should an osteoblastoma. Osteoblastomas commonly occur in the posterior elements of the vertebral bodies, and about half of the cases demonstrate speckled calcifications (Fig. 34.24). A classic radiology differential is that of an expansile lytic lesion of the posterior elements of the spine, which includes osteoblastoma, ABC, and tuberculosis.

Discriminator. Mentioned when ABC is mentioned (especially in the posterior elements of the spine).

METASTATIC DISEASE AND MYELOMA

Metastatic disease should be considered for any lytic lesion—benign or aggressive in appearance—in a patient over the age of 40. Metastatic diseases can appear perfectly benign radiographically (Fig. 34.25), so it is not valid to say, "Since this lesion looks benign, it should not be a metastatic disease. Most metastatic diseases have an aggressive appearance and will not be in the FEGNOMASHIC differential, but a significant number appear benign. In fact, metastatic diseases can have any radiographic appearance, therefore, any bone lesion in a patient over the age of 40 should have metastatic diseases as a consideration, unless trauma or arthritis is the primary concern.

For statistical purposes I do not mention metastatic diseases in a patient under the age of 40. I will be correct more than 99% of the time using 40 as a cut-off age. Otherwise, metastatic diseases would have to be mentioned in every single case of a lytic lesion, and I am trying to find ways to limit the list of differential possibilities. I am not saying that metastatic diseases do not occur in patients under the age of 40, only that I am willing to miss them (unless given a history of a known primary neoplasm).

Although myeloma most commonly presents as a diffuse permeative process in the skeleton (Fig. 34.26), it can present as either a solitary lesion (Fig. 34.27) or as multiple lytic lesions. Bubbly, lytic bone lesions of myeloma are more correctly called plasmacytomas. I try to mention plasmacytoma separately from metastatic disease because it can occur in a slightly younger population (age above 35 years is my cut-off) and can precede clinical or hematologic evidence of myeloma by 3 to 5 years. In general, there is no harm in lumping all metastatic disease, including myeloma, into one group and using greater than age 40 as the limiting factor.

Virtually any metastatic process can present as a lytic, benign-appearing lesion; therefore, it serves no purpose to try to guess the source of the metastatic disease from its appearance. In general, lytic expansile metastatic diseases tend to come from thyroid and

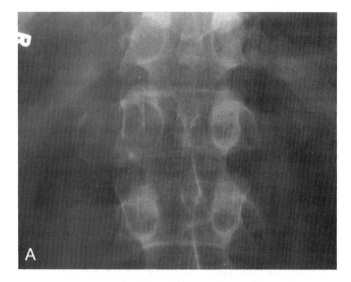

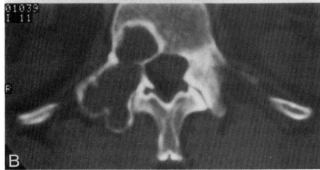

Figure 34.24. Osteoblastoma. A lytic expansile lesion involving the right T-12 pedicle and transverse process is seen on this anteroposterior plain film in (*A*), which is seen on the CT scan (*B*), to extend into the vertebral body. It has intact cortices and contains some calcified matrix. This is a classic example of an osteoblastoma of the spine.

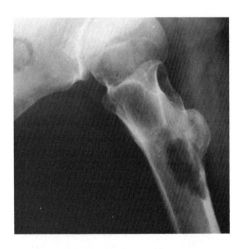

Figure 34.25. Metastatic Disease. A well-defined lytic lesion is seen in the proximal femur in this 50-year-old patient who has pain associated with this lesion. Biopsy showed this to be a renal metastasis. A significant number of metastatic lesions can have a completely benign appearance, as in this example.

renal tumors (Fig. 34.28). The only metastatic lesion that is said to *always* be lytic is renal cell carcinoma.

Discriminator. Must be over age 40.

ANEURYSMAL BONE CYST

Aneurysmal bone cysts are the only lesions I know of that are named for their radiographic appearance. They are virtually always aneurysmal, or expansile (Figs. 34.29 and 34.30). Rarely, an ABC will present before it is expansile, but that is unusual enough not to worry about. Aneurysmal bone cysts primarily occur in patients who are under the age of 30, although occasionally one will be encountered in older patients. I use bony expansion and age below 30 as fairly rigid guidelines, and seldom miss the diagnosis of ABC.

Aneurysmal bone cysts are, like giant cell tumors, somewhat controversial. There are apparently two types of ABCs: a primary type and a secondary type. The secondary type occurs in conjunction with another lesion or from trauma, whereas a primary ABC has no known cause or association with other lesions. Secondary ABCs have been said to occur with giant cell tumors, osteosarcomas, and almost any other lesion. I have seen dozens of ABCs and have seen only one in association with another lesion, so I doubt that this occurs very often. As to occurring after trauma, I do not understand why they would be age-limited if trauma were causative. Also, malignant tumors were once thought to occur after trauma because of the frequent association of a history of antecedent trauma with malignant bone tumors. This is not seriously considered today and is thought to be coincidental. I suspect that ABCs and trauma are also coincidental, but this is mere speculation.

Aneurysmal bone cysts typically present because of pain. They can occur anywhere in the skeleton, and there is no location that would make them more highly ranked in the differential diagnosis. As with os-

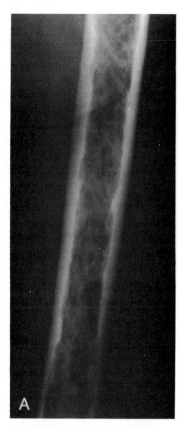

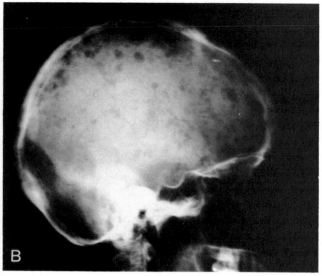

Figure 34.26. Multiple Myeloma. A. A diffuse permeative pattern is present throughout the femur in this patient with multiple myeloma. **B.** A lateral skull film shows a typical presentation of multiple myeloma in the skull with multiple small holes throughout the calvarium, which are well defined.

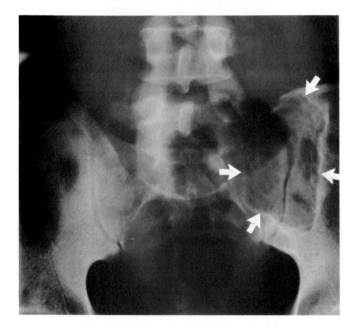

Figure 34.27. Plasmacytoma. A large, well-defined lytic lesion is seen in the left ilium (*arrows*) in this patient with multiple myeloma. This is a common location for a plasmacytoma. Like metastases, plasmacytomas often have a completely benign appearance.

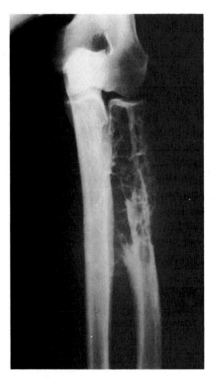

Figure 34.28. Metastatic Disease. An expansile lesion with a soap-bubble appearance is present in the proximal radius in a patient with renal cell carcinoma. An expansile lytic lesion is a common finding with renal or thyroid metastatic disease.

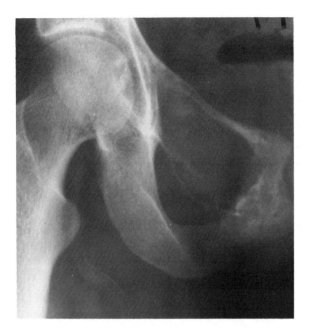

Figure 34.29. Aneurysmal Bone Cyst. An expansile lytic lesion is present in the superior pubic ramus in this 20-year-old patient who presents with pain. This is a fairly typical appearance for an ABC.

teoblastoma, they often occur in the posterior elements of the spine.

Discriminators. 1. Must be expansile. 2. Must be under age 30.

SOLITARY BONE CYST

Solitary bone cysts are also called simple bone cysts or unicameral bone cysts. They are not necessarily unicameral (one compartment), however. This is the only lesion in FEGNOMASHIC that is always central in location (Fig. 34.31). Many of the other lesions may be central, but a solitary bone cyst can be excluded if it is not. It is one of the few lesions that does not occur most commonly around the knees. Two-thirds to three-fourths of these lesions occur in the proximal humerus (Fig. 34.32) and proximal femur (Fig. 34.33). Applying this rule by itself is not that helpful, or one-third to one-fourth of the lesions would be missed.

Solitary bone cysts are usually asymptomatic unless fractured, which is a common occurrence. Even when pathologic fractures occur, they rarely form periostitis. A classic radiographic finding for a solitary bone cyst is the fallen fragment sign (Fig. 34.32). This occurs when a piece of cortex breaks off following a fracture in a solitary bone cyst, and the piece of cortical bone sinks to the gravity-dependent portion of the lesion. This has not been described in any other lesion, and indicates a fluid-filled cystic lesion, rather than a lesion filled with matrix.

Solitary bone cysts occur almost exclusively in young patients under the age of 30. Although long

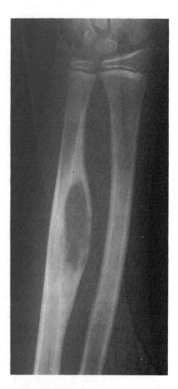

Figure 34.30. Aneurysmal Bone Cyst. A well-defined expansile lesion is seen in the midshaft of the ulna in a child who presents with pain in this region. This is a characteristic appearance for an ABC.

bones are most commonly involved, solitary bone cysts have been described in almost every bone in the body. They begin at the physeal plate in long bones and grow into the shaft of the bone; therefore, they are not epiphyseal lesions. They can, however, extend up into an epiphysis after the plate closes, but this is unusual. A fairly common location is in the calcaneus, where they have a characteristic location adjacent to the inferior surface of the calcaneus (Fig. 34.34).

Discriminators. 1. Must be central. 2. Must be under age 30. 3. No periostitis.

HYPERPARATHYROIDISM (BROWN TUMORS)

Brown tumors of hyperparathyroidism (HPT) can have almost any appearance, from a purely lytic lesion (Fig. 34.35) to a sclerotic process. Generally, when the patient's HPT is treated, the brown tumor undergoes sclerosis and will eventually disappear. If a brown tumor is going to be considered in the differential diagnosis, additional radiographic findings of HPT should be seen. Subperiosteal bone resorption is pathognomonic for HPT and should be searched for in the phalanges (particularly in the radial aspect of the middle phalanges) (Fig. 34.35), distal clavicles (resorption), medial aspect of the proximal tibias, and sacroiliac joints. If the physes are open they should have a frayed, ragged appearance, as in rickets, due to the effect of parathormone. Osteoporosis or osteosclerosis

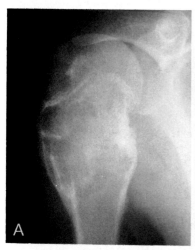
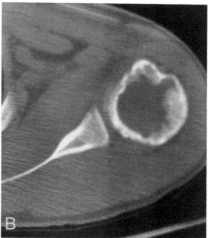

Figure 34.31. Solitary Bone Cyst. A plain film (**A**) and a CT scan (**B**) of the proximal humerus show a central, well-defined lytic lesion in this young person, which is typical in location and appearance for a solitary bone cyst. Note on the CT the central location of this lesion, which is characteristic.

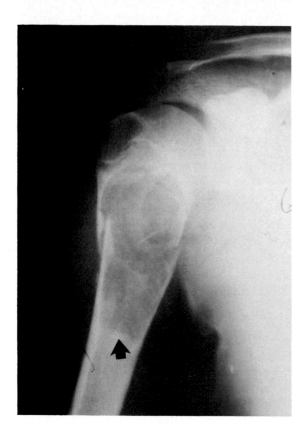

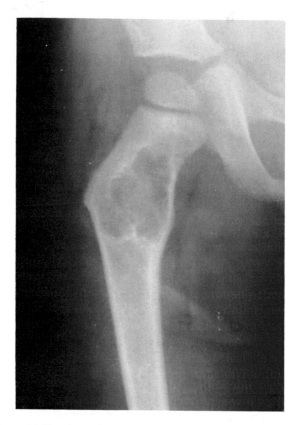

Figure 34.32. Solitary Bone Cyst. A well-defined lytic lesion is present in the proximal humerus in this child who suffered a fracture through the lesion. The location and central appearance, as well as the age of the patient, are characteristic for a solitary bone cyst. A piece of cortical bone has broken off and descended through the serous fluid contained within the lesion and can be seen in the dependent portion of the lesion (*arrow*) as a fallen fragment sign. A fallen fragment sign is said to be pathognomonic for a unicameral bone cyst.

Figure 34.33. Solitary Bone Cyst. A well-defined lytic lesion, which is central in location, is seen in the proximal femur in this child. This is characteristic for a solitary bone cyst.

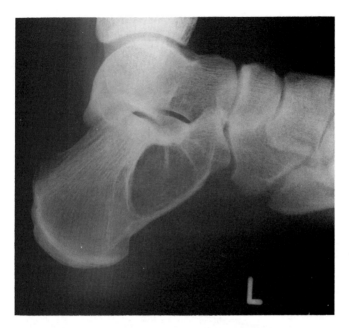

Figure 34.34.   Solitary Bone Cyst. A well-defined lytic lesion is seen in the calcaneus abutting the inferior surface, which is typical in location and appearance for a solitary bone cyst. A solitary bone cyst in the calcaneus occurs almost exclusively in this location and is not subject to pathologic fracture as readily as when they occur in the proximal femur and humerus.

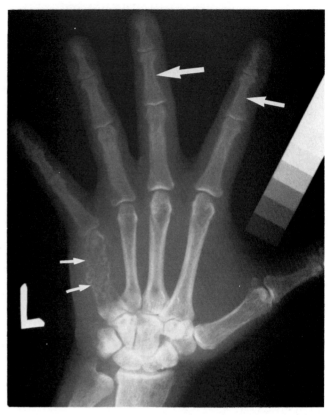

Figure 34.35.   Brown Tumor. An expansile lytic lesion is seen in the fifth metacarpal (*small arrows*), and a second, smaller lytic lesion is seen in the proximal portion of the fourth proximal phalanx. This patient can be noted to have subperiosteal bone reabsorption, best seen in the radial aspect of the middle phalanges (*large arrows*), which makes the diagnosis of hyperparathyroidism with multiple brown tumors most likely.

might suggest that renal osteodystrophy with secondary HPT is present, but subperiosteal resorption must be present, or brown tumor can be safely excluded from the differential.

Most authorities believe that brown tumors occur most commonly in primary HPT; however, because we see so many more patients with secondary HPT, more brown tumors are seen in patients with secondary rather than primary HPT.

Discriminator. Must have other evidence of HPT.

INFECTION

Unfortunately, there is no reliable way to radiographically exclude a focus of osteomyelitis. It has a protean radiographic appearance, and can occur at any location and in a patient of any age. It may or may not be expansile, have a sclerotic or nonsclerotic border, or have associated periostitis (3). Therefore, infection will be in almost every differential diagnosis of a lytic lesion, which is acceptable, since it is one of the most common lesions encountered. Soft-tissue findings such as obliteration of adjacent fat planes are notoriously unreliable and even misleading, as tumors and EG can do the same thing.

When osteomyelitis occurs near a joint, if the articular surface is abutted, invariably the joint will be involved and show either cartilage loss or an effusion (Fig. 34.36), or both. This finding is not particularly helpful, since any lesion can cause an effusion, but it

is occasionally useful in ruling out osteomyelitis when no effusion is present and the lesion abuts the articular surface.

If a bony sequestrum is present, osteomyelitis should be strongly considered (Fig. 34.37). As mentioned previously, the only lesions described that demonstrate sequestra are infection, EG, and fibrosarcoma, with osteoid osteoma sometimes mimicking a sequestum. The finding of a sequestrum in osteomyelitis can be significant for treatment in that it usually requires surgical removal rather than antibiotics alone since a sequestrum is a focus of devitalized bone that does not have a blood supply and will not be effectively treated with parenteral medication. For this reason, CT is routinely recommended when osteomyelitis is considered.

Discriminators. None.

CHONDROBLASTOMA

Chondroblastomas are rare lesions, but are among the easiest lesions for radiologists to deal with because they occur only in the epiphyses (Fig. 34.38) (a handful of cases have been reported in the metaphy-

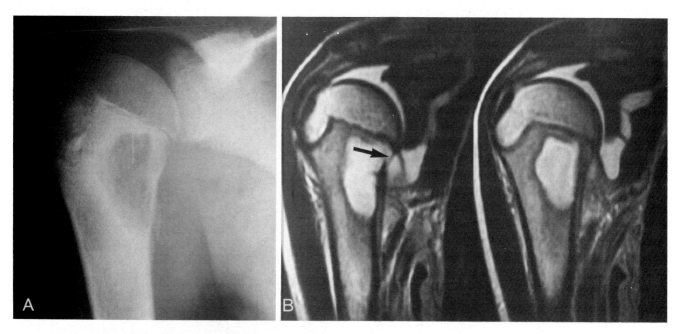

Figure 34.36. Brodie's Abscess. A. A plain film of the proximal humerus in this child with shoulder pain reveals a well-defined lytic lesion in the medial metaphysis. **B.** A T2-weighted MR of the humerus shows the lesion to have high signal and an associated joint effusion. The probable site of connection to the joint can be seen (arrow), which likely represents a draining abscess. Aspiration of the joint fluid revealed pus. This is a large focus of osteomyelitis or Brodie's abscess. (Case courtesy of Rick Harnsberger, M.D., Salt Lake City, UT.)

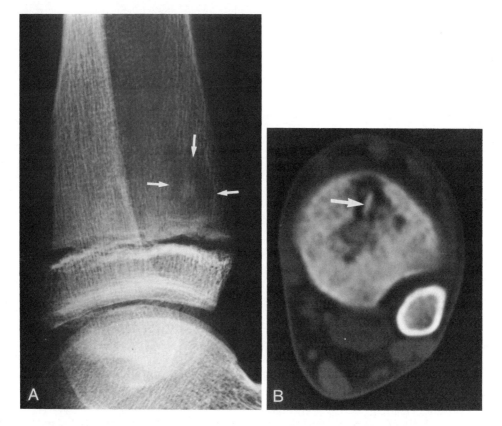

Figure 34.37. Osteomyelitis. A. A lytic lesion is present in the distal tibia, which is only faintly seen on the plain film (arrows). **B.** A CT scan through this area reveals a lytic lesion that contains a calcific density within (arrow), which is a bony sequestrum. In retrospect, the sequestrum can be faintly seen on the original plain film. This is an area of osteomyelitis with a bony sequestration.

Figure 34.38.   Chondroblastoma. A. A plain film in this young patient shows a well-defined lytic lesion in the medial femoral condyle. **B.** A sagittal T1-weighted MR through the medial knee joint reveals a fairly homogeneous lesion that abuts the articular surface. Biopsy showed this to be a chondroblastoma.

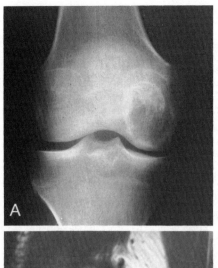

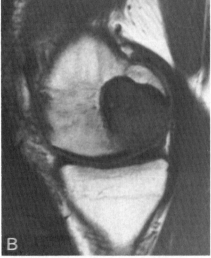

ses but this is rare) and they occur almost exclusively in patients under the age of 30. From 40 to 60% demonstrate calcification, so absence of calcification is not helpful. Presence of calcification is helpful as long as it is certain that it is not detritus or sequestra from infection or EG, both of which can occur in the epiphyses.

The differential diagnosis of a lytic lesion in the epiphysis of a patient under the age of 30 is simple: (*a*) infection (most common), (*b*) chondroblastoma, and (*c*) giant cell tumor (it has its own diagnostic criteria so it can usually be definitely ruled out or in). This is an old, classic differential and probably encompasses 98% of epiphyseal lesions.

A caveat on epiphyseal lesions is to always consider the possibility of a subchondral cyst or geode (Fig. 34.39), which has been described in four disease processes: (*a*) degenerative joint disease (must have joint space narrowing, sclerosis, and osteophytes), (*b*) rheumatoid arthritis, (*c*) CPPD (calcium pyrophosphate dihydrate crystal disposition disease) or pseudogout, and (*d*) avascular necrosis. Be certain no joint pathology that might indicate one of these processes is present, or an unnecessary biopsy of a geode

might be performed on the basis of the differential of an epiphyseal lesion.

Apophyses are identical to epiphyses as far as the differential diagnosis of lytic lesions, with the exception of geodes, which only occur adjacent to articular surfaces. The carpal bones, the tarsal bones, and the patella have a tendency to behave like epiphyses in their differential diagnosis of lesions. Therefore, a lytic lesion in these areas has a similar differential diagnosis as an epiphyseal lesion.

Discriminators.   1. Must be under age 30. 2. Must be epiphyseal.

CHONDROMYXOID FIBROMA

Like the osteoblastoma, the chondromyxoid fibroma is such a rare lesion that failure to mention it is probably not going to result in missing more than one in a lifetime. Why include it then? I recommend not including it, but it is part of the classic FEGNOMASHIC differential. If it is mentioned, at least know what it looks like. Basically, chondromyxoid fibromas resemble NOFs. Unlike NOFs, however, they can be seen in a patient of any age. Chondromyxoid fibromas often extend into the epiphyses (Fig.

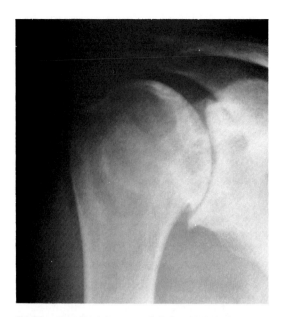

Figure 34.39. Geode. A large, well-defined lytic lesion in the proximal humerus is present, which is associated with marked degenerative disease of the glenohumeral joint. When definite degenerative joint disease is present and associated with a lytic lesion, the lytic lesion should be considered to be a geode. A biopsy was performed, which confirmed this to be a geode, or subchondral cyst; however, the biopsy could have been avoided.

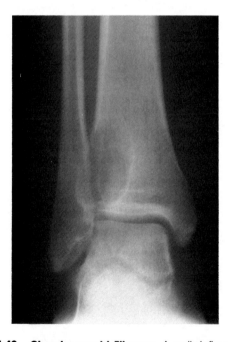

Figure 34.40. Chondromyxoid Fibroma. A well-defined lytic lesion in the distal tibia that extends slightly into the epiphysis is noted on this anteroposterior plain film. A nonossifying fibroma could certainly have this appearance; however, this underwent biopsy and was found to be a chondromyxoid fibroma. Chondromyxoid fibromas often will extend into the epiphysis, as in this example, whereas NOFs usually will not.

34.40), whereas NOFs rarely do. They can present with pain, also, which will not occur with an NOF.

They have been reported to progress from a benign process to an aggressive and even malignant lesion, but this is extremely rare. Even though chondromyxoid fibromas are cartilaginous lesions, calcified cartilage matrix is virtually never seen radiographically.

Discriminator. 1. Mention when an NOF is mentioned. 2. No calcified matrix.

SUMMARY

That, in essence, is the differential diagnosis for a benign cystic lesion of bone. It is probably 98% accurate, which is good enough for most radiologists. To increase the accuracy to 99% it would be necessary to add many uncommon or rare lesions, and the whole process would become too confusing for most radiologists to learn and apply. If there is a favorite lesion that is not in this list, by all means add it. Likewise, if the list is already too cumbersome, forget about osteoblastoma and chondromyxoid fibroma. I am unable to make it much simpler than that and still be reasonably accurate.

Some of the lesions I have purposefully omitted are intraosseous ganglion, pseudotumor of hemophilia, hemangioendothelioma, ossifying fibroma, intraosseous lipoma, glomus tumor, neurofibroma, plasma cell granuloma, and schwannoma. Others could be added to this list, of course, but are best left to the pathologist—not the radiologist—for the diagnosis.

There are several features that are somewhat useful in separating the various lesions in FEGNOMASHIC. For instance, if the patient is under the age of 30, be sure to consider *EG, chondroblastoma, NOF, solitary bone cyst,* and *ABC* (Table 34.2). If the patient is over 30, those five lesions can probably be excluded. Note that this is not a differential diagnosis for lesions in patients under the age of 30; it simply means these entities should not be mentioned in older patients. Under the age of 30 other lesions, such as fibrous dysplasia and infection, must also be mentioned.

There are a few lytic lesions that have no good discriminators other than age, and therefore, must be mentioned routinely. I call these lesions "automatics" because one should automatically mention them regardless of the location or appearance of the lesion. *Infection* and *E.G.* must be mentioned under the age of 30, while *metastatic diseases* and *infection* must be included in any differential in a patient over the age of 40 (Table 34.3). These lesions have a protean radiographic appearance and should be mentioned not only in the benign, cystic differential, but also for an aggressive lesion.

If periostitis or pain is present (assuming no trauma, which can be a foolhardy assumption), you can exclude *fibrous dysplasia, solitary bone cyst, NOF,* and *enchondroma* (Table 34.4). If the lesion is epiphyseal, the differential is *infection, giant cell tu-*

Table 34.2. Lesions in Patients Under 30 Years of Age

EG
ABC
NCF
Chondroblastoma
Solitary bone cyst

Table 34.3. "Automatics"

Under age 30
  Infection
  EG
Over age 40
  Infection
  Metastatic diseases and myeloma

Table 34.4. Lesions That Have No Pain or Periostitis

Fibrous dysplasia
Enchondroma
NOF
Solitary bone cyst

Table 34.5. Epiphyseal Lesions

Infection
Giant cell tumor
Chondroblastoma
Geode

Table 34.6 Differential for Rib Lesions

Fibrous dysplasia
ABC
Metastatic diseases and myeloma
Enchondroma and EG

Table 34.7. Multiple Lesions (FEEMHI)

Fibrous dysplasia
EG
Enchondroma
Metastatic diseases and myeloma
Hyperparathyroidism (brown tumors)
Infection

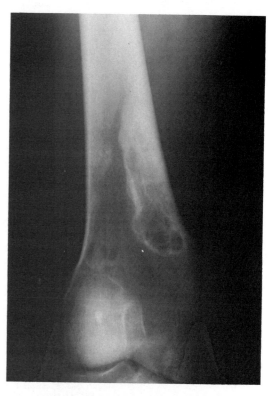

Figure 34.41. Healing Nonossifying Fibroma. A plain film of the femur in this 15-year-old patient reveals several mixed lytic, sclerotic lesions in the diametaphyseal region, which are well-defined. The large lesion has diffuse sclerosis in its proximal two-thirds. These represent NOFs that are starting to sclerose and disappear.

Figure 34.42. Giant Bone Island. A large sclerotic lesion is present in the right supraacetabular region of the ilium, which represents a giant bone island. The slightly feathered margins of the trabeculae blending in with the normal bone, and the long axis of the lesion being in the direction of primary weight bearing, are characteristic for a bone island.

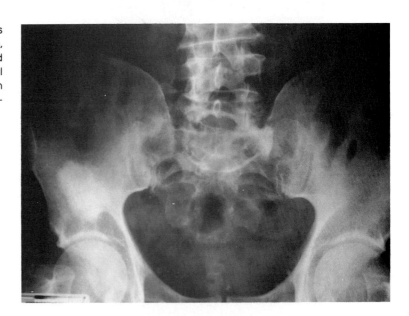

mor, *chondroblastoma* (and do not forget *geodes*) (Table 34.5). If the patient is over 40 years of age, add metastatic diseases and myeloma and remove chondroblastoma from the epiphyseal list.

The epiphyseal differential tends to apply also to the tarsal bones (especially the calcaneus), the carpal bones, and the patella. In the calcaneus, a unicameral bone cyst should also be considered, and has a characteristic appearance and location (Fig. 34.34). Apophyses are "epiphyseal equivalents" and have the same differential as epiphyses. The difference between an epiphysis and an apophysis is that epiphyses contribute to the length of a bone, whereas apophyses serve as ligamentous attachments.

A classic differential for benign, cystic rib lesions is the mnemonic FAME, in which F = *fibrous dysplasia*, A = *ABC*, M = *metastatic diseases* and *myeloma*, and E = *enchondroma* and *EG* (Table 34.6).

If there are multiple lytic lesions present, FEEMHI is a useful menemonic of the lesions in FEGNOMASHIC, which can be multiple. F = *fibrous dysplasia*, E = MDu*enchondroma*, E = *E.G.*, M = *metastatic diseases* and *myeloma*, H = *hyperparathyroidism* (brown tumor), and I = *infection* (Table 34.7).

A few findings that just do not seem to narrow the differential diagnosis are presence or absence of a soft-tissue mass, expansion of the bone (except it must be present in an ABC), a sclerotic or nonsclerotic border (except it must be nonsclerotic in giant cell tumor), presence or absence of bony struts or compartments in the lesion, and size of the lesion.

If calcified matrix is identified in a lesion, it is tempting to narrow the differential to either the osteoid series or the chondroid series of lesions, depending on the character of the matrix. Be careful of this. Very few radiologists can reliably differentiate chondroid from osteoid matrix. Routine calcification of a lesion or debris, detritus, or sequestrations in osteomyelitis can mimic chondroid or osteoid calcification and be misleading. The only lesion that must exhibit calcified matrix is the enchondroma (except in the phalanges). Chondroblastomas and osteoblastomas demonstrate calcified matrix about half the time, and chondromyxoid fibromas never have radiographically demonstrable calcified matrix.

DIFFERENTIAL DIAGNOSIS OF A SCLEROTIC LESION

Many lytic lesions spontaneously regress and are not usually seen in patients over the age of 30. When these lesions regress, they often fill in with new bone and have a sclerotic or blastic appearance. Therefore, when a sclerotic focus is identified in a 20- to 40-year-old patient, especially if it is an asymptomatic, incidental finding, the following lesions should be considered: NOF (Fig. 34.41), EG, aneurysmal bone cyst, solitary bone cyst, and chondroblastoma. Several other lesions should be included that can also appear sclerotic: fibrous dysplasia, osteoid osteoma, infection, brown tumor (healing), and perhaps a giant bone island (Fig. 34.42). In any patient over the age of 40, the number-one possibility should be metastatic disease.

References

1. David R, Oria R, Kumar R, et al. Radiologic features of eosinophilic granuloma of bone. Pictorial essay. AJR 1989;153:1021–1026.
2. Dahlin D. Giant cell tumor of bone: highlights of 407 cases. AJR 1985;144:955–960.
3. Gold R, Hawkins R, Katz R. Pictorial essay. Bacterial osteomyelitis: findings on plain radiography, CT, MR, and scintigraphy. AJR 1991;157:365–370.

35

Malignant Bone and Soft-Tissue Tumors

Clyde A. Helms

RADIOGRAPHIC FINDINGS

Malignant bone tumors, thankfully, are not very common. Nevertheless, every radiologist should be able to recognize them and give a useful differential diagnosis. First, how does one recognize a malignant tumor and differentiate if from a benign process? This can be difficult and oftentimes impossible. Recognizing that it is *aggressive* is usually easy, but saying that it is *malignant* is another matter altogether. Processes such as infection and eosinophilic granuloma can mimic malignant tumors and are, of course, benign. They will often be included in the differential diagnosis of an aggressive lesion along with malignant tumors. What radiologic plain film criteria are useful for determining malignant versus benign? Standard textbooks give four aspects of a lesion to be examined: (*a*) cortical destruction, (*b*) periostitis, (*c*) orientation or axis of the lesion and, (*d*) zone of transition. Let me discuss each of these criteria and show why only the last one—the zone of transition—is accurate to a 90% plus rate. It is important to recognize

that these are plain film criteria and do not apply to computed tomography (CT) or magnetic resonance imaging (MR) in many instances.

Cortical Destruction

Benign fibroosseous lesions and cartilaginous lesions often have part of their noncalcified matrix (fibrous matrix or chondroid matrix, both of which are radiolucent on plain films) replacing cortical bone, which can give the false impression of cortical destruction on plain films (Fig. 35.1) or CT. Also, benign processes such as infection and eosinophilic granuloma can cause extensive cortical destruction and mimic a malignant tumor. It is well known that aneurysmal bone cysts cause such thinning of the cortex as to make the cortex radiographically undetectable (Fig. 35.2). For these reasons, cortical destruction can occasionally be misleading. Cortical destruction always makes one think of a malignant lesion when using the "gestalt approach," but the lesion must also have other criteria for a malignant process, such as a wide zone of transition.

Periostitis

Periosteal reaction occurs in a nonspecific manner whenever the periosteum is irritated, whether it is irritated by a malignant tumor, a benign tumor, infection, or trauma. Callus formation in a fracture is actually just periosteal reaction of the most benign type. Periosteal reaction occurs in two types: benign or aggressive, based more on the timing of the irritation rather then whether it is a malignant or benign process causing the periostitis. For example, a slow-growing benign tumor will cause thick, wavy, uniform or dense periostitis (Fig. 35.3**A**) because it is a low-grade chronic irritation that gives the periosteum time to lay down thick new bone and remodel into more normal cortex. A malignant tumor causes a periosteal reaction that is high-grade and more acute, hence, the periosteum does not have time to consolidate. It appears lamellated (onionskinned) (Fig. 35.3**B**) or amorphous or even sunburst-like. If the irritation stops or diminishes, the aggressive periostitis will solidify and appear benign. Therefore, when periostitis is seen, the radiologist should try to characterize it into either a benign (thick, dense, wavy) type or an aggressive (lamellated, amorphous, sunburst) type. Unfortunately, judging the lesion by its periostitis can be very misleading. First, it takes considerable experience to accurately characterize periostitis because many times the reaction is not clearly benign or aggressive. Second, many benign lesions cause

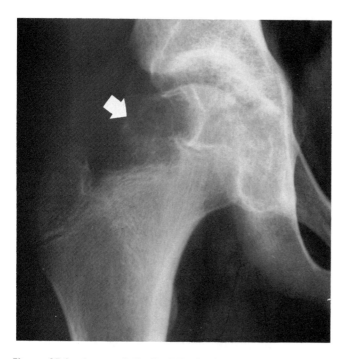

Figure 35.1. Apparent Cortical Destruction. This benign chondroblastoma has noncalcified chondroid tissue replacing cortical bone in the proximal femur (*arrow*) which gives this lesion a destructive appearance. This is an example of cortical replacement, rather than cortical destruction, which can be very confusing if one uses cortical destruction as an aggressive or malignant key. Note in this example that the zone of transition is narrow, as one would expect in a benign lesion such as this.

aggressive periostitis, such as infection, eosinophilic granuloma, aneurysmal bone cysts, osteoid osteomas, and even trauma. Seeing *benign* periostitis, however, can be very helpful because malignant lesions will not cause benign periostitis. Some investigators with great experience in dealing with malignant bone tumors state that the only way benign periostitis can occur in a malignant lesion is if there is a concomitant fracture or infection. Exceptions to this are extremely uncommon.

Orientation or Axis of the Lesion

This is a very poor determinant of benign versus aggressive lesions and rarely helps determine into which category the lesion should be placed. It has been said that if a lesion grows in the long axis of a long bone, rather than is circular, it is benign. There are simply too many exceptions for this to be helpful. For example, Ewing's sarcoma, an extremely malignant lesion, usually has its axis along the shaft of a long bone. Conversely, many fibrous cortical defects are circular, yet totally benign. Thus, the axis of the lesion is not helpful in assessing benignity versus malignancy.

Zone of Transition

This is without question the most reliable plain film indicator for benign versus malignant lesions. Unfortunately, it also has some drawbacks, which I will point out. The zone of transition is the border of the lesion with the normal bone. It is said to be "narrow" if it is so well defined it can be drawn with a fine-point pen (Fig. 35.4). If it is imperceptible and cannot be clearly drawn at all, it is said to be "wide" (Fig. 35.5). Obviously, all shades of gray lie in between, but most lesions can be characterized as having either a narrow or wide zone of

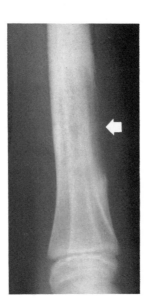

Figure 35.2. Aneurysmal Bone Cyst. This benign lesion has thinned the cortex to such a degree as to make it imperceptible (*arrow*). As in Figure 35.1, this could be misconstrued as cortical destruction, giving the false impression of a malignant or very aggressive lesion.

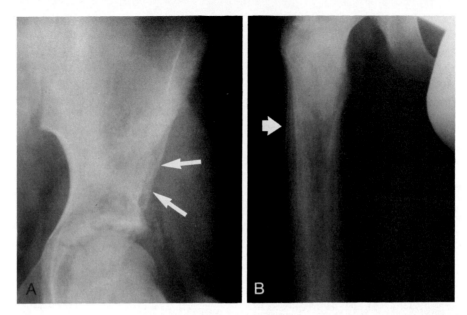

Figure 35.3. Benign Periostitis. A. Thick, wavy periostitis (*arrows*) along the ilium in a child with a permeative lesion in the pelvis is characteristic for infection or eosinophilic granuloma. Ewing's sarcoma was initially considered in the differential; however, the benign periostitis would make a malignant lesion very unlikely. Biopsy showed this lesion to be eosinophilic granuloma. **B. Aggressive Peri-** **ostitis.** Lamellated or onion-skin periostitis (*arrow*) is characteristic of an aggressive process such as in this patient with Ewing's sarcoma of the femur. Again, this aggressive type of periostitis could conceivably occur in a benign process such as infection or eosinophilic granuloma.

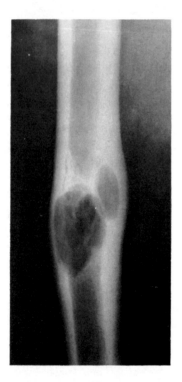

Figure 35.4. Narrow Zone of Transition. When the margins of a lesion can be drawn with a fine-point pen, as in this example, it is said to be a narrow zone of transition, which is characteristic of a benign lesion. A narrow zone of transition may or may not have a sclerotic border. This is a nonossifying fibroma.

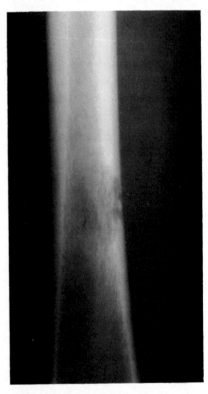

Figure 35.5. Wide Zone of Transition. A lytic, permeative process is seen in the midshaft of the femur in this patient that on biopsy was found to be a malignant fibrous histiocytoma. The zone of transition in this lesion is said to be wide as it cannot be easily drawn with a fine-point pen. A permeative lesion such as this, by definition, has a wide zone of transition.

Table 35.1. Age of Patients with Malignant Tumors

1–30	Ewing's sarcoma, ostogenic sarcoma
30–40	Giant cell tumor, parosteal sarcoma, fibrosarcoma, malignant fibrous histiocytoma, reticulum cell sarcoma
Over 40	Chondrosarcoma, metastatic disease, myeloma

transition. If the lesion has a sclerotic border it, of course, has a narrow zone of transition. If a lesion has a narrow zone of transition, it is a benign process.

The exceptions to that are rare. If a lesion has a wide zone of transition it is aggressive, although not necessarily malignant. As with aggressive periostitis, many benign lesions as well as malignant lesions can cause a wide zone of transition. A few of the same processes that can cause aggressive periostitis and thereby mimic a malignant tumor can have a wide zone of transition (i.e., infection and eosinophilic granuloma). They are aggressive in their radiographic appearance because they are usually fast-acting, aggressive lesions. The zone of transition is usually easier to characterize than the periostitis, plus it is always present to evaluate, whereas, many lesions, benign or malignant, have no periostitis. For these reasons, the zone of transition is the most useful indicator of whether a lesion is benign or malignant.

A lesion consisting of multiple small holes is said to be "permeative" (see Chapter 38 for the difference between a permeative and a pseudopermeative lesion). It has no perceptible border and therefore has a wide zone of transition. Round cell tumors such as multiple myeloma, reticulum cell sarcoma (primary lymphoma of bone), and Ewing's sarcoma are typical of this type of lesion. However, infection and eosinophilic granuloma can have this same appearance.

Once it is decided that a particular lesion is most likely malignant, the differential is fairly straightforward. First, the list of malignant tumors is relatively short, and, second, most tumors follow somewhat strict age groupings. Jack Edeiken (1), one of the preeminent bone radiologists of our era, evaluated 4000 malignant bone tumors and found that they could be diagnosed correctly 80% of the time just by using the patient's age! He basically divides the tumors into decades of when they usually affect a patient. For example, osteosarcoma and Ewing's sarcoma are the only childhood primary malignant tumors of bone, and after the age of 40 only metastatic disease, myeloma, and chondrosarcoma are common (Table 35.1). Although there are certainly outliers that are uncommon, these age guidelines are extremely useful. It is inappropriate to mention Ewing's sarcoma in a 40-year-old patient or metastatic disease in a 15-year-old patient, unless there is a known primary tumor. In fact, *any* bone lesion, regardless of its appearance, could be a metastatic le-

sion and would be suspicious in a patient with a known primary tumor.

Magnetic Resonance Imaging

While plain films are the best modality for characterizing a bony lesion, i.e., being able to distinguish benign from malignant and generating a differential diagnosis, MR is without question the imaging procedure of choice for determining the extent of a lesion, both in the skeleton and in the soft tissues. For this reason if resection of a tumor is contemplated, MR should be performed.

In assessing benignity versus malignancy MR is somewhat controversial (2). Benign lesions tend to be well marginated, have uniform, homogeneous signal, do not encase neurovascular structures, and do not invade bone. Malignant lesions tend to have irregular margins, inhomogeneous signal, and may encase neurovascular structures or invade bone.

Although almost all tumors will have low signal on T1-weighted images, which become very high in signal intensity with T2 weighting (as will fluid collections), there are a few exceptions. Fibrosarcomas, malignant fibrous histiocytomas, and desmoid tumors can occasionally demonstrate low signal on both T1- and T2-weighted sequences. Any tumor with calcification will be low in signal on both T1- and T2-sequences.

In some instances MR will characterize the lesion better than plain films and allow a specific diagnosis to be made. Lipomas are easily diagnosed with MR by their homogeneous high signal on T1-weighted images and sharp margins whether they are intraosseous (Fig. 35.6) or in the soft tissues (Fig. 35.7). Hemangiomas and arteriovenous malformations most commonly have mixed high and low signal on both sequences because of the combination of fatty elements and blood (Fig. 35.8). They characteristically have low-signal serpiginous vessels visible.

The finding of a low signal mass on T1-weighted images that is high in signal on T2-weighted images is suspicious for a tumor, but this is a very nonspecific finding and needs to be correlated clinically. Intramuscular injection sites can mimic soft-tissue tumors (Fig. 35.9), as can any area of soft-tissue trauma. Many malignant tumors exhibit high signal radiating from involved bone which is soft-tissue edema and virtually indistinguishable from tumor spread.

TUMORS

Osteosarcoma

The most common malignant primary bone tumor is an osteosarcoma. They occur almost exclusively in children and young adults (under the age of 30). Some

Figure 35.6.   Intraosseous Lipoma. A. A coronal proton density image (TR 2000; TE 20) of the shoulder shows a barely discernible lesion in the upper humerus (*arrows*) that blends in with the normal fatty marrow. **B.** The T2* image (MPGR; TR 600; TE 20; θ 30°) more readily reveals the lesion and again shows it having signal characteristics similar to that of the subcutaneous fat. This is virtually pathognomonic for a fatty lesion, in this case an intraosseous lipoma.

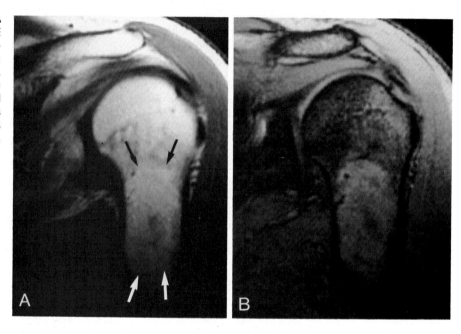

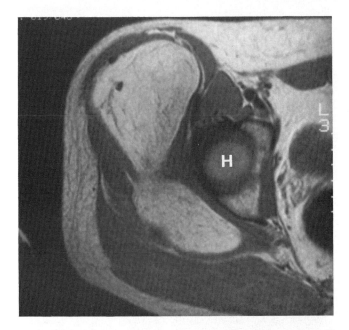

Figure 35.7. Lipoma. This axial proton-density image (TR 2000; TE 20) through the pelvis shows a large bilobed lesion lateral to the hip (*H*) which has sharp margins and signal characteristics similar to the subcutaneous fat. This is a lipoma. Lipomas will usually contain a small amount of low signal linear tissue, as in this example, which should not be cause to consider this lesion malignant.

texts describe a second peak of osteosarcoma around the 6th decade, but this is probably because of secondary osteosarcoma in Paget's disease and because of prior radiation. Although osteosarcoma typically occurs toward the end of a long bone, it may occur anywhere in the skeleton with enough frequency that location is not a helpful discriminator. These lesions are usually destructive, with obvious sclerosis present from either tumor new bone formation or reactive sclerosis (Fig. 35.10); however, on occasion an osteosarcoma can be entirely lytic. These are usually telangiectatic osteosarcomas. There are many different types and classifications of osteosarcomas but it serves little purpose for the radiologist to try to distinguish between most of them. Magnetic resonance imaging of an osteosarcoma generally reveals a large soft-tissue component with heterogeneous high and low signal on both T1- and T2-weighted images (Fig. 35.11).

Parosteal Osteosarcoma

A type of osteosarcoma that should be distinguished from the central osteosarcoma, however, is

Figure 35.8. Hemangioma. A. A T1-weighted axial image (TR 900; TE 30) through the midthighs shows a lesion with mixed high and low signal in the lateral part of the left thigh. **B.** A T2-weighted image (TR 2000; TE 70) shows most of the lesion with high signal; however some linear, serpiginous low signal structures can be appreciated. This is typical for a hemangioma. Mixed fatty and vascular tissues cause high signal on both T1- and T2-weighted images, and the vessels often are seen as serpiginous low-signal structures.

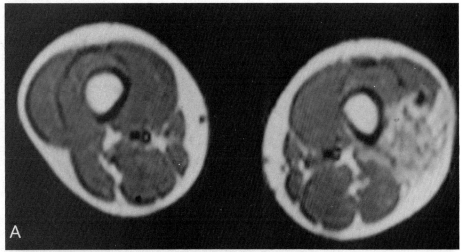

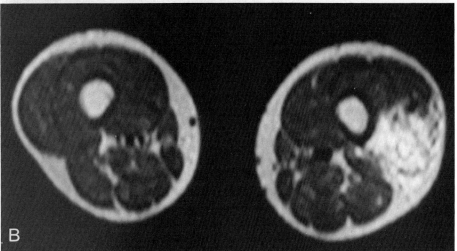

Figure 35.9. Intramuscular Injection Sites. Proton density (**A**) (TR 2000; TE 20) and T2-weighted (**B**) (TR 2000; TE 70) axial images through the left thigh of a child show a mass in the anterior thigh that resembles a typical soft-tissue tumor. This, however, is an intramuscular injection site.

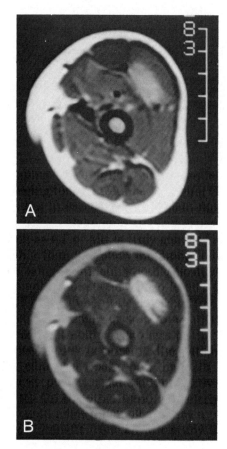

the parosteal osteosarcoma. A parosteal osteosarcoma originates from the periosteum of the bone and grows outside the bone (Fig. 35.12). It often wraps around the diaphysis without breaking through the cortex at all. It occurs in an older age group than the central osteosarcomas and is not as aggressive or as deadly as long as it has not extended into the medullary portion of the bone. Treatment used to consist of merely shaving the tumor off the bone it was arising from, however, recurrence rates were so high that now wide-bloc excisions are performed. Once a parosteal osteosarcoma violates the cortex of the adjacent bone it is considered to be as aggressive as a central osteosarcoma and is treated in a similar fashion, i.e., amputation or radical excision. Therefore, the radiologist needs to evaluate the lesion for invasion of the adjacent cortex to help determine treatment and prognosis. This is best done with CT or MR (Fig. 35.12*B* and *C*). A common location for parosteal osteosarcomas to arise from is the posterior femur, near the knee.

A lesion that can mimic an early parosteal osteosarcoma in this location is a cortical desmoid tumor. A cortical desmoid tumor is an avulsion injury that is totally benign but can appear somewhat aggressive. Unfortunately, it can appear malignant histologically, so biopsy can lead to disastrous consequences. Ampu-

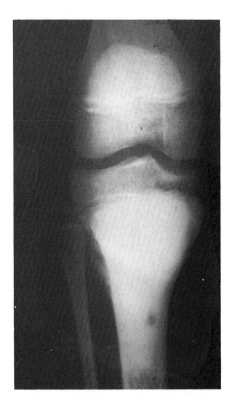

Figure 35.10. Osteosarcoma. A densely sclerotic lesion in the proximal tibia of a child is noted, which is characteristic for an osteogenic sarcoma.

Figure 35.11. Osteosarcoma. A proton density (**A**) (TR 2000; TE 20) and T2-weighted (**B**) (TR 2000; TE 60) image of the thighs in this teenager shows a lesion in the right femur, which is surrounded by a huge soft-tissue mass. The soft-tissue mass has mixed high and low signal on both imaging sequences and is very inhomogeneous. A biopsy revealed this to be an osteosarcoma.

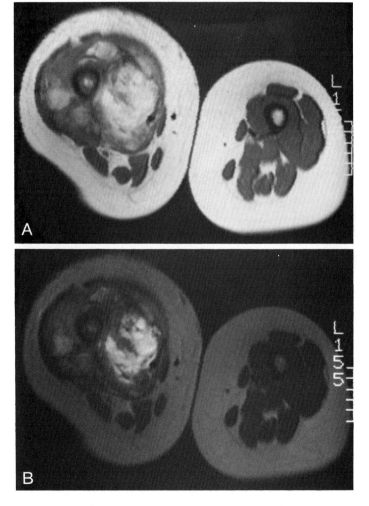

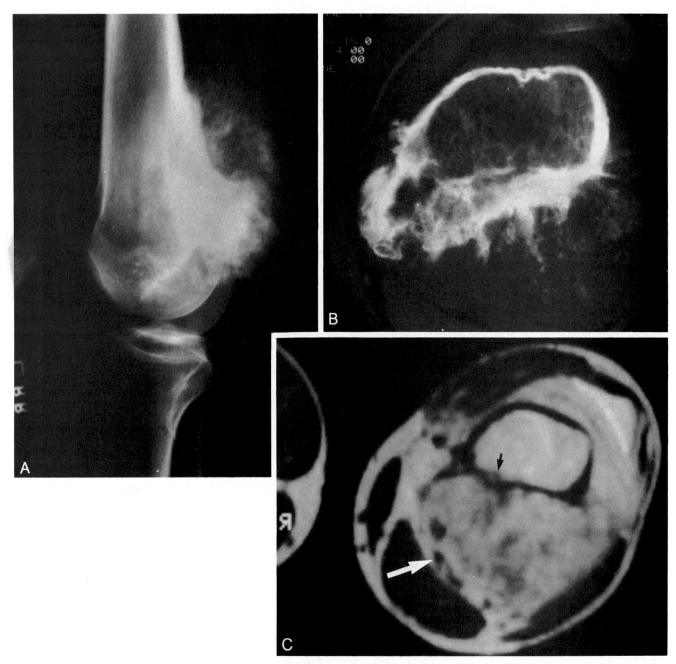

Figure 35.12.   Parosteal Osteosarcoma. A. A lateral plain film of the knee shows a bony lesion emanating from the posterior cortex of the distal femur with a large, calcified soft-tissue mass. Note that the densest calcification is central, and the periphery is only faintly calcified, characteristics that are typical for a parosteal osteosarcoma. **B.** A CT through the lesion reveals the tumor to be invading the medullary portion of the bone. This is a poor prognostic sign and is essential information to the surgeon. **C.** A T2-weighted axial MR (TR 2000; TE 60) through another parosteal osteosarcoma shows this lesion to have only minimal breakthrough into the medullary portion of the bone (*small arrow*) and shows the vessels posteriorly displaced (*large arrow*) but not encased by the tumor.

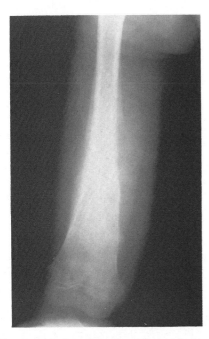

Figure 35.13. Ewing's Sarcoma. An anteroposterior plain film of the femur of a child shows a predominantly sclerotic process with large amounts of sunburst periostitis in the diaphysis, which on biopsy was found to be Ewing's sarcoma.

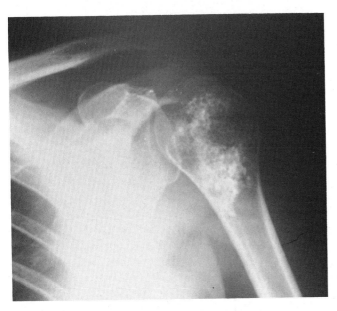

Figure 35.14. Chondrosarcoma. Typical snowflake, or popcorn-like, amorphous calcification in the proximal humerus is seen, which is typical of an enchondroma. This patient, however, had pain associated with this lesion and on biopsy this was found to be a chondrosarcoma. (Case courtesy of Dr. Tomas Jimenez-Robinson, Rio Piedras, Puerto Rico)

tations for benign cortical desmoid tumors that were confused for malignancies have occurred.

Another lesion that can be confused for a parosteal osteosarcoma is an area of myositis ossificans. Like cortical desmoid tumors, areas of myositis ossificans

can be histologically confused for malignancies with disastrous consequences. Therefore, differentiation is, of course, vital. Fortunately, differentiation between parosteal osteosarcoma and myositis ossificans is usually easily done radiographically (See Chapter 39 for differential points between parosteal osteosarcoma and myositis ossificans, and cortical desmoid tumors.)

Ewing's Sarcoma

The classic Ewing's sarcoma is a permeative (multiple small holes) lesion in the diaphysis of a long bone in a child (Fig. 35.3B). In fact, however, only about 40% of these tumors occur in the diaphysis, with the remainder being metaphyseal, diametaphyseal, and in flat bones. They do tend to be primarily in children and adolescents, although a significant number occur in patients in their 20s, especially in flat bones. Although most often permeative in appearance, they can elicit reactive new bone that can give the lesion a partially sclerotic or "patchy" appearance. Ewing's sarcomas often have an onion-skin type of periostitis, but can also have periostitis that is sunburst or amorphous in character (Fig. 35.13). Rarely, if ever, will a Ewing's sarcoma have benign-appearing periostitis (thick, uniform, or wavy).

If benign periostitis is present, other lesions should be considered instead, such as infection and eosinophilic granuloma. The classic differential diagnosis for a permeative lesion in a child is Ewing's sarcoma, infection, and eosinophilic granuloma. These three entities can appear radiologically identical. Ewing's sarcoma should be removed from the differential diagnosis if definite benign periostitis or a sequestration is present. The presence or absence of a soft-tissue mass is not helpful in distinguishing between these three lesions. The presence of symptoms is not helpful, as all three entities can be symptomatic.

Chondrosarcoma

Chondrosarcomas have a protean appearance that makes it difficult, at times, to make the diagnosis with any assurance. They most commonly occur in patients over the age of 40. Chondrosarcoma rarely occurs in children, although occasionally one will be encountered from malignant degeneration of an osteochondroma. It can be extremely difficult to histologically differentiate a low-grade chondrosarcoma from an enchondroma. The diagnosis of chondrosarcoma usually initiates radical excision and therapy, although it is debatable (and somewhat controversial) as to whether a low-grade chondrosarcoma is even a malignant tumor. For these reasons, the diagnosis of "possible chondrosarcoma" should be reserved for those lesions that are painful (Fig. 35.14) or that

Figure 35.15.   Chondrosarcoma. A large soft-tissue mass with amorphous, irregular calcification is seen in a lesion arising from the ilium on this CT of the pelvis. This is typical for a chondrosarcoma.

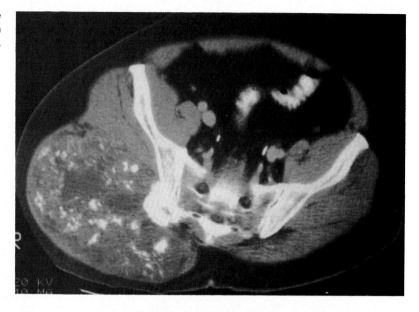

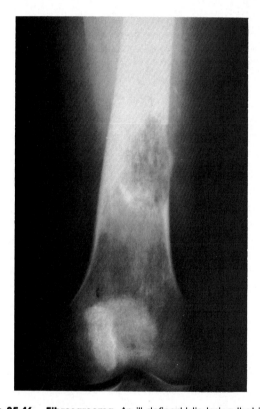

Figure 35.16.   Fibrosarcoma. An ill-defined lytic lesion that is permeative or moth-eaten in appearance is seen in the diaphysis of the femur which on biopsy was shown to be a fibrosarcoma.

show definite aggressive characteristics, such as periostitis and destruction. The truth of the matter is neither radiologists nor pathologists can distinguish between enchondromas and low-grade chondrosarcomas.

Chondrosarcoma should be considered in the diagnosis any time there is a bony or soft-tissue mass with amorphous, snowflake calcification in an older

patient (over 40) (Fig. 35.15). Without the presence of calcified chondroid matrix, the lesion is indistinguishable from any other aggressive lytic lesion, such as metastatic disease, plasmacytoma, fibrosarcoma, malignant fibrous histocytoma, or infection. Usually the radiologist can only give a long differential diagnosis such as this, which is entirely acceptable. The lesion will have to undergo biopsy at any rate, so it is not necessary for the radiologist to make the diagnosis. This is true for most malignant tumors.

Malignant Giant Cell Tumor

Approximately 20% of giant cell tumors are malignant. Unfortunately, there does not seem to be any way to foretell which giant cell tumor will become malignant. Radiologically, the benign and malignant giant cell tumors appear identical. Histologically, the benign and malignant giant cell tumors are the same. If metastases (usually to the lung) occur, or if a previously resected giant cell tumor recurs, it is considered by most oncologists to be malignant. Malignant giant cell tumors tend to occur primarily in the 4th decade of life.

Fibrosarcoma

Fibrosarcomas are lytic malignant tumors that do not produce osteoid or chondroid matrix. They usually do not cause reactive new bone, and, therefore, are almost always lytic in appearance. This lytic appearance may take any form, from permeative (Fig. 35.16) to moth-eaten, to a fairly well-defined area of lysis (Fig. 35.17). The age range for fibrosarcoma is quite broad, but they tend to predominate in the 4th

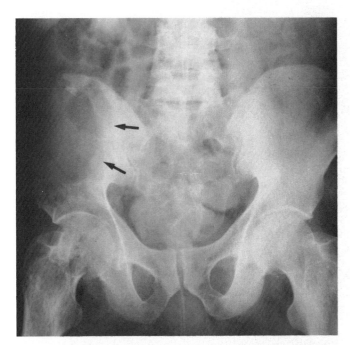

Figure 35.17. Fibrosarcoma. A large, lytic, destructive process of the entire right iliac wing (*arrows*) is noted, which is fairly well defined. On biopsy this was shown to be a fibrosarcoma. Fibrosarcomas can be very slow growing and will occasionally have a narrow zone of transition such as this.

decade. This is one of the few malignant tumors that can, on occasion, have a bony sequestrum.

Malignant Fibrous Histiocytoma

These tumors were originally classified as fibrosarcomas by most pathologists, but have come into their own grouping in the past decade. Radiologically they appear identical to fibrosarcomas: lytic lesions with variations extending from permeative (Fig. 35.18) to fairly well-defined. Like fibrosarcomas, they may, on occasion, have a bony sequestrum.

Desmoid Tumor

A desmoid tumor (not to be confused with a cortical desmoid; see Chapter 39) is a half-grade fibrosarcoma. It has also been called a desmoplastic fibroma or aggressive fibromatosis. These lesions, like fibrosarcoma, are lytic, but are usually fairly well defined because of their slow growth. They often have benign periostitis present that has thick spicules or "spikes." They usually have a multilocular appearance with thick bony septa (Fig. 35.19). They are slow growing and do not metastasize, but can exhibit inexorable tumor extension into surrounding soft tissues with devastating results. Like fibrosarcoma and malignant fibrous histiocytomas, these lesions can exhibit a bony sequestrum.

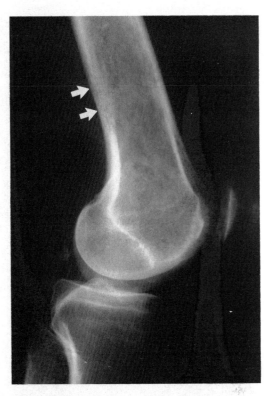

Figure 35.18. Malignant Fibrous Histiocytoma. A moth-eaten or permeative process in the distal femur with some involvement of the posterior cortex (*arrows*) is seen on this lateral x-ray. In a patient under the age of 30, a Ewing's sarcoma, eosinophilic granuloma, or infection would be the differential diagnosis. In a patient over the age of 30, infection and malignant fibrous histiocytoma would be more common. A reticulum cell sarcoma could have a similar appearance.

Reticulum Cell Sarcoma (Primary Lymphoma of Bone)

This is a rare neoplasm that has a radiologic appearance identical to Ewing's sarcoma, i.e., a permeative or moth-eaten pattern (Fig. 35.20). Reticulum cell sarcoma tends to occur in an older age group than Ewing's sarcoma, and, whereas Ewing's sarcomas are typically systemically symptomatic, the reticulum cell sarcoma patient is often asymptomatic. In fact, it is said to be the only malignant tumor that can involve a large amount of bone while the patient is asymptomatic.

Metastatic Disease

Metastatic lesions must be included in *any* differential diagnosis of a bone lesion in a patient over the age of 40. They can have virtually any appearance. They can mimic a benign lesion or an aggressive primary bone tumor. It can be difficult, if not impossible, to judge the origin of the tumor from the appearance of the metastatic focus, although some appearances are fairly characteristic. For instance, multiple scle-

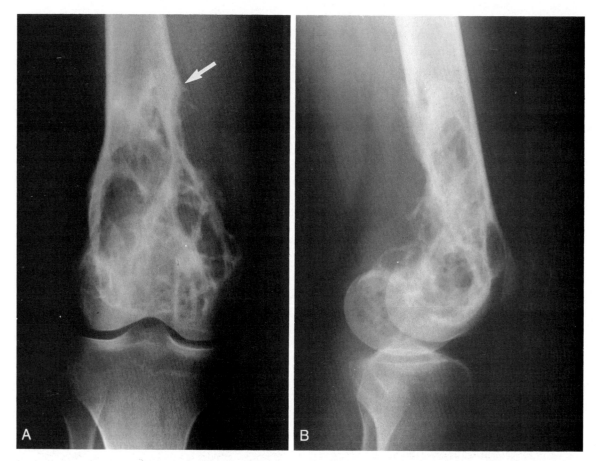

Figure 35.19. Desmoid Tumor. A multilocular, heavily septated, destructive, lytic lesion of the distal femur is noted in these antero-posterior (**A**) and lateral (**B**) plain films of the femur, which is fairly characteristic for a desmoid tumor. The thick septa and narrow zone of transition are characteristic of a benign process, whereas the Codman's triangle (*arrow*) and large amount of bony destruction indicate an aggressive process.

rotic foci in a male are most likely prostatic metastases (Fig. 35.21), although lung, bowel, or almost any other metastatic tumor could present like this. In a female, the same picture would most likely be from breast metastases. Although nearly every metastatic bone lesion can be either lytic or blastic, the only primary tumor that virtually never presents with blastic metastatic disease is renal cell carcinoma. The classic differential diagnosis for an expansile, lytic metastasis is renal cell or thyroid carcinoma (Fig. 35.22).

Myeloma

Like metastases, myeloma should only be considered in a patient over the age of 40, although some radiologists use age 35 for the lower limits of myeloma. Myeloma typically has a diffuse permeative appearance (Fig. 35.23) that can mimic a Ewing's sarcoma or reticulum cell sarcoma. Because of the age criteria, Ewing's sarcoma and myeloma are not in the same differential, however. Myeloma frequently involves the calvarium (Fig. 35.24). Rarely, myeloma can present with multiple sclerotic foci resembling diffuse metastatic disease. Myeloma is one of the only lesions

that is not characteristically hot on a radionuclide bone scan, therefore, radiologic "bone surveys" are performed in place of radionuclide bone scans when evidence of myeloma is found clinically. Occasionally myeloma will present with a lytic bone lesion called a plasmacytoma. This lesion can mimic any lytic bone lesion, benign or aggressive, in its appearance; it can precede other evidence of myeloma by up to 3 years.

Soft-Tissue Tumors

There is no authoritative, useful differential diagnosis for soft-tissue tumors, whether or not there is calcification, bony destruction, fat plane involvement, or whatever. The two most common soft-tissue tumors, **fibrosarcoma** and **liposarcoma**, should be mentioned as the most likely possibilities for any soft-tissue tumor, but any cell type can produce a benign or malignant tumor and mimic any other soft-tissue tumor. A lipoma, obviously, can be separated out by the appearance of fat, but a liposarcoma may or may not have fat present. There are at least three subtypes of liposarcomas, two of which have only small amounts of fat present. Therefore, one is generally left

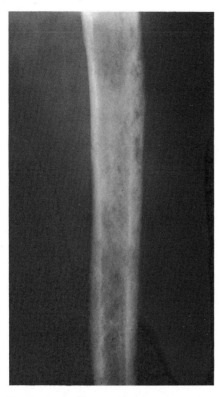

Figure 35.20.   Reticulum Cell Sarcoma. A diffuse permeative pattern is seen throughout the humerus in this 35-year-old patient which is characteristic of reticulum cell sarcoma.

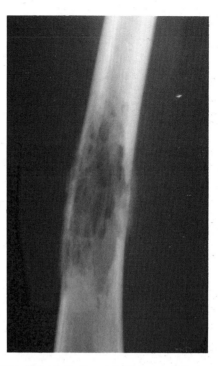

Figure 35.22.   Metastatic Renal Cell Carcinoma. A lytic lesion in the diaphysis of the femur is noted, which is typical for renal cell carcinoma. Up to one-third of renal cell carcinomas present initially with a bony metastasis. Renal cell carcinoma virtually never presents with a blastic metastastic focus.

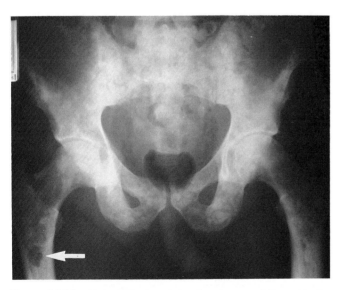

Figure 35.21.   Metastatic Prostate Carcinoma. Diffuse blastic matastases are seen throughout the pelvis and proximal femurs with a lytic, distructive lesion seen in the right proximal femur (arrow). Prostate metastases tend to be blastic, but can occasionally be lytic.

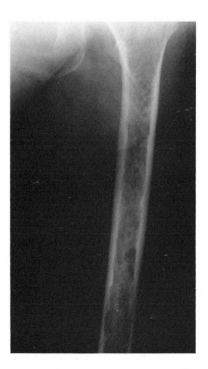

Figure 35.23.   Multiple Myeloma. A diffuse, moth-eaten pattern is seen throughout the diaphysis of the femur in this 45-year-old patient which is characteristic for myeloma. Reticulum cell sarcoma could have a similar appearance.

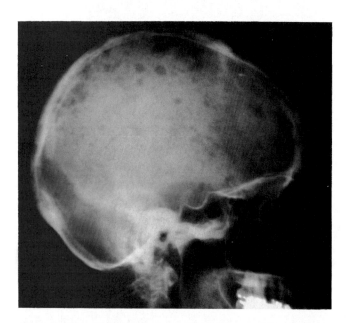

Figure 35.24.   Multiple Myeloma. A lateral view of the skull shows multiple lytic lesions in the calvarium, which is a characteristic appearance of multiple myeloma.

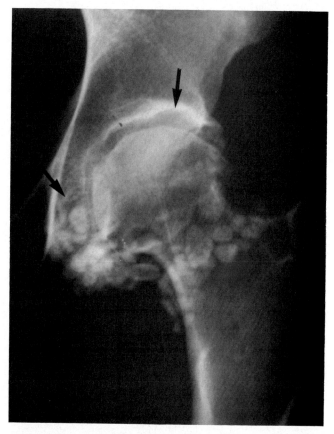

Figure 35.25.   Synovial Osteochondromatosis. Multiple calcific loose bodies in a hip joint, as in this example, are virtually pathognomonic for synovial osteochondromatosis. Notice the erosions in the acetabulum (*arrows*). In up to 30% of cases, the loose bodies are nonossified, in which cases this process is indistinguishable from PVNS.

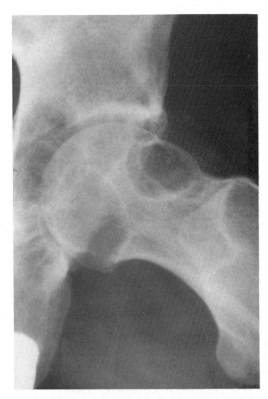

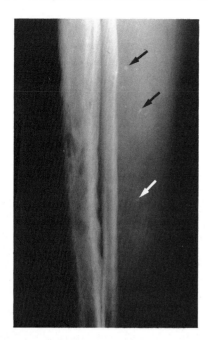

Figure 35.28. Hemangioma. Multiple irregular lytic lesions, predominantly cortical in nature, are seen in the tibia in this patient with a soft-tissue mass. Cortical holes such as this occur almost exclusively in radiation and soft-tissue hemangioma. Note the phleboliths in the posterior soft-tissues (*arrows*) which are often seen in hemangioma and make this an easy diagnosis.

Figure 35.26. Pigmented Villondular Synovitis. Large erosions in the femoral head and acetabulum are characteristic for PVNS; however, nonossified synovial osteochondromatosis could present, such as this.

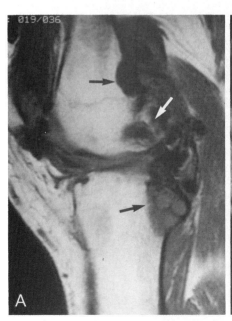

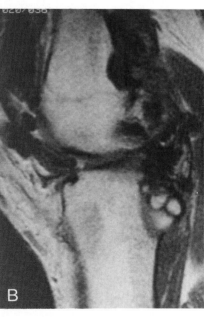

Figure 35.27. Pigmented Villondular Synovitis. Proton-density (**A**) (TR 1500; TE 20) and T2-weighted (**B**) (TR 1500; TE 60) sagittal images of the knee in this patient with painful swelling show diffuse low signal throughout the synovium and eroding into the bone (*arrows*). The low signal on both T1- and T2-weighted images is typical for hemosiderin deposits in PVNS.

to giving descriptions of size and extent of the tumor and letting the pathologist determine the diagnosis.

Synovial sarcomas, or synoviomas, only rarely originate in a joint. They are often adjacent to joints, but probably arise from synovial tissue in tendon sheaths rather than in joints themselves. There are no malignant tumors that routinely need to be considered in the differential diagnosis of joint lesions.

Synovial osteochondromatosis is a benign joint lesion that probably occurs from metaplasia of the synovium and leads to multiple calcific loose bodies in a joint. This can histologically mimic a chondrosar-

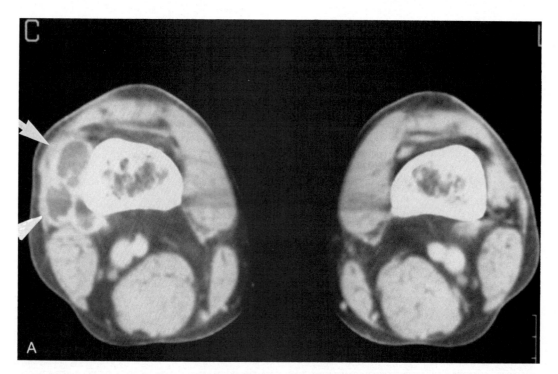

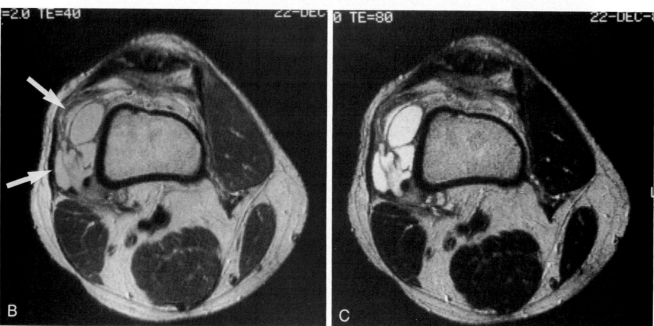

Figure 35.29. Atypical Synovial Cyst. A. A CT scan through the distal femurs in a patient with a soft-tissue mass around the right knee shows a multilocular soft-tissue mass adjacent to the distal right femur (*arrows*). **B.** A proton-density MR (TR 2000; TE 20) through the same area shows intermediate intensity signal in a homogeneous multilocular soft-tissue mass (*arrows*). **C.** A T2-weighted image (TR 2000; TE 60) shows high-intensity signal in the lesion, which is typical for fluid, although a tumor could have these signal characteristics This was an atypical synovial cyst arising from the knee joint.

coma, and therefore is best diagnosed radiographically, since it has a pathognomonic radiographic appearance (Fig. 35.25). Up to 30% of the time the loose bodies do not calcify, however, and it then can mimic pigmented villonodular synovitis (PVNS).

Pigmented villonodular synovitis is a benign synovial soft-tissue process that causes joint swelling and pain, and, occasionally, joint erosions (Fig. 35.26). It virtually never has calcifications associated with it. The MR appearance of PVNS is characteristic. Marked low signal lining the synovium is seen on T1- and T2-weighted images because of the hemosiderin deposits (Fig. 35.27). Chronic bleeding into a joint, so-called hemosiderotic arthritis, could have a similar appearance, but is even more rare than PVNS.

Hemangiomas will often have phleboliths associated with them, and often cause cortical holes in adjacent bone that can mimic a permeative or moth-eaten pattern (Fig. 35.28), a "pseudopermeative" pattern.

The true permeative pattern of round cell lesions occurs in the intramedullary or endosteal part of the bone and can be differentiated from a "pseudopermeative" pattern by the intact cortex.

Atypical synovial cysts, such as Baker's cysts around the knee, can present as a soft-tissue mass and result in an unnecessary biopsy. On CT these lesions may not be appreciated as fluid-filled lesions and their association with a joint can be easily overlooked. Magnetic resonance imaging will demonstrate a very high signal intensity with T2 weighting that is very homogeneous and often septated (Fig. 35.29).

References

1. Edeiken J. Roentgen diagnosis of diseases of bone. 3rd ed. Baltimore: Williams & Wilkins, 1981.
2. Berquist T, Ehman R, King B, Hodgman C, Ilstrup D. Value of MR imaging in differentiating benign from malignant soft-tissue masses: study of 95 lesions. AJR 1990;155: 1251–1255.

36
Trauma

Clyde A. Helms

SPINE
HAND AND WRIST
ARM
PELVIS
LEG

Most of the differential diagnoses in skeletal radiology that I use are geared to be 95% inclusive, that is, the correct diagnosis will be mentioned 95% of the time. The yield can be increased by lengthening the list, but if the list gets too long it can be unwieldy and less useful for the clinician. In trauma cases, however, being right 95% of the time is not good enough. Missing the correct diagnosis 5% of the time is unacceptable. Fractures simply should not be missed.

Before starting with specific examples, a few key points should be kept in mind concerning radiology of trauma. First, have a high index of suspicion. Every radiologist in the world has missed fractures on x-rays because they were not sufficiently attuned to the fact that there might be a fracture present. Oftentimes, the history is either nonexistent or misleading and the anatomic area of concern is therefore overlooked. When in doubt, examine the patient! Orthopaedic surgeons rarely miss seeing fractures on x-rays because they have examined the patient, they know where the patient hurts, and they have a high index of suspicion. Second, always get two x-rays at 90° to one another in every trauma case. A high percentage of fractures are seen only on one view (the anteroposterior or the lateral) and will therefore be missed unless two views are routinely obtained. Third, once a fracture is identified, do not forget to look at the rest of the film. About 10% of all cases have a second finding that often is as significant or even more so than the initial finding. Many fractures have associated dislocation, foreign bodies, or additional fractures, so be sure to examine the entire film.

Finally, do not hesitate to obtain a computed tomography (CT) scan or a magnetic resonance imaging (MR) study if the plain films fail to confirm what is believed to be present clinically. Magnetic resonance imaging is being used more frequently as a primary imaging tool for trauma, replacing CT or radionuclide studies in cases where the plain films are negative or equivocal. Make sure that an expensive examination such as CT or MR is truly going to affect patient care rather than just show an abnormality, and then have the same treatment whether positive or negative. For example, there is no reason to do a CT scan or an MR study to find a subtle or occult fracture of the radial head in the elbow because the patient is going to have a posterior splint regardless of the results of the advanced study (assuming the patient had trauma to the elbow, has pain, and the plain film shows a displaced posterior fat pad indicative of fluid in the joint). On the other hand, an elderly patient who has hip pain following a fall and has a negative plain film would benefit from an MR study because his treatment will depend on whether or not an occult fracture is present.

SPINE

The cervical spine is one of the most commonly filmed parts of the body in a busy emergency department and can be one of the most difficult examinations to interpret. One of the most important pieces of information for the radiologist to have is the clinical history. If the patient has been involved in an automobile accident and has no neck pain, it is extremely unlikely that a fracture is present. So-called "precautionary" x-rays are not justified. On the other hand, if the plain films are negative in a trauma victim who has neck pain or neurologic deficits, obtain a CT scan (1).

Usually, a cross-table lateral view of the C-spine is obtained first, so as to not unduly move the patient who might have a cervical fracture. If the lateral C-spine appears normal, the remainder of the C-spine series, including flexion and extension views (if the patient can cooperate) is obtained.

What does one look for on the lateral C-spine? First, make certain that all seven cervical vertebral bodies can be visualized. A large number of fractures are missed because the shoulders obscure the lower C-spine levels (Fig. 36.1). If the entire cervical spine is not visualized, repeat the film with the shoulders lowered.

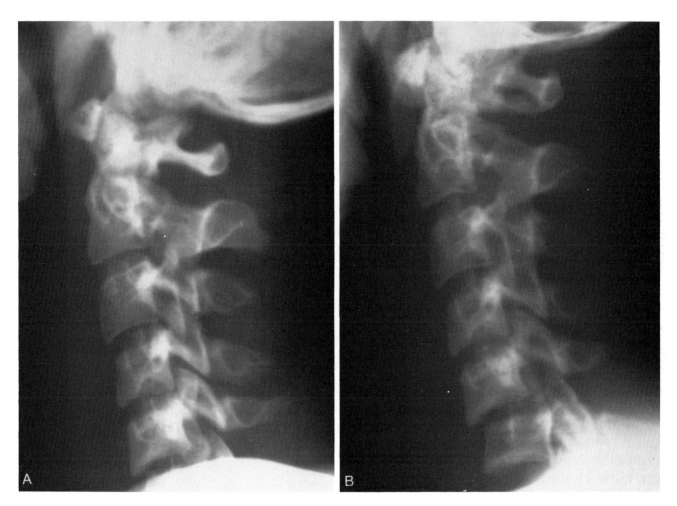

Figure 36.1.   Shoulders Obscuring C5-6 Dislocation. This patient presented to the emergency department following an injury suffered while diving into a shallow swimming pool. He had neck pain but no neurologic deficits. **A.** The initial x-ray obtained of the C-spine was interpreted as within normal limits. However, only five cervical vertebrae are visible because of high-riding shoulders. **B.** A repeat examination with the shoulders lowered reveals a dislocation of C-5 on C-6. To visualize C-7, the shoulders were lowered even further. The C-7 vertebral body must be visualized on every lateral C-spine examination in a trauma setting.

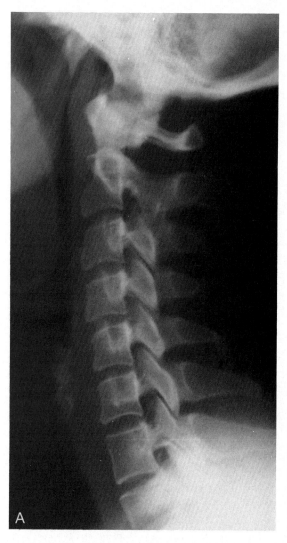

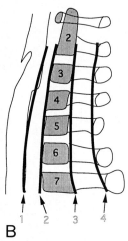

Figure 36.2.   Normal Lateral Cervical Spine. A. Lateral x-ray of a normal cervical spine. **B.** Diagrammatic representation of a lateral C-spine showing four parallel lines that should be observed in every lateral C-spine examination. Line 1 is the soft-tissue line that is closely applied to the posterior border of the airway through the first four or five vertebral body segments and then widens around the laryngeal cartilage and runs parallel to the remainder of the cervical vertebrae. Line 2 demarcates the anterior border of the cervical vertebral bodies. Line 3 is the posterior border of the cervical vertebral bodies. Line 4 is drawn by connecting the junction of the lamina at the spinous process, which is called the spinolaminal line. It represents the posterior extent of the central canal which contains the spinal cord itself. These lines should be generally smooth and parallel with no abrupt step-offs.

Next, evaluate five parallel (more or less) lines for step-offs or discontinuity as follows (Fig. 36.2):

Line number 1 is the prevertebral soft tissue and extends down the posterior aspect of the airway; it should be several millimeters from the first three or four vertebral bodies and then moves further away at the laryngeal cartilage. It should be less than one vertebral body width from the anterior vertebral bodies from C-3 or C-4 to C-7, and it should be smooth in its contour.

Line 2 follows the anterior vertebral bodies and should be smooth and uninterrupted. Anterior osteophytes can encroach on this line and extend beyond it and should therefore be ignored in drawing this line. Interruption of the anterior vertebral body line is a sign of a serious injury (Fig. 36.1**B**).

Line 3 is similar to the anterior vertebral body line (line 2) except that it connects the posterior vertebral bodies. Like line 2, it should be smooth and uninterrupted, and any disruption signifies a serious injury.

Line 4 connects the posterior junction of the lamina with the spinous processes and is called the spi-

nolaminal line. The spinal cord lies between lines 3 and 4; therefore, any offset of either of these lines could mean a bony structure is impinging the cord. It takes very little force against the cord to cause severe neurologic deficits, and any bony structure lying on the cord must be recognized as soon as possible.

Line 5 is not really a line so much as a collection of points—the tips of the spinous processes. They are quite variable in their size and appearance, although C-7 is consistently the largest. A fracture of one of the spinous processes, by itself, is not a serious injury, but it occasionally heralds other, more serious injuries.

After visually inspecting the above-described five lines on the lateral C-spine, then inspect the Cl-2 area a little more closely. Make certain that the anterior arch of C-1 is no greater then 2.5 mm from the dens (Fig. 36.3). Any greater separation than this (except in children where up to 5.0 mm can be normal) is suspicious for disruption of the transverse ligament between C-1 and C-2 (Fig. 36.4).

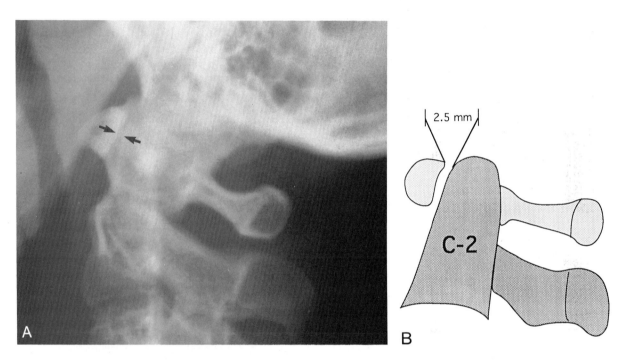

Figure 36.3.   Normal C-1 and C-2. A lateral x-ray (**A**) and drawing (**B**) of the upper cervical spine showing the normal distance of the anterior arch of C-1 less than 2.5 mm in distance from the odontoid process (dens) of C-2 (*arrows*).

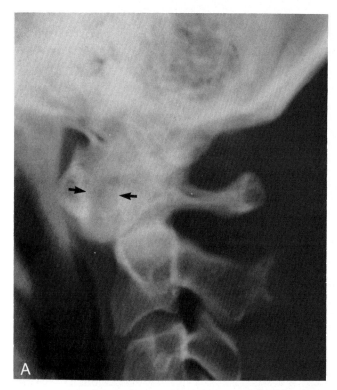

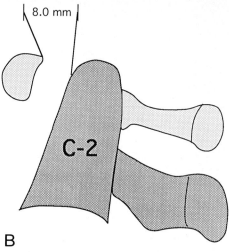

Figure 36.4. C1-2 Dislocation. A lateral x-ray (**A**) and drawing (**B**) of the upper cervical spine in a patient who suffered trauma to the neck shows the anterior arch of C-1 is 9 mm anterior to the odontoid process of C-2 (*arrows*). This is diagnostic of a dislocation of C-1 on C-2 and indicates rupture of the transverse ligaments that normally hold these vertebral segments together.

The disc spaces are examined next to see that there is no inordinate widening or narrowing, either of which could indicate an acute traumatic injury. If a disc space is narrowed it will usually be secondary to degenerative disease, but make certain that associated osteophytosis and sclerosis are present before diagnosing degenerative disease.

The above examination of the lateral C-spine can be done in less than 1 minute. If it is normal, then the remainder of the examination can be completed, in-cluding flexion and extension views. It is imperative that the patient initiate the flexion and extension without help from the technician or anyone else. A patient, if conscious and semialert, will not injure himself or herself with voluntary flexion and extension, and will have muscle guarding preventing motion if there is an injury present. Even gentle pressure to aid in flexion or extension can cause severe injury if a fracture or dislocation is present.

A few examples of fractures, dislocations, and other abnormalities are illustrated in the following paragraphs.

Jefferson Fracture. A blow to the top of the head, such as when an object falls directly on the apex of the skull, can cause the lateral masses of C-1 to slide apart, splitting the bony ring of C-1. This is called a Jefferson fracture (Fig. 36.5). It nicely illustrates how a bony ring will not break in just one place, but must break in several places. This is a rule that is seldom violated. All of the vertebral rings, when fractured, must fracture in two or more places. The bony rings of the pelvis behave similarly.

Computed tomography is excellent at demonstrating the complete bony ring of C-1 and shows the fractures, as well as any associated soft-tissue mass, much better than plain films. In diagnosing a Jefferson fracture on plain film the lateral masses of C-1 must extend beyond the margins of the C-2 body (Fig. 36.5**A**). Just seeing asymmetry of the spaces on either side of the dens is not enough to make the diagnosis as this can be normally asymmetric with rotation or with rotatory fixation of the atlantoaxial joint.

Rotatory fixation of the atlantoaxial joint is a somewhat controversial, little understood process where the atlantoaxial joint becomes fixed and the C1-C2 bodies move en mass instead of rotating on one another. It is easily diagnosed with open-mouth odontoid views. In the normal odontoid view, the spaces lateral to the dens (odontoid) are equal. With rotation of the head to the left the space on the left widens, and with rotation to the right the space on the right widens. With rotatory fixation, one of the spaces is wider than the other and stays wider even with rotation of the head to the opposite side (Fig. 36.6). This is a relatively innocuous malady that by itself is usually treated with a soft cervical collar and/or gentle traction. It is rarely associated with disruption of the transverse ligaments at C1-2 (diagnosed by an increase of greater than 2.5 mm in the space between the anterior arch of C1 and the dens), however, and when it is, it is then a serious problem. It usually presents spontaneously or following very mild trauma such as an unusual sleeping position.

"Clay-shoveler's" Fracture. Another relatively innocuous injury is a fracture of the C-6 or C-7 spinous process called a "clay-shoveler's" fracture. Sup-

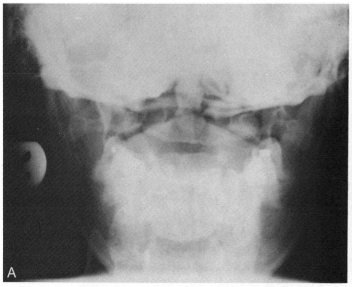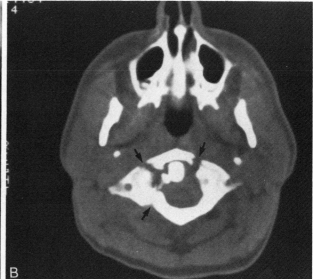

Figure 36.5. Jefferson Fracture. A. An AP open-mouth odontoid view is suspicious for the lateral masses of C-1 being laterally displaced on the body of C-2. However, because of overlying structures, this is difficult to appreciate. **B.** Therefore, a CT examination was obtained and shows multiple fracture sites in the C-1 ring (*arrows*). This is called a Jefferson fracture. Computed tomography should be routinely used in spinal trauma because of frequent shortcomings of plain films.

posedly, workers shoveling sticky clay would toss the shovel full of clay over their shoulders; once in a while the clay would stick to the shovel, causing the ligaments attached to the spinous processes (supraspinous ligaments) to undergo a tremendous force, pulling on the spinous process and avulsing it. This can occur at any of the lower cervical spinous processes (Fig. 36.7).

"Hangman's" Fracture. A "hangman's" fracture is an unstable, serious fracture of the upper cervical spine that is caused by hyperextension and distraction (such as hitting one's head on a dashboard). This is a fracture of the posterior elements of C-2 and, usually, displacement of the C-2 body anterior to C-3 (Fig. 36.8). These patients actually do better than one might think. They often escape neurologic impairment because of the fractured posterior elements of C-2 that, in effect, causes a decompression and takes pressure off the injured area.

Flexion-teardrop Fracture. Severe flexion of the cervical spine can cause a disruption of the posterior ligaments with anterior compression of a vertebral body. This is called a flexion "teardrop" fracture (Fig. 36.9). A teardrop fracture is usually associated with spinal cord injury, often from the posterior portion of the vertebral body being displaced into the central canal.

Unilateral Locked Facets. Severe flexion associated with some rotation can result in rupture of the apophyseal joint ligaments and facet joint dislocation. This can result in locking of the facets in an overriding position that, in effect, causes some stabilization to protect against further injury. This is called unilat-

eral locked facets (Fig. 36.10). It occasionally occurs bilaterally.

"Seatbelt Injury." "Seatbelt injury" is seen secondary to hyperflexion at the waist (as occurs in an automobile accident while restrained by a lap belt). This causes distraction of the posterior elements and ligaments and anterior compression of the vertebral body. It usually involves the T-12, L-1, or L-2 levels. Several variations of this injury can occur: a fracture of the posterior body is called a Smith fracture and a fracture through the spinous process is called a Chance fracture. Horizontal fractures of the pedicles, laminae, and transverse processes can also occur (Fig. 36.11).

Spondylolysis. A somewhat controversial spinal abnormality that may or may not be caused by trauma is spondylolysis. Spondylolysis is a break or defect in the pars interarticularis portion of the lamina (Fig. 36.12). On oblique views, the posterior elements form the figure of a "Scottie dog" with the transverse process being the nose, the pedicle forming the eye, the inferior articular facet being the front leg, the superior articular facet representing the ear, and the pars interarticularis (the portion of the lamina that lies between the facets) equivalent to the neck of the dog. If a spondylolysis is present, the pars interarticularis, or the neck of the dog, will have a defect or break. It often looks as if the Scottie dog has a collar around the neck.

The cause of a spondylolysis is said by some investigators to be congenital and by others to be posttraumatic. Many believe this is a stress-related injury from infancy that develops when toddlers try to walk and repeatedly fall on their buttocks, sending stress to

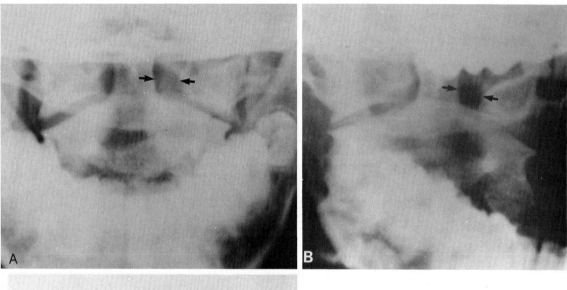

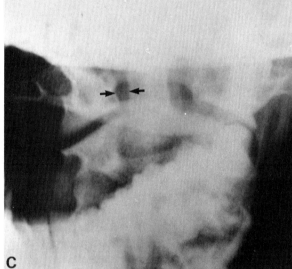

Figure 36.6.   Rotary Fixation of the Atlantoaxial Joint. This patient presented to the emergency department with pain and decreased motion in the cervical spine. **A.** An AP open-mouth odontoid view shows the space on the left side of the odontoid between the odontoid and the lateral mass of C-1 (*arrows*) is wider than the corresponding space on the right side. This is often due to rotation. Therefore, open-mouth odontoid views with right and left obliquities were obtained. **B.** This view shows rotation of the patient's head to the left, which causes the space on the left side of the odontoid process (*arrows*) to be wider than that on the right, which is appropriate. **C.** This view, however, shows that when the patient turns the head to the right the space on the right (*arrows*) does not get wider than the space on the left. This is diagnostic of rotary fixation of the atlantoaxial joint.

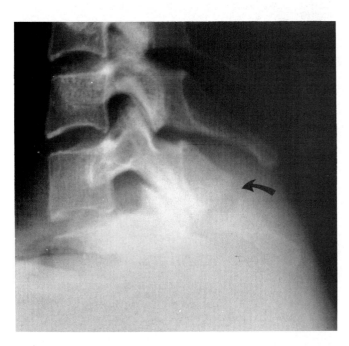

Figure 36.7. Clay Shoveler's Fracture. A nondisplaced fracture of the C-7 spinous process (*arrow*) is noted which is diagnostic of a clay shoveler's fracture.

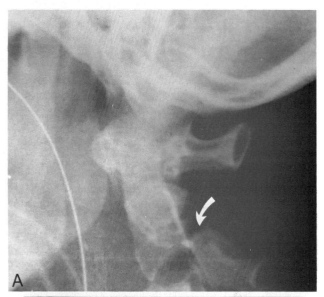

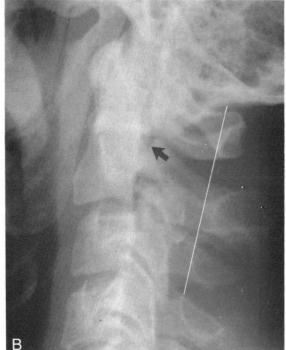

Figure 36.8. Hangman's Fracture. A. Lateral films of a patient with a hangman's fracture shows an obvious example of the posterior elements of the CT vertebral body fractured and displaced inferiorly (*arrow*). **B.** This view shows a very subtle fracture through the posterior elements of C-2 (*arrow*) in another patient. A line drawn through the spinolaminal lines of the posterior elements shows the C-2 spinolaminal line to be offset posteriorly in this example.

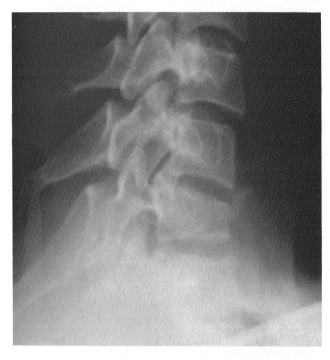

Figure 36.9.   Flexion Teardrop Fracture. This patient suffered a hyperflexion injury in an automobile accident and presented to the emergency department with severe neurologic deficits. A lateral x-ray of the lower cervical spine shows wedging anteriorly of the C-7 vertebral body with some displacement of the posterior vertebral line at C-7 into the central canal. A small avulsion fracture off the anterior body is also noted.

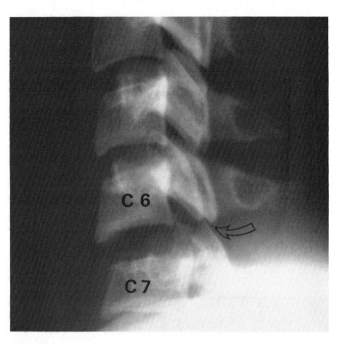

Figure 36.10.   Unilateral Locked Facets. The C6-7 disc space is abnormally widened and the C-7 vertebra is posteriorly located in relation to C-6. Also note the C-7 facets, which are dislocated and locked on the C-6 facets (*arrow*). When the facets are perched in this manner, it is termed "locked facets," which are unilateral in this example.

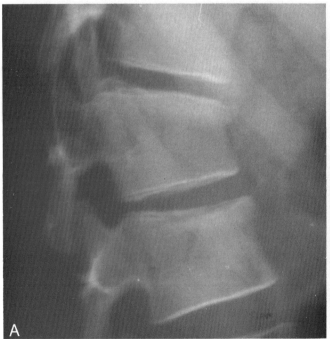

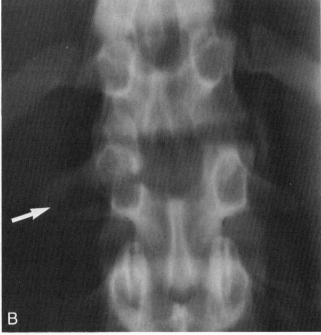

Figure 36.11.   Seatbelt Fracture. Hyperflexion at the waist can cause anterior wedging of the vertebral body in the lower thoracic or upper lumbar region as shown in **A**. By itself, although painful, it is somewhat innocuous; however, **B** shows a horizontal fracture through the right transverse process and pedicle (*arrow*) due to ex-

treme traction during the flexion injury. When fracture of the posterior elements occurs, this injury is considered to be unstable and potentially debilitating. Any anterior wedging injury to a vertebral body should have the posterior elements of that level closely inspected.

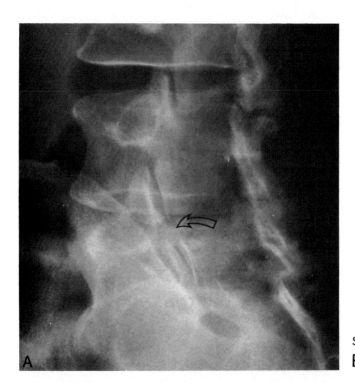

A

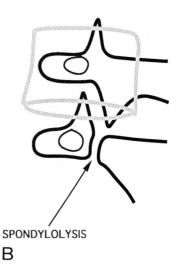

B

Figure 36.12. Spondylolysis. A. An oblique plain film of the lumbar spine shows a defect in the neck of the Scottie dog at L-5 (*arrow*) which is diagnostic of a spondylolysis. **B.** A drawing of an oblique view of the lumbar spine shows how a spondylolysis appears as a "collar" around the Scottie dog's neck.

SPONDYLOLYSIS

their lower lumbar spine. The significance of spondylolysis is just as controversial as its etiology. More and more clinicians are coming to the viewpoint that a spondylolysis is an incidental finding with no clinical significance in most cases. Certainly some patients have pain related to a spondylolysis and get relief following surgical stabilization. It is important to identify spondylolysis preoperatively in patients undergoing lumbar discectomy so the possibility of clinical symptoms from the spondylolysis that can mimic disc symptoms can be evaluated. Although plain films can usually show spondylolysis, CT will show it to better advantage, as well as demonstrate any associated disc disease. Magnetic resonance will show spondylolysis, but it can be difficult to see and is easily overlooked with this method.

If spondyloysis is bilateral and the vertebral body in the more cephalad position slips forward on the more caudal body, spondylolisthesis is said to be present (Fig. 36.13). Spondylolisthesis may or may not be symptomatic and by itself has no clinical significance. If severe it can cause neuroforaminal stenosis and can impinge on the nerve roots in the central spinal canal. If it is symptomatic it can be stabilized surgically.

HAND AND WRIST

Several seemingly innocuous fractures in the hand require surgical fixation rather than just casting and, therefore, should be recognized by the radiologist as serious injuries.

Bennent's Fracture. One such fracture is a fracture at the base of the thumb into the carpomet-

acarpal joint, a Bennent's fracture (Fig. 36.14). Because of the insertion of the strong thumb adductors at the base of the thumb, it is almost impossible to keep the metacarpal from sliding off its proper alignment. It almost always requires internal fixation. The radiologist occasionally has to remind a nonorthopaedic practitioner of this, as well as closely examine the alignment of a Bennent's fracture in plaster that has not been internally fixed with wires.

A comminuted fracture of the base of the thumb that extends into the joint has been termed a Rolando fracture (Fig. 36.15), and a fracture of the base of the thumb that does not involve the joint has been called a pseudo-Bennent's fracture.

Mallet finger or baseball finger is an avulsion injury at the base of the distal phalanx (Fig. 36.16) where the extensor digitorum tendon inserts. With the extensor tendon inoperative, the distal phalanx flexes without opposition, which can result in a flexion deformity and inability to extend the distal phalanx if not properly treated.

A fracture at the volar aspect of the base of the interphalangeal and metacarpophalangeal joints from an avulsion of the volar plate can appear innocent but often requires surgical intervention. The volar plate is a dense fibrocartilaginous band that covers the joint on the volar aspect and can get interposed in the joint once it is torn, often requiring surgical removal.

"Gamekeeper's Thumb." Another innocent-appearing fracture that often requires internal fixation is an avulsion on the ulnar aspect of the first metacarpophalangeal joint (Fig. 36.17); this is where the ul-

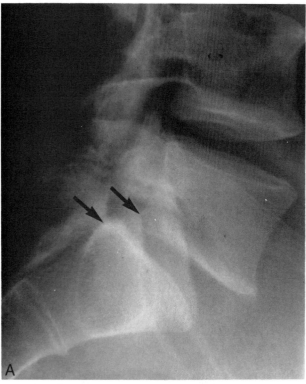

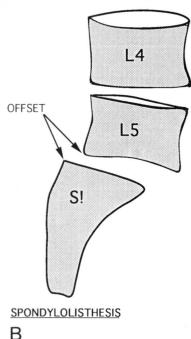

SPONDYLOLISTHESIS

B

Figure 36.13.   Spondylolisthesis. A. A lateral plain film of the lumbar spine shows that the L-5 vertebral body is slightly anteriorly offset on the S1 body as noted by the posterior margins (*arrows*). **B.** The drawing illustrates this more clearly. Since this offset is less than 25% as measured by the length of the S1 endplate, it is termed a "grade 1" spondylolisthesis. A grade 2 offset is more than 25% but less than 50% of the length of the S1 endplate.

nar collateral ligament of the thumb inserts. If the ulnar collateral ligament is torn, normal function of the thumb can be impaired and this can have a serious

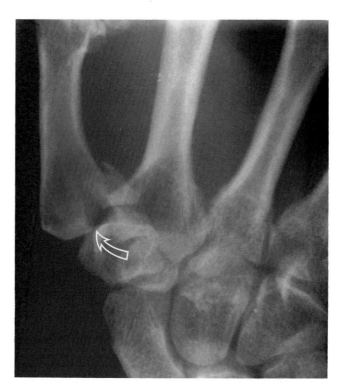

Figure 36.14.   Bennent's Fracture. A small corner fracture of the base of the thumb is noted which involves the articular surface of the base of the thumb (*arrow*); this is a serious injury that almost always requires internal fixation.

result if not properly treated. This injury is called a "gamekeeper's thumb" because of the propensity of English game wardens to acquire it from breaking rabbits' necks between their thumb and forefinger. A more current scenario is falling on a ski pole and having the pole jam into the webbing between the thumb and index finger. This avulsion injury usually requires pinning to fix the ligament securely.

Lunate/perilunate Dislocation. A fall on the outstretched arm can result in any number of wrist fractures and dislocations. One serious such injury is the lunate/perilunate dislocation. This occurs when the ligaments between the capitate and the lunate are disrupted, allowing the capitate to dislocate from the cup-shaped articulation of the lunate. This is best seen on lateral views. Ordinarily, on the lateral view the capitate should be seen seated in the cup-shaped lunate (Figs. 36.18 and 36.19**A**). In a dorsal dislocation (the capitate occasionally dislocates volarly, but this is uncommon), the capitate and all of its surrounding bones, including the metacarpals, come to lie dorsal to a line drawn through the radius and the lunate (Figs. 36.19**B** and 20). If the capitate then pushes the lunate volarly and tips it over, the line drawn up through the radius shows the lunate volarly displaced and the line goes through the capitate. This has been termed a "lunate dislocation" (Figs. 36.19**C** and 36.21). Failure to diagnose and treat this disorder can

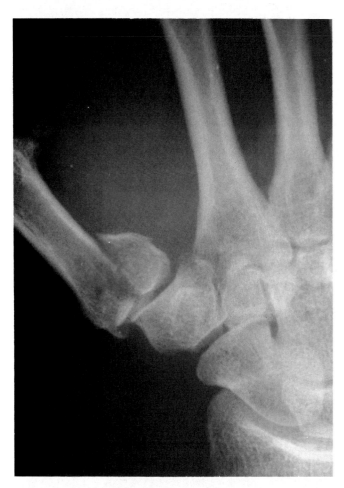

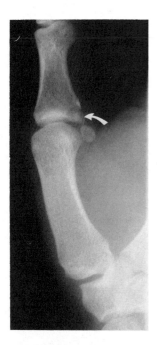

Figure 36.17. Gamekeeper's Thumb. A small avulsion injury on the ulnar aspect of the first metacarpophalangeal joint (*arrow*) is diagnostic of a gamekeeper's thumb. This is the insertion site for the ulnar collateral ligament and usually requires internal fixation.

Figure 36.15. Rolando Fracture. A comminuted fracture of the base of the thumb that extends into the articular surface is a more serious type of Bennent's fracture, which has been termed a Rolando fracture.

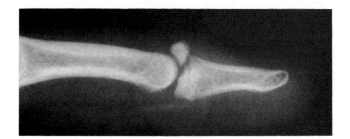

Figure 36.16. Mallet Finger. A small avulsion injury is noted at the base of the distal phalanx, which is where the extensor digitorum tendon inserts. This is termed a mallet finger or baseball finger since it is often caused by a baseball striking the distal phalanx and causing the avulsion.

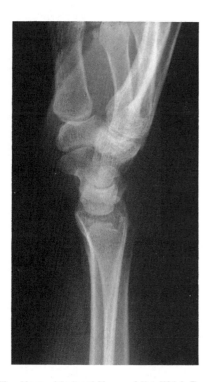

Figure 36.18. Normal Lateral X-ray of the Wrist. The normal lateral view should show the lunate seated in the distal radius and the capitate seated in the lunate. A line drawn up through the radius should connect all three structures. Compare this x-ray with the drawing in Figure 36.19**A**.

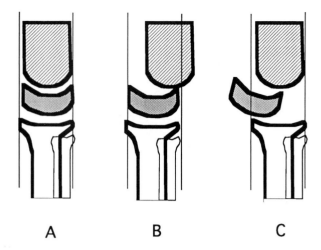

A   B   C

Figure 36.19.   Perilunate and Lunate Dislocations. Schematic depiction of normal lateral wrist (**A**), perilunate dislocation (**B**), and lunate dislocation (**C**). (Dorsal is to the right).

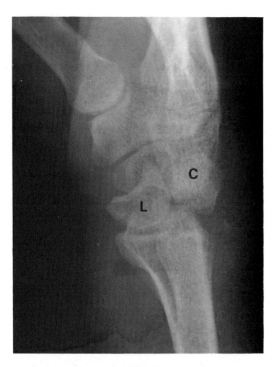

Figure 36.20.   Perilunate Dislocation. Although the lunate (L) is normal in relation to the distal radius, the capitate (C) and the remainder of the wrist are dorsally displaced in relation to the lunate. Compare this x-ray with the drawing in Figure 36.19**B**.

result in permanent median nerve impairment as it can get impinged by the volarly displaced lunate.

A lunate or perilunate dislocation can be diagnosed on an AP view of the wrist by noting a triangular or "pie-shaped" lunate (Fig. 36.21**B**). Ordinarily, the lunate has a rhomboid shape on the AP view, with the upper and lower borders parallel.

Several fractures are known to be associated with a perilunate dislocation, the most common of which is a transscaphoid fracture. The capitate, radial styloid, and triquetrum are also known to frequently fracture when a perilunate dislocation occurs.

Hook of the Hamate Fracture. One of the most difficult wrist fractures to radiologically identify is a fracture of the hook of the hamate. A special view, the carpal tunnel view, should be obtained when trying to see the hook of the hamate. This view is obtained with the wrist (palm down) flat on an x-ray plate and the fingers pulled dorsally. The x-ray beam is angled about 45°, parallel to the palm of the hand so the carpal tunnel is in profile. The hook of the hamate is seen as a bony protuberance off the hamate on the ulnar aspect of the carpal tunnel. A fractured hook of the hamate is often identified with the carpal tunnel view (Fig. 36.22) but can occasionally be very difficult to visualize. A CT scan will often show an obvious fracture that the plain film does not (Fig. 36.23) and should be considered in any possible carpal fracture when plain films are not diagnostic.

A fracture of the hook of the hamate most commonly occurs from a fall on the outstretched hand. A clinical setting that has gained attention in sports medicine circles is that of a professional athlete who participates in an activity where the butt of a club, bat, or racket is held in the palm of the hand. Overswinging can result in the butt of the club levering off the hook of the hamate. This has been seen in profes-

sional baseball players, tennis players, and golfers. Why professionals? Amateurs usually are not strong enough to exert enough force to lever the hook off, and if they do will usually terminate that activity, allowing healing, whereas a professional continues participation, which can lead to a nonunion of the fracture.

Rotary subluxation of the navicular is another wrist injury seen after a fall onto the outstretched hand. This results from rupture of the scapholunate ligament, which allows the scaphoid (navicular) to rotate dorsally. On an AP wrist plain film, a space is seen between the navicular and the lunate (Fig. 36.24) where ordinarily they are closely opposed. This has been called the "Terry Thomas" sign after the famous British actor with a gap between his two front teeth.

Navicular Fracture. A fracture of the navicular is a potentially serious injury because of the high rate of avascular necrosis that occurs with this injury. When avascular necrosis occurs, it usually requires surgical intervention with bone grafting to obtain healing. This fracture can be very difficult to detect initially, therefore, whenever a fracture of the navicular is clinically suspect (trauma with pain over the snuffbox of the wrist), the wrist should be casted and repeat x-rays obtained in 1 week. Often the fracture is then visualized because of the disuse osteoporosis and hyperemia around the fracture site.

If avascular necrosis of the navicular develops, it is the proximal fragment that undergoes necrosis be-

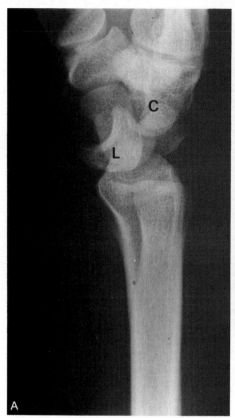

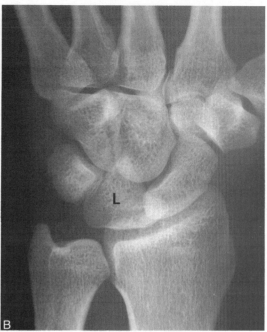

Figure 36.21. Lunate Dislocation. A. The lateral x-ray of the wrist shows the lunate (*L*) tipped off of the distal radius, whereas the capitate (*C*) seems to be normally aligned in relation to the radius, yet is dislocated from the lunate. Compare this with the drawing in Figure 36.19**C**. The AP view shows a pie-shaped lunate (*L*) rather than a lunate with a more rhomboid shape. A pie-shaped lunate on the AP view is diagnostic of a perilunate or lunate dislocation.

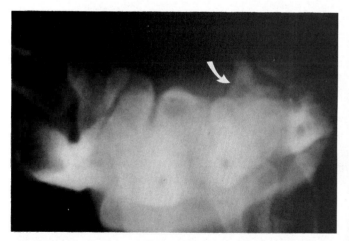

Figure 36.22. Fracture of the Hook of the Hamate. The hook of the hamate is seen on a carpal tunnel view in this patient and has an area of sclerosis with a faint cortical break (*arrow*). This represents a fracture at the base of the hook of the hamate.

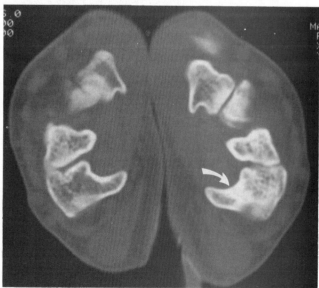

Figure 36.23. A CT of a Fractured Hamate. A CT scan through the wrist in this patient shows a faint lucency surrounded by sclerosis in the left hamate (*arrow*), which represents a fracture through the base of the hook of the hamate with moderate reactive sclerosis. This could not be seen in the plain films, even in retrospect.

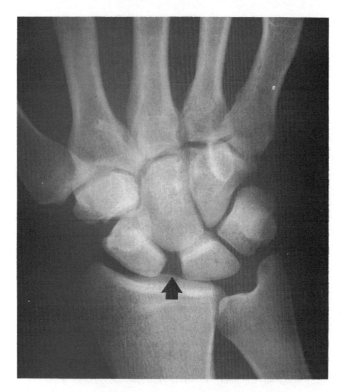

Figure 36.24.   Rotatory Subluxation of the Navicular. An AP view of the wrist shows a gap or space between the navicular and the lunate (*arrow*). This is abnormal and represents the "Terry Thomas" sign, which means the scapholunate ligament is ruptured. This is diagnostic of a rotatory subluxation of the navicular.

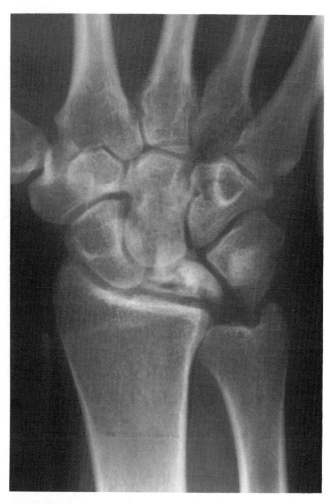

Figure 36.26.   Kienbock's Malacia. An AP view of the wrist reveals the lunate to be sclerotic and abnormal in shape. The lunate has collapsed because of aseptic necrosis. This is known as Keinbock's malacia. Note that the ulna is shorter than the radius, this is termed negative ulnar variance, that is often associated with Kienbock's malacia.

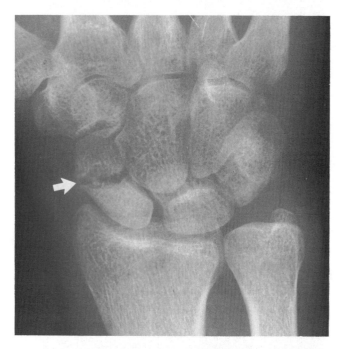

Figure 36.25.   Avascular Necrosis of the Navicular. An AP view of the wrist shows a fracture through the waist of the navicular (*arrow*). The proximal half of the navicular is slightly sclerotic in relation to the remainder of the carpal bones, which indicates avascular necrosis of the proximal half.

cause the blood supply to the navicular begins distally and runs proximally. A fracture with disruption of the blood supply thus leaves the proximal pole without a vascular supply; hence, it dies. Avascular necrosis is diagnosed by noting increased density of the proximal pole of the navicular as compared with the remainder of the carpal bones (Fig. 36.25).

Avascular necrosis can occur in other carpal bones, most commonly the lunate. This is called Kienbock's malacia and is most often caused by trauma, although some investigators claim it is idiopathic. It is diagnosed by noting the increased density to the lunate bone, which may or may not go on to collapse and fragmentation (Fig. 36.26). It often requires surgical bone grafting and occasionally removal or proximal carpal row fusion. It has a high association with a discrepancy between the length of the radius and the ulna as seen at the radiocarpal joint. If the ulna is shorter than the radius, it is termed "negative ulnar

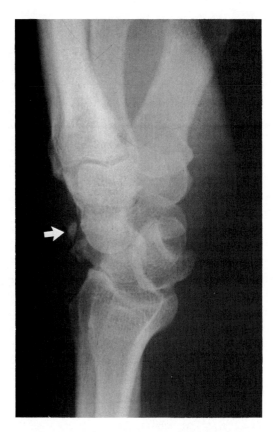

Figure 36.27. Triquetral Fracture and Perilunate Dislocation. A perilunate or lunate dislocation is present (it is difficult to classify exactly which has occurred since both the lunate and the capitate are out of their normal position). A small avulsion is seen on the dorsum of the wrist (*arrow*), which is virtually diagnostic of an avulsion off the triquetrum. It is often associated with a lunate or perilunate dislocation.

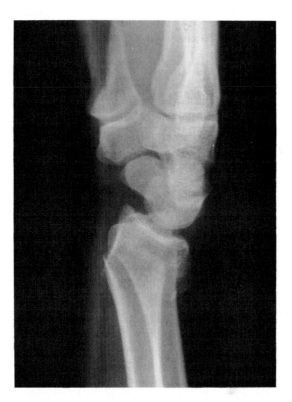

Figure 36.28. Colle's Fracture. A fracture of the distal radius with dorsal angulation is noted, which has been termed a Colle's fracture.

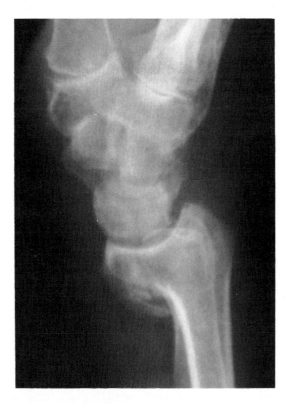

Figure 36.29. Smith's Fracture. A fracture of the distal radius with volar angulation such as this is called a Smith's fracture. This is a much less common injury than the Colle's fracture, shown in Figure 36.28.

variance" and there is an increased incidence of Kienbock's malacia (Fig. 36.26). If the ulna is longer than the radius, it is termed "positive ulnar variance" and there is an increased incidence of triangular fibrocartilage tears.

A common avulsion fracture in the wrist is a triquetral fracture. It is best seen on a lateral film, which shows a small chip of bone off the dorsum of the wrist (Fig. 36.27). This is virtually pathognomonic of an avulsion from the triquetrum.

ARM

Colle's Fracture.   One of the most common fractures of the forearm is a fracture of the distal radius and ulna following a fall on an outstretched arm. This results in a dorsal angulation of the distal forearm and wrist and is called a Colle's fracture (Fig. 36.28). When the fracture angulates volarly it is called a Smith's fracture (Fig. 36.29). A Smith's fracture is a much less common occurrence than a Colle's fracture. Sometimes the radius and ulna suffer a traumatic insult and the force on the bones causes bending instead of a frank fracture. This has been termed a

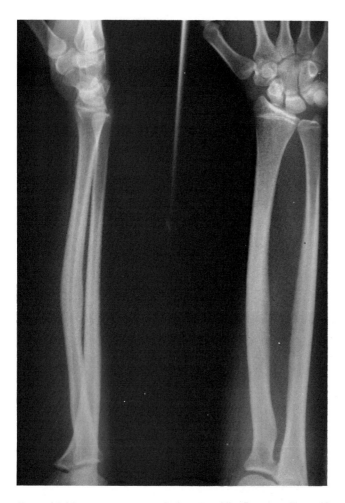

Figure 36.30.   Plastic Bowing Deformity of the Forearm. These AP and lateral views of the forearm of a child show the radius to be abnormally bowed anteriorly. This has been termed a plastic bowing deformity of the forearm and occurs only in children.

"plastic bowing deformity of the forearm" (Fig. 36.30) and is often treated by breaking the bones under anesthesia and resetting them. Left untreated, a plastic bowing deformity can result in reduced supination and pronation.

Monteggia Fracture.   The forearm is a two-bone system that has some of the same properties as a ring-bone. As mentioned previously, a solid ring cannot break in only a single place, it must break in at least two points. In the forearm, a fracture of one bone should be accompanied by a fracture of the other. If the second fracture is not present a dislocation of the nonfractured bone usually occurs. The most common example of this is a fracture of the ulna with a dislocation of the proximal radius (Fig. 36.31). This is called a Monteggia fracture. It has also been termed a "nightstick" injury, from a policeman hitting someone with a nightstick. The person being hit instinctively raises the arm for protection and the nightstick falls on the ulna, fracturing it and dislocating the radial

head. The dislocated radial head can be missed clinically and develop into aseptic necrosis with subsequent elbow dysfunction. Therefore, whenever the forearm is fractured, the elbow must be examined to exclude a dislocation.

Galleazzi Fracture.   A fracture of the radius with dislocation of the distal ulna is called a Galleazzi fracture (Fig. 36.32). This is much less common than a Monteggia fracture and, because the deformity of the dislocated ulna is usually obvious, it is rarely missed clinically.

A helpful indicator of a fracture about the elbow is a displaced posterior fat pad. Ordinarily the posterior fat pad is not visible on a lateral view of the elbow because it is tucked away in the olecranon fossa of the distal humerus. When the joint becomes distended with blood secondary to a fracture, the posterior fat pad is displaced out of the olecranon fossa and is visible on the lateral view (Fig. 36.33**A**). Therefore, in the setting of trauma, a visible posterior fat pad indicates a fracture. In an adult (epiphyses closed) the fracture site is almost always the radial head (Fig. 36.33**B**). In a child (epiphyses open) it is usually indicative of a supracondylar fracture (Fig. 36.34).

Often, the fracture itself is not visualized and extraordinary steps are taken by clinicians and radiologists alike to demonstrate the fracture. These steps include oblique views, special radial head views, tomograms, and even CT scans or MR studies. These are absurd attempts to document pathology that will be treated identically whether or not it is radiographically recorded. As long as there is no obvious deformity or loose body, it does not matter if the fracture is definitely identified or not in a patient with a post-traumatic painful elbow and a visible posterior fat pad. An infection, an arthritide, or any elbow effusion could cause a joint effusion and a displaced posterior fat pad, but the clinical setting would not be to rule out a fracture.

The anterior fat pad also gets displaced with a joint effusion. Ordinarily it is visible as a small triangle just anterior to the distal humeral diaphysis on a lateral film (Fig. 36.35). With an effusion it gets displaced superiorly and outward from the humerus and has been called a "sail sign" since it resembles a spinnaker sail (Figs. 36.33 and 36.34).

Shoulder dislocations are generally easily diagnosed, both clinically and radiographically. The most common shoulder dislocation is the anterior dislocation. It is at least 10 times more common than a posterior dislocation. For all practical purposes, anterior and posterior dislocations are the only two types of shoulder dislocations to be concerned with.

An anterior dislocation occurs when the arm is forcibly externally rotated and abducted. This is commonly seen when football players "arm tackle," when

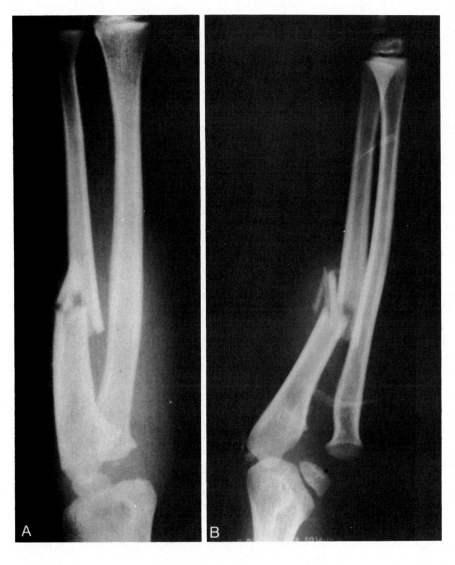

Figure 36.31. Monteggia Fracture. A blow to the forearm such as with a policeman's night stick can result in a fracture of the ulna (**A**). Although the head of the radius appears normally placed in **A**, the lateral examination shown in **B** reveals the head of the radius to be displaced. Failure to recognize this abnormality can result in death of the radial head with subsequent elbow dysfunction. This illustrates the importance of always obtaining two views of a bone following trauma.

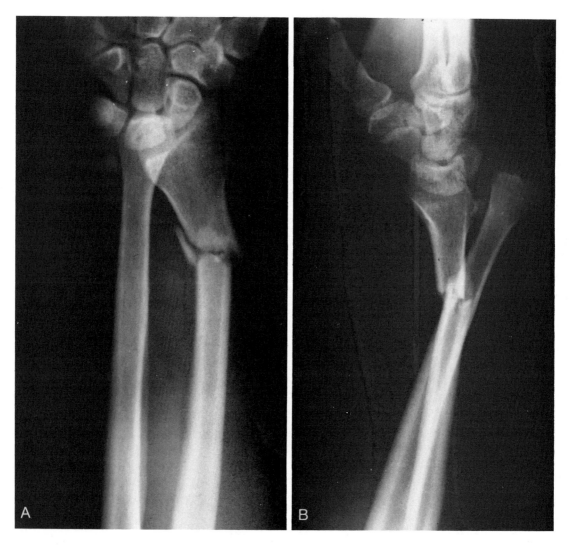

Figure 36.32.   Galleazzi Fracture. A. A fracture of the distal radius in this patient is seen on the AP view without a definite fracture of the ulna. **B.** This view shows an obvious dislocation of the distal ulna, which would almost certainly not be missed clinically. This has been termed a Galleazzi fracture and is much less common than the Monteggia fractures.

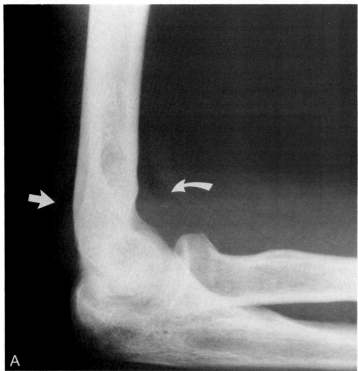

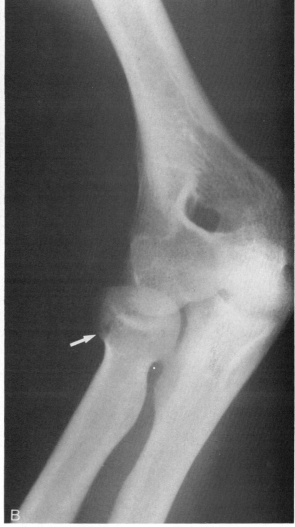

Figure 36.33.   Displaced Elbow Fat Pads. A. On the lateral view of this elbow the posterior fat pad is faintly visible (*arrow*) and the anterior fat pad is elevated and anteriorly displaced (*curved arrow*). These findings indicate a fracture about the elbow that in an adult should be in the radial head. **B.** An oblique view shows the fracture of the radial head (*arrow*). Even without seeing the fracture on the x-rays, it should be surmised to be present when the posterior fat pad is visualized in the setting of trauma. The elevated and displaced anterior fat pad has been termed a "sail sign."

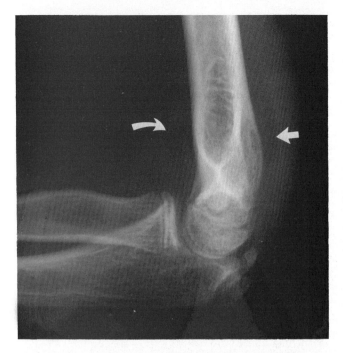

Figure 36.34. Displaced Elbow Fat Pads. A lateral view of the elbow in this child shows a posterior fat pad (*arrow*) and a sail sign anteriorly (*curved arrow*). This is indicative of a fracture about the elbow, which in a child (epiphyses are open) usually means a supracondylar fracture.

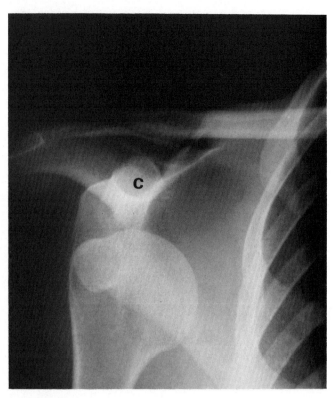

Figure 36.36. Anterior Shoulder Dislocation. An AP view of the right shoulder shows the humeral head to lie medial to the glenoid and inferior to the coracoid process (C). This is diagnostic of an anterior dislocation of the shoulder.

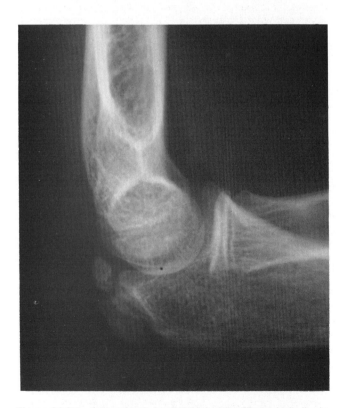

Figure 36.35. Normal Anterior Fat Pad of the Elbow. Note the lucency just anterior to the humerus of this normal elbow and compare this with the sail sign of the anterior fat pads in Figures 36.33 and 36.34.

kayakers "brace" with the paddle above their heads and allow their arms to get too far posterior, when skiers plant their uphill pole and get it stuck, and from other similar athletic positions. Radiographically, the diagnosis is easily made on an AP shoulder film: the humeral head is seen to lie inferiorly and medial to the glenoid (Fig. 36.36). The humeral head often impacts on the inferior lip of the glenoid causing an indentation on the posterosuperior portion of the humeral head; this is called a "Hill-Sachs" deformity. The presence of a Hill-Sachs deformity is said to indicate a greater likelihood of recurrent dislocation, and some surgeons use it as an indicator to surgically intervene to prevent a recurrence. A bony irregularity or fragment off the inferior glenoid, which occurs from the same mechanism as the Hill-Sachs deformity, is called a "Bankhart" deformity. It is not seen radiographically as often as the Hill-Sachs deformity.

A posterior dislocation can be a difficult diagnosis to make both clinically and radiographically. An AP view may look completely normal, or nearly so. On the AP view of a normal shoulder the humeral head should slightly overlap the glenoid (Fig. 36.37), forming what has been called a "crescent sign." In a patient with a posterior dislocation, this crescent of bony overlap is usually absent and a small space is

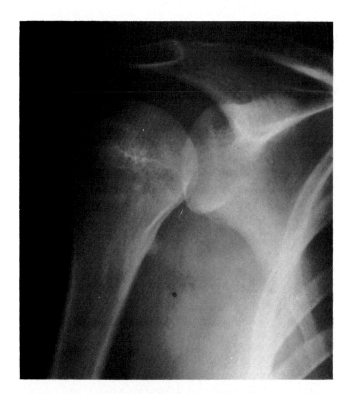

Figure 36.37. Normal AP View of the Shoulder. Note in this example of a normal shoulder that the humeral head slightly overlaps the glenoid, which has been termed the crescent sign.

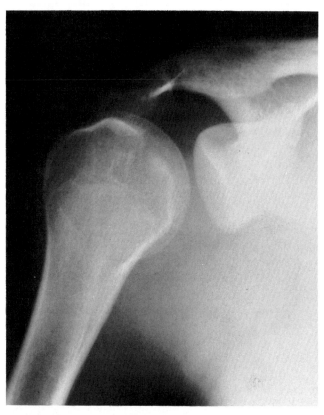

Figure 36.38. Posterior Shoulder Dislocation. Note that the humeral head in this patient is slightly displaced from the glenoid on the AP view. This is termed absence of the crescent sign and is often seen with a posterior dislocation. Compare this with the normal shoulder in Figure 36.37.

seen between the glenoid and the humeral head (Fig. 36.38).

The best way to unequivocally diagnose a dislocated shoulder is to obtain a transscapular view. An axillary view will show basically the same thing but requires the patient to move the arm and shoulder, which can be painful and may even redislocate the shoulder if it has spontaneously reduced itself. The transscapular view is obtained by angling the x-ray beam across the shoulder in the same plane as the blade of the scapula. This gives an en face view of the glenoid, and the humeral head can easily be related to it as either normal, anterior (Fig. 36.39), or posterior. Because of frequently overlapping ribs and clavicles, the exact anatomy is often difficult to discern on the transscapular view. To find the glenoid one has to find the coracoid, the spine of the acromion, and the blade of the scapula. These three structures all lead to the glenoid and form a "Y" around it. All that is necessary to find the center of the glenoid is to find two of those bony landmarks, usually the coracoid and the blade of the scapula. The humeral head can then be found and its position determined.

An entity that can be mistaken for a dislocated shoulder is a traumatic hemarthrosis, which displaces the humeral head inferolaterally on the AP film (Fig. 36.40). Since the anterior dislocation displaces inferomedially, it should not be confused with this. The posterior dislocation will easily be excluded by looking at a transscapular view. This has been termed a "pseudo-dislocation." It should be recognized so that attempts to "reduce" the "dislocation" are not made. Also, it can foretell a subtle or occult humeral head fracture.

If a fracture is suspected about the shoulder and the plain films are negative or equivocal, a CT scan should be performed. A complex joint such as the shoulder or hip is best examinal with CT scanning when the full extent of the fracture needs to be identified (Fig. 36.41).

PELVIS

Fractures of the pelvis, and especially those involving the acetabulum, can be difficult to evaluate completely with plain films alone. Computed tomography scanning should be considered in almost all acetabular fractures because of the possibility of free fragments and subtle fractures that plain films do not show (Fig. 36.42).

Sacral fractures are said to occur in half of the cases that have pelvic fractures. They can be difficult to see on even the best of films because the sacrum is often hidden by bowel gas. In looking for sacral fractures,

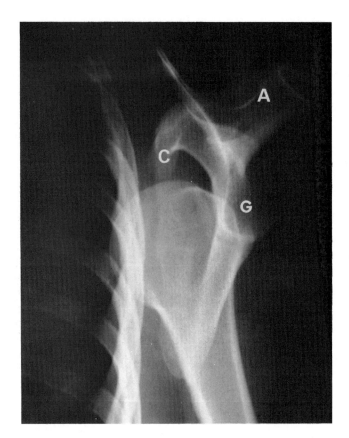

Figure 36.39. Transcapular View of an Anterior Dislocation. This transcapalur view of the shoulder is obtained by aiming the x-ray beam parallel to the shoulder blade. The coracoid process (C) can be seen anteriorly and the spine of the acromion (A) can be seen posteriorly. Both of these structures extend inwardly and meet at the glenoid (G). The humeral head is seen in this example to lie anterior to the glenoid.

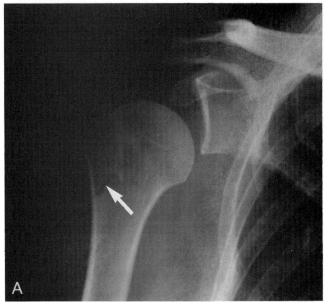

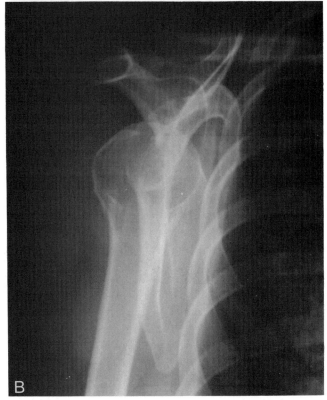

Figure 36.40. Pseudodislocation of the Shoulder. A. An AP view of the shoulder in this patient who had trauma to the shoulder shows the humeral head to be inferiorly placed in relation to the glenoid with absence of the normal crescent sign. A dislocation was suspected. **B.** The transscapular lateral film, however, reveals the humeral head to be normally placed over the glenoid. This is a pseudodislocation due to a hemarthrosis. A search for an occult fracture should be made. In this case a fracture can be seen in **A** (*arrow*), which caused bleeding into the joint.

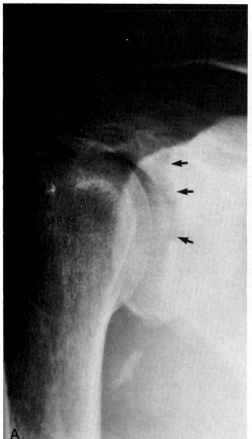

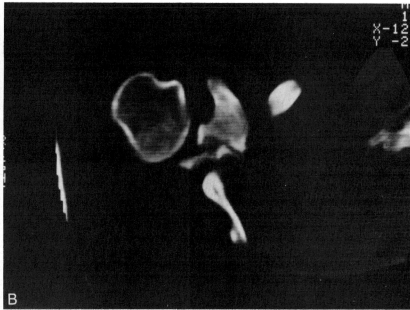

Figure 36.41. Fracture of the Glenoid. A. An AP view of the shoulder demonstrates a faint lucency indicative of a fracture of the glenoid (*arrows*) with a fragment of bone seen inferior to the joint. **B.** The full extent of the fracture cannot be appreciated until the CT is examined. On the CT scan the fracture can be seen to extend fully through the scapula and is seen to be slightly displaced in the articular portion.

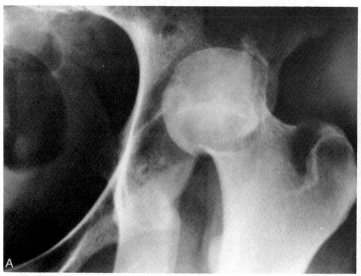

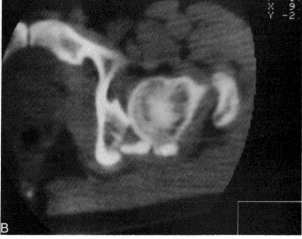

Figure 36.42. Dislocation of the Hip. A. An AP plain film of the left hip shows dislocation of the femoral head, which lies slightly superior to the acetabulum. **B.** Fractures are easily identified on the CT scan. A cortical break through the articular surface of the posterior acetabulum as well as the dislocation is identified.

one should examine the arcuate lines of the sacrum bilaterally to see if they are intact. Fractures often interrupt these lines and, because of the side-to-side asymmetry, can therefore be easily identified (Fig. 36.43).

Sacral stress fractures in patients who are osteoporotic or who have undergone radiation therapy can present as patchy or linear sclerosis on the sacral

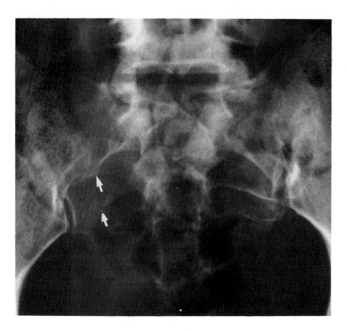

Figure 36.43.   Fracture of the Sacrum. An AP view of the sacrum in this patient shows normal arcuate lines on the left side of the sacrum that are interrupted on the right side (*arrows*). Interruption of these lines indicates a fracture through this portion of the sacrum.

ala that may or may not show cortical disruption on plain films (Fig. 36.44**A**). These should be differentiated from metastatic disease because of their characteristic location, appearance, history of prior radiation, and by seeing a cortical break. Computed tomography will usually, but not always, demonstrate cortical disruption (Fig. 36.44**B**). These fractures have a characteristic appearance on radionuclide bone scans (Fig. 36.45**A**), which is termed the "Honda sign" because of its appearance to the logo of the car. The Honda sign is seen only with bilateral stress fractures; unilateral fractures will have increased radionuclide uptake throughout one sacral ala. Magnetic resonance imaging will demonstrate an area of diffuse low signal on T1-weighted images corresponding to the area of involvement (Fig. 36.45**B**). Sacral stress fractures have also been termed "insufficiency fractures," indicating that the underlying bone is abnormal, similar to a pathologic fracture.

Avulsion injuries affect the pelvis quite often and should be easily recognized by radiologists. On occasion, an avulsion injury can have an aggressive appearance and, if not diagnosed radiographically, a biopsy might be performed. This can be calamitous as avulsion injuries have been known to mimic malignant lesions histologically, with a misdiagnosis leading to radical treatment (Fig. 36.46). Therefore, when an avulsion injury is a consideration, it becomes a "do not touch" lesion (see Chapter 39). Common sites for pelvic avulsions include the ischium, the superior and inferior anterior iliac spines (Fig. 36.47), and the iliac

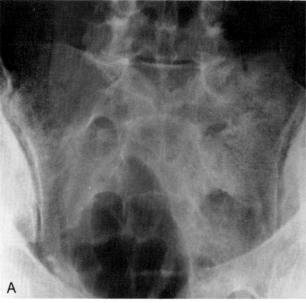

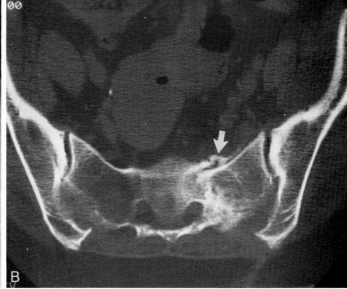

Figure 36.44.   Sacral stress fracture. A. Faint sclerosis is noted in the left part of the sacrum as compared with the right in this patient complaining of pelvic pain. A radionuclide bone scan showed increased isotope uptake on the left half of the sacrum and meta-

static disease was postulated. **B.** A CT scan through this region which demonstrates a cortical disruption (*arrow*) indicative of a fracture. This is a characteristic plain film and CT appearance of a stress fracture of the sacrum.

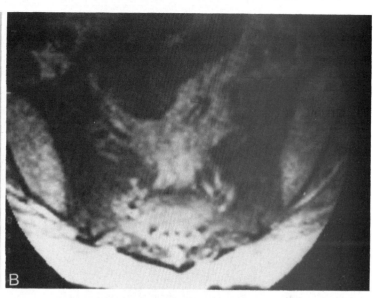

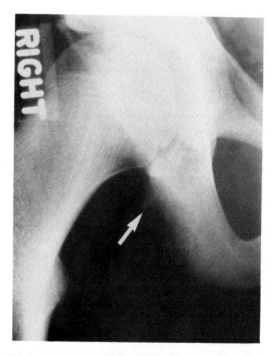

Figure 36.45. Sacral Stress Fracture. A. A radionuclide bone scan in an osteoporotic patient with pelvic pain shows a classic Honda sign seen with bilateral sacral stress fractures. **B.** A T1-weighted coronal MR in this patient shows diffuse low signal throughout the sacrum adjacent to the sacroiliac joints bilaterally. This represents edema and hemorrhage in the fractures and corresponds to the bone scan Honda sign.

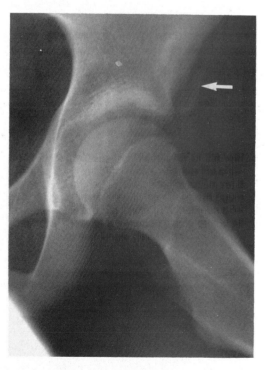

Figure 36.46. Avulsion Off The Ischium. An AP view of the pelvis shows an area of cortical disruption and periostitis at the right ischium (*arrow*) in a patient complaining of pain at this site. These findings are characteristic for an ischial avulsion and should not undergo biopsy.

Figure 36.47. Rectus Femoris Avulsion. An AP plain film of the left hip shows a faint calcific density superior to the acetabulum (*arrow*), which is characteristic for an avulsion of the rectus femoris muscle from the anterior inferior iliac spine.

crest. These injuries are said to be fairly common in long jumpers, sprinters, hurdlers, gymnasts, and cheerleaders.

Another area in the pelvis that can demonstrate radiologic findings as a result of stress is the symphysis pubis. In ultramarathoners, cross-country skiers, soccer players, and other athletes the symphysis can be affected by degenerative joint disease (DJD) or osteoarthritis. (Fig. 36.48). The hallmarks of DJD are sclerosis, joint space narrowing, and osteophytosis. In certain joints, however, erosions can occur as a result of DJD. These joints include the temporomandibular

joint, the acromioclavicular joint, the symphysis pubis, and the sacroiliac joint.

When the sacroiliac joints are involved with DJD, this can closely resemble an HLA-B27 spondyloarthropathy (Fig. 36.49) and lead to erroneous diagnosis and treatment. Large osteophytes can develop across the sacroiliac joints and mimic sclerosis or even a tumor (Fig. 36.50).

LEG

Overt fractures in the femur and lower leg are, for the most part, straightforward and deserve no special radiologic treatment for fear of missing subtle abnormalities.

Stress fractures, however, need to be considered in anyone with hip or leg pain, as overlooking the diagnosis can lead to a complete fracture. The most serious stress fracture, and fortunately, one of the rarest, is the femoral neck stress fracture (Fig. 36.51). Many of these progress to complete fractures (Fig. 36.52) that, with continued weight bearing, can displace; therefore, these are very serious lesions.

Stress fractures also occur in the distal diaphysis of the femur and, the proximal, middle, and distal thirds of the tibia. All of these stress fractures need to be treated with the utmost caution since complete fractures are not uncommon with continued stress (Fig. 36.53). Sclerosis in a weight-bearing bone that has a horizontal or oblique linear pattern should be considered a stress fracture until proven otherwise. A history of repetitive stress is not always obtained, so the diagnosis should not depend solely on the history.

A stress fracture occasionally will appear somewhat aggressive with aggressive periostitis and no definite linearity to the sclerosis (Fig. 36.54**A**). If this is mistaken for a tumor and undergoes biopsy, it can be confused with a malignancy, with subsequent radical therapy. These should, therefore, not undergo biopsy

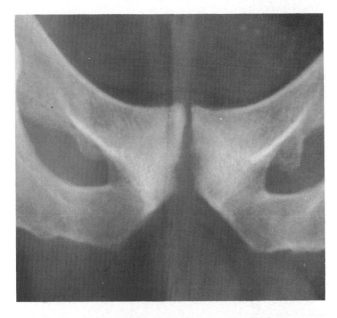

Figure 36.48. Osteoarthritis of the Symphysis Pubis. Sclerosis with erosion is noted at the symphysis in this ultramarathoner complaining of severe pubic pain. This is characteristic of DJD or osteoarthritis at this site in such an overuse setting. Erosions are ordinarily not seen in DJD, except in certain joints such as the symphysis pubis, sacroiliac, and the acromioclavicular.

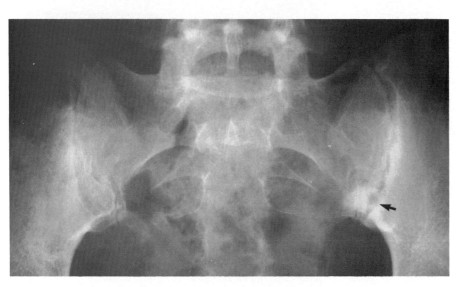

Figure 36.49. Osteoarthritis of the Sacroiliac Joint. Sclerosis and erosions (*arrow*) are seen in the left sacroiliac joint in this young, professional dancer. Although this has the appearance of an inflammatory arthritis, this is also seen in DJD or osteoarthritis secondary to overuse.

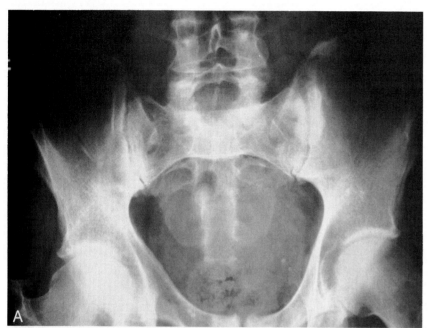

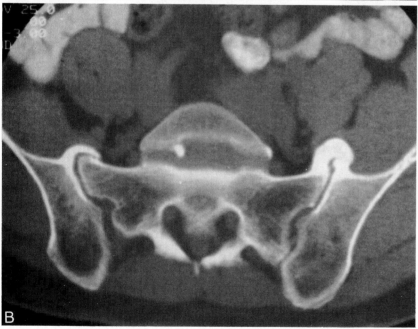

Figure 36.50.   Sacroiliac Osteophytes. A. An AP view of the pelvis in this marathoner shows dense sclerosis over both sacroiliac joints. **B.** A CT scan through this area demonstrates dense, bridging osteophytes, characteristic of DJD.

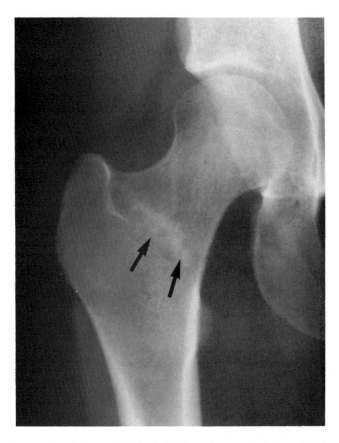

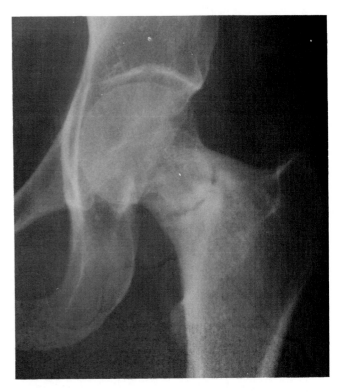

Figure 36.52.   Stress Fracture of the Femoral Neck. A linear lucency with surrounding sclerosis is seen in the femoral neck in this jogger with hip pain. This is a severe femoral neck stress fracture.

Figure 36.51.   Femoral Stress Fracture. An area of linear sclerosis (*arrows*) is seen at the base of the femoral neck in a runner with hip pain. This is diagnostic of a stress fracture of the femur. (Case courtesy of Dr. David Simms, Wichita, KS).

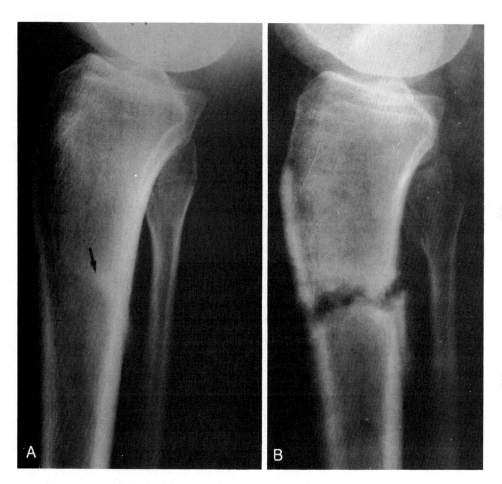

Figure 36.53. Stress Fracture of the Proximal Tibia. A. A faint linear sclerotic area (*arrow*) is seen, which is characteristic for a stress fracture of the proximal tibia. **B.** This view shows the result of continued exercise in this patient: a complete fracture of the tibia and of the proximal fibula.

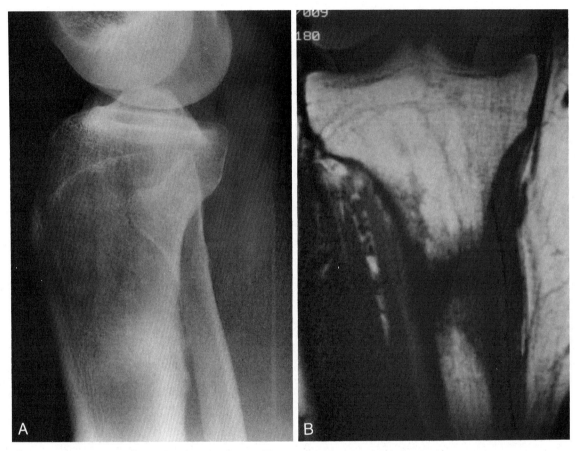

Figure 36.54. Stress Fracture of the Tibia. A. An irregular focus of sclerosis is seen in the posterior proximal tibia with adjacent periostitis. There was concern that this might represent a primary bone tumor and the surgeons recommended a biopsy. **B.** An MR scan was performed, however, which shows a linear low signal area running obliquely across the tibia on this T1-weighted coronal image, which is characteristic for a stress fracture. No significant soft-tissue mass was found. The patient's recent history included an increase in his jogging. A stress fracture was diagnosed based on these images.

under any circumstance. If the clinical presentation is unusual for a stress fracture and the plain films are not diagnostic, take additional films 1 or 2 weeks later. Computed tomography and MR sometimes will better delineate the lesion (Fig. 36.54**B**), and should show normal soft tissues. Stress fractures can be difficult to diagnose radiologically early on but should be straightforward after several weeks.

One final stress fracture that deserves mention because it is frequently misdiagnosed clinically and overlooked radiographically is the calcaneal stress fracture (Fig. 36.55). It is often clinically misdiagnosed as a "heel spur" or plantar fasciitis, and can be a somewhat subtle radiographic finding.

Hip Fracture. Overt fractures in the lower extremity are uncommonly missed on radiographs; however, a few exceptions should be noted. Hip fractures in the elderly population can be very difficult to detect (Fig. 36.56) and a high index of suspicion should be maintained. A negative plain film in an elderly patient with hip pain following trauma (even relatively mild trauma) does not exclude a femoral neck fracture. Magnetic resonance imaging has been shown to be very useful in demonstrating femoral neck fractures that are occult (Fig. 36.57).

Tibial Plateau Fracture. Another fracture that can be difficult to exclude on routine plain films is a tibial plateau fracture. A cross-table lateral plain film should be obtained in cases of knee trauma to look for

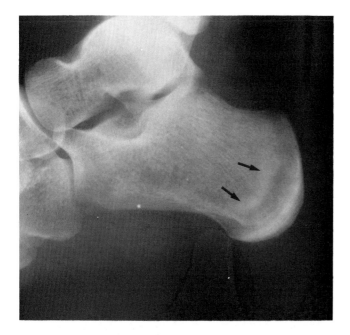

Figure 36.55.   Calcaneal Stress Fracture. A linear band of sclerosis is seen in the posterior calcaneus (*arrows*), which is diagnostic for a stress fracture of the calcaneus.

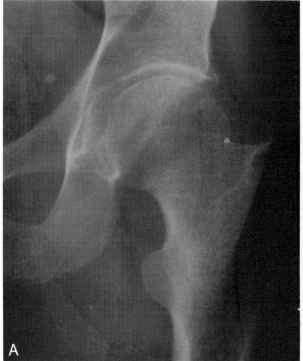
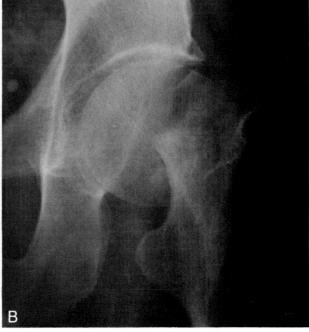

Figure 36.56.   Fracture of the Hip. A. An AP view of the hip was obtained in an elderly man following a fall. It was interpreted as normal and the patient was dismissed from the emergency department. Two weeks later the patient returned to the emergency department unable to walk and another x-ray (**B**) was obtained. It shows a complete fracture through the femoral neck. In retrospect, the fracture can be faintly seen in **A** and should have been picked up initially. Fractures of the hip in the elderly can be very difficult to see and should be diligently searched for with additional views when the clinical setting is appropriate.

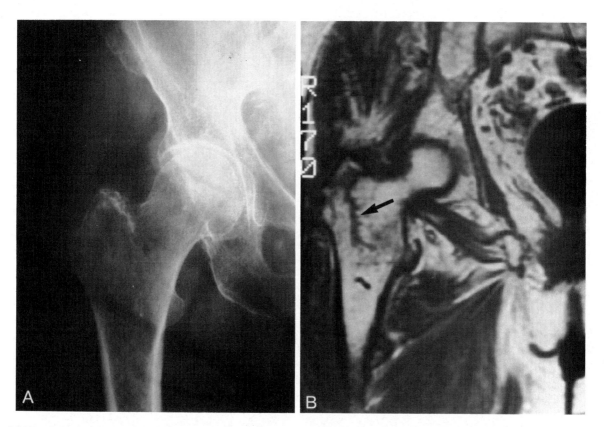

Figure 36.57.   Occult Fracture of the Hip. A. An AP plain film in an elderly patient with hip pain after a fall appears normal. **B.** A coronal T1-weighted MR was obtained because of the clinical suspicion of a fracture and shows linear low signal in the intertrochanteric region (*arrow*) confirming the fracture.

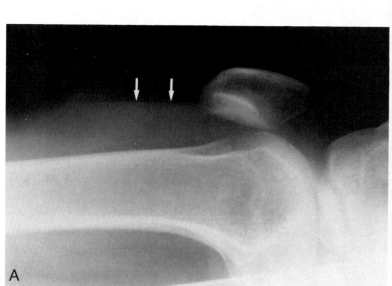

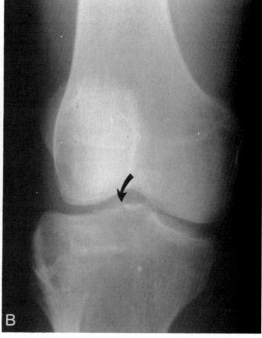

Figure 36.58.   Tibial Plateau Fracture. A. A cross-table lateral plain film of the knee reveals a fat-fluid level (*arrows*), which indicates a fracture with fatty marrow leaking into the joint. **B.** An AP view shows a barely discernible fracture (*arrow*) near the tibial spines, indicative of a tibial plateau fracture.

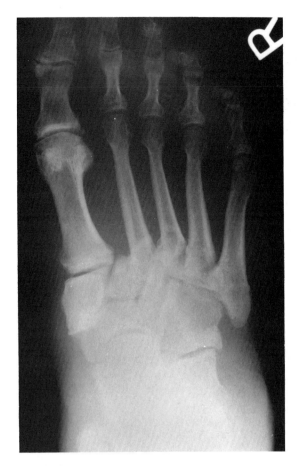

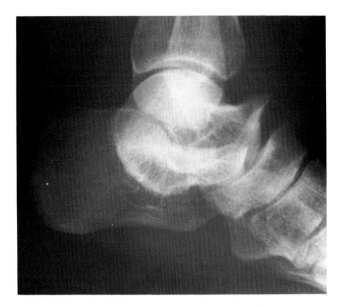

Figure 36.61. Calcaneal Fracture. Boehler's angle in this calcaneus is less than 20° which is indicative of a fracture of the calcaneus.

Figure 36.59. Lisfranc Fracture. An AP view of the foot in this patient shows a space between the first and second metatarsals with the base of the second metatarsal displaced off the second cuneiform. This is indicative of a Lisfranc fracture dislocation.

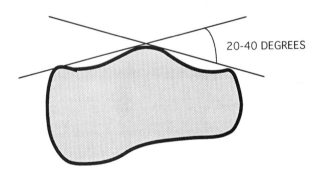

Figure 36.60. Boehler's Angle in a Normal Calcaneus. This drawing depicts the normal calcaneus with a line across the anterior process extending to the apex of the calcaneus intersecting with a line from the posterior portion of the calcaneus to the apex. This is termed Boehler's angle, and when it becomes flattened or less than 20°, a calcaneal fracture should be diagnosed.

a fat-fluid level (Fig. 36.58); this indicates a fracture that allows fatty marrow to leak into the knee joint. In the appropriate clinical setting, tomograms or CT may be necessary to make the diagnosis.

Lisfranc Fracture. A serious fracture in the foot that can be missed radiographically when little or no displacement occurs is the so-called Lisfranc fracture (Fig. 36.59). It is named after a surgeon in Napoleon's army who would do forefoot amputations in patients with gangrenous toes following frostbite. The Lisfranc fracture is a fracture-dislocation of the tarsometatarsals. If the dislocation is slight it can be easily overlooked. A key to normal alignment is that the medial border of the second metatarsal should always line up with the medial border of the second cuneiform. If it does not, a Lisfranc fracture-dislocation should be suspected. This fracture is seen most commonly in patients who catch the forefoot in something such as a hole in the ground, or a horseback rider falling and hanging by the forefoot in the stirrups. It is commonly seen as a neurotrophic or Charcot joint in diabetics.

Fracture of the calcaneus can be difficult to appreciate on routine radiographs. Boehler's angle is a normal anatomic landmark that should be looked for in every foot film when trauma has occurred (Fig. 36.60). If this angle is narrower than 20° it indicates a compression of the calcaneus, as seen in jumping injuries (Fig. 36.61).

This is a fairly simplified overview of some commonly overlooked fractures and dislocations and should not be interpreted as a substitute for the more complete texts listed in the bibliography (2, 3).

References

1. Vandemark R. Radiology of the cervical spine in trauma patients: practice pitfalls and recommendations for improving efficiency and communication. AJR 1990;155:465–472.
2. Rogers LF. Radiology of skeletal trauma. New York: Churchill Livingstone, 1982.
3. Rockwood CA Jr, Green DP, Bucholz RW. Fractures in adults. 3rd ed. Philadelphia: JB Lippincott, 1991.

37

Arthritis

Clyde A. Helms

OSTEOARTHRITIS
RHEUMATOID ARTHRITIS
HLA-B27 SPONDYLOARTHROPATHIES
CRYSTAL-INDUCED ARTHRITIS
   Gout
   Pseudogout (CPPD)
COLLAGEN-VASCULAR DISEASES
SARCOID
HEMOCHROMATOSIS
MULTICENTRIC RETICULOHISTIOCYTOSIS
NEUROPATHIC OR CHARCOT JOINT
HEMOPHILIA, JRA, AND PARALYSIS
SYNOVIAL OSTEOCHONDROMATOSIS
PIGMENTED VILLONODULAR SYNOVITIS (PVNS)
SUDECK'S ATROPHY
JOINT EFFUSIONS
AVASCULAR NECROSIS

OSTEOARTHRITIS

Osteoarthritis, or degenerative joint disease (DJD), is the most common arthritide. It is believed to be caused by trauma—either overt or as an accumulation of microtrauma over the years, although there is also an hereditary form that occurs primarily in middle-aged women called primary osteoarthritis. The hallmarks of DJD are ***joint space narrowing, sclerosis,*** and ***osteophytosis*** (Table 37.1 and Fig. 37.1). If all three of these findings are not present on the radiograph, another diagnosis should be considered. Joint space narrowing is the least specific finding of the three, yet it is virtually always present in DJD. Unfortunately, it is also seen in almost every other joint abnormality.

Sclerosis should be present in varying amounts in all cases of DJD unless severe osteoporosis is present. Osteoporosis will cause the sclerosis to be diminished. For instance, in long-standing rheumatoid arthritis in which the cartilage has been destroyed, DJD often occurs with very little sclerosis. Osteophytosis will be diminished in the setting of osteoporosis also.

Otherwise, sclerosis and osteophytosis should be prominent in DJD.

The only disorder that will cause osteophytes without sclerosis or joint space narrowing is diffuse idiopathic skeletal hyperostosis (1). This is a common bone-forming disorder that at first glance resembles DJD except there is no joint space narrowing (or disc space narrowing in the spine) and there is no sclerosis (Fig. 37.2). Diffuse idiopathic skeletal hyperostosis is not believed to be caused by trauma or stress as is DJD and is not painful or disabling as DJD can be. Millions of dollars per year are awarded to federal employees upon retirement for "disability" payments for supposed DJD acquired on their jobs when in fact they have diffuse idiopathic skeletal hyperostosis and are misdiagnosed.

Osteoarthritis is divided into two types: primary and secondary. Secondary osteoarthritis is what radiologists refer to when speaking of DJD. It is, as mentioned, secondary to trauma of some sort. It can occur in any joint in the body but is particularly common in the hands, knees, hips, and spine.

Primary osteoarthritis is a familial arthritis that affects middle-aged females almost exclusively and is seen only in the hands. It affects the distal interphalangeal joints, the proximal interphalangeal joints, and the base of the thumb in a bilaterally symmetrical fashion (Fig. 37.3). If it is not bilaterally symmetric, the diagnosis of primary osteoarthritis should be questioned.

A type of primary osteoarthritis that can be very painful and debilitating is erosive osteoarthritis. It has the identical distribution mentioned for primary osteoarthritis, but is associated with severe osteoporosis of the hands as well as erosions. It is uncommon and radiologists generally see little of this disorder. It is also called Kellgren's arthritis.

There are a few exceptions to the classic triad of findings seen in DJD (sclerosis, narrowing, and osteophytes). Several joints also exhibit erosions as a manifestation of DJD: the *temporomandibular joint*, the *acromioclavicular joint*, the *sacroiliac joints*, and the *symphysis pubis* (Table 37.2). When erosions are seen in one of these joints, DJD must be considered or inappropriate treatment may be instituted (Fig. 37.4).

Table 37.1. Hallmarks of DJD

Joint space narrowing
Sclerosis
Osteophytes

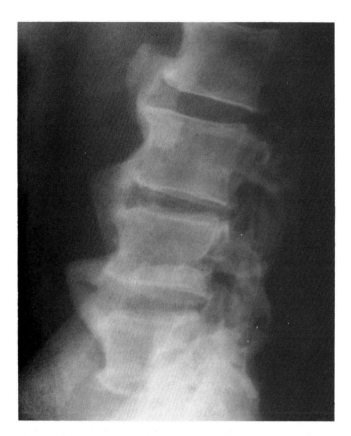

Figure 37.2. Diffuse Idiopathic Skeletal Hyperostosis. A lateral view of the lumbar spine shows extensive osteophytosis without significant disc space narrowing or sclerosis. This is a classic picture for diffuse idiopathic skeletal hyperostosis.

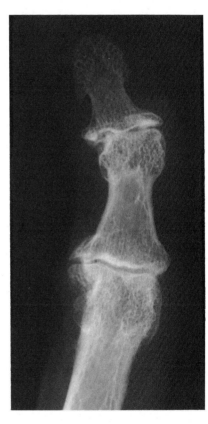

Figure 37.1. Osteoarthritis (DJD). A plain film of a finger with osteoarthritis (DJD) of the distal and proximal interphalangeal joints. Both joints demonstrate joint space narrowing, subchondral sclerosis, and osteophytosis which are hallmarks of degenerative joint disease.

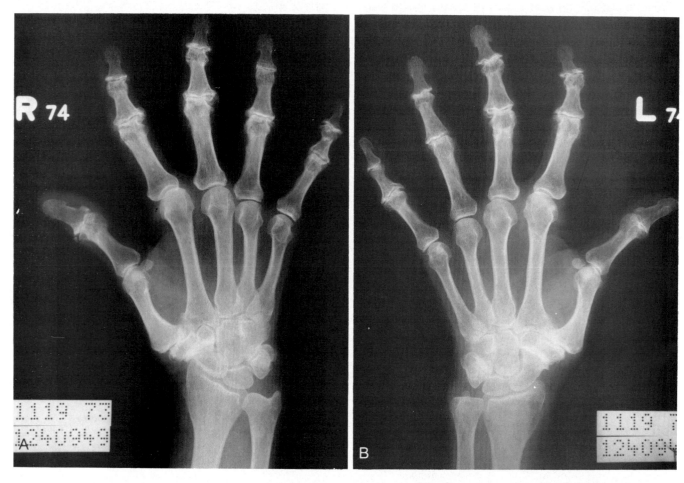

Figure 37.3.   Primary Osteoarthritis. Bilateral hand films (**A** and **B**) in a patient with primary osteoarthritis. Present are classic findings of osteophytosis, joint space narrowing and sclerosis at the distal inter- phalangeal joints, the proximal interphalangeal joints, and at the base of the thumb. This is bilaterally symmetric, which is typical for primary osteoarthritis.

A subchondral cyst, or geode (taken from the geologic term used when a volcanic rock has a gas pocket that leaves a large cavity in the rock), is often found in joints affected with DJD. Geodes are cystic formations that occur around joints in a variety of disorders (including, in addition to **DJD**, **rheumatoid arthritis**, **calcium syrophosphate dihydrate crystal deposition disease (CPPD)**, and **avascular necrosis** (Table 37.3) (2). Presumably, one method of geode formation is that synovial fluid is forced into the subchondral bone, causing a cystic collection of joint fluid. Another etiology is following a bone contusion in which the contused bone forms a cyst. They rarely cause problems by themselves but are often misdiagnosed as something more sinister (Fig. 37.5).

RHEUMATOID ARTHRITIS

Rheumatoid arthritis is a connective tissue disorder of unknown etiology that can affect any synovial

Table 37.2.   Joints That Have Erosions As a Feature of DJD

Sacroiliac
Acromioclavicular
Temporomandibular
Symphysis pubis

Table 37.3.   Diseases in Which Geodes Are Found

DJD
Rheumatoid arthritis
CPPD
AVN

joint in the body. The radiographic hallmarks are **soft-tissue swelling**, **osteoporosis**, **joint space**

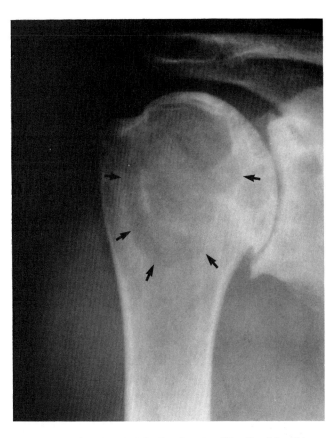

Figure 37.5.   Subchondral Cyst or Geode of the Shoulder. This patient has marked DJD of the shoulder with joint space narrowing, sclerosis, and osteophytosis. A large lytic process (*arrows*) is seen in the humeral head, which is a subchondral cyst or geode often seen in association with DJD. Because of the DJD in the shoulder, a biopsy to rule out a more sinister lesion in the humeral head should be avoided.

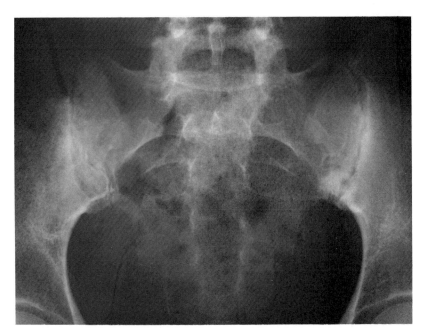

Figure 37.4. Osteoarthritis of the SI Joint. A young woman who is a professional dancer complained of left-sided hip pain. An AP film of the pelvis demonstrated left SI joint sclerosis, joint irregularity, and erosions. A complete workup to rule out an HLA B-27 spondyloarthropathy was negative and no laboratory or clinical evidence for infection was found. Her clinical history pointed to this being completely occupation-related and an aspiration biopsy to rule out infection was therefore not performed. This is not an unusual appearance for DJD of the SI joints.

narrowing, and **_marginal erosions_**. In the hands it is classically a **_proximal_** process that is **_bilaterally symmetric_** (Table 37.4 and Fig. 37.6). There are so many exceptions to these rules, however, that I have come to regard them as no better than 80% accurate. Rheumatoid arthritis has a large variety of appearances and can be very difficult to diagnose with any degree of assurance from its radiographic appearance alone.

Rheumatoid arthritis in large joints is fairly characteristic in that it causes marked joint space narrowing and is associated with osteoporosis. Erosions may or may not be present and tend to be marginal, that is, away from the weight-bearing portion of the joint. In the hip, the femoral head tends to migrate axially whereas in osteoarthritis it tends to migrate superolaterally (Figs. 37.7 and 37.8). In the shoulder, the humeral head tends to be "high-riding" (Fig. 37.9). Other things to think of when confronted with a high-riding shoulder are a torn rotator cuff and CPPD (Table 37.5).

When rheumatoid arthritis is long-standing it is not unusual for secondary DJD to superimpose itself on the findings one would expect with rheumatoid arthritis. This picture of DJD differs somewhat from that usually seen in that the sclerosis and osteophytes are considerably diminished in severity as compared with the joint space narrowing (Fig. 37.10).

HLA-B27 SPONDYLOARTHROPATHIES

A group of diseases that was formerly known as "rheumatoid variants" is now known as the seronegative, HLA-B27-positive spondyloarthropathies. These disorders are all linked to the HLA-B27 histocompatibility antigen. Included in this group of diseases are ankylosing spondylitis, inflammatory bowel disease, psoriatic arthritis, and Reiter's syndrome. They are characterized by bony ankylosis, proliferative newbone formation, and predominantly axial (spinal) involvement.

One of the more characteristic findings in these disorders is that of syndesmophytes in the spine. A syndesmophyte is a paravertebral ossification that resembles an osteophyte except that it runs vertically while an osteophyte has its orientation in a horizontal axis. Sometimes it can be difficult to decide if a particular paravertebral ossification is an osteophyte or a syndesmophyte based on its orientation alone (Fig. 37.11). Bridging osteophytes and large syndesmophytes can have a similar appearance, with both having an orientation halfway between vertical and horizontal. How should one evaluate those cases? Look at the other vertebral bodies and use the ossifications on

Table 37.4.   Hallmarks of Rheumatoid Arthritis

Soft-tissue swelling
Osteoporosis
Joint space narrowing
Marginal erosions
Proximal distribution (hands)
Bilaterally symmetric

Figure 37.6.   Rheumatoid Arthritis. An erosive arthritis affecting primarily the carpal bones and the metacarpophalangeal joints is seen that has associated osteoporosis and soft-tissue swelling (note the soft-tissue over the ulnar styloid processes). It is a bilaterally symmetric process in this patient, which is classic.

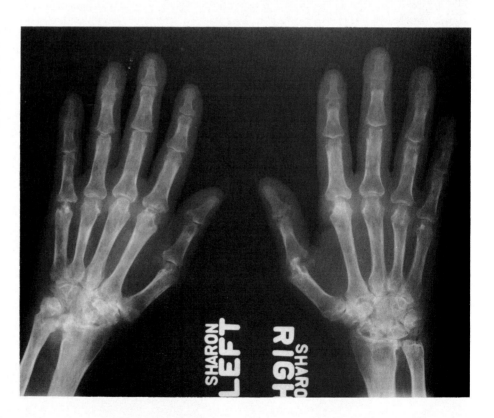

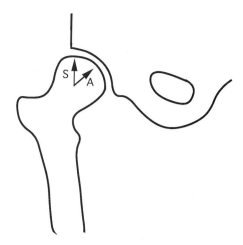

Figure 37.7. **Migration of the Femoral Head.** A drawing of the hip showing routes of migration of the femoral head. Osteoarthritis of the hip tends to cause superior (S) migration of the femoral head in relation to the acetabulum, whereas rheumatoid arthritis tends to cause axial (A) migration of the femoral head in relation to the acetabulum.

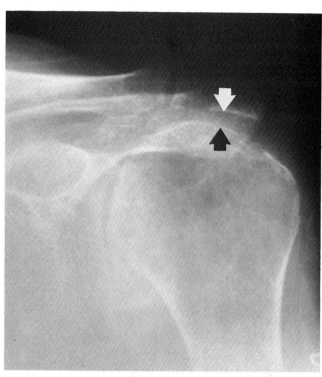

Figure 37.9. **Rheumatoid Arthritis in the Shoulder.** An AP view of the shoulder in this patient with rheumatoid arthritis shows that the distance between the acromion and the humeral head is diminished (*arrows*). Ordinarily this space is about 1 cm in width to allow the rotator cuff to pass freely beneath the acromion. This is a common finding in rheumatoid arthritis as well as CPPD.

Table 37.5. **Causes of High-riding Shoulder**

Rheumatoid arthritis
CPPD
Torn rotator cuff

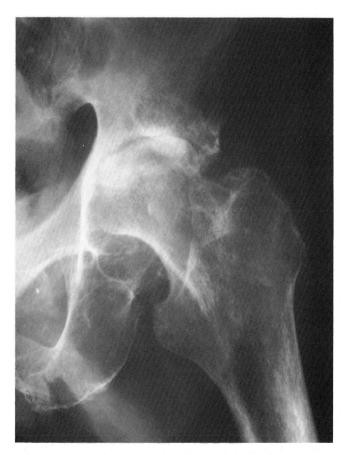

Figure 37.8. **Rheumatoid Arthritis of the Hip.** Note the severe joint space narrowing in this patient with rheumatoid arthritis. The femoral head has migrated in an axial direction with fairly concentric joint space narrowing. Minimal secondary degenerative changes have occurred as noted by the sclerosis in the superior portion of the joint; however, these have been diminished somewhat by the osteoporosis that usually accompanies rheumatoid arthritis.

them to determine if they are osteophytes or syndesmophytes. If no other level is involved, one might not be able to tell one from the other.

Syndesmophytes are classified as to whether they are marginal and symmetric or nonmarginal and asymmetric. A marginal syndesmophyte has its origin at the edge or margin of a vertebral body and extends to the margin of the adjacent vertebral body. They are invariably bilaterally symmetric as viewed on an AP spine film. Ankylosing spondylitis classically has marginal, symmetric syndesmophytes (Fig. 37.12). Inflammatory bowel disease has an identical appearance when the spine is involved. Nonmarginal, asymetric syndesmophytes are generally large and bulky. They emanate from the vertebral body away from the endplate or margin and are unilateral or asymmetric as viewed on an AP spine film (Figs. 37.11 and 37.13). Psoriatic arthritis and Reiter's syndrome classically have this type of syndesmophyte.

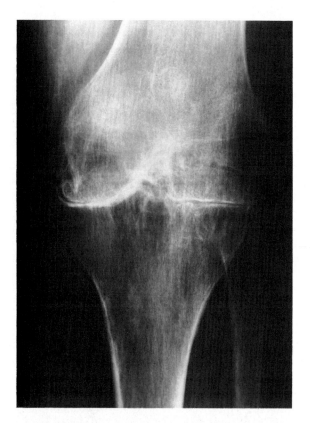

Figure 37.10.   Secondary Degenerative Disease in the Knee in a Patient with Rheumatoid Arthritis. This patient has a history of long-standing rheumatoid arthritis. An AP view of the knee shows severe osteoporosis and joint space narrowing. Secondary DJD is occurring as evidenced by the sclerosis and osteophytosis; however, these findings are out of proportion to the severe joint space narrowing. When DJD narrows a joint to this extent, the osteophytosis and sclerosis are invariably much more pronounced.

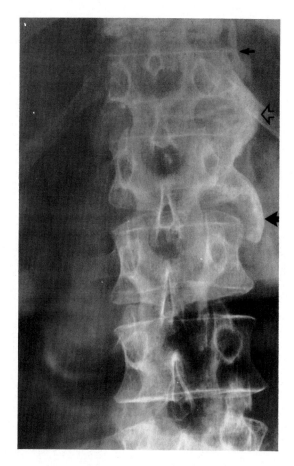

Figure 37.11. Psoriasis with Syndesmophytes. The large paravertebral ossification on the left side of the T12-L1 disc space (*open arrow*) is difficult to differentiate between an osteophyte and a syndesmophyte. Either could have this appearance. However, the paravertebral ossification at the left L1-2 disc space (*large solid arrow*) definitely has a vertical rather than a horizontal orientation, as does the faint ossification seen at the T11-T12 disc space (*small solid arrow*). These definitely represent syndesmophytes. Therefore, it makes sense to logically assume that the ossification at the T12-L1 disc space is almost certainly a syndesmophyte as well. This patient has large nonmarginal, asymmetric syndesmophytes, which are typical of psoriatic arthritis or Reiter's disease. This patient has psoriasis.

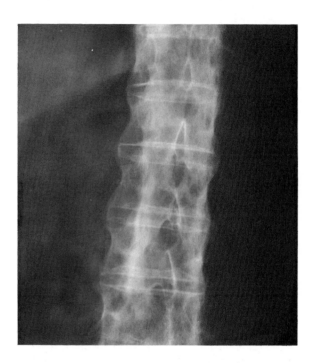

Figure 37.12. Marginal, Symmetric Syndesmopyhtes in Anky-losing Spondylitis. Bilateral marginal syndesmophytes are seen bridging the disc spaces throughout the lumbar spine in this patient. This is a so-called "bamboo spine" and is classic for ankylosing spon-dylitis and inflammatory bowel disease.

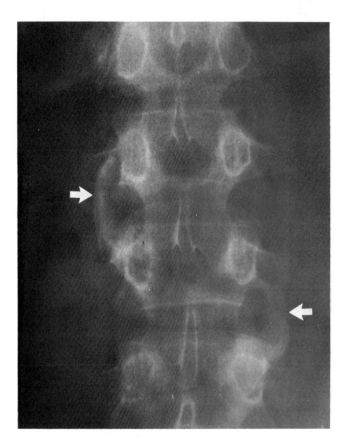

Figure 37.13. Syndesmophytes in Psoriatic Arthritis. Large, bulky, nonmarginal, asymmetric syndesmophytes (*arrows*) are seen in this patient with psoriatic arthritis.

Figure 37.14. Ankylosing Spondylitis. Bilateral symmetric, SI joint sclerosis and erosions are seen in this patient with ankylosing spondylitis. Inflammatory bowel disease could have a similar appearance. Although this is classic for these two disorders, it would not be that unusual for psoriatic disease or Reiter's syndrome to also have this appearance. Although less likely, it would be possible for infection and even DJD to be bilateral in this fashion.

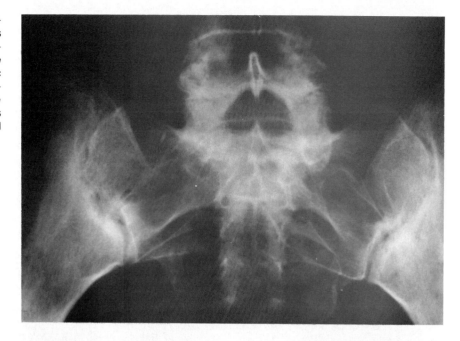

Figure 37.15. Fusion of the SI Joints in Ankylosing Spondylitis. Bilateral complete fusion of the SI joints in this patient with ankylosing spondylitis makes the SI joints totally indistinguishable. Inflammatory bowel disease could have a similar appearance.

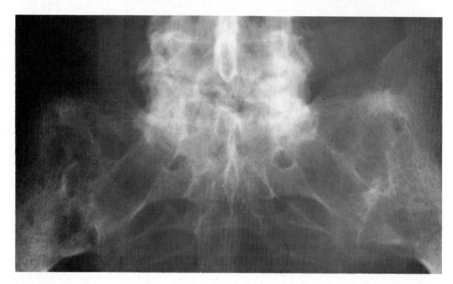

Involvement of the sacroiliac (S-I) joints is common in the HLA-B27 spondyloarthropathies. The patterns of involvement, like the patterns of involvement of the spine, are somewhat typical for each disorder. Ankylosing spondylitis and inflammatory bowel disease typically cause bilaterally symmetric SI joint disease, which is initially erosive in nature and progresses to sclerosis and fusion (Figs. 37.14 and 37.15). It is extremely unusual to have asymmetric or unilateral SI joint disease in these two disorders.

Reiter's syndrome and psoriatic arthritis can exhibit unilateral or bilateral SI joint involvement. It seems that it is bilateral about 50% of the time. It is often asymmetric when it is bilateral, but exact symmetry can be difficult to assess; therefore, when it is definitely bilateral and not clearly asymmetric, consider the SI joints to be in the bilateral symmetric cat-

egory. This means that if there is bilateral, symmetric SI joint disease it could be caused by any of the four HLA-B27 spondyloarthropathies. If there is unilateral (or clearly asymmetric) SI joint involvement, one can exclude ankylosing spondylitis and inflammatory bowel disease and consider Reiter's syndrome or psoriatic disease. In this latter example one would have to also consider infection and DJD (remember that DJD can cause erosions in the SI joints) (Table 37.6 and Figs. 37.4 and 37.16).

Computed tomography can be very helpful in examining the SI joints and is considered by many to be the diagnostic procedure of choice because of the unobstructed view of the entire joint (Fig. 37.17).

Large-joint involvement with the HLA-B27 spondyloarthropathies is uncommon (except for ankylosing spondylitis) but when it does occur, the arthropathy

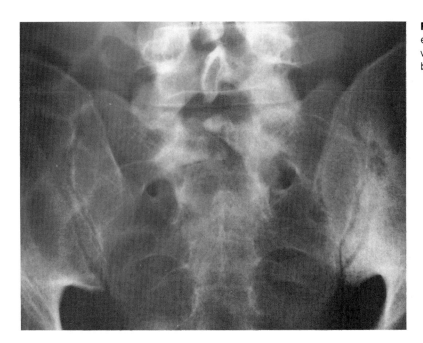

Figure 37.16. Psoriasis with SI Joint Disease. Unilateral SI sclerosis and erosions are seen in this patient with psoriasis. Ankylosing spondylitis and inflammatory bowel disease virtually never have this appearance.

Table 37.6. Causes of Sacroiliac Joint Disease

Ankylosing spondylitis
Inflammatory bowel disease
Psoriasis
Reiter's syndrome
Infection
DJD

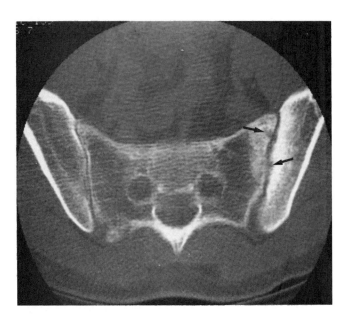

Figure 37.17. Computed Tomography of the SI Joints in Psoriasis. A computed tomography scan through the SI joints in this patient with psoriasis shows unilateral SI joint sclerosis and erosions (*arrows*), typical for psoriasis or Reiter's disease.

will resemble rheumatoid arthritis (Fig. 37.18). The hips are involved in up to 50% of the patients with ankylosing spondylitis.

Small-joint involvement, specifically in the hands and feet, is not common in ankylosing spondylitis and inflammatory bowel disease. Psoriasis causes a distinctive arthropathy that is characterized by its distal predominance, proliferative erosions, soft-tissue swelling, and periostitis. Proliferative erosions are different from the clean-cut, sharply marginated erosions seen in all other erosive arthritides in that they have fuzzy margins with wisps of periostitis emanating from them (Fig. 37.19**A**). The severe forms are often associated with bony ankylosis across joints (Fig. 37.19**B**) and arthritis mutilans deformities. A fairly common finding is a calcaneal heel spur that has fuzzy margins as opposed to the well-corticated heel spur seen in DJD or posttrauma (Fig. 37.20).

Reiter's syndrome causes identical changes in every respect to psoriasis with the exception that the hands are not as commonly involved as the feet. The interphalangeal joint of the great toe is a commonly affected location in Reiter's disease (Fig. 37.21).

CRYSTAL-INDUCED ARTHRITIS

The crystal-induced arthritides include primarily gout and pseudogout (CPPD). Ochronosis and Wilson's disease are so rare that they will not be covered.

Gout

Gout is a metabolic disorder that results in hyperuricemia and leads to monosodium urate crystals being deposited in various sites in the body, especially joint cartilage. The actual causes of the hyperuricemia are myriad and include heredity.

The arthropathy caused by gout is very characteristic radiographically. It takes 4–6 years for gout to

Figure 37.18. Ankylosing Spondylitis with Hip Disease. An AP view of the pelvis in this patient with ankylosing spondylitis shows bilateral complete fusion of the SI joints. Concentric left hip joint narrowing is present with axial migration of the femoral head. This would be a typical finding in rheumatoid arthritis or, as in this example, in ankylosing spondylitis. Note the secondary DJD changes in the left hip as well.

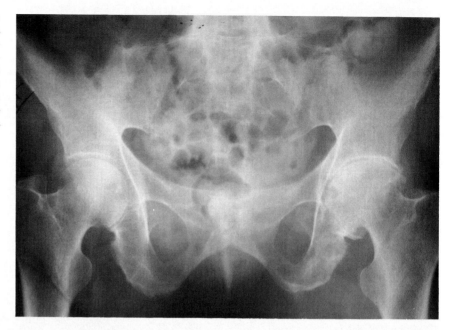

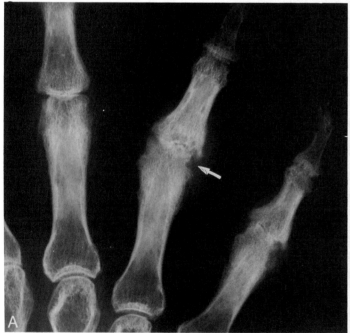

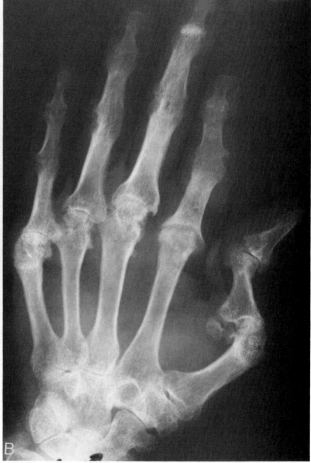

Figure 37.19. Psoriatic Arthritis. A. Cartilage loss at the proximal interphalangeal joints of the third, fourth, and fifth digits in this hand is apparent, with erosions noted most prominently in the third digit (arrow). These erosions are not sharply demarcated but are covered with fluffy new bone. These are termed "proliferative erosions." Note also the periostitis along the shafts of each of the proximal phalanges. **B.** Advanced psoriatic arthritis. Fusion or ankylosis is apparent across the proximal interphalangeal joints of the second through the fifth digits. Several of the distal interphalangeal joints are also ankylosed. Severe joint space narrowing at the metacarpophalangeal joints is noted. This distal arthridite is typical for psoriatic arthritis in advanced stages.

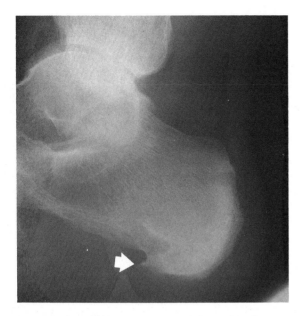

Figure 37.20. Reiter's Syndrome. A lateral view of a calcaneus in a patient with Reiter's syndrome shows poorly defined new bone on the posteroinferior margin of the calcaneus with a calcaneal spur (*arrow*) which is also poorly defined. This is typical of psoriatic or Reiter's disease as opposed to the well-formed calcaneal spur in DJD.

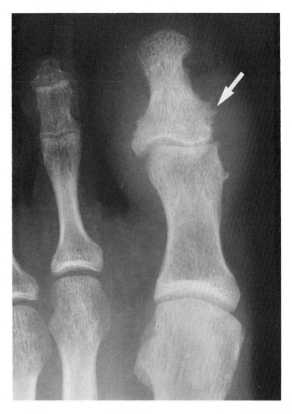

Figure 37.21. Reiter's Syndrome. An AP view of the large toe in a patient with Reiter's disease shows fluffy periostitis (*arrow*) in the erosions adjacent to the interphalangeal joint of the great toe. Marked soft-tissue swelling is also present throughout the great toe. These changes are typical in appearance and location for Reiter's disease or psoriasis.

cause radiographically evident disease and most patients are treated successfully long before the destructive arthropathy occurs; therefore, gouty arthritis is not commonly encountered.

The classic radiographic findings in gout are ***well-defined erosions***, often with sclerotic borders or overhanging edges; ***soft-tissue nodules*** that calcify in the presence of renal failure; and a ***random distribution*** in the hands ***without marked osteoporosis*** (Table 37.7 and Fig. 37.22). Even though erosions with overhanging edges occur with gout, they can occur in other disorders as well and are by no means pathognomonic. The sclerotic margins of the erosions are rarely seen in any other arthritide; therefore, this is a very useful differential point. Gout typically affects the metatarsophalangeal joint of the great toe (Fig. 37.23). In the advanced stages it can be very deforming (Fig. 37.24). Patients with gout often have chondrocalcinosis because they have a predisposition for pseudogout (CPPD). Up to 40% of the patients with gout concomitantly have CPPD.

Pseudogout (CPPD)

Calcium pyrophosphate dihydrate crystal deposition disease has a classic triad: pain, cartilage calcification, and joint destruction. The patient may have any combination of one or more of this triad at any one time. Each of these will be dealt with individually in some detail, but note that two of the three are radiographic findings. This is a disorder that is best diagnosed radiographically.

Table 37.7. Hallmarks of Gout

Well-defined erosions (sclerotic margins)
Soft-tissue nodules
Random distribution
No osteoporosis

The pain of CPPD is nonspecific. It can mimic that of gout (hence the term pseudogout) or infection or just about any arthritis. It typically is intermittent over a large number of years until DJD occurs and becomes the main cause of pain.

Cartilage calcification, known as chondrocalcinosis, can occur in any joint but tends to affect a few select sites in most patients. These are the medial and lateral compartments of the ***knee*** (Fig. 37.25), ***the triangular fibrocartilage of the wrist*** (Fig. 37.26), and the ***symphysis pubis*** (Table 37.8). Chondrocalcinosis in these areas is virtually diagnostic of CPPD (3). When CPPD crystals occur in the soft tissues, such as in the rotator cuff of the shoulder, an x-ray cannot differentiate between CPPD and calcium hydroxyapatite, which occurs in calcific tendinitis. Calcium hydroxyapatite does not occur in the joint cartilage except in extremely unusual cases; therefore,

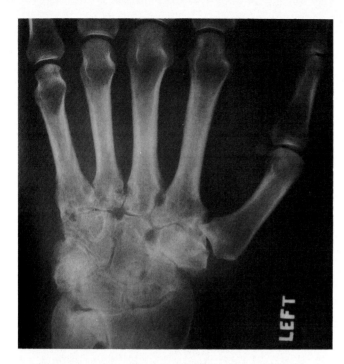

Figure 37.22. Gout. Sharply marginated erosions, some with a sclerotic margin, are noted throughout the carpus and proximal metacarpals. These erosions are classic in gout. Note the absence of marked demineralization.

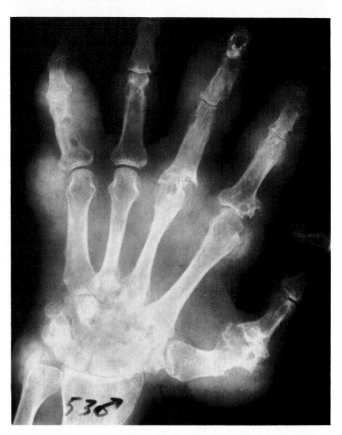

Figure 37.24. Advanced Gout. Marked diffuse and focal soft-tissue swelling is present throughout the hand and wrist in this patient with long-standing gout. Destructive, large, well-marginated erosions, some with overhanging edges, are noted near multiple joints. The focal areas of soft-tissue swelling are called tophi, some of which are calcified. These only calcify with coexistent renal disease.

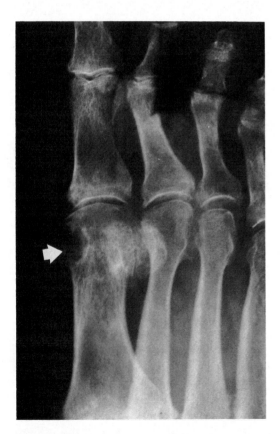

Figure 37.23. Gout. A sharply marginated erosion with an overhanging edge (*arrow*) and a sclerotic margin is seen in the metatarsophalangeal in the great toe in this patient with gout. This appearance and location are classic for gout, whereas psoriasis and Reiter's disease usually involve the interphalangeal joint and do not have erosions that are this sharply marginated.

all chondrocalcinosis can be considered to be secondary to CPPD.

The joint destruction or arthropathy is virtually indistinguishable from DJD. In fact, it *is* DJD. It is caused by CPPD crystals eroding the cartilage. There are a few features of the DJD caused by CPPD that will help distinguish it from DJD caused by trauma or overuse, however. The main difference is one of location. The CPPD has a proclivity for the ***shoulder***, the ***elbow*** (Fig. 37.27), the ***radiocarpal joint*** in the wrist (Fig. 37.28), and the ***patellofemoral joint*** of the knee (Table 37.9). These are areas not normally involved by DJD of wear and tear (such as in the distal interphalangeal joints of the hand, the hip, and the medial compartment of the knee). When DJD is seen in the joints that CPPD tends to involve, a search for chondrocalcinosis should be made. If necessary, a joint aspiration for CPPD crystals may be required to confirm the diagnosis.

Occasionally, the arthropathy of CPPD causes such severe destruction that a neuropathic or Charcot joint is mimicked on the x-ray. This has been termed a pseudo-Charcot joint. It is not a true Charcot joint because of the presence of sensation (4).

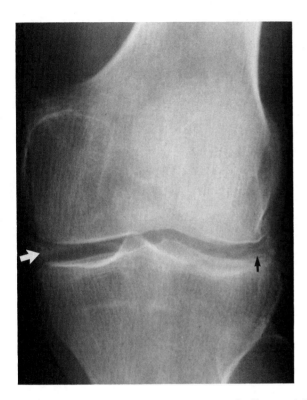

Figure 37.25. Chondrocalcinosis in the Knee. Cartilage calcification known as chondrocalcinosis is seen in the fibrocartilage (*white arrow*) and in the hyaline articular cartilage (*black arrow*) in this patient with CPPD.

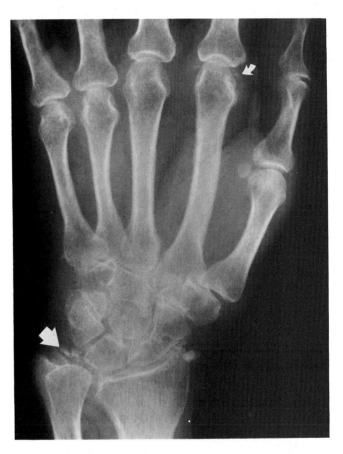

Figure 37.26. Chondrocalcinosis in the Wrist. This patient with CPPD exhibits chondrocalcinosis in the triangular fibrocartilage of the wrist (*large arrow*). A small amount of chondrocalcinosis is also seen in the second metacarpophalangeal (*small arrow*). Triangular ligament calcification is one of the more common locations for chondrocalcinosis to occur.

Table 37.8. Most Common Location of Chondrocalcinosis in CPPD

Knee
Triangular fibrocartilage of wrist
Symphysis pubis

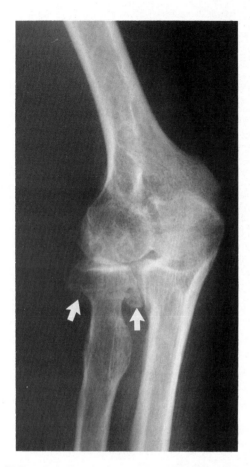

Figure 37.27.   Calcium Pyrophosphate Dihydrate Deposition Disease Arthropathy. Degenerative joint disease of the elbow is seen in this patient with CPPD. Note the joint space narrowing with minimal sclerosis and large osteophytes (*arrows*). Osteophytes of this nature are termed "drooping" osteophytes and are often seen in CPPD. The elbow is an unusual place for DJD to occur except in the setting of CPPD.

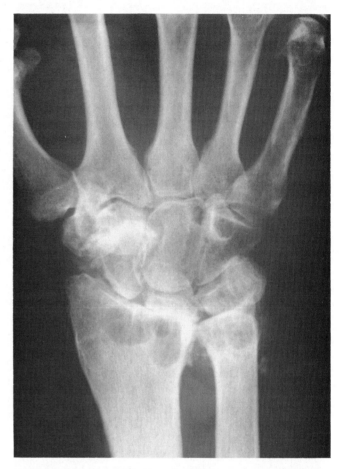

Figure 37.28.   Calcium Pyrophosphate Dihydrate Crystal Deposition Disease Arthropathy. Marked DJD at the radiocarpal joint is seen in this patient with CPPD. Severe joint space narrowing and sclerosis with large subchondral cysts or geodes are all hallmarks of DJD. This is an unusual location for DJD except in the setting of CPPD.

Table 37.9.   Most Common Location of Arthropathy in CPPD

Shoulder
Radiocarpal joint
Patellofemoral joint
Elbow

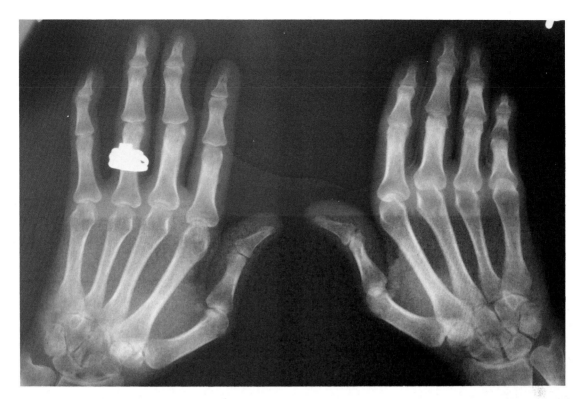

Figure 37.29. Systemic Lupus Erythematosus. Marked soft-tissue wasting, as noted by the concavity in the hypothenar eminence, with ulnar deviation of the phalanges, seen primarily in the right hand, are hallmarks of systemic lupus erythematosus.

Table 37.10. Diseases with High Association with CPPD

Primary hyperparathyroidism
Gout
Hemochromatosis

There are three diseases that have a high degree of association with CPPD. These are ***primary hyperparathyroidism***, ***gout***, and ***hemochromatosis*** (Table 37.10). This is not a differential diagnosis for chondrocalcinosis. These are diseases that tend to occur at the same time that CPPD occurs. If the patient has one of these three disorders he or she is more likely to have CPPD than is a nonaffected person. There is probably no good reason to work up every patient with chondrocalcinosis for one of the three associated diseases since they are so uncommon and CPPD is extremely common.

COLLAGEN-VASCULAR DISEASES

Scleroderma, systemic lupus erythematosus, dermatomyositis, and mixed connective tissue disease are all grouped together as collagen-vascular diseases. The striking abnormality in the hands in each of these disorders is osteoporosis and soft-tissue wasting. Systemic lupus erythematosus characteristically has severe ulnar deviation of the phalanges (Fig. 37.29). Erosions are generally not a feature of these disorders. Soft-tissue calcifications are typically present in scleroderma (Fig. 37.30) and dermatomyositis. The calcifications in scleroderma are typically subcutaneous, whereas in dermatomyositis they are intramuscular in location. Mixed connective tissue disease is an overlap of scleroderma, systemic lupus erythematosus, polymyositis, and rheumatoid arthritis. It has a myriad of radiographic findings.

SARCOID

Sarcoidosis is a disease that causes deposition of granulomatous tissue in the body, primarily in the lungs, but also in the bones. In the skeletal system it has a predilection for the hands where it causes lytic destructive lesions in the cortex. These often have a so-called "lace-like" appearance, which is characteristic (Fig. 37.31). It can have associated skin nodules in the hands.

HEMOCHROMATOSIS

Hemochromatosis is a disease of excess iron deposition in tissues throughout the body leading to fibrosis and eventual organ failure. Twenty to 50% of patients with hemochromatosis have a characteristic arthropathy in the hands that should suggest the diagnosis. The classic radiographic changes are essentially DJD, which involves the second through the fourth metacarpophalangeal joints (Fig. 37.32). Up to 50% of the patients with hemochromatosis also have

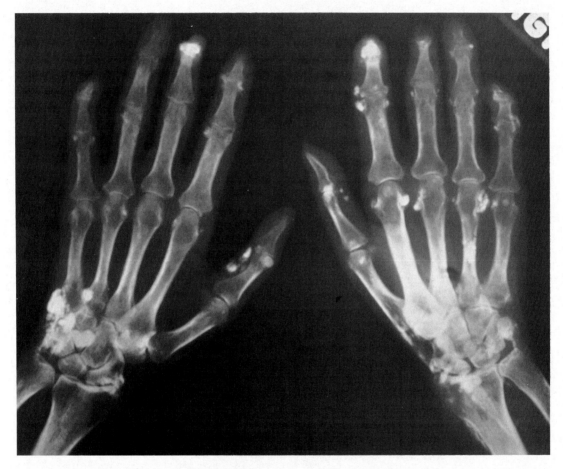

Figure 37.30.   Scleroderma. Diffuse subcutaneous soft-tissue calcification is seen throughout the hands and wrists in this patient with scleroderma. Soft-tissue wasting and osteoporosis are also present, as well as bone loss in multiple distal phalanges secondary to the vascular abnormalities often present in this disease.

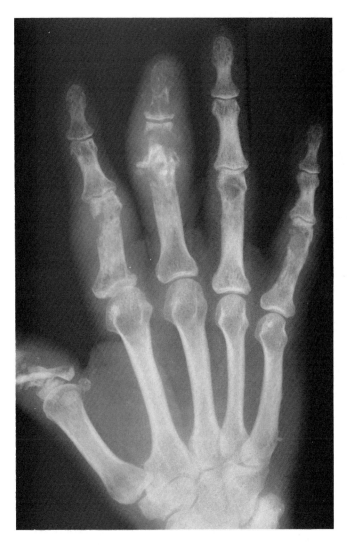

Figure 37.31. Sarcoid. An AP view of the hand in this patient with sarcoid demonstrates classic changes of bony involvement with this granulomatous process. Note the "lace-like" pattern of destruction seen most prominently in the proximal phalanges and in the distal third phalanx. Soft-tissue swelling and some areas of severe bony dissolution are also noted, which occur in more advanced patterns of sarcoid. These changes are typically limited to the hands but can rarely occur in other parts of the skeleton.

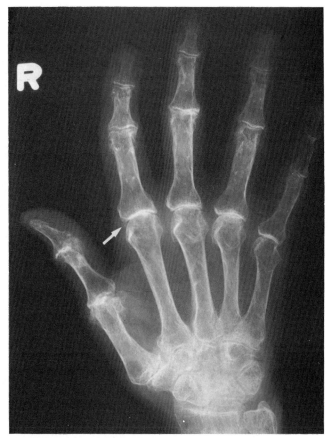

Figure 37.32. Hemochromatosis. An AP view of the hand in this patient with hemochromatosis shows severe joint space narrowing throughout the hand, which is most marked at the metacarpophalangeal joints. Associated sclerosis at the metacarpophalangeal joints with large osteophytes seen off the metacarpal heads suggests DJD. These are very unusual joints for DJD to occur in, yet this is the classic appearance of hemochromatosis. No chondrocalcinosis is seen in the triangular cartilage in this patient; hovever, a small amount of chondrocalcinosis can be seen at the second metacarpophalangeal (*arrow*). Fifty percent of patients with hemochromatosis also have CPPD.

Figure 37.33. Multicentric Reticulohistiocytosis. An AP view of the hand in this patient reveals multiple soft-tissue nodules seen best in the second digits bilaterally with diffuse erosions that are sharply demarcated and strikingly bilaterally symmetric. There is little or no osteoporosis. These changes are classic for multicentric reticulohistiocytosis.

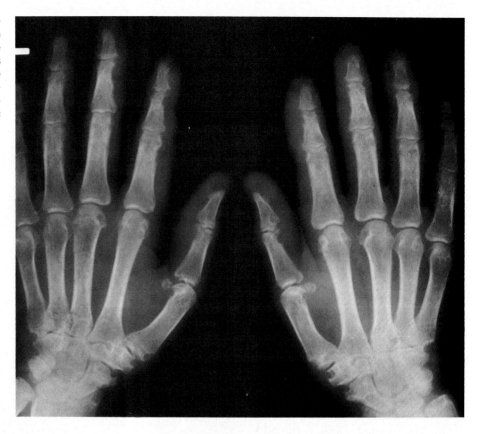

Table 37.11. Hallmarks of a Neuropathic Joint

Joint destruction
Dislocation
Heterotopic new bone formation

CPPD; therefore, a search should be made for chondrocalcinosis. Another finding that is often seen in hemochromatosis is called "squaring" of the metacarpal heads. They appear enlarged and block-like as a result of the large osteophytes commonly seen in this disorder. The osteophytes are often said to be "drooping" because of the unusual way they hang off the joint margin.

MULTICENTRIC RETICULOHISTIOCYTOSIS

Multicentric reticulohistiocytosis is a very rare disorder that is also called lipoid dermatoarthritis. It is a disease of cutaneous xanthomas that are associated with a mutilating arthritis of the hands, which is very characteristic (5). Multiple erosions, predominantly in the phalanges, are found that are strikingly bilaterally symmetric and not associated with osteoporosis (Fig. 37.33). Rheumatoid arthritis usually is mentioned in the differential diagnosis because of the erosions and bilateral symmetry; however, the distal distribution and lack of osteoporosis are against rheumatoid. Multicentric reticulohistiocytosis can proceed to an arthritis mutilans or can spontaneously arrest.

NEUROPATHIC OR CHARCOT JOINT

The radiographic findings for a Charcot joint are characteristic and almost pathognomonic. A classic triad has been described that consists of *joint destruction*, *dislocation*, and *heterotopic new bone* (Table 37.11 and Fig. 37.34).

Joint destruction is seen in every type of arthritis and therefore seems very nonspecific; however, nothing causes as severe destruction in a joint as a Charcot joint. Progressive joint destruction occurs in a neuropathic joint because the joint is rendered unstable by inaccurate muscle action and is unprotected by intact nerve reflexes. Early in the development of a Charcot joint, the joint destruction may merely appear to be joint space narrowing. It is extremely difficult to make the diagnosis this early. In the spine, instead of joint space destruction there is disc space destruction (Fig. 37.35).

Dislocation, like joint destruction, can be present in varying degrees. Early on the joint may have subluxation instead of dislocation.

Heterotopic new bone has also been termed "debris" or "detritus" and consists of soft-tissue calcification or clumps of ossification adjacent to the joint. It too can be present in varying amounts.

The most commonly seen Charcot joint today is in the foot of a diabetic. The disease typically affects the first and second tarsometatarsal joints in a fashion similar to a Lisfranc fracture (Fig. 37.36).

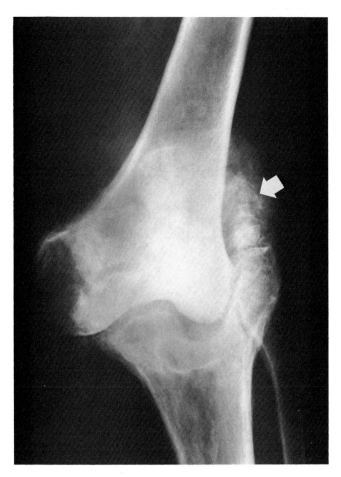

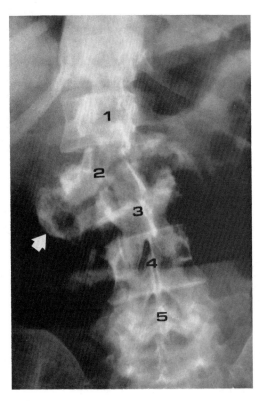

Figure 37.35.   Charcot Spine. An AP view of the spine in this para-plegic patient shows severe destruction of the L-2 and L-3 vertebral bodies and the intervening disc space, heterotopic new bone (*arrow*), and malalignment or dislocaton. Numbers indicate lumbar vertebrae.

Figure 37.34.   Charcot Joint. An AP view of the knee in this patient with tabes dorsalis shows the classic changes of a neuropathic or Charcot joint. Note the severe joint destruction, the subluxation, and the heterotopic new bone (*arrow*).

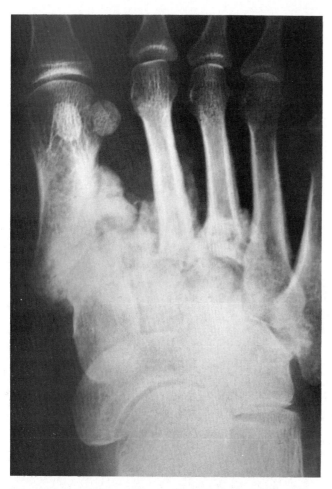

Figure 37.36.   Lisfranc Charcot Joint. Dislocation of the second and third metatarsals along with joint destruction and large amounts of heterotopic new bone are present in the foot of this diabetic patient. These findings are classic for a Charcot joint, which has been termed a Lisfranc fracture-dislocation. It is most commonly seen secondary to trauma rather than as a Charcot joint but is the most common neuropathic joint seen today.

Tabes dorsalis from syphilis is rarely seen today. More commonly seen is a Charcot joint in a patient with paralysis who continues to use the affected limb for support. A Charcot joint that is also seen on occasion is the so-called pseudo-Charcot joint in CPPD.

HEMOPHILIA, JUVENILE RHEUMATOID ARTHRITIS, AND PARALYSIS

Why would clinically disparate entities like paralysis, juvenile rheumatoid arthritis (JRA), and hemophilia be covered in the same section? Because they are usually radiographically indistinguishable.

The classic findings for JRA and hemophilia are **overgrowth of the ends of the bones** (epiphyseal enlargement) associated with **gracile diaphyses** (Fig. 37.37). Joint destruction may or may not be present. A finding that is purported to be classic for JRA and hemophilia is widening of the intercondylar

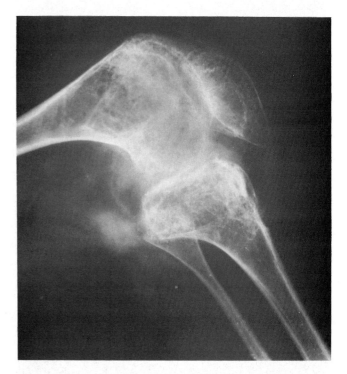

Figure 37.37.   Juvenile Rheumatoid Arthritis. A lateral view of the knee in this patient with JRA shows the classic findings of overgrowth of the ends of the bones and associated gracile diaphyses. These changes can also be seen in hemophilia or paralysis patients.

notch of the knee. This sign can be quite variable and difficult to use. It is rarely present when the other classic signs are not also present and obvious.

Another process that can mimic the findings in JRA and hemophilia is a joint that has undergone disuse from paralysis (Fig. 37.38). It has always been said that the reason the epiphyses are overgrown in JRA and hemophilia is because of the hyperemia; however, many other things cause hyperemia without affecting the size of the epiphyses (such as rheumatoid arthritis and infection). The thing that JRA, hemophilia, and paralysis all have in common is disuse. This is most likely what causes the overgrowth of the ends of the bones seen in all three of these disorders.

SYNOVIAL OSTEOCHONDROMATOSIS

Synovial osteochondromatosis is a relatively common disorder caused by a metaplasia of the synovium, resulting in deposition of foci of cartilage in the joint. Most of the time these cartilaginous deposits calcify and are readily seen on an x-ray (Fig. 37.39). It is most commonly seen in the knee, hip, and elbow. Up to 30% of the time the cartilaginous deposits do not calcify. In these cases all that is seen on the x-ray is a joint effusion, unless erosions or joint destruction occurs (Fig. 37.40).

The calcifications begin in the synovium and then tend to shed into the joint where they can cause symptoms of free fragments or "joint mice." They then em-

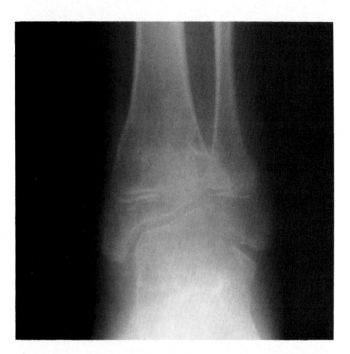

Figure 37.38.   Muscular Dystrophy Simulating JRA or Hemophilia. An AP view of the ankle in this patient with muscular dystrophy shows subtle changes of overgrowth of the distal tibia and fibular epiphyses. Marked tibiotalar slant, which can also be present in JRA or hemophilia, is also present.

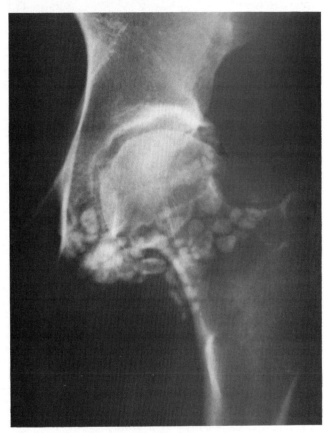

Figure 37.39.   Synovial Osteochondromatosis. An AP view of the hip in this patient with left hip pain shows multiple calcified loose bodies in the hip joint, which is virtually diagnostic of synovial osteochondromatosis.

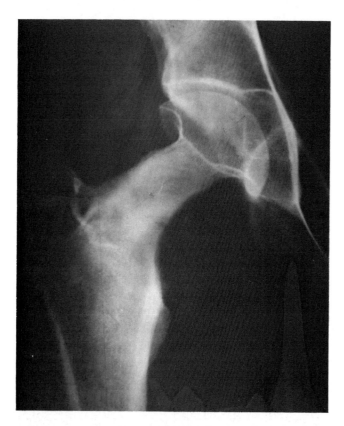

Figure 37.40.   Synovial Osteochondromatosis without Calcification. An AP view of the hip in this patient shows the femoral neck to be eroded with the femoral head having an "apple core" appearance. This has occurred from the pressure erosion of multiple nonossified loose bodies in the joint. This is nonossified synovial osteochondromatosis (which is probably more properly termed "synovial chondromatosis"). It usually does not cause this degree of bony erosion and is indistinguishable from pigmented villonodular synovitis.

bed into the synovium and tend not to be free in the joint after a while. It is usually necessary to perform a complete synovectomy to relieve the symptoms.

PIGMENTED VILLONODULAR SYNOVITIS

Pigmented villonodular synovitis is a rare, chronic, inflammatory process of the synovium that causes synovial proliferation. A swollen joint with lobular masses of synovium occurs and causes pain and joint destruction (Fig. 37.41). It rarely, if ever, calcifies. It has been termed "giant cell tumor of tendon sheath and tendon sheath xanthoma" when it occurs in a tendon sheath, which is not unusual. Joints with PVNS look radiographically identical to noncalcified synovial osteochondromatosis, yet they are much less common. Therefore, whenever pigmented villonodular synovitis is a consideration, mention synovial osteochondromatosis (noncalcified). Pigmented villonodular synovitis has a characteristic appearance on magnetic resonance imaging (MR) with low-signal hemosiderin seen lining the synovium on both T1- and T2- weighted images (Fig. 37.42).

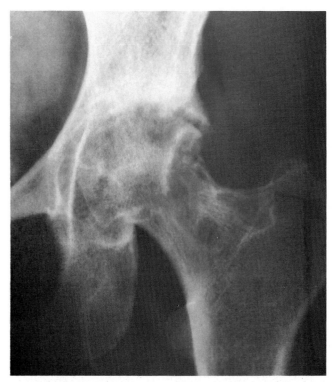

Figure 37.41.   Pigmented Villonodular Synovitis. An AP view of the hip in this patient shows joint space destruction and bony erosions throughout the femoral head and neck. Pigmented villonodular synovitis or synovial chondromatosis could have this appearance.

SUDECK'S ATROPHY

Also known as shoulder-hand syndrome and reflex sympathetic dystrophy, Sudeck's atrophy is a poorly understood joint affliction that typically occurs after minor trauma to an extremity, resulting in pain, swelling, and dysfunction. Severe, patchy osteoporosis and soft-tissue swelling are seen radiographically (Fig. 37.43). It typically affects the distal part of an extremity such as a hand or foot, yet intermediate joints such as the knee and hip are believed by some to occasionally be involved. The pain usually subsides but the osteoporosis may persist. The swelling, with time, will subside and the skin may become atrophic. It is important for the radiologist to recognize the aggressive osteoporosis in this disorder and differentiate it from disuse osteoporosis so the treating physician can begin aggressive physical therapy.

JOINT EFFUSIONS

Most joint effusions are clinically obvious and do not require radiographic validation. The elbow is an exception. In the setting of trauma to the elbow an effusion indicates a fracture. The radiographic signs of an elbow effusion are generally clearly seen (displaced fat pads, as described in Chapter 36) and have proven to be valid. Clinical determination of an elbow effu-

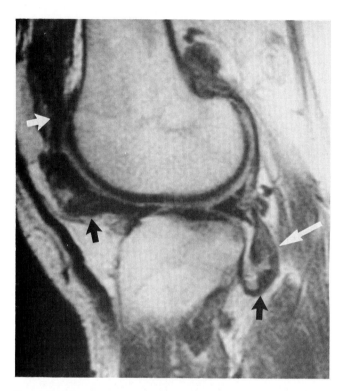

Figure 37.42.   Pigmented Villonodular Synovitis. A sagittal T2-weighted MR (TR 1500; TE 60) in a knee with pigmented villonodular synovitis shows low signal masses of tissue in the joint (*arrows*) with only a small amount of high signal joint fluid visible. This is a characteristic appearance of pigmented villonodular synovitis with MR.

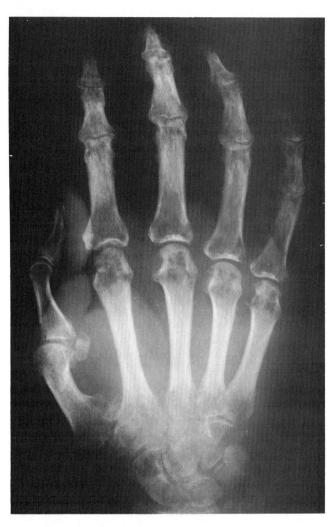

Figure 37.43.   Sudeck's Atrophy. Diffuse soft-tissue swelling and marked osteoporosis that is so aggressive it has a spotty or permeative appearance is noted around all of the joints in the hand. This patient has severe hand pain and dysfunction following minor trauma. This is characteristic of Sudeck's atrophy.

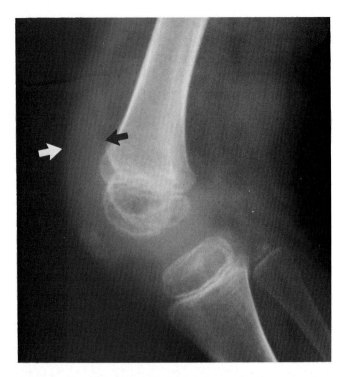

Figure 37.44.   Knee Joint Effusion. This patient has joint fluid in the knee, with widely displaced fat pads. The suprapatellar fat pad (*white arrow*) is more than 5 mm from the anterior suprafemoral fat pad (*black arrow*), which indicates a joint effusion. The suprapatellar fat pad is difficult to see in this example.

sion can be difficult; therefore, the radiologist can be very helpful in this area.

Clinical determination of a hip effusion is also very difficult. The presence of a hip effusion can be valuable in certain clinical settings. For instance, a patient with pain in the hip and an effusion should have the joint aspirated to rule out an infection. If only pain were present, an aspiration would probably not be performed. The radiology literature mentions displacement of the fat stripes about the hip as being an indicator for an effusion, but this has been proved to be unfounded. The only fat pad around the hip that gets displaced with an effusion is the obturator internus, and it is uncommonly seen.

The radiographic sign for a knee effusion that seems to be the most reliable is the measurement of the distance between the suprapatellar fat pad and the anterior femoral fat pad (Fig. 37.44). A distance between these two fat pads of more than 10 mm is definite evidence for an effusion. A distance of less than 5 mm is normal. A distance of 5–10 mm is equivocal. It does not make any difference if there is an effusion in the knee—the patient gets treated the same, regardless. If it were vital to the patient one could aspirate the joint or perform an MR study to find out. I should point out that an MR should never be performed just to see if there is fluid in the joint.

Shoulder effusions are very difficult to detect unless they are massive enough to displace the humeral head inferiorly, as with a fracture and hemarthrosis (see Chapter 36). Fortunately, as with most other joints, treatment is not based solely on the presence or absence of an effusion, so it hardly matters. The same is true in the ankle, wrist, and smaller joints.

AVASCULAR NECROSIS

Avascular necrosis (AVN), or aseptic necrosis, can occur around almost any joint for a host of reasons including steroids, trauma, a variety of underlying disease states, and even idiopathically. It is often seen in renal transplant patients.

The hallmark of AVN is increased bone density at an otherwise normal joint. Increased density at a narrowed joint usually indicates DJD; however, if either osteophytes or joint space narrowing are absent, another disorder should be considered.

The earliest sign of AVN is a joint effusion. This often is not visible radiographically or is so nonspecific that it does not help with the diagnosis unless the clinical setting had already raised suspicion for AVN. The next sign for AVN is a patchy or mottled density (Fig. 37.45). In the knee this density increase can occur throughout an entire condyle, while in the hip it often involves the entire femoral head. Next, a subchondral lucency develops that forms a thin line along the articular surface (Fig. 37.46). This lucent line has been described as being an early indicator for AVN when in fact it is a late finding. Also, the lucent line stage is often not present in the evolution of AVN. Therefore, using the lucent line as one of the main criteria for AVN can lead to missing early findings in some cases and missing the diagnosis completely in others.

The final sign in AVN is collapse of the articular surface and joint fragmentation (Fig. 37.47). I must stress that these changes all occur on only one side of a joint, which makes for an easy diagnosis since almost everything else around joints involves both sides of the joint.

Magnetic resonance imaging is extremely useful in evaluating AVN. It is the most sensitive imaging study available, often showing AVN when plain films or radionuclide scans are normal (6). In the hip AVN typically has an area of low or mixed signal on T1-weighted images that is located in the anterosuperior portion of the femoral head (Figs. 37.48 and 37.49). If the anterior portion of the femoral head is not involved, the diagnosis of AVN should be questioned, as it is very rare to present otherwise.

A form of AVN that is smaller and more focal than that just described is osteochondritis dissecans. It is believed to be caused by trauma, although others believe it is primarily idiopathic. It occurs most often in

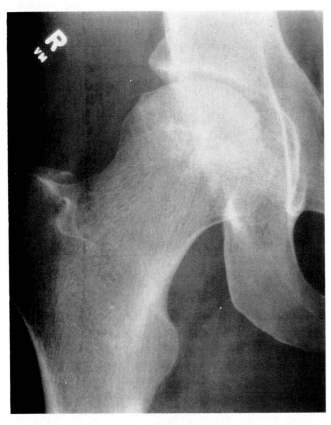

Figure 37.45. Early Avascular Necrosis of the Hip. Patchy sclerosis is present in the femoral head in this patient with a renal transplant and avascular necrosis of the right hip. No subchondral lucency or articular surface irregularity in the weight-bearing region is yet present, with the exception of a small cortical irregularity seen laterally.

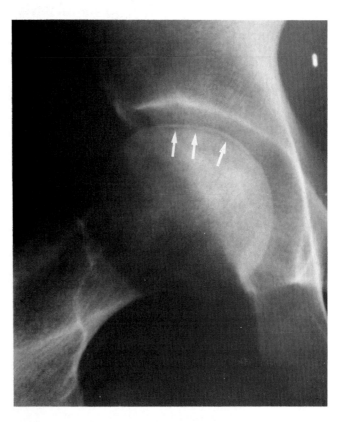

Figure 37.46. Avascular Necrosis of the Hip. A definite subchondral lucency (*arrows*) is seen in the weight-bearing portion of this hip with AVN. Patchy sclerosis throughout the femoral head is also noted.

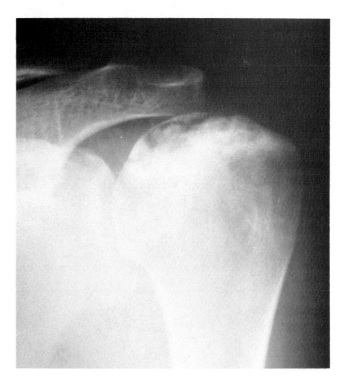

Figure 37.47. Avascular Necrosis of the Shoulder. Articular surface collapse is present in this shoulder with long-standing AVN. Dense bony sclerosis is also present.

Figure 37.48. Avascular Necrosis of the Hip. An axial T1-weighted image (TR 600; TE 20) of the hips shows a focal area of abnormality in the left femoral head (*arrow*), which is characteristic for AVN. The low signal serpigenous border is a typical finding, as is the anterior location.

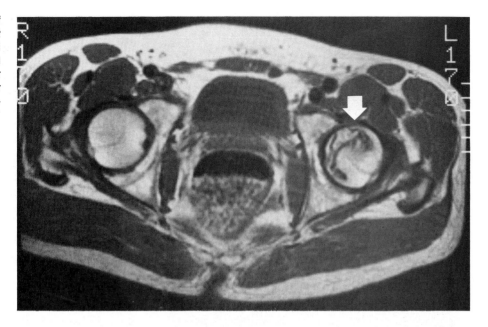

Figure 37.49.   Avascular Necrosis of the Hip. A coronal T1-weighted image (**A**) (TR 600; TE 20) and a coronal GRASS image (**B**) (TR 500; TE 15; θ 15°) show bilateral AVN that is more advanced in the left hip. The T1-weighted image (**A**) shows diffuse low signal intensity in the femoral necks which increases on the GRASS T2* image (**B**). This is typical for edema or hyperemia seen in AVN. Note the bilateral joint effusions seen as high signal on the T2* image (**B**).

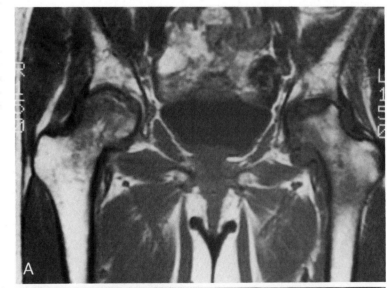

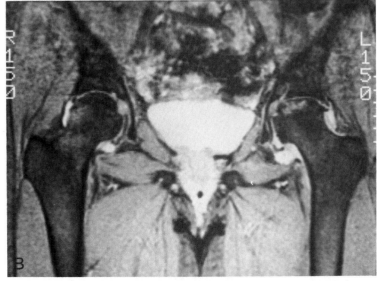

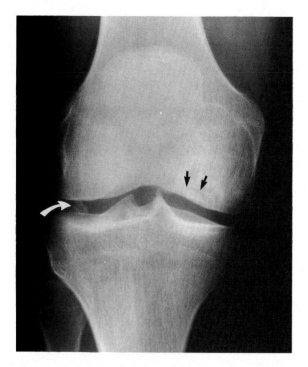

Figure 37.50.   Osteochondritis Dissecans. A small focal area of avascular necrosis in the medial epicondyle of the femur (*black arrows*) is present, which is an area of osteochondritis dissecans. Part of the area of AVN has shed a bony fragment (*white arrow*) that is loose in the joint, which is known as a joint mouse.

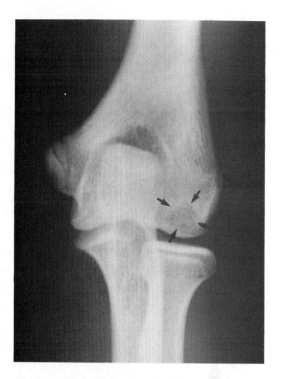

Figure 37.52.   Osteochondritis Dissecans of the Elbow. The third most common site for osteochondritis dissecans is in the capitellum of the elbow. The faint lucency seen in this capitellum (*arrows*) was at first believed to be a chondroblastoma or an area of infection.

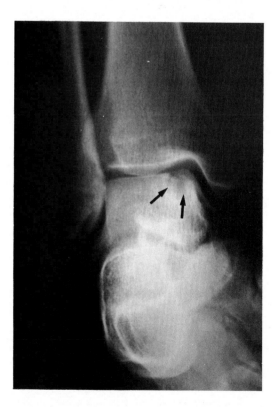

Figure 37.51.   Osteochondritis Dissecans of the Talus. A focal area of AVN in the talus as seen here (*arrows*) is called osteochondritis dissecans. The talus is the second most common site after the knee and, as in the knee, can cause a joint mouse, or loose body in the joint.

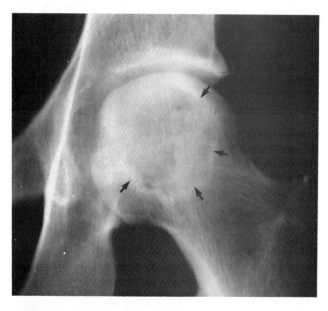

Figure 37.53.   Geode in the Hip. A large cystic lesion (*arrows*) is seen in this patient with AVN of the hip. Note the adjacent patchy sclerosis, indicative of avascular necrosis. A subchondral cyst or geode should be considered any time a lytic lesion is found around a joint.

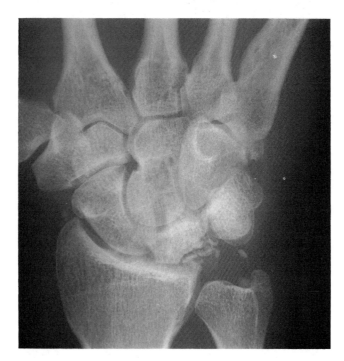

Figure 37.54. Kienbock's Malacia. Avascular necrosis of the lunate, Kienbock's malacia, is demonstrated in this patient's wrist. The increased density and partial fragmentation of the lunate are characteristic for AVN. Also, note the slightly shortened ulna (in comparison with the radius), which is called negative ulnar variance. Negative ulnar variance is said to have a high association with Kienbock's malacia.

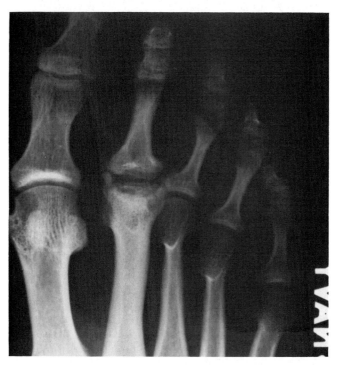

Figure 37.56. Freiberg's Infraction. Flattening, collapse, and sclerosis of the second metatarsal head, as seen in this patient, is typical of AVN or Freiberg's infraction. It can also involve the second, third, or fourth metatarsal heads. Note the compensatory hypertrophy of the cortex of the second metatarsal, which is invariably found with this disorder.

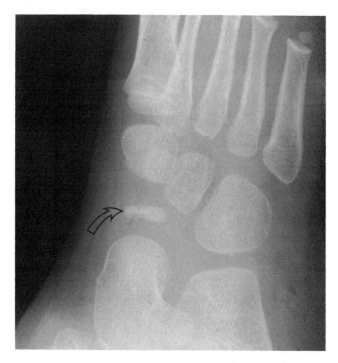

Figure 37.55. Kohler's Disease. Flattening and sclerosis of the tarsal navicular (*arrow*) in children is thought by many to be AVN and is called Kohler's disease. Others have found this to be an asymptomatic normal variant bone and believe that it is an incidental finding.

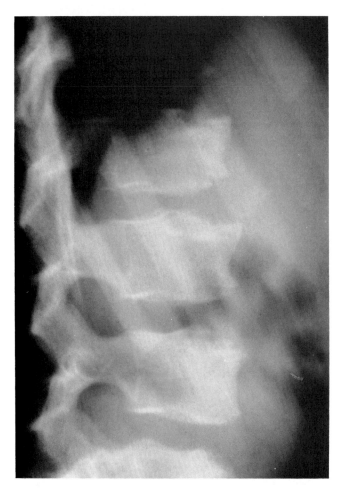

Figure 37.57. Scheuermann's Disease. Avascular necrosis of the apophyseal rings of the vertebral bodies is called Scheuermann's disease. He originally described a painful kyphosis with multiple vertebral bodies involved. It is most commonly seen without kyphosis or pain and with only a few vertebral bodies involved.

the knee at the medial epicondyle (Fig. 37.50). It also is frequently seen in the dome of the talus (Fig. 37.51) and occasionally in the capitellum (Fig. 37.52). Osteochondritis dissecans frequently leads to a small fragment of bone being sloughed off and becoming a free fragment in the joint, a "joint mouse" (Fig. 37.50).

Avascular necrosis is one of the disorders around joints in which subchondral cysts or geodes can occur. It is the only one of the four disorders (rheumatoid arthritis, DJD, and CPPD being the others) that can have an essentially normal joint and have a geode (Fig. 37.53). The other abnormalities will have joint space narrowing and/or osteophytes, osteoporosis, chondrocalcinosis, or other findings.

A host of names have been ascribed to epiphyseal avascular necrosis, usually with the eponym being the first person to describe the disorder. These are believed to be idiopathic for the most part, but can also occur secondary to trauma. A few of the more common epiphyses involved are the following: the carpal lunate, Kienbock's malacia (Fig. 37.54); the tarsal na-

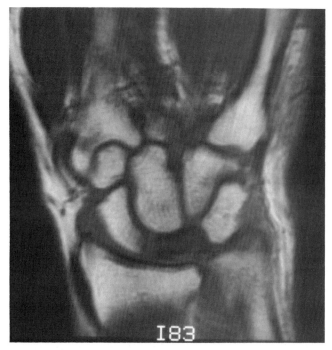

Figure 37.58. Kienbock's Malacia. A T1-weighted (TR 600; TE 20) coronal MR of the wrist shows low signal throughout the lunate, which is characteristic for AVN of the lunate, Kienbock's malacia.

vicular, Kohler's disease (Fig. 37.55); the metatarsal heads, Freiberg's infraction (Fig. 37.56); the femoral head, Legg-Perthe's disease; the ring epiphyses of the spine, Scheurmann's disease (Fig. 37.57); and the tibial tubercle, Osgood-Schlatter's disease, also called surfer's knees. Magnetic resonance imaging can be very useful in identifying AVN in these sites. It shows diffuse low signal on T1-weighted images that involves the entire area of avascular necrosis (Fig. 37.58).

References

1. Resnick D, Shaul S, Robins J. Diffuse idiopathic skeletal hyperostosis with extraspinal manifestations. Radiology 1975;115:513–524.
2. Resnick D, Niwayama G, Coutts R. Subchondral cysts (geodes) in arthritic disorders: pathologic and radiographic appearance of the hip joint. AJR 1977;128:799–806.
3. Resnick D, Niwayama G, Goergen T, et al. Clinical, radiographic and pathologic abnormalities in calcium pyrophosphate dihydrate deposition disease (CPPD): pseudogout. Radiology 1977;122:1–15.
4. Helms CA, Chapman GS, Wild JH. Charcot-like joints in calcium pyrophosphate dihydrate deposition disease. Skeletal Radiol 1981;7:55–58.
5. Gold R, Metzger A, Mirra J, Weinberger H, Killebrew K. Multicentric reticulohistiocytosis (lipoid dermatoarthritis). An erosive polyarthritis with distinctive clinical, roentgenographic, and pathologic features. AJR 1975;124:610–624.
6. Mitchell D, Kressel H, Arger P, Dalinka M, Spritzer C, Steinberg M. Avascular necrosis of the femoral head: morphologic assessment by MR imaging, with CT correlation. Radiology 1986;161:739–742.

38

Metabolic Bone Disease

Portions of this chapter were adapted from an earlier work by the author, *Fundamentals of Skeletal Radiology*, 1989, Philadelphia, W. B. Saunders Company. Reprinted by permission.

Clyde A. Helms

OSTEOPOROSIS

Osteoporosis is defined as diminished bone *quantity* in which the bone is otherwise normal. This contrasts to osteomalacia in which the bone quantity is normal but the *quality* of the bone is abnormal in that it is not normally mineralized. Osteomalacia results in excess nonmineralized osteoid. It is not possible in most cases to distinguish between osteoporosis and osteomalacia on plain films; hence, many prefer the term "osteopenia" for the plain film finding of diminished mineralization.

The causes of osteoporosis are myriad, the most common of which is primary osteoporosis (so-called senile osteoporosis or osteoporosis of aging). This is seen most commonly in postmenopausal females and is a major health concern because of the increase of vertebral body and hip fractures in this patient population. Another name for this type of osteoporosis is primary osteoporosis.

Secondary osteoporosis implies that an underlying disorder, such as thyrotoxicosis or renal disease, has caused the osteoporosis. Only about 5% of the cases of osteoporosis are of the secondary type. The differential diagnosis for secondary osteoporosis is quite long and probably should not be memorized. One cannot even be sure if it is osteoporosis or osteomalacia based on the plain films; therefore, the differential for presumed osteoporosis would have to include the causes of osteomalacia.

The main radiographic finding in osteoporosis is thinning of the cortex. Although this can be seen in any bone, it is most reliably demonstrated in the second metacarpal at the middiaphysis. The normal metacarpal cortical thickening should be approximately one-fourth to one-third the thickness of the metacarpal (Fig. 38.1). In osteoporosis this cortical thickness is decreased (Fig. 38.2). The metacarpal cortex (and all bony cortices, for that matter) decreases in thickness normally with age, and is thinner in females than in males of the same age. Several tables have been published that give the normal metacarpal cortical measurement that have age and sex adjustments to allow the determination of normal. Unfortunately, these only determine the mineralization of the peripheral skeleton and do not seem to relate to whether or not vertebral body or hip fractures will occur.

Measurement of the bone mineral content in the axial skeleton can be done by one of several methods that use computed tomography to assess the bone quantity in the spine. There is much debate over which method is superior and even whether or not knowing the bone mineral content is clinically more helpful than just knowing the age and sex of the patient, which is fairly accurate for predicting the bone-mass quantity. Most agree that knowing the axial bone mineral measurement does not help predict which patients are at risk for vertebral body and hip fractures.

Exercise and proper diet seem to help delay the onset of primary osteoporosis.Calcium additives have not been shown to reverse the process of primary osteoporosis. Estrogen clearly plays a role in alleviating postmenopausal osteoporosis, yet its use in a widespread manner is somewhat controversial.

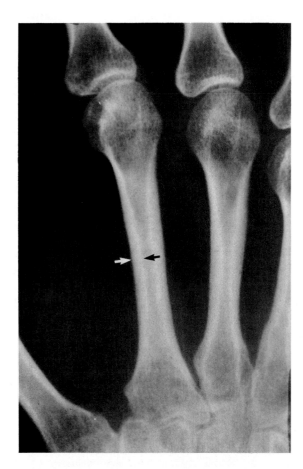

Figure 38.1. Normal Mineralization. The cortical width (*arrows*) at the midsecond metacarpal in this patient with normal mineralization is greater than one-third of the total width of the metacarpal.

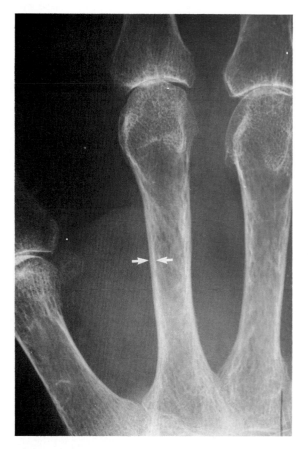

Figure 38.2. Osteoporosis. Severe cortical narrowing (*arrows*) at the midsecond metacarpal cortex is seen in this patient with severe osteoporosis. Note the intracortical tunneling that occurs in more aggressive forms of osteoporosis.

A type of osteoporosis that can be seen in a patient of any age is disuse osteoporosis. It results from immobilization from any cause, most commonly following treatment of a fracture. The radiographic appearance of disuse osteoporosis is different from primary osteoporosis in that it occurs somewhat more rapidly and gives the bone a patchy appearance (Fig. 38.3). This is from osteoclastic resorption in the cortex causing intracortical holes. If allowed to continue with disuse, the bone would resemble any bone with marked osteoporosis, i.e., severe cortical thinning.

Occasionally, aggressive osteoporosis from disuse can mimic a permeative lesion such as a Ewing's sarcoma or multiple myeloma because of the multiple cortical holes that project over the medullary space, thus resembling a medullary permeative process (Fig. 38.4). The way to differentiate a true intramedullary permeative process from an intracortical process such as osteoporosis is to observe the cortex and see if it is solid or riddled with holes (Fig. 38.5). If the cortex is solid, one can assume the permeative process is emanating from the medullary space (Fig. 38.6); if the cortex has multiple small holes, assume the permeative pattern is from the cortical process. I call a permeative

appearance that is secondary to cortical holes a "pseudopermeative" process to distinguish it from a true permeative process (1).

Other causes for a pseudopermeative process include hemangioma and radiation. A hemangioma can cause cortical holes in two ways: from focal hyperemia causing focal osteoporosis, or by the blood vessels themselves tunneling through the cortex (Fig. 38.7). Radiation can cause cortical holes in bone and mimic a permeative pattern because of the death of cortical osteocytes, which can result in large lacunae in the cortex (Fig. 38.8). The cortical holes from radiation can be large, in which case they would not be confused with a true permeative process, but they can also be small and resemble an aggressive lesion.

If a permeative lesion is found, the differential diagnosis is usually an aggressive process such as Ewing's sarcoma, infection, or eosinophilic granuloma in a young person (under age 30) or multiple myeloma, metastatic carcinomatosis, or primary lymphoma of bone in an older patient. If, however, the permeative pattern is a result of cortical holes, i.e., a pseudopermeative pattern, the differential diagnosis is considerably less sinister: *aggressive osteoporosis,*

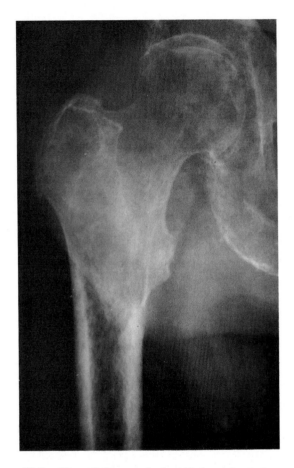

Figure 38.3. Disuse Osteoporosis. A mottled, patchy appearance is present in the proximal right femur in this patient with aggressive disuse osteoporosis secondary to an amputation. Note the mottled, irregular cortex seen in the femoral shaft, which is representative of cortical holes that can be seen in aggressive osteoporosis.

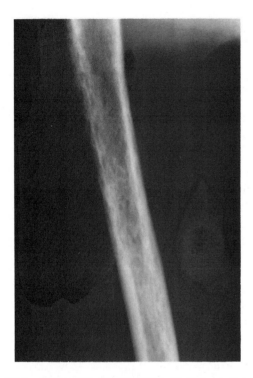

Figure 38.4. Aggressive Osteoporosis. Multiple small holes are seen in the cortex and overlying the medullary space in the proximal humerus of this patient who has suffered a stroke. This represents aggressive osteoporosis from disuse and is mimicking an aggressive permeative process. However, these holes are almost entirely within the cortex of the bone.

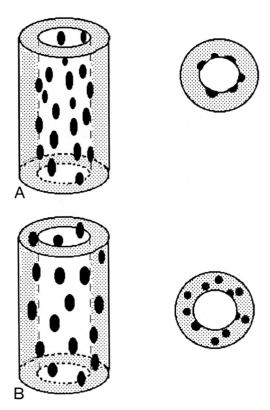

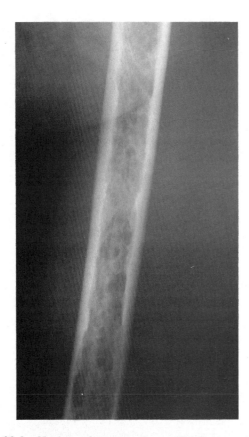

Figure 38.5.   Differentiation of Permeative Process. A. Schematic of a permeative lesion. A true permeative process has multiple small holes secondary to endosteal involvement with sparing of the cortex. This represents a marrow process. **B.** Schematic of a pseudopermeative process. A pseudopermeative process such as osteoporosis has multiple small cortical holes that are then superimposed over the marrow, giving a similar appearance to a permeative process.

Figure 38.6.   Myeloma Causing a Permeative Process. A diffuse permeative process throughout the femur is seen in this patient with myeloma. Note that the cortex is solid, although the endosteum has some scalloping. This is a true permeative process.

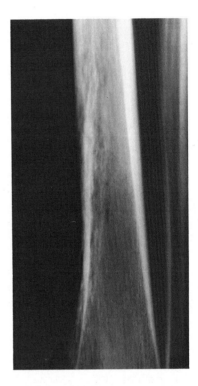

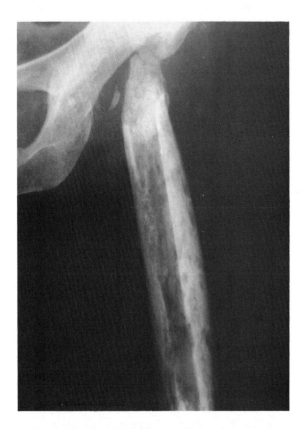

Figure 38.7.   Pseudopermeative Process Secondary to Hemangioma. A permeative pattern is seen in the distal tibia in this patient with pain and swelling. It was thought to represent a Ewing's sarcoma and a biopsy was performed with subsequent heavy loss of blood. This was found to be a hemangioma. An examination of the cortex demonstrates that the medial aspect is diffusely riddled with cortical holes as compared with the lateral aspect. The endosteum laterally also is completely spared, making a marrow process very unlikely. Hemangioma, radiation, and osteoporosis can cause a pseudopermeative process, although in this example, osteoporosis and radiation would be unlikely because of its focal nature.

Figure 38.8.   Pseudopermeative Pattern Secondary to Radiation. This patient had a fibrosarcoma treated with excision of the femoral head and subsequent radiation. A follow-up film shows a diffuse permeative pattern throughout the proximal femur. Since the cortex is riddled with holes, it was thought that this was secondary to radiation rather than tumor recurrence. This is a pseudopermeative appearance secondary to radiation.

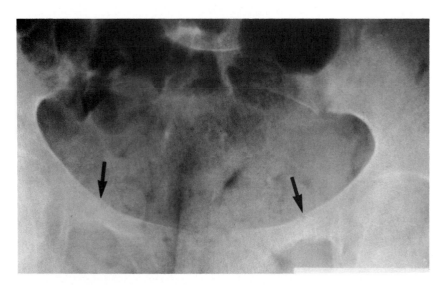

Figure 38.9.   Looser's Fractures in Osteomalacia. Bilateral pubic rami fractures (*arrows*) are faintly identified in this patient with osteomalacia secondary to phenytoin (Dilantin) therapy. These are called Looser's fractures and are pathognomonic for osteomalacia, although they are uncommonly seen.

Table 38.1.   Differential Diagnosis of Pseudopermeative Pattern

Aggressive osteoporosis
Hemangioma
Radiation

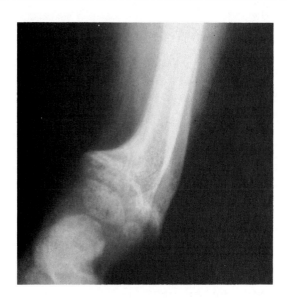

Figure 38.10.   Rickets. Osteomalacia in children is called rickets and is identified by fraying and splaying of the epiphyses as well as bending of the bone secondary to softening. This patient had renal osteodystrophy.

hemangioma, or *radiation changes*. This differential diagnosis does not arise often but is very useful when it does (Table 38.1).

OSTEOMALACIA

Osteomalacia is the result of too much nonmineralized osteoid. The most common cause is renal osteodystrophy. The radiographic findings are almost identical to those of osteoporosis and, for the most part, the two disorders are indistinguishable. The only findings that are pathognomonic for osteomalacia are Looser's fractures, which are fractures through large osteoid seams (Fig. 38.9). They are extremely uncommon, but tend to occur in the femur, pelvis, and scapula.

In children, osteomalacia is called rickets. It causes the epiphyses to become flared and irregular and the long bones undergo bending from the bone softening (Fig. 38.10). As in adults, the most common cause is renal disease, although other causes such as biliary disease and dietary insufficiencies are occasionally seen.

HYPERPARATHYROIDISM

Hyperparathyroidism (HPT) occurs from excess parathyroid hormone (PTH). Parathyroid hormone causes osteoclastic resorption in bone, which leads to osteoporosis and osteomalacia. Primary HPT is caused by parathyroid adenomas and hyperplasia. Up to 40% of patients with primary HPT will demonstrate skeletal abnormalities radiographically. The most common cause of HPT is from renal disease, which leads to secondary HPT. Secondary HPT is because of the parathyroids secreting excess PTH in response to the hypocalcemia that occurs.

The radiographic sign that is pathognomonic for HPT is subperiosteal bone resorption. It is seen most commonly on the radial aspect of the middle phalanges of the hand (Fig. 38.11), but can be seen in any long bone in the body. It is commonly seen on the medial aspect of the proximal tibia, at the sacroiliac joints (Fig. 38.12), and in the distal clavicle.

Other radiographic findings include osteosclerosis, usually diffuse, but often involving the spine in a manner resembling the stripes on rugby jerseys, hence, the name "rugger jersey spine" (Fig. 38.13). Brown tumors are cystic lesions that are often expan-

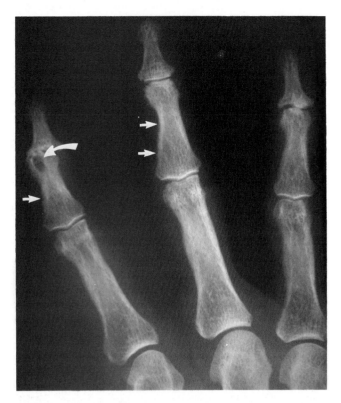

Figure 38.11. Hyperparathyroidism. Subperiosteal bone resorption can be seen at the radial aspect of the middle phalanges (*straight arrows*), which is pathognomonic for HPT. The lytic lesion seen in the distal middle phalanx (*curved arrow*) may be a small Brown tumor.

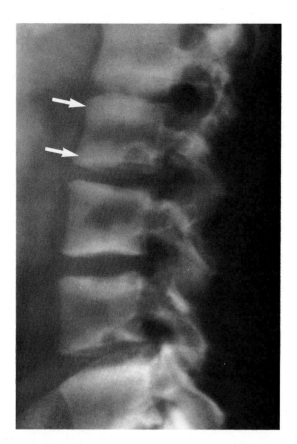

Figure 38.13. Hyperparathyroidism. Sclerotic bands present at the vertebral body endplates (*arrows*) are characteristic of a rugger jersey spine. This is seen in HPT.

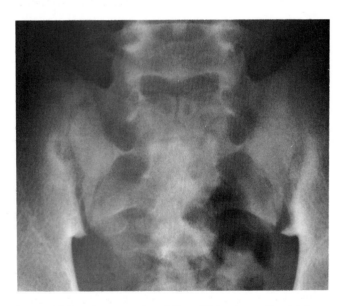

Figure 38.12. Hyperparathyroidism. Bilateral sacroiliac joint erosive changes with sclerosis are present in this patient with renal osteodystrophy and secondary hyperparathyroidism. Bilateral sacroiliac joint changes such as this are often seen with HPT.

sile and aggressive in appearance (Fig. 38.14). They were once said to be more common in primary HPT, but are seen more commonly associated with second-ary HPT today because of the overwhelming preponderance of patients with secondary disease as compared with primary disease. A Brown tumor can have a variety of appearances, so the only thing characteristic about it is that it is associated with subperiosteal bone resorption. If the underlying HPT is treated, the subperiosteal resorption may disappear before the Brown tumor does. This is not commonly seen, however.

Metabolic bone surveys (plain films of the hands, spine, and long bones) were once routinely obtained in patients to look for subperiosteal bone resorption, Brown tumors, osteosclerosis, calcifications, and Looser's fractures. They are no longer recommended, however, as the yield of positive findings is extremely low, and rarely will a positive finding affect treatment. In place of the metabolic bone survey it is now recommended that plain films of the hands be obtained to look for subperiosteal resorption (2). A radionuclide bone scan can be obtained in selected cases, which will show increased radionuclide uptake by Brown tumors and Looser's fractures. Also, investigation of causes of hypercalcemia, which can be caused by metastatic disease or metabolic bone disease, should include a bone scan (3).

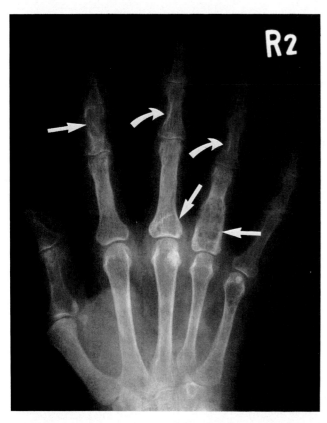

Figure 38.14. Brown Tumors in HPT. Several lytic lesions are present in the phalanges (*straight arrows*) in this patient with HPT; these are Brown tumors. Note the subperiosteal bone resorption in the radial aspect of the middle phalanges (*curved arrows*), which is pathognomonic for HPT.

HYPOPARATHYROIDISM

Hypoparathyroidism occurs because of a deficiency of the parathyroid glands to secrete normal amounts of PTH. Few skeletal changes occur in hypoparathyroidism. The calvarium on occasion will show thickening, and calcification in the basal ganglia of the brain has been described.

PSEUDOHYPOPARATHYROIDISM AND PSEUDOPSEUDOHYPOPARATHYROIDISM

Pseudohypoparathyroidism is caused by a congenital failure of tissues to respond to PTH. The parathyroid glands are normal in these cases. Treating these patients with PTH is of no help since the problem lies in the end organs, not the parathyroid glands. A characteristic appearance is seen in these patients: obesity, round facies, short stature, and brachydactyly (Fig. 38.15). The tubular bones of the hands and feet are often all short. In pseudopseudohyparathyroidism there is no parathyroid abnormality and no end organ problem; these patients merely resemble patients with pseudohypoparathyroidism. In summary, hypoparathyroidism is a parathyroid gland problem,

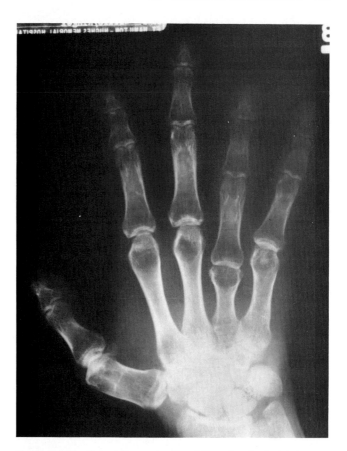

Figure 38.15. Pseudohypoparathyroidism. Brachydactyly is present in several of the metacarpals in this patient with pseudohypoparathyroidism. A short fourth metacarpal as seen here is a frequent finding in this entity.

pseudohypoparathyroidism is an end organ problem, and pseudopseudohypoparathyroidism is a mimicker of pseudohypoparathyroidism morphologically.

PITUITARY GLAND HYPERFUNCTION

A secreting adenoma or hyperplasia of the anterior lobe of the pituitary gland will result in accelerated bone growth. If it occurs before the epiphyses close, it causes giantism. If it occurs after the epiphyses are closed, the result is acromegaly.

Acromegaly has several characteristic radiographic features in the skeletal system. The skull film invariably shows calvarial thickening, enlarged sinuses, and an enlarged sella turcica. The jaw is prognathic. The terminal tufts of the distal phalanges become hypertrophied and have a so-called "spade" appearance (an appearance not unlike a spade or shovel) (Fig. 38.16). The joint spaces are occasionally minimally enlarged because of hypertrophy of the hyaline articular cartilage. Early degenerative joint disease ensues because the cartilage itself is abnormal. The soft-tissues also hypertrophy, with various measurements of soft-tissue thickening employed by some as an indicator for acromegaly. For instance, thicken-

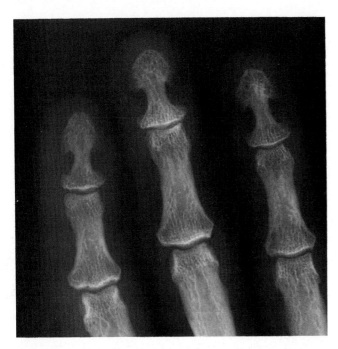

Figure 38.16. Acromegaly. Enlargement of the distal tufts in the phalanges (so-called "spade tufts") are characteristic for acromegaly.

ing of the heel pad adjacent to the calcaneus has been used as a sign of acromegaly.

THYROID GLAND HYPERFUNCTION

In children, hyperthyroidism can result in increased skeletal maturation; however, this is seldom marked. A rare manifestation of hyperthyroidism in adults is thyroid acropachy. This occurs only after prior thyroidectomy and the cause is unknown. A characteristic appearing periostitis occurs in the metacarpals and phalanges of the hands and feet (Fig. 38.17). It invariably involves the ulnar aspect of the fifth metacarpal, a useful differential point that can be used to tell thyroid acropachy from other causes of diffuse periostitis such as hypertrophic pulmonary osteoarthropathy and pachydermal periostitis, a rare form of idiopathic periostitis and skin thickening.

THYROID GLAND HYPOFUNCTION

Decreased thyroid secretion, or cretinism, results in delayed skeletal maturation in children. Delay in ossification of epiphyseal centers with occasional appearance of "stippled" epiphyses is seen. A delay in epiphyseal closure also occurs, in some instances with failure of epiphyseal closure noted in the 3rd and 4th decade.

OSTEOSCLEROSIS

The radiographic finding of diffuse increased bone density, osteosclerosis, is somewhat uncommon, yet

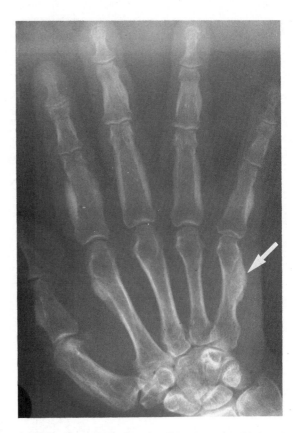

Figure 38.17. Thyroid Acropachy. Extensive periostitis is noted in the metacarpals and phalanges in this patient with thyroid acropachy. It is characteristic to have marked involvement of the ulnar aspect of the fifth metacarpal (*arrow*) in this entity.

Table 38.2. Differential Diagnosis of Diffuse Bony Sclerosis (Dense Bones)

Renal osteodystrophy
Sickle cell disease
Myelofibrosis
Osteopetrosis
Pyknodysostosis
Metastatic carcinoma
Mastocytosis
Paget's disease
Athletes
Fluorosis

every radiologist must have a differential diagnosis for this process. Fortunately, it is a rather short differential and there are criteria to narrow down the list of possibilities.

The list of diseases that can cause diffuse osteosclerosis is quite long, but a list that includes 95–98% of the pathologic processes is all that is really necessary. The entities I include in the differential diagnosis of diffuse osteosclerosis are listed in Table 38.2.

The mnemonic I use to remember them is "*Regular Sex Makes Occasional Perversions Much More Pleasurable And Fantastic.*" I will cover each of these topics in generalities, trying to point out the features of

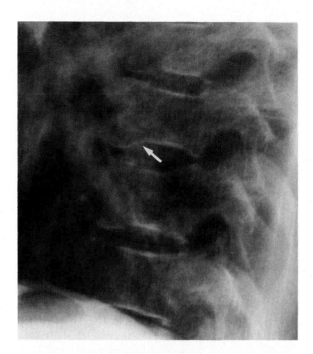

Figure 38.18. Sickle Cell Disease. Step-off deformities (*arrow*) are seen in the endplates of several vertebral bodies in this patient with sickle cell disease. They are also called fish vertebrae.

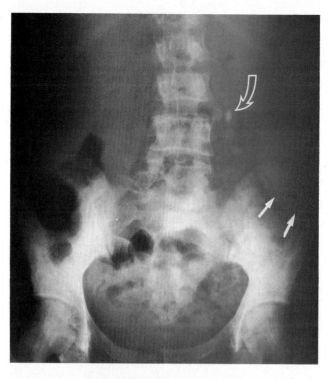

Figure 38.19. Myelofibrosis. Diffuse increased bone density is seen throughout the pelvis and spine in this patient with my-elofibrosis. The spleen is markedly enlarged (*straight arrows*), and opaque iron tablets (*curved arrow*) can be seen, which were taken for the anemia that is often found in this disorder.

each that should be looked for to allow inclusion or exclusion from the differential.

Renal Osteodystrophy

Anything that causes HPT can cause osteosclerosis, but renal disease is by far the most common disease in which osteosclerosis is seen. Although the most common presentation of renal osteodystrophy is osteopenia, about 10–20% of the patients with renal osteodystrophy will exhibit osteosclerosis, and the reasons for it are unknown. As mentioned previously, the sine qua non of renal osteodystrophy is subperiosteal bone resorption, seen earliest and most reliably at the radial aspect of the middle phalanges of the hands. Without this finding, osteosclerosis caused by renal disease should not be entertained.

Sickle Cell Disease

Like renal osteodystrophy, the underlying cause of dense bones in sickle cell disease is unknown. It only occurs in a small percentage of patients. Additional signs to look for are bone infarcts and step-off deformities of the vertebral body endplates (Fig. 38.18). These are also called "fish" vertebrae after their appearance like the vertebrae found in fish. Avascular necrosis of the hip is frequently an accompanying finding.

Myelofibrosis

Also called agnogenic myeloid metaplasia, my-elofibrosis is a disease caused by progressive fibrosis of the marrow in patients over 50 years of age. It leads to anemia with marked splenomegaly and extramedullary hematopoiesis. Whenever osteosclerosis is seen in a patient over the age of 50, a search should be made for a large spleen and extramedullary hematopoiesis (Fig. 38.19).

Osteopetrosis

This is a hereditary abnormality that results in extremely dense bones throughout the skeleton (Fig. 38.20). There are congenita and tarda forms, with different degrees of severity in each. The congenita form occurs at birth and can be lethal. Anemia, jaundice, hepatosplenomegaly, and infections are often present in this form. The tarda form is seen in older children and adults and has milder clinical problems. The tarda form may be so mild that it has no clinical findings. Although uncommon, it is not so rare that one will never see a case; therefore, it should be included in this differential diagnosis. A characteristic finding is the so-called "bone-in bone" appearance often seen in the vertebral bodies in which the vertebrae have a small replica of the vertebral body inside the normal

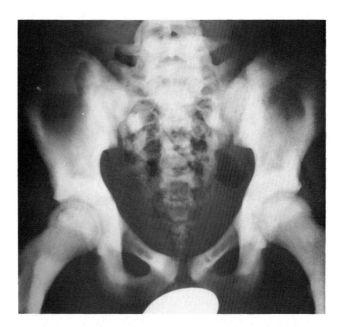

Figure 38.20.   Osteopetrosis. Marked, diffuse bony sclerosis is seen throughout the skeleton in this patient with osteopetrosis.

one. Also characteristic are the "sandwich vertebrae" in which the endplates are densely sclerotic, giving the appearance of a sandwich (Fig. 38.21). The sandwich vertebrae appearance resembles a rugger jersey spine, but can be differentiated by being much denser and more sharply defined.

Pyknodystosis

This is the other congenital abnormality with dense bones that should be considered in the differential diagnosis of osteosclerosis. It is seen less commonly than osteopetrosis. These patients are typically short and have hypoplastic mandibles. The distinguishing radiographic finding that is essentially pathognomonic is acroosteolysis with sclerosis. The distal phalanges often have the appearance of chalk that has been put into a pencil sharpener: they are pointed and dense (Fig. 38.22). No other disease process has this appearance. Another name for this disorder is Toulouse-Lautrec syndrome, named for the famous artist who was afflicted with pyknodysostosis.

Metastatic Carcinoma

Only rarely will diffuse metastatic carcinoma cause a problem in diagnosis. I have seen only a handful of cases where diffuse metastatic carcinoma mimicked diffuse osteosclerosis, and in every case the primary tumor was either prostate or breast carcinoma. If cortical destruction or a lytic component is present, it simplifies the differential diagnosis, so a search should be made for these.

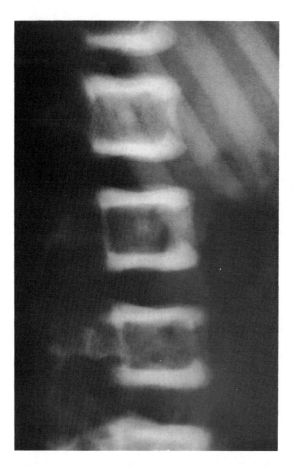

Figure 38.21.   Sandwich Vertebrae. Dense bands of sclerosis parallel to the endplates are seen in this patient with osteopetrosis. These are called sandwich vertebrae, which are much more distinct than the dense bands of sclerosis seen in a rugger jersey spine (see Fig. 38.13).

Mastocytosis

This is another rare disorder that can cause uniform increased bone density. Unfortunately, there are no other plain film findings that might help with the diagnosis. Patients with this disease have thickened small bowel folds with nodules but, of course, to see them, an upper gastrointestinal contrast study must be performed (Fig. 38.23). Urticaria pigmentosa is a characteristic skin lesion found in these patients.

Paget's Disease

Diffuse Paget's disease that could be confused with one of the other diseases in the differential diagnosis of generalized osteosclerosis is very rare. Paget's disease classically causes bony enlargement (Fig. 38.24), but this is not always present. It occurs most commonly in the pelvis (Fig. 38.25) where it has been said the iliopectineal line on the pelvic brim must be thickened if Paget's disease is present. In fact, the iliopectineal line is usually, but not always, thickened.

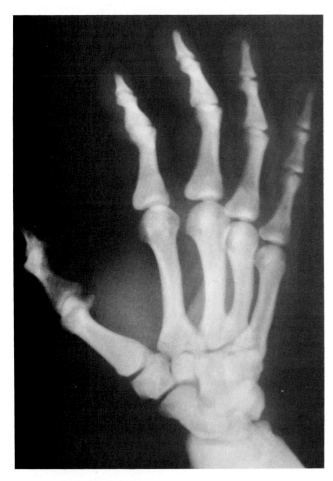

Figure 38.22.   Pyknodysostosis. Diffuse, dense sclerosis is seen throughout the hand and wrist in this patient with pyknodysostosis. Note the absent distal phalangeal tufts that appear pointed and sclerotic, which is virtually pathognomonic for pyknodysostosis.

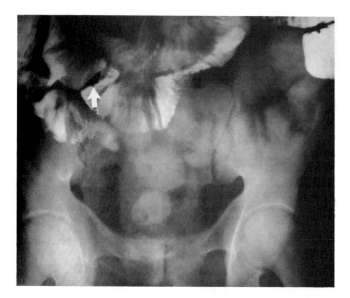

Figure 38.23.   Mastocytosis. Uniform increased bone density is seen throughout the pelvis in this patient with mastocytosis. Small bowel thickened folds with nodules (*arrow*) can be seen in this barium study; these are often found in mastocytosis.

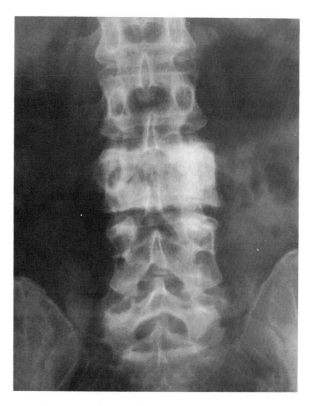

Figure 38.24.   Paget's Disease. Dense, bony sclerosis with overgrowth of the vertebral body is seen at the L-3 vertebra in this patient with Paget's disease. The left L-3 pedicle is markedly dense and enlarged.

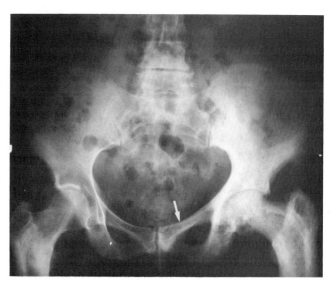

Figure 38.25.   Paget's Disease. Bony sclerosis with some bony enlargement is seen in the left pelvis and proximal femur of this patient and is characteristic of Paget's disease. Note the cortical thickening of the left superior pubic ramus (*arrow*), which is called thickening of the iliopectineal line and is commonly seen in Paget's disease.

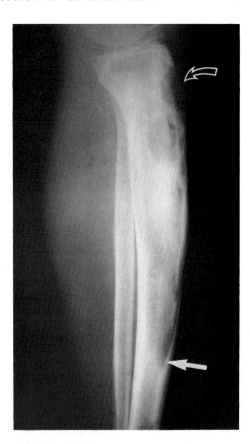

Figure 38.26. Paget's Disease. A lytic process involving the proximal two-thirds of the tibia is noted and has a blade of grass or flame-shaped leading edge (*straight arrow*), which is characteristic for Paget's disease. This represents the lytic phase of Paget's disease. The sclerotic phase of Paget's disease can be seen in the midportion of this lesion, and an area of probable sarcomatous degeneration can be seen in the proximal tibia (*curved arrow*) where apparent cortical destruction is noted. This represents all three phases or stages of Paget's disease.

Paget's disease can occur in any bone in the body, including the smaller bones of the hands and feet.

Paget's disease has three distinct phases visible radiographically: a lytic phase, a sclerotic phase, and a mixed lytic-sclerotic phase. The lytic phase often has a sharp leading edge called a "flame-shaped" or "blade of grass" leading edge (Fig. 38.26). In a long bone, with

the sole exception being the tibia, Paget's disease always starts at the end of the bone; therefore, if a lesion is present in the middle of a long bone and does not extend to either end, one can safely exclude Paget's disease.

Athletes

Plain film radiographs of professional athletes quite often demonstrate increased cortical thickness and apparent diffuse osteosclerosis to the point of appearing pathologic. Undoubtedly, increased stress causes hypertrophy of bone as well as muscle. The increased density in these otherwise normal subjects is occasionally misinterpreted as abnormal, with extensive workups and even bone biopsy resulting.

Fluorosis

This is a rare disorder that is usually a result of chronic intake of fluoride in certain geographic areas where large amounts of fluoride are present in the drinking water. It can also be a result of long-term therapy with sodium fluoride for osteoporosis.

A radiographic finding that patients with fluorosis often have is ligamentous calcification. Calcification of the sacrotuberous ligament is said to be characteristic for fluorosis.

SUMMARY

There are other categories of disease that could be covered in a chapter on metabolic bone disease, but most of the remaining disorders are exceedingly rare and not likely to be seen by most radiologists on a routine basis.

References

1. Helms C, Munk P. Pseudopermeative skeletal lesions. Br J Radiol 1990;63:461–467.
2. Cooper KL. Radiology of metabolic bone disease. Endocrinol Metab Clin North Am 1989;18:955–976.
3. McAfee JG. Radionuclide imaging in metabolic and systemic skeletal diseases. Semin Nucl Med 1987;17:334–349.

39

Skeletal "Don't Touch" Lesions

Clyde A. Helms

POSTTRAUMATIC LESIONS
NORMAL VARIANTS
OBVIOUSLY BENIGN LESIONS

Skeletal "don't touch" lesions are those processes that are so radiographically characteristic that a biopsy or additional diagnostic tests are unnecessary. Not only does the biopsy result in unnecessary morbidity and cost, but in some instances, as will be mentioned, a biopsy can also be frankly misleading and lead to additional unnecessary surgery.

Most radiology training stresses giving a differential diagnosis of a lesion, leaving it up to the clinician to decide between the various entities. For the "don't touch" lesions, however, a differential list is inappropriate as that often makes the next step in the decision-making process a biopsy. Because these lesions do not need to undergo biopsy for a final diagnosis, a radiologic diagnosis should be made without a list of differential possibilities. These lesions can be classified into three categories: (*a*) posttraumatic lesions, (*b*) normal variants, and (*c*) lesions that are real but obviously benign.

POSTTRAUMATIC LESIONS

Myositis ossificans is an example of a lesion that should not undergo biopsy because its aggressive histologic appearance can often mimic a sarcoma (1). Unfortunately, radical surgery has been performed based on the histologic appearance of myositis ossificans when the radiologic appearance was diagnostic. The typical radiologic appearance of myositis ossificans is circumferential calcification with a lucent center (Fig. 39.1). This is often best appreciated on a computed tomography (CT) scan. (Fig. 39.2). A malignant tumor that mimics myositis ossificans has an ill-defined periphery and a calcified or ossific center (Fig. 39.3). Periosteal reaction can be seen with myositis ossificans or with a tumor. Occasionally, the peripheral calcification of myositis ossificans can be too faint to appreciate; in these

cases, a computed tomography scan should help, or delayed films 1 or 2 weeks later are recommended. Biopsy should be avoided when myositis ossificans is a clinical consideration.

Avulsion Injury. Another posttraumatic entity in which a biopsy can be misleading is any avulsion injury (2, 3). These injuries can have an aggressive radiographic appearance, but because of their characteristic location at ligament and tendon insertion sites (e.g., anterior-inferior iliac spine or ischial tuberosity) they should be recognized as benign. (Figs. 39.4 and 39.5). Again, delayed films of several weeks will usually allow the problem case to become more radiographically clear. Biopsy can lead to the mistaken diagnosis of a sarcoma and should therefore be avoided. Any area undergoing healing can have a high nuclear/chromatin ratio and a high mitotic figure count, thereby occasionally simulating a malignancy histologically.

Cortical desmoid is a process on the medial supracondylar ridge of the distal femur that is considered by many to be the result of an avulsion of the adductor magnus muscle. It occasionally simulates an aggressive lesion radiographically and histologically can look malignant (4). In many instances, biopsy has led to amputation for this benign, radiographically characteristic lesion. (Fig 39.6 and 39.7). Cortical desmoids occur only on the posteromedial epicondyle of the femur. They may or may not be associated with pain and can have increased radionuclide uptake on a bone scan. They may or may not exhibit periosteal new bone and usually occur in young people. Biopsy should be avoided in all cases.

Trauma can lead to large, cystic geodes or subchondral cysts near joints and can be mistaken for other lesions, resulting in a biopsy being ordered. Although the biopsy specimen is not likely to mimic a malignant process, it is nevertheless avoidable. Because geodes from degenerative disease almost always are associated with additional findings such as joint space narrowing, sclerosis, and osteophytes, a diagnosis should be made radiographically (Fig. 39.8). However, on occasion the additional findings are subtle and can be missed (Fig. 39.9). Geodes can also occur in the setting of calcium pyrophosphate dihydrate

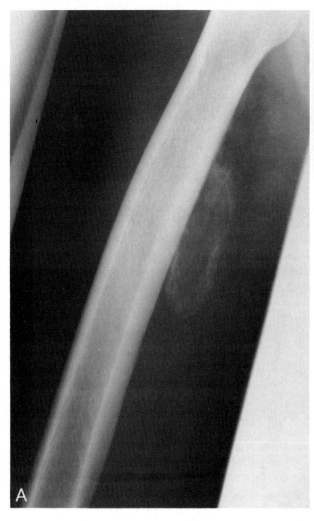

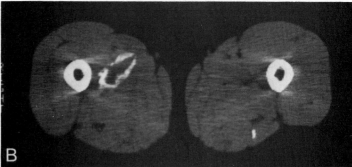

Figure 39.1. Myositis Ossificans. A. A plain film of the femur in this patient who presented with a soft-tissue mass shows a calcific density adjacent to the posterior cortex of the femur, which is calcified primarily in its periphery. It is difficult on the plain film alone to definitely say that this is peripheral, circumferential calcification; therefore, the computed tomographic scan shown in **B** is helpful in showing that the calcification is unequivocally peripheral in nature. This is virtually diagnostic of myositis ossificans.

crystal disease, CPPD, rheumatoid arthritis, and avascular necrosis (5, 6).

Discogenic Vertebral Sclerosis. An entity that is often confused for metastatic disease to the spine is discogenic vertebral disease. It can mimic metastatic disease very closely, and unless the radiologist is familiar with this process, it can lead to an unnecessary biopsy (7). Discogenic vertebral disease most often is sclerotic and focal (Fig. 39.10). It is always adjacent to the endplate, and the associated disc space should be narrow. Osteophytosis is invariably present. It really is a variant of a Schmorl's node and should not be confused with a metastatic focus. On occasion it can be lytic or even mixed lytic/sclerotic. The typical clinical setting is a middle-aged woman with chronic low back pain. Old films often confirm the benign nature of this process. In the setting of disc space narrowing and osteophytosis, focal sclerosis adjacent to an endplate should not undergo biopsy.

Fracture. Occasionally, a fracture will be the cause of extensive osteosclerosis and periostitis, which can mimic a primary bone tumor (Fig. 39.11).

Lack of immobilization can result in exuberant callus which can be misinterpreted as aggressive periostitis or even tumor new bone. Results of a biopsy in such a case might resemble a malignant lesion; therefore, any case associated with trauma should be carefully reviewed for a fracture.

Pseudodislocation of the Humerus. Another traumatic process that can be misdiagnosed radiologically, leading to inappropriate treatment and morbidity, is a pseudodislocation of the humerus (Fig. 39.12). This results from a fracture with hemarthrosis, which causes distension of the joint and migration of the humeral head inferiorly (8). An axial or transcapular view shows it is not anteriorly or posteriorly dislocated (the usual forms of shoulder dislocation) but merely inferiorly subluxated. On an anteroposterior view, it can mimic a posterior dislocation in that the normal superimposition of the humeral head and the glenoid is missing. Often, attempts are made to "relocate" the humeral head, which, of course, are both fruitless (since it is not dislocated) and painful. A fracture is invariably present, and if not seen on the initial films it should be sought after with additional

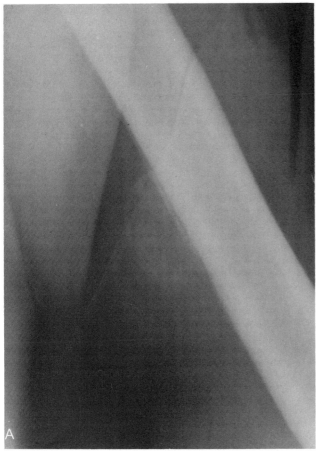

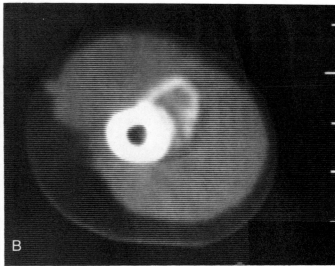

Figure 39.2.   Myositis Ossificans. A. Hazy calcification is seen adjacent to the humeral shaft with underlying periosteal reaction noted. It is difficult to ascertain whether or not the calcification is circumferential. **B.** A computed tomography scan through this mass shows that the calcification is unequivocally circumferential in nature, making the diagnosis of myositis ossificans a certainty.

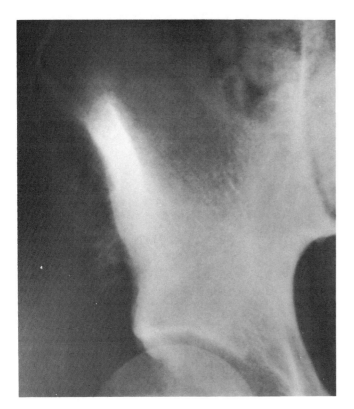

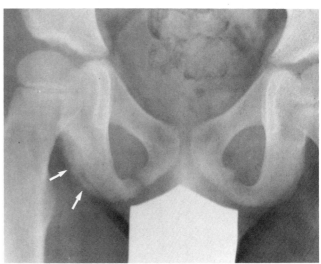

Figure 39.4.   Avulsion Injury. Cortical irregularity (*arrows*) at the ischial tuberosity in this patient with pain over this region raises the question of possible tumor. This is a classic appearance, however, for an avulsion injury from this region and a biopsy should be avoided.

Figure 39.3.   Osteogenic Sarcoma. Hazy, ill-defined calcification is seen adjacent to the iliac wing in this patient, which can be ascertained from the plain film as to definitely not being circumferential in nature. Even though a prior history of trauma was obtained in this case, myositis ossificans is not a consideration with this appearance of calcification. Biopsy showed this to be an osteogenic sarcoma.

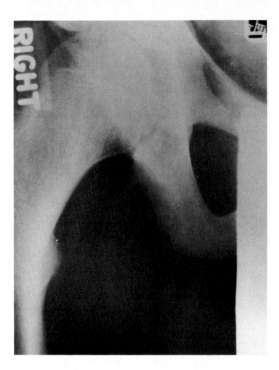

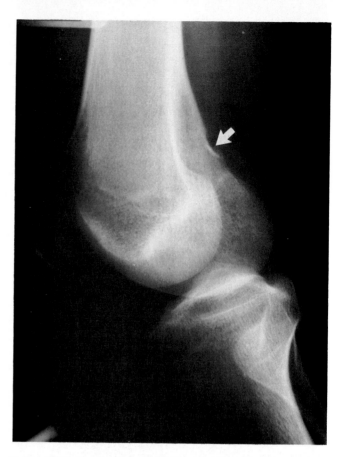

Figure 39.5. Avulsion Injury. Cortical irregularity with a Codman's triangle of periostitis is seen along the ischial tuberosity that was at first thought to represent a malignancy. Because of the characteristic location, an avulsion injury was considered and the lesion was observed. It healed without sequella. (Case courtesy Dr. John Wilson, San Francisco, CA).

Figure 39.7. Cortical Desmoid. A well-defined cortical defect is seen in the posterior distal femur (*arrow*), which is a common appearance for a fairly well-healed cortical desmoid.

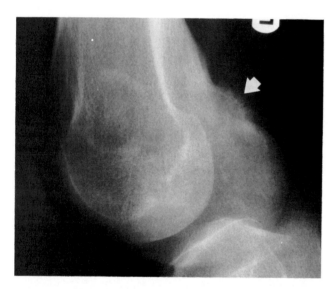

Figure 39.6. Cortical Desmoid. A focal cortical irregularity in this patient is seen in the posterior aspect of the femur (*arrow*) with adjacent periostitis noted. Although a tumor such as an early parosteal osteosarcoma could perhaps have this appearance, this is a characteristic location and appearance for a cortical desmoid and should not undergo biopsy.

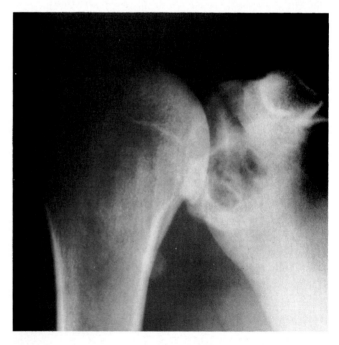

Figure 39.8. Geode. A large cystic lesion was found in the shoulder in this middle-aged weight lifter, and the possibility of a metastatic process was considered. Because the humeral head has sclerosis and osteophytosis as well as a loose body in the joint, degenerative disease of the shoulder was diagnosed; this makes the cystic lesion almost certainly a geode or subchondral cyst.

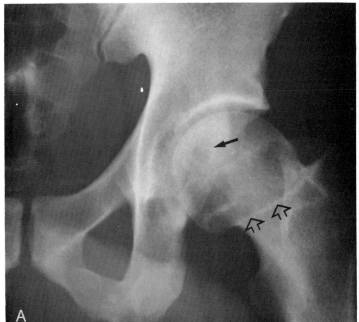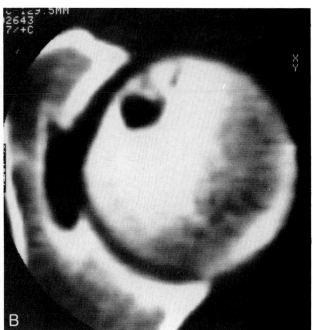

Figure 39.9. Geode. A. A cystic lesion was noted in the femoral head (*arrows*) of a young male with a painful hip. **B.** A computed tomography scan through this area shows the subarticular nature and adjacent sclerosis. The differential diagnosis of infection, eosinophilic granuloma, and chondroblastoma was given. A ring of osteophytes (*open arrowheads*) was noted in retrospect on the plain film **(A)** in the subcapital region, which indicates degenerative disease of the hip. Degenerative joint disease is extremely unusual in a 20-year-old healthy male; however, it makes the lytic lesion in the femoral head almost certainly a subchondral cyst or geode. This was an active soccer player who had been playing with pain in his hip for several years following an injury that had caused the degenerative disease. Unfortunately, a biopsy was performed anyway and a subchondral cyst or geode was confirmed.

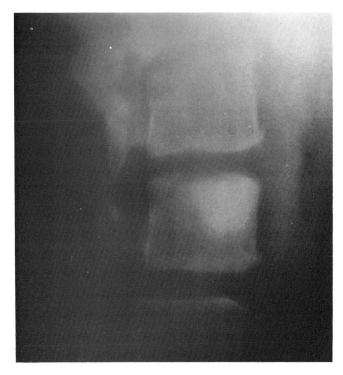

Figure 39.10. Discogenic Vertebral Sclerosis. This patient has sclerosis on the inferior portion of the L-4 vertebral body associated with minimal osteophytosis and joint space narrowing at the adjacent disc space. This is the classic appearance for discogenic vertebral sclerosis, and a biopsy to rule out metastatic disease should not be performed.

Figure 39.11.   Fracture Mimicking Osteosarcoma. A. This 16-year-old patient had experienced pain around the knee for 2 weeks prior to these x-rays. The knee films showed diffuse sclerosis and extensive periostitis about the distal femur, which is thought to be characteristic for an osteogenic sarcoma. The periosteal reaction, however, was thought to be much too thick, dense, and wavy to represent malignant type of periostitis. **B.** A small offset of the epiphysis can be seen (*arrow*), which indicates an epiphyseal slippage consistent with a Salter epiphyseal fracture. This child had fallen off a bicycle and fractured the femur, yet continued to be active. The lack of immobility caused exuberant periostitis or callus with a large amount of reactive sclerosis, all of which mimicked an osteogenic sarcoma.

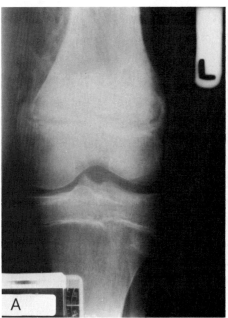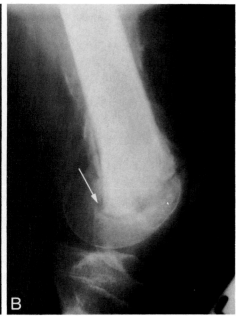

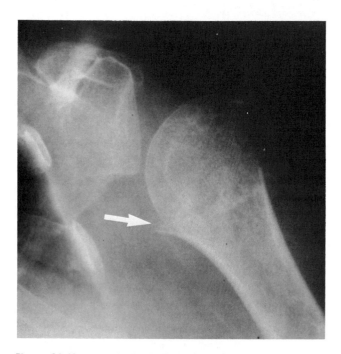

Figure 39.12.   Pseudodislocation of the Shoulder. The humeral head in this patient is inferiorly placed in relation to the glenoid, which is the characteristic location when a hemarthrosis is present. A minimally displaced fracture of the neck of the humerus with avulsion of the greater tuberousity has occurred (*arrow*), causing the hemarthrosis.

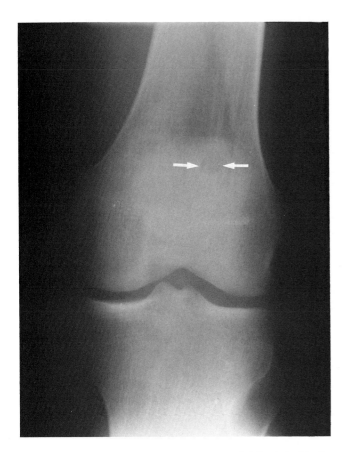

Figure 39.13. Dorsal Defect of the Patella. A lytic defect in the upper outer quadrant of the patella was seen in this patient (*arrows*), which is characteristic for a normal variant called dorsal defect of the patella. It occurs only in the upper outer quadrant and should be asymptomatic.

views. The transcapular or the axial view is the key to making the diagnosis of a pseudodislocation. If necessary, the joint can be aspirated to confirm the presence of a bloody effusion and to show the normal position of the humeral head when fluid has been removed from the joint.

NORMAL VARIANTS

Dorsal Defect of the Patella. A normal variant that has been described in the patella that can be mistaken for a pathologic process is a lytic defect in the upper, outer quadrant called a dorsal defect of the patella (Fig. 39.13) (9). It can mimic a focus of infection, osteochondritis dissecans, or a chondroblastoma. It is a normal developmental anomaly, however, and because of its characteristic location it should not undergo biopsy. On magnetic resonance imaging (MR) it will have an appearance similar to many other bony lesions, i.e., low signal on T1-weighted images and high signal on T2-weighted images (Fig. 39.14). Hence, MR is useful for identifying the lesion but not for characterizing it.

Pseudocyst of the Humerus. Another entity often confused for a lytic pathologic lesion is a pseudocyst of the humerus (Fig. 39.15). This is merely an anatomic variant caused by the increased cancellous bone in the region of the greater tuberosity of the humerus that gives this region a more lucent appearance on radiographs (10, 11). With hyperemia and disuse caused by rotator cuff problems or any other shoulder disorder, this area of lucency may appear strikingly more lucent and mimic a lytic lesion. Many of these have mistakenly undergone biopsy, and several have even had repeat biopsies after the initial pathology report stated "normal bone, no lesion in specimen." Because of the associated hyperemia from the shoulder disorder (be it rotator cuff injury or whatever), a bone scan can show increased radionuclide uptake and thus sway the surgeon to perform a biopsy of this normal variant. It is radiographically characteristic in its location and appearance and should not undergo biopsy. Although other lesions, such as a chondroblastoma, infection, or even a metastatic focus, could occur in a similar location, they do not have quite the same appearance as a pseudocyst of the humerus.

Os Odontoideum. A normal variant of the cervical spine that may, in fact, be posttraumatic is an os odontoideum (12). It is an unfused dens that may move anterior to the C-2 body with flexion and can mimic a fractured dens (Fig. 39.16). Many of these require surgical fixation; some surgeons fuse every case, feeling that they are all unstable. Radiologists should recognize that this process is not acute, and thus save the patient halo fixation and possible immediate surgical intervention. Most of these cases are seen following trauma and, if no neurologic deficits are present, these patients can be seen electively and spared the horrors associated with treatment of the acutely fractured cervical spine. The radiologic signs for recognizing an os odontoideum are the smooth, often well-corticated, inferior border of the dens and the hypertrophied, densely corticated anterior arch of C-1 (13). This latter finding presumably represents compensatory hypertrophy and indicates a long-standing condition.

OBVIOUSLY BENIGN LESIONS

Multiple real lesions exist that should be recognized radiographically as benign and left alone. These are lesions that should be diagnosed by the radiologist, not the pathologist. Listing a differential in these cases often spurs the surgeon to a biopsy, when, in fact, no biopsy should be necessary.

Nonossifying Fibroma. Perhaps the most often encountered lesion in this category is the nonossifying fibroma. Nonossifying fibroma is identical to a fibrous cortical defect, but the term is usually reserved

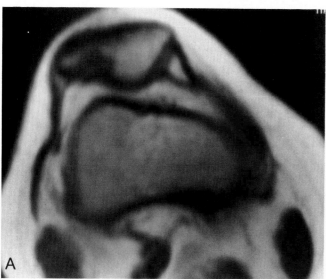

Figure 39.14. Dorsal Defect of the Patella. A. An axial T1-weighted MR shows a focal area of low signal in the patella in a subarticular location in the lateral facet of the patella. **B.** The axial T2-weighted image shows high signal in the lesion. This is typical in location and appearance for a dorsal defect of the patella.

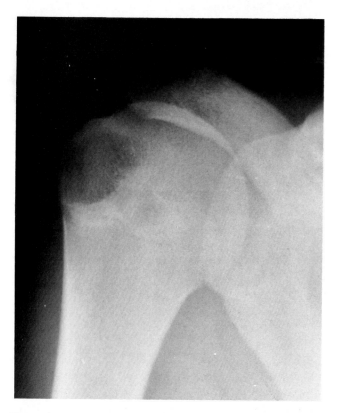

Figure 39.15. Pseudocyst of the Humerus. A well-defined lytic process is seen in the greater tuberosity, which was thought to represent a lytic lesion. This patient was symptomatic and had increased radionuclide uptake on isotope bone scan. This is a characteristic location and appearance, however, for a pseudocyst of the humerus, which merely represents decreased cortical bone in this region. This becomes more pronounced when pain in the shoulder is present and hyperemia or disuse osteoporosis occurs.

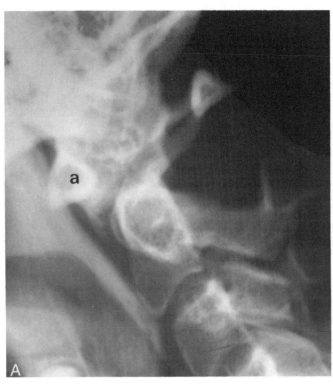

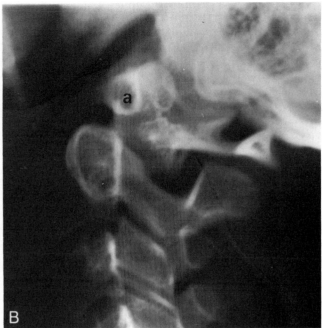

Figure 39.16.   Os Odontoideum. Flexion (**A**) and extension (**B**) views show the anterior arch (*a*) of the C-1 vertebrae has moved markedly anterior in relation to the body of C-2 in flexion. The odontoid or dens is difficult to see but appears to be separated from the body of C-2. Because of the smooth borders of the separated dens and because of the cortical hypertrophy of the anterior arch of C-1, this can safely be called an os odontoideum, which is a congenital or long-standing posttraumatic abnormality rather than an acute fracture. Obviously, patients with this condition should have no neurologic problems, yet in many instances are still believed to be unstable and are surgically fused. This, however, can be done on an elective basis.

for defects larger than 2 cm. They are, classically, lytic lesions located in the cortex of the metaphysis of a long bone and have a well-defined, often sclerotic, scalloped border with slight cortical expansion (Fig. 39.17). They are almost exclusively found in patients under the age of 30; hence, the natural history of the lesion is involution. As they involute they fill in with new bone, giving it a sclerotic appearance (Fig. 39.18); thus, they can have some increased radionuclide activity on bone scans. They are most often mistaken for an area of infection, eosinophilic granuloma, fibrous dysplasia, or aneurysmal bone cyst. They are asymptomatic and have never been reported to be associated with malignant degeneration. On occasion, a pathologic fracture can occur through these lesions, but most surgeons do not advocate prophylactic curettage to prevent fracture, as with unicameral bone cysts. Nonossifying fibromas can be quite large but invariably have a benign appearance (Fig. 39.19), and biopsy should be avoided. The asymptomatic nature should help differentiate them from most of the other lesions in the differential diagnosis and thereby preclude even giving a differential diagnosis. On occasion they are found to be multiple, yet each lesion is so characteristic they should be easily diagnosed.

Bone islands are not a radiographic dilemma when they are 1 cm or less in size. Occasionally, however, they grow to golf ball size or larger and mimic sclerotic metastases (Fig. 39.20). They are always asymptomatic. Radiographically, two signs can be found to help distinguish giant bone islands from metastases. First, bone islands usually are oblong with their long axis in the axis of stress on the bone, e.g., in a long bone they align themselves along the axis of the diaphysis. Second, the margins of a bone island, if examined closely, will show bony trabeculae extending from the lesion into the normal bone in a spiculated fashion (14). This is characteristic of a bone island and helpful in differentiating it from a more aggressive process.

Unicameral bone cysts are often prophylactically curettaged and packed so as to prevent fracture with subsequent deformity. When these cysts occur in the calcaneus, however, they should be left alone. They always occur in the anterior-inferior portion of the calcaneus (Fig. 39.21), an area that does not receive undue stress. In fact, a pseudotumor of the calcaneus is seen in the identical position because of the absence of stress and resulting atrophy of bony trabeculae (Fig. 39.22). These lesions are asymptomatic, only rarely fracture, and should not suffer the same

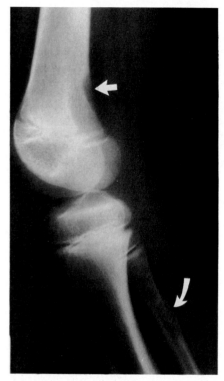

Figure 39.17. Nonossifying Fibroma. A well-defined, slightly expansile, lytic lesion is seen in the fibula (*curved arrow*); this is characteristic for a nonossifying fibroma. A second lytic lesion is seen in the posterior distal femur (*straight arrow*), which is also typical in appearance for a nonossifying fibroma.

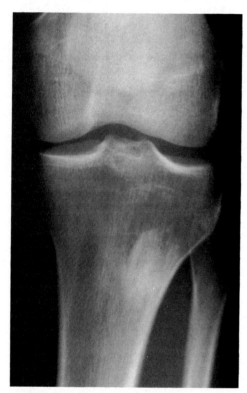

Figure 39.18. Healing Nonossifying Fibroma. A minimally sclerotic process is seen in the proximal tibia, which was thought by the surgeons to represent a focus of infection or an osteoid osteoma, even though the patient was asymptomatic. This is a characteristic appearance for a disappearing or healing nonossifying fibroma and should not undergo biopsy.

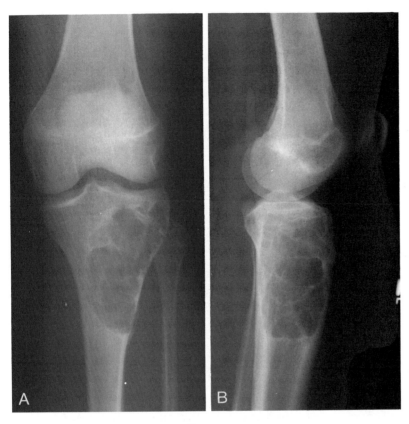

Figure 39.19. Nonossifying Fibroma. A large, well-defined, minimally expansile lytic lesion of the proximal tibia is present, which is characteristic for a nonossifying fibroma. Even though the patient was asymptomatic, biopsy was performed and the diagnosis confirmed. (Case courtesy Dr. Larry Yeager, Redwood City, CA.)

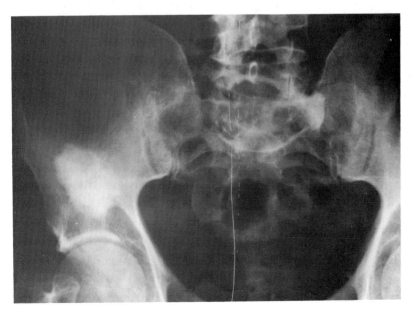

Figure 39.20. Giant Bone Island. A large sclerotic focus is seen in the right iliac wing. Note how the lesion is somewhat spherical or oblong in the lines of trabecular stress, which is characteristic for a bone island. This patient was asymptomatic and had no evidence of a primary carcinoma.

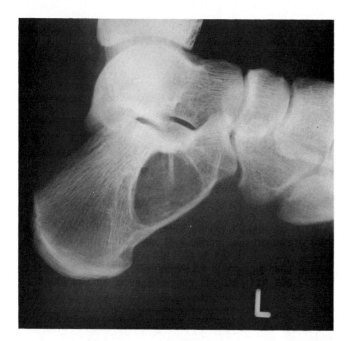

Figure 39.21.   Unicameral Bone Cyst. A well-defined lytic lesion on the anterior-inferior portion on the calcaneus, as in this example, is virtually pathognomonic for a unicameral bone cyst or simple bone cyst. Because this is an area of diminished stress, it is thought not to be necessary to prophylactically curettage and pack this lesion in an effort to avoid a pathologic bone fracture, which is often done in the femur and humerus with unicameral bone cysts.

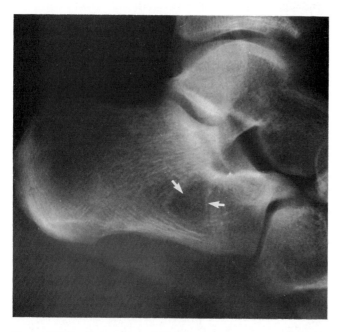

Figure 39.22.   Pseudocyst of the Calcaneus. An area of radiolucency is seen on the anterior-inferior portion of the calcaneus (*arrows*) similar to the example in Figure 39.21, but not as well defined. This is a pseudocyst similar to the pseudocyst of the humerus that results from diminished stress through this region.

fate as their counterparts in long bones, i.e., surgical removal.

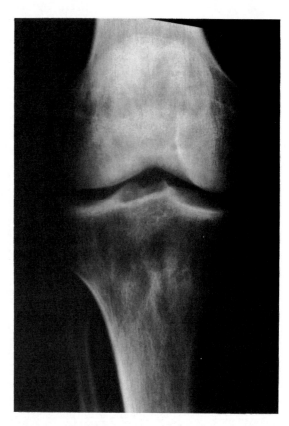

Figure 39.23.   Early Bone Infarct. Patchy demineralization is seen in the distal femur and proximal tibia in this patient with systemic lupus erythematosus. The opposite leg was similarly involved. This is characteristic for early bone infarcts and should not be confused with infection or metastatic disease.

Bone Infarction.   Early in the course of its development a bone infarct can have a patchy, or a mixed lytic-sclerotic pattern, or even resemble a permeative process (Fig. 39.23) (15). In a patient with bone pain and a permeative bone lesion, many aggressive disorders head the differential list and a biopsy soon ensues. If this process can be noted to be multiple and in the diametaphyseal region of a long bone, especially if the patient has an underlying disorder such as sickle cell anemia or systemic lupus erythematosus, areas of early bone infarction should be considered. In some cases the characteristic MR appearance of an infarct may save a patient from biopsy when the plain films are equivocal (Fig. 39.24).

CONCLUSION

These are but a few of the many examples in skeletal radiology where the well-trained radiologist can be of invaluable assistance to the clinician and the patient by helping avert a needless biopsy. Dozens of other examples are nicely shown in normal variant textbooks, which are widely available. Because of the potential harm in performing a needless biopsy, the above examples are stressed. When these lesions are

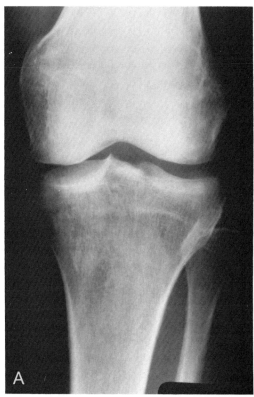
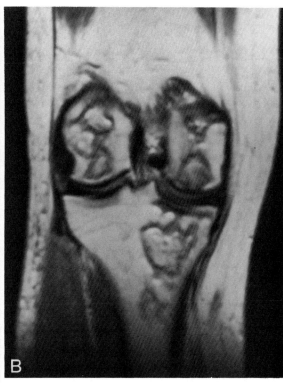

Figure 39.24.   Bone Infarct. A. A plain film of the knee shows a permeative pattern in the proximal tibia, which was at first thought to be infection or a primary tumor. **B.** A T1-weighted coronal MR shows the characteristic serpigenous border seen with bone infarct in the tibia and in the femur. Magnetic resonance imaging can on occasion better characterize the ill-defined early bone infarct, as in this example. This patient has systemic lupus erythematosus.

encountered by the radiologist, a differential diagnosis should not be offered, as it will often lead the surgeon to a biopsy in an attempt to get a diagnosis. A biopsy in many of these entities is not only unnecessary but can be misleading.

References

1. Murray R, Jacobson H. The radiology of skeletal disorders. 2nd ed. New York: Churchill Livingstone, 1977:603.
2. Wootton J, Cross M, Holt K. Avulsion of the ischial apophysis. J Bone Joint Surg 1990;72B:625–627.
3. Schneider R, Kaye J, Ghelman B. Adductor avulsive injuries near the symphisis pubis. Radiology 1976;120:567–569.
4. Barnes G, Gwinn J. Distal irregularities of the femur simulating malignancy. AJR 1974;122:180–185.
5. Ostiere S, Seeger L, Eckardt J. Subchondral cysts of the tibia secondary to osteoarthritis of the knee. Skel Radiol 1990;19:287–289.
6. Resnick D, Niwayama G, Coutts R. Subchondral cysts (geodes) in arthritic disorders: pathologic and radiographic appearance of the hip joint. AJR 1977;128:799–806.
7. Martel W, Seeger J, Wicks J, Washburn R. Traumatic lesions of the discovertebral junction in the lumbar spine. AJR 1976;127:457–464.
8. Helms C, Richmond B, Sims R. Pseudodislocation of the shoulder: a sign of an occult fracture. Emerg Med 1986;18:237–241.
9. Johnson JF, Brogdon BG. Dorsal effect of the patella: incidence and distribution. AJR 1982;139:339–340.
10. Helms C. Pseudocyst of the humerus. AJR 1979;131:287–292.
11. Resnick D, Cone R. The nature of humeral pseudocysts. Radiology 1984;150:27–28.
12. Minderhoud J, Braakman R, Penning L. Os odontoideum: clinical, radiological, and therapeutic aspects. J Neurol Sci 1969;8:521–544.
13. Holt RG, Helms CA, Munk PL, Gillespy T 3rd. Hypertrophy of C-1 anterior arch: useful sign to distinguish os odontoideum from acute dens fracture. Radiology 1989;173:207–209.
14. Onitsuka H. Roentgenologic aspects of bone islands. Radiology 1977;124:607–612.
15. Munk PL, Helms CA, Holt RG. Immature bone infarcts: findings on plain radiographs and MR scans. AJR 1989;152:547–549.

40
Miscellaneous Bone Lesions

Clyde A. Helms

There are a host of bony conditions, diseases, and syndromes that do not fit conveniently into any of the preceding chapters, yet should be given some mention in an attempted overview of musculoskeletal radiology. These are listed alphabetically for lack of a more scientific basis.

ACHONDROPLASIA

The most common cause of dwarfism is achondroplasia, a congenital, hereditary disease of failure of endochondral bone formation. The femurs and humeri are more profoundly affected than the other long bones, although the entire skeleton is abnormal. The spine typically has narrowing of the interpedicular distances in a caudal direction (Fig. 40.1), the opposite of normal where the interpedicular distances get progressively wider as one proceeds down the spine. The long bones are short but have normal width, giving them a thick appearance.

AVASCULAR NECROSIS

The term "avascular necrosis" (AVN) refers to the lack of blood supply with subsequent bone death and ensuing bony collapse in an articular surface. The etiology of AVN is an extensive differential that most commonly includes *trauma, steroids, aspirin, renal disease, collagen vascular diseases, alcoholism,* and *idiopathic* causes (Table 40.1) (1). The radiographic appearance ranges from patchy sclerosis (Fig. 40.2**A**) to articular surface collapse and fragmentation (Fig. 40.3). Just prior to collapse, a subchondral lucency is occasionally seen (Fig. 40.4); however, this is a late and inconstant sign of AVN. Magnetic resonance imaging (MR) is extremely valuable in demonstrating the presence and extent of AVN (Fig. 40.2**B**), even when plain films are apparently normal. Magnetic resonance imaging is currently considered to be the most efficacious way to evaluate a joint for AVN (2). It is useful not only in AVN of the hip, but also in the knee, wrist, foot, and ankle.

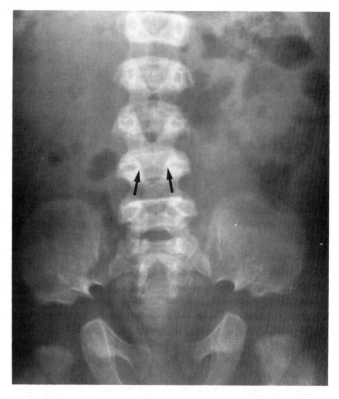

Figure 40.1. Achondroplasia. An anteroposterior plain film of the spine in this patient with achondroplasia demonstrates narrowing of the interpedicular distance (*arrows*) in a caudal direction, which is characteristic of this disorder. Ordinarily, the interpedicular distance widens in each vertebra in a caudal direction.

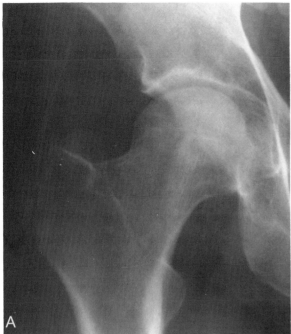

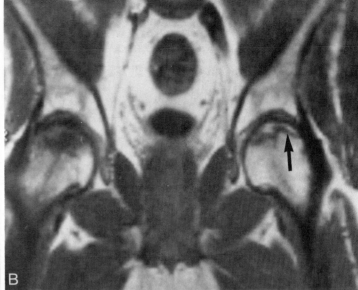

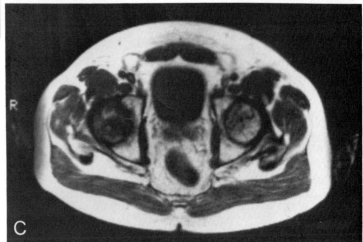

Figure 40.2.   Avascular Necrosis. A. A plain film of the hip in this patient with AVN shows faint, patchy sclerosis throughout the femoral head. This is a relatively early plain film finding for AVN. Coronal (**B**) and axial (**C**) MR images in the same patient, which are T1-weighted (TR 500; TE 28), show typical findings in AVN. Diffuse low signal in the right hip is noted, which is more extensive involvement than the left. The left hip has a low signal serpigenous rim (*arrow*), which is characteristic for AVN.

Table 40.1.   Common Causes of AVN

Trauma
Steroids
Renal disease
Collagen vascular diseases
Alcoholism
Idiopathic causes

HYPERTROPHIC PULMONARY OSTEOARTHROPATHY

Hypertrophic pulmonary osteoarthropathy is manifested by clubbing of the fingers and periostitis, usually in the upper and lower extremities (Fig. 40.5), which may or may not be associated with bone pain. It is most commonly seen in patients with lung cancer, but many other etiologies have been reported, including bronchiectasis, gastrointestinal disorders, and liver disease. The actual mechanism of formation of periostitis secondary to a distant malignancy or other process is unknown. The differential diagnosis for periostitis in a long bone without an underlying bony abnormality would include *hypertrophic pulmonary osteoarthropathy, venous stasis, thyroid acropachy, pachydermoperiostosis,* and *trauma* (Table 40.2).

MELORHEOSTOSIS

Melorheostosis is a rare, idiopathic disorder characterized by thickened cortical new bone that accumulates near the ends of long bones, usually only on one side of the bone, and has an appearance likened to "dripping candle wax" (Fig. 40.6). It can affect several adjacent bones and can be symptomatic.

MUCOPOLYSACCHARIDOSES (MORQUIO'S, HURLER'S, AND HUNTER'S SYNDROMES)

The mucopolysaccharidoses are a group of inherited diseases characterized by abnormal storage and

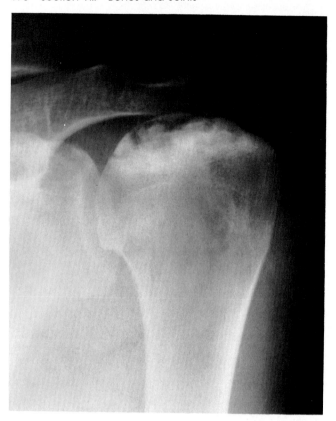

Figure 40.3. Avascular Necrosis. An anteroposterior plain film of the shoulder reveals articular surface collapse in this patient who was treated with steroids for systemic lupus erythematosus. This is an advanced stage of AVN.

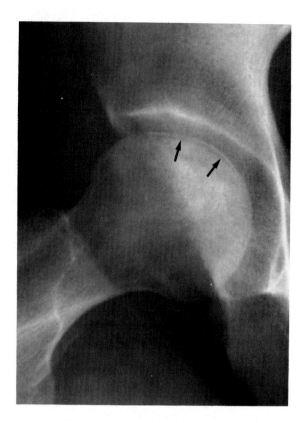

Figure 40.4. Avascular Necrosis. An anteroposterior frog-leg lateral view of the hip in this patient with sickle cell disease shows a subchondral lucency (*arrows*) and patchy sclerosis in the femoral head, indicative of AVN. This is a relatively advanced stage of AVN. The subchondral lucency is often better demonstrated with the frog-leg lateral view.

excretion in the urine of various mucopolysaccharidoses such as keratin sulfate (Morquio's) and heparan sulfate (Hurler's). These patients have short stature, primarily from shortened spines, and characteristic plain film findings. In the spine, patients with Morquio's have platyspondyly (generalized flattening of the vertebral bodies) with a central anterior projection or "beak" off the vertebral body, as viewed on a lateral plain film (Fig. 40.7). Hurler's and Hunter's show platyspondyly with a beak that is anteroinferiorly positioned (Fig. 40.8). The pelvis in these disorders is similar in appearance to that of achondroplasts with wide, flared iliac wings and broad femoral necks. A characteristic finding in the hands is a pointed proximal fifth metacarpal base that has a notch appearance to the ulnar aspect (Fig. 40.9).

MULTIPLE HEREDITARY EXOSTOSIS

Also known as diaphyseal aclasia, this is not a uncommon hereditary disorder that seems to affect multiple members of a family with multiple osteochondromas, or exostoses. An osteochondroma is a cartilage-capped bone outgrowth that may be pedunculated or sessile in appearance. In the multiple hereditary form, the knees are virtually always involved (Fig. 40.10). The

incidence of malignant degeneration in this population has been reported to be as high as 20%. As with solitary osteochondromas, the more axially situated lesions are more prone to undergo malignant degeneration, while the more peripheral lesions are less likely to do so. The proximal femurs are frequently involved and have a characteristic appearance (Fig. 40.11).

OSTEOID OSTEOMA

The etiology of osteoid osteoma is unknown. It may be an infection (bacterial or viral) or a slow-growing tumor, but nobody knows. It is a painful lesion that occurs almost exclusively in patients under the age of 30 and is treated successfully with surgical excision.

Radiographically, an osteoid osteoma is said to have a classic appearance, but in fact, it has many different appearances, which can make diagnosis difficult (3). The classically described radiographic appearance is a cortically based sclerotic lesion in a long bone that has a small lucency within it that is called the nidus (Fig. 40.12**A**). It is the nidus that causes the pain and the surrounding reactive sclerosis. If the nidus is surgically removed, complete cessation of pain is the rule. Com-

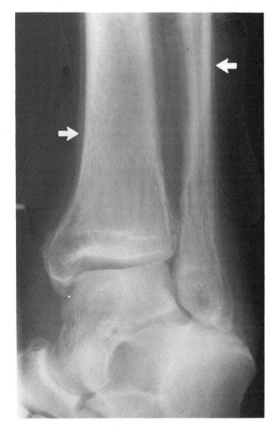

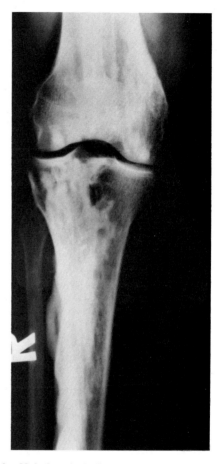

Figure 40.5. Hypertrophic Pulmonary Osteoarthrosis. Periostitis can be seen along the shafts of the distal tibia and fibula (*arrows*) in this patient with bronchogenic carcinoma and leg pain. This is characteristic for hypertrophic pulmonary osteoarthrosis.

Figure 40.6. Melorheostosis. Dense, wavy, new bone is seen adjacent to the lateral tibial cortex, which has a dripping candle wax appearance, which is classic for melorheostosis. A similar pattern can be seen in the medial aspect of the distal femur.

Table 40.2.   Periostitis without Underlying Bony Lesions

Trauma
Hypertrophic pulmonary osteoarthropathy
Venous stasis
Thyroid acropachy
Pachydermoperiostosis

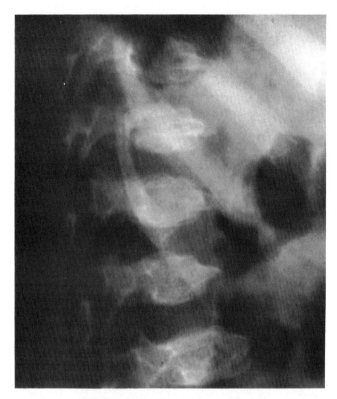

Figure 40.7. Morquio's Syndrome. A lateral plain film of the spine reveals a central beak or anterior bony projection off the vertebral bodies in this patient with Morquio's syndrome.

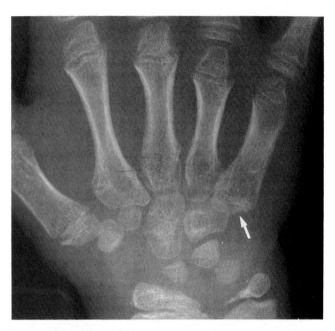

Figure 40.9. Hurler's Syndrome. An anteroposterior plain film of the hand in this patient with Hurler's syndrome shows a notch (*arrow*) at the base of the fifth metacarpal, which is a characteristic finding in all of the mucopolysaccharidoses.

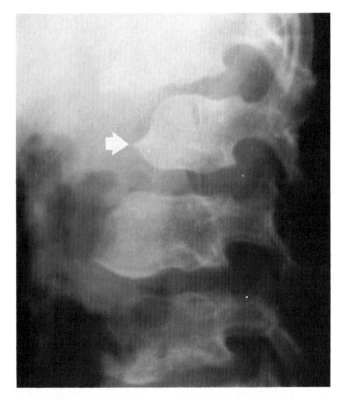

Figure 40.8. Hurler's Syndrome. A lateral plain film of the spine in this patient with Hurler's syndrome shows an inferiorly placed bony projection extending anteriorly off the vertebral bodies (*arrow*).

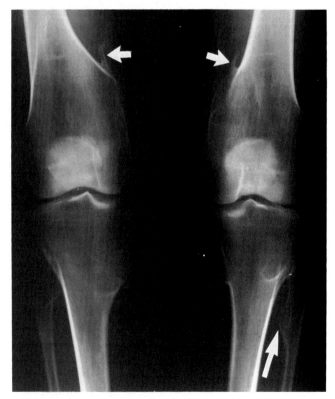

Figure 40.10. Multiple Hereditary Exostosis. The knees are involved in virtually every case of multiple hereditary exostosis. They typically show not only multiple exostoses (*arrows*), but marked undertubulation in the metaphyses.

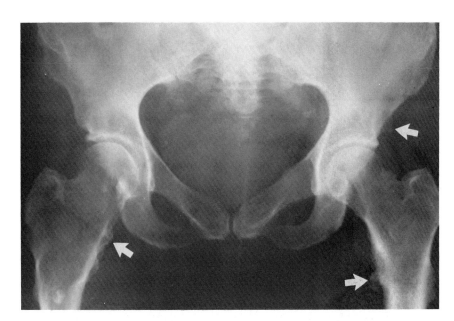

Figure 40.11. Multiple Hereditary Exostosis. The femoral necks are often involved in multiple hereditary exostosis. They will show undertubulation, as in this example, and usually have one or more exostoses (*arrows*).

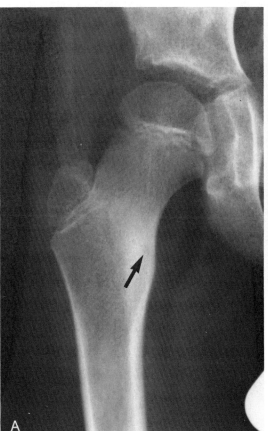

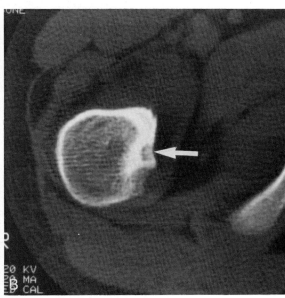

Figure 40.12. Osteoid Osteoma. A. An anteroposterior plain film of the femur in a child with hip pain shows an area of sclerosis medially near the lesser trochanter with a small lucency (*arrow*), which is the nidus of an osteoid osteoma. Osteomyelitis could have this identical appearance. **B.** A computed tomograpy scan of the femur shows the sclerosis medially and the lucent nidus (*arrow*) to better advantage. The computed tomography scan gives the surgeon a more precise anatomic location of the nidus than the plain film.

puted tomography is often very helpful in demonstrating the exact location of the nidus (Fig. 40.12**B**).

If the nidus of an osteoid osteoma is located in the medullary rather than the cortical portion of a bone, or if it is located in a joint, there is much less reactive sclerosis present. This gives the lesion a different overall appearance than the more common cortical lesion in that it does not appear as sclerotic. Up to 80%

of osteoid osteomas are located intracortically, with the remainder being in the intramedullary part of a bone. Rarely, an osteoid osteoma will present in the periosteum, causing tremendous periostitis.

The nidus itself is usually lucent but often develops some calcification within it. It then has the appearance of a sequestrum, as is seen in osteomyelitis. If the nidus calcifies completely, it blends in with the

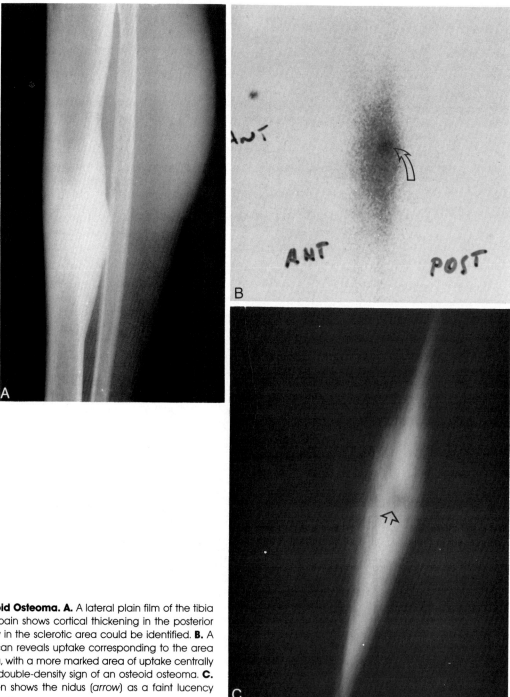

Figure 40.13.   Osteoid Osteoma. A. A lateral plain film of the tibia in this child with leg pain shows cortical thickening in the posterior diaphysis. No lucency in the sclerotic area could be identified. **B.** A radionuclide bone scan reveals uptake corresponding to the area of sclerosis in the tibia, with a more marked area of uptake centrally (*arrow*), which is the double-density sign of an osteoid osteoma. **C.** The surgical specimen shows the nidus (*arrow*) as a faint lucency within the sclerotic bone.

surrounding sclerosis and cannot be seen on most radiographs. Therefore, the diagnosis of an osteoid osteoma is in no way dependent on seeing a nidus.

Because an osteoid osteoma resembles osteomyelitis, regardless of the appearance of the nidus, it can be difficult to differentiate the two radiographically. In fact, it cannot be done with plain films, computed tomography, or MR. However, because the nidus is extremely vascular, it avidly accumulates radiopharmaceutical bone-scanning agents. An osteoid osteoma

will have an area of increased uptake corresponding to the area of reactive sclerosis but, in addition, will demonstrate a second area of increased uptake corresponding to the nidus (Fig. 40.13). This has been termed the "double-density" sign (4). In contrast, osteomyelitis has a photopenic area corresponding to the plain film lucency that represents an avascular focus of purulent material. The natural history of an osteoid osteoma is presumed to be spontaneous regression since they are rarely seen over the age of 30.

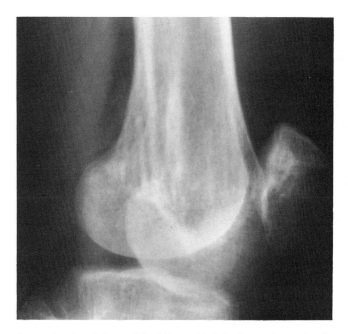

Figure 40.14. Osteopathia Striata. Multiple linear dense streaks are seen in the distal femur, which are characteristic of osteopathia striata.

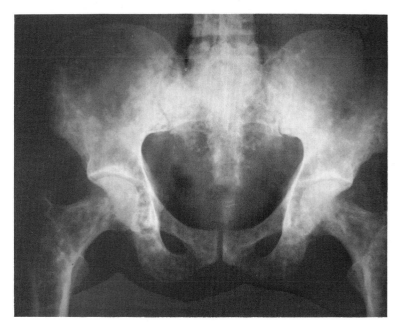

Figure 40.15. Osteopoikilosis. An anteroposterior view of the pelvis reveals multiple small, round sclerotic foci throughout the pelvis and femurs. This is diagnostic of osteopoikilosis. Metastatic disease is occasionally mistaken for this disorder.

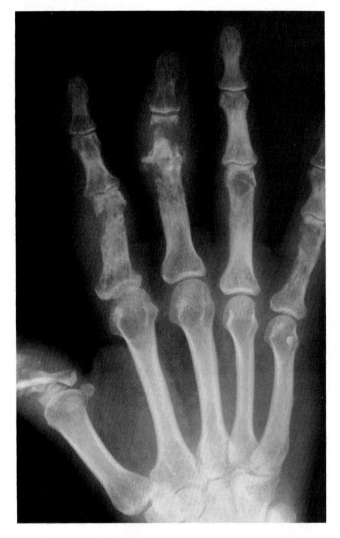

Figure 40.16.   Sarcoid. An anteroposterior plain film of the hands in a patient with sarcoidosis shows multiple lytic lesions, many of which demonstrate a lace-like pattern.

Figure 40.17. Idiopathic Transient Osteoporosis of the Hip. A. A plain film of a 40-year-old male with left hip pain shows osteoporosis involving the left hip, with no other abnormalities seen. **B.** A T1-weighted (TR 700; TE 12) coronal MR done at the same time as the plain film shows low signal in the superior portion of the left femoral head. This is a characteristic appearance for AVN, but is a nonspecific finding. Clinically, this patient had no underlying causes for AVN, and he was treated conservatively. **C.** Seven months later, after near total cessation of the hip pain, a repeat MR (TR 600;TE 20) shows no abnormality in the hip. This is consistent with idiopathic transient osteoporosis of the hip.

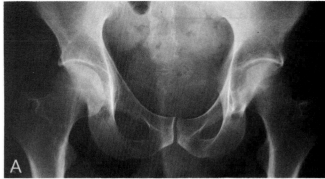

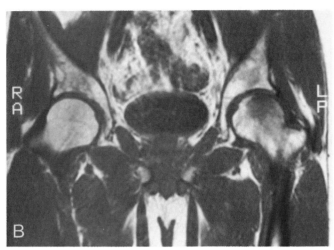

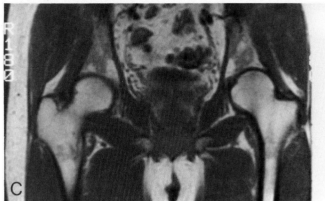

OSTEOPATHIA STRIATA

Also known as Voorhoeve's disease, this disorder is manifested by multiple 2–3 mm thick linear bands of sclerotic bone aligned parallel to the long axis of a bone (Fig. 40.14). It usually affects multiple long bones and is asymptomatic; hence, it is usually an incidental finding.

OSTEOPOIKILOSIS

Osteopoikilosis is an hereditary, asymptomatic disorder that is usually an incidental finding of multiple small (3–10 mm) sclerotic bony densities affecting primarily the ends of long bones and the pelvis (Fig. 40.15). It has no clinical significance other than that it can be confused for diffuse osteoblastic metastases.

PACHYDERMOPERIOSTOSIS

Pachydermoperiostosis is a rare, familial disease that is manifested by thickening of the skin of the extremities and face and clubbing of the fingers. it seems to be more common in black patients. The periosteal reaction is similar to that of hypertrophic pulmonary osteoarthropathy, but pachydermoperiostosis is rarely painful.

SARCOIDOSIS

Sarcoidosis is a noncaseating granulomatous disease that primarily affects the lungs. When the mus-culoskeletal system is involved, the hands are mainly affected, with the spine and long bones only infrequently involved. Sarcoid causes a characteristic "lace-like" pattern of bony destruction in the hands (Fig. 40.16). Multiple phalanges are typically affected in either one or both hands. It is so radiographically characteristic that there is almost no differential diagnosis for this pattern.

TRANSIENT OSTEOPOROSIS OF THE HIP

This poorly understood disorder is an idiopathic process that begins with a painful hip with no underlying disorder or other findings other than osteoporosis, which is limited to the painful hip. Some believe it is early AVN; however, this has not been conclusively proved. Its appearance on MR is similar to early AVN (5) in that low signal on T1-weighted images is seen throughout the femoral head and neck (Fig. 40.17). Transient osteoporosis of the hip invariably is self-limited with full resolution. It tends to occur more often in males.

References

1. Mankin H. Nontraumatic necrosis of bone (osteonecrosis). N Engl J Med 1992;326:1473–1479.
2. Mitchell D, Kressel H, Arger P, Dalinka M, Spritzer C, Steinberg M. Avascular necrosis of the femoral head: morphologic assessment by MR imaging, with CT correlation. Radiology 1986;161:739–742.

3. Marcove R, Heelan R, Huvos A, Healey J, Lindeque B. Osteoid osteoma. Diagnosis, localization, and treatment. Clin Orthop 1991;267:197–201.
4. Helms CA, Hattner RS, Vogler JB III. Osteoid osteoma: radionuclide diagnosis. Radiology 1984;151:779–784.
5. Takatori Y, Kokubo T, Ninomiya S, Nakamura T, Okutsu I, Kamogawa M. Transient osteoporosis of the hip. Magnetic resonance imaging. Clin Orthop 1991;271:190–194.

41

Magnetic Resonance Imaging of the Knee

Clyde A. Helms

TECHNIQUE
MENISCI
CRUCIATE LIGAMENTS
COLLATERAL LIGAMENTS
PATELLA
BONY ABNORMALITIES

Magnetic resonance imaging (MR) of the knee has developed into one of the most frequently requested examinations in radiology. This is because of its inherent accuracy in depicting internal derangements and allowing the orthopaedic surgeons to use the study as a road map for subsequent therapeutic arthroscopic procedures. Also, it has a very high negative predictive value; therefore, a normal MR knee examination is highly accurate in excluding an internal derangement (1, 2).

TECHNIQUE

The proper imaging protocol is essential for a high diagnostic accuracy rate. If the appropriate sequences are obtained, an accuracy of 90–95% can be expected. A sagittal T1-weighted (or proton-density) sequence is essential for examining the menisci. Four or 5-mm thick slices with a relatively small field of view and at least a 192 matrix are recommended. The knee should be imaged using a dedicated knee coil and externally rotated about 5–10° (do not exceed 10°) to put the anterior cruciate ligament in the plane of imaging. T2 spin-echo or T2* GRASS (gradient recalled acquisition in the steady state) sagittal images are obtained primarily to examine the cruciate ligaments. With T2-weighted spin-echo images, meniscal tears may be difficult to see; however, they will be picked up on the proton-density images.

Coronal images are obtained to examine the collateral ligaments and to look for meniscocapsular separations. These abnormalities can generally only be seen with T2-weighted images. T1-weighted coronal images are therefore a waste of time as there is nothing to be seen on these images that cannot be equally well seen on the sagittal images or the T2 or T2* coronal images. T2* GRASS coronal images or repeating the sagittal spin-echo sequences in the coronal plane are imperative. The coronal images are rarely useful for seeing a meniscal tear that cannot be appreciated on the sagittal images.

Axial images are obtained primarily for use by the technicians as a scout view. They can also be utilized for viewing the patellofemoral cartilage and for examining a medial patellar plica. As in the coronal images, to afford an opportunity to see any pathology. T2-weighted or T2* images must be obtained. Because it takes too long to obtain another full spin-echo sequence with proton-density and T2-weighted images, a T2* GRASS sequence is recommended.

MENISCI

The normal meniscus is a fibrocartilagenous, C-shaped structure that is uniformly low in signal on both T1- and T2-weighted sequences (Fig. 41.1). With T2* sequences, the menisci will usually demonstrate some internal signal. With T1-weighted images, any signal within the meniscus is abnormal, except in children, where some signal is normal and represents normal vascularity.

Meniscal Degeneration. Meniscal signal that does not disrupt an articular surface is representative of intrasubstance degeneration (Fig. 41.2), which is myxoid degeneration of the fibrocartilage. It most likely represents aging and normal wear and tear. It is not thought to be symptomatic, and cannot be diagnosed clinically or with arthroscopy. Some choose, therefore, not to mention intrasubstance degeneration in the radiology interpretation. A grading scale for meniscal signal that is widely used is the following (Fig. 41.3): Grade 1, rounded or amorphous signal that does *not* disrupt an articular surface; Grade 2, linear signal that does *not* disrupt an articular surface; and Grade 3, rounded or linear signal that disrupts an articular surface (Fig. 41.4). Grades 1 and 2 are intrasubtance degeneration and should not be reported as "grade 1 or 2 tears." The term "tear" often leads to an unnecessary arthroscopy (arthroscopy is not indicated for intrasubstance degeneration). Grade 3 is a meniscal tear.

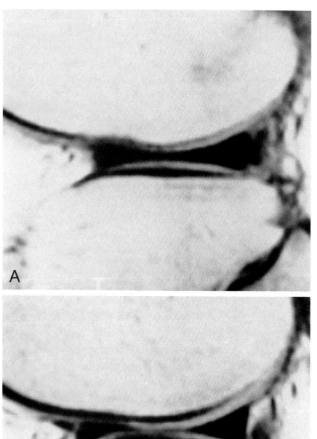

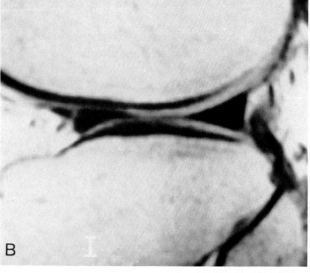

Figure 41.1.   Normal Meniscus. A. A T1-weighted sagittal image (TR 600; TE 30) through a normal lateral meniscus demonstrates uniform low signal in the meniscus. This is a section through the body of the meniscus as it has a bowtie configuration. Two sections of the body should be seen in each meniscus with 4- or 5-mm thick slices. **B.** In the same T1-weighted sequence, this sagittal image demonstrates uniform low signal in the anterior and posterior horns of this normal lateral meniscus.

Mensical Tear.   When high signal in a meniscus disrupts the superior or inferior articular surface, a meniscal tear is diagnosed (Fig. 41.4). Meniscal tears have many different configurations and locations; an oblique tear extending to the inferior surface of the posterior horn of the medial meniscus is the most common type. In a small but significant percentage of cases, it can be virtually impossible to be certain if meniscal high signal disrupts an articular surface. In these cases it is recommended that the surgeon be advised that it is too close to call. The surgeon can then

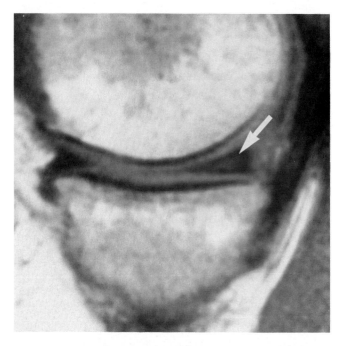

Figure 41.2.   Intrasubstance Degeneration. Faint intermediate signal can be seen in the posterior horn of this meniscus (*arrow*) that does not disrupt the articular surface of the meniscus. This is intrasubstance degeneration.

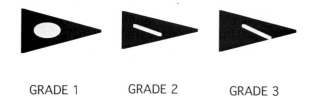

GRADE 1   GRADE 2   GRADE 3

Figure 41.3.   Grading Scale for Menisci. A schematic of the MR grading scale for meniscal abnormalities. Grade 1 is rounded or amorphous signal in the meniscus that does not disrupt an articular surface. Grade 2 is linear signal that does not disrupt an articular surface. Grades 1 and 2 represent intrasubstance degeneration. Grade 3 is signal that does disrupt an articular surface and indicates a meniscal tear.

rely on his or her clinical expertise to decide if arthroscopy is warranted and, if it is, the MR will guide the surgeon to where the questionable tear is located. If these equivocal cases are excluded, the remaining cases will have an extremely high accuracy rate.

Bucket-handle Tear.   Another very common meniscal tear is a bucket-handle tear. This is a vertical longitudinal tear that can result in the inner free edge of the meniscus becoming displaced into the intercondylar notch (Fig. 41.5). It is most easily recognized by observing on the sagittal images that only one image is present that has the bowtie appearance of the body segment of the meniscus (Fig. 41.6). Normally, two contiguous sagittal images with a bowtie shape are seen because the normal meniscus is 10–12 mm in width and the sagittal images are 4–5 mm in thickness. On the coronal images, a bucket-handle

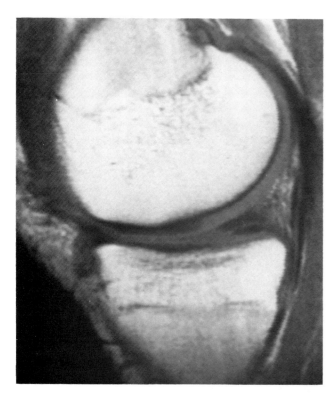

Figure 41.4.   Meniscal Tear. This T1-weighted sagittal image (TR 600; TE 30) shows linear high signal in the posterior horn of the meniscus that disrupts the inferior articular surface. This is the appearance of a meniscal tear.

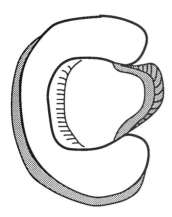

Figure 41.5.   Bucket-handle Tear. This drawing illustrates a bucket-handle tear with the torn free edge of the meniscus displaced as the handle of the bucket.

tear may reveal the meniscus to be shortened and truncated; however, often the torn meniscus remodels and truncation cannot be appreciated. The displaced inner edge of the meniscus (the "handle" of the bucket) is often seen in the intercondylar notch on sagittal or coronal views (Fig. 41.7); however, it can occasionally be difficult to find the displaced meniscal fragment.

Discoid Meniscus. A discoid meniscus is a large meniscus that can have many different shapes —lens-shaped, wedged, flat, and others. It is not known if it is congenital or acquired, but most are found in children or young adults. It is seen laterally in up to 3% of the population, with a discoid medial meniscus being much less common. A discoid meniscus is thought to be more prone to tear than a normal meniscus, and can be symptomatic even without being torn. Although they are easily identified on coronal images by noting meniscal tissue extending into the tibial spines at the intercondylar notch (Fig. 41.8), they are most reliably diagnosed by noting more than two consecutive sagittal images that show the meniscus with a bowtie appearance (Fig. 41.9) (3).

Transverse Ligament. The lateral meniscus often has what appears to be a tear on the anterior horn near its upper margin, which is a pseudotear from the insertion of the transverse ligament (Fig. 41.10). This can easily be differentiated from a real tear by following it medially across the knee in Hoffa's fat pad where it inserts into the anterior horn of the medial meniscus. The function of the transverse ligament is unknown.

CRUCIATE LIGAMENTS

Anterior Cruciate Ligament. The normal anterior cruciate ligament (ACL) is seen in the intercondylar notch as a linear, predominantly low signal structure on T1-weighted images; it often shows some linear striations near its insertion onto the medial tibial spine when viewed on sagittal images (Fig. 41.11). When torn, the ACL is most often simply not visualized, although sometimes the actual disruption will be seen (Fig. 41.12). T2-weighted or T2*-weighted images are imperative for obtaining the highest accuracy in diagnosing ACL tears, as fluid and hemorrhage will often obscure the ligament on T1-weighted images. Partial tears or strains of the ACL are manifested by high signal within an otherwise intact ligament.

Posterior Cruciate Ligament. The normal posterior cruciate ligament (PCL) is a gently curved, homogeneously low signal structure (Fig. 41.13) that is infrequently torn and even less frequently repaired by surgeons. When torn, it takes on diffuse intermediate signal throughout (Fig. 41.14). Most orthopaedic surgeons do not even inspect the PCL at arthroscopy and do not repair it when torn because it rarely is a cause of instability.

Meniscofemoral Ligament. A low signal round structure is often seen just anterior or posterior to the PCL, as seen in the sagittal views. A loose body or a free fragment of a piece of torn meniscus can have this appearance (Fig. 41.15), but it is most commonly due to a meniscofemoral ligament that extends obliquely across the knee from the medial femoral condyle to the posterior horn of the lateral meniscus. If it

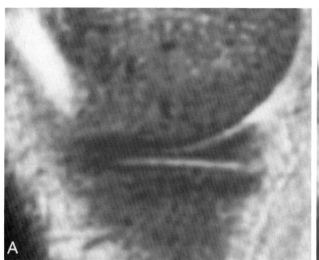

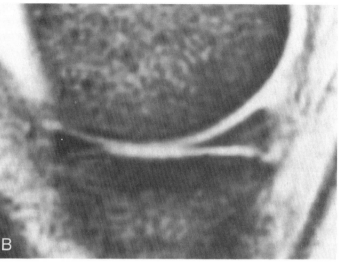

Figure 41.6.   Bucket-handle Tear. Sagittal T1-weighted images (TR 600; TE 30) through the medial meniscus at its most medial aspect reveal one bowtie, indicative of the body of the meniscus (**A**) with the adjacent image (**B**) having apparent normal anterior and pos-terior horns. However, since there should be two consecutive sagittal images with a bowtie configuration, this indicates a bucket-handle tear.

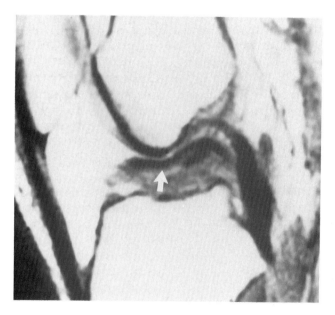

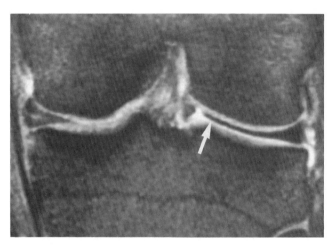

Figure 41.8.   Discoid Lateral Meniscus. A coronal GRASS image (TR 500; TE 30; θ, 30°) through the intercondylar notch shows a large lateral meniscus with meniscal tissue extending into the notch medi-ally (*arrow*).

Figure 41.7.   Displaced Fragment in Bucket-handle Tear. A sagit-tal T1-weighted image (TR 600; TE 30) through the intercondylar notch in a patient with a bucket-handle tear reveals the displaced free fragment or handle (*arrow*) just anterior to the PCL.

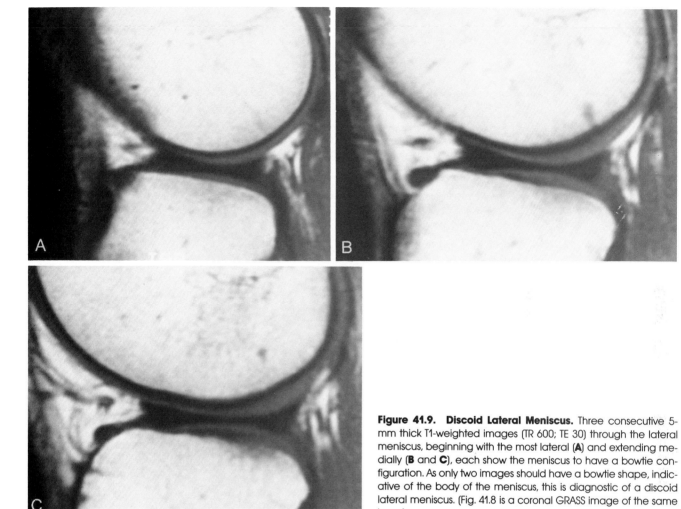

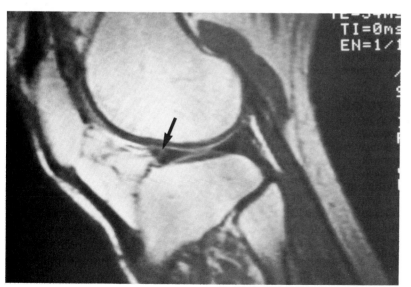

Figure 41.9. Discoid Lateral Meniscus. Three consecutive 5-mm thick T1-weighted images (TR 600; TE 30) through the lateral meniscus, beginning with the most lateral (**A**) and extending medially (**B** and **C**), each show the meniscus to have a bowtie configuration. As only two images should have a bowtie shape, indicative of the body of the meniscus, this is diagnostic of a discoid lateral meniscus. (Fig. 41.8 is a coronal GRASS image of the same knee.)

Figure 41.10. Pseudotear from a Transverse Ligament. A sagittal T1-weighted image (TR 600; TE 30) through the lateral meniscus shows linear high signal through the upper anterior horn (*arrow*), which resembles a tear. This is the insertion of the transverse ligament onto the meniscus.

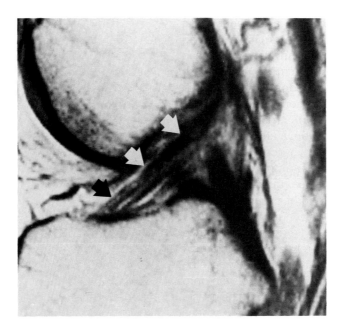

Figure 41.11. Normal ACL. A sagittal T1-weighted image (TR 600; TE 30) through the intercondylar notch shows the normal appearance of the ACL (*arrows*).

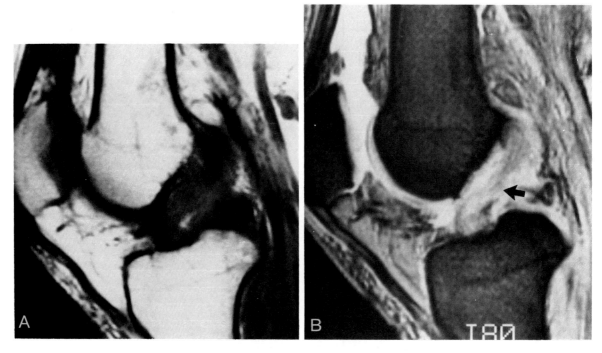

Figure 41.12. Torn ACL. A. A sagittal T1-weighted image (TR 600; TE 30) through the intercondylar notch does not reveal any structure that resembles a normal ACL. This is a common MR appearance of a torn ACL. **B.** A sagittal GRASS image (TR 500; TE 30; θ 30°) in the same knee shows fibers of the torn ACL that are disrupted centrally (*arrow*).

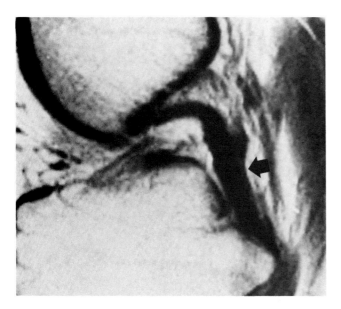

Figure 41.13. Normal PCL. A sagittal T1-weighted image (TR 600; TE 30) through the intercondylar notch shows the appearance of the normal PCL with its characteristic uniform low signal (*arrow*).

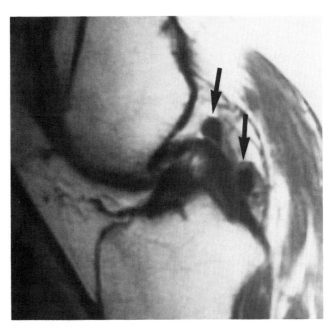

Figure 41.15. Free Fragment of a Torn Meniscus. A sagittal T1-weighted image (TR 600; TE 30) through the intercondylar notch in this patient with a torn meniscus shows two rounded low signal structures (*arrows*) that are free fragments of meniscal tissue. A meniscofemoral ligament of Wrisberg could have the appearance of either of these loose bodies.

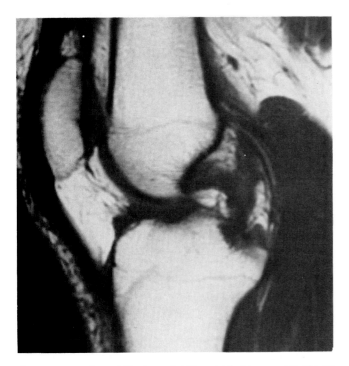

Figure 41.14. Torn PCL. A sagittal T1-weighted image (TR 600; TE 30) through the intercondylar notch reveals the PCL to have diffuse intermediate signal throughout. This is typical for a torn PCL.

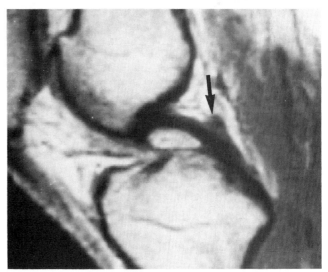

Figure 41.16. Ligament of Wrisberg. A sagittal T1-weighted image (TR 600; TE 30) through the intercondylar notch shows a rounded low signal structure posterior to the PCL, which is the meniscofemoral ligament of Wrisberg (*arrow*).

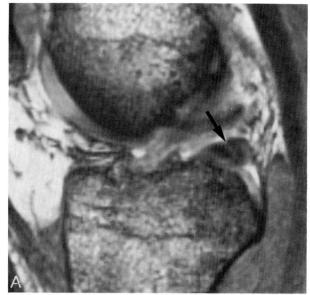

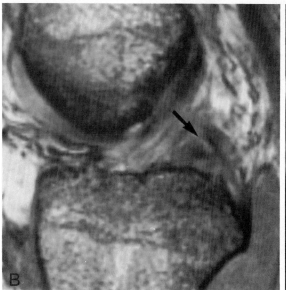

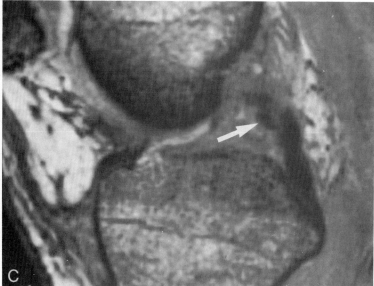

Figure 41.17.   Pseudotear from Ligament of Humphry insertion.
A. A sagittal three-dimensional volume image (TR 500; TE 15; θ 30°) through the lateral meniscus reveals an apparent tear of the posterior horn (*arrow*). **B.** On the adjacent image, 3 mm more medially the "tear" seems to widen (*arrow*) as the meniscus becomes less well seen. **C.** On the next adjacent image, medially a ligament of Humphry (*arrow*) is seen anterior to the PCL. Note that the ligament of Humphry is a continuation of the structure seen on the prior image and extends into the upper part of the posterior horn of the lateral meniscus in **A.**

passes in front of the PCL, it is called the ligament of Humphry, and if it passes behind the PCL, it is called the ligament of Wrisberg (Fig. 41.16). One or the other of these ligaments is present in up to 72% of all knees.

The insertion of the ligament of Humphry or Wrisberg onto the lateral meniscus can produce a pseudotear similar to that caused by the transverse ligament on the anterior horn of the lateral meniscus (Fig. 41.17). Prior to calling a tear on the upper aspect of the posterior horn of the lateral meniscus, care must be taken to look for a meniscofemoral ligament to be certain it is not a pseudotear from the ligament's insertion. Similarly, prior to calling a loose body in front of or behind the PCL, care must be taken to try to follow the structure across to the lateral meniscus to determine if it is a meniscofemoral ligament.

COLLATERAL LIGAMENTS

Medial Collateral Ligament.   The medial collateral ligament (MCL) originates on the medial femoral condyle and inserts on the tibia. It is closely applied to the joint and is intimately associated with the medial joint capsule and the medial meniscus. The MCL is uniformly low in signal on T1 and T2 or T2* sequences. Injuries to the MCL usually occur from a valgus stress to the lateral part of the knee (such as a "clipping" injury in football). A grade 1 injury represents a mild sprain and is diagnosed on MR by noting fluid or hemorrhage in the soft tissues medial to the MCL. The ligament is otherwise normal. A grade 2 injury is a partial tear and is seen as high signal in and around the MCL on T2 or T2* coronal sequences. The ligament is intact, although the deep or superficial fibers may show minimal disruption (Fig. 41.18). A grade 3 injury is a com-

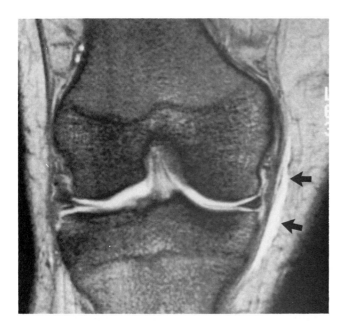

Figure 41.18.   Partial Tear of the MCL. A GRASS coronal image (TR 500; TE 15; θ 30°) reveals high signal adjacent to the MCL (*arrows*), which represents edema and hemorrhage from a partial tear or sprain of the MCL. The MCL is clearly intact; hence, a complete tear is easily excluded.

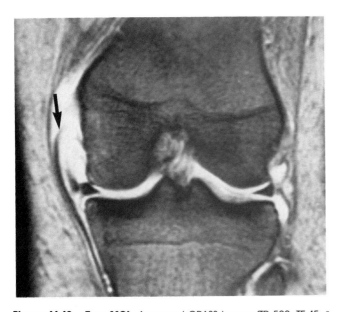

Figure 41.19.   Torn MCL. A coronal GRASS image (TR 500; TE 15, θ 30°) shows a large joint effusion with the MCL disrupted proximally (*arrow*). In addition, joint fluid can be seen extending between the medial meniscus and the MCL, which indicates a meniscocapsular separation. Neither of these diagnoses could be made on the T1-weighted coronal images.

plete disruption of the MCL. It can be best appreciated on T2 or T2* images (Fig. 41.19).

A meniscocapsular separation occurs when the medial meniscus is torn from its attachment to the joint capsule. It occurs most commonly at the site of the MCL and often occurs concomitantly with an MCL in-

jury. It is easily recognized on a T2 or T2* coronal image by noting joint fluid extending between the medial meniscus and the capsule (Fig. 41.20). It is essential to use T2 or T2* sequences as a T1-weighted image will not detect the fluid between the meniscus and the capsule.

Lateral Collateral Ligament. The lateral collateral ligament consists of three parts. The most posterior structure is the tendon of the biceps femoris, which inserts onto the head of the fibula. Next, anterior to the biceps is the true lateral collateral ligament, also called the fibulocollateral ligament, which extends from the lateral femoral condyle to the head of the fibula. The biceps and the fibulocollateral ligament usually join and insert onto the head of the fibula as a conjoined tendon. Anterior to the fibulocollateral ligament is the iliotibial band, which extends into the fascia more anteriorly and blends into the lateral retinaculum on the patella. The lateral collateral ligament is infrequently torn.

PATELLA

Chondromalacia Patella. The patellar cartilage commonly undergoes degeneration causing exquisite pain and tenderness. This is called chondromalacia patella. It can be diagnosed on sagittal images but is generally more easily identified on axial images. Since hyaline articular cartilage has the same signal intensity as joint fluid on T1-weighted sequences, T2 or T2* sequences are necessary to diagnose chondromalacia patella in most instances.

Chondromalacia patella begins with focal swelling and degeneration of the cartilage. This can be seen as low or high signal foci in the cartilage. As it progresses, it causes thinning and irregularity of the articular surface of the cartilage, and finally underlying bone is exposed. This final stage occurs more commonly from trauma than from wear and tear (Fig. 41.21).

Patellar Plica. A normal structure that is seen in over half of the population is the medial patellar plica. It is an embryologic remnant from when the knee was divided into three compartments. It is a thin, fibrous band that extends from the medial capsule toward, and sometimes onto, the medial facet of the patella (Fig. 41.22). A suprapatellar and infrapatellar plica also exist. The medial patellar plica can, on rare occasions, thicken and cause clinical symptoms indistinguishable from a torn meniscus; this has been termed "plica syndrome." An abnormal plica can be easily removed arthroscopically.

BONY ABNORMALITIES

Contusions. The most frequently encountered bony abnormality seen with MR is a contusion. A con-

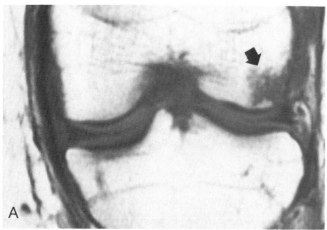
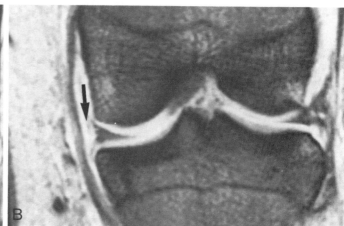

Figure 41.20.   Meniscocapsular Separation. A. A T1-weighted coronal image (TR 600; TE 30) reveals a contusion of the lateral femoral condyle (*arrow*), indicative of a valgus strain, which is often associated with a MCL tear. The MCL appears normal on this image; however, the linear low signal in the soft tissues just adjacent to the MCL is suggestive of fluid. This would indicate a partial tear or sprain of the MCL. **B.** A coronal GRASS image (TR 500; TE 15; θ 30°) in the same knee reveals fluid between the medial meniscus and the MCL (*arrow*), which is diagnostic for a meniscocapsular separation. Faint high signal in the MCL and adjacent to it indicates a partial tear. A T2 or T2* sequence in the coronal plane is necessary to see these abnormalities.

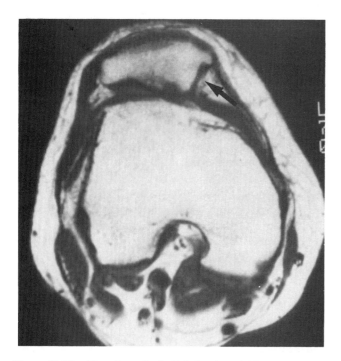
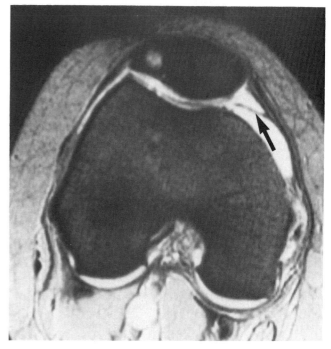

Figure 41.21.   Chondromalacia Patella. An axial T1-weighted image (TR 600; TE 30) through the patella shows virtually no cartilage covering the medial facet (*arrow*). Subchondral sclerosis and an irregular articular surface can be noted in the lateral facet. These changes indicate severe chondromalacia patella. T2-weighted images are recommended to see more subtle changes in the articular cartilage.

Figure 41.22.   Plica. An axial GRASS image (TR 500; TE 15; θ 30°) through the patella shows a low signal linear structure (*arrow*) extending from the medial capsule toward the medial facet of the patella. This is a medial patellar plica that is not abnormally thickened. Without the joint effusion or the T2-weighted image, the plica would not be visualized.

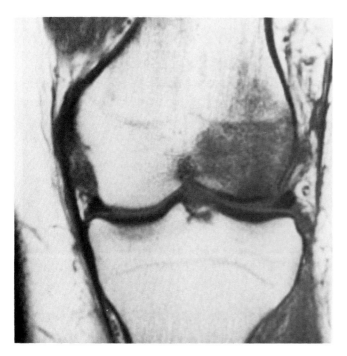

Figure 41.23. Contusion. A coronal T1-weighted image (TR 600; TE 30) shows a focus of low signal in the lateral femoral condyle, which is subarticular. This is a characteristic appearance for a severe bone contusion.

tusion represents microfractures from trauma (4). They are also called bone bruises. They are easily identified on T1-weighted sequences as subarticular areas of inhomogeneous low signal (Fig. 41.23). With T2 weighting, a contusion will show increased signal for several weeks, depending on its severity. It can be difficult to see increased signal with T2* images because of the susceptibility artifacts of the bone seen with T2* images. Contusions can progress to osteochondritis dissecans if they are not treated with diminished weight bearing; hence, an isolated bone contusion, with no other internal derangement, is a serious finding that requires protection.

A commonly seen contusion is one that occurs on the posterior part of the lateral tibial plateau (Fig. 41.24). it is invariably associated with a torn ACL. Acute ACL tears have been reported to have this type of contusion in over 90% of cases (5).

Fractures. Magnetic resonance imaging is useful in examining fractures about the knee. Tibial plateau fractures can be imaged precisely with computed tomography; however, MR allows the soft tissues to be seen in addition to any bony abnormalities. A fracture that occurs that is almost always associated with an internal derangement is the Segond fracture. It is a

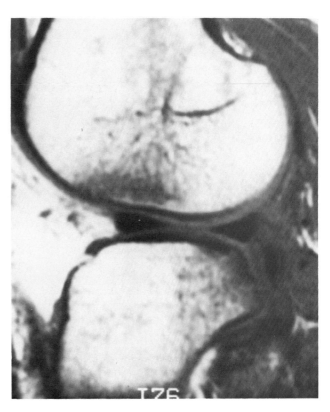

Figure 41.24. Contusion. A sagittal T1-weighted image through the lateral compartment shows irregular low signal in a subarticular location of the posterior tibial plateau and in the anterior part of the lateral femoral condyle. These findings are characteristic for bone contusions. This distribution of contusions in the posterior lateral tibial plateau and anterior in the lateral femoral condyle is almost always associated with a torn ACL.

small bony fragment pulled off the posterior lateral tibial joint line by an avulsion of the lateral joint capsule. It is almost always associated with an ACL tear.

References

1. Crues JI, Mink J, Levy T, Lotysch M, Stoller D. Meniscal tears of the knee: accuracy of MR imaging. Radiology 1987;164:445–448.
2. Mink JH, Deutsch AL. Magnetic resonance imaging of the knee. Clin Orthop 1989;244:29–47.
3. Silverman J, Mink J, Deutsch A. Discoid menisci of the knee; MR imaging appearance. Radiology 1989;173:351–354.
4. Mink JH, Deutsch AL. Occult cartilage and bone injuries of the knee: detection, classification, and assessment with MR imaging. Radiology 1989;170:823–829.
5. Murphy B, Smith R, Uribe J, Janecki C, Hechtman K, Mangasarian R. Bone signal abnormalities in the posterolateral tibia and lateral femoral condyle in complete tears of the anterior cruciate ligament: a specific sign? Radiology 1992;182:221–224.

42

Magnetic Resonance Imaging of the Shoulder

Clyde A. Helms

Magnetic resonance imaging (MR) of the shoulder is a still-evolving examination for its diagnostic utility for abnormalities of the rotator cuff and the glenoid labrum. It has been shown by some investigators to have a high degree of accuracy (1–4), while others report a barely acceptable rate of accuracy. Although there is currently some controversy over its utility, MR of the shoulder is nevertheless replacing standard arthrography and computed tomographic (CT) arthrography for examining the rotator cuff and the glenoid labrum.

ANATOMY

The rotator cuff is comprised of the tendons of four muscles that converge on the greater and lesser tuberosities of the humerus: the supraspinatus, infraspinatus, subscapularis, and teres minor (Fig. 42.1). Of these, the supraspinatus most commonly causes clinically significant problems, and is the one that is most commonly surgically treated. The supraspinatus tendon lies just superior to the scapula and inferior to the acromioclavicular (AC) joint and acromion. It inserts into the greater tuberosity of the humerus. Two to three centimeters proximal to its insertion is a section of the tendon called the "critical zone." This area is reported to have decreased vascularity and is therefore less likely to heal following trauma. The critical zone of the supraspinatus tendon is where most rotator cuff tears occur.

The glenoid labrum is a fibrocartilaginous ring that surrounds the periphery of the bony glenoid of the scapula. It serves as an attachment site for the cap-

sule and broadens the base of the glenohumeral joint to allow increased stability. Tears of the glenoid labrum most commonly occur from, and result in, dislocations of the humerus.

ROTATOR CUFF

The rotator cuff commonly suffers from what has been termed "impingement syndrome." Impingement of the critical zone of the supraspinatus tendon occurs from abduction of the humerus, which allows the tendon to be impinged between the anterior acromion and the greater tuberosity. The tendon can also be impinged by the undersurface of the AC joint if downward-pointing osteophytes or a thickened capsule is present. Other theories exist for impingement syndrome, including natural degeneration from aging and a predisposition for the critical zone to undergo degeneration due to decreased blood supply. Most investigators agree that whatever the cause, the natural course of impingement syndrome is a complete, or full-thickness, tear of the rotator cuff.

The rotator cuff is best seen on oblique coronal images that are aligned parallel to the supraspinatus muscle (Fig. 42.2). Both T1- and T2-weighted sequences are mandatory. Multiple acceptable variations of imaging sequences are available to demonstrate the normal and abnormal structures that can be seen in the oblique coronal plane. The most com-

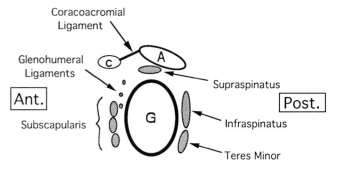

Figure 42.1. Schematic of Shoulder Anatomy. This drawing shows the rotator cuff muscles in a sagittal plane (anterior is on the left). (C, coracoid; A, acromion; G, glenoid.)

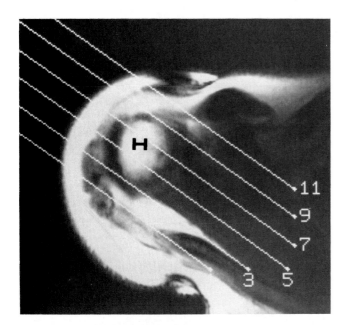

Figure 42.2. Scout View for Oblique Coronal Images. This axial image through the supraspinatus shows the cursors angled along the plane of the supraspinatus muscle (anterior on top) *H,* humeral head.

monly employed protocol is a spin-echo proton-density and T2-weighted sequence. Some prefer to use a spin-echo T1-weighted image in conjunction with a GRASS or other type of T2* sequence. The slice thickness should be no greater than 5 mm, and 3 mm is preferable. As with most joint imaging, a small field of view (16–20 cm) is recommended. A dedicated shoulder coil or a surface coil placed anteriorly over the shoulder is necessary, although no particular type of shoulder coil appears to be clearly superior.

In examining the rotator cuff, the most anterior oblique coronal images will show the critical zone of the supraspinatus tendon. A useful landmark for noting the supraspinatus tendon is the AC joint, which is an anterior structure and usually easily located. The infraspinatus tendon is seen on the more posterior images and can easily be mistaken for the tendon of the supraspinatus. The supraspinatus tendon can be differentiated from that of the infraspinatus by noting the more horizontal course of the supraspinatus as compared with the infraspinatus, which runs obliquely inferiorly to superiorly.

The normal supraspinatus tendon is said to be uniformly low in signal on all pulse sequences (Fig. 42.3). Unfortunately, this is not always the case. In fact, it usually has some intermediate-to-high signal in the critical zone, which causes much confusion. If the signal in the critical zone gets brighter on the T2-weighted images, it is abnormal and represents either tendinitis or a partial tear (severe tendinitis) (Fig. 42.4). However, if it disappears or has the same signal intensity as the adjacent muscle on T2-weighted se-

quences, it may represent one of many different processes:

1. Partial volume averaging of peritendinous fat can cause some high signal in the supraspinatous tendon on the oblique coronal images; this does not get brighter on T2-weighted images.
2. If the plane of the oblique coronal images is slightly off of the plane of the tendon, muscle slips can be partially volume averaged, which may appear as relatively high signal on T1-weighted images but will not get brighter with T2-weighted images.
3. The so-called "magic angle" effect can cause apparent high signal in a tendon that lies at 55° to the bore of the magnet (as does the critical zone of the supraspinatus tendon) (5). This high signal will not be seen on T2-weighted images (or any sequence with a long TE). This is believed to be a common cause of high signal in the critical zone on T1-weighted images.
4. Myxoid and fibrillar degeneration of the supraspinatus tendon are commonly found in autopsy specimens that increase with age. The majority of asymptomatic shoulders in patients over the age of 50 are believed to have some tendon degeneration in the supraspinatus; this has been termed "tendonopathy." This is seen as high signal in the critical zone on T1-weighted images that does not increase with T2 weighting (6). It has not been determined if this can be symptomatic.

Because high signal can be seen in the critical zone of the supraspinatus in a variety of normal situations, how can one differentiate the normal from the abnormal? As long as the T2-weighted images do not show the signal getting brighter, it probably does not matter. Tendon degeneration (tendonopathy) can be seen in asymptomatic shoulders of all ages; hence, it needs to be correlated with the clinical picture. If the signal gets brighter on T2-weighted images it must be considered pathologic—either tendinitis or a partial tear. If, in addition, fluid is present in the subacromial bursa, a small full-thickness tear should be mentioned as a possibility even if a definite tendon disruption cannot be seen. A small amount of fluid can be seen in the subacromial bursa because of a partial tear, but if a substantial amount of fluid is found, a full-thickness tear is almost certainly present.

If disruption of the supraspinatus tendon can be seen, obviously a full-thickness tear is present. In these cases fluid is invariably present in the subacromial bursa (Fig. 42.5). Care should be made to look for retraction of the supraspinatus muscle, as marked retraction will obviate some types of surgery.

Thus, three categories exist for the appearance of the supraspinatus tendon. (*a*) High signal on T1-

Figure 42.3. Normal Supraspinatus Tendon. A T1-weighted (TR 600; TE 30) oblique coronal image shows a normal supraspinatus tendon (*arrow*) with uninterrupted low signal extending from the musculotendinous junction to the insertion on the greater tuberosity.

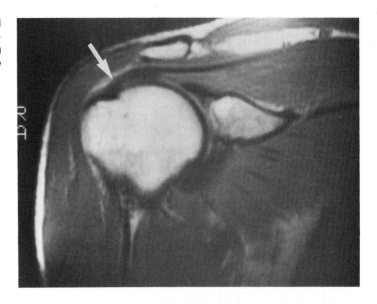

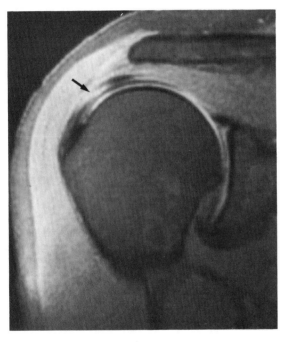

Figure 42.4. Partial Tear of the Supraspinatus Tendon. A T1-weighted (TR 700; TE 20) oblique coronal image with fat saturation shows high signal in the critical zone of the supraspinatus tendon (*arrow*) with the tendon appearing very irregular. A small amount of fluid is seen in the subacromial bursa. Arthroscopy confirmed a partial tear on the bursal side of the supraspinatus tendon.

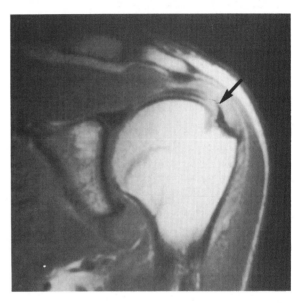

Figure 42.5. Torn Supraspinatus Tendon. An oblique coronal proton-density image (TR 1500; TE 20) shows disruption of the supraspinatus tendon (*arrow*) and a large amount of fluid in the subacromial bursa, which is seen surrounding the torn tendon.

weighted images that does not get brighter on T2-weighted images. This can represent one of several processes in a normal tendon or myxoid degeneration, also called tendonopathy. This should basically be considered "normal" as it has not been proved that tendonopathy is symptomatic. (*b*) High signal on T1-weighted images that gets brighter on T2-weighted sequences. Little or no fluid is present in the subacromial bursa. This represents tendinitis or a partial tear. (*c*) If tendon disruption and/or a large amount of

fluid is present in the subacromial bursa with high signal in the critical zone on T1- and T2-weighted images, a full-thickness tear should be diagnosed.

BONY ABNORMALITIES

The undersurface of the anterior acromion and the AC joint should be examined for osteophytes or irregularities that can be responsible for impingement syndrome (Fig. 42.6). In the proper clinical setting an anterior acromioplasty will relieve the symptoms of impingement syndrome and prevent a more serious full-thickness rotator cuff tear. It is imperative that the surgeon also remove any AC joint undersurface ir-

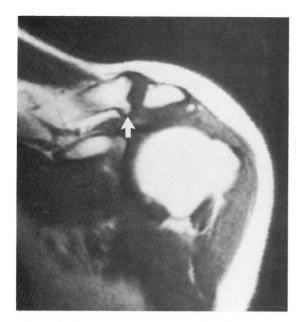

Figure 42.6. Acromioclavicular Joint Osteophytes. An oblique coronal T1-weighted image (TR 600; TE 30) reveals osteophytes extending inferiorly off the AC joint (arrow). This is a common source of impingement on the supraspinatus tendon.

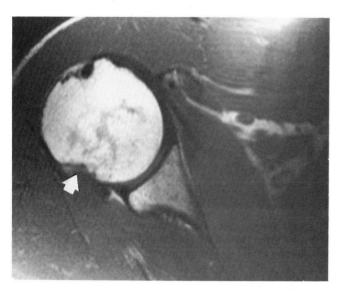

Figure 42.7. Hill-Sachs Lesion. An axial T1-weighted image (TR 600; TE 30) through the superior portion of the humeral head shows a posterior impaction (arrow) caused by the glenoid labrum during an anterior dislocation of the humerus. This has been termed a Hill-Sachs lesion.

regularity, if present, or a failed surgery can be expected.

Abnormalities of the humeral head include sclerosis and cystic changes about the greater tuberosity, which are commonly present in patients with impingement syndrome and rotator cuff tears. Bony impaction on the posterosuperior aspect of the humeral head can be seen in patients with anterior instability of the humeral head. This is called a Hill-Sachs lesion

and is best identified on the superior-most two or three axial images (Fig. 42.7). The normal humeral head should be round on the superior slices; any irregularity seen posteriorly is abnormal.

GLENOID LABRUM

Tears of the glenoid labrum cause glenohumeral joint instability. They are commonly caused by dislocations, but less traumatic episodes, such as repeated trauma from throwing, can result in labral tears. Torn or detached labra are often repaired arthroscopically with good results.

The glenoid labrum is best imaged on axial T2-weighted or T2*-weighted images. T1-weighted axial images are not necessary to diagnose labral abnormalities and can be omitted from the shoulder protocol.

The normal labrum is a triangular-shaped low-signal structure as viewed on an axial image, with the anterior labrum usually larger than the posterior labrum (Fig. 42.8). The anterior labrum is much more commonly involved with tears than the posterior, and the superior labrum is even less commonly involved. The superior labrum is evaluated on the oblique coronal views.

If no joint effusion is present, a labral tear can be difficult to see unless it is quite severe. If joint fluid extends between the bony glenoid and the base of the labrum, a torn labrum is present. Tears in the body of the labrum are diagnosed by noting fluid extending into the labrum or by truncation of the labrum (Fig. 42.9). The attachment of the glenohumeral ligaments to the labrum can cause a linear high signal that can mimic a tear (Fig. 42.10), so care must be taken to be certain high signal fluid is actually present in the tear (7).

BICEPS TENDON

The long head of the biceps tendon runs in the bicipital groove between the greater and lesser tuberosities and inserts onto the superior labrum. It can be impinged by an abnormal acromion in the same way the supraspinatus tendon is impinged, resulting in tenosynovitis or tendinitis. In tenosynovitis, fluid can be seen in the tendon sheath surrounding an otherwise normal tendon. Because fluid in the glenohumeral joint can normally fill the biceps tendon sheath, this diagnosis is difficult to make with MR alone. If the tendon is enlarged and/or has signal within it, tendinitis is present (Fig. 42.11). If the tendon is not seen on one or more of the axial images, it is disrupted or dislocated. Dislocation is uncommon, but when it occurs the tendon can be seen to lie anteromedial to the joint.

Figure 42.8.   Normal Labrum. An axial T2* GRASS image (TR 600; TE 30; Θ 20°) shows a normal anterior (*black arrow*) and posterior (*white arrow*) glenoid labrum. The anterior labrum is usually larger than the posterior labrum.

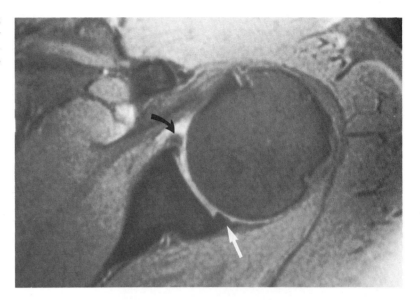

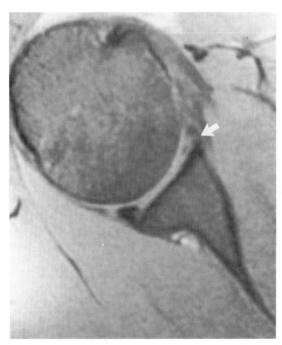

Figure 42.9.   Torn Labrum. An axial T2* GRASS image (TR 500; TE 9; Θ 20°) shows disruption of the anterior labrum (*arrow*). Note the normal posterior labrum for comparison.

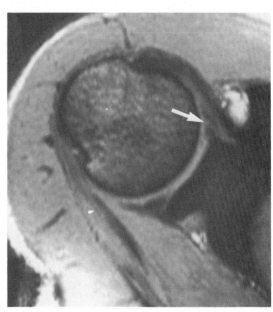

Figure 42.10.   Insertion of Glenohumeral Ligament. This axial T2* GRASS image (TR 600; TE 15; Θ 70°) reveals linear intermediate signal extending obliquely across the anterior labrum (*arrow*), which simulates a tear. This is the insertion of the middle glenohumeral ligament onto the labrum.

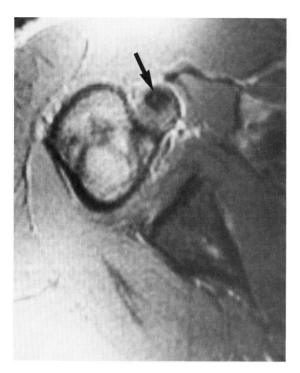

Figure 42.11. Biceps Tendinitis. An axial T2* GRASS image (TR 600; TE 30; Θ 30°) shows the biceps tendon (*arrow*) to be swollen and filled with high signal, indicating tendinitis.

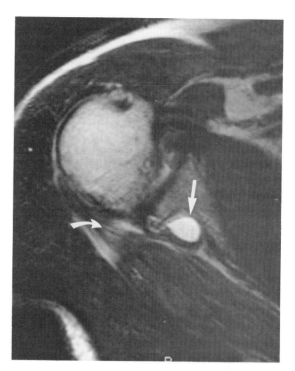

Figure 42.12. Ganglion in Spinoglenoid Notch. An axial T2 image (TR 1850; TE 80) reveals a large high-signal mass posterior to the scapula in the spinoglenoid notch (*arrow*). This is a ganglion that has impressed the suprascapular nerve, causing shoulder pain and atrophy of the infraspinatus muscle. Note the high signal in the infraspinatus muscle (*curved arrow*), which indicates fatty infiltration from atrophy.

SUPRASCAPULAR NERVE ENTRAPMENT

The suprascapular nerve is made up of branches from the C-4, C-5, and C-6 roots of the brachial plexus. It runs superior to the scapula, from anterior to posterior, just medial to the coracoid process. It gives off a branch that innervates the supraspinatus muscle as it courses posteriorly in the suprascapular notch, and then innervates the infraspinatus muscle after it runs through the spinoglenoid notch in the posterior scapula. It can easily be entrapped by a tumor or a ganglion as it runs above the scapula because it is bounded superiorly by a transverse ligament both anteriorly and posteriorly. A fairly common finding is a ganglion in the spinoglenoid notch that impresses the infraspinatus portion of the nerve with resultant pain and atrophy of the supraspinatus muscle (Fig. 42.12). This is most commonly seen in males who are athletic, particularly weight lifters. The ganglion can be percutaneously drained with computed tomography guidance or surgically removed. They can also spontaneously rupture, which results in cessation of symptoms (8).

References

1. Burk DJ, Karasick D, Kurtz AB, et al. Rotator cuff tears: prospective comparison of MR imaging with arthrography, sonography, and surgery. AJR 1989;153:87–92.
2. Evancho AM, Stiles RG, Fajman WA, et al. MR imaging diagnosis of rotator cuff tears. AJR 1988;151:751–754.
3. Farley T, Neumann C, Steinbach L, Jahnke A, Petersen S. Full-thickness tears of the rotator cuff of the shoulder: diagnosis with MR imaging. AJR 1992;158:347–351.
4. Zlatkin MB, Iannotti JP, Roberts MC, et al. Rotator cuff tears: diagnostic performance of MR imaging. Radiology 1989;172:223–229.
5. Erickson S, Cox I, Hyde J, Carrera G, Strandt J, Estowski L. Effect of tendon orientation on MR imaging signal intensity: a manifestation of the "magic angle" phenomenon. Radiology 1991;181:389–392.
6. Kjellin I, Ho CP, Cervilla V, et al. Alterations in the supraspinatus tendon at MR imaging: correlation with histopathologic findings in cadavers. Radiology 1991;181:837–841.
7. Kaplan P, Bryans K, Davick J, Otte M, Stinson W, Dussault R. MR imaging of the normal shoulder: variants and pitfalls. Radiology 1992;184:519–524.
8. Fritz R, Helms C, Steinbach L, Genant H. Suprascapular nerve entrapment: evaluation with MR imaging. Radiology 1992;182:437–444.

43

Magnetic Resonance Imaging of the Foot and Ankle

Clyde A. Helms

Magnetic resonance imaging (MRI) is playing an increasingly important role in the examination of the foot and ankle (1). Orthopaedic surgeons and podiatrists are learning that critical diagnostic information can be obtained in no other way and are relying on MR for many therapeutic decisions.

TENDONS

One of the more common reasons to perform MR of the foot and ankle is to examine the tendons. Although multiple tendons course through the ankle, only a few are routinely affected pathologically. These are primarily the flexor tendons, located posteriorly in the ankle. The extensor tendons, located anteriorly, are rarely abnormal. Only those tendons that are more commonly seen to be abnormal will be discussed in detail.

Tendons can be directly traumatized or be injured from overuse. Either etiology can result in (a) *tenosynovitis*, which is seen on MR as fluid in the tendon sheath with the underlying tendon appearing normal; (b) *tendinitis* or a partial tear, which is seen as focal or fusiform swelling of the tendon with signal within the tendon that gets bright on T2- or T2*-weighted images; thinning or attenuation of the tendon is a more severe form of tendinitis that can be recognized on MR; and (c) *tendon rupture*, which is best identified on axial images by noting the absence of a tendon on one or more images. Complete tendon disruption

can be difficult to see on sagittal or coronal images because of the tendency for tendons to run oblique to the plane of imaging. An exception to this is the Achilles tendon, which is usually best seen on a sagittal image (2).

It is important to distinguish between tendinitis and a complete disruption as surgical repair is often warranted for the latter and not for the former. It is often difficult to make the distinction clinically.

Achilles Tendon

The Achilles tendon does not have a sheath associated with it, therefore, tenosynovitis does not occur. Tendinitis is commonly seen in the Achilles tendon; however, it is such an easy clinical diagnosis that MR is usually not necessary. Complete disruption is commonly seen in athletes and in males around the age of 40. It is also commonly associated with other systemic disorders that cause tendon weakening, such as rheumatoid arthritis, collagen vascular diseases, crystal deposition diseases, and hyperparathyroidism.

Achilles tendon disruption can be treated surgically or by placing the patient in a cast with equinus positioning (marked plantar flexion) for several months. It is controversial as to which treatment is superior, with both methods of treatment seemingly working well. Magnetic resonance imaging is being used by many surgeons to help decide if surgery should be performed. If a large gap is present (Fig. 43.1), some surgeons feel surgery should be performed for reapposition of the torn ends of the tendon; whereas, if the ends of the tendon are not retracted, nonsurgical treatment is preferred. No papers have been published to show that this is, in fact, scientifically valid.

Posterior Tibial Tendon

The posterior tibial tendon is the most medial and the largest, except for the Achilles, of the flexor tendons (Fig. 43.2). The flexor tendons are easily remembered and identified by using the mnemonic "Tom, Dick, and Harry," with Tom representing the posterior *t*ibial tendon, Dick the flexor *d*igitorum longus

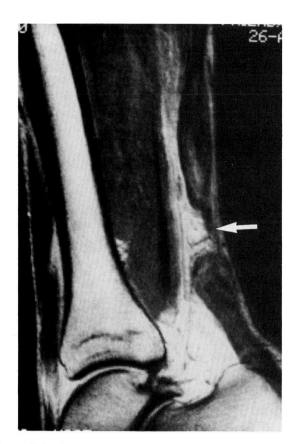

Figure 43.1.   Torn Achilles Tendon. A sagittal T1-weighted image (TR 600; TE 30) reveals the Achilles tendon to be torn with a 2-cm gap. Only a thin remnant of the tendon remains intact across the gap (*arrow*). Note the high signal in the swollen ends of the separated tendon, indicative of hemorrhage and edema.

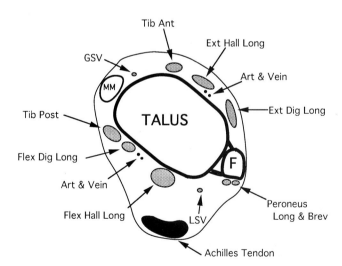

Figure 43.2.   Schematic of Axial Ankle Anatomy. This drawing of the tendons around the ankle at the level of the tibiotalar joint shows the relationship of the flexor tendons posteriorly and the extensor tendons anteriorly. (*F*, fibula; *MM*, medial malleolus; *GSV*, greater saphenous vein; *LSV*, lesser saphenous vein.)

tendon, and Harry the flexor *h*allucis longus tendon. The posterior tibial tendon inserts onto the navicular, second to fourth cuneiforms, and the bases of the sec-

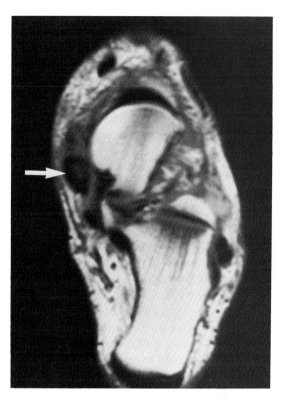

Figure 43.3.   Posterior Tibial Tendon Tendinitis. A proton-density (TR 2000; TE 20) axial image through the ankle at the level of the midcalcaneus shows the posterior tibial tendon (*arrow*) swollen and containing high signal. This is the appearance of marked tendinitis.

ond to fourth metatarsals. As it sweeps under the foot it provides some support for the longitudinal arch; hence, problems in the arch or plantar fascia can sometimes lead to stress on the posterior tibial tendon with resulting tendinitis or even rupture. Posterior tibial tendinitis and rupture are commonly encountered in rheumatoid arthritis.

Differentiation of tendinitis from tendon rupture can be difficult clinically, and MR has become very valuable for making this distinction (3). Most surgeons will operate on a disrupted posterior tibial tendon, whereas nonoperative therapy is usually preferred for tendinitis.

Posterior tibial tendinitis is seen on axial T1-weighted images as swelling and/or signal within the normally low signal tendon on one or more images (Fig. 43.3). T2- or T2*-weighted images show the signal in the tendon getting brighter. Tendon disruption is diagnosed by noting the absence of low signal tendon on one or more axial images. This typically occurs just at or above the level of the tibiotalar joint.

Flexor Hallucis Longus Tendon

The flexor hallucis longus (FHL) tendon is easily identified near the tibiotalar joint because it is usually the only tendon at that distal level that has muscle still attached. In the foot the FHL can be seen beneath

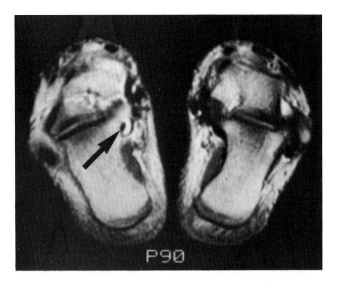

Figure 43.4. Flexor Hallucis Longus Tenosynovitis. A T2-weighted (TR 2000; TE 80) axial image of both ankles in this ballet dancer with a painful right ankle reveals fluid in the tendon sheath around the flexor hallucis longus tendon (*arrow*). This needs to be correlated with the clinical examination as fluid can normally extend into the tendon sheath of the flexor hallucis longus tendon from the tibiotalar joint in up to 20% of normal patients.

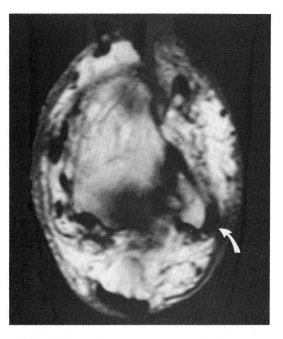

Figure 43.5. Dislocated Peroneus Longus Tendon. An axial T1-weighted image (TR 600; TE 30) in this skier who injured the ankle in a fall shows a low signal rounded structure (*arrow*) lateral to the lateral malleolus. This is a dislocated peroneus longus tendon.

the sustentaculum talus, which it uses as a pulley to plantar flex the foot.

The FHL is known as the Achilles tendon of the foot in ballet dancers because of the extreme flexion positions they employ. Ballet dancers often will have tenosynovitis of the FHL, seen on MR as fluid in the sheath surrounding the tendon (Fig. 43.4). Care must be taken to have clinical correlation, as fluid can be seen in the FHL tendon sheath from a connection to the ankle joint, which has an effusion in up to 20% of normal patients. Rupture of the FHL is rare.

Peroneus Tendons

The peroneus longus and peroneus brevis tendons can be seen posterior to the distal fibula, to which they are bound by a thin fibrous structure, the superior retinaculum. The fibula serves as a pulley for the tendons to work as the principal everter of the foot. The tendons course close together adjacent to the lateral aspect of the calcaneus until a few centimeters below the lateral malleolus where they separate, with the peroneus brevis tendon inserting onto the base of the fifth metatarsal and the peroneus longus tendon crossing under the foot to the base of the first metatarsal. Avulsion of the base of the fifth metatarsal from a pull by the peroneus brevis tendon is known as a "dancer's fracture" or a Jones fracture.

Disruption of the superior retinaculum, often seen in skiing accidents (4), can result in displacement of the peroneus tendons (Fig. 43.5) and must be surgically corrected. It often occurs with a small bony avulsion, called a flake fracture, off the fibula.

Entrapment of the peroneus tendons in a fractured calcaneus or fibula can occur, and is easily diagnosed with MR. This can be a difficult diagnosis to make clinically. Complete disruption of the peroneal tendons is uncommon, but is easily noted with MR.

AVASCULAR NECROSIS

Avascular necrosis commonly occurs in the foot and ankle. The talar dome is the second most common location of osteochondritis dissecans (the knee is the most common site). Magnetic resonance is useful in identifying and staging osteochondritis dissecans. Even when not apparent on plain films, magnetic resonance imaging can show osteochondritis dissecans as a focal area of low signal in the subarticular portion of the talar dome on T1-weighted images. On T2- or T2*-weighted images, if high signal is seen surrounding the dissecans fragment in the bone at the bed of the fragment, or throughout the fragment (Fig. 43.6), it is most likely an unstable fragment. If the fragment has become displaced and lies in the joint as a loose body, MR can sometimes be useful to localize it; however, loose bodies in any joint can be exceedingly difficult to find.

Diffuse low signal throughout a tarsal bone on T1-weighted images is typical for avascular necrosis. This occasionally occurs in the tarsal navicular (Fig. 43.7). Magnetic resonance imaging can be useful in making this diagnosis when plain films are normal or equivocal.

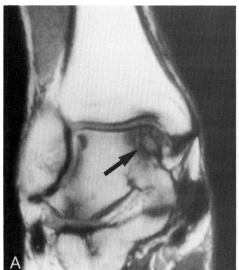
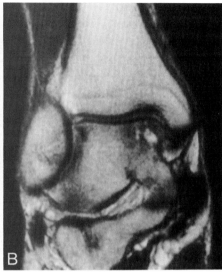

Figure 43.6. Unstable Osteochondritis Dissecans of the Talus. A. A proton-density (TR 2000; TE 20) coronal image through the talus shows a focus of low signal in the medial subarticular part of the talus (*arrow*). This is a characteristic appearance for osteochondritis dissecans. **B.** A T2-weighted (TR 2000; TE 80) image shows high signal throughout the focus of osteochondritis dissecans, which indicates an unstable fragment.

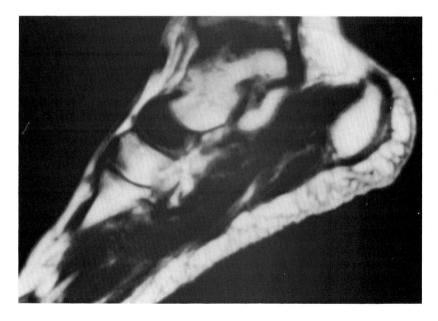

Figure 43.7. Avascular Necrosis of the Tarsal Navicular. A T1-weighted (TR 600; TE 30) sagittal image of the ankle in this patient with pain on the dorsum of the foot shows diffuse low signal throughout the tarsal navicular. This is a characteristic appearance for avascular necrosis and will often precede any plain film findings.

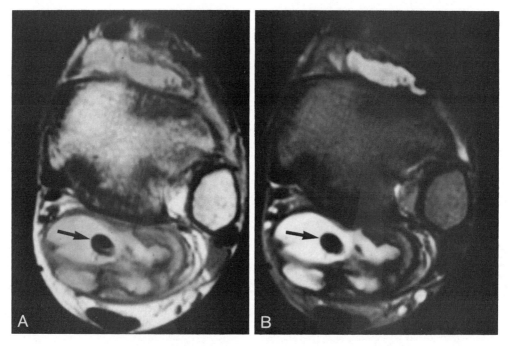

Figure 43.8. Giant Cell Tumor of Tendon Sheath. Axial proton-density (**A**) and T2 weighted (**B**) images reveal a mass surrounding the flexor hallucis longus tendon (*arrows*), which is confined by the tendon sheath. Although high signal fluid is present, large amounts of low signal material is lining the distended tendon sheath. This low signal is hemosiderin, which is typically found in a giant cell tendon of tendon sheath. Pigmented villonodular synovitis in a joint has an identical appearance.

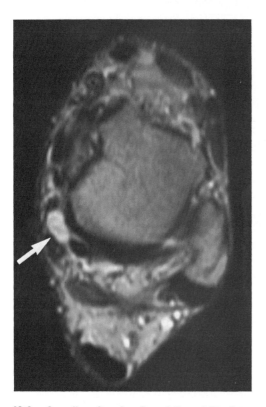

Figure 43.9. Ganglion Causing Tarsal Tunnel Syndrome. A T2-weighted (TR 2000; TE 70) axial image of the ankle in a patient complaining of pain and paresthesia on the plantar aspect of the foot shows a high signal mass (*arrow*) lying between the flexor digitorum tendon anteriorly and the flexor hallucis longus tendon posteriorly. This is the position of the tibial nerve that can be impinged by a mass, such as in this case, resulting in tarsal tunnel syndrome. This was a small ganglion. (Case courtesy Dr. Rick Mitchell, Fullerton, CA).

TUMORS

There are a few tumors that have a predilection for the foot and ankle (5). Up to 16% of synovial sarcomas occur in the foot. Desmoid tumors are commonly seen in the foot. Giant cell tumors of tendon sheath (also called xanthomas and pigmented villonodular synovitis) are often found in the tendon sheaths of the foot and ankle (Fig. 43.8). They are characterized by marked low signal in the synovial lining and in the tendons on T1- and T2-weighted images, just as pigmented villonodular synovitis appears in a joint.

The differential diagnosis for calcaneal tumors is similar to that of the epiphyses—giant cell tumor, chondroblastoma, and infection—with a unicameral bone cyst added.

Soft-tissue tumors in the medial aspect of the foot and ankle can press on the posterior tibial nerve, resulting in tarsal tunnel syndrome (6). Clinically, patients with tarsal tunnel syndrome present with pain and paresthesia in the plantar aspect of the foot. In the aforementioned mnemonic, "Tom, Dick, and Harry," the "and" is for artery, nerve, and vein. It is the position of the posterior tibial nerve. The nerve is easily compressed in the tarsal tunnel, which is bounded medially by the flexor retinaculum, a strong fibrous band that extends across the medial ankle joint for about 5–7 cm in a superior-to-inferior direction. Ganglions and neural tumors, both of which can look similar on T1- and T2-weighted images, often lie in the tarsal tunnel (Fig.

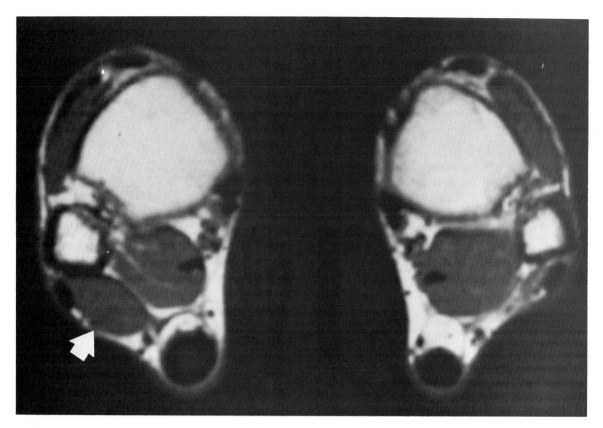

Figure 43.10. Anomalous Muscle. An axial T1-weighted image of both ankles in this patient complaining of a mass in the right ankle shows an anomalous muscle (*arrow*) lateral to the flexor hallucis longus muscle that is responsible for the mass the patient feels.

43.9) and compress the posterior tibial nerve, resulting in pain and paresthesia on the plantar aspect of the foot extending into the toes. Tarsal tunnel syndrome often occurs secondary to trauma, fibrosis, or idiopathically, all of which may not respond to surgical intervention; hence, MR is valuable in delineating a treatable lesion in many cases.

Anomalous muscles in the foot or ankle are reported to be present in up to 6% of the population. These can be mistaken for a tumor and biopsy may be performed unnecessarily. Magnetic resonance imaging will show these "tumors" to have imaging characteristics identical to normal muscle (Fig. 43.10) and to be sharply circumscribed. Accessory soleus and peroneus brevis muscles are the most common accessory muscles encountered around the foot and ankle.

LIGAMENTS

Magnetic resonance imaging is not the best way to diagnose ankle ligament abnormalities. The clinical evaluation is usually straightforward and no diagnostic imaging of any type is necessary. Nevertheless, in clinically equivocal cases or when the examination is ordered for other reasons, the ligaments can be clearly evaluated with high-quality MR in most instances (7).

The deltoid ligament lies medially as a broad band beneath the tendons. Although it is often seen on coronal images deep to the posterior tibial tendon, it has a variable anatomic position and is not well studied with MR.

The lateral complex is made up of two parts: a superior group, the anterior and posterior tibiofibular ligaments that make up part of the syndesmosis (Fig. 43.11), and an inferior group, the anterior and posterior talofibular ligaments and the calcaneofibular ligament (Fig. 43.12). The anterior and posterior tibiofibular ligaments can be seen on axial images at or slightly above the tibiotalar joint. The anterior and posterior talofibular ligaments are seen on the axial images just below the tibiotalar joint and emanate from a concavity in the distal fibula called the malleolar fossa (Fig. 43.12**B**). The most commonly torn ankle ligament is the anterior talofibular ligament. It is easily identified when a joint effusion is present because it makes up the anterior capsule of the joint (Fig. 43.13). The anterior talofibular ligament is usually torn without other ligaments being involved; however, if the injury is severe enough, the next ligament to tear is the calcaneofibular ligament. Finally, with very severe trauma, the posterior talofibular ligament will tear.

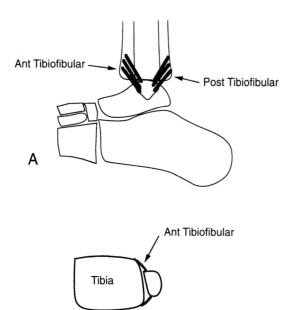

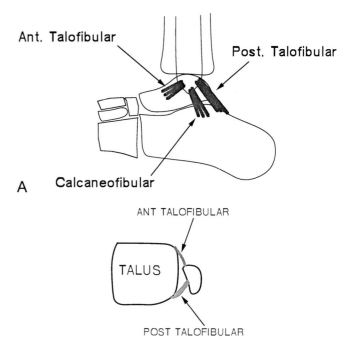

Figure 43.11.   Schematic of Lateral Collateral Ligaments. A. This drawing of the ankle in a lateral view shows how the anterior and posterior tibiofibular (*tib-fib*) ligaments extend off the fibula and course superiorly to the tibia. **B.** A drawing in the axial plane shows that the fibula has a flat or convex surface at the origin of these ligaments.

Figure 43.12.   Schematic of Lateral Collateral Ligaments. A. This drawing of the ankle in a lateral view shows how the anterior and posterior talofibular ligaments, and the calcaneofibular ligament extend off the fibula and course inferiorly. These ligaments arise off of the fibula more distally than the anterior and posterior tibiofibular ligaments. **B.** A drawing in the axial plane shows that the anterior and posterior talofibular ligaments arise from the level of the distal fibula, which has a concave medial surface, the malleolar fossa.

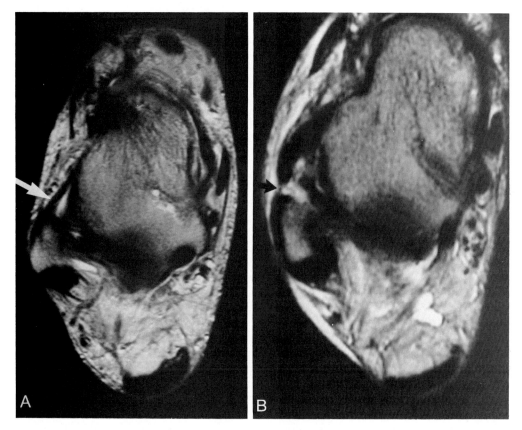

Figure 43.13. Anterior Talofibular Ligament. A. An axial T2-weighted image (TR 4000; TE 76) through the distal fibula at the level of the malleolar fossa (the concave medial surface of the fibula) shows an intact anterior talofibular ligament (*arrow*) that makes up part of the joint capsule at this level. Note the high signal joint fluid adjacent to the ligament. **B.** This axial T2-weighted image (TR 3200; TE 100) at the level of the malleolar fossa reveals a thickened anterior talofibular ligament that has a disruption (*arrow*). The marked thickening of the ligament indicates a chronic process. (Case courtesy of Dr. Jerrold Mink, Los Angeles, CA.)

Figure 43.14.   Posterior Tibiofibular Ligament and Loose Body. A sagittal T2* GRASS image (TR 500; TE 15; θ 30°) through the midankle in a patient with occasional locking and a plain film (not shown) that demonstrates a calcified loose body near the posterior talus reveals two apparent loose bodies. The more posterior one (*large arrow*) matches the calcified loose body on the plain film. The other one (*small arrow*) is not a loose body but is the posterior tibiofibular ligament, which often resembles a loose body on sagittal T2-weighted images.

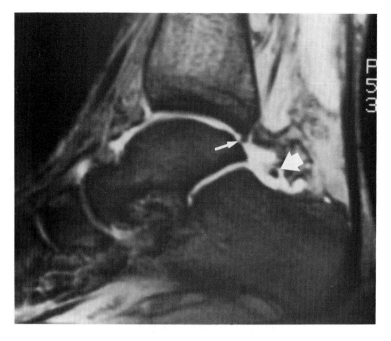

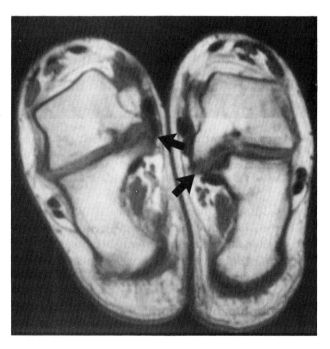

Figure 43.15.   Tarsal Coalition. An axial T1-weighted image in a patient with painful flat feet shows bilateral talocalcaneal coalition (*arrows*) which is primarily fibrous. The normal joint space is irregular and widened bilaterally. In cases of suspected coalition, both ankles should be imaged as coalition often occurs bilaterally.

On sagittal T2- or T2*-weighted images, the posterior tibiofibular ligament can mimic a loose body in the joint (Fig. 43.14). This pitfall is probably the most clinically important piece of ankle ligament information in this section, as unnecessary surgery for a presumed loose body can occur because of failure to recognize the normal anatomy.

BONY ABNORMALITIES

Tarsal coalition is a common cause of a painful flatfoot. It occurs most commonly at the calcaneonavicular joint and the middle facet of the talocalcaneal joint (Fig. 43.15). Up to 80% of patients with tarsal coalition have bilateral coalition. It can be difficult (or impossible) to see the coalition on plain films; however, computed tomography and MR will show bony coalition with a high degree of accuracy. The coalition can also be fibrous or cartilaginous, however. In these cases, secondary findings, such as joint space irregularity at the affected joint or degenerative joint disease at nearby joints that are subjected to accentuated stress, can be seen. For now, MR does not appear to have superiority to computed tomography for tarsal coalition.

Fractures of the foot and ankle are usually well documented with plain films. Stress fractures, however, can be difficult to radiographically or clinically diagnose, and can mimic more sinister abnormalities. Magnetic resonance imaging will show stress fractures as linear low signal on T1-weighted images with high signal on T2 weighting (Fig. 43.16).

Magnetic resonance imaging has had mixed reviews when used for diagnosing osteomyelitis in the foot. In diabetic patients with foot infections, it is important to diagnose osteomyelitis as the treatment is often much more aggressive, including amputation, than if the bone is not involved. Unfortunately, MR is not highly accurate in this regard. If the marrow appears normal, MR is highly accurate in predicting no osteomyelitis; however, if low signal is present in the marrow around a joint, osteomyelitis may or may not

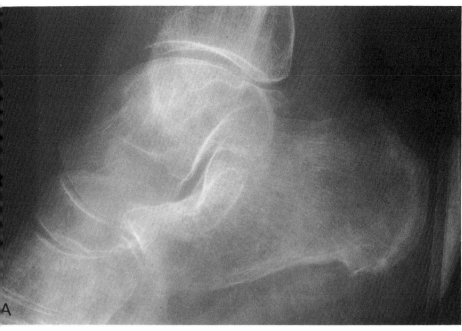

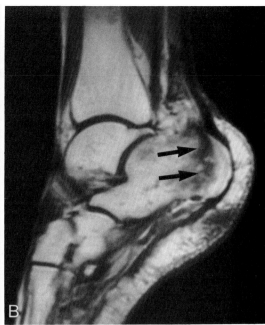

Figure 43.16. Calcaneal Stress Fracture. A 70-year-old patient with a prior history of lung cancer presented with heel pain and a normal plain film (**A**). A bone scan showed diffuse increased radionuclide uptake throughout the posterior calcaneus. A sagittal T1- weighted MR (**B**) revealed a linear area of low signal (*arrows*), which is characteristic for a stress fracture. Metastatic disease would not have this appearance.

be present. Low signal can be caused by edema or hyperemia without infection. Magnetic resonance imaging is therefore very sensitive but not very specific in diagnosing osteomyelitis in the foot and ankle (8).

References

1. Kneeland J, Macrandar S, Middleton W, Cates J, Jesmanowicz A, Hyde J. MR imaging of the normal ankle: correlation with anatomic sections. AJR 1988;151:117–126.
2. Quinn S, Murray W, Clark R, Cochran C. Achilles tendon: MR imaging at 1.5 T. Radiology 1987;164:767–770.
3. Rosenberg Z, Cheung Y, Jahss M, Noto A, Norman A, Leeds N. Rupture of posterior tibial tendons: CT and MR imaging with surgical correlation. Radiology 1988;169:229–236.
4. Oden R. Tendon injuries about the ankle resulting from skiing. Clin Orthop 1987;216:63–69.
5. Keigley B, Haggar A, Gaba A, Ellis B, Froelich J, Wu K. Primary tumors of the foot: MR imaging. Radiology 1989;171:755–759.
6. Erickson S, Quinn S, Kneeland J, et al. MR imaging of the tarsal tunnel and related spaces: normal and abnormal findings with anatomic correlation. AJR 1990;155:323–328.
7. Erickson S, Smith J, Ruiz M, et al. MR imaging of the lateral collateral ligament of the ankle. AJR 1991;156:131–136.
8. Erdman W, Tamburro F, Jayson H, Weatherall P, Ferry K, Peshock R. Osteomyelitis: characteristics and pitfalls of diagnosis with MR imaging. Radiology 1991;180:533–539.

Section IX PEDIATRIC RADIOLOGY

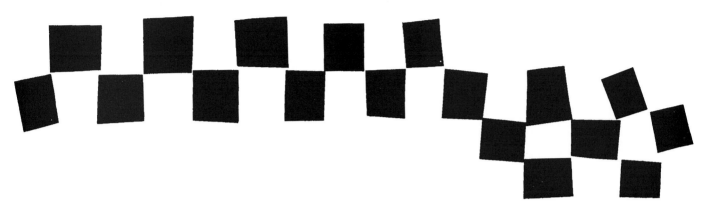

44

Pediatric Chest

Susan D. John
Leonard E. Swischuk

Table 44.1. Focal Alveolar Consolidation

Bacterial pneumonia
  <2 years of age—*H. influenzae*
  >2 years or age—*S. pneumoniae*
                  M. pneumoniae
                  Staphylococcus
Nonbacterial infection
  Tuberculosis
  Actinomycosis
Pulmonary infarction
Pulmonary contusion

PULMONARY INFILTRATIVE PATTERNS

Pulmonary infiltrates in children are classified in the same way as in adults as being either primarily alveolar or interstitial. It should also be noted whether the infiltrates are focal or diffuse and unilateral or bilateral. Some infiltrates occur in a central or parahilar distribution, whereas others are predominantly peripheral or basal in location. Mixed patterns also occur. An understanding of the causes of these various patterns is necessary in order to provide a useful interpretation of lung infiltrates in children.

Alveolar Patterns

Alveolar Consolidation occurs when the alveoli are filled with some substance, usually fluid. When such a consolidation is focal, the fluid most often is exudate due to bacterial pneumonia (Table 44.1). The most common organism varies with the age of the child: *Haemophilus influenzae* is most common before 2 years of age and *Streptococcus pneumoniae* is most common in older children. Staphylococcal and mycoplasmal pneumonias are also fairly common causes of focal consolidating pneumonias, and although infections with Gram-negative organisms occur, they are not very common in children. Primary tuberculosis should be considered, particularly when the infiltrate is accompanied by hilar lymphadenopathy.

Atelectasis. An important observation when faced with a focal lung consolidation is the presence or absence of volume loss. If volume loss is present, the consolidation is much more likely to be due to atelectasis, which is a very common occurrence in childhood viral respiratory tract infections. Generally, volume loss will not be seen with a bacterial pneumonia until it begins to resolve (Fig. 44.1). Atelectasis is also very common in patients with acute asthma (Fig. 44.2). The clinical presentation in such patients is often very helpful, for consolidations that occur in a patient with symptoms of acute asthma (i.e., wheezing) are much more likely to be due to atelectasis. Pneumonia in a patient with asthma does not result in an asthma attack, but rather has the same clinical symptoms as in any other child (i.e., high fever, cough, chest pain). Other causes of focal lung consolidations are much less common in children and include fungal infection, tuberculosis, pulmonary infarction, contusion, and other causes of focal pulmonary hemorrhage.

Multiple Patchy Lung Opacities can be seen with a wide variety of conditions (Table 44.2). Once again, these opacities reflect filling of the alveolar space with either exudate, edema, or blood. If patchy infiltrates

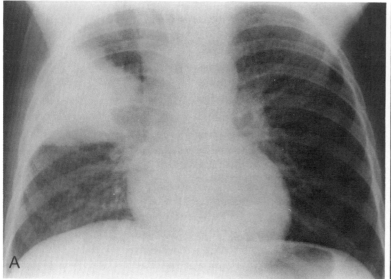

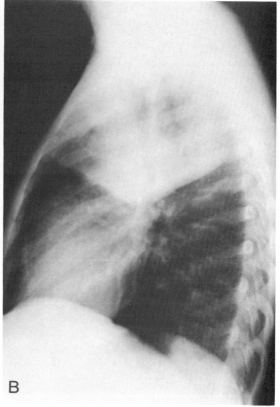

Figure 44.1.   Bacterial Pneumonia. A. and **B.** A typical alveolar consolidation in the right upper lobe. Note that the fissures are not displaced, indicating that there is little volume loss.

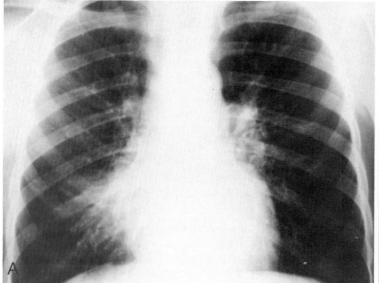

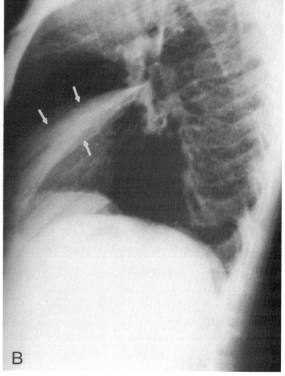

Figure 44.2.   Acute Asthma. A. Opacity silhouettes the right heart border on the posteroanterior view. **B.** Lateral view shows displacement of the horizontal and oblique fissures (*arrows*), indicating right middle lobe atelectasis.

Table 44.2. Multiple Patchy Lung Opacities

Infection
   Staphylococcus
   Mycoplasma
   Fungal
   Opportunistic organisms
Aspiration
   Hydrocarbon ingestion
   Near drowning
Immune-mediated pneumonitis
   Milk allergy
   Hypersensitivity pneumonitis
Pulmonary hemorrhage
Pulmonary edema

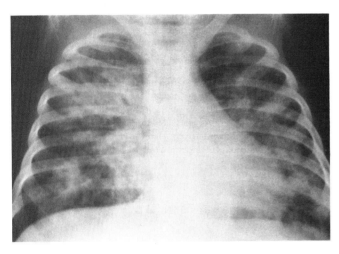

Figure 44.3. Staphylococcal Pneumonia. Note the typical multiple, bilateral alveolar opacities.

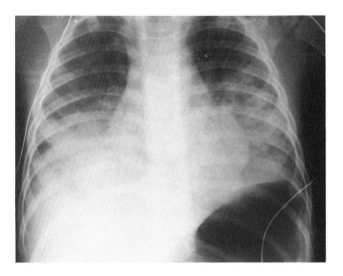

Figure 44.4. Hydrocarbon Aspiration. Typical patchy alveolar opacities are seen in the lung bases bilaterally in this child who ingested kerosene.

are confined to one lobe, a bacterial or *Mycoplasma* infection is the most likely cause. Multiple bilateral alveolar infiltrates suggest bacterial infection (most commonly, *Staphylococcus*) (Fig. 44.3) or fungal dis-

ease. Opportunistic infections in immunocompromised patients are much more likely to be multiple and bilateral. Pneumonias due to aspiration tend to present with multiple patchy pulmonary opacities. The pneumonitis associated with hydrocarbon ingestion typically occurs in the medial portions of the lung bases (Fig. 44.4). Other less common causes of patchy alveolar opacities include milk allergy, hypersensitivity pneumonitis, uremic lung disease, near drowning, and pulmonary hemorrhage (i.e., idiopathic pulmonary hemosiderosis).

Interstitial Patterns

Pulmonary infections that primarily involve the bronchi and peribronchial interstitium (e.g., viruses, *Mycoplasma pneumoniae*, pertussis, *Chlamydia*) are often associated with areas of segmental or subsegmental atelectasis that can also appear as patchy pulmonary opacities. These are often clustered around the lung hila, unlike bacterial infections which tend to lie more peripherally. Nevertheless, atelectasis and patchy pneumonia may be indistinguishable unless the atelectasis is seen to resolve rapidly on a repeat chest radiograph.

Parahilar Peribronchial Opacity. Abnormal parahilar peribronchial opacity due to bronchial and peribronchial inflammation and edema occurs commonly in children because of conditions associated with bronchitis and peribronchitis (Table 44.3). This pattern is best described as ill-defined increased soft-tissue density in the parahilar regions that sometimes has a shaggy appearance (Fig. 44.5), and because viral infections are most common, it is most often seen with these infections (1). Bilateral hilar adenopathy and scattered areas of subsegmental atelectasis are common associated findings (Fig. 44.6), and overall this pattern is very different from the more peripheral alveolar opacification that is most often seen with bacterial pneumonias. However, it should be noted that a superimposed bacterial pneumonia can develop later in the course of a viral lower respiratory tract infection. *Mycoplasma pneumoniae* infections also commonly produce this pattern and when one encounters parahilar peribronchial infiltrates that are unusually severe or that persist over an extended period of time one might consider the diagnosis (2). *Chlamydia trachomatis* pneumonitis has a similar appearance and usually occurs just after the newborn period (Fig. 44.7). Pertussis infections also produce this pattern, and on a more chronic basis one should consider such conditions as asthma, cystic fibrosis (see Fig. 44.18), immunologic deficiency diseases, and chronic aspiration.

Hazy, reticular, or reticulonodular opacities that occur diffusely in the lungs indicate lung pathology that is primarily interstitial and, therefore, the causes

Table 44.3. Parahilar Peribronchial Opacity

Acute—
  infection
  Viral
  Mycoplasma
  Chlamydia
  Pertusssis
Chronic
  Asthma
  Cystic fibrosis
  Immunologic deficiency disease
  Chronic aspiration

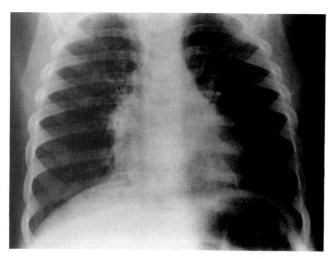

Figure 44.5. Adenovirus Infection. Bilateral parahilar peribronchial infiltrates are typical of viral lower respiratory tract infections.

include basically the same conditions that cause parahilar peribronchial infiltrates (Table 44.4). The most common causes of an interstitial pattern in the lungs of a child is once again either a viral or *Mycoplasma* infection (Fig. 44.8). In general, bacterial infections of the lung do not have this appearance, except in the newborn period where bacterial pneumonia can present as diffuse haziness or reticulonodularity. Fungal infections, such as *Histoplasma capsulatum* and *Coccidioides immitis*, can also occasionally result in an interstitial pattern.

Pulmonary edema, when it is confined to the interstitial space, also can produce hazy lungs, but more often creates a reticular pattern in the lungs. Cardiogenic pulmonary edema occurs when the pulmonary venous pressures are elevated because of left-sided myocardial failure or congenital lesions that cause impeded blood flow through the left side of the heart (e.g., pulmonary vein atresia, cor triatriatum, hypoplastic left heart syndrome). Overall, however, noncardiogenic causes of pulmonary edema are probably more common in children, and, in this regard, one of the most common causes of pulmonary edema in children is acute glomerulonephritis. Sodium and fluid

retention due to the renal disease leads to hypervolemia, which can then result in cardiomegaly and pulmonary vascular congestion with edema. The radiographic appearance in such patients can be virtually indistinguishable from those patients with edema caused by cardiac failure (Fig. 44.9). Other noncardiogenic causes of pulmonary edema in children are more or less the same as those that occur in adults, including near drowning, increased intracranial pressure, inhalation injuries, drug overdose, and adult respiratory distress syndrome.

Other less common causes of a diffuse interstitial pattern in the lungs include a variety of systemic diseases and a few primary lung conditions. Pulmonary lymphangiectasia is a rare condition that consists of dilated lymphatic channels secondary to either abnormal embryonic development of the lymphatic system or obstruction of lymphatic drainage. The dilated lymphatics result in a coarsely nodular or reticular pattern in the lungs, usually in a newborn (Fig. 44.10). Pulmonary hemangiomatosis is a similar but very rare condition. Recurrent hemorrhage into the lungs in patients with idiopathic pulmonary hemosiderosis eventually leads to a chronic diffuse haziness or reticularity of the lungs. The reticuloendothelioses can involve the lungs with an interstitial pattern that often is more prominent in the upper lung zones. The lung volumes are normal or increased, which differs from most other fibrotic conditions in which the lung volumes tend to be decreased.

Interstitial lung disease that predominates in the lower lobes can be seen with conditions such as tuberous sclerosis, connective tissue diseases, and the various types of primary interstitial pneumonitides (e.g., desquamative, lymphocytic, etc.). Leukemia, lymphoma, and lymphatic metastases to the lungs can also cause a reticular or reticulonodular infiltrative pattern in children. Mycoplasmal pneumonitis sometimes presents as a unilobar reticular pattern (Fig. 44.11).

Miliary Nodules. Occasionally, interstitial disease can result in tiny nodules (less than 5 mm in diameter), known as a miliary pattern (Table 44.5). This pattern in children is most often due to hematogenous dissemination of tuberculosis or histoplasmosis (Fig. 44.11), although viral pneumonitis, idiopathic pulmonary hemosiderosis, and metastatic disease can all have this appearance (Fig. 44.12).

ABNORMALITIES OF AERATION

Pulmonary aeration abnormalities are best evaluated on the chest radiograph by observing the following criteria: (*a*) the relative size of a lung or hemithorax, (*b*) the degree of radiolucency of the lung, and (*c*) the pulmonary vascularity or blood flow to the lung. Bilateral smallness of the lungs is commonly due to less than complete inspiration, as the technical diffi-

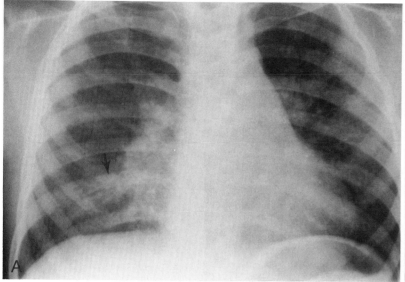

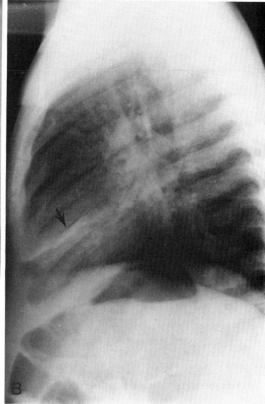

Figure 44.6. Viral Lower Respiratory Tract Infection with Atelectasis. A. and **B.** The typical parahilar peribronchial infiltrates are accompanied by right middle lobe atelectasis (*arrows*) and possible right hilar adenopathy.

Table 44.4. Hazy, Reticular, or Reticulonodular Patterns

Infection
  Viral
  Mycoplasma
  Fungal
Pulmonary edema
  Heart disease
  Acute renal failure
  Near drowning
  Increased intracranial pressure
  Inhalation injury
  Drug overdose
  "Adult" respiratory distress syndrome
Pulmonary lymphangiectasia/hemangiomatosis
Idiopathic pulmonary hemosiderosis
Interstitial pneumatosis
Histiocytosis X
Tuberous sclerosis
Connective tissue diseases
Malignancy
  Leukemia/lymphoma
  Lymphangitic metastasis

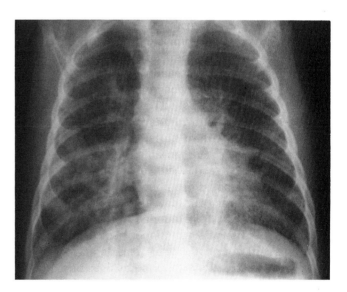

Figure 44.7. Chlamydia Pneumonitis. Prominent parahilar peribronchial infiltrates with slight nodularity are seen in the lung bases. The appearance is similar to that seen with viral infections.

culties of obtaining good inspiratory chest films in children are not insignificant. In such cases, the lungs can appear quite opaque or the pulmonary vascularity may seem prominent, but one should be cautious in trying to interpret such a film. The lungs may also appear small if the diaphragm is elevated either because of neuromuscular abnormality or to the pres-

ence of large masses or fluid collections in the abdomen. Infrequently, inspiratory obstruction of the trachea can lead to bilateral underaeration of the lungs. Such obstruction is most often due to intratracheal masses, foreign bodies, or extrinsic compression of the trachea by anomalous vascular structures. A hyperlucent but small hemithorax usually signifies

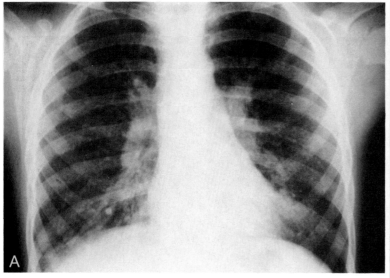

Figure 44.8. Viral Lower Respiratory Tract Infection. A. A reticulonodular pattern is accompanied by parahilar peribronchial infiltrates in this patient with an influenza A infection. **B.** Note the prominent reticulonodular pattern caused by herpes pneumonia in an immunosuppressed patient.

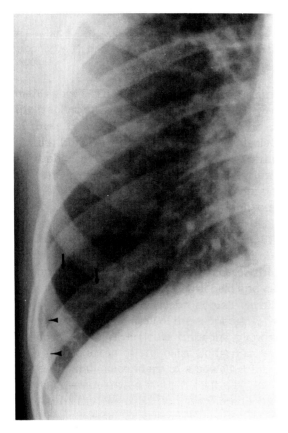

Figure 44.9. Acute Glomerulonephritis. Note the prominent interstitial markings (*arrows*) due to pulmonary edema and a small pleural effusion (*arrowheads*).

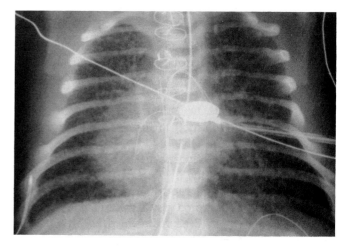

Figure 44.10. Pulmonary Lymphangiectasia. Note the diffuse reticulonodular pattern throughout both lungs due to dilated lymphatics in the interstitium. Dextrocardia is also present. The patient underwent surgical repair of total anomalous pulmonary venous return, type I.

Table 44.5. Miliary Nodules

Infection
   Tuberculosis
   Histoplasmosis
   Viral
Idiopathic pulmonary hemosiderosis
Metastatic disease

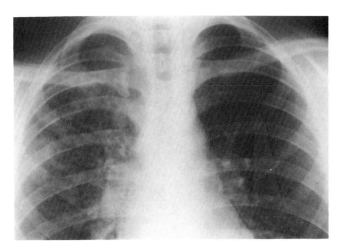

Figure 44.11. Mycoplasma Pneumonia. Note the reticulonodular pattern that involved only the right upper lobe in this patient with positive immunoglobulin titers for *Mycoplasma*.

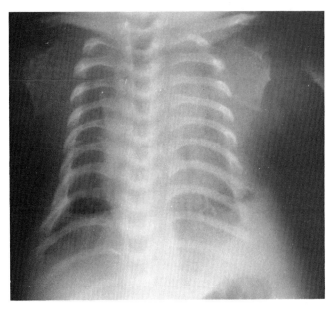

Figure 44.13. Lung Hypoplasia. The very small thoracic cage caused by rib shortening in this thanatophoric dwarf is associated with marked lung hypoplasia.

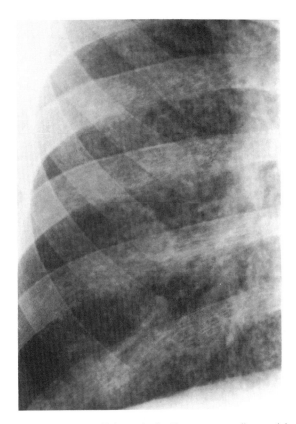

Figure 44.12. Miliary Tuberculosis. The numerous tiny nodules in the lungs of this immunosuppressed patient represent hematogenous dissemination of tuberculosis.

some degree of pulmonary hypoplasia, either congenital or acquired.

Pulmonary Hypoplasia

Congenital pulmonary hypoplasia is associated with hypoplasia or the abscence of the ipsilateral pulmonary artery; thus, the pulmonary vessel branches will be diminished in size on the radiographs. Con-

genital lung hypoplasia is sometimes associated with congenital heart disease, most often tetralogy of Fallot or persistent truncus arteriosus. Typically, in cases of tetralogy of Fallot, it is the left lung that is hypoplastic. In other patients, congenital lung hypoplasia is often asymptomatic and may not be noted until later in life.

Pulmonary hypoplasia in the neonate can be unilateral or bilateral. Bilateral pulmonary hypoplasia is most often the result of compression of the lungs during fetal development. Congenital dysplasias or syndromes that are associated with short ribs and a small thoracic cage compressing the lungs (e.g., asphyxiating thoracic dystrophy, thanatophoric dwarfism, Ellis-van Creveld syndrome) are associated with hypoplastic lungs (Fig. 44.13). The degree of hypoplasia in such infants is often severe and it is the main factor leading to the demise of these infants. Chromosomal abnormalities such as the trisomies are also associated with hypoplastic lungs and, in some infants, hypoplasia is "primary" and unexplained.

The most common cause of intrathoracic compression of the fetal lungs is that which occurs secondary to congenital diaphragmatic hernias. Although the hernia itself is most often unilateral, the increased volume of the thorax on the side of the hernia very frequently leads to secondary compression of the contralateral lung, resulting in asymmetric but bilateral lung hypoplasia (Fig. 44.14). The degree of hypoplasia in such patients varies in severity; the earlier in gestation that the hernia occurs, the more severely hypoplastic the lungs will be. Pulmonary insufficiency in these patients is the most significant cause of morbid-

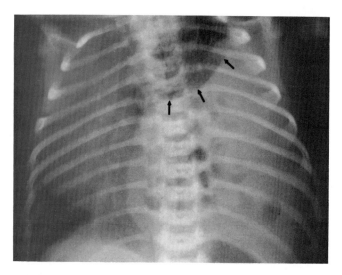

Figure 44.14.   Congenital Diaphragmatic Hernia. Multiple air- and fluid-filled loops of bowel in the left hemithorax displace the mediastinum into the right hemithorax. Note the small, hypoplastic left lung (*arrows*).

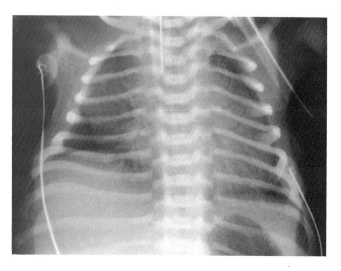

Figure 44.15.   Lung Hypoplasia. Bilateral hypoplastic lungs in this newborn infant were the result of oligohydramnios due to leaking amniotic membranes.

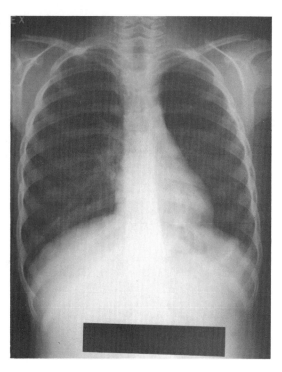

Figure 44.16.   Swyer-James Lung. Note that the left lung is small and relatively hyperlucent when compared with the right lung. The left pulmonary vascularity is decreased.

ity and mortality, and infants with less severely hypoplastic lungs can now be supported with artificial ventilation or extracorporeal membranous oxygenation (ECMO) until their lungs develop enough to permit survival. Other causes of intrathoracic compression leading to bilateral pulmonary hypoplasia include bilateral chylothorax, large intrathoracic cysts or tumors (e.g., neuroblastoma, teratoma, cystic adenomatoid malformation), or marked cardiomegaly.

Extrathoracic compression of the fetal lungs is most often due to oligohydramnios, which can result from renal or urinary tract abnormalities in the fetus or to a variety of causes of abnormal amniotic fluid production or leakage (Fig. 44.15). The classic example of pulmonary hypoplasia caused by oligohydram-

nios occurs in Potter's syndrome due to bilateral renal agenesis. Congenital cystic disease of the kidneys and obstructive uropathy (e.g., posterior urethral valves, prune belly syndrome) can have a similar result. Extrathoracic compression of the fetal lungs can also be caused by neuromuscular abnormalities with persistent elevation of the diaphragm or prolonged distension of the abdomen by large abdominal masses or ascites.

Swyer-James Syndrome. The Swyer-James lung is an acquired hypoplastic lung that develops following a severe inflammatory insult resulting in an obliterative bronchiolitis with bronchiolar obstruction, bronchiectasis, and distal air space destruction (Fig. 44.16). In these cases, air enters the lung by way of the air-drift phenomenon but becomes trapped because of the bronchiolar obstruction. This air trapping results in a lung that changes very little in size between inspiration and expiration. This is an important feature that classically distinguishes the hypoplastic Swyer-James lung from the congenitally hypoplastic lung, although it is not clearly present in all cases. Radionuclide ventilation-perfusion studies can be used to verify the expiratory airway obstruction as well as the diminished perfusion of the hypoplastic lung. Finally, it should be noted that although classically the Swyer-James lung is clear and hyperlucent, some patients show a reticular pattern in the hypoplastic lung, which is probably due to fibrosis. Other causes of a unilateral small

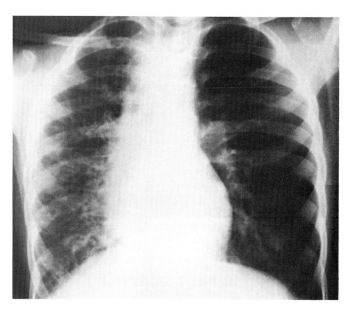

Figure 44.17. Unilateral Pulmonary Vein Atresia. The right lung is small with a diffuse reticularity that is very likely due to fibrosis from prolonged pulmonary edema and/or infection in this patient with pulmonary vein atresia on the right.

Table 44.6. Bilateral Lung Hyperinflation

Diffuse peripheral obstruction
  Viral bronchitis/bronchiolitis
  Asthma
  Cystic fibrosis
  Immunologic deficiency diseases
  Chronic aspiration
  Graft vs. host disease
Central obstruction
  Extrinsic
    Vascular anomalies
    Mediastinal masses
  Intrinsic
    Tracheal foreign body
    Tracheal neoplasm/granuloma

reticular lung include acquired hypoplasia due to radiation therapy or unilateral pulmonary vein atresia or stenosis (Fig. 44.17). The reticularity of the lung in pulmonary vein atresia is due to a combination of interstitial pulmonary edema, fibrosis, and dilated interstitial lymphatics.

Bilateral Lung Hyperinflation

Bilateral overaeration of the lungs is most often caused by airway obstruction that can be either central or diffuse and peripheral (Table 44.6).

Small Airway Obstruction. Obstructive emphysema secondary to widespread small airway obstruction is much more common and classically occurs with viral bronchitis and bronchiolitis, asthma, and cystic fibrosis. Acute bronchiolitis in infants often is accompanied by severe air trapping and overinflation of the lungs with little or no other visible pulmonary abnormality. Infants with cystic fibrosis can present with an appearance identical to bronchiolitis (3), and this diagnosis should be considered in any infant who presents with multiple episodes of bronchiolitis (Fig. 44.18). Hyperinflation tends to be less severe in older children with viral lower respiratory tract infections, but the mechanism (i.e., mucosal edema and bronchospasm secondary to inflammation) is the same. Similar peripheral small airway obstruction with parahilar peribronchial infiltrates is seen with certain immunologic deficiency diseases, chronic aspiration, and graft versus host disease.

Central Airway Obstruction leading to bilateral overaeration of the lungs is less common than peripheral obstruction. Intratracheal lesions such as foreign bodies, neoplasms, granulomas, and intrinsic stenoses of the trachea are all rather rare. More commonly, tracheal obstruction is due to extrinsic compression as might occur with mediastinal masses such as cysts, neoplasms, adenopathy, and a variety of congenital vascular abnormalities. Most commonly, these latter abnormalities involve a vascular ring composed either of a double aortic arch or a right aortic arch with an aberrant left subclavian artery combined with a ligamentum arteriosum. A right-sided aortic arch is the key radiographic clue to the presence of one of these lesions, as it will be present in both (Fig. 44.19). Most cases of double aortic arch consist of a large posterior, right-sided arch and a small anterior, left-sided arch that encircle the esophagus and trachea. Classically, the diagnosis is verified by barium esophagram, which shows a reverse S-shaped indentation of the esophagus caused by compression by the encircling aortic arches (Fig. 44.20). Lateral radiographs may also demonstrate the tracheal narrowing and posterior compression.

Similar radiographic abnormalities are seen when the ring consists of a right ascending aortic arch, an aberrant left subclavian artery that passes posterior to the esophagus, and a ligamentum arteriosum or persistent ductus arteriosus stretching from the left subclavian artery to the pulmonary artery anterior to the trachea. The precise anatomy in each of these anomalies can be beautifully demonstrated by magnetic resonance imaging (MR) (Fig. 44.19) (4). The pulmonary sling anomaly is a rare condition that may also result in tracheal compression and bilateral hyperaeration of the lungs. In this condition, the left pulmonary artery arises from the right pulmonary artery and as it courses toward the left lung it passes between the trachea and esophagus, and compresses the trachea posteriorly.

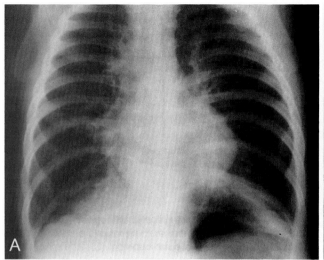

Figure 44.18. Cystic fibrosis. A. The early stages of this disease are often manifest only by parahilar peribronchial infiltrates and hyperinflation of the lungs. This appearance resembles that seen with viral lower respiratory tract infections or bronchiolitis. **B.** Later, the characteristic changes of end-stage cystic fibrosis are seen, including bronchial wall thickening, bronchiectasis, and persistent atelectasis.

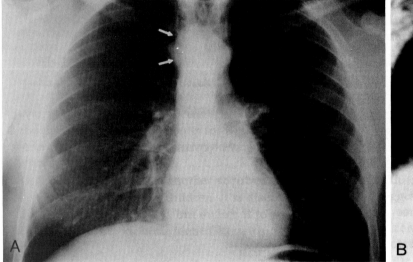
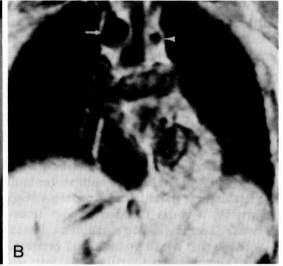

Figure 44.19. Double Aortic Arch. A. Note the large right-sided aortic arch displacing the trachea to the left (*arrows*). A smaller nodular opacity is seen to the left of the tracheal shadow. **B.** Coronal MR clearly defines the large right aortic (*arrow*) and the smaller left arch (*arrowhead*), which encircle and compress the trachea.

Asymmetric/Unilateral Aeration Abnormalities

Pulmonary aeration abnormalities are frequently asymmetric or unilateral. A large, hyperlucent hemithorax most often indicates overinflation of an entire lobe or lung. This hyperaeration may be due either to obstructive emphysema (Table 44.7) or to compensatory overinflation resulting from decreased volume of the contralateral lung. The pulmonary vascularity in the hyperinflated lung can often be used to help determine if the overinflation is obstructive or compensa-

tory. Generally, obstructive emphysema will result in diminished size of the pulmonary vessels because of compression and hypoxia-induced reflex arterial spasm (Fig. 44.21). On the other hand, the blood vessels to a compensatorily hyperinflated lung will be normal or even increased. If doubt remains, the combination of inspiratory and expiratory frontal views of the chest can be helpful. The general rule is that the lung that does not change or changes the least in volume is the abnormal lung (Fig. 44.22). This holds true whether the lung is obstructed and overinflated, or it is small due to atelectasis or hypoplasia. The

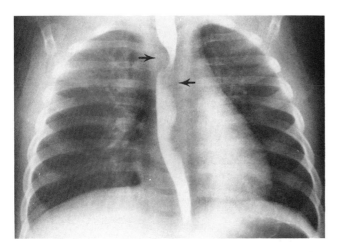

Figure 44.20. Double Aortic Arch. The encircling aortic arches compress the esophagus, creating a reverse-S configuration (*arrows*). Note that the right arch is higher and more prominent than the left.

Table 44.7. Unilateral Obstructive Emphysema

Bronchial foreign body
Mucous plug
Congenital lobar emphysema
Bronchial stenosis/atresia
Tuberculosis
Vascular anomalies
Mediastinal masses

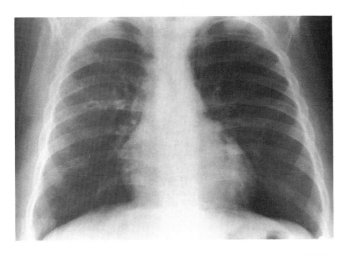

Figure 44.21. Obstructive Emphysema of the Left Lung. Note the small size of the pulmonary vessels on the left when compared with those on the right. The bronchial obstruction was due to a mucous plug in this patient with viral bronchitis.

same principle applies if fluoroscopy is performed. The only exception is mild congenital pulmonary hypoplasia, which can be associated with relatively normal lung dynamics.

Congenital Lobar Emphysema. The best-known cause of unilateral obstructive emphysema in the neonate is congenital lobar emphysema. This con-

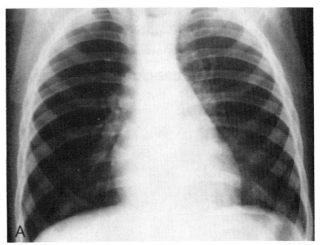

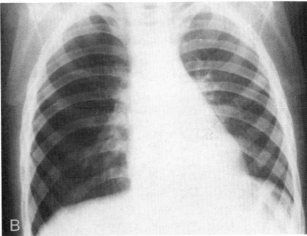

Figure 44.22. Bronchial Foreign Bodies on the Right. A. On inspiration, the right lung is slightly larger and more radiolucent than the left. **B.** With expiration, the left lung decreases in size, but the right lung remains overinflated. This indicates obstructive emphysema on the right, in this case due to pieces of walnut in the right mainstem bronchus.

dition consists of obstructive emphysema of a single lobe of the lung, most commonly the left upper, right upper, and right middle lobes, in this order. Usually emphysema is the result of segmental bronchial cartilage underdevelopment, which leads to expiratory airway collapse and a ball-valve type of obstruction. Early in the newborn period, the obstructed lobe may be opaque because of delayed clearance of fluid that has accumulated distal to the obstruction. Gradually, the fluid clears and the involved lobe becomes air-filled and overinflated (Fig. 44.23). When the enlargement of the emphysematous lobe is severe, it can occupy the entire hemithorax and erroneously lead to the appearance of a pneumothorax or of emphysema of the entire lung. Careful inspection, however, may reveal the collapsed, compressed adjacent lobes of the ipsilateral lung, confirming the diagnosis (Fig. 44.24). A similar appearance can occur in the rare case of bronchial stenosis or atresia. Classically, an oval opacity is

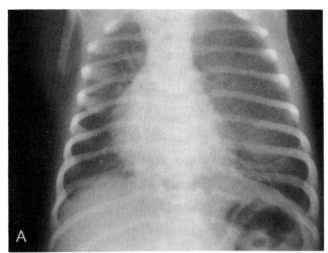

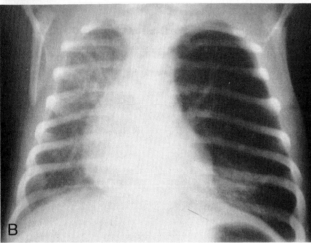

Figure 44.23.   Congenital Lobar Emphysema. A. Initially, the left upper lobe was large and hazy because of fluid trapped in the obstructed lung. **B.** A later film shows that the fluid has cleared, leaving a typical overinflated left upper lobe with compressive atelectasis of the left lower lobe.

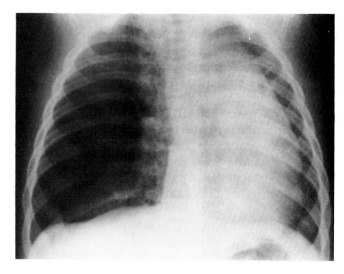

Figure 44.24.   Congenital Lobar Emphysema of the Right Middle Lobe. Note the overinflated middle lobe causing compression of the right upper and lower lobes and shift of the mediastinum to the left.

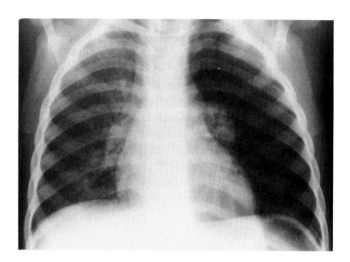

Figure 44.25.   Primary Tuberculosis. Note the left hilar adenopathy and obstructive emphysema of the left lung due to tuberculous granulomas of the left main bronchus.

seen adjacent to the overinflated lung near the hilum, representing a collection of mucus (mucocele) within the obstructed bronchus.

Endobronchial Lesions.   In older infants and children, obstructive emphysema is most often due to an endobronchial foreign body or a mucous plug (Fig. 44.21). Mucous plugs most often are seen in asthmatics and in children with viral lower respiratory tract infections. Other less common causes of unilateral obstructive emphysema include endobronchial masses such as tuberculous granulomas (Fig. 44.25) and extrinsic compressing lesions such as anomalous blood vessels and mediastinal tumors and cysts. Pneumothorax can lead to a large hyperlucent hemithorax that mimics obstructive emphysema of the lung. At times, particularly in supine patients, the free air may lie entirely along the anterior surface of the lung and no free lung edge will be visible. Clues to the presence of such an anterior pneumothorax include increased

radiolucency of the hemithorax and sharpness of the mediastinal border on the side of the pneumothorax (Fig. 44.26). In newborn infants, such a pneumothorax can compress the normal thymus gland, creating a mediastinal "pseudomass." Rarely, an air-filled lung cyst, or pneumatocele, or a markedly dilated stomach that has herniated into the chest through a diaphragmatic hernia can occupy an entire hemithorax, rendering it hyperlucent.

PULMONARY CAVITIES

Cavities that occur in the lungs of children are most often inflammatory or postinflammatory. Lung abscesses usually are a complication of a bacterial pneumonia and are frequently multiple. The wall of an

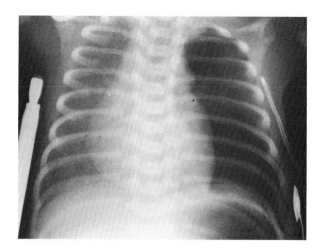

Figure 44.26. Pneumothorax in a Neonate. A left anterior pneumothorax causes increased radiolucency of the left lung and increased sharpness of the left heart border. Because the infant is supine, the free air lies anteriorly and a lateral lung edge is not visualized.

abscess is thick and irregular, and some contain air-fluid levels (Fig. 44.27). An abscess can also form distal to a bronchial obstruction, which in children is often due to a retained foreign body. Cavitary tuberculosis is rare in childhood and echinococcal cysts are rare outside of endemic areas.

Pneumatocele. Thin-walled lung cavities in children most often are pneumatoceles, which also most commonly result from pulmonary infections. Staphylococcal pneumonia is classically associated with pneumatocele formation, although they can occur with other infections, including tuberculosis (Fig. 44.28). Pneumatoceles develop from a bronchial obstruction that leads to air trapping and alveolar rupture, and occasionally such pneumatoceles can become large and cause significant mass effect. More often, however, the pneumatoceles remain relatively small and resolve spontaneously. Occasionally, pneumatoceles can rupture, leading to pneumothorax or pneumomediastinum. Other causes of pneumatoceles in children include blunt chest trauma (Fig. 44.29), hydrocarbon pneumonitis, and Langerhans' cell histiocytosis. True congenital lung cysts are uncommon. These cysts are usually thin-walled and more commonly occur in the lower lobes. Such cysts are often asymptomatic unless they become infected or undergo rapid expansion with the development of a tension phenomenon.

Cystic adenomatoid malformation is a rare congenital lesion of the lung that is characterized by abnormal lung tissue containing dysplastic adenomatous tissue within communicating cysts of variable sizes. The radiographic appearance of these lesions can vary from a predominantly solid lesion with multiple tiny cysts to multiple large thin-walled cysts that

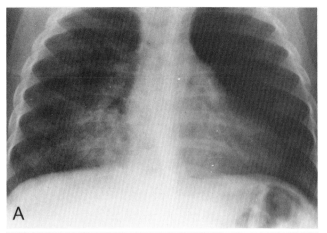

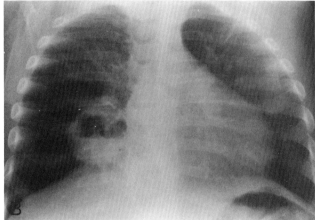

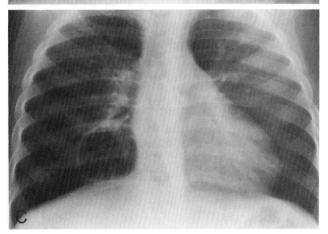

Figure 44.27. Pulmonary Abscess. A. A typical bacterial pneumonia is seen in the right middle lobe. **B.** Later, cavitation has developed in the central portion of the pneumonia and an air-fluid level is evident. This is a typical appearance for a lung abscess. **C.** With healing, the thick walls of the abscess become thin.

can mimic congenital lobar emphysema (Fig. 40.30) (5). In the newborn period, the cysts usually are fluid-filled and the lesion has the appearance of a solid mass. With time, air replaces the fluid and small cysts become apparent. These cysts gradually enlarge and can cause enough mass effect to lead to respiratory

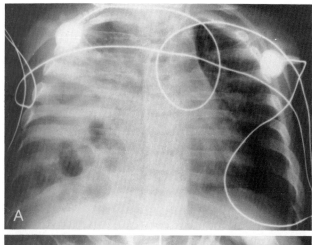

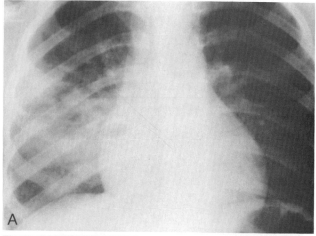

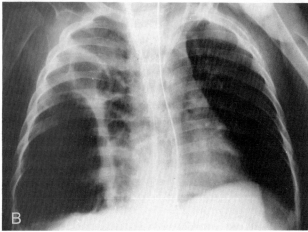

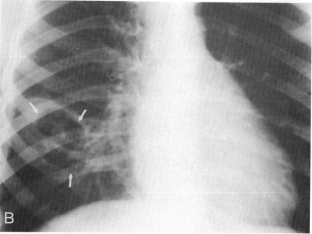

Figure 44.28. Postinflammatory Pneumatocele. A. Note the early pneumatocele formation in the right lung due to progressive primary tuberculosis. **B.** A later radiograph shows marked enlargement of the pneumatoceles.

Figure 44.29. Posttraumatic Pneumatocele. A. A motor vehicle accident resulted in a right lung contusion. **B.** After the contusion resolves, a thin-walled pneumatocele remains (*arrows*).

distress. The malformation is usually unilateral and can affect any portion of the lung.

Congenital Diaphragmatic Hernia. Air-filled loops of bowel in a congenital diaphragmatic hernia can resemble the multiple cysts of cystic adenomatoid malformation. An important clue to the correct diagnosis of diaphragmatic hernia is the absence or paucity of gas-filled bowel loops within the abdomen (Fig. 44.31). Congenital diaphragmatic hernias most often occur through the foramen of Bochdalek, which lies posteriorly and medially in each hemidiaphragm. Left-sided hernias are much more common, but right-sided Bochdalek hernias do occur. Hernias through the foramen of Morgagni, which lies anteriorly, are less common and usually are less severe. Infants with large diaphragmatic hernias usually present with severe respiratory distress immediately after birth. Compression of the ipsilateral lung in utero causes it to be hypoplastic, and often the contralateral lung is also small. The patients are profoundly hypoxic, and persistent fetal circulation due to hypoxia-induced pulmonary hypertension usually further compromises

the infant's condition. Even with early diagnosis and surgery, the mortality of this condition remains high. Extracorporeal membrane oxygenation has been helpful in some patients by circumventing the problem of pulmonary hypertension and, consequently, the right-to-left shunting of blood away from the lungs.

LUNG DISEASE IN THE NEONATE

The conditions leading to respiratory distress in the newborn infant are numerous and can be divided basically into those treated medically and those requiring surgical intervention. Surgical conditions consist primarily of congenital and developmental abnormalities that result in a space-occupying lesion within the chest (e.g., diaphragmatic hernia, congenital lobar emphysema, chylothorax, pneumothorax, cystic adenomatoid malformation). Most of these conditions have been covered in other parts of this chapter. This section will deal with pulmonary parenchymal disease of the newborn.

Idiopathic respiratory distress syndrome (hyaline membrane disease) is one of the most common causes

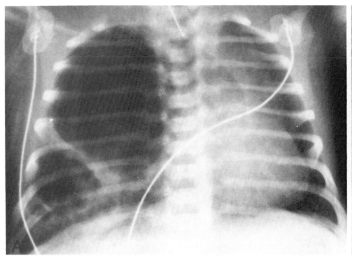

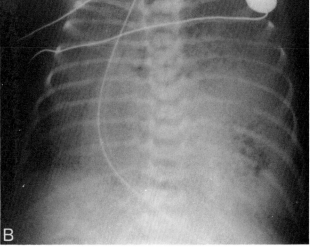

Figure 44.30. Cystic Adenomatoid Malformation. A. Note the multiple air-filled cysts of widely variable size that expand the right lung and shift the mediastinum to the left. **B.** In this patient, the con-genital malformation is predominantly solid or fluid-filled, with multiple, small air-filled cysts of varying sizes. Note that the mass in the left lung displaces the mediastinum and nasogastric tube to the right.

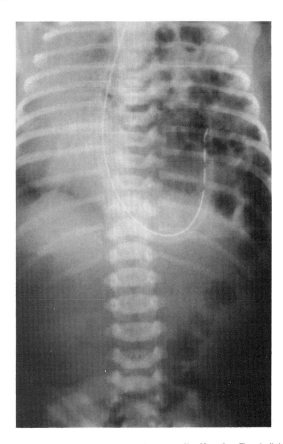

Figure 44.31. Congenital Diaphragmatic Hernia. The left hemithorax is filled with multiple air-filled loops of bowel, displacing the mediastinum to the right. The course of the nasogastric tube and the absence of normal bowel loops are clues to the diagnosis.

of respiratory distress in the newborn infant. This condition is most commonly seen in premature infants; however, it occasionally occurs in term infants of diabetic mothers. In both cases, immaturity is the main predisposing factor. The primary abnormality is a lack

of surfactant normally produced by the type II alveolar cells. This substance is responsible for decreasing the surface tension of the alveoli; when absent, the alveoli are poorly distensible and remain collapsed. A cycle of hypoxia, acidosis, and diminished perfusion results. Clinically, these infants present with respiratory distress within the first few hours after birth.

The classic radiographic findings of hyaline membrane disease consist of lungs that are small in volume and have a finely granular pattern with air bronchograms that extend into the lung periphery (Fig. 44.32). The granular pattern basically reflects the histologic findings of distended alveolar ducts and terminal bronchioles superimposed over generalized alveolar collapse. When the alveolar and terminal bronchials overdistend, small, round, 1–2 mm bubbles result. During expiration, the air bronchograms and granular pattern disappear and the lungs become totally opaque.

Similar lung opacities can be seen with neonatal pneumonia, pulmonary lymphangiectasia, neonatal-retained fluid syndrome, and congenital heart abnormalities associated with severe pulmonary venous obstruction. However, unlike patients with hyaline membrane disease, the lung volumes in these conditions are normal to increased (Fig. 44.33). In a few cases of neonatal pneumonia, the lung pattern is indistinguishable from respiratory distress syndrome. Until recently, the primary form of therapy of this condition consisted of positive pressure-assisted ventilation, which attempts to force air deeper into the respiratory tree and alveoli. Although in some patients the use of assisted ventilation significantly improves oxygenation, in others, the elevated airway pressures result in complications due to air leakage from the distended terminal airways. Air dissects through the

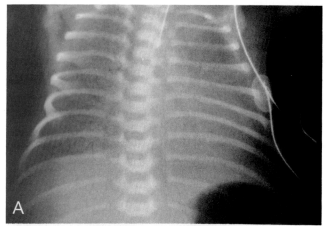

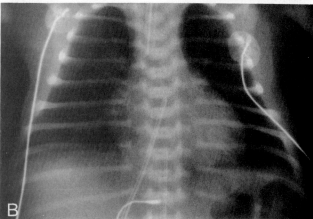

Figure 44.32.   Hyaline Membrane Disease. A. Shortly after birth, the lungs are small and diffusely opaque with air bronchograms that extend into the periphery of the lung. This is a typical appearance for hyaline membrane disease. **B.** After several treatments with endotracheal surfactant, the lung volumes have dramatically improved and the lung opacity has virtually disappeared.

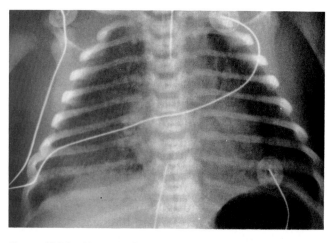

Figure 44.33.   Neonatal Pneumonia. The lungs are diffusely hazy with a granular appearance that is similar to that seen with hyaline membrane disease. Note, however, that the lungs are normal in volume.

interstitium and lymphatics (pulmonary interstitial emphysema), creating a radiographic pattern of ser-

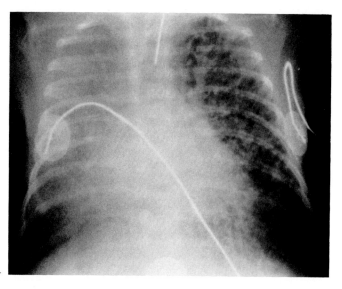

Figure 44.34.   Pulmonary Interstitial Emphysema. Serpiginous bubbles of interstitial air extend to the periphery of the left lung. The interstitial air causes the lung to be stiff and hyperexpanded, even during expiration.

piginous bubbles that extends all the way to the lung periphery (Fig. 44.34). Unlike the air bronchogram of uncomplicated hyaline membrane disease, the bubbles of pulmonary interstitial emphysema do not collapse upon expiration.

Pneumomediastinum and pneumothorax are other common complications of positive pressure ventilation. Air can also dissect into the pericardium and peritoneum, and occasionally air embolism can develop with devastating consequences. The hypoxemia associated with the respiratory distress syndrome sometimes leads to persistent patency of the ductus arteriosus, and often radiographic changes are the first clue to this complication. Suggestive findings include lungs that are large and increasingly opaque with loss of the granular pattern, cardiomegaly, and pulmonary vascular congestion (Fig. 44.35). The increased lung opacity is due to pulmonary edema. Neurogenic pulmonary edema, due to cerebral hypoxic injury and hemorrhage, is a common noncardiac cause of pulmonary edema in the premature infant.

Bronchopulmonary Dysplasia.   Continued use of positive pressure-assisted ventilation and high O_2 concentrations can damage the lung parenchyma and result in bronchopulmonary dysplasia (6). The damage probably results from a combination of oxygen toxicity and mechanical damage to the alveolar cells and bronchiolar mucosal cells, eventually leading to fibrosis. In the early stages of the disease, the radiographs show little abnormality other than those caused by the underlying lung disease, most often hyaline membrane disease. In many cases, an early diffuse haziness or reticulonodularity develops, which most likely is due to interstitial pulmonary edema. In

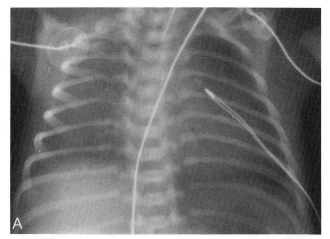

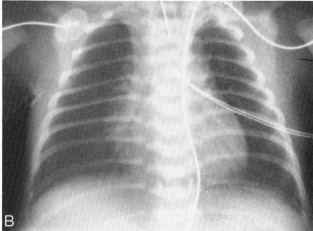

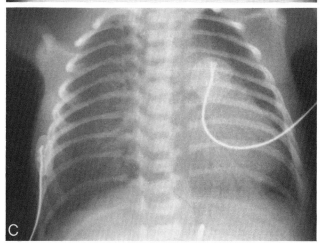

Figure 44.35. Patent Ductus Arteriosus in a Premature Infant with Hyaline Membrane Disease. A. Early films showed typical small granular lungs due to hyaline membrane disease. **B.** Following surfactant therapy, the lungs increased in volume and became clear. **C.** A few days later, the heart has enlarged and, although the lungs have increased in volume, they have also become more opaque. The lung opacity represents pulmonary edema due to the development of a patent ductus arteriosus.

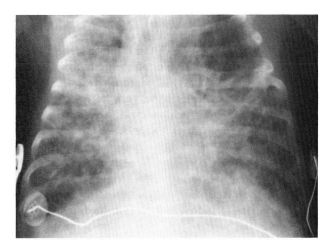

Figure 44.36. Bronchopulmonary Dysplasia. Note the coarse reticularity of the lungs with multiple various-sized bubbles and scattered areas of atelectasis. This pattern is typical of the uneven aeration seen with severe bronchopulmonary dysplasia.

initial damage and prolonged ventilatory therapy results in the more characteristic uneven pattern of aeration of the alveolar groups. Alternating areas of overdistension and collapse of alveolar groups give the appearance of bubbles that are variable in size and tend to be larger in the lung bases (Fig. 44.36). Unlike the fixed bubbles of pulmonary interstitial emphysema, the bubbles of bronchopulmonary dysplasia collapse on expiration.

Other patients with advanced bronchopulmonary dysplasia demonstrate streaky opacities that radiate from the hila and scattered patchy opacities because of atelectasis. In most patients, the radiographic abnormalities undergo gradual clearing during the early years of life. Pulmonary function abnormalities often persist after the chest radiograph has returned to normal. These infants often suffer from reactive airway disease and/or frequent or severe viral lower respiratory tract infections. The increasing use of intratracheal surfactant therapy for hyaline membrane disease may potentially decrease the incidence of many of the complications previously associated with this condition (7, 8).

Wilson-Mikity Syndrome. The Wilson-Mikity syndrome is a condition that also occurs in premature infants and radiographically resembles bronchopulmonary dysplasia. Unlike bronchopulmonary dysplasia, however, this syndrome does not necessarily develop following high oxygen concentrations or positive pressure ventilation. Most infants are clinically normal during the first few days of life, but develop the symptoms of cyanosis, respiratory distress with retractions, and apnea during the 2nd to 4th weeks of life. Radiographically, the lungs are usually clear until the onset of symptoms, at which time a reticulonodular pattern develops diffusely in the lungs (Fig. 44.37).

some patients, the lungs heal at this stage and never progress to the typical bubbly appearance of the later stages of bronchopulmonary dysplasia. More severe

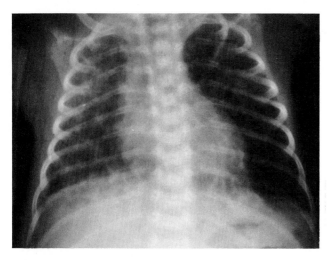

Figure 44.37. Wilson-Mikity Syndrome. Note the diffuse lung reticularity and early bubble formation. This appearance is virtually indistinguishable from that seen in patients with bronchopulmonary dysplasia.

Table 44.8. Diffusely Hazy or Reticular Lungs (Neonate)

Decreased lung volumes
   Poor inspiration
   Hyaline membrane disease
Normal-to-increased lung volumes
   Retained fluid
   Aspiration (amniotic fluid/meconium)
   Pneumonia
   Pulmonary edema
   Pulmonary lymphangiectasia

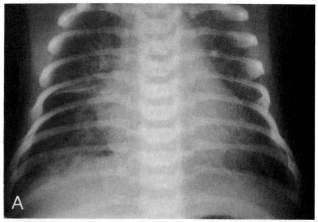

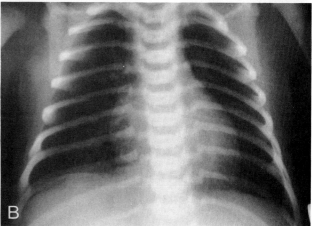

Figure 44.38. Retained Fluid Syndrome. A. On the 1st day of life, the lungs of this term newborn show diffuse haziness, streaky parahilar opacities, and bilateral pleural effusions. **B.** The following day, all of these abnormalities had resolved, which is the typical sequence of events in an infant with retained lung fluid.

Focal areas of hyperaeration and atelectasis are seen that tend to progress to larger cyst-like areas. This pattern of alternating collapse and hyperaeration of the alveolar groups is thought to be due to immaturity and uneven maturation of the alveoli. Unlike bronchopulmonary dysplasia, pulmonary fibrosis does not occur and pulmonary hypertension is uncommon in the Wilson-Mikity syndrome. The lungs eventually return to normal in surviving infants.

Retained Lung Fluid. A pattern of diffuse haziness or reticularity in a newborn infant with normal-sized lungs can be seen in a variety of abnormal conditions (Table 44.8). In an otherwise normal term neonate, particularly those delivered by cesarean section, this pattern often represents retained lung fluid. Other associated radiographic findings include streaky parahilar opacities, hyperinflation of the lungs, and pleural effusions. The lung findings are usually bilateral; however, in a few cases, right-sided predominance is seen. In most infants with the retained fluid syndrome (transient respiratory distress of the newborn), both the symptoms and the radio-

graphic abnormalities clear rapidly within the first 24–48 hours of life (Fig. 44.38). A similar reticular pattern in the lungs of a newborn can occur with pneumonia or with pulmonary edema (Fig. 44.39).

Meconium Aspiration. Intrauterine fetal distress can lead to the passage of meconium in utero, which can then be aspirated into the tracheobronchial tree. Classically, the aspirated meconium particles cause obstruction of the small peripheral bronchioles, resulting in unevenly distributed areas of subsegmental atelectasis with areas of alternating overdistension. This creates a coarsely reticulonodular or nodular appearance of the lungs (Fig. 44.40). In some infants, more fluid and debris than meconium is aspirated. In such cases, rapid radiographic clearing can be seen with little residual air trapping. In more severe cases, the air trapping can result in complications such as pneumothorax and pneumomediastinum. Because of the resulting hypoxia, persistent fetal circulation is also a common complication (see "Patent Ductus Artesiosus"). Treatment most often

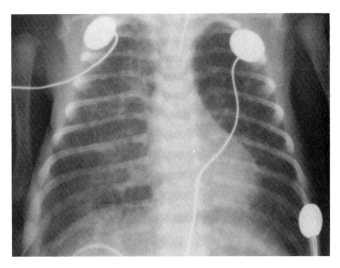

Figure 44.39. Neonatal Pneumonia. Note the diffuse reticular pattern throughout the lungs of this patient with neonatal pneumonia. Early alveolar changes are present in the central regions of the right lung.

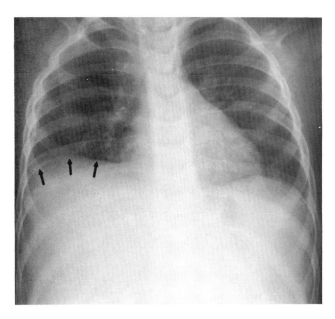

Figure 44.41. Right Pleural Effusion in a Patient with Nephrotic Syndrome. Note the flattened and laterally displaced curvature of the right hemidiaphragm (*arrows*), indicating the presence of subpulmonic pleural fluid.

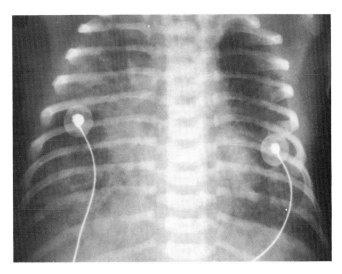

Figure 44.40. Meconium Aspiration. Note a typical coarse, reticulonodular pattern throughout both lungs.

consists of endotracheal suctioning and the administration of humidified oxygen.

Pulmonary Lymphangiectasia. A coarse, reticulonodular pattern is also seen in infants with pulmonary lymphangiectasia. This is a rare condition that can occur as an isolated abnormality or can be associated with congenital heart disease or generalized lymphangiectasia (Fig. 44.10). The isolated form of the disease is thought to result from abnormal pulmonary lymphatic development, resulting in dilated and obstructed lymphatic channels. The lungs often are hyperinflated and pleural effusions may also occur. Lymphangiectasia associated with congenital heart disease usually is seen with one of the conditions leading to severe pulmonary venous obstruction (i.e., hypoplas-

tic left heart syndrome, total anomalous pulmonary venous return type III, or pulmonary vein atresia).

ECMO. Extracorporeal membrane oxygenation is becoming more widely used for the support of infants with life-threatening respiratory disease. The technique consists of a bypass of the pulmonary blood flow through a semipermeable silicon membrane. The procedure interrupts the cycle of pulmonary hypertension and persistent fetal circulation (right-to-left shunting) and diminishes the damaging effect of high oxygen concentrations and barotrauma to the lungs. Extracorporeal membrane oxygenation is most commonly used in patients with congenital diaphragmatic hernia, hyaline membrane disease, meconium aspiration syndrome, and neonatal sepsis and pneumonia. While on the extracorporeal circuit, the lungs invariably become completely opaque (9). This is an expected occurrence because the lungs are collapsed. Occasionally, pleural effusions will also be present but are not radiographically detectable because of the opacity of the lungs. In such cases, the lungs often fail to reexpand despite increasing ventilator pressures, and ultrasound can be used to identify the pleural fluid.

PLEURAL THICKENING AND EFFUSIONS

Generalized thickening of the pleural space because of the accumulation of fluid has the same configurations in children as in adults. The most easily recognized pattern is thickening along the lateral and apical portions of the lung. Subpulmonic collections can mimic an elevated diaphragm, but characteristic

Figure 44.42.   Chylothorax. Ultrasound easily identifies fluid in the pleural space (*arrow*). *F*, pleural fluid; *D*, diaphragm; *L*, liver; *A*, ascites.

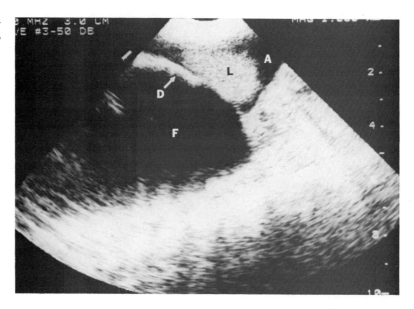

Table 44.9.   Pleural Effusions

Unilateral
   Pneumonia/empyema
   Chylothorax
   Iatrogenic
   Trauma
   Intraabdominal inflammation
   Intrathoracic neoplasm
   Ruptured aneurysm of ductus arteriosus
Bilateral
   Renal disease
   Lymphoma
   Neuroblastoma
   Congestive heart failure
   Collagen vascular diseases
   Fluid overload

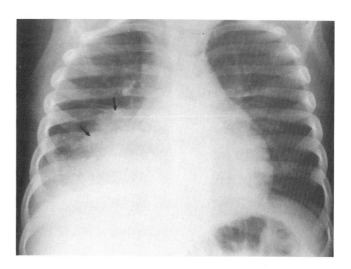

Figure 44.43.   Pneumococcal Pneumonia with Associated Pleural Effusion. Note a right pleural effusion that partially obscures the consolidating pneumonia of the right middle lobe (*arrows*).

flattening and laterally displaced curvature of the dome are clues to the presence of subpulmonic pleural fluid (Fig. 44.41). When a totally opaque hemithorax of normal or increased volume is encountered, the opacity is nearly always due to a large collection of pleural fluid. Opacification of an entire lung by pneumonia is very unusual in children, however, occasionally a large cyst or intrathoracic mass can occupy most of the hemithorax. In such cases one should look for residual radiolucency in the costophrenic angle, which does not occur when pleural fluid is the cause of total opacification of a hemithorax. The presence of pleural fluid can be easily verified by ultrasound (Fig. 44.42). The type of fluid in the pleural space (serous effusion, inflammatory exudate, chyle, or blood) cannot be determined radiographically.

Unilateral Pleural Effusions are most commonly associated with a pneumonia in the ipsilateral lung (Fig. 44.43 and Table 44.9). Such effusions are often transudates, but empyema is the best possibility if the collection is large (Fig. 44.44). Empyemas most often occur with staphylococcal, *Haemophilus*, and pneumococcal pneumonias, but serous effusions may be seen with a variety of infections, including mycoplasma. Infections below the diaphragm can also result in pleural effusions, particularly subphrenic abscesses or pancreatitis. Rarely, a unilateral effusion will accompany an intrathoracic tumor that involves the pleura (Fig. 44.45).

Bilateral Serous Pleural Effusions are most commonly seen in patients with renal diseases such as acute glomerulonephritis or nephrotic syndrome. The next most common cause of bilateral effusions is lymphoma (usually non-Hodgkin's) (Fig. 44.46) or neuroblastoma in the abdomen or chest. Congestive heart

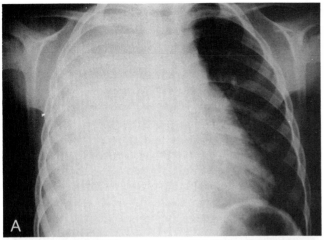

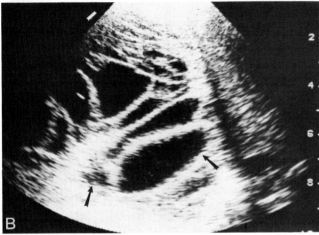

Figure 44.44. Empyema. A. The entire right hemithorax is opacified with shift of the mediastinum to the left. **B.** Ultrasound confirms a large collection of fluid (pus) in the right pleural space with multiple thick septations (*arrows*).

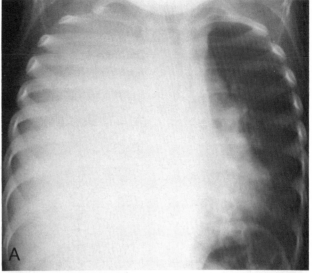

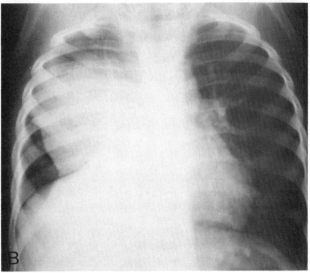

Figure 44.45. Pleural Effusion Associated with a Thoracic Neoplasm. A. Pleural fluid causes complete opacification of the right hemithorax and shift of the mediastinum to the left. **B.** Upon drainage of the effusion, a large right intrathoracic mass (teratoma) becomes apparent.

failure, collagen vascular diseases, and fluid overload may also result in pleural effusions.

Hemothorax is usually the result of trauma, either due to direct chest wall trauma with or without rib fractures or to aortic rupture from a deceleration injury. Occasionally, bleeding disorders can also result in hemothorax. Rarely, an aneurysm of the ductus arteriosus can rupture and bleed into the pleural space.

Chylothorax. The most common cause of massive pleural effusion in the neonate is chylothorax. Chylous effusions are usually unilateral and more commonly occur on the right (Fig. 44.47), but bilateral chylothoraces occur. The cause of chylothorax is unknown, but the most likely possibilities are a traumatic tear or a congenital defect of the thoracic duct. Chylous effusions can occasionally result from superior vena cava thrombosis, and such effusions are more difficult to manage. Most chylothoraces resolve following thoracentesis, although occasionally chest tube drainage is required. Pulmonary lymphangiecta-

sia is a rare cause of chylothorax. Finally, note that another relatively common cause of pleural fluid is iatrogenic and related to complications of indwelling catheters in thoracic vessels (10, 11).

LUNG MASSES

The most common pulmonary mass in children is actually not a true mass but is a pseudomass caused by a spherical pneumonia (Fig. 44.48). Such an appearance is not uncommon at certain stages of pneumonia in children. Pulmonary abscess can also have a mass-like appearance, usually with central cavitation. In regard to true pulmonary masses, postinflammatory granulomas are the most common and are usually due to tuberculosis or fungal infections. Such

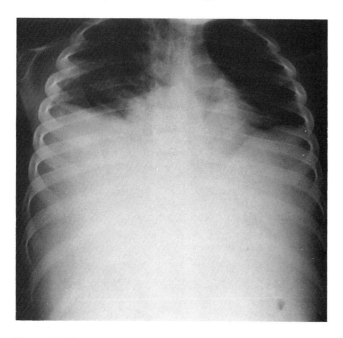

Figure 44.46. Bilateral Pleural Effusions—Lymphoma. Note the large bilateral subpulmonic pleural effusions in a patient with abdominal non-Hodgkin's lymphoma.

granulomas are usually small and very often are calcified (Fig. 44.49). Plasma cell granuloma, or postinflammatory pseudotumor, is a reactive lesion that develops from a healing pneumonia. Calcifications in such nodules are uncommon and the lesion gradually resolves over a period of years. Nodules have also been reported following atypical measles pneumonia. Many childhood pulmonary masses are congenital or developmental in origin.

Bronchogenic Cysts are cysts that are lined with respiratory epithelium and filled with mucoid liquid. They can occur in the lung parenchyma or in the mediastinum, and a subcarinal location is very common (Fig. 40.50). Some are connected to the bronchial tree and thus are air-filled.

Pulmonary Sequestration is one of several developmental bronchopulmonary foregut malformations (12). Sequestration is a mass of lung tissue that lacks a connection to the bronchial tree and is supplied by abnormal vessels extending from the descending aorta. Classically, sequestrations have been divided into those that are covered by their own pleura (extralobar) or by the pleura of the adjacent normal lung (intralobar). Sequestrations most often occur as a triangular or oval-shaped mass in the medial and basal portion of a lung, more commonly on the left (Fig. 44.51**A**). Not uncommonly, some air will be present within the sequestration because of collateral air drift. This lesion is usually clinically silent until it becomes infected, and the most common presentation is that of recurrent pneumonia. The diagnosis is assured by demonstrating the abnormal blood supply.

This can sometimes be achieved by ultrasound or computed tomography (CT) (13); however, MR and angiography best demonstrate the abnormal vessels (Fig. 44.51, **B** and **C**).

Rare Pulmonary Masses. Other causes of a pulmonary mass are rare and usually have few distinguishing features. If one encounters a mass connected to an unusually large vessel, the diagnosis of a pulmonary arteriovenous malformation is likely. A central, oval-shaped nodule associated with overaeration of the involved lobe suggests the diagnosis of a mucocele in a patient with bronchial atresia. Primary lung tumors are rare and the majority are benign. Pulmonary hamartoma is a benign congenital tumor that occasionally contains characteristic flocculent calcifications. Rarely, laryngeal papillomas can spread into the trachea and the lungs. Primary pulmonary malignancies are very rare and include sarcomas, primitive neuroectodermal tumors, and squamous cell carcinoma. Pulmonary blastoma is a rare neoplasm composed of both epithelial and mesenchymal elements. These tumors can be either solid or cystic.

By far the most common malignant neoplasm in the lung during childhood is metastatic, whether single or multiple. The most common childhood tumors to metastasize to the lungs are Wilms' tumor, Ewing's sarcoma, osteosarcoma, and rhabdomyosarcoma. Other masses and nodules that can be multiple include granulomas (most often fungal), abscesses, hemangiomas, and Wegener's granulomatosis. Cavitary nodules are characteristic of septic emboli, Wegener's granulomatosis, laryngeal papillomatosis, sarcoidosis, and metastases.

MEDIASTINAL AND HILAR MASSES

The division of the mediastinum into anterior, middle, and posterior compartments is the most useful scheme for categorizing mediastinal masses in both children and adults. This discussion will use an arbitrary system based on the division of the chest into roughly thirds on the lateral view.

Thymus Gland. The thymus gland is the primary normal structure residing in the anterior mediastinum and is also the most common cause of an apparent anterior mediastinal mass. The normal thymus gland can vary widely in its appearance and sometimes causes considerable confusion in interpreting an infant or young child's chest radiograph. The gland is commonly very prominent at birth and frequently remains easily visible up to about 2 years of age. Not uncommonly, the gland remains visible in an older child.

On posteroanterior chest radiographs, the thymus gland typically causes smooth bilateral widening of the superior mediastinum. The gland overlies and silhouettes the upper cardiac borders, although some-

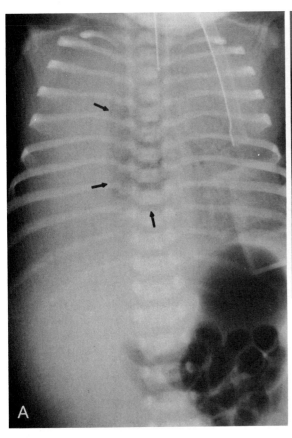

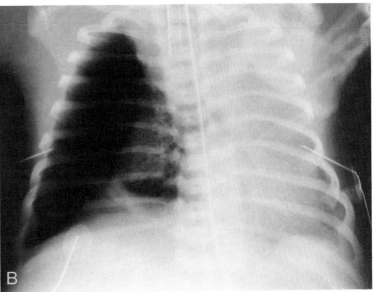

Figure 44.47. Neonatal chylothorax. A. The right hemithorax is opaque and the mediastinum is shifted into the left chest. Note the small right lung (*arrows*). **B.** After the chylous effusion is drained, the hypoplastic right lung becomes more clearly visible.

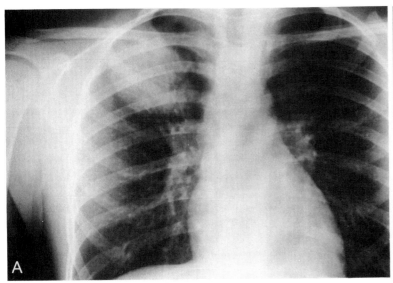

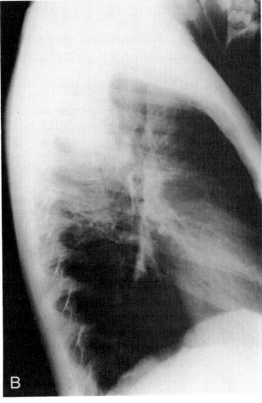

Figure 44.48. Round Pneumonia. A and **B**. This pneumonia of the right upper lobe has a round, mass-like configuration on both views.

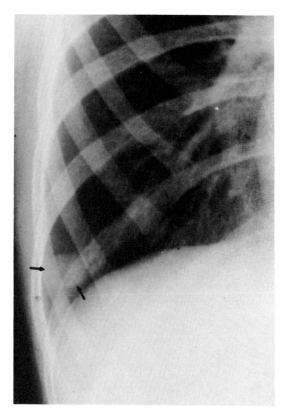

Figure 44.49.   Histoplasma Granuloma. Note the small, round, well-defined mass in the right costophrenic angle (*arrows*).

times a small notch is visible at the junction between the thymus and the heart (Fig. 44.52, **A** and **B**). The border of the thymus gland also sometimes has a slightly wavy contour due to compression by the overlying ribs (Fig. 44.52**C**). In other cases, one thymic lobe will appear more prominent than the other and tends to have a triangular configuration that has been called the "sail" sign (Fig. 44.52**D**). This appearance is more commonly seen on the right and may be mistaken for lung pathology (i.e., lobar consolidation), particularly if the patient is in slightly right-sided rotated position. On the lateral view of the chest, the thymus lies over the anterosuperior portion of the cardiac silhouette in the retrosternal space (Fig. 44.52**E**).

The normal thymus gland can occasionally acquire more unusual configurations. For example, thymic tissue may extend high into the superior mediastinum, the lower neck, or posteriorly, between the innominate and left brachiocephalic arteries. However, only rarely do any of these atypical positions result in symptoms. Stress atrophy of the thymus is an interesting phenomenon that can occur secondary to almost any type of illness or to the use of steroids. The thymus can rapidly shrink in size during illness, only to return to normal size after the infant has recovered. Occasionally, rebound hypertrophy follows stress atrophy.

When stress atrophy of the thymus gland is severe, the mediastinum will appear very narrow, suggesting the absence or hypoplasia of thymus gland (Fig. 44.53). The distinction between thymic atrophy and aplasia becomes important in infants who are suspected of having certain immunologic disorders. The best known of these disorders is the DiGeorge syndrome, which, in its most severe form, consists of thymic aplasia, absence of the parathyroid glands, cardiovascular anomalies (especially those involving the aortic arch), and a variety of other congenital anomalies. This syndrome is caused by the faulty development of the third and fourth pharyngeal pouches. In infants, ultrasound can be helpful in identifying the presence of a small thymus gland that is not apparent radiographically (14).

A large thymus gland is nearly always a normal gland in an infant. Leukemia or lymphoma can infiltrate the thymus gland, sometimes causing massive enlargement (Fig. 44.54). Thymic cysts are uncommon developmental lesions that are best seen with ultrasound. They appear as well-defined, round, anechoic lesions, unless they have been complicated by hemorrhage or infection. When this occurs, echogenic material or debris will be seen within the cyst. Spontaneous hemorrhage into the thymus gland has also been described in newborn infants. When pneumothorax is present in a neonate (unilateral or bilateral), the thymus gland can become compressed and elevated by the free air, creating a pseudomass in the superior mediastinum (Fig. 44.55). This mass-like compression of the thymus gland may be a clue to a subtle anterior pneumothorax.

When thymic abnormalities are suspected and cannot be evaluated adequately by ultrasound, either CT or MR may be used (15). The thymic lobes should have a smooth, somewhat triangular shape with homogeneous texture (Fig. 44.56). Bulging or convexity of the borders of the thymus gland should suggest the possibility of pathologic enlargement, particularly if adjacent structures such as the trachea or the great vessels are displaced or compressed. Primary neoplasms or cysts produce focal alterations of attenuation or signal intensity, whereas infiltration by leukemia or lymphoma or hemorrhage results in a more diffuse and heterogenous parenchymal pattern. Overall, MR probably is best in defining whether a thymus gland is normal or abnormal.

Anterior Mediastinal Masses. The same imaging approach can be used to evaluate any mediastinal mass, the majority of which in the anterior mediastinum in children are tumors. The most common are dermoids and teratomas. Strictly speaking, dermoids are generally benign tumors comprised only of ectodermal elements, whereas teratomas contain elements from all dermal layers. Teratomas commonly

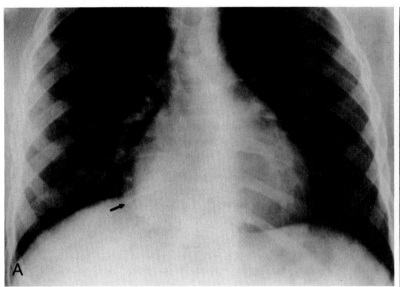

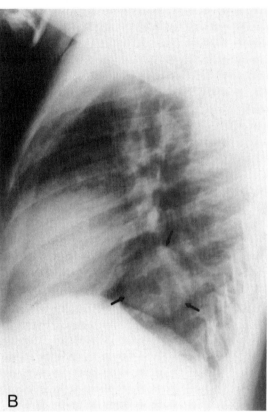

Figure 44.50.   Bronchogenic Cyst. A. A rounded opacity peeks out from behind the right heart border (*arrows*). **B.** A lateral view more clearly shows the round, well-defined cyst (*arrows*).

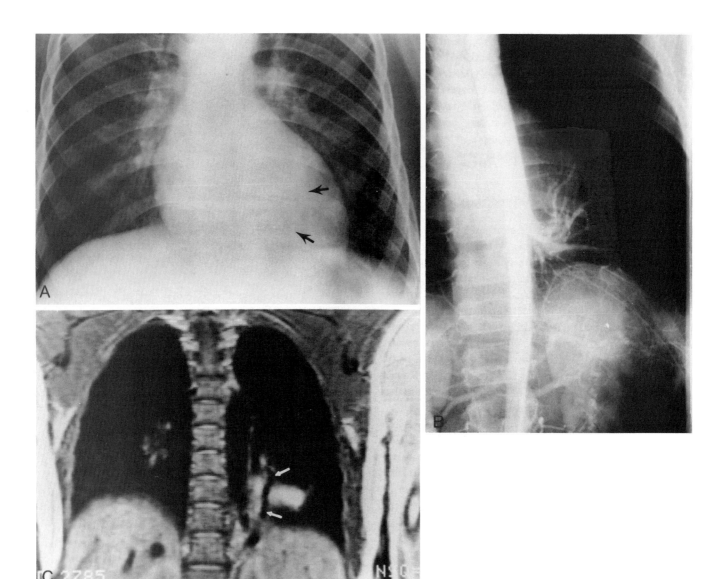

Figure 44.51. Pulmonary Sequestration. A. A poorly defined opacity is seen through the cardiac silhouette on the left (*arrows*). **B.** Angiography demonstrates the abnormal vessels arising from the descending aorta that supply the sequestrated lung tissue. **C.** Coronal MR images in another patient with a left lower lobe sequestration. The sequestration appears as a high-intensity mass associated with a large abnormal vessel (*arrows*).

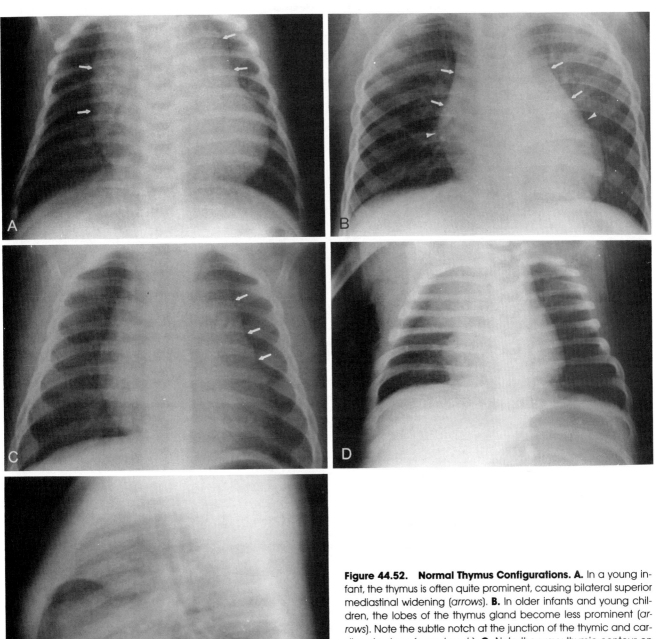

Figure 44.52. Normal Thymus Configurations. A. In a young infant, the thymus is often quite prominent, causing bilateral superior mediastinal widening (*arrows*). **B.** In older infants and young children, the lobes of the thymus gland become less prominent (*arrows*). Note the subtle notch at the junction of the thymic and cardiac shadows (*arrowheads*). **C.** Note the wavy thymic contour on the left due to compression by the ribs (*arrows*). **D.** The right thymic lobe is prominent in this patient with a configuration that has been likened to a sail. **E.** Note the straight inferior border of the thymus glands which lies in the retrosternal space on the lateral view.

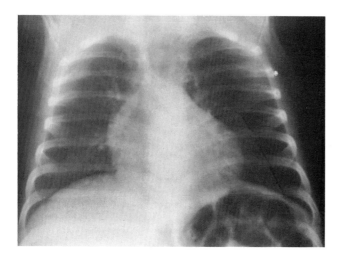

Figure 44.53.   Stress Atrophy of the Thymus. Note the narrow superior mediastinum due to absence of a thymic shadow in this infant suffering from failure to thrive.

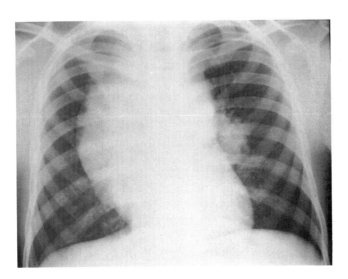

Figure 44.54.   Hodgkin's Lymphoma. Note the massive thymic enlargement due to lymphomatous involvement.

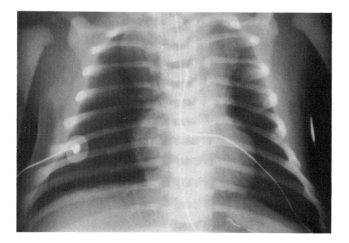

Figure 44.55.   Thymic Pseudomass. Note that the thymus gland is elevated and compressed by the bilateral anterior pneumothoraces, creating the appearance of a superior mediastinal mass.

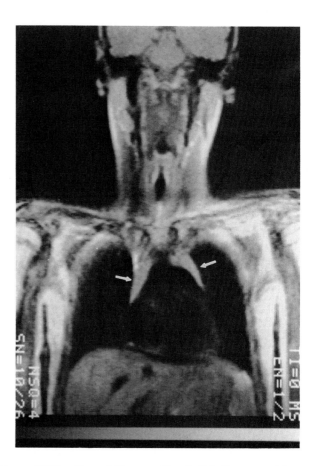

Figure 44.56.   Normal Thymus Gland—MR. The normal thymus gland is elegantly demonstrated on this coronal MR image in an older child (*arrows*).

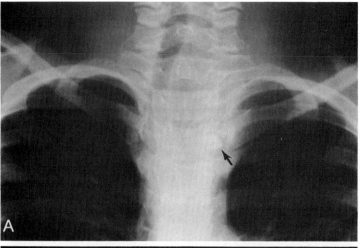

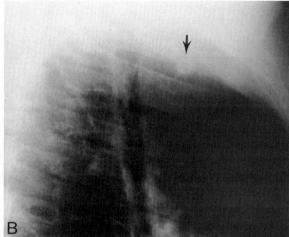

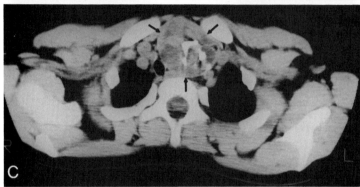

Figure 44.57. **Mediastinal Teratoma. A.** Note the superior mediastinal mass that displaces the trachea to the right. A tooth-like calcification is noted within the mass (*arrow*). **B.** Lateral view shows the anterior location of the mass and the calcification (*arrow*). **C.** A CT scan reveals the heterogenous nature of this teratoma (*arrows*), which contains dense calcifications and hypodense areas representing fat.

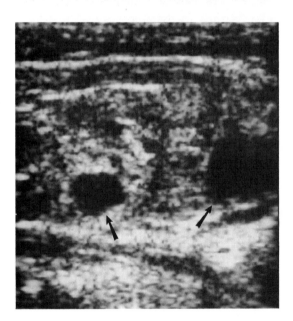

Figure 44.58. **Thyroid Cyst.** Ultrasound demonstrates colloid cysts (*arrows*) in the thyroid gland of a patient with multinodular goiter due to congenital dyshormonogenesis. Note the inhomogenous texture of the gland, a common finding in diffuse thyroid disease.

contain calcifications that are probably best demonstrated by CT (Fig. 44.57). Other less common neoplasms found in the anterior mediastinum include thyroid tumors, hemangiomas, and cystic hygromas (usually extending from the neck). Ultrasound is an excellent means of evaluating an enlarged thyroid gland and easily differentiates cysts from neoplasms (Fig. 44.58). Cystic hygroma is a congenital malformation of lymphatic origin, and again, ultrasound is an ideal imaging modality for showing the multiloculated cystic nature of these lesions (Fig. 44.59) (16). Hemangiomas tend to be more echogenic on ultrasound, although small cystic areas representing vascular lakes are often seen in the cavernous type of hemangioma. Blood flow within hemangiomas is sometimes demonstrable with color flow Doppler imaging.

Middle Mediastinal Masses. Normal structures in the middle mediastinum from which masses can arise include the heart and great vessels, the esophagus, the airway, and lymph nodes. Lymphadenopathy is by far the most common middle mediastinal mass. Focal, inflammatory lymphadenopathy is much more common than neoplastic disease, but when massive adenopathy is seen, lymphoma or leukemia should be given primary consideration, for these tumors are not uncommon in the middle mediastinum (Fig. 44.60). Mediastinal lymph node enlargement can also occur in histiocytosis X.

Hilar lymph node enlargement may accompany mediastinal adenopathy or may occur alone. Bilateral hilar adenopathy most commonly is the result of viral

Figure 44.59. Lymphangioma. Ultrasound shows the characteristic multicystic appearance of a lymphangioma.

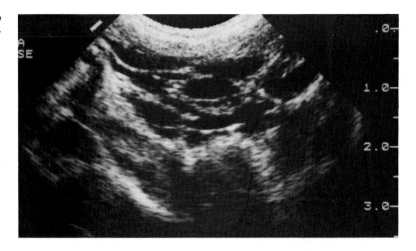

lower respiratory tract infections in children, although mycoplasmal, fungal, and tuberculous infections must also be considered (Fig. 44.61). Noninflammatory hilar lymph node enlargement occurs with lymphoma, histiocytosis X, and metastatic disease. Sarcoidosis and Wegener's granulomatosis are rare causes of adenopathy in children.

When unilateral hilar lymphadenopathy is encountered, one should strongly suspect primary tuberculosis. Lymphadenopathy is the most common radiographic finding of primary tuberculosis in children (17) and often is associated with an area of opacity within the ipsilateral lung parenchyma (the so-called Ghon complex) (Fig. 44.62). The lung opacity can be due to either atelectasis or alveolar infiltrate. Unilateral lymphadenopathy is also frequently seen with mycoplasma or fungal infections of the lung and occasionally is seen with a bacterial pneumonia. Unilateral lymphadenopathy due to a viral infection is uncommon. Neoplastic lymph node enlargement can be unilateral as well as bilateral.

Cystic masses in the middle mediastinum can be associated with either the airway or the esophagus. Bronchogenic cysts usually have a smooth, round appearance and commonly occur around the carina (Fig. 44.63) (18). Esophageal duplication cysts are developmental abnormalities due to abnormal division of the neurenteric complex during fetal development. Those that are not connected to the spinal canal tend to lie in the middle mediastinum. These cysts usually do not communicate with the esophagus but can be shown to displace and compress the esophagus on contrast studies. In some cases, gastric mucosa will be present in the cyst lining, and this can lead to ulceration and hemorrhage.

Enlargement of vascular structures that reside in the middle mediastinum can also give the appearance of a mass. Aortic aneurysms are rare in childhood, except for those associated with trauma or with connective tissue disorders such as the Marfan or Ehler-Danlos syndromes. In the newborn infant, a small bump can be seen along the upper descending aorta, which is caused by a dilated infundibulum of the ductus arteriosus after closure (Fig. 44.64). Normally this "ductus bump" disappears in the first weeks of life; enlargement or persistence of this bump in later infancy suggests the presence of an aneurysm of the ductus arteriosus. Enlargement of the aorta and the main pulmonary artery will be addressed later in this chapter.

A mass-like appearance along the upper left cardiac border can be caused by herniation of the left atrial appendage through a partial pericardial defect or a coronary artery aneurysm. Coronary artery aneurysms are most likely to occur in children with periarteritis nodosa or the mucocutaneous lymph node syndrome. Enlargement of the azygos vein may present as a mass in the right paratracheal region. In children, this most often occurs when increased volumes of blood are returning to the heart through the azygos vein, such as with total anomalous pulmonary venous return to the azygos vein or absence of the inferior vena cava with azygos continuation.

Posterior mediastinal masses are largely of neurogenic origin. Close inspection of the vertebra and posterior ribs may reveal pedicular erosion, interpedicular or rib space widening, and bone erosions, all of which are clues to the presence of a mass extending into the spinal canal. In such cases, the mass is most often a neoplasm of the neuroblastoma-ganglioneuroma group (Fig. 44.65). These tumors are probably congenital in origin and arise in paraspinal sympathetic nerve tissue. Primary thoracic neuroblastoma is not uncommon and has a more favorable prognosis than neuroblastoma, which originates in the abdomen. Intrathoracic neuroblastoma can also be seen with secondary spread of an abdominal neuroblastoma. Ganglioneuroma is the benign counterpart of neuroblastoma and the two lesions cannot be reliably distinguished from one another radiographically. Cal-

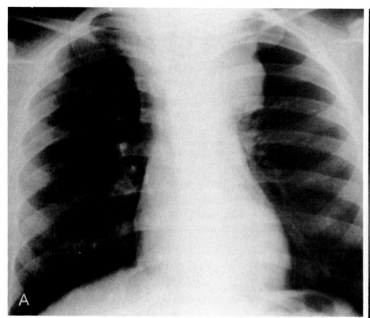

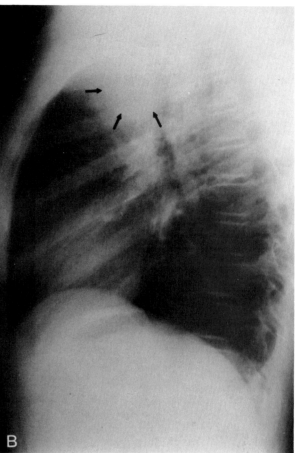

Figure 44.60.   Histocytic Lymphoma. A. The large left para-tracheal mass represents lymphadenopathy due to lymphoma. **B.** Lateral view shows the middle mediastinal location of this mass (*arrows*).

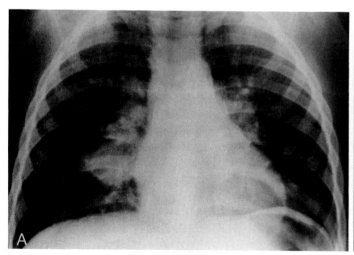

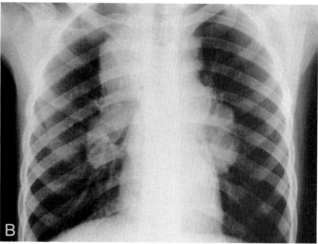

Figure 44.61.   Bilateral Hilar Adenopathy. A. Note the prominent nodular, hilar opacities representing lymph nodes in this patient with primary tuberculosis. **B.** The bilateral hilar and paratracheal masses represent lymphadenopathy due to Hodgkin's lymphoma.

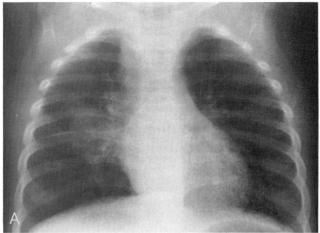

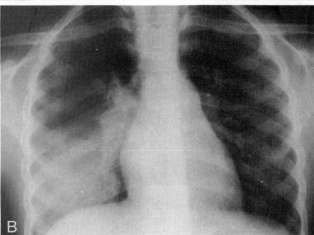

Figure 44.62.   Unilateral Hilar Adenopathy. A. Right hilar adenopathy and adjacent parenchymal opacity comprise the typical Ghon complex of primary tuberculosis. **B.** Note the right hilar adenopathy associated with a bacterial pneumonia.

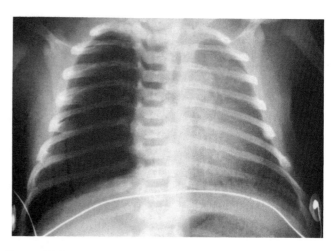

Figure 44.64.   Ductus Bump. The prominent "bump" that is seen along the upper descending aorta represents the dilated infundibulum of the ductus arteriosus in this newborn infant.

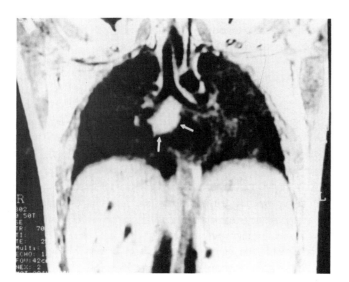

Figure 44.63.   Bronchogenic Cyst. Coronal MR demonstrates a high intensity, fluid-filled cyst in a characteristic subcarinal location (*arrows*).

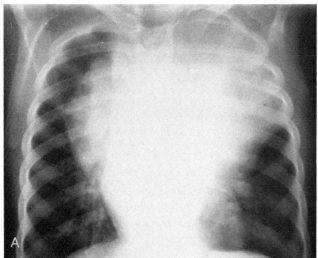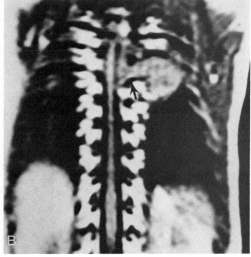

Figure 44.65.   Thoracic Neuroblastoma. A. Note the large mediastinal mass. Thinning of the posterior and medial portion of the left second rib and widening of the T2-3 rib space localizes this mass in the posterior mediastinum and suggests possible intraspinal exten- sion. **B.** Coronal MR of a different patient with a left posterior mediastinal mass demonstrating extension of the tumor into the spinal canal (*arrow*).

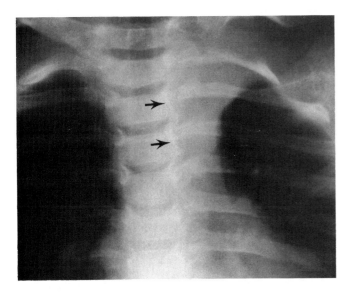

Figure 44.66.   Neurofibromatosis. Note the soft-tissue mass in the superior and posterior mediastinum on the left that deforms the left pedicles of several of the upper thoracic vertebrae (*arrows*).

cifications may be seen in both lesions, and it is believed that some neuroblastomas can mature to ganglioneuromas.

Neurofibromas also occur in the posterior mediastinum and often cause widening of adjacent intervertebral foramina (Fig. 44.66). These tumors can be solitary but more often occur with the neurofibromatosis syndrome. Anterior thoracic meningoceles can create a similar radiographic appearance and also often occur in patients with neurofibromatosis. Neurenteric cysts are a form of enteric duplication cysts that communicate with the spinal canal. The cysts lie in the posterior mediastinum and are almost always associ- ated with vertebral anomalies. Spinal cord anomalies may also be present, and MR is the procedure of choice for evaluating this condition. A posterior mediastinal inflammatory mass occasionally accompanies inflammatory conditions of the spine. Rare causes of a posterior mediastinal mass include lymphangioma, teratoma, lymphoma, and sarcoma. Diaphragmatic hernias through the foramen of Bochdalek and pulmonary sequestration often present as masses in the inferior portion of the posterior mediastinum adjacent to the diaphragm.

CONGENITAL HEART DISEASE

A wide variety of imaging modalities are now available for diagnosing and evaluating congenital heart disease in children. Classically, most of these conditions required angiocardiography; however, many congenital cardiac abnormalities can now be diagnosed noninvasively by echocardiography and MR (19). Perhaps the radiologist's most important role is the identification and classification of cardiovascular abnormalities by plain radiography. Although the specific diagnosis often will not be apparent on the plain films, a systematic approach to plain film interpretation will allow one to place the abnormality in one of several groups of lesions. This section will provide a framework for the development of an organized scheme for radiographic evaluation of congenital heart disease.

A recommended scheme of interpretation begins with the assessment of the pulmonary vascularity (20). Vascular patterns can be placed in one of three broad groups: increased (congested), decreased, and normal (Table 44.10). If the vascularity is determined

Table 44.10.   Pulmonary Vascular Patterns

Increased vascularity (active) without cyanosis
    ASD
    VSD
    Patent ductus arteriosus
    Aortic-pulmonary window
    Ruptered aneurysm of sinus of Valsalva
    Coronary artery fistula
    Partial anomalous pulmonary venous return
Increased vascularity (active) with cyanosis
    Total anomalous pulmonary venous return (types I, II)
    Persistent truncus arteriosus
    Complete endocardial cushion defect
    Transposition of the great vessels complex
    Single ventricle (without pulmonary stenosis)
Increased vascularity (passive)
    Total anomalous pulmonary venous return (type III)
    Pulmonary vein atresia
    Hypoplastic left heart syndrome (in failure)
Decrease vascularity
    Tetralogy of Fallot
    Pseudotruncus arteriosus
    Hypoplastic right heart syndrome (right-to-left shunt)
        Tricuspid atresia
        Pulmonary atresia
        Tricuspid stenosis
        Hypoplastic right ventricle
    Ebstein's anomaly
    Uhl's anomaly
    Trilogy of Fallot
    Single ventricle or transposition of great vessels with pulmonary
        stenosis or atresia
    Tricuspid or pulmonary insufficiency with right-to-left shunt
Normal vascularity
    Left heart lesions
        Coarctation of the aorta
        Interrupted aortic arch
        Hypoplastic left heart syndrome (before failure develops)
        Mitral stenosis and insufficiency
        Aortic stenosis and insufficiency
        Cor triatriatum
    Right heart lesions (without right-to-left shunt)
        Pulmonary stenosis or insufficiency
        Tricuspid insufficiency
    Endomyocardial abnormalities
        Endocardial fibroelastosis
        Cardiomyopathy
        Aberrant left coronary artery

to be increased, one should attempt to further distinguish congestion that is active from that which is passive.

Active congestion occurs whenever the amount of blood flowing through the pulmonary vasculature has increased. This occurs in those conditions that result in left-to-right shunting and in those in which there is preferential blood flow into the lower pressure pulmonary circulation. Left-to-right shunts do not become radiographically apparent until the output of the right ventricle is approximately two and a half times greater than that of the left ventricle. At this point, the pulmonary vessels become increased in diameter and are visible farther than usual into the periphery of the lungs (Fig. 44.67**A**). The vessels may appear tortuous but the margins remain relatively distinct. In borderline cases, the diameter of the right descending pulmonary artery can be helpful; if the measurement of this artery is less than that of the trachea, a left-to-right shunt is unlikely.

Passive congestion of the pulmonary vasculature reflects elevation of the pulmonary venous pressure, which can result from obstruction or dysfunction of the left side of the heart. As venous pressure increases and the veins dilate, edema fluid leaks into the perivascular interstitial tissues, causing the margins of the vessels to become less distinct on the chest radiograph (Fig. 44.67**B**). As pulmonary venous hypertension increases, alveolar pulmonary edema and pleural effusions can develop. In patients with large left-to-right shunts and associated left heart failure, a mixed pattern of passive and active congestion occurs.

Decreased pulmonary vascularity indicates diminished blood flow to the lungs, most often due to obstruction of the right ventricular pulmonary outflow tract and associated right-to-left shunts. Oligemia causes the lungs to appear more radiolucent than usual and the vessels are uniformly thin and wispy (Fig. 44.67**C**). A diminished caliber of the peripheral two-thirds of the pulmonary arteries combined with prominence of the central pulmonary arteries is characteristic of pulmonary arterial hypertension due to increased pulmonary vascular resistance.

Normal pulmonary vascularity is usually seen in patients with uncomplicated valvular disease, coarctation of the aorta, and mild forms of cardiomyopathy. As these conditions become more severe, congestive heart failure eventually can develop, but before that time, the vessels usually retain a normal contour and diameter.

Asymmetry of the blood flow to the lungs occasionally occurs, and is most commonly seen in tetralogy of Fallot, persistent truncus arteriosus, and valvular pulmonic stenosis. In tetralogy of Fallot, it is the blood flow to the left lung that tends to be diminished when compared with the right. Blood flow to either lung can be decreased in persistent truncus arteriosus, and occasionally the flow to only one lobe of the lung will be decreased. In valvular pulmonic stenosis, the abnormal valve tends to direct the blood flow preferentially into the left pulmonary arterial system. Although this can cause enlargement of the main left pulmonary artery and a generalized increase of blood flow to the left lung, on a practical basis, this is seldom apparent on the radiographs of children with this condition. Alteration of the pulmonary vasculature due to aeration abnormalities of one lung (i.e., obstructive emphysema, atelectasis) has been discussed previously.

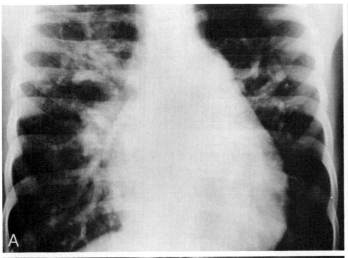

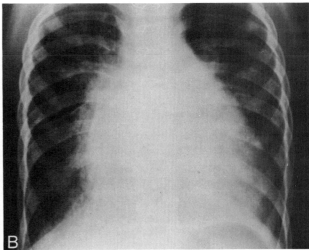

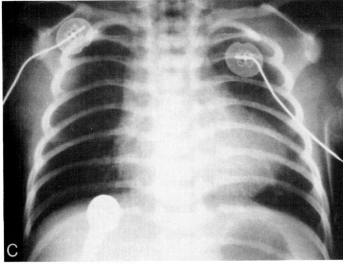

Figure 44.67. Pulmonary Vascular Patterns. A. *Active congestion*—note the large but distinct pulmonary vessels extending into the periphery of the lung due to left-to-right shunting in a patient with a large VSD. **B.** *Passive congestion*—passive vascular congestion due to mitral insufficiency results in indistinctness of the pulmonary vascular markings. **C.** *Decreased vascularity* in a patient with tetralogy of Fallot. Note the right aortic arch and the charactertistic "boot" cardiac configuration due to right ventricular hypertrophy.

Pulmonary Artery. An enlarged pulmonary artery is seen in all conditions that display generalized increased pulmonary blood flow (e.g., left-to-right shunts), in valvular pulmonic stenosis due to poststenotic dilation (Fig. 44.68), and in pulmonary valve insufficiency due to increased right ventricular output. Often in infants and children, an enlarged pulmonary artery will also be higher in position than a normal pulmonary artery and can sometimes be mistaken for a large aortic knob. A small or absent pulmonary artery shadow occurs when the main pulmonary artery is underdeveloped or in an abnormal position. Those conditions with decreased blood flow due to pulmonary outflow tract obstruction generally demonstrate a flat or concave appearance in the normal location of the pulmonary artery. A similar appearance occurs in conditions characterized by an abnormal position of the pulmonary artery, such as persistent truncus arteriosus or transposition of the great vessels.

Aorta. Evaluation of the aorta should include estimation of size, position, and contour abnormalities.

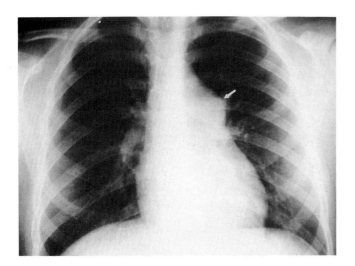

Figure 44.68. Pulmonary Artery Enlargement. Poststenotic dilation of the pulmonary artery is seen in this patient with valvular pulmonic stenosis (*arrow*).

The next step in the scheme of radiographic interpretation of congenital heart disease involves assessment of the main pulmonary artery and aorta.

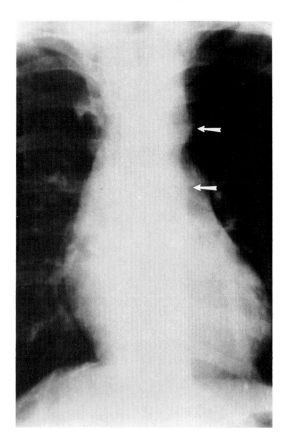

Figure 44.69. Coarctation of the Aorta. Note pre- and post-stenotic dilation of the aorta creating the characteristic figure-3 sign (arrows).

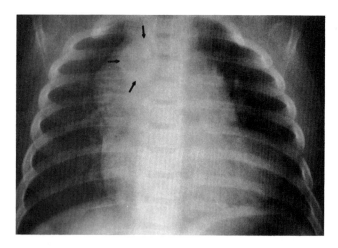

Figure 44.70. Tetralogy of Fallot. A prominent right-sided aortic arch can be seen displacing the distal trachea to the left (arrows). Right aortic arch is a relatively common finding in patients with tetralogy of Fallot.

The aorta may appear small because of hypoplasia, such as that which occurs in the hypoplastic left heart syndrome, and with certain left-to-right shunts (e.g., atrial septal defect (ASD), ventricular septal defect (VSD)). The size of the aorta is best assessed in the region of the aortic knob, but the aorta in children normally is smaller than in adults and a truly small aorta may be difficult to verify radiographically. On the other hand, a prominent aortic knob in infants and children is very often abnormal. Enlargement of the ascending aorta and the aortic knob is most often the result of poststenotic dilation due to valvular aortic stenosis or increased aortic blood flow that is seen with aortic valve insufficiency, left-to-right shunting at the great vessels level (e.g., patent ductus arteriosus, persistent truncus arteriosus), and severe tetralogy of Fallot. Generalized aortic enlargement can occur with systemic hypertension. The most common abnormality of the contour of the aorta is the notching that occurs at the site of coarctation of aorta. Dilation of the aorta proximal and distal to the coarctation results in the characteristic "figure-3" sign (Fig. 44.69)

Right-sided Aortic Arch. A right-sided aortic arch is most often an isolated anomaly; however, it can also accompany congenital heart disease. In a large percentage of cases, the congenital heart lesion will be either persistent truncus arteriosus or tetralogy of Fallot. A right aortic arch can often be seen as a bulge or fullness in the right paratracheal region, slightly above the usual level of a normal left-sided aortic arch. The trachea, which normally lies slightly to the right of the midline, will be displaced to the left by a right aortic arch (Fig. 44.70). A barium esophagram can confirm the diagnosis by demonstrating a right-sided indentation. A right-sided aortic arch may also be a clue to the presence of a vascular ring such as a double aortic arch or aberrant left subclavian artery with an encircling ligamentum arteriosum. In such cases, the barium swallow reveals opposing indentations in the barium-filled esophagus in a "reverse-S" configuration (see Fig. 44.20).

Cardiomegaly is an important indicator of cardiac disease in children and often accompanies congenital heart disease. Unfortunately, the estimation of cardiac enlargement in children is necessarily somewhat subjective and measurements such as the cardiothoracic ratio are usually not particularly helpful. Beware of the normally prominent thymus gland overlying the heart, and films taken in a poor degree of inspiration that can erroneously suggest cardiac enlargement. The configurations due to enlargement of specific cardiac chambers are the same as those seen in adults. Generalized cardiomegaly with a globular appearance suggests pericardial fluid; this finding can be easily confirmed with ultrasound (Fig. 44.71). Pericardial effusions in children most commonly accompany viral infections or rheumatic fever. Other causes include acute or chronic renal failure, collagen vascular diseases, bacterial infections, and, rarely, tuberculosis, fungal infections, and pericardial metastases. Blood in the pericardial space is usually the result

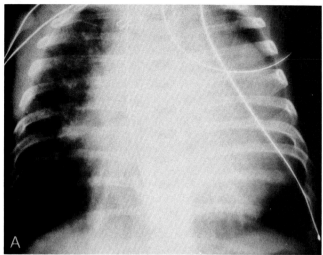

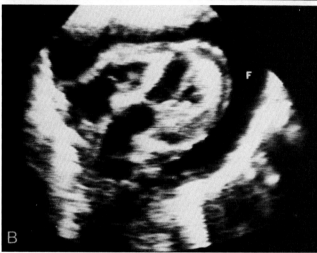

Figure 44.71. Pericardial Effusion. A. The cardiac silhouette is markedly enlarged and has a rounded, globular appearance due to a pericardial effusion that developed following open heart surgery. **B.** Ultrasound is the best method for verifying pericardial fluid (F).

of trauma. Generalized cardiac enlargement also occurs with a variety of conditions that result in increased blood volumes and elevated cardiac outputs. These conditions include acute and chronic renal diseases, inappropriate secretion of antidiuretic hormone, large arteriovenous fistulae, chronic anemias (especially sickle cell disease and thalassemia), and hyperthyroidism.

Acyanotic Heart Disease with Increased Pulmonary Vascularity (Active)

Actively increased pulmonary vascularity in the absence of cyanosis most often occurs when a defect is present that allows oxygenated blood from the left side of the heart or the aorta to be shunted back to the right side of the heart or the pulmonary circulation. Because no desaturated blood is shunted into the systemic circulation, cyanosis does not occur. The in-

creased blood volumes recirculating through the right side of the heart and the pulmonary circulation results in increased size of the pulmonary vessels and cardiac enlargement. The most common conditions in this category are VSD, ASD, and patent ductus arteriosus. Although the definitive diagnosis of these lesions is made by echocardiography or angiocardiography, radiographs sometimes provide clues to the correct diagnosis.

Ventricular septal defect is the most common congenital heart abnormality after bicuspid aortic valve. Although it can accompany many of the cyanotic forms of congenital heart disease, it also frequently occurs as an isolated anomaly. The defects are categorized according to their location within the ventricular septum. The majority of defects occur in the membranous portion of the septum at the site of fusion of the membranous and muscular portions and are thus called perimembranous defects. Defects in the muscular portion of the septum are less common and tend to be smaller and less hemodynamically significant than the perimembranous type of defect. The third type of defect is uncommon and develops high in the membranous portion of the intraventricular septum because of abnormal development of the conus portion of the truncus arteriosus. This type is most often seen with persistent truncus arteriosus or tetralogy of Fallot.

Clinically, newborns with VSD are usually asymptomatic and often a murmur will not be detected until after the newborn period. This delayed manifestation of left-to-right shunting is the result of the normal phenomenon of postnatal pulmonary vascular involution. In the fetus, the walls of the pulmonary arteries are thicker than in postnatal life, resulting in increased pulmonary vascular resistance and relative right ventricular hypertrophy. Because of the elevated pulmonary vascular pressure, blood flow through the lungs (and, hence, through the septal defect) is inhibited. This situation persists in the postnatal period. During the first days or weeks of life, the pulmonary vascular resistance diminishes, eventually allowing left-to-right shunting to occur across the septal defect. In some instances, this normal sequence of involution fails to occur. Such infants are cyanotic due to right-to-left shunting across the ductus arteriosus; this condition has been called the persistent fetal circulation syndrome. In patients with moderate-to-large VSDs, symptoms usually develop within the first 2 years of life. Small defects can close spontaneously.

The characteristic radiographic findings in VSD consist of pulmonary artery enlargement, increased pulmonary vascularity, and cardiomegaly that is predominantly left-sided (Fig. 44.72). Increased pulmonary venous return results in volume overload of the left atrium and ventricle, leading to their dilation.

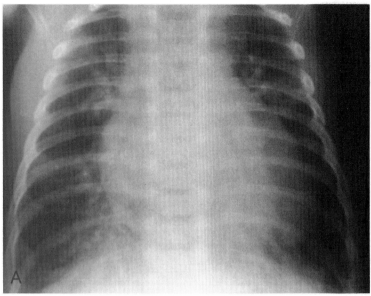

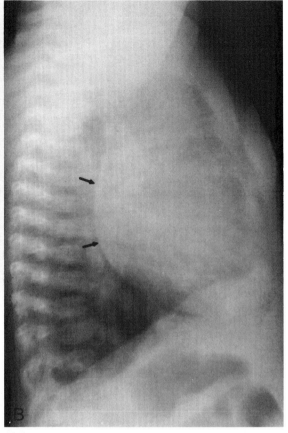

Figure 44.72. Ventricular Septal Defect. A. Cardiac enlargement that is predominantly left-sided and increased pulmonary vascularity are characteristic of VSD. **B.** Lateral view demonstrates left atrial enlargement (*arrows*).

Left ventricular dilation causes a "drooping" shape of the left cardiac border. Left atrial enlargement is best seen on the lateral or left anterior oblique view as a bulge along the upper posterior cardiac border that causes posterior displacement of the esophagus and the left mainstem bronchus. If the shunt is large, biventricular dilation enlargement occurs.

Atrial septal defect is much less common than VSD. The most common type of ASD is that which occurs centrally at the fossa ovalis, the so-called ostium secundum defect. Because the shunt with ASD is a low-pressure shunt, these children seldom develop symptoms in infancy or early childhood. If the shunt persists as the child grows older, the risk of developing pulmonary hypertension increases. As the pressure in the right side of the heart rises, the shunt becomes balanced and eventually reverses to a right-to-left shunt. This phenomenon is referred to as Eisenmenger's physiology, and can be seen with any left-to-right shunt.

Unlike VSD, the left atrium is not enlarged in patients with ASD because of rapid shunting of blood away from the left atrium into the right side of the heart. Typically, the right atrium is enlarged, causing prominence of the right cardiac border on the frontal view (Fig. 44.73). On the lateral view, right ventricular enlargement produces fullness in the retrosternal space. In both ASD and VSD, the aorta is rather small,

as the shunt is below the level of the great vessels and thus diverts blood away from the aorta.

The ostium primum type of ASD (or endocardial cushion defect) is an abnormality caused by abnormal development of the primitive endocardial cushions that normally form the interatrial and interventricular septa and atrioventricular valves. This condition commonly occurs in trisomy 21. The specific malformation and resultant hemodynamics in this condition vary widely and range from two separate atrioventricular valves with a low ASD and a VSD of variable size to the complete form that consists of a common atrioventricular ring with a five-leaflet valve. The mitral valve is deformed (cleft) and abnormally positioned and results in elongation of the left ventricular outflow tract, creating a "goose neck" appearance on angiography (Fig. 44.74).

The partial form of this abnormality behaves hemodynamically as a simple atrial left-to-right shunt with only mild degrees of mitral or tricuspid insufficiency. The clinical course of the complete form, however, is much more severe. The shunts are large and usually bidirectional because of the abnormal valve development and, therefore, the patients are cyanotic and tend to develop pulmonary hypertension and congestive heart failure early. Radiographically, these patients present with marked cardiomegaly with right

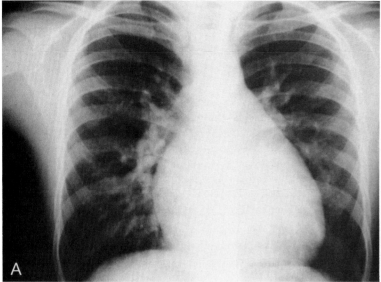

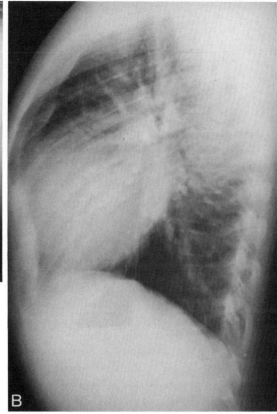

Figure 44.73. Atrial Septal Defect. A. Note the characteristic cardiomegaly, mild right atrial enlargement, and increased pulmonary vascularity in ASD. **B.** Lateral view shows a normal left atrium and fullness in the retrosternal region due to right ventricular enlargement.

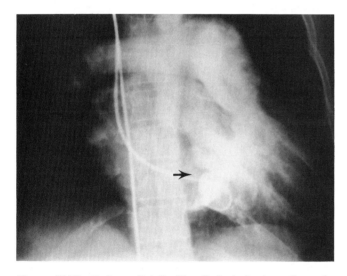

Figure 44.74. Endocardial Cushion Defect. Angiocardiography demonstrates the cleft mitral valve (*arrow*) and the elongated left ventricular outflow tract (goose-neck deformity).

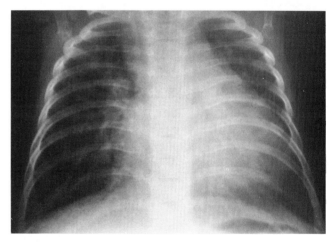

Figure 44.75. Endocardial Cushion Defect. Note the marked cardiomegaly, right atrial enlargement, and increased pulmonary vascularity, typical of this condition.

atrial and right ventricular predominance and pulmonary vascular engorgement (Fig. 44.75).

Patent Ductus Arteriosus (PDA). The ductus arteriosus is a normal structure that connects the pulmonary artery and aorta in fetal life. Normally, this structure begins to close immediately after birth, but in some infants closure is delayed. Such delayed closure and patency are common complications of hypoxia in the premature infant. In other infants, the cause of persistent patency is unknown, and usually these infants develop symptoms within the first 1 or 2 years of life. Blood is shunted from the aorta through the ductus to the pulmonary artery, resulting in increased blood volumes flowing through the left side of the heart. Consequently, the left atrium, left ventricle, and pulmonary artery become dilated and enlarged. Active pulmonary vascular engorgement occurs and increased outflow from the left ventricle also leads to enlargement of the proximal aorta, a feature that dif-

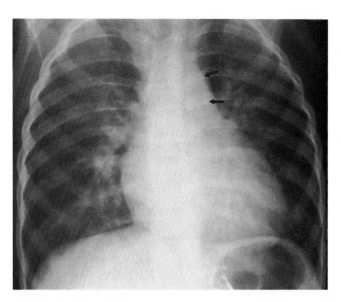

Figure 44.76. Patent Ductus Arteriosus. The heart is enlarged with left-sided prominence and increased pulmonary vascularity. Note the prominent aorta (arrows).

fers from the small aorta that is seen with ASD and VSD (Fig. 44.76). In young infants with large shunts, the cardiomegaly tends to be more generalized and often the size of the aorta is difficult to evaluate because of overlying thymus. Patent ductus arteriosus is easily demonstrable at angiography and also can easily be diagnosed by echocardiography.

Aortic pulmonary window is a rare condition that is very similar to patent ductus arteriosus, both hemodynamically and radiographically. The abnormality results from failure of complete division of the primitive truncus arteriosus, which leaves a communication between the aorta and the pulmonary artery just above the valves. Other rare conditions that result in shunting of blood from the aorta to the pulmonary artery and the right side of the heart include rupture of an aneurysm of the sinus of Valsalva and fistulas between the coronary arteries and the coronary sinus, pulmonary artery, or right cardiac chambers.

Cyanotic Heart Disease with Increased Pulmonary Vascularity (Active)

This category consists of a group of complex heart abnormalities whose common feature is the admixture of oxygenated and deoxygenated blood that is then circulated systemically, resulting in cyanosis. The most common diseases in this group are persistent truncus arteriosus, total anomalous pulmonary venous return (types I and II), the complete endocardial cushion defect complex, single ventricle (without pulmonary stenosis), and the transposition of the great vessels complexes.

Transposition anomalies of the great vessels include a complex group of lesions that consist of abnor-

mal anterior-to-posterior positioning of the aorta and pulmonary artery and variable abnormalities of the relationship between the ventricles and the atria and their connections to the great vessels. Complete transposition of the great vessels is the most common form of cyanotic congenital heart disease with increased pulmonary blood flow. In this condition, the anterior-to-posterior relationship of the aorta and pulmonary artery are reversed so that the aorta arises from the heart anteriorly and the pulmonary artery is posterior. The ventricles generally lie in their normal position, and thus the transposed great vessels arise from the incorrect ventricle (ventriculoarterial discordance). This results in two separate circulations, one through the pulmonary circulation and the other systemic.

Communications must exist between these two circulations for the infant to survive, and these communications are most commonly a VSD, ASD, or PDA. Bidirectional shunting occurs through these communications, allowing adequate mixing of the blood if the shunts are large enough. If no pulmonary stenosis is present, blood tends to flow preferentially into the low-resistance pulmonary circulation. This results in increased pulmonary venous return and pronounced diastolic or volume overloading, and congestive heart failure develops in the first weeks of life. The prognosis is more favorable in those cases with associated pulmonary stenosis.

Radiographically, cardiomegaly develops in the first few days of life with an oval or egg-shaped configuration (Fig. 44.77). The superior mediastinum and base of the heart are narrow because of a combination of thymic atrophy and the abnormal positioning and alignment of the aorta and pulmonary artery. Both active and passive pulmonary vascular congestion can be seen. On lateral views of the chest, the anteriorly displaced aorta causes increased opacity in the retrosternal region. Angiocardiography establishes the diagnosis (Fig. 44.77).

In corrected transposition of the great vessels, ventricular inversion (left-to-right reversal) accompanies the transposed positions of the aorta and pulmonary artery. This causes the aorta to lie anterior and to the left, and thus the condition is often called L-transposition. Ordinary transposition is referred to as D-transposition. Blood circulates normally through the heart to the pulmonary and systemic circulation (right atrium to left ventricle to pulmonary artery, and left atrium to right ventricle to aorta), even though the connections between the ventricles and aorta and pulmonary artery are switched. In these cases, atrioventricular discordance is present, which means that the anatomic right ventricle functions as a left ventricle and vice versa. Patients with the simple form of this condition tend to be asymptomatic, but in many pa-

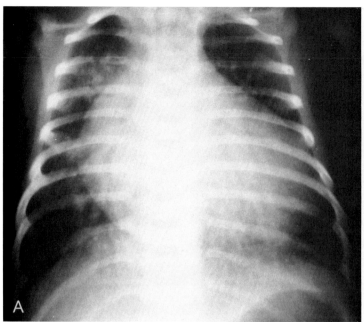

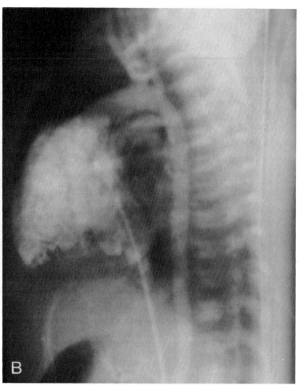

Figure 44.77. Transposition of the Great Vessels. A. The heart is enlarged with a typical "egg" shape. Note the narrow superior mediastinum and increased pulmonary vascularity. **B.** Angiocardiography shows the aorta arising anteriorly from the right ventricle.

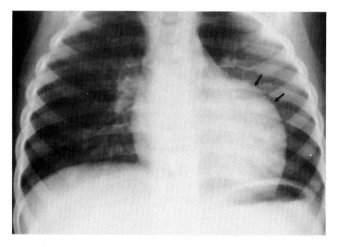

Figure 44.78. Congenitally Corrected Transposition. The transposed aorta arising from the inverted right ventricle on the left causes characteristic prominence along the upper left cardiac border (arrows).

tients other cardiac defects coexist (e.g., VSD, pulmonary stenosis, conduction defects). The diagnosis is suggested radiographically by a characteristic prominence along the upper left cardiac border that is due to the right ventricular outflow tract and the left-sided aorta (Fig. 44.78).

Double-outlet right ventricle (DORV) can, for convenience sake, be considered with transposition. It is also characterized by an aorta that is anterior and arises from the right ventricle. The pulmonary artery, however, also empties the right ventricle, either

originating entirely from the right ventricle (type I DORV) or overriding a high VSD and draining both the left and right ventricles (type II DORV or the Taussig-Bing anomaly). The hemodynamics of this condition are similar to those of the complete form of transposition of the great vessels. Radiographic findings are also similar. However, because the aorta and pulmonary artery tend to be oriented in a more side-to-side fashion, the cardiac waist is usually of normal or even increased width, unlike the narrow waist seen in transposition of the great vessels (TGV).

Total anomalous pulmonary venous return is a condition in which the pulmonary veins, instead of emptying normally into the left atrium, return blood to the right side of the heart via the right atrium, coronary sinus, or a systemic vein. This anomaly can occur in conjunction with a variety of other major cardiac defects, but this discussion will refer only to the isolated form. The best-known classification of the types of total anomalous pulmonary venous return was described by Darling et al. as types I–IV. In all types, the pulmonary veins converge into a single common vein before emptying into the anomalous site. In type I total anomalous pulmonary venous return, the most common form, the abnormal vein empties into a large supracardiac vein (the persistent left superior vena cava or vertical vein, the left brachiocephalic vein, the right superior vena cava or the azygos vein). In the type II anomaly, the common vein drains into the coronary sinus or directly into the right atrium. In the type III anomaly, the common

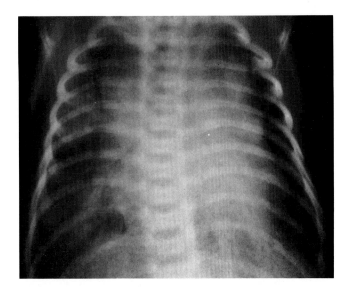

Figure 44.79. Total Anomalous Pulmonary Venous Return—Type I. The characteristic snowman or figure-8 configuration results from cardiomegaly combined with prominence of the superior mediastinum due to the anomalous pulmonary vein.

vein travels through the esophageal hiatus to empty into the portal vein or, less commonly, an abdominal systemic vein.

Total anomalous pulmonary venous return types I and II overload the right side of the heart, causing dilation of the right atrium, right ventricle, and pulmonary artery and engorgement of the pulmonary vessels. Some communication with the left side of the heart is mandatory for survival and this usually occurs in the form of an ASD or patent foramen ovale. The classic radiographic configuration of the type I anomaly is the "snowman" heart, so named because of prominence of the superior mediastinum due to a large, inverted U-shaped vessel that empties into the superior vena cava (Fig. 44.79). This configuration is only present when the abnormal common pulmonary vein enters the persistent left superior vena cava or vertical vein. In the other forms of the type I anomaly and in the type II anomaly, the cardiac configuration is less specific. Type II findings resemble those of the transposition complex of lesions, and in the type I anomaly, if the abnormal vein empties into the azygos vein, it will be dilated.

The type III form of total anomalous venous return is hemodynamically and radiographically distinct from the other forms of this disease. Although blood is once again directed incorrectly to the right side of the heart, the length and small caliber of the common vein increases the resistance to flow and creates pulmonary venous obstruction. Radiographically, the pulmonary vessels are thin with hazy margins caused by associated pulmonary interstitial edema and passive vascular engorgement (Fig. 44.80). The heart does not enlarge. The differential diagnosis

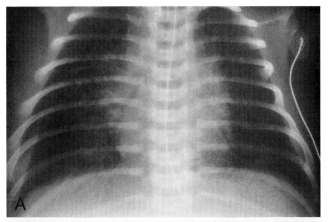

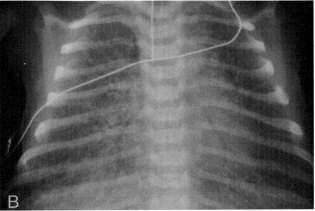

Figure 44.80. Total Anomalous Pulmonary Venous Return—Type III. A. Note that the heart is normal in size with thin and somewhat indistinct pulmonary vessels due to passive vascular congestion. A prominent interstitial pattern in the lungs represents pulmonary edema, and bilateral pleural effusions are also present. **B.** Another patient with more severe pulmonary edema. Once again note the normal heart size.

includes other congenital heart diseases that cause increased pulmonary venous pressures early in infancy, predominantly the hypoplastic left heart syndrome and pulmonary vein atresia.

Persistent truncus arteriosus is an anomaly that occurs when the primitive truncus arteriosus fails to divide normally into the aorta and pulmonary arteries. The result is that both vessels are drained by a single vessel that overrides a high VSD. The best-known classification of the variations of this anomaly is probably that of Collett-Edwards, which is based on the site of origin of the pulmonary artery. This has more recently been modified to exclude the type IV anomaly in which the blood flow to the pulmonary arteries is derived from systemic collaterals (Fig. 44.81). The degree of cyanosis is variable in these patients and the symptoms depend largely on the amount of pulmonary blood flow. Most often the chest radiograph shows cardiomegaly and active pulmonary vascular congestion. In most forms of this condition, concavity is seen at the usual site of the main pulmo-

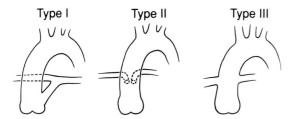

Type I   Type II   Type III

Figure 44.81. Persistent Truncus Arteriosus. These diagrams illustrate the basic forms of the original Collett-Edwards classification of persistent truncus arteriosus.

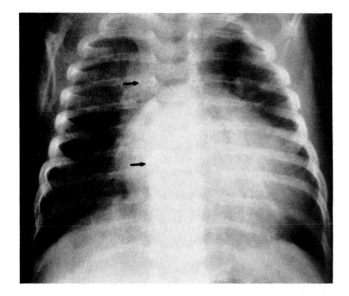

Figure 44.82. Persistent Truncus Arteriosus. Note the cardiomegaly and increased pulmonary vascularity associated with absence of a normal pulmonary artery shadow. Combined with a right-sided aorta (*arrows*), these findings strongly suggest the diagnosis.

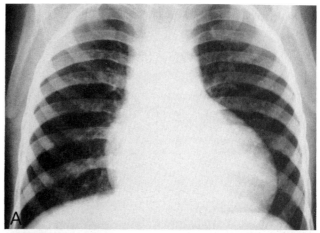

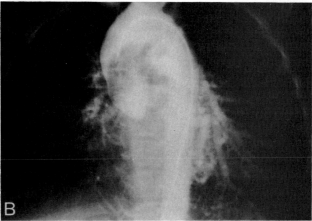

Figure 44.83. Pulmonary Atresia with VSD and Systemic Collaterals (Pseudotruncus Arteriosus). A. Radiograph shows cardiomegaly and absence of a normal pulmonary artery shadow. **B.** With angiocardiography, the tortuous primitive collaterals that supply the lungs can be seen.

nary artery. The presence of a concave pulmonary artery in a patient with active pulmonary vascular congestion strongly suggests this diagnosis, particularly if a right aortic arch is present, which occurs in approximately 30% of the cases (Fig. 44.82). The aorta (truncus) is often dilated with a high arch and an elevated left pulmonary artery.

Pseudotruncus Arteriosus. The form of persistent truncus arteriosus that was classified by Collett and Edwards as type IV is now generally considered to be a distinct anomaly rather than a variation of truncus arteriosus. In this anomaly, the blood supply to the lungs occurs through primitive collaterals originating from the descending aorta. Therefore, this condition is now often referred to as pulmonary atresia with VSD and systemic collaterals, or a form of pseudotruncus arteriosus. The radiographic findings are similar to those in true persistent truncus arteriosus (Fig. 44.83). Angiocardiography provides the diagnosis and also helps to determine whether or not the pulmonary arteries converge into a common vessel. This is significant in that those patients with confluent pulmonary arter-

ies are more likely to be surgically correctable. Patients with tetralogy of Fallot in which the pulmonary artery is severely stenotic or atretic are hemodynamically similar; however, blood is supplied to the pulmonary circulation by a patent ductus arteriosus rather than systemic collateral vessels (Fig. 44.84). These patients also often were referred to in the past as those with pseudotruncus arteriosus.

Single ventricle refers to a group of anomalies in which one ventricle is rudimentary, leaving the other large ventricle as the only functional ventricle. An underdeveloped right ventricle is most common. The connections between the atrioventricular valves, the aorta, and the pulmonary artery to the ventricles are variable. Transposition of the great vessels often accompanies single ventricle, but pulmonary valve stenosis and pulmonary artery atresia also are common and are more significant, associated lesions. If no pulmonary stenosis is present, mixing of saturated and unsaturated blood occurs in the single chamber, and the radiographs show cardiomegaly and pulmonary vascular en-

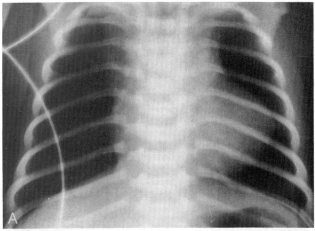

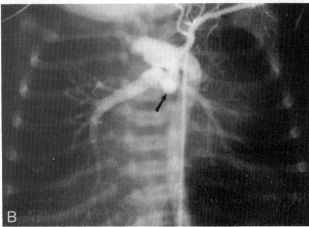

Figure 44.84.   Severe Tetralogy of Fallot with Pulmonary Atresia.
A. The heart is enlarged and the pulmonary vascularity is diminished.
B. Aortogram identifies the patent ductus arteriosus (*arrow*), which
supplies blood from the aorta to the pulmonary arterial system.

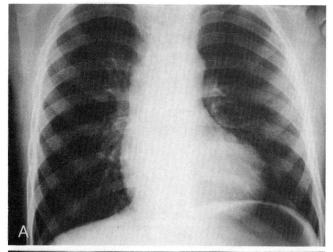

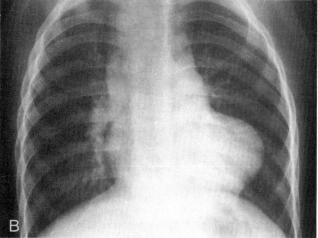

Figure 44.85.   Tetralogy of Fallot. A. Note the upwardly displaced
cardiac apex due to right ventricular hypertrophy and concave pulmonary artery shadow. **B.** Another patient with a characteristic boot-
shaped heart and right-sided aortic arch.

gorgement. When pulmonary stenosis is present, blood
flow to the lungs is diminished and cyanosis is more
severe. Echocardiography is usually diagnostic; however, sometimes angiocardiography or MR is needed for
complete demonstration of the anatomy.

Decreased Pulmonary Vascularity

A decreased pulmonary vascular pattern usually indicates a condition in which the flow through the
right side of the heart is obstructed. This obstruction
can occur anywhere from the tricuspid valve to the
pulmonary arteries. Often an intracardiac right-to-left
shunt is also present, which varies with the severity of
right ventricular outflow obstruction.

Tetralogy of Fallot is the most common cardiac
anomaly to cause a pattern of diminished pulmonary
vascularity and is the most common cause of cyanotic
congenital heart disease. The classic components of
this anomaly are (*a*) a high VSD, (*b*) pulmonary stenosis (usually infundibular, with or without valvular stenosis), (*c*) right ventricular hypertrophy, and (*d*) an
aorta that overrides the VSD. A right aortic arch occurs
in approximately 25% of cases and pulmonary artery
coarctations, hypoplasia, or absence are common.

The degree of pulmonary stenosis is the most critical component of this anomaly. Severe stenosis leads
to marked right-to-left shunting and aortic enlargement, causing greater overriding. Greater right-to-left
shunting results in a more severe cyanosis. Those patients with only mild pulmonary stenosis are usually
acyanotic and virtually asymptomatic (i.e., the so-
called "pink" or "balanced" tetralogy of Fallot).

Patients with moderate-to-severe forms of this
anomaly have a fairly characteristic radiographic appearance. The pulmonary vascularity is decreased
with a shallow or concave pulmonary artery shadow.
Right ventricular hypertrophy does not generally
cause overall enlargement of the cardiac silhouette;
however, often the cardiac apex will be displaced laterally and superiorly, creating the classic "boot-shaped"
heart (Fig. 44.85). Unequal pulmonary blood flow due

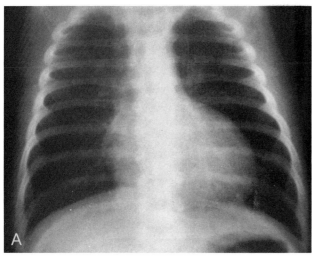 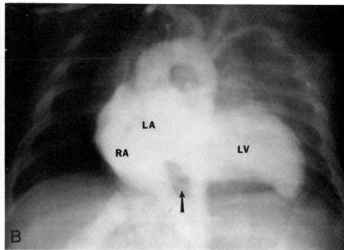

Figure 44.86. Tricuspid Atresia. A. In this patient, typical findings of left ventricular and right atrial enlargement and a concave pulmonary artery segment are seen. Note the decreased pulmonary vascularity. **B.** Angiocardiography shows contrast in the right atrium (*RA*), left atrium (*LA*), and enlarged left ventricle (*LV*). A bare area is seen due to lack of filling of a normal right ventricle (*arrow*).

to pulmonary artery hypoplasia or atresia (most commonly on the left) is not an uncommon finding.

A right-sided aortic arch occurs in approximately 25% of cases of tetralogy of Fallot and can be a useful discriminator from other conditions producing decreased pulmonary vascularity. Right aortic arch is uncommon in other conditions with right ventricular outflow obstruction except for persistent truncus arteriosus with generally decreased pulmonary blood flow. Therefore, the combination of a right aortic arch and decreased pulmonary vascularity is highly suggestive of tetralogy of Fallot, followed by persistent truncus arteriosus.

Hypoplastic Right Heart. The hypoplastic right heart syndrome consists primarily of tricuspid atresia and pulmonary atresia. Rarely, isolated hypoplasia of the right ventricle occurs. The common features of all of these conditions include a small right ventricle and right-to-left shunting through an ASD, resulting in cyanosis. In tricuspid atresia, the right atrioventricular valve is absent. In order for blood to reach the left side of the heart, it must pass from the right atrium to the left atrium through an ASD. A VSD also is often present, which allows some blood to pass into the hypoplastic right ventricle, but this usually is hemodynamically insignificant. A PDA can also be present.

In most cases of tricuspid atresia, nonspecific cardiomegaly and diminished pulmonary vascularity are seen radiographically. The pulmonary artery shadow is flat or concave, and right atrial enlargement varies, depending on the size of the ASD (i.e., more right atrial enlargement accompanies a small ASD) (Fig. 44.86). Less commonly, tricuspid atresia is accompanied by transposition of the great vessels. When this occurs, the pulmonary artery drains the left ventricle and, if no pulmonary stenosis is present, the pulmonary vascularity is engorged.

Pulmonary atresia, when accompanied by an intact ventricular septum, is also considered a part of the hypoplastic right heart syndrome. In most cases, the pulmonary valve is atretic and the right ventricle and tricuspid valve are hypoplastic. Less commonly, the right ventricle is near normal in size and the tricuspid valve more normal. In such cases, blood that enters the right ventricle has no recourse but to be regurgitated back into the right atrium, resulting in marked right atrial enlargement (Fig. 44.87). In either case, survival requires that a patent ductus arteriosus be present to shunt blood into the pulmonary circulation. Prostaglandin E_1 is now used to help maintain ductal patency until surgery can be performed.

In patients with pulmonary atresia accompanied by a VSD, the right ventricle is not hypoplastic. This situation occurs both in severe tetralogy of Fallot (pulmonary atresia with PDA, VSD, and an overriding aorta) and pulmonary atresia with VSD and systemic collaterals (the old type IV truncus arteriosus of Collete and Edwards). The most significant difference between these two conditions is the derivation of pulmonary blood flow. In severe tetralogy of Fallot, blood reaches the lungs through a long, tortuous, "wandering" patent ductus arteriosus. The other form of pulmonary atresia with VSD relies on primitive systemic collaterals that transport blood from the aorta to the pulmonary artery branches. The radiographic appearance of these conditions has been discussed in previous sections.

Right ventricular hypoplasia as an isolated abnormality is rare. When this occurs, the radiographic findings are similar to those seen in the other conditions included under the hypoplastic right heart syndrome.

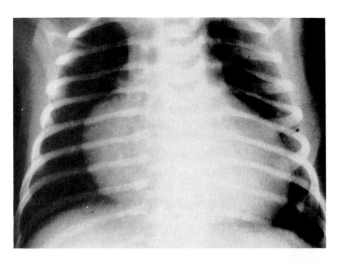

Figure 44.87.   Pulmonary Atresia with Intact Ventricular Septum. In this patient, a nearly normal-sized right ventricle is present. Because of regurgitation of blood flowing into the right ventricle, marked right atrial enlargement occurred.

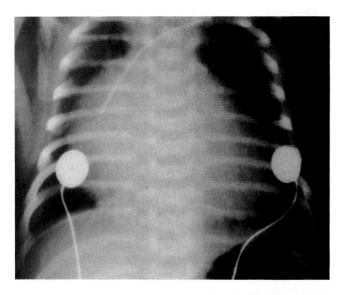

Figure 44.88.   Ebsteins Anomaly. Note the severe cardiomegaly with marked right atrial enlargement. The pulmonary vascularity typically is decreased.

Ebstein's anomaly and Uhl's anomaly are other conditions characterized by abnormalities of the right ventricle. *Ebstein's anomaly* consists of a malformed, enlarged tricuspid valve that is displaced downward, resulting in atrialization of a large portion of the right ventricle. The true right ventricle is very small, and the atrialized portion has abnormal musculature, contracts ineffectively, and results in functional obstruction to right atrial emptying. Atrial right-to-left shunting occurs and results in cyanosis in the more severely affected patients. Clinical symptoms and radiographic findings vary, depending on the degree of downward displacement of the tricuspid valve. The usual radiographic findings consist of cardiomegaly that is mainly right-sided, decreased pulmonary vascularity, and a

flattened pulmonary artery shadow (Fig. 44.88). Occasionally, the small displaced right ventricle is seen as a bulge along the upper left cardiac border, causing a squared cardiac appearance.

Uhl's anomaly is a rare anomaly consisting of focal or complete absence of the right ventricular myocardium. The very thin, poorly contractile right ventricle functionally impairs the flow of blood through the right side of the heart. The clinical and radiographic findings are similar to those of Epstein's anomaly.

Normal Pulmonary Vascularity

Congenital cardiac anomalies that are typically characterized by normal pulmonary vascularity consist predominantly of abnormalities of the cardiac valves and the great vessels. The majority of these anomalies cause left-sided obstruction. When a concomitant left-to-right shunt is present, cardiac failure develops early and, of course, the pulmonary vascularity is no longer normal. In the absence of a left-to-right shunt, such lesions can be present for many years without causing left ventricular failure.

Congenital cardiac valve stenosis most commonly affects the aortic or pulmonary valves. Congenital mitral or tricuspid stenosis is rare. The radiographic findings in these conditions in children are similar to those seen in adults, and consist mainly of hypertrophy of the ventricle that ejects blood through the stenotic valve and poststenotic dilation of the aorta or pulmonary artery, respectively (Fig. 44.89). In general, ventricular hypertrophy does little to change the size of the cardiac silhouette but, with time, can alter the shape of the heart. Left ventricular hypertrophy causes a more rounded appearance of the left cardiac border, and right ventricular hypertrophy produces fullness in the retrosternal region on the lateral view and lateral displacement of the cardiac apex on the posteroanterior view. In valvular pulmonic stenosis, poststenotic dilation of the pulmonary artery is often accompanied by prominence of the left pulmonary artery and increased pulmonary blood flow to the left lung. This phenomenon most likely results from preferential flow through the stenotic valve into the left pulmonary artery. However, it is less commonly observed on the x-rays of children than adults, for the findings take time to develop.

Aortic and pulmonary stenosis may also occur above or below the valve. Subvalvular is more common than supravalvular aortic stenosis, and the subvalvular narrowing can be due either to a discrete diaphragm or disproportionate hypertrophy of the intraventricular septum in the subaortic region. Supravalvular aortic stenosis is most often associated with Williams syndrome (idiopathic hypercalcemia of infancy) (Fig. 44.90) The features of this syndrome include supravalvular aortic stenosis and

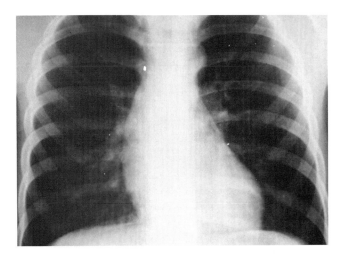

Figure 44.89. Aortic Valve Stenosis. The ascending aorta and aortic arch are prominent in this 5-year-old child with congenial aortic stenosis.

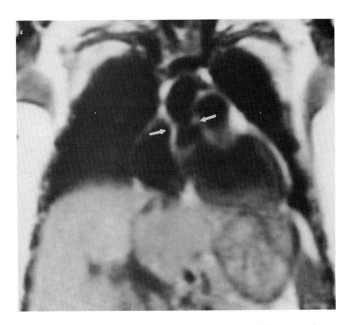

Figure 44.90. Supravalvular Aortic Stenosis (Williams Syndrome). Coronal MR demonstrates the short-segment narrowing of the aorta just above the sinus of Valsalva (*arrows*).

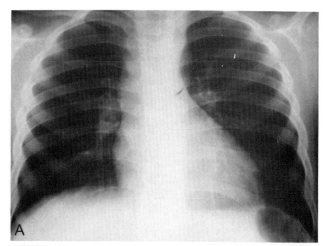

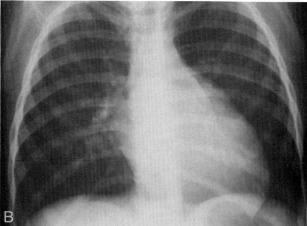

Figure 44.91. Congenital Valvular Insufficiency. A. Note the dilation of the left ventricle and the ascending aorta, which are characteristic of aortic valve insufficiency. **B.** Note the left atrial and left ventricular dilation in a patient with congenital mitral insufficiency.

other systemic and pulmonary vascular stenoses, facial dysmorphism, mental and growth retardation, and hypercalcemia that is possibly due to abnormal regulation of vitamin D metabolism. Subvalvular (infundibular) pulmonary stenosis is the form of stenosis most often seen in tetralogy of Fallot. Supravalvular pulmonary stenosis usually consists of multiple areas of narrowing in the peripheral pulmonary artery. Unlike the valvular forms of aortic and pulmonary stenosis, the subvalvular and supravalvular forms are usually not associated with poststenotic great vessel dilation.

Valvular Insufficiency. Isolated congenital insufficiency of any of the cardiac valves is a very rare occurrence; however, sometimes valvular insufficiency accompanies other cardiac anomalies. In general, valvular insufficiency causes dilation of the cardiac chambers or vessels on both sides of the involved valve (Fig. 44.91). The resulting cardiac configurations are the same as those seen in adults with valvular insufficiency.

Coarctation of the aorta occurs in two distinct forms: the juxtaductal (adult) type, which lies at or just distal to the level of the ductus arteriosus, and the rarer preductal (infantile) form, which generally is a long-segment narrowing. Coarctation of the aorta often is associated with other cardiac anomalies, most commonly bicuspid aortic valve, patent ductus arteriosus, or VSD. Patients with the preductal form of coarctation undergo a more severe clinical course, frequently developing congestive heart failure during the first month of life. Patients with the juxtaductal form usually remain asymptomatic until later in childhood, except in those cases with an associated left-to-right shunt. Older children usually present with hyperten-

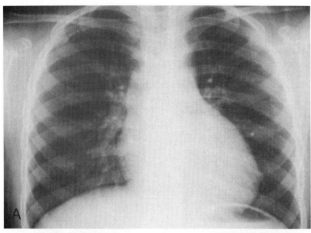

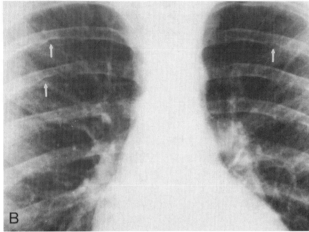

Figure 44.92. Coarctation of the Aorta. A. Note the typical rounded prominence of the left cardiac border due to left ventricular hypertrophy. The figure-3 sign is difficult to see in this patient. **B.** Note the small notches along the inferior edges of some of the upper ribs bilaterally (*arrows*).

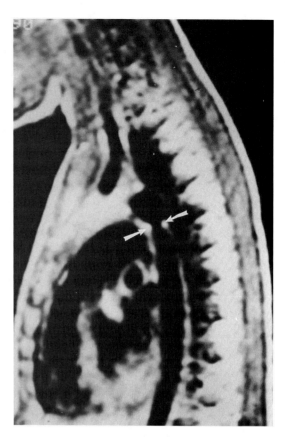

Figure 44.93. Coarctation of the Aorta. A slightly oblique sagittal MR image clearly shows the area of coarctation (*arrows*).

sion, discrepancies between the blood pressure in the upper and lower extremities, or a heart murmur.

In juxtaductal coarctation of the aorta, the aortic narrowing leads to pressure overloading and hypertrophy of the left ventricle. The heart usually is normal in size; however, eventually some rounding and prominence of the left cardiac border can develop. Pre- and poststenotic dilation of the aorta commonly occurs and is responsible for the so-called figure-3 sign (Fig. 44.92**A**). In some cases, the poststenotic dilation can extend along the entire thoracic portion of the descending aorta. Progressive collateral circulation develops, usually involving the intercostal arteries. It is the dilation of these arteries that eventually causes a notching along the inferior edge of the posterior ribs, most often from T-4 to T-8 (Fig. 44.92**B**). This finding usually is not visible until the patient is at least 7 or 8 years of age. Coarctation of the aorta is now frequently diagnosed by echocardiography and further definition of the anatomy is achieved by MR (Fig. 44.93).

Hypoplastic left heart syndrome consists of a variety of lesions characterized by some degree of underdevelopment of the left side of the heart. The anomalies range from isolated atresia of the ascending aorta or aortic or mitral valves, to aortic and mitral valve atresia combined with marked hypoplasia of the left atrium, left ventricle, and ascending aorta. In all cases, blood flow through the left heart is severely impaired and a patent ductus arteriosus is necessary to allow blood to reach the systemic circulation. Although the heart size and pulmonary vascularity can appear normal in the first few hours of life, cardiomegaly and congestive heart failure usually develop within the first 2 days. At this point, the pulmonary vasculature becomes passively congested and often a diffusely hazy or reticular pattern develops in the lungs (Fig. 44.94). This is due to interstitial pulmonary edema and resembles that which is seen in other causes of severe pulmonary venous obstruction such as pulmonary vein atresia and total anomalous pulmonary venous return type III. The diagnosis can usually be accomplished by echocardiography.

Cor triatriatum is a rare anomaly that also presents in early infancy with pulmonary venous obstruction. In this anomaly, the pulmonary veins empty into a common vein, which is abnormally incorporated into the left atrium. A partial membrane at this site cre-

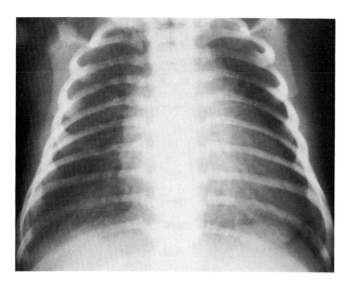

Figure 44.94. Hypoplastic Left Heart Syndome. Note the cardiomegaly and passive pulmonary vascular congestion. These findings usually develop within the first few days of life.

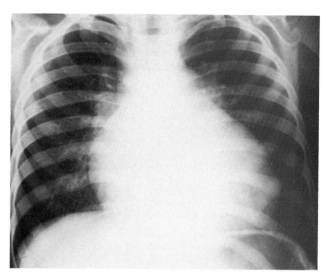

Figure 44.95. Cardiomyopathy. Note the marked cardiomegaly with left-sided predominence and early passive vascular congestion in this child with idiopathic cardiomyopathy.

ates an extra chamber along the superior and dorsal aspect of the left atrium and variably obstructs venous emptying into the left atrium. The usual radiographic findings consist primarily of cardiomegaly and passive venous congestion without evidence of left atrial enlargement.

Primary abnormalities of the myocardium can also present with a normal pulmonary vascular pattern. Cardiomyopathies may accompany a variety of conditions in children. These include bacterial or viral infections, autoimmune diseases, toxic insults, and hereditary neuromuscular diseases. Asymmetric septal hypertrophy is an unusual form of cardiomyopathy that is associated with subvalvular hypertrophic aortic stenosis. Radiographic findings of cardiomyopathy include cardiomegaly that may be generalized or predominantly left-sided (Fig. 44.95). The pulmonary vascularity remains normal until congestive heart failure develops. Endocardial fibroelastosis is a condition in which the left ventricular myocardium becomes markedly thickened and contains increased amounts of elastic and fibrous tissue. This results in marked left ventricular and left atrial enlargement. Radiographically, the heart has a rounded configuration because of the thickened myocardium (Fig. 44.96). The enlarged left ventricle often encroaches on the right ventricle and impairs right ventricular function as well. The left ventricle also can cause left lower lobe atelectasis by compression of the left lower lobe bronchus. Congestive heart failure usually occurs early in infancy in these patients.

Cardiac Malpositions

Cardiac malpositions are a confusing group of abnormalities and a detailed description of these condi-

tions will not be attempted here. Nevertheless, mastery of the terminology used to describe these conditions can help provide a basic understanding of the anatomy involved. Dextrocardia implies a heart that lies to the right of the spine because of primary malpositioning during development. Levocardia is the normal position of the heart, to the left of the spine. When faced with cardiac malpositioning, one must then determine the position of the abdominal organs (i.e., the abdominal situs). In general, the right atrium will lie on the same side as the liver and the left atrium will lie on the side opposite the liver. Situs solitus refers to the "normal" position of the viscera, that is, the liver on the right and the stomach on the left. The reversed position is referred to as visceral situs inversus.

Inversion refers to positioning of anatomic structures, usually from right-to-left and vice versa, and thus a dextroposed heart can be either inverted or noninverted (i.e., the atria and ventricles are inverted or noninverted). The atria and ventricles can be inverted simultaneously or separately, and are referred to as concordant if they remain normally related to each other (i.e., the left atrium is connected to the left ventricle and the right atrium to the right ventricle). If the left atrium is connected to the right ventricle or vice versa, the condition is referred to atrioventricular discordance.

Mirror-image Dextrocardia. The most common type of cardiac malposition is referred to as mirror-image dextrocardia. In these patients, the cardiac chambers are completely inverted and the cardiac apex points to the right. Normal anteroposterior chamber relationships are preserved and there is no discordance. Visceral situs inversus is present and

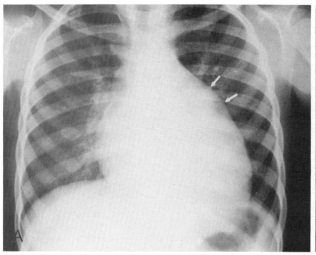

Figure 44.96.   Endocardial Fibroelastosis. A. Note enlargement of the left atrium (*arrows*) and left ventricle. **B.** Another patient with a markedly enlarged left ventricle that has resulted in left lower lobe atelectasis (*arrows*).

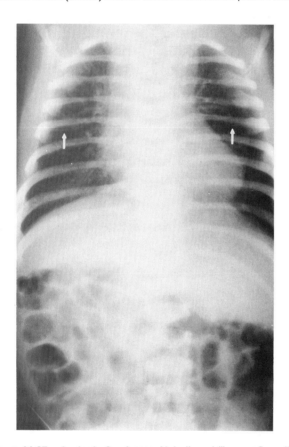

Figure 44.97.   Asplenia Syndrome. Note the midline configuration of the liver. Bilateral horizontal lung fissures are faintly seen (*arrows*).

the incidence of congenital heart disease in such patients is only slightly greater than that in patients with complete situs solitus.

Dextroversion refers to right-sided rotation of the cardiac position so that the right atrium and ventricle become more posterior and the left atrium and ventricle lie anterior. Chamber inversion does not occur in this condition. Visceral situs solitus or inversus can be present, and in either case congenital cyanotic heart disease is frequent. Other variations of dextroposition are relatively rare.

Asplenia-polyspenia   Syndromes. Visceral heterotaxia and congenital heart disease are common components of the cardiosplenic (asplenia-polysplenia) syndromes. The asplenia (Ivemark's) syndrome is usually associated with more severe forms of congenital heart disease than the polysplenia syndrome. The liver often lies in the midline, and intestinal malrotation commonly occurs. For simplicity's sake, the asplenia syndrome can be thought of as bilateral right-sidedness (i.e., absent spleen, bilateral three-lobed lung, bilateral superior vena cava) (Fig. 44.97) and polysplenia resembles bilateral left-sidedness (i.e., multiple spleens, bilateral bilobed lungs, interrupted inferior vena cava with azygous continuation, biliary atresia). Situs inversus with levocardia is a rare situation. Systemic venous abnormalities and congenital heart disease with right ventricular outflow track obstruction are common associated abnormalities.

Positional abnormalities of the aorta and great vessels are common and the components of these anomalies are highly variable. The most important vascular anomalies are those that produce symptoms, mainly those of airway obstruction. These conditions were discussed previously.

References

1. Swischuk LE, Hayden CK, Jr. Lower respiratory tract infection in children (Is roentgenographic differentiation possible?). Pediatr Radiol 1986;16:278–284.
2. Guckel C, Benz-Bohm G, Widemann B. Mycoplasmal pneumonias in childhood: roentgen features, differential diagnosis and review of the literature. Pediatr Radiol 1989;19:499–503.

3. Amodio JB, Berdon WE, Abramson SJ. Cystic fibrosis in childhood: pulmonary, paranasal sinus, and skeletal manifestations. Semin Roentgenol 1987;22:125–135.

4. Lowe GM, Donaldson JS, Backer CL. Vascular rings: 10-year review of imaging. Radiographics 1991;11:637–646.

5. Rosado-de-Christenson ML, Stocker JT. From the archives of the AFIP congenital cystic adenomatoid malformation. Radiographics 1991;11:865–886.

6. Fitzgerald P, Donoghue V, Gorman W. Bronchopulmonary dysplasia: a radiographic and clinical review of 20 patients. Br J Radiol 1990;63:444–447.

7. Bick U, Muller-Leisse C, Troger J. Therapeutic use of surfactant in neonatal respiratory distress syndrome: correlation between pulmonary x-ray changes and clinical data. Pediatr Radiol 1992;22:169–173.

8. Wood BP, Sinkin RA, Kendig JW, Notter RH, Shapiro DL. Exogenous lung surfactant: effect on radiographic appearance in premature infants. Radiology 1987;165:11–13.

9. Gross GW, Cullen J, Kornhauser MS. Thoracic complications of extracorporeal membrane oxygenation: findings on chest radiographs and sonograms. AJR 1992;158:353–358.

10. Amodio JB, Abramson SJ, Berdon WE, Solar C, Markowitz R, Kasznica J. Iatrogenic causes of large pleural fluid collections in the premature infant: ultrasonoic and radiographic findings. Pediatr Radiol 1987;17:104–108.

11. Goutail-Flaud MF, Sfez M, Berg A, et.al. Central venous catheter-related complications in newborns and infants: a 587-case survey. J Pediatr Surg 1991;26:645–650.

12. John PF, Beasley SW, Mayne V. Pulmonary sequestration and related congenital disorders: a clinico-radiological review of 41 cases. Pediatr Radiol 1989;20:4–9.

13. West MS, Donaldson JS, Shkolnik A. Pulmonary sequestration: diagnosis by ultrasound. J Ultrasound Med 1989;8:125–130.

14. Han BK, Babcock DS, Oestreich AE. Normal thymus in infancy: sonographic characteristics. Radiology 1989;170:471–474.

15. Siegel MJ, Glazer HS, Wiener JI, Molina PL. Normal and abnormal thymus in childhood: MR imaging. Radiology 1989;172:367–371.

16. Liu P, Daneman A, Stringer DA. Real-time sonography of mediastinal and juxtamediastinal masses in infants and children. J Can Assoc Radiol 1988;39:190–202.

17. Leung AN, Müller NL, Pineda PR, FitzGerald JM. Primary tuberculosis in childhood: radiographic manifestations. Radiology 1992;182:87–91.

18. DuMontier CM, Graviss ER, Siberstein MJ, McAllister WH. Bronchogenic cysts in children. Clin Radiol 1985;36:431–436.

19. Bisset GS, III. Magnetic resonance imaging of congenital heart disease in the pediatric patient. Radiol Clin North Am 1991;29:279–291.

20. Swischuk LE, Stansberry SD. Pulmonary vascularity in pediatric heart disease. J Thorac Imag 1989;4:1–6.

45

Pediatric Abdomen and Pelvis

Susan D. John
Leonard E. Swischuk

GASTROINTESTINAL TRACT

Gastrointestinal Obstruction

Congenital gastrointestinal (GI) obstructions are an important consideration in infants and children, as opposed to in adults. For the most part, congenital obstructions present early in life, usually in the first 30 days. Indeed, many present within the first 1 or 2 days of life and, by the same token, acquired obstructions usually present later. This mixture of etiologies, especially as related to small bowel and colonic obstruction, has lead us to consider these obstructions under four basic age-group categories (Table 45.1).

Many imaging modalities are now available for evaluating disease processes in general, but no matter which modality is used to investigate GI obstruction, the basic job of the imager is to determine the location or level of obstruction and, if possible, the cause. In this regard, even in this day of sophisticated imaging it is the plain abdominal film, with decubitus or upright augmentation, that provides the most information.

For purposes of organization of GI obstructions, it is often helpful to consider them on the basis of the anatomic divisions of the GI tract. In other words, are they hypopharyngeal upper esophageal, esophageal, gastric, duodenal, small intestinal, or colonic? Determination of the site of obstruction depends upon noting the most distal extent of the air-filled, abnormally distended portion of the GI tract. Wherever the abnormally distended air column ends, most likely, is the level of obstruction.

HYPOPHARYNGEAL/UPPER ESOPHAGEAL OBSTRUCTION

A variety of hypopharyngeal masses obviously can produce obstruction to swallowing, but this is not a common problem in the pediatric age group. In children, the most common cause of hypopharyngeal/upper esophageal obstruction is a spastic cricopharyngeus muscle. Even this condition, however, is not very common and, furthermore, there is debate as to whether a prominent cricopharyngeus muscle indentation alone always is symptomatic. When it is associated with symptoms, the cause often is underlying brain stem disease, but in other cases the spasm is idiopathic. In refractory cases, surgical division of the muscle may be required.

Table 45.1. Most Common Causes of GI Tract Obstruction by Age

Age	Cause of Obstruction
0–1 Month	Congenital anomalies
	Atresia/stenosis
	Malrotation/volvulus
	Hirschsprung's disease
	Meconium plug or small left colon syndrome
	Meconium ileus
1–6 Months	Hernias
6 Months–3 years	Intussusception
3 Years and older	Perforated appendicitis
	Adhesions
	Regional enteritis

Figure 45.1. Esophageal Atresia. A. Frontal view demonstrating the blind, air-filled upper esophageal pouch (*arrows*). Note gas within the stomach and intestines. This latter finding indicates the presence of an associated lower tracheoesophageal fistula. **B.** Lateral view in another patient demonstrates the typical air-filled pouch (*arrows*). A catheter is present in the pouch. Note that the trachea is being compressed by the pouch.

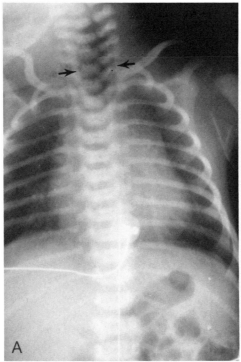
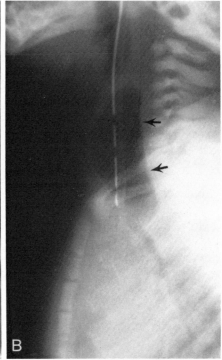

Table 45.2. Causes of Esophageal Obstruction

Congenital atresia/stenosis
Web/diverticulum
Foreign body
Stricture (peptic, caustic)
Extrinsic compression (cysts, neoplasms, vascular)
Achalasia

Difficulties with swallowing also can occur with inflammatory processes such as epiglottitis, retropharyngeal abscess, tonsillar abscess, and any number of tumors or cysts that might occur in this area. Rarely, one might encounter a pharyngeal diverticulum that may be so large that it produces obstruction. These diverticula can be congenital or iatrogenic due to perforation of the hypopharynx during intubation. Since intubation is so common these days, the incidence of iatrogenic diverticula has increased. All of these diverticula are best demonstrated with barium swallow.

ESOPHAGEAL OBSTRUCTIONS

Esophageal Atresia and Tracheo esophageal Fistula. The most common congenital obstruction of the esophagus is esophageal atresia (Table 45.2). The site of obstruction usually is in the upper third of the esophagus, and the air-filled esophageal pouch is classic (Fig. 45.1). Because the pouch is chronically distended in utero (swallowed amniotic fluid), it acts as a mass and causes pressure on the adjacent trachea with resultant focal tracheomalacia. The severity of this latter problem is variable, but when severe, respiratory difficulty can persist even after repair of the esophageal problem.

Esophageal atresia frequently is associated with tracheoesophageal fistula and, most commonly, the fistula extends from the trachea, just above the carina, to the distal esophageal pouch. The fistula allows air to enter the stomach and intestines, in some cases in large volumes. The fact that air is present in the stomach is important in differentiating esophageal atresia without fistula from esophageal atresia with fistula. Without a fistula there is no way for air to get into the stomach or intestines. The proximal, obstructed esophageal pouch can be demonstrated with barium but only small volumes, introduced with a nasoesophageal tube, should be utilized. Fistulae also occur to the upper pouch, but very rarely.

Esophageal atresia is more common in trisomy 21 than in the regular patient population and, in some cases, can be associated with vertebral anomalies. It is also associated with duodenal atresia and imperforate anus. Esophageal atresia results from faulty separation of the GI tract from the neurenteric tube and subsequent faulty canalization of the esophagus. As a result, one may encounter a variety of communications between the esophageal pouch and the spine, ranging from fibrous bands to actual fistulae. If the communication involutes at either end and only the central portion remains, a neurenteric cyst results. Conversely, if an esophageal communication persists, a diverticulum is formed and a spinal communication leads to a

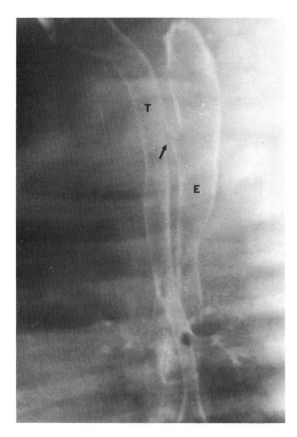

Figure 45.2. Tracheoesophageal Fistula. Note the trachea (*T*), esophagus (*E*), and the slanted fistula (*arrow*) between these two structures.

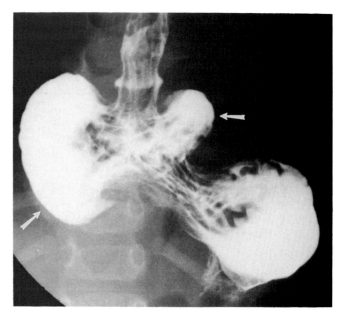

Figure 45.3. Intrathoracic Stomach. Note the large herniated portion of the stomach (*arrows*).

meningocele. This same phenomenon occurs between the trachea and esophagus, for with faulty separation of these two structures one also can end up with a fistula, fibrous band, or diverticulum. Isolated tracheoesophageal fistulae are located high in the esophagus and usually are identified with barium swallow (Fig. 45.2). They are the third most common abnormality in the esophageal atresia-tracheoesophageal fistula group of lesions.

Congenital Esophageal Stenosis. A far less common cause of congenital esophageal obstruction is congenital stenosis. In these cases, the problem once again arises from faulty tracheal and esophageal separation where tracheobronchial cartilage remnants remain in the wall of the esophagus. On barium swallow, small diverticula (mucous glands) can be seen in the areas of stenosis. Congenital stenosis of the esophagus secondary to a so-called intrathoracic stomach is not truly a congenital lesion. Even though seen at birth, this condition lies more in the realm of acquired disease for it represents the aftermath of chronic intrauterine herniation of the stomach (hiatus hernia) into the thoracic cavity, gastroesophageal, reflux, and subsequent peptic esophageal stricture (Fig. 45.3). Other uncommon congenital causes of esophageal obstruction include esophageal webs and

diverticula. Esophageal obstruction also can result from a variety of extrinsic lesions that produce pressure on the esophagus. These include a variety of vascular rings and anomalies, mediastinal cysts, and tumors.

Acquired esophageal obstructive lesions are primarily either strictures or foreign bodies. Esophageal neoplasms are extremely rare in infants and children and malignant neoplasms are virtually unheard of. In terms of acquired esophageal strictures, the most common are the result of peptic or caustic injury to the esophagus.

Peptic esophagitis is associated with gastroesophageal reflux and can be seen with or without a hiatus hernia. However, it might be noted that although gastroesophageal reflux is very common in infants, peptic esophagitis with stricture is a relatively uncommon complication. It is important to note that gastroesophageal reflux may be primary (chalasia) and due to a lax gastroesophageal sphincter, or secondary to a gastric outlet obstruction. In the latter cases, the cause of obstruction (pylorospasm, pyloric stenosis, gastric diaphragm, gastric ulcer disease, etc.) must be identified and treated for reflux to stop. Gastroesophageal reflux is best identified with 24-hour pH monitoring, but this procedure often is cumbersome. The next most sensitive study is nuclear scintigraphy (Fig. 45.4) and third is the barium upper GI series. Ultrasound also can demonstrate gastroesophageal reflux, but is not commonly utilized.

Peptic esophageal strictures usually are short and located in the distal third of the esophagus. This is not always true, and the occasional case of Barrett esophagus with a high stricture also can be encoun-

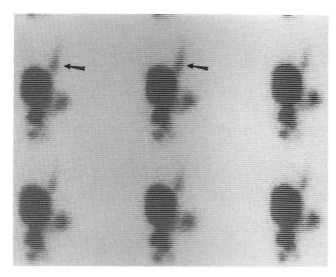

Figure 45.4. Gastroesophageal Reflux. Note reflux into the esophagus (*arrows*). Note that on all of these frames the degree of reflux varies.

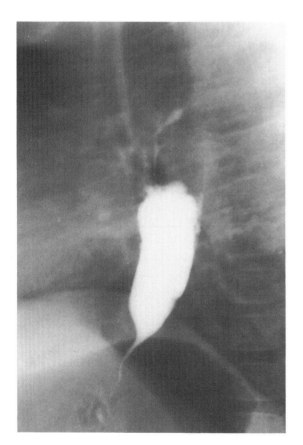

Figure 45.5. Peptic Stricture. Note the beak-like narrowing of the distal esophagus (*arrow*). The findings mimic those of achalasia.

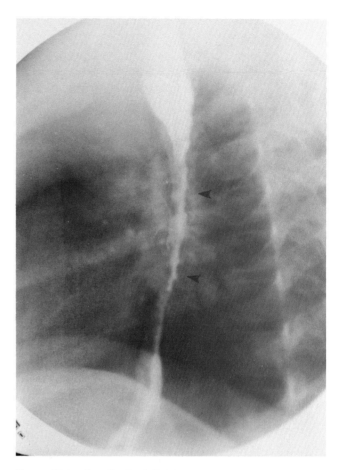

Figure 45.6. Caustic (Lye) Stricture. Note the characteristic long segment irregular configuration of the stricture (*arrows*).

Caustic esophagitis with stricture usually results from accidental ingestion of alkaline substances such as sodium hydroxide, potassium hydroxide (lye), or alkaline disk batteries. Disk batteries can become lodged in the esophagus and leak their alkaline contents, producing deep burns of the mucosa and submucosa. It is important to appreciate that all alkaline burns cause deep penetrating injury to the esophagus and, for this reason, stricture is common. Acids, even those swallowed in significant quantities, tend to produce more superficial burns; therefore, while mucosal injury may be extensive, deep mural injury with subsequent fibrotic stricture is less common.

Radiographically, lye strictures lead to long areas of irregular narrowing (Fig. 45.6). However, if the burn is due to an ingested battery or medication (aspirin, tetracycline, Clinitest tablets) a more focal burn and stricture will be seen. Acquired esophageal stricture also can be seen with epidermolysis bullosa, an hereditary condition characterized by inflammatory skin and mucosal lesions that can heal with fibrosis and stricture formation.

Acute Esophagitis. Esophageal obstruction due to acute inflammatory disease without stricture also can be seen. Acute inflammation with spasm can

tered. Peptic strictures may be irregular, but, in other cases, surprisingly smooth, and may mimic the findings of achalasia (Fig. 45.5). Achalasia is an uncommon cause of esophageal obstruction in infancy and children.

Table 45.3.   Causes of Gastric Obstruction

Atresia/antral diaphragm
Duplication cyst
Pylorospasm
Hypertrophic pyloric stenosis
Gastritis/ulcer disease
Volvulus
Microgastria

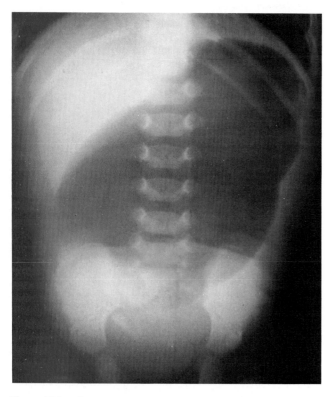

Figure 45.7.   Gastric Atresia. Typical findings consist of an air-filled stomach, with no air distal to this point.

be seen with monilial, herpetic, or peptic esophagitis. Monilial and herpetic esophagitis are becoming a more common problem now that the number of human immunodeficiency virus (HIV)-positive patients is increasing. The findings of acute esophagitis are discussed later in this chapter.

GASTRIC OBSTRUCTION

Congenital obstructing lesions of the stomach are far less common than are congenital obstructing lesions elsewhere in the GI tract. For the most part, these obstructions consist of gastric atresia, gastric diaphragms, and duplication cysts (Table 45.3). The latter must be critically located in the antrum or be very large to result in obstruction. They are often best demonstrated with ultrasound where they appear sonolucent with a wall that demonstrates both mucosal and muscular layers (see Fig. 45.70).

Gastric Atresia.   With gastric atresia, no air is seen distal to the stomach (Fig. 45.7) and the problem is believed to arise from a vascular insult to the stomach in utero. In some cases atresia takes the form of a gastric diaphragm or membrane and, if incomplete, some gas will be seen distal to the obstructing web. Gastric atresia has an increased incidence in patients with congenital epidermolysis bullosa and, as in the esophagus, the problem is one of stricturing after the initial inflammatory insult to the mucosa. In the newborn infant, if obstruction of the stomach is complete and air does not pass into the duodenum, usually no further contrast studies are required. However, if obstruction is incomplete, ultrasound or an upper GI series can be used to identify an incomplete diaphragm. Gastric volvulus is an uncommon cause of gastric obstruction, as is microgastria. Microgastria frequently is associated with other anomalies of other systems and is a common association with the polysplenia and asplenia syndromes. In terms of acquired gastric obstructions, the most common problems are pylorospasm and hypertrophic pyloric stenosis.

Pylorospasm should probably not be thought of as a primary disease process, but rather as a reactive problem to some type of insult to the gastric mucosa (ulceration, inflammation, etc.) or indirect muscle contracture from some other cause of stress. Mucosal inflammation is often due to simple milk allergy, while in other cases frank peptic ulceration can be seen. Most often no abnormality of the gastric mucosa is identified and simple pylorospasm is the problem. The condition currently is usually identified with real-time ultrasound, which demonstrates persistent spasm of the antropyloric region. Neither the mucosa or underlying muscle are thickened, in most cases, but occasionally minimal thickening of the outer circular muscle can be seen (Fig 45.8). Eventually, and intermittently, the antropylorus opens and gastric contents are allowed to pass into the duodenum. The findings also can be demonstrated with upper GI series, but ultrasound usually suffices. In simple cases, if no predisposing cause such as ulcer disease is identified, antispasmodic therapy can be helpful.

Hypertrophic Pyloric Stenosis is now generally considered to be an acquired condition that, in some cases, may be related to prolonged pylorospasm. This condition most often develops between 2 and 8 weeks of age and is characterized by hypertrophy of the pyloric muscle. In the past, the entity was diagnosed with a barium upper GI series but currently, and certainly in the future, it will be diagnosed almost exclusively with ultrasound. With ultrasound the elongated pyloric canal and thickened, hypoechoic pyloric muscle are characteristic on both longitudinal and cross-sectional scans (Fig. 45.9). The pyloric muscle measures 3 mm or more in thickness while the pyloric ca-

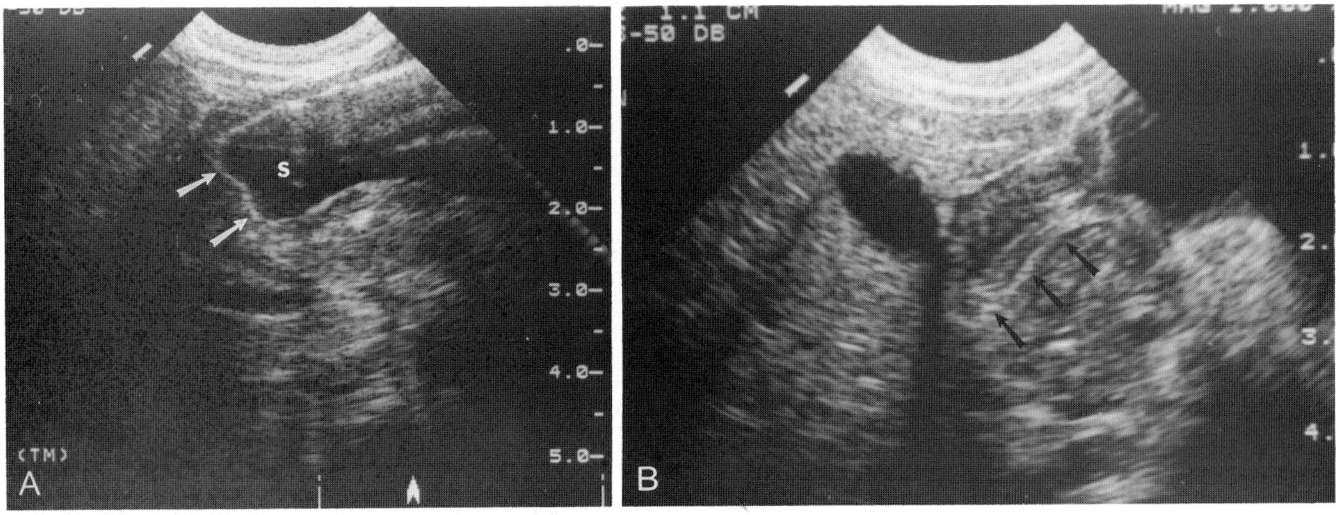

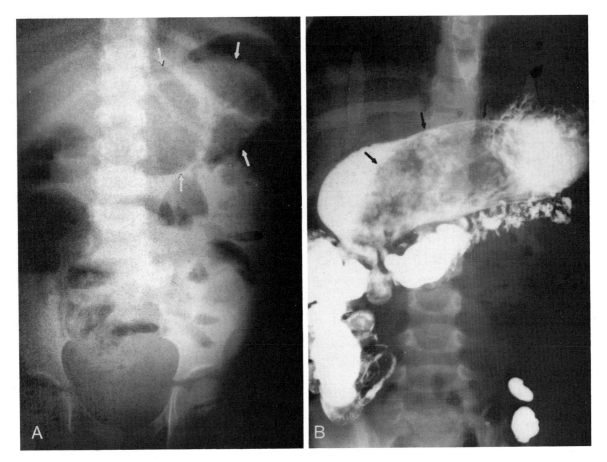

Figure 45.11. Overdistended Stomach Artefact. A. Note the overdistended, fluid-filled stomach (*S*) with a rather straight-appearing distal end (*arrows*). The pyloric canal is not visualized because it is posteriorly directed. **B.** With some of the fluid removed, the abnormal antropyloric canal (*arrows*) now is visualized. The partially empty stomach allows the pylorus to rotate anteriorly from its posterior position.

Figure 45.12.   Bezoar. A. Note the filling defect (*arrows*) in the stomach. **B.** Upper GI series demonstrates the filling defect (*arrows*), characteristic of a bezoar.

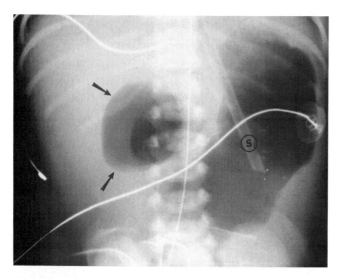

Figure 45.13.   Duodenal Atresia. The findings are those of a classic double-bubble sign consisting of the distended duodenal bulb (arrows) and stomach (S).

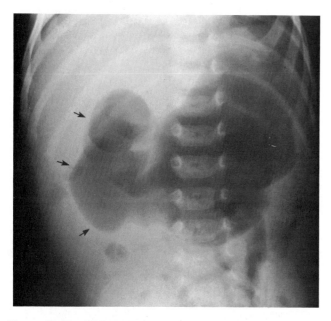

Figure 45.14.   Midgut Volvulus. The characteristically distended descending duodenum (arrows) is seen. The duodenal bulb and stomach also are distended, but the remainder of the intestine shows sparse gas.

ten appears as an oblique indentation of the third or fourth portion of the duodenum. In such cases, confirmation of the presence of midgut volvulus can be accomplished with a barium enema but, commonly, with a little time (5–10 minutes) some barium will pass through the obstruction and outline a corkscrew appearance of the small bowel (Fig. 45.15**C**). In such cases, volvulus should be assumed. Naturally, the small bowel will be malpositioned and lie in the right or right midabdomen rather than in its usual left upper quadrant position. Bowel edema due to venous stasis may also be encountered.

Before leaving the topic of midgut volvulus, it should be noted that not all cases demonstrate high duodenal obstruction. Indeed, in some cases volvulus is intermittent and gas can be seen throughout the GI tract, although the intestine usually is dilated. Nevertheless, most cases demonstrate obstruction of the third to fourth portions of the duodenum and midgut volvulus should be presumed present until proven otherwise. In terms of other conditions that might produce similar findings, one is left primarily with duodenal webs and diaphragms. Other congenital abnormalities leading to obstruction at this level are rather uncommon. Occasionally, an adjacent enteric cyst might be the cause and, rarely, the so-called preduodenal portal vein may be encountered.

Duodenal Hematoma.   Of the acquired causes of duodenal obstruction, perhaps duodenal hematoma is most common. Hematomas usually result from blunt abdominal trauma and can be detected with ultrasound or upper GI series (Fig. 45.16). Although blunt abdominal trauma in general is common in childhood, the commonest cause of duodenal hematoma in childhood is the battered child syndrome. These patients also may sustain trauma to the pancreas followed by posttraumatic pancreatitis.

Obstruction of the duodenum secondary to peptic ulcer disease is not nearly as common in children as it is in adults. Tumors of any type are rare in the duodenum, but any benign or malignant tumor can lead to obstruction. In addition, tumors adjacent to the duodenum such as those occurring in the pancreas, gallbladder, or liver can produce obstruction. The findings in these patients are no different from those seen in adults.

SMALL INTESTINAL OBSTRUCTION

Small intestinal obstruction in the neonate and young infant is more likely to be congenital in nature while, in the older child, acquired problems are more common (Table 45.5). In addition, congenital small bowel obstructions occur less commonly in the proximal small bowel than in the distal small bowel.

Jejunal Atresia.   With proximal obstruction, one usually is dealing with jejunal atresia. Plain films demonstrate a variable number of distended loops of jejunum (Fig. 45.17) and often no further contrast studies are required. A variation of intestinal atresia is the so-called apple peel small bowel, where diffuse atresia of the small bowel is present in the form of multiple sites of severe stenosis. This condition tends to be familial. Segmental volvulus of the small bowel can occur anywhere along its length, but is uncommon. Similarly, internal hernias are rare.

Ileal Atresia/Meconium Ileus.   In the distal small bowel, most problems occur in the immediate neonatal period rather than later in infancy and child-

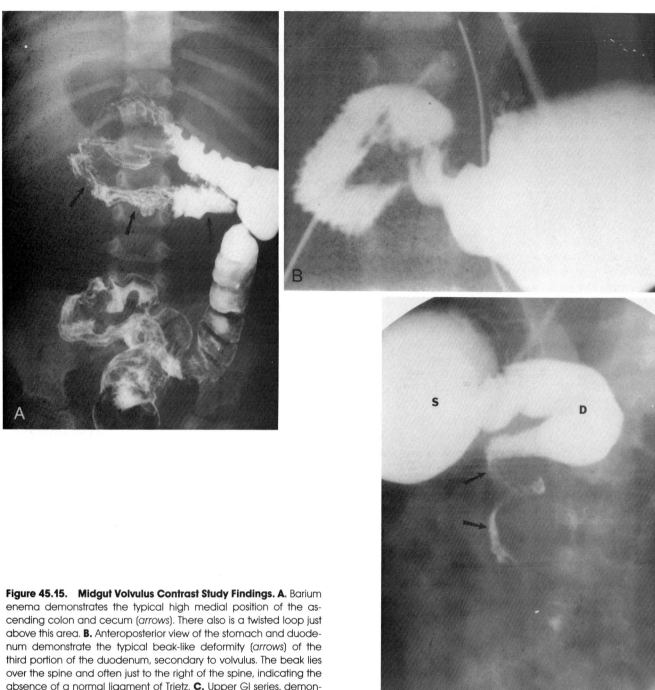

Figure 45.15. Midgut Volvulus Contrast Study Findings. A. Barium enema demonstrates the typical high medial position of the ascending colon and cecum (*arrows*). There also is a twisted loop just above this area. **B.** Anteroposterior view of the stomach and duodenum demonstrate the typical beak-like deformity (*arrows*) of the third portion of the duodenum, secondary to volvulus. The beak lies over the spine and often just to the right of the spine, indicating the absence of a normal ligament of Trietz. **C.** Upper GI series, demonstrating typical spiraling of the small bowel (*arrows*). *D*, Descending duodenum; *S*, stomach.

hood. In the neonate, one is usually dealing with problems such as distal ileal atresia or meconium ileus. In both conditions, contrast studies reveal a characteristic generalized microcolon. With meconium ileus, one may see meconium plugs in the distal small bowel (Fig. 45.18) and, with ileal atresia, air-fluid levels on plain films are more common. It is important to distinguish between the two conditions, for ileal atresia is a surgical problem while meconium ileus can often be treated with water-soluble contrast enema. When performing water-soluble contrast enemas, it is important to have the contrast material reflux into the terminal ileum and outline, as well as lubricate, the inspissated meconium balls. Meconium ileus is the earliest manifestation of cystic fibrosis and should not be confused with the meconium plug syndrome. On plain films, when one notes grossly distended loops of intestine with bubbly appearing intestinal contents, one should be highly suspicious of the presence of meconium ileus (Fig. 45.18). Although

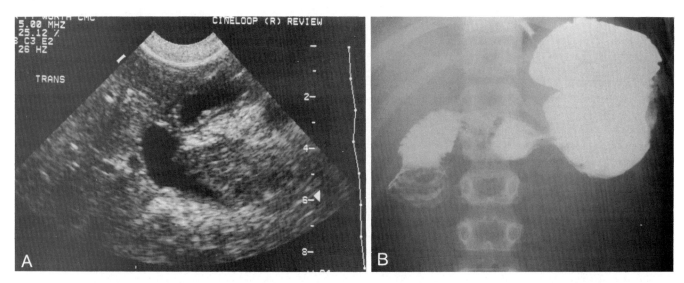

Figure 45.16. Duodenal Hematoma. A. Ultrasonographic features demonstrating the echogenic hematoma (*arrows*) producing obstruction of the duodenum (*D*). *S*, stomach. **B.** Upper GI series in an-other patient demonstrates the typical intramural filling defect of the hematoma (*arrows*).

Table 45.5. Causes of Small Intestinal Obstruction

Atresia/stenosis
Meconium ileus
Incarcerated hernia
Intussusception
Perforated appendicitis

this pattern can be seen with any low small bowel or colonic obstruction, it is most commonly seen with meconium ileus.

Meconium Plug Syndrome. In the neonate it is difficult to separate distal small bowel obstruction from colonic obstruction and usually the entities are handled together. Once the pattern of numerous distended loops of intestine is seen, suggesting the possibility of low small bowel or colonic obstruction, one must push on to a contrast study of the colon. With the meconium plug syndrome, also known as the small left colon syndrome, a dilated colon full of meconium with an empty distal descending colonic segment is characteristic (Fig. 45.19). In other cases, the empty segment is not nearly as long. This condition is the result of functional immaturity of the colon and is seen both in normal, usually large, babies and in infants delivered of diabetic mothers. The problem is transient and can often be treated by rectal stimulation or repeated saline enemas. In more persistent cases, an enema using contrast that contains the detergent Tween 80 (such as Gastrografin) can be used to irritate the colon enough to produce defecation.

Hirschsprung's Disease. The primary differential diagnosis of the meconium plug syndrome is Hirschsprung's disease and, indeed, only biopsy or follow-up of the patients can distinguish between the

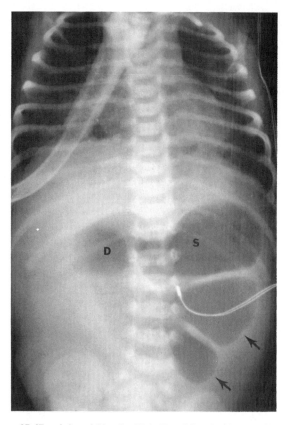

Figure 45.17. Jejunal Atresia. Note the distended loops of the upper intestine (*arrows*). No air is present distal to this area. *D*, duodenum; *S*, stomach.

two conditions in the neonate. Meconium plug syndrome resolves with no further problems. Additional contrast enema findings in patients with Hirschsprung's disease include a tortuosity or corrugation of the narrowed aganglionic segment of the colon (Fig. 45.20). In addition, there may be delayed evacuation

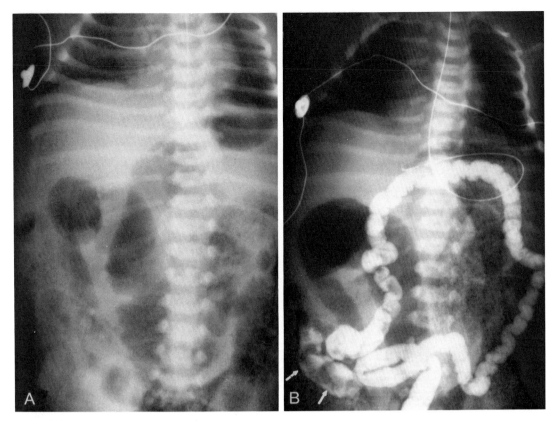

Figure 45.18.   Meconium Ileus. A. Note the soap-bubble effect of air mixed with meconium in the numerous distended loops of intestine. **B.** Contrast enema demonstrates a typical microcolon with re-

flux into the terminal ileum, which is filled with pellets of meconium (*arrows*).

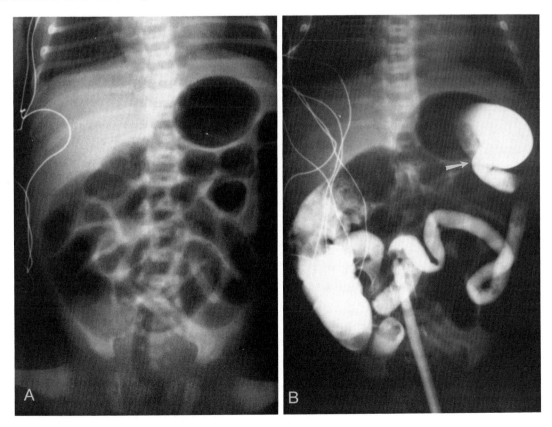

Figure 45.19.   Meconium Plug Syndrome (Small Left Colon Syndrome). A. Note the numerous loops of distended intestine. Also, note air in the relatively narrow rectosigmoid colon. **B.** Contrast en-

ema demonstrates the small left colon and characteristic transition zone (*arrow*). These findings mimic those of Hirschsprung's disease.

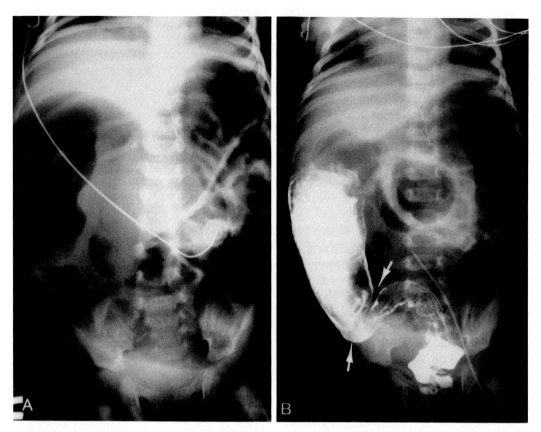

Figure 45.20.   Hirschsprung's Disease.   A. Plain film demonstrates an enormously distended colon. Note that there is no gas in the rectum. **B.** Contrast study demonstrates a narrowed rectum and sigmoid, with a classic transition zone (*arrows*). The colon above this area is dilated. It is not unusual for the sigmoid colon to flop over to the right side in infants.

of the barium, usually well beyond 24 hours. Nonetheless, in any given case the diagnosis finally is accomplished with rectal biopsy. Necrotizing enterocolitis is an uncommon but serious complication of Hirschsprung's disease. It is usually due to stasis colitis.

Incarcerated Inguinal Hernia.   After the neonatal period, perhaps the most common cause of low intestinal obstruction, in infants under 18 months, is an incarcerated inguinal hernia. The findings of intestinal obstruction on plain films are characteristic, and the key to diagnosis of the condition is visualization of a unilaterally prominent inguinal canal or actual loops of air-filled bowel in the scrotum (Fig. 45.21). Ultrasound can help in detecting the incarcerated intestine in those cases where the findings are equivocal.

Intussusception.   Shortly after the 1st year of life, intussusception becomes an increasingly important acquired cause of intestinal obstruction. Ileocolic intussusception is the most common type. Lead points such as diverticula, polyps, or tumors are more commonly encountered in neonates and in older children. In most cases, intussusception is idiopathic. It is believed that redundant, inflamed mucosa or lymph nodes act as the lead point.

The abdominal radiographs in patients with intussusception may be normal or may demonstrate obvious intestinal obstruction. In approximately half the cases, one may see the head of the intussusceptum on plain films (Fig. 45.22**A**). Regardless of what is seen on the plain films, if there is strong clinical suspicion of intussusception, one should proceed with ultrasound and then a contrast or air enema. Not all agree that ultrasound is required, but it is a very effective imaging modality for the demonstration of intussusception. Characteristically, one will see an oval mass in longitudinal section and a round mass in cross-section. Variable concentric rings, fluid in the lumen and even a sonolucent edematous outer ring, will be seen (Fig. 45.22**B**). The findings result from the indrawing of a portion of bowel into the adjacent and more distal portion of bowel (usually ileum telescopes into colon), and the findings represent layers of intestine alternating with layers of mesentery. Color flow Doppler ultrasound recently has been utilized to determine viability of the head of the intussusception, but bowel ischemia and perforation still are more often assessed clinically and radiographically. Nonsurgical reduction should be attempted in any case as long as there is no evidence of free air or peritonitis (Fig. 45.22**C**). It should be noted that small amounts of free fluid are

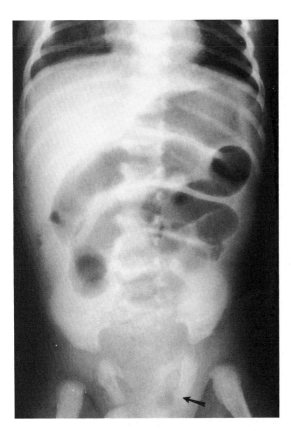

Figure 45.21. Inguinal Hernia. Note the numerous loops of distended intestine, signifying the presence of an intestinal obstruction. Also note air in the hernia or over the left inguinal region (*arrow*).

commonly seen with ultrasound in intussusception and are not a contraindication for nonsurgical reduction.

A variety of methods may be used for demonstration and reduction of intussusception. Barium was almost exclusively used for hydrostatic reduction in the past, but this method now is losing popularity and probably eventually will be abandoned. The main disadvantage of barium is that if perforation occurs, barium leaks into the peritoneal cavity, and peritonitis results. We have used Gastrografin diluted 5:1 for years and have found it satisfactory, but currently air reduction is very popular (2, 3). Recent studies have observed that with air, one is able to generate greater pressures in the colon than one was able to do with barium. The pressure generated depends both on the viscosity of barium but also the height of the barium column. We have always placed our Gastrografin column to 4–5 feet and have experienced reduction rates of 80–90%. It has been shown that the Gastrografin column needs to be elevated to this level to equal the 120 mm Hg pressure generated with air pumps.

In cases of intussusception that are refractory to hydrostatic or air reduction, repeated attempts and the use of sedation are often helpful. Overall, the only contraindication to nonsurgical reduction of intus-

susception is the presence of free air or signs and symptoms of peritonitis. The duration of symptoms and the presence of small bowel obstruction are not generally considered deterrents. Reintussusception occurs in approximately 5–10% of cases and nonsurgical reduction may be attempted at least once.

Appendicitis. After about 2 years of age, perforated appendicitis becomes an increasingly common cause of intestinal obstruction and in later childhood it is the primary cause. With acute, nonperforated appendicitis there is no obstruction, but once the appendix perforates, obstruction gradually develops, due to a combination of functional obstruction and abscess formation (Fig. 45.23). These patients often improve symptomatically and often it is difficult to convince oneself clinically that perforated appendicitis is present. Nevertheless, radiographic evidence of low intestinal obstruction in the older child should be considered to be caused by perforated appendicitis until proven otherwise, and one may proceed to a number of other imaging studies to make the diagnosis. Plain films may show the presence of a right lower quadrant mass, but free air is usually not seen. Abscesses can be demonstrated with either ultrasound or computerized tomography (CT). In some cases, barium enema is useful and demonstrates the abscess adhering to various portions of the GI tract.

Regional Enteritis. Another relatively common cause of low small bowel obstruction is regional enteritis. These patients often mimic those with chronic appendiceal abscess. Ultrasonographically, the thickened loop of small bowel often can be identified but it is contrast studies that provide the definitive findings. These findings are no different from those seen in adults and consist of a variety of configurations including the string sign, linear ulcers, and a deformed, narrowed terminal ileocecal region. Other problems in this area, such as tuberculosis, lymphoma, and *Yersinia* colitis, are much less common but produce findings that may be difficult to differentiate from regional enteritis.

COLONIC OBSTRUCTION

Congenital obstructions of the colon are more common than acquired obstructions (Table 45.6). The meconium plug syndrome and neonatal Hirschsprung's disease have been discussed in previous sections. Hirschsprung's disease in later infancy and childhood is less difficult to diagnose, than in the neonatal period. Characteristically, the narrowed distal aganglion segment is visualized and leads to a zone of transition beyond which the proximal dilated colon is seen (Fig. 45.24). Functional megacolon is quite common in childhood and is associated with spasm of the puborectalis muscle. These cases may be difficult to differentiate from so-called low-segment Hirsch-

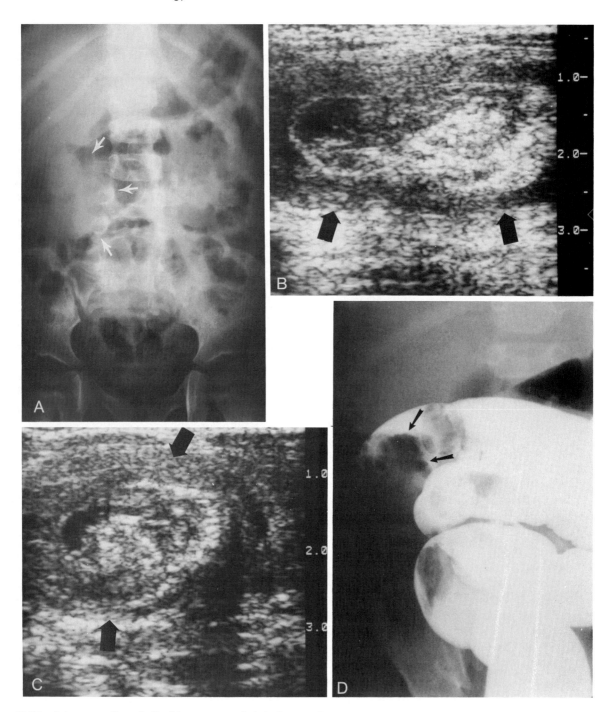

Figure 45.22. Intussusception. A. On this near-normal plain film, note the suggestion of a soft-tissue mass in the right upper quadrant (*arrows*). **B.** Ultrasonogram, longitudinal view through the intussusception, demonstrates the typical oval configuration (*arrows*). **C.** Cross-sectional view showing concentric rings of the intussusception. Some hypoechoic fluid is present in the lumen on both views (*arrows*). **D.** Subsequent contrast enema demonstrates the typical appearance of the intussusception (*arrows*).

sprung's disease. In many instances, the puborectalis muscle spasm is secondary to anal fissures; in other instances, it is idiopathic. The characteristic indentation by the puborectalis sling provides the major clue to the presence of functional or psychogenic megacolon (Fig. 45.25). These patients can store considerable volumes of stool in their colon. Colon atresia occurs in the neonatal period and is relatively rare.

Usually, there is massive distension of the colon proximal to the area of atresia or stenosis (Fig. 45.26).

Imperforate or Ectopic Anus is a common cause of obstruction in the neonate. This anomaly can range from simple anal atresia to arrest of the colon as it descends through the puborectalis sling, with fistula formation from the arrested hindgut to some part of the genital or urinary tract. In females, the fistula

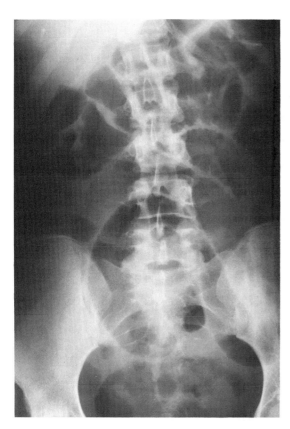

Figure 45.23. Perforated Appendicitis. Note the numerous loops of distended small bowel with a general paucity of gas in the right lower quadrant. There is also scoliosis with concavity to the right. A functional small bowel obstruction is present.

Table 45.6. Causes of Colonic Obstruction

Atresia/stenosis
Meconium plug syndrome (small left colon)
Hirschsprung's disease
Functional megacolon
Ectopic (imperforate) anus
Inflammatory stricture
Volvulus
Trauma
Neoplasm

from the blind-ending distal colon can empty into the bladder, uterus, or vagina. In males, it tends to enter into the urethra but can also enter the bladder. In both sexes it can enter the perineum. Many of these patients have associated sacral and urinary tract anomalies (Fig. 45.27**A**) and in complicated cases, congenital abnormalities such as hydrometrocolpos and persistent cloaca are seen.

Once imperforate anus is encountered, it is important to identify other anomalies, especially of the genitourinary tract, and to determine the level of the fistula. Ultrasound can be utilized to demonstrate the end of the pouch (Fig. 45.27**B**), the fistula may be injected directly, or the fistula may opacify during retro-

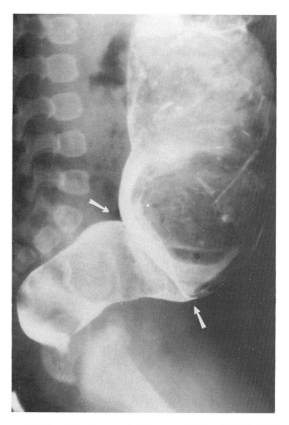

Figure 45.24. Hirschsprung's Disease (Older Child). Note the characteristic transition zone (*arrows*) between the dilated feces-filled colon above and the relatively narrowed rectum below.

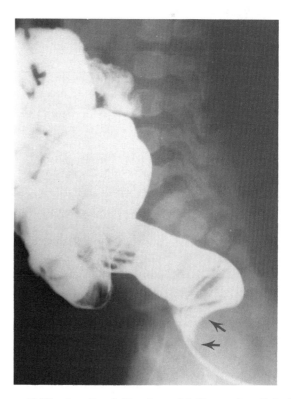

Figure 45.25. Functional (Psychogenic) Megacolon. Note the typical pronounced indentation of the posterior rectum (*arrows*) by the puborectalis sling.

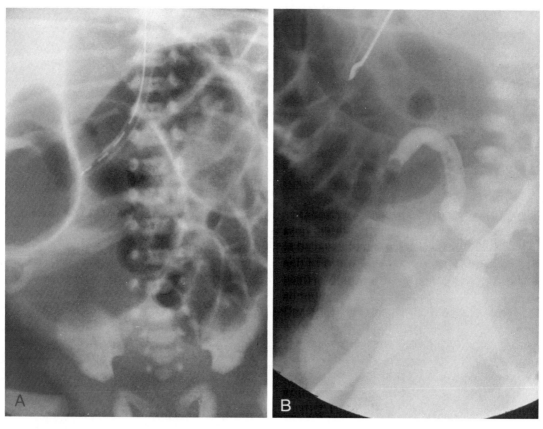

Figure 45.26. Colon Atresia. A. There are numerous loops of distended intestine in this patient and the two or three largest ones are in the midabdomen and on the right. **B.** Retrograde contrast study demonstrates the blind-ending microcolon (*arrows*). The distended air-filled colon is proximal to this area.

grade voiding cystourethrography, which usually is performed in these patients. In females, flush retrograde vaginography may be required. If it is determined that the fistula empties above the puborectalis sling, then it can be presumed that the puborectalis muscle is hypoplastic and that continence will be difficult to accomplish with any type of surgical procedure. If the fistula empties distal to the puborectalis sling, the puborectalis muscle is more developed and continence is more likely. The "M" line of Cremin has been utilized to determine the level at which the blind pouch ends (Fig. 45.28). This line is drawn perpendicular to the long axis of the ischia, and passes through the junction between the middle and lower third of the ischia. If the blind pouch and fistula end above the line, the fistula is considered high. If it ends below the line, it is considered low, and if it ends at the line, it is considered intermediate. Intermediate fistulae usually pose the same problems as high fistulae.

Acquired Causes of Colonic Obstruction are relatively uncommon except for perforated appendicitis and regional enteritis. Inflammatory strictures associated with ulcerative colitis and necrotizing enterocolitis also can be encountered. These usually tend to be smooth and appear much the same as they do in adults. They may be single or multiple. Tumors of the colon generally are uncommon and the findings are similar to those seen in adults. Trauma to the colon, producing obstruction, most commonly is seen with motor vehicle accidents or the battered child syndrome, the latter being more common.

Sigmoid and cecal volvulus are much less common in children than in adults, but the findings are exactly the same. Volvulus tends to occur more frequently in bedridden patients than in normal patients and has a higher incidence in retarded children.

Inflammation and Infection

ESOPHAGUS

Inflammation of the esophagus is encountered with peptic esophagitis, caustic material ingestion, viral infections, and monilial infection. The latter two conditions are becoming more common as the HIV-positive population grows. With monilial esophagitis, mucosal irregularities are seen, and intense spasm of the esophagus leading to a so-called pseudodiverticulum configuration can occur. Viral (usually herpes) esophagitis, causes small superficial ulcers, best demonstrated with double contrast studies. These ulcers can be diffuse or focal and may result in intense spasm with severe dysphagia.

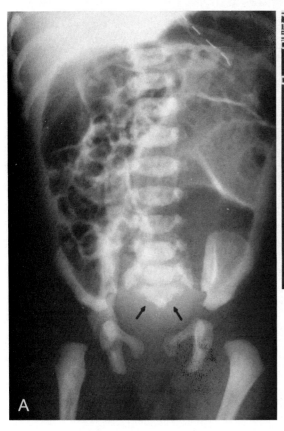

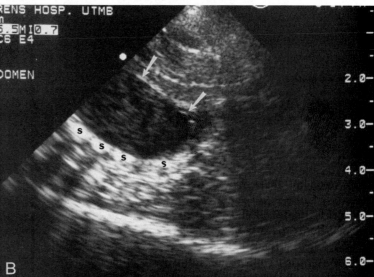

Figure 45.27. Imperforate Anus. A. There are two or three loops of distended colon on the right; small bowel gas also is visualized. The sacrum (*arrows*) is underdeveloped. **B.** Sagittal ultrasonogram in another infant demonstrates the distended distal pouch (*arrows*) that overlies the sacral segments (*S*). The pouch ends at the lower most sacral segment.

Peptic esophagitis tends to involve the lower third of the esophagus but, with severe reflux, may involve the entire esophagus. Findings consist of thickening of the esophageal wall, stiffening of the esophagus, and lack of normal peristaltic activity. Ulcerations may be seen and, in some cases, the ulcers may be deep (Fig. 45.29). Nonfibrotic narrowing occurs in the early stages but later fibrotic stricturing results.

With caustic ingestion, extensive esophageal burns are the rule and, in fact, the esophagus may be denuded. Indeed, perforation into the mediastinum can occur. Contrast studies are not generally performed in the acute stage of caustic injury but later, as esophageal strictures develop, contrast studies are the rule (Fig. 45.6).

STOMACH

Peptic gastritis is the most common inflammatory condition of the stomach, even in infants and young children. The findings are no different from those seen in adults; superficial ulcerations and delicate, edematous, cobblestoned appearance of the mucosa are especially well demonstrated with double contrast studies. When frank ulcers occur, again, these appear no different than in adults. Milk allergy is another common cause of gastritis in infants, and commonly leads to vomiting and bleeding. On upper GI series these patients demonstrate, for the most part, only in-

tense antropyloric spasm but with ultrasonography, thickening of the mucosa can be detected, as with any type of gastritis. Patients on steroid therapy are especially prone to develop these changes.

Ingestion of caustic substances that are acidic are more likely to result in gastritis than esophagitis. This is especially true when large volumes of high-specific gravity acids are ingested. However, overall caustic injuries are more likely to involve the esophagus than the stomach because the ingestion of acids is far less common than alkaline agents.

DUODENUM

The most common, inflammatory process involving the duodenum in infants and children is peptic ulcer disease. As in adults, an ulcer crater is sometimes, but not always, visualized. Children tend to present with bleeding due to peptic ulcer disease more often than adults. It is important to realize that peptic ulcer disease is probably more common in children than is generally believed.

SMALL BOWEL

Simple viral gastroenteritis is the most common inflammatory condition of the small bowel. On ultrasound, thickened mucosa is seen along with dilated fluid-filled loops. Upper GI series are seldom performed in these patients. Plain abdominal films may

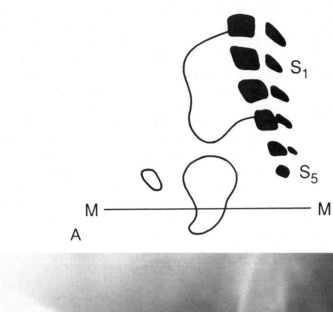

A

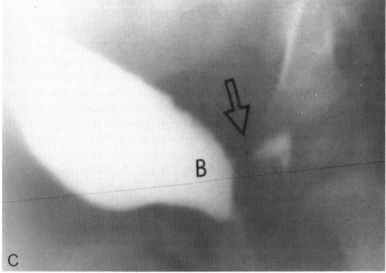

C

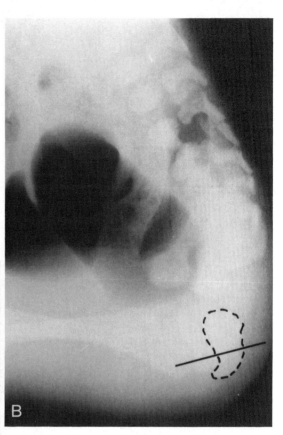

B

Figure 45.28. Imperforate Anus—Cremin's M Line. A. The M line is drawn horizontally through the junction of the middle and lower thirds of the ischium (*M*). S_1, S_5, sacral segments. The line demarcates the level of the puborectalis sling. **B.** Inverted film in another infant demonstrates the distal air-filled pouch of the hindgut. Note the position of the M line. The pouch ends well above the M line, indicating a high imperforate anus. **C.** The same patient, demonstrating a fistula (*arrow*) from the bladder (*B*) to the rectum.

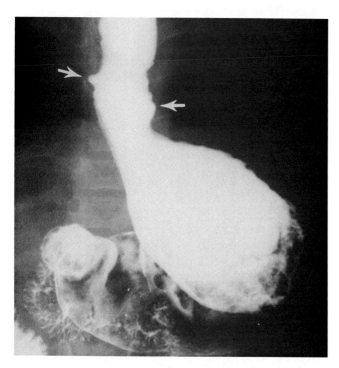

Figure 45.29. Peptic Esophagitis. Inflammation of the distal esophagus causes narrowing, mucosal irregularity, and ulcers (arrows).

show extensive accumulations of gas within the GI tract, and the sheer volume of the gas may at first erroneously suggest mechanical obstruction.

The next most common inflammatory condition in the small bowel is regional enteritis. The terminal ileum is the primary site of involvement, and regional enteritis of the proximal small bowel, stomach, or esophagus are rather rare. The radiographic findings are no different from those seen in adults and consist of a variable length of narrowed irregular terminal ileum, with or without linear ulcers and sinus tracts (Fig. 45.30, **A** and **B**). The transmural bowel wall thickening common in these patients is readily demonstrable with ultrasound (Fig. 45.30**C**). Clinically, these patients may mimic those with appendicitis, especially chronic perforated appendicitis. Tuberculous and *Yersinia* enterocolitis can mimic the findings of regional enteritis, but are rare on this continent.

COLON

Almost every condition that produces colitis in the adult can produce colitis in infants and children: ulcerative colitis, regional enteritis, amebic colitis, and pseudomembranous colitis. Almost any form of colitis, on ultrasound, manifests in thickening of the mucosa.

Necrotizing Enterocolitis, on the other hand, is almost exclusively a pediatric problem and is most commonly seen in premature infants. Its etiology lies in hypoxia and hypoperfusion of the gut and the clinical

findings tend to mimic those of sepsis. However, the passage of blood per rectum is more common with necrotizing enterocolitis. Initially these patients demonstrate dilated loops of bowel, both small bowel and colon, but the hallmark of the disease is pneumatosis cystoides intestinalis (Fig. 45.31, **A** and **B**). Pneumatosis results from destruction of the mucosa and passage of gas produced by bacterial (*Escherichia coli*) superinfection into the bowel wall, and in some cases into the portal venous system (Fig. 45.31**B**). Pneumatosis cystoides intestinalis may appear as linear, curvilinear, or bubbly-to-granular collections of air. In the past, the presence of portal vein gas was considered a dire prognostic sign, but currently, with aggressive treatment, it is of less concern. Many patients later develop strictures. Necrotizing enterocolitis is treated medically by withholding feedings, administering antibiotics, and blood transfusions, if necessary. Surgical intervention is necessary when perforation or peritonitis occurs. In addition, when fixed dilated loops are seen, these loops are presumed to be ischemic and nonviable and also should prompt surgical intervention. Free air, indicating intestinal perforation, is best demonstrated with cross-table lateral or lateral decubitus views of the abdomen.

Typhlitis. Another inflammatory process of the colon, occurring primarily in patients with leukemia, is typhlitis. In this condition, the patients are severely neutropenic and a necrotizing enterocolitis localized to the cecal region develops. The findings may mimic those of acute appendicitis or acute regional enteritis. The clinical setting should suggest the correct diagnosis. Ultrasonographically, the mucosa is thickened (4) and with barium enema a variety of cecal deformities including thumb printing, spasm, and mucosal irregularity are seen (Fig. 45.32).

Appendicitis, after gastroenteritis, is the most common inflammatory process in the abdomen of infants and children. Not all cases present with classic symptoms, nor do all present with classic radiographic findings. In nonperforated appendicitis the abdomen often is relatively airless, and one or two loops of air-filled small bowel or cecum in the right lower quadrant may be seen. Scoliosis with concavity to the right usually is present and there may be poor visualization of the ipsilateral psoas muscle. This is not due to edema but rather to distortion of muscle edge by the spasm. Such distortion causes the lateral edge of the muscle to disappear. Fecaliths are seen in approximatly 50% of cases of appendicitis, and when a fecalith is identified in a patient with a clinically acute abdomen, appendicitis should be presumed. On the other hand, some fecaliths are silent and there is debate as to whether elective prophylactic appendectomy should be performed when they are encountered.

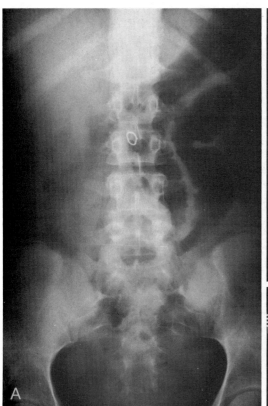

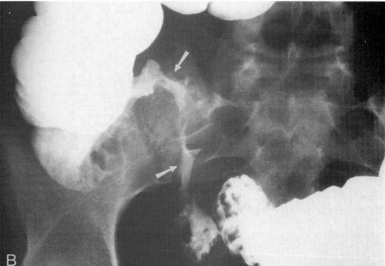

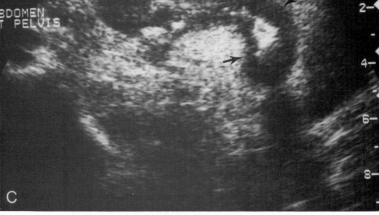

Figure 45.30.   Regional Enteritis. A. Plain radiograph shows two dilated, obstructed small bowel loops with a paucity of gas in the right side of the abdomen. **B.** Barium enema demonstrates the markedly narrowed and irregular terminal ileum (*arrows*). Note that the tip of the cecum is also involved. **C.** Note the transmural hypoechoic thickening of the wall of the terminal ileum (*arrows*).

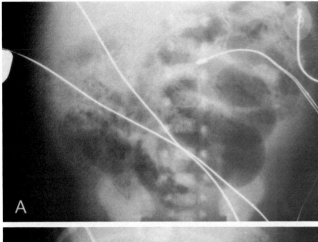

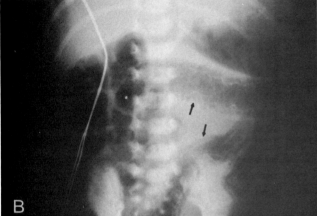

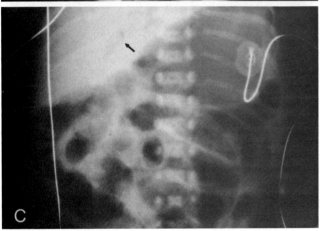

Figure 45.31.   Necrotizing Enterocolitis. A. Note the multiple loops of distended bowel. The bubbly and linear radiolucencies in the bowel wall represent pneumatosis intestinalis (*arrows*). **B.** Another patient with marked pneumatosis of the wall of the colon (*arrows*). **C.** Note the branching radiolucencies overlying the liver, representing air within the portal venous system (*arrow*).

Ultrasonographically, acute appendicitis manifests in a distended, fluid-filled, swollen appendix with variable destruction of the mucosa (Fig. 45.33**A**). The appendix measures 6 mm or more in diameter but is of variable length (5–7). It is tender and noncompressible. When perforation occurs, the appendix decompresses and is more difficult to detect with ultra-

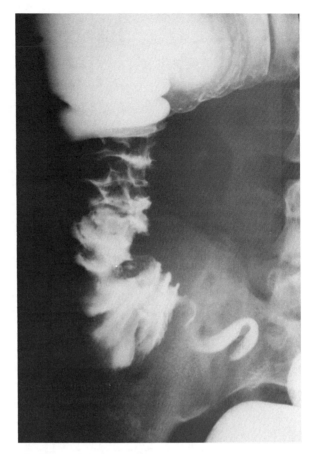

Figure 45.32.   Typhilitis. Note the spasm, thumbprinting, and mucosal thickening involving the cecum.

sound (8). Fecaliths, both calcified and noncalcified, are readily demonstrated with ultrasound.

With perforation of the appendix, clinical findings improve but never become normal. The radiograph, however, usually becomes distinctly abnormal, as the generalized inflammatory process in the area of perforation tends to cause functional obstruction of the small bowel (Fig. 45.23). If abscesses develop they usually are best detected with ultrasound or CT. Ultrasonographically, appendiceal abscesses may be entirely hypoechoic or virtually solid. Most, however, show a mixed echopattern and some are exceptionally well defined and smooth (Fig. 45.34). Barium enema studies are employed in those cases where the diagnosis is in doubt; it demonstrates plastering of the inflammatory process to various portions of the colon and adjacent small bowel.

PERITONITIS

Bacterial Peritonitis.   The causes of bacterial peritonitis in children, for the most part, are similar to those of adults and include perforated appendicitis and generalized sepsis. Children with nephrotic syndrome are more prone to develop generalized bacterial peritonitis. The presence of free fluid in the abdomen

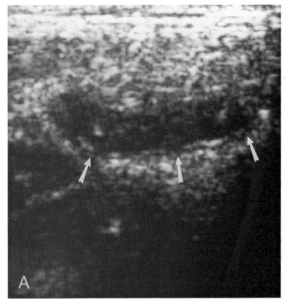

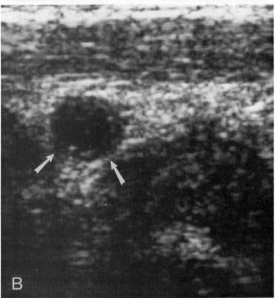

Figure 45.33. Acute Appendicitis—Ultrasound Findings. A. A longitudinal image of the appendix demonstrating the fluid-filled lumen (*arrows*), which could not be compressed. **B.** The appendix in cross-section. Note the areas of decreased echogenicity of the mucosal lining of the appendix (*arrows*).

is the main imaging finding, and ultrasound is the best method for identifying and quantitating such fluid.

Meconium Peritonitis is a condition of the newborn period that results from intrauterine GI perforation. The perforation is either a result of a fetal bowel obstruction or intrauterine ischemia of the intestines leading to necrosis. Obstructive lesions are probably more common and the cause is often either atresia of the distal small bowel or colon or obstruction and/or volvulus associated with meconium ileus. In some patients, active perforation remains after birth and the

patient presents with a clinical picture of peritonitis. In other cases, the perforation seals off in utero, and the extruded meconium is often palpated as an abdominal mass. This meconium sometimes calcifies and can be identified on plain films. The calcified meconium appears as scattered amorphous or curvilinear calcifications throughout the peritoneal cavity (Fig. 45.35**A**). In addition, the meconium sometimes enters the scrotum through a patent processus vaginalis. Residual cystic masses of meconium can also be identified sonographically (Fig. 45.35**B**). When calcifications are also present, they create multiple scattered, bright echoes and the appearance has been likened to a "snowstorm." The calcifications slowly disappear with age, although some patients may develop bowel obstruction later in childhood due to adhesions.

LIVER AND BILIARY SYSTEM

Cholecystitis is more common than generally believed in the pediatric population. The findings are exactly the same as those in adults. The inflamed gallbladder is distended, usually shows a thickened wall, and may show surrounding edema (9). Cholecystitis occurs in normal individuals but is also seen in patients who are HIV-positive. Gallstones also are more common than generally appreciated in infants and children. Many gallstones are due to the presence of a hemolytic anemia, but others have the same etiology as in adults.

Ascending Cholangitis can occur at any age group and the findings are no different from those seen in adults. However, it might be noted that ascending cholangitis, due to abnormal pancreatic duct insertion into the common bile duct, has been considered a strong etiologic factor in the development of choledochal cysts in infancy.

Hepatitis and Biliary Atresia. Hepatitis is not uncommon in children, but there are few imaging findings. If the liver is very edematous, it may appear hypoechoic on ultrasound. Hepatitis in the newborn is related to infection with a specific virus (e.g., hepatitis B virus, cytomegalovirus) or is associated with familial or metabolic conditions that result in cholestatic jaundice (e.g., α_1-antitrypsin deficiency, Byler disease), but most often the term "neonatal hepatitis" is used to refer to idiopathic cholestatic jaundice in the newborn. This condition is generally considered to be closely related to biliary atresia and, together, neonatal hepatitis and biliary atresia account for most cases of cholestatic jaundice in the newborn period. Diffuse extrahepatic bile duct atresia is believed by some to be the result of chronic cholangiohepatitis, probably caused by viral infection. Less common forms of biliary atresia include intrahepatic ductal

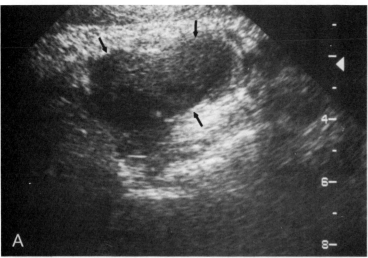

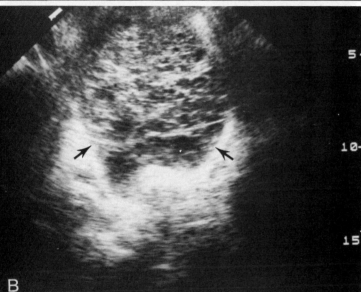

Figure 45.34. Abscesses Secondary to Perforated Appendicitis. A. Note the oval-shaped complex fluid collection (*arrows*) that was found in the right lower quadrant. **B.** This abscess developed postappendectomy and demonstrates a large amount of echogenic debris within the abscess fluid (*arrows*).

atresia and focal atresia of the bile ducts, which is presumably due to an intrauterine vascular insult.

In the workup of neonatal cholestatic jaundice, it is of considerable importance to distinguish between neonatal hepatitis and biliary atresia, for idiopathic cholestatic jaundice is usually treated medically but extrahepatic bile duct atresia requires prompt surgical correction. Ultrasound alone usually does not provide sufficient information to distinguish the two conditions and sonography primarily is used to exclude other causes of obstructive jaundice such as choledochal cysts, inspissated bile syndrome, or obstructing masses or gallstones. Although the gallbladder is often small or absent in patients with extrahepatic biliary atresia, in approximately 20% of cases a normal gallbladder is seen. Hepatobiliary scintigraphy using ^{99m}Tc-iminodiacetate (IDA) analogs often provides useful information (10, 11) (Fig. 45.36). In the early stages of extrahepatic biliary atresia, hepatocyte function is normal; therefore, the liver will show normal tracer uptake but no excretion into the bile ducts and GI tract. The demonstration of tracer activity within the GI tract strongly supports the diagnosis of neonatal hepatitis and virtually excludes the possibility of extrahepatic biliary atresia. Phenobarbital is sometimes administered prior to the examination to enhance the biliary excretion of the isotope and improve the discriminatory value of the examination. The definitive diagnosis of biliary atresia is usually made by liver biopsy and intraoperative cholangiography.

PANCREATITIS

Blunt abdominal trauma is the most common cause of pancreatitis in childhood, and the most common cause of such trauma is the battered child syndrome. Ultrasonographically, the pancreas often is entirely normal. In other cases it is enlarged and hypoechoic. If an actual pancreatic fracture or lacera-

Figure 45.35.   Meconium Peritonitis. A. Numerous amorphous calcifications are seen scattered throughout the peritoneal cavity. **B.** Ultrasound revealed a hypoechoic mass (*M*), representing residual meconium in the peritoneal cavity. Note the scattered echogenic calcifications adjacent to the mass (*arrows*).

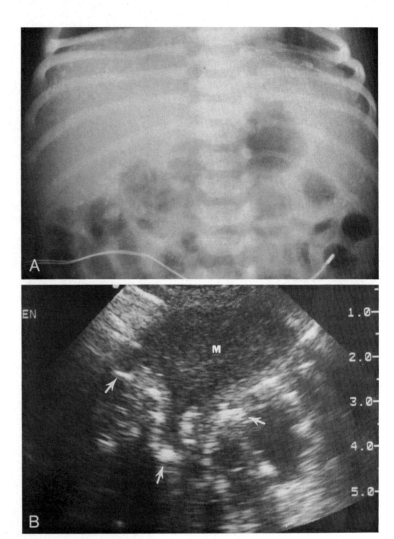

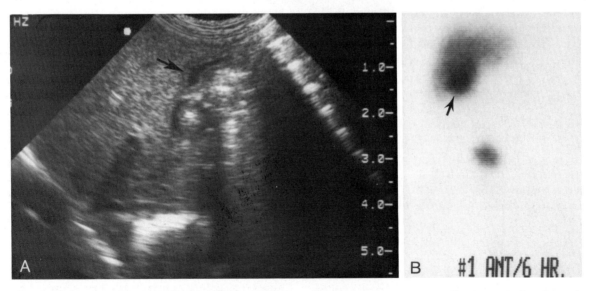

Figure 45.36.   Neonatal Hepatitis. A. Ultrasound identified a small gallbladder (*arrow*) and no evidence of dilated bile ducts. **B.** Nuclear scintigraphy favors hepatitis, demonstrating delayed excretion of the tracer and a small amount of activity in the GI tract (*arrow*).

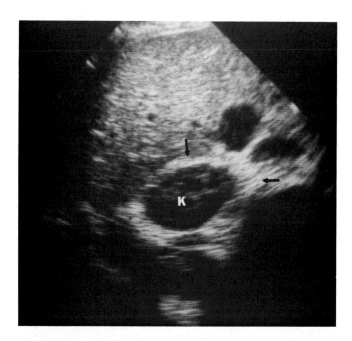

Figure 45.37. Pancreatitis. Note the prominent echogenicity of the perirenal fat (*arrows*). K, kidney.

Table 45.7. Causes of GI Bleeding

Peptic ulcer disease
Enterocolitis
    Necrotizing enterocolitis
    Milk allergy
    Hirschsprung's disease
    Regional enteritis
    Ulcerative colitis
Hemorrhagic gastritis of the newborn
Anal fissures
Bleeding disorders
Henoch-Schönlein purpura
Hemolytic uremic syndrome
Juvenile polyps
Meckel's diverticulum
Intussusception
Portal vein thrombosis

tion is encountered, the laceration itself is hypoechoic. This finding also is clearly demonstrable with CT. The gold standard for the detection of acute pancreatitis is the serum amylase level. In more severe cases, peripancreatic extravasation of lipase may cause lipolysis and increased echogenicity of otherwise undetectable fat. Infants and children do not have a great deal of abdominal fat; therefore, when echogenic fat is seen between the right lobe of the liver and the right kidney in a patient with suspected pancreatitis, the diagnosis should be strongly suggested (Fig. 45.37). Severe, emphysematous pancreatitis is not common in children, but complications such as chronic relapsing pancreatitis and pancreatic duct ectasia can occur. Pancreatic pseudocysts are the most common complication of pancreatitis, and ultra-

sound is very useful for both detection and follow-up of such pseudocysts (Fig. 45.38).

MESENTERIC ADENITIS

This condition is difficult to diagnose because it mimics appendicitis. Until ultrasound was available, acutely enlarged lymph nodes were not routinely identified in the abdomen. More recently, enlarged lymph nodes in the right lower quadrant, the usual site of mesenteric adenitis, have been readily delineated and, in the absence of an abnormal appendix, should suggest the diagnosis (Fig. 45.39). These lymph nodes are larger than normal and with color flow Doppler ultrasound, increased blood flow can be demonstrated. The usual form of mesenteric adenitis is a self-limiting condition with no complications. So-called giant mesenteric adenitis can produce a mass-like lesion in the right lower quadrant with considerable distortion of the terminal ileum and cecum.

Gastrointestinal Bleeding

The causes of GI bleeding in patients in the pediatric age group are numerous and vary widely, depending upon the age of the patient (Table 45.7). In the neonate, inflammatory conditions are relatively common and include necrotizing enterocolitis, milk allergy, and the enterocolitis that sometime accompanies Hirschsprung's disease. Ulcer disease and hemorrhagic gastritis are not uncommon in the newborn and are often associated with hypoxemia and/or sepsis. Anal fissures are a common cause of rectal bleeding.

In older infants and children, peptic ulcer disease is an important cause of upper GI tract bleeding and is probably more common in children than has been previously realized. Coagulopathies and other bleeding disorders can occasionally result in intestinal hematomas and bleeding. Henoch-Schönlein purpura is a condition due to a vasculitis of unknown etiology that mainly affects the skin, GI tract, joints, and kidneys. In approximately one-half of cases, crampy abdominal pain and intestinal bleeding occur. Ultrasound is a fairly sensitive method for detecting the affected loops of bowel (12), which usually demonstrate segmental and circumferential thickening of the bowel wall (Fig. 45.40). It is not uncommon for the abdominal symptoms to precede the more characteristic skin rash. Bloody diarrhea is also a common component of the hemolytic uremic syndrome in young children, and GI bleeding may also be the presenting symptom in patients with unsuspected portal vein thrombosis.

Rectal bleeding in older children is most often due to juvenile polyps. Such polyps are thought to be inflammatory and most commonly occur in the rectum and sigmoid colon, although other parts of the colon

Figure 45.38. Pancreatic Pseudocyst. Posttraumatic pancreatitis in this battered child was complicated by the development of a large lobulated pseudocyst (C). *P,* pancreas.

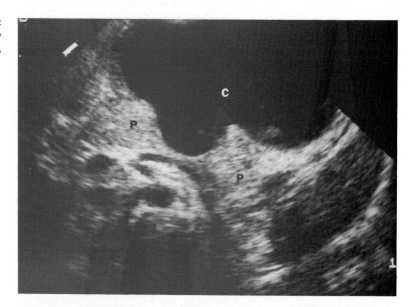

Figure 45.39. Mesenteric Adenitis. Note the multiple enlarged, hypoechoic lymph nodes (*arrows*) that were seen on ultrasound of the right lower quadrant.

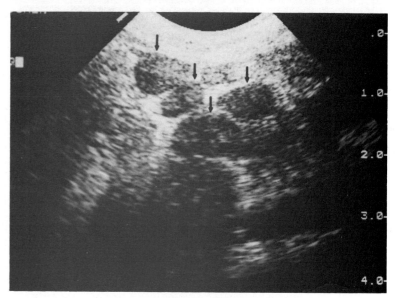

can also be affected. Painless rectal bleeding also may occur with Meckel's diverticulum, and in some cases the bleeding may be profuse. Meckel's diverticulum arises from the antimesenteric border of the ileum, approximately 80 cm from the ileocecal valve. Twenty to 30% of these diverticula contain ectopic gastric or pancreatic tissue that may be complicated by ulceration, hemorrhage, and perforation. Although a barium small bowel examination can sometimes demonstrate the diverticulum, the best initial examination to identify a bleeding Meckel's diverticulum is a ^{99m}Tc pertechnate scan. The tracer localizes in the ectopic gastric mucosa (Fig. 45.41); therefore, the examination may miss diverticula that do not contain such mucosa. Intussusception is an important cause of painful hematochezia in young children, and inflammatory bowel disease such as regional enteritis also causes GI bleeding.

GENITOURINARY TRACT

Normal Anatomy

Neonatal kidneys are proportionately larger and more lobulated than kidneys in older children and adults. In addition, on ultrasound the medullary pyramids usually are quite hypoechoic and, in the early days of ultrasound, falsely suggested cystic kidney (Fig. 45.42**A**). In addition, the renal parenchyma in infants under 2 or 3 months of age normally is more echogenic than in older children and adults. Indeed, it approaches the echogenicity of the liver (Fig. 45.42**B**). Otherwise, the kidneys appear the same as in adults.

Newborn female infants generally have a prominent uterus as a result of estrogen secretion by the mother (Fig. 45.43**A**). The uterus remains enlarged for 2 or 3 months and then involutes and remains small until

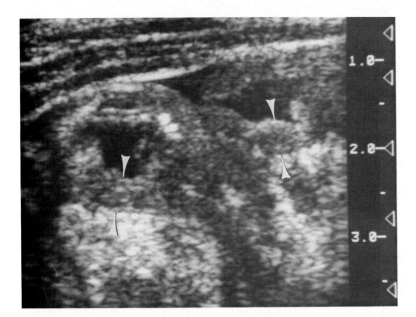

Figure 45.40. Henoch-Schönlein Purpura—Ultrasound Findings. Note the marked echogenic thickening of the bowel wall due to mucosal and submucosal edema and hemorrhage (*arrows*).

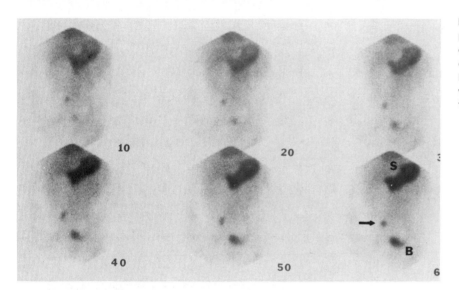

Figure 45.41. Meckel's Diverticulum. A scan performed with ⁹⁹ᵐTc-pertechnate shows an abnormal collection of tracer in the right lower quadrant (*arrow*), the intensity of which parallels that of the stomach (*S*). Gastric mucosa within the diverticulum is responsible for the tracer localization. *B*, bladder.

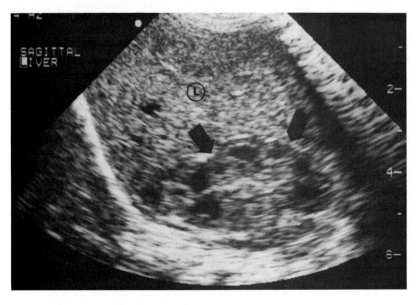

Figure 45.42. Normal Neonatal Kidney. Note the lobulated appearance of the kidney (*arrows*) and the sonolucent medullary pyramids, which often are misinterpreted for cysts. Echogenicity of the kidney is similar to that of the liver (*L*) and is normal.

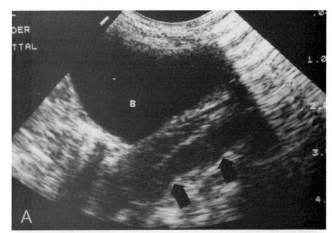

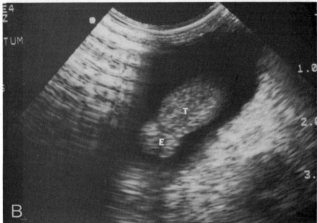

Figure 45.43. Genital Tract. A. Normal prominent uterus in neonate. Note the prominent, enlarged uterus *(arrows)* in this newborn female infant. *B,* bladder. **B.** Prominent epididymis in neonate. Note the testicle *(T)* and prominent epididymis *(E)*. The testicle is surrounded by a hydrocele.

puberty. In males, the main difference in the genital tract is that the epididymis in neonates and young infants is larger than in older children and adults (Fig. 45.43**B**). Apart from these differences, the anatomic features of the genitourinary tract in infants and children is about the same as in adults.

Urinary Tract Infections

Urinary tract infection is a common problem in infants and children; it is more common in females. Usually due to an ascending infection originating in the lower urinary tract, if unchecked, the infection can lead to chronic reflux, scarring, and general growth impairment of the kidneys. In neonates, urinary tract infection more often accompanies generalized sepsis, and the infection usually is hematogenous. In older infants and children, in both females and males, obstructive uropathy can lead to urinary tract infection. This is perhaps more common a problem in males. Isolated cystitis is not an uncommon problem and may be bacterial or viral. It is manifest

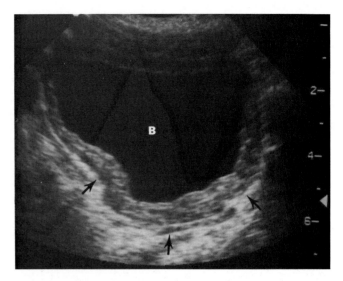

Figure 45.44. Cystitis. Note the thickened bladder wall *(arrows)*. The bladder *(B)* is filled with anechoic urine.

primarily by thickening of the mucosa of the bladder, which is best demonstrated with ultrasound and cystourethrography (Fig. 45.44).

Lobar Nephronia (Acute Bacterial Focal Nephritis). In most cases of urinary tract infection without obstructive uropathy, the kidneys are normal. One may rarely encounter a focal nephritis (lobar nephronia) and, in these cases, an echogenic area may be defined with ultrasound. Such areas often are best demonstrated with glomerular imaging agents such as ^{99m}Tc glucoheptonate and ^{99m}Tc 2,3-dimercaptosuccinic acid (DMSA). Lobar nephronia, however, is not the most common problem, and indeed tends to be a one-time event. More commonly, the problem is repetitive and refractory urinary tract infection, and in such a case one should look for underlying reflux and/or structural abnormality.

Reflux Nephropathy. Sterile, familial reflux is said to lead to renal growth impairment, scarring, and atrophy; most often, however, such renal damage occurs when infection also is present. In familial or sporadic sterile reflux, the problem is believed to be due to abnormal insertion of the ureter into the bladder, resulting in the so-called golf hole orifice. For this reason, it has been suggested that siblings of patients with refractory reflux be evaluated for the presence of reflux whether they are infected or not.

With both the golf hole ureteral orifice and infection, reflux results from the abnormal insertion of the distal ureter into the bladder. Normally, the ureter inserts at a slant and, as the bladder distends and its wall stretches, a valve-like mechanism compresses the distal ureter and thus prevents reflux. With the congenital golf hole urethral orifice, the ureter enters more horizontally (Fig. 45.45) and the valve-like mechanism is lost. With infection, the abnormal entry

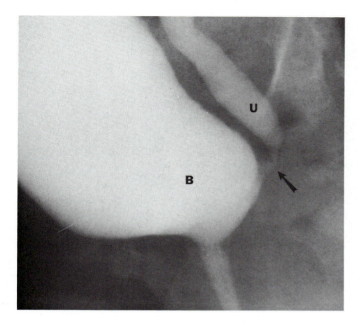

Figure 45.45. Horizontal Ureteral Insertion with Reflux. Note the horizonal insertion of the distal ureter (*arrow*) into the bladder (*B*). The ureter (*U*) is dilated because of reflux.

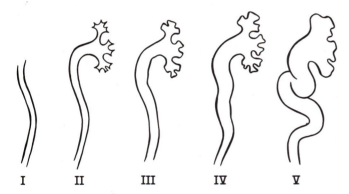

I   II   III   IV   V

Figure 45.46. Classification of Reflux. Grade I occurs into the distal ureter. Grade II into the upper collecting system with no dilation of the upper tract. Grade III reflux shows similar findings, but there is mild blunting of the calyces. All of these findings are exaggerated in Grade IV reflux, where considerable hydroureter and calyceal dilatation occur. Grade V reflux occurs when the ureter is massively dilated and tortuous and the upper tract are markedly dilated. (International classification modified after Levit SB. Medical versus surgical treatment of primary vesicoeueteral reflux: report of the International Reflux Study Committee. Pediatrics 1981;67:392–400.)

of the ureter results from bladder wall thickening. The same phenomenon occurs with the so-called Hutch diverticulum, a periureteral bladder diverticulum that is associated with vesicoureteral reflux and infection.

Urinary tract reflux can be evaluated both with voiding cystourethrography and nuclear scintigraphy (13, 14). The latter is more sensitive, but provides no anatomic definition, while the former provides precise anatomic definition. Since evaluation of the urethra is not usually important in females and important in

males only with the first episode of infection (i.e., to rule out posterior urethral valves, etc.), nuclear scintigraphy often is favored, except for the first study in males. Reflux often is graded from I through V (Fig. 45.46). Grade I reflux is of questionable significance and occurs only into the ureter. Grade II reflux reaches the kidney, but there is no dilation of the collecting system. Grade III reflux requires the presence of distension of the collecting system, while grade IV reflux is indicative of gross dilation of the urinary tract. Marked tortuosity of the ureter with gross hydroureter and hydronephrosis signify the presence of grade V reflux. Grades I through III reflux patterns usually can be treated medically with prolonged prophylactic administration of antibiotics. Grades IV and V reflux usually require surgical correction with tailoring and/or reimplantation of the ureter.

Renal Abscess is relatively uncommon in children but is very adequately demonstrated with both ultrasonography and CT (Fig. 45.47). The features are those of a round or oval cystic-like structure that may contain echogenic debris. Multiple renal abscesses are less common but can be seen, especially in immunocompromised patients and particularly in those with HIV infection. These patients also are prone to fungal infection, including candidiasis. Fungal infection can lead to complete impaction of the calyces, pelvis, and ureter and result in anuria. Hydropyonephrosis is uncommon but is readily demonstrated with ultrasound, where the dilated renal pelvis and calyces will be seen to contain abundant debris.

Renal Parenchymal Disease

A number of parenchymal conditions can be encountered in childhood, and virtually all lead to increased ultrasonographic echogenicity of the renal parenchyma (Fig. 45.48). Interestingly enough, however, in acute glomerulonephritis, the ultrasonographic echogenicity of the kidneys usually is normal. Similarly, in the nephrotic syndrome echogenicity is relatively normal in most cases, but the kidneys frequently appear plump and swollen. In the neonatal period, acute tubular necrosis can transiently produce marked echogenicity of the kidneys. The condition is self-limiting but common and can involve the tubules in the cortex, or appear only in the medulla (Fig. 45.46, **B** and **C**). There is little point in elaborating on the various conditions that can produce increased echogenicity of the kidneys in childhood as they are the same as in adulthood, and eventually renal biopsy is required for diagnosis.

Occasionally, a sonographic pattern of hyperechogenicity involving only the renal medullary pyramids is encountered. Most conditions causing this appearance are associated with hypercalciuria and include renal tubular acidosis, long-term furosemide

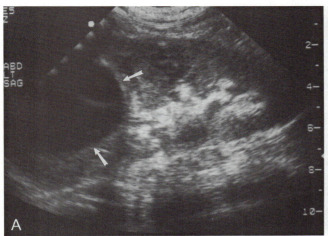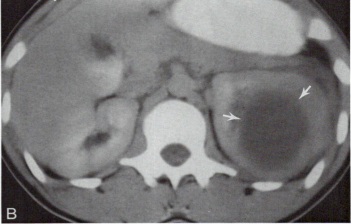

Figure 45.47. Renal Abscess—Ultrasound Findings. A. Note the anechoic abscess (*arrows*) in the upper pole of the left kidney. **B.** A CT study with contrast enhancement also demonstrates the abscess (*arrows*) in the generally enlarged left kidney. Compare with the normal right kidney on the other side.

therapy, medullary sponge kidney, Bartter's syndrome, and other hypercalcemic states such as hyperparathyroidism and Williams syndrome (15). A similar appearance has also been seen in the transient renal insufficiency of infancy and sickle cell hemoglobinopathy.

Hydronephrosis

Hydronephrosis can result from obstructive uropathy, ureterovesicular reflux, or simple volume overload of the collecting system. The latter is rare and occurs with Bartter's syndrome, diabetes insipidus, and psychogenic water drinking. Reflux has been discussed earlier in this chapter. Urinary tract obstruction can be located anywhere from the renal pelvis to the urethra, and perhaps the most common site is at the ureteropelvic junction. Ureteropelvic junction obstruction is congenital in origin and usually results from a short stenotic area of the ureter just at the ureteropelvic junction. It is believed to result from an intrauterine vascular insult and may be bilateral or unilateral. Characteristically, there is calyceal and renal pelvic dilation with no dilation of the ureter (Fig. 45.49**A**). The problem is vividly demonstrated with any imaging modality but is most often first identified with ultrasound. The degree of obstruction can be assessed with furosemide washout nuclear scintigraphy (Fig. 45.49, **B to D**). Stenosis of the ureter distal to the ureteropelvic junction is uncommon. Total megaureter usually results from stenosis of the distal ureter just as it enters the bladder or from gross reflux. With gross reflux, the distal ureter is widely patent, while with primary megaureter it is narrowed (Fig. 45.50). Hydronephrosis secondary to lower urinary tract problems will be discussed later in this chapter. However, the most common cause is posterior urethral valves in males.

Renal Anomalies of Position and Number

Incomplete duplication and positional abnormalities of the kidneys, such as ectopic and horseshoe kidneys, appear no different than they do in adults. They are readily demonstrated with ultrasound, occasionally with CT, and often, for confirmation, with retrograde pyelography. There is, however, one entity that is of prime consideration, as it most commonly presents in infancy. The problem consists of a completely duplicated kidney and ureter associated with ectopic positioning of the ureter from the upper kidney and a ureterocele (i.e., ectopic ureterocele). Simple ureteroceles also occur in children, but ectopic ureterocele is more common and usually occurs in females. The upper kidney may be hydronephrotic (Fig. 45.51**A**) or atrophic, and when atrophic may be difficult to visualize. However, the typical, round, oval, or lobulated ureterocele is classic (Fig. 45.51**B**). The ureterocele may be flaccid or turgid, and when flaccid can be made to disappear with the pressures generated during voiding cystourethrography. Therefore, ultrasound is the modality of choice for demonstration of the ureterocele, while cystourethrography and retrograde pyelography are utilized to evaluate the ureters. With the cystogram, reflux into the lower pole ureter may be seen (Fig. 45.51**C**), while with retrograde pyelography the dilated, tortuous, obstructed ectopic ureter is defined. The ectopic ureter most commonly inserts into the bladder but can insert into the urethra, or even the vagina, leading to chronic dribbling.

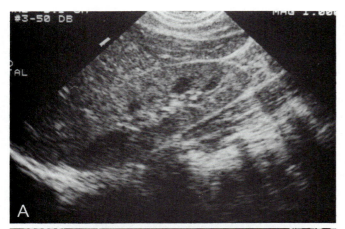

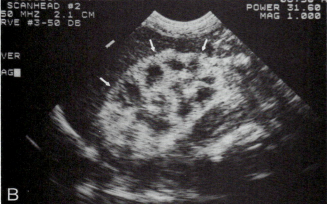

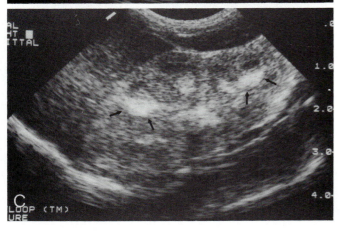

Figure 45.48. Diffuse Renal Parenchymal Disease. A. Increased echogenicity of the renal cortex (*arrows*) in a patient with hemolytic uremic syndrome. **B.** Generally increased echogenicity of a neonatal kidney (*arrows*) due to acute tubular necrosis. Note the sonolucent medullary pyramids. **C.** In this neonate, medullary necrosis is manifest by increased echogenicity of the medullary pyramids (*arrows*). Both with neonatal cortical and medullary necrosis, the problem usually is transient.

Renal Vascular Disease

Renal vein disease is more common than renal artery disease in children. Renal vein thrombosis is most common in the neonatal period and is the result of dehydration and/or sepsis. Indeed, these are the common denominators for most cases of renal vein thrombosis throughout the pediatric age group. Renal vein thrombosis also commonly is seen with the nephrotic syndrome due to the hypercoagulable state of these patients. In any case, the findings are no different than those seen in adults and consist of enlargement of the kidney, loss of its normal architecture on ultrasonography, and the presence of a thrombus in the inferior vena cava and the renal veins. Ultrasonography with color flow Doppler usually provides the diagnosis. Renal arterial disease also can be evaluated with color flow Doppler ultrasound, but eventually usually requires arteriography. Congenital stenoses of the renal arteries are uncommon in childhood, but do occur. Such stenoses are not an uncommon feature of neurofibromatosis. Renal artery thrombosis is generally uncommon in the pediatric age group.

Renal Agenesis, Hypoplasia, and Atrophy

Unilateral renal agenesis, hypoplasia, or atrophy may be entirely asymptomatic or associated with systemic hypertension. Bilateral renal agenesis results in Potter's syndrome. Because of the renal agenesis there is decreased output of urine, oligohydramnios, and fetal compression by the uterus, leading to the characteristic deformities and hypoplastic lungs of the Potter's syndrome. The hypoplastic lungs result from compression of the fetal thorax and, for this reason, the condition usually is lethal. At birth, the infant presents with severe respiratory distress and refractory pneumothoraces. When imaging these infants it is important to note that the adrenal glands often appear relatively large and lose their usual triangular shape, and may be mistaken for normal kidneys (Fig. 45.52).

Renal atrophy usually results from long-standing urinary tract infection and reflux. The greatest risk exists when reflux occurs under the age of 2 years. It seems that later in childhood, even though reflux and infection may be present, there is much less of a chance for renal damage resulting in hypoplasia to occur. Atrophy also can result from a vascular insult to the kidney, but not nearly as often as from infection and reflux.

Renal Cystic Disease

The classification of renal cystic disease constantly undergoes change, but basically one is dealing with simple renal cysts, infantile and juvenile (autosomal recessive) cystic disease, adult or autosomal dominant renal cystic disease, multicystic dysplastic kidney, multilocular cystic disease, medullary cystic disease, and a few miscellaneous entities (16). Because of the common use of ultrasound in the investigation of re-

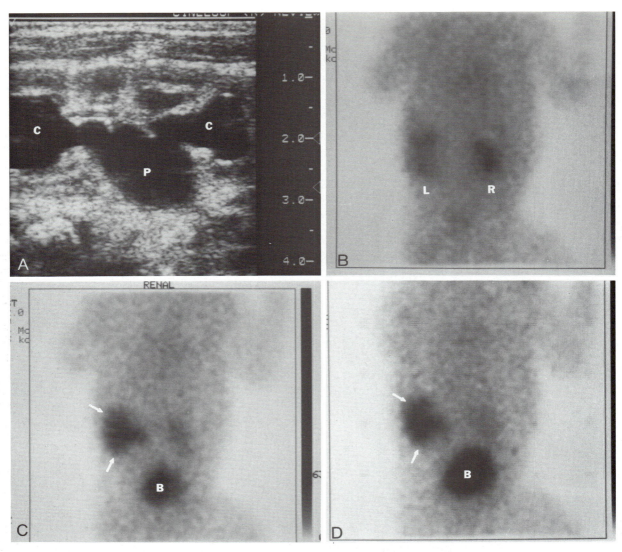

Figure 45.49. Ureteropelvic Junction Obstruction. A. Sonogram demonstrating a dilated renal pelvis (*P*) and markedly dilated renal calyces (*C*). **B.** Nuclear scintigraphy, early phase, demonstrates activity in both the right (*R*) and left (*L*) kidneys. Note that there is less activity in the left kidney. **C.** Fifteen minutes later, there is marked accumulation of radioactive tracer in the left kidney (*arrows*); some is now accumulating in the bladder (*B*). The right kidney has washed out and is normal. **D.** After the administration of furosemide there is no activity seen in the right kidney, increased activity is seen in the bladder (*B*), and there is persistent marked activity in the obstructed left kidney (*arrow*).

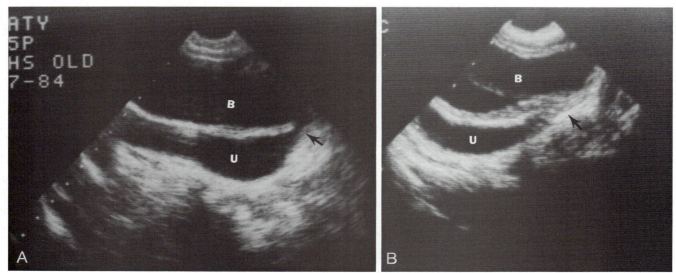

Figure 45.50. Megaureter. A. Primary megaureter can be diagnosed when the dilated ureter (*U*) demonstrates a persistently spastic distal segment (*arrow*). *B*, urinary bladder. **B.** Refluxing ureter demonstrates similar dilation of the ureter (*U*), but the distal end is open (*arrow*). *B*, urinary bladder. (From Hayden CK Jr, Swischuk LE. Pediatric ultrasonography, 2nd ed. Baltimore: Williams & Wilkins, 1992.

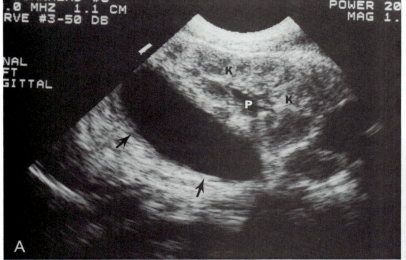

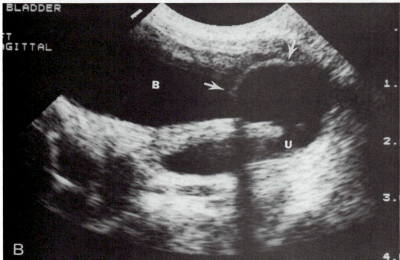

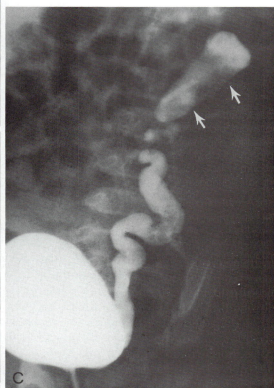

Figure 45.51. Ectopic Ureterocele. A. Sagittal sonogram through the left kidney demonstrates a hydronephrotic upper pole (*arrows*) and a compressed lower renal segment (*K*). *P*, renal pelvis. **B.** Sagittal sonogram through the urinary bladder (*B*) demonstrates the distended ureterocele (*arrows*) projecting into the bladder base. Note the dilated ureter (*U*) as it inserts into the ureterocele. **C.** Cystogram demonstrates reflux into the tortuous ureter, which then leads to the dilated upper segment (*arrows*). This is the same segment as demonstrated in the upper pole of the kidney in **A.**

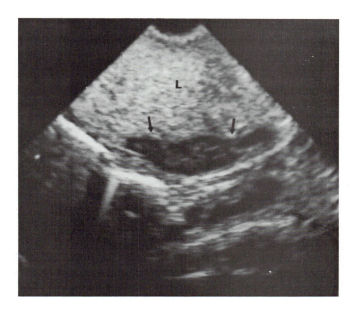

Figure 45.52. Renal Agenesis. In this patient with bilateral renal agenesis (Potter's syndrome), the large but normal adrenal gland (*arrows*) may erronously suggest the presence of a kidney. *L*, liver.

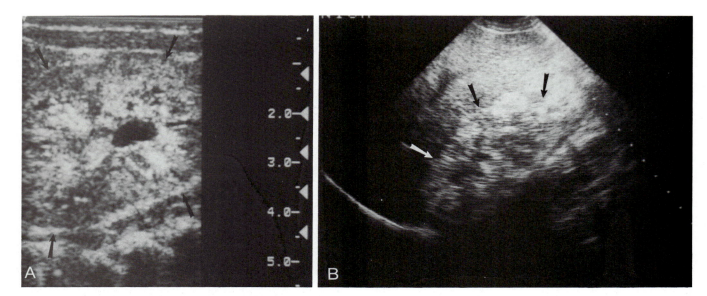

Figure 45.53. Polycystic Kidney Disease. A. Infantile polycystic kidney disease (autosomal recessive). Note the enlarged echogenic kidney (*arrows*) with suggestion of radiating dilated tubules and small scattered cysts. **B.** Juvenile polycystic kidney disease (autosomal recessive). Note the enlarged and highly echogenic kidney (*arrows*). Individual tubular structures and cysts generally are not visualized.

nal disease in general, it is realized that simple renal cysts are more common in infancy and childhood than previously suspected. Their identification and appearance is the same as in adults.

Autosomal Recessive (Infantile) Polycystic Kidney Disease is characterized by bilaterally enlarged kidneys with dilated renal tubules. These are arranged in a radiating pattern and can be identified with ultrasound. In the past, delayed intravenous pyelography was required for their demonstration. Sonographically, these kidneys are echogenic and, depending upon the degree of tubular dilation, the tubules may be identified as individual structures (Fig. 45.53**A**). In the juvenile form of this disease, the kidneys usually are markedly echogenic (Fig. 45.53**B**) but the individual dilated tubules are less distinct. Hepatic fibrosis is common in this disease and, in the juvenile form, usually predominates, leading to liver cirrhosis and varices. Conversely, the patients presenting in infancy demonstrate more severe renal disease.

Autosomal Dominant (Adult) Polycystic Kidney Disease may also present in the neonatal period with bilateral renal enlargement and marked echogenicity of the kidneys. The dilated tubules characteristic of the recessive form are not identified. One may occasionally identify a few small cysts scattered throughout the kidney (Fig. 45.54**A**). Later in life these cysts become larger and variable in size (Fig. 45.54, **B** and **C**). This condition is associated with cystic disease of other organs, primarily the liver and pancreas, and, as opposed to infantile polycystic kidney disease, renal function in childhood is normal.

Multicystic Dysplastic Kidney is the most common form of cystic disease to present in the neonatal period. Usually it is unilateral but can be bilateral or even segmental. This condition is entirely asymptomatic and discovered only because of a palpable abdominal mass. Characteristically, numerous small-to-large cysts are identified in the kidney with variable amounts of intervening dysplastic renal parenchyma (Fig. 45.55). These kidneys, in the past, were routinely removed, but currently the tendency to watch them for involution is common. Multicystic dysplastic kidneys are believed to result from an early fetal insult to the ureteropelvic junction resulting in fetal hydronephrosis, destruction of the kidney, and eventual cystic dysplasia. If the obstruction occurs later in gestation, some renal parenchyma remains and the problem manifests as giant hydronephrosis. The two entities, however, are intimately related.

Multilocular Cystic Disease of the kidney is a segmental entity that is closely related to Wilms' tumor. Other names for this condition include multilocular cysts, benign nephroma, cystic hamartoma, cystic lymphangioma, and cystic Wilms' tumor. The typical appearance of this form of cystic kidney disease is a unilateral mass composed of multiple cysts separated by very thin septae. In addition, a characteristic crescent of normal residual renal tissue can be seen (Fig. 45.56).

Medullary sponge kidney seldom presents in childhood and when it does, the findings are no different from those seen in adulthood. However, medullary cystic disease (familial nephronophthisis) frequently presents in infancy and early childhood. It is charac-

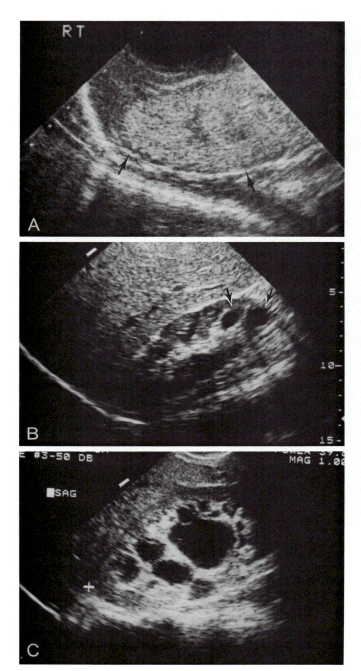

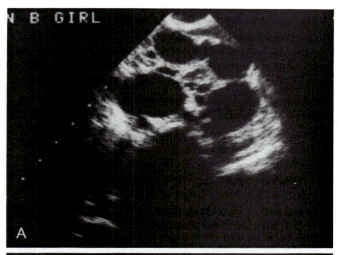

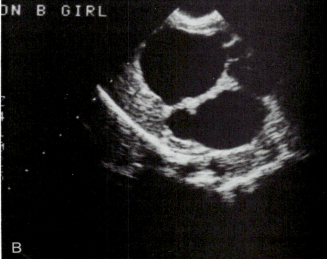

Figure 45.55. Multicystic Dysplastic Kidney. A. The entire kidney in this infant has been replaced by variable-sized sonolucent cysts. **B.** On another view, some of these cysts appear much larger. Note that there is considerable intervening soft tissue present.

Figure 45.54. Adult Polycystic Kidney Disease (Autosomal Dominant). A. In the neonate, these kidneys often appear enlarged and diffusely echogenic (*arrows*). Small cysts may be seen, generally under 3 or 4 mm in diameter. **B.** Findings in an older child, demonstrating two small cysts (*arrows*) in the lower pole of the right kidney. **C.** On the left, however, there are numerous variable-sized cysts throughout the entire kidney.

terized by small, echogenic kidneys with a few scattered medullary or corticomedullary cysts (Fig. 45.57). Glomerulocystic disease, a rare entity, manifests in enlarged echogenic kidneys whose renal function remains intact.

Multiple renal cysts can also be seen in a variety of syndromes such as tuberous sclerosis, Conradi's disease, Zellweger's syndrome, and Turner's syndrome.

Urinary Tract Calcifications

Renal calculi are more common in infants and children than originally believed. In the past it was believed that some underlying metabolic abnormality had to be present before renal stones would develop. This has been proven to be untrue and many children have renal calculi without underlying metabolic disease. The identification and other features of these calculi are no different in children than in adults. Intravenous pyelography often is used to define these calcifications if they produce hydronephrosis and renal colic, but they also can be identified with ultrasound. Diffuse nephrocalcinosis often is seen with

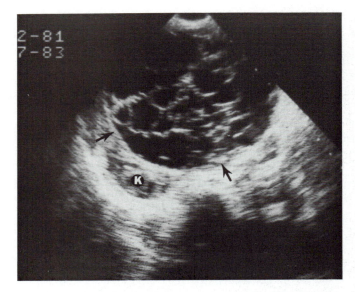

Figure 45.56.   Multilocular Cystic Disease (Cystic Wilms' Tumor). Note the large cystic lesion of the kidney (*arrows*). There is very little intervening soft tissue between the various cysts. In addition, the cysts are more uniform in size. Note the compressed crescent of normal kidney parenchyma (*K*).

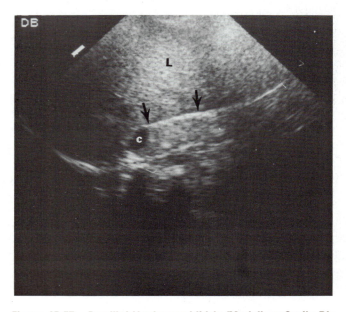

Figure 45.57.   Familial Nephronophthisis (Medullary Cystic Disease). Note the small echogenic kidney (*arrows*) with no semblance of normal architecture. A small cyst (*C*) is seen in its upper pole. *L*, liver.

renal tubular acidosis (distal tubules), chronic glomerulonephritis, or oxalosis, but can occur with any cause of systemic hypercalcemia. Nephrocalcinosis can appear smooth and homogenous throughout the parenchyma or be more punctate.

Large Kidneys

Unilateral enlargement of a kidney usually results from hydronephrosis, multicystic dysplastic kidney, renal vein thrombosis, or renal tumors. Bilateral renal enlargement can be seen with hydronephrosis, polycystic kidney disease, storage diseases, and with certain glomerulonephropathies, including the nephrotic syndrome. Bilateral renal enlargement due to neoplasms is less common, although leukemia or lymphoma may infiltrate the renal parenchyma.

Nephroblastomatosis. Small islands of primitive metanephric blastema, which are thought to be the precursor of Wilm's tumor, commonly exist in the kidneys of the fetus and newborn infant. These small collections of primitive cells usually spontaneously regress by 4 months of age. A diffuse and proliferative form of persistent renal blastema can also occur and is referred to as nephroblastomatosis. The abnormal tissue can occur as multifocal discrete nodules within the renal parenchyma or may completely replace the renal cortex. The classic appearance of nephroblastomatosis on CT or intravenous pyelogram is that of bilateral lobulated and enlarged kidneys with marked compression, stretching, and distortion of the pelvicalyceal structures (Fig. 45.58). Sonographically, these kidneys appear as enlarged lobular, echogenic kidneys or as enlarged kidneys with diffuse hypoechoic thickening of the cortex. Small, focal deposits are often difficult to visualize by ultrasound and are better evaluated with contrast-enhanced CT (17).

Bladder and Urethral Abnormalities

Cystitis and vesicoureteral reflux have been discussed earlier in this chapter and this section deals primarily with other abnormalities of the bladder and urethra. Bladder tumors are relatively uncommon in children, but can be seen. Often these are rhabdomyosarcomas, and in males, commonly are from the prostate gland. Generally they present early in infancy and are quite large. Diverticula of the bladder can take the form of a persistent urachal remnant over the dome of the bladder, Hutch diverticula at the ureterovesicle junction (associated with reflux), or generalized diverticula due to chronic obstruction or neurologic disease. Bladder diverticula also are a common feature of the cutis laxa syndrome. Extrophy of the bladder is readily recognized clinically and radiographic findings consist primarily of widening of the symphysis pubis and splaying of the pelvic bones.

Prune Belly Syndrome. A large, patulous bladder is often seen in the prune belly (Eagle-Barrett) syndrome. Clinically, these patients demonstrate absence of the abdominal musculature, and it has been suggested that the muscular abnormality may be secondary to chronic intrauterine abdominal distension.

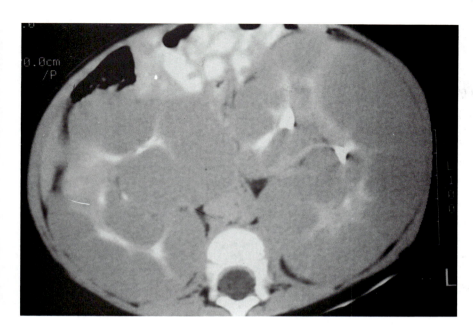

Figure 45.58. Nephroblastomatosis. In this condition, the kidneys are massively enlarged with lobulated thickening of the parenchyma and stretching and compression of the collecting structures.

The enlarged bladder is associated with marked vesicoureteral reflux and hydronephrosis, due to either anatomic or functional obstruction of the urethra. Cystography demonstrates the large, floppy bladder and massively dilated ureters (Fig. 45.59). Urachal remnants extending from the dome of the bladder are also common. This condition is almost exclusively a problem of male infants.

Posterior Urethral Valve. The most common cause of urethral obstruction in infants is a posterior urethral valve. Again almost exclusively a problem of male infants, it usually takes the form of a type I valve with obstruction below the verumontanum. In this condition, abnormal migration and insertion of the urethrovaginal folds result in a sail-like valve that leads to antigrade obstruction of the posterior urethra. The obstruction causes marked dilation of the posterior urethra, and bladder hypertrophy and trabeculation with associated vesicoureteral reflux (Fig. 45.60**A**). The type III valve, which is a transverse diaphragm of the posterior urethra, is less common but can also produce obstruction (Fig. 45.60**B**). The type II valve is rare and of questionable significance, or indeed, existence. Anterior urethral valves are less common.

Other causes of urethral obstruction, both congenital and acquired, are relatively infrequent in infants and children. However, functional obstruction secondary to a neurogenic bladder is common. The problem is no different than in adults, with some of the bladders appearing large and atonic, and others small, spastic, and contracted. These latter bladders show marked trabeculation and thickening of the bladder wall.

Ambiguous Genitalia

Ambiguous genitalia result from a number of states. Perhaps the most common cause is adrenal hyperplasia, where a normal female undergoes masculinization of the external genitalia. The clitoris enlarges but the vagina and uterus are present. The main role of imaging in intersex states centers around demonstrating the presence or absence of a vagina and uterus. This is best accomplished with ultrasonography, although retrograde vaginography may be required in some cases. In complex cases, virtually every orifice available on the perineum should be injected with contrast. Once the anatomy of the reproductive organs is known, attention is focused on the urinary tract. It is important to determine whether a urogenital sinus is present. In these cases, both the urethra and vagina empty into the sinus (Fig. 45.61). All of these features are important for surgical treatment and gender assignment, but a detailed discussion of the problem is beyond the scope of this book (18).

Testicular Abnormalities

The most common cause of a scrotal mass in childhood is a hydrocele (Fig. 45.62). Hydroceles may be congenital or may develop an association with testicular inflammation, trauma, or torsion. Ultrasound readily demonstrates the normal testicle surrounded by fluid. Inflammatory conditions of the testicles (epididymoorchitis) manifest in enlargement of the testicle and increased blood flow on color Doppler ultrasound imaging. The identification of such blood flow can help to distinguish orchitis from acute testicular torsion; an enlarged and inflamed testicle sec-

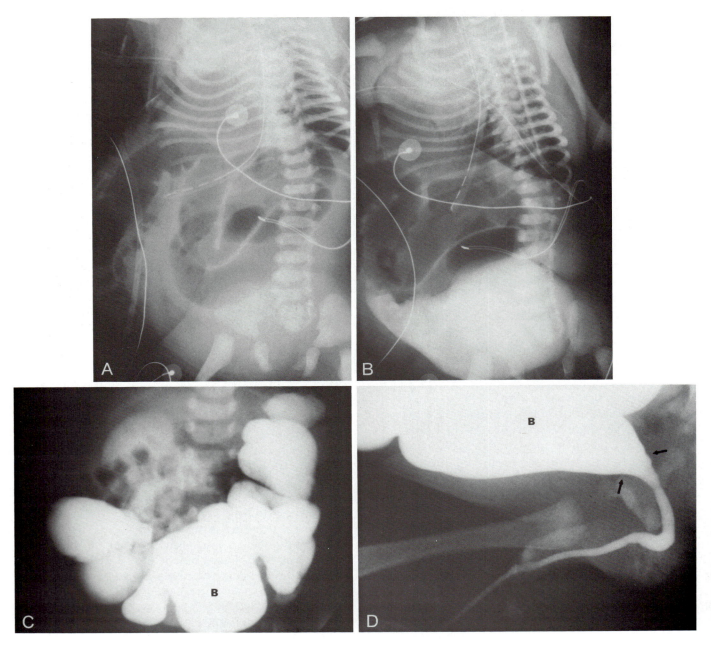

Figure 45.59.   Prune Belly Syndrome (Eagle-Barrett Syndrome).
A. Plain film demonstrates the large floppy abdomen. **B.** Retrograde cystogram demonstrates the large floppy urinary bladder in the lower abdomen. **C.** Another patient with a large bladder (*B*) and massive reflux into grossly dilated ureters and upper collecting systems on both sides. **D.** Lateral view of the bladder demonstrates the characteristic cone-shaped posterior urethra-bladder neck region (*arrows*). *B,* urinary bladder.

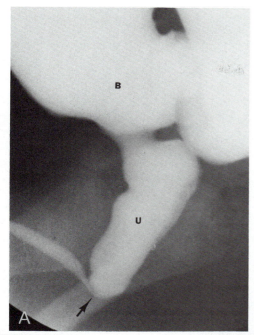

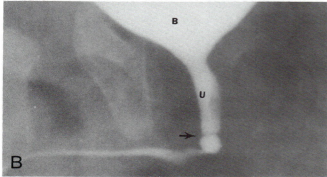

Figure 45.60. Posterior Urethral Valve. A. Typical sail, type I valve, producing obstruction of the distal posterior urethra (*arrow*). The valve itself is seldom visualized. *U*, dilated posterior urethra; *B*, urinary bladder. There also is massive reflux into the dilated ureters posterior to the bladder. **B.** Type III valve. Note the characteristic thin diaphram (*arrow*) in the distal posterior urethra. *U*, urethra; *B*, bladder.

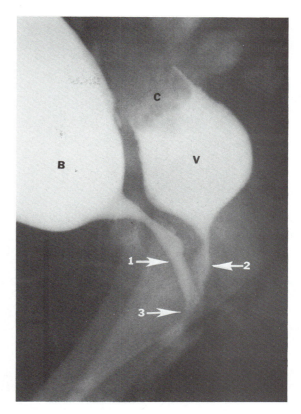

Figure 45.61. Urogenital Sinus. Note the urinary bladder (*B*), vagina (*V*), and the cervix (*C*). Also note the *arrows* showing the urethra (*1*), fistula (*2*), from the vagina to the short urogenital sinus (*3*).

ondary to testicular torsion demonstrates decreased blood flow within the testicle. The surrounding epididymis and tissues may demonstrate increased flow in cases of torsion, but the testicle itself will demonstrate decreased or absent flow (19, 20). Classically, testicular torsion is diagnosed with nuclear scintigraphy by lack of isotope accumulation within the testicle.

Congenital absence of the testis is uncommon, and usually nonpalpable testis is caused by an undescended testis. Most undescended testicles can be found in the inguinal region and are easily identified by ultrasound. Magnetic resonance imaging (MR) can also be used to detect a nonpalpable testis (Fig. 45.63)

and is particularly well suited for testicles that reside in the pelvis (21).

Testicular tumors are uncommon in childhood. The most common neoplasm is the infantile embyronal (yolk-sac) carcinoma. Although ultrasound can be used to verify the solid nature of a testicular mass, testicular tumors generally cannot be differentiated from one another sonographically.

ABDOMINAL MASSES

Abdominal masses are common in infants and children, and in most cases imaging plays an important role in the diagnosis and/or management of these masses. Plain radiographs are frequently obtained in the initial workup and, although they are seldom diagnostic, they can sometimes provide clues to the location of the mass and the presence of calcifications. Ultrasound is generally accepted as the most valuable procedure for the initial evaluation of pediatric abdominal masses. Ultrasound easily differentiates cystic from solid masses and commonly suggests the organ of origin and the diagnosis. Nevertheless, further imaging is often obtained, particularly in those cases in which the mass is large or poorly defined or in a location that is obscured by bowel gas. In such cases, either CT or MR can be used; CT is often favored when

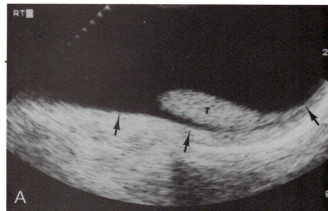

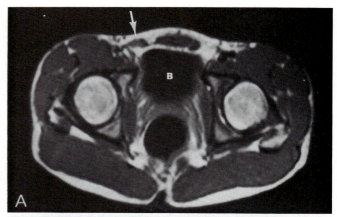

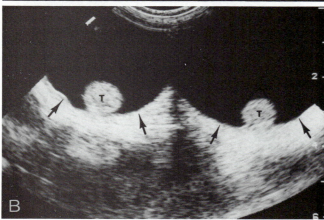

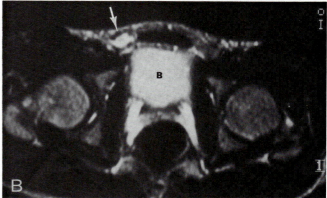

Figure 45.62.   Hydrocele. A. Lateral view demonstrates the large anechoic hydrocele (*arrows*) with the testicle (*T*) lying on its floor. **B.** Cross-sectional view demonstrates bilateral hydroceles (*arrows*). *T*, testicles.

Figure 45.63.   Ectopic Testicle. A. T1-weighted axial view of the inguinal region demonstrates the low-signal testicle (*arrow*) in the inguinal canal. *B*, urinary bladder. **B.** T2-weighted image demonstrates the testicle to be of high signal intensity (*arrow*). *B*, urinary bladder.

the mass is of renal origin, but MR is becoming increasingly popular. Angiography and radionuclide studies have limited applications.

True abdominal masses in children consist of a wide variety of cysts, neoplasms, and congenital and developmental abnormalities, and the location and ultrasound characteristics of the mass often determine the imaging approach. In addition to true masses, one should be aware of several common pseudomasses. A fluid-filled stomach, urinary bladder, or a loop of intestine is a common cause of a mass-like appearance on abdominal radiographs. The true nature of such masses is usually apparent when one is aware of their appearance, but when in doubt, ultrasound can be used for verification. Structures outside the abdomen, such as large skin lesions, umbilical hernias, and meningomyelocele, can also mimic an abdominal mass radiographically.

Renal and Adrenal Masses

The most common abdominal masses in infants and children are of renal origin and consistent primarily of kidneys that are enlarged due to hydronephrosis or cystic renal disease. These conditions are easily diagnosed with ultrasound and have been discussed earlier in this chapter. Simple cysts of the kidney are relatively uncommon in children. The sonographic findings of an anechoic mass with a thin, well-defined wall and through transmission are characteristic (22). Such cysts are usually of little consequence to the patient and rarely require further imaging.

Wilms' Tumor. A solid renal mass most commonly represents a neoplasm, and Wilms' tumor is the most common renal neoplasm of childhood. Wilms' tumor arises from the primitive metanephric epithelium and demonstrates widely varied histologies that have been classified into favorable and unfavorable groups. The survival rates in patients with Wilms' tumor are likewise widely variable, ranging from as high as 90% for tumors with favorable histology to very low survival in patients with the uncommon sarcomatous subtypes (clear cell sarcoma, malignant rhabdoid tumor). Most often, Wilms' tumor presents as a non-tender, rapidly growing, unilateral abdominal mass in

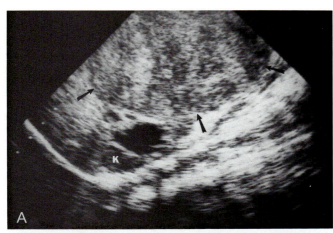

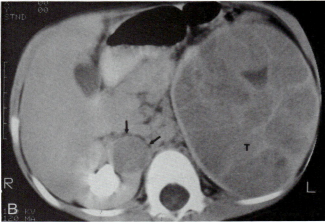

Figure 45.64.   Wilms' Tumor. A. Ultrasound demonstrates a large mass (*arrows*) with a heterogenous echotexture arising from the kidney (*K*). Note the hydronephrosis of the involved kidney. **B.** A CT scan shows the large, partially cystic Wilms' tumor (*T*) on the left, and identifies a smaller tumor mass in the contralateral kidney (*arrows*).

a young child with a mean age of presentation of 3 years. Aniridia, hemihypertrophy, Beckwith-Wiedemann syndrome, and the Drash syndrome have all been associated with Wilms' tumor. Wilms' tumor also arises with greater frequency in horseshoe and fused kidneys than in normal kidneys. Bilateral tumors are found in approximately 10% of patients, and bilateral disease seems to be associated with a better prognosis.

On ultrasound, Wilms' tumor characteristically is a well-defined, predominantly solid mass arising from the kidney (Fig. 45.64**A**). Frequently, hypoechoic or anechoic areas are present within the tumor because of necrosis. Hydronephrosis of the involved kidney is also commonly seen. Evaluation of the inferior vena cava and right atrium is important because this tumor has a propensity to extend into the renal vein and then into these structures. This can also be easily accomplished with ultrasonography.

Imaging in addition to ultrasound is obtained in most cases of Wilms' tumor, especially in those cases

where the tumor is large and the classic "claw sign" of an intrarenal mass is not clearly seen. In these cases, either CT or MR can be used. Such studies are also useful for excluding a mass in the contralateral kidney, which can occasionally be small and difficult to identify with ultrasound (Fig. 45.64**B**). Calcification is uncommon in Wilms' tumor, but occasionally amorphous calcifications occur.

Mesoblastic Nephroma.   The most common renal tumor of the neonate is mesoblastic nephroma. Like Wilms' tumor, mesoblastic nephroma probably also arises from the metanephric blastema, although it is most often a benign tumor. Sonographically, this tumor is indistinguishable from Wilms' tumor.

Other renal tumors are relatively rare in children. Renal cell carcinoma is very rare in young children, although it sometimes occurs in older children and adolescents. Like Wilms' tumor, renal cell carcinoma usually presents as an asymptomatic abdominal mass, although hematuria is sometimes present and frequently is gross. Hypertension is less common with renal cell carcinoma than with Wilms' tumor. The imaging characteristics of renal cell carcinoma are indistinguishable from Wilms' tumor. Angiomyolipoma is a benign tumor composed of immature blood vessels, muscle, and fat. This neoplasm is commonly associated with tuberous sclerosis. Other primary renal tumors are exceedingly rare. Metastatic disease to the kidneys is uncommon, although direct invasion of the kidneys by neuroblastoma is known to occur. Renal infiltration by leukemia or lymphoma may also occur.

One should be aware that infection can sometimes mimic a renal mass, usually in the form of a renal abscess or focal bacterial nephritis (lobar nephronia). These conditions were discussed earlier in the chapter.

Adrenal Hemorrhage.   Suprarenal masses most often arise from the adrenal gland and characteristically cause downward and outward displacement of the ipsilateral kidney. In the newborn, the most common cause of adrenal enlargement is adrenal hemorrhage. The exact cause of adrenal hemorrhage is not known; however, predisposing factors include large babies (e.g., infants of diabetic mothers, Beckwith-Wiedemann syndrome), obstetric trauma, neonatal sepsis, and hypoxia. Small hemorrhages may go unnoticed, but more commonly the infants present with an abdominal mass, jaundice, and anemia. Hemorrhage occurs more frequently on the right and is occasionally bilateral. Although adrenal hemorrhage most often occurs in the neonatal period, older children may develop adrenal hemorrhage due to trauma, meningococcemia, or anticoagulant therapy.

Ultrasound is an ideal modality for evaluating adrenal hemorrhage (23). The normal adrenal gland in the newborn is larger and more easily visualized than that

Figure 45.65.   Normal Adrenal Gland. Note the characteristic "Y" shape (*arrow*) of the normal adrenal gland sitting astride the kidney (*K*).

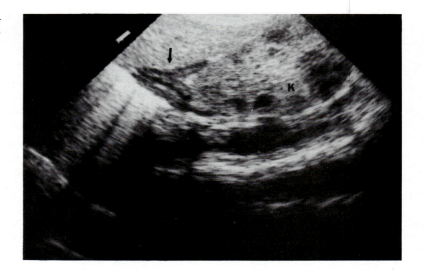

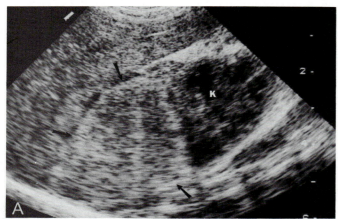

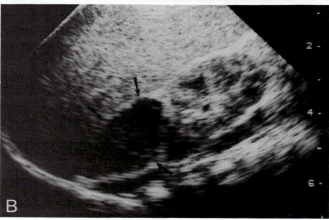

Figure 45.66.   Adrenal Hemorrhage—Ultrasound Findings. A. In the early stages, hemorrhage into the adrenal gland presents as an echogenic suprarenal mass (*arrows*) that displaces the kidney inferiorly (*K*). **B.** As the hemorrhage resolves, the clot becomes smaller and hypoechoic to anechoic (*arrows*).

of the adult. Sonographically, the gland appears as an inverted V-shaped structure superior to the upper pole of the kidney, with an echogenic central region and a peripheral hypoechoic zone (Fig. 45.65). Adre-

nal hemorrhage results in enlargement of the gland and loss of the characteristic V shape. Initially, the hematoma resembles a solid, highly echogenic mass (Fig. 45.66). As the hemorrhage begins to resolve, it becomes increasingly hypoechoic, starting in the central region and progressing peripherally. In most cases, the hematoma decreases in size within the 1st week and sometimes calcifies. The calcifications begin around the rim of the gland, but eventually a small, completely calcified gland remains. Although severe life-threatening adrenal hemorrhage can occur, most infants are not significantly affected by the hemorrhage and adrenal insufficiency rarely develops. Occasionally, adrenal hemorrhage may be complicated by compression of the ipsilateral kidney or by ipsilateral renal vein thrombosis. Rarely, the adrenal hemorrhage may become infected, creating an adrenal abscess.

Neuroblastoma.   The most common tumor arising from the adrenal gland is neuroblastoma, a neoplasm of neural crest origin (24–26). Neuroblastoma belongs to a group of related tumors that range from the benign ganglioneuroma to the malignant and aggressive neuroblastoma. Neuroblastoma may also arise from sympathetic ganglia in the retroperitoneum, posterior mediastinum, the neck, or the pelvis. This is predominantly a neoplasm of early childhood presenting in children less than 5 years of age.

Children with neuroblastoma most often present with advanced disease and large abdominal masses. The presenting symptoms are often related to metastatic disease or intraspinal extension. In contrast to Wilms' tumor, neuroblastomas are usually poorly marginated masses that frequently extend across the midline and into the chest. In some cases, the ipsilateral kidney is invaded, and when this occurs, the tumor can be mistaken for an intrarenal mass. Calcifications are much more common in neuroblastoma than in

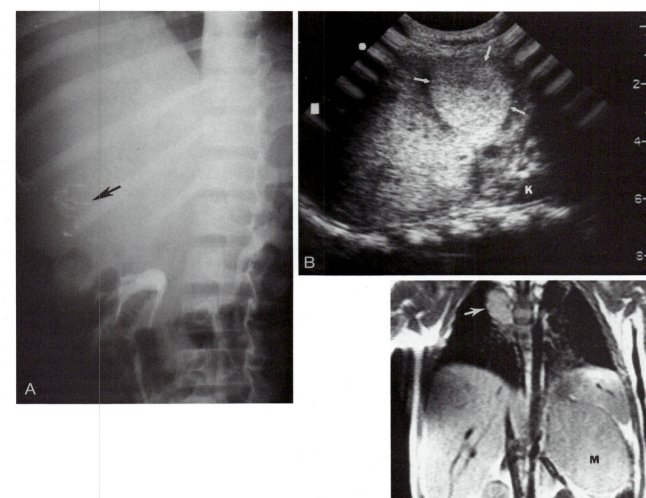

Figure 45.67 Neuroblastoma. A. Radiograph shows a large soft-tissue mass that displaces the right kidney inferiorly. Note the irregular, amorphous calcifications within the mass (*arrow*). **B.** On ultrasound, the mass demonstrates moderate echogenicity. Note the characteristic echogenic nodule within the mass (*arrows*). *K*, kidney. **C.** Magnetic resonance imaging also shows the large mass (*M*), displacing the left kidney. A second tumor mass is identified adjacent to the spine in the right upper hemithorax (*arrow*).

Wilms' tumor, with an incidence as high as 50–75% of cases (Fig. 45.67**A**).

As with other abdominal masses, ultrasound is an excellent screening examination for neuroblastoma. The ultrasound characteristics of this tumor are somewhat variable, but most neuroblastomas appear echogenic and heterogenous in texture. In some cases, a characteristic echogenic nodule can be identified within the larger part of the tumor mass (Fig. 45.67**B**). Because neuroblastoma is usually large and tends to invade surrounding structures, additional imaging is usually required to define the margins and extent of the tumor mass.

Both CT and MR can be used to better define the extent of neuroblastoma involvement and to detect metastatic deposits and intraspinal extension (Fig.

45.67**B**). Neuroblastoma frequently metastasizes to the liver and lymph nodes. Bone marrow infiltration also commonly occurs, and changes in marrow intensity in the vertebra and extremities is demonstrated on MR (27). Magnetic resonance imaging is also capable of demonstrating encasement and/or displacement of blood vessels by the tumor.

Skeletal metastases are also common with neuroblastoma; therefore, bone scintigraphy should also be included in the workup of this tumor. More recently, ^{131}I-meta-iodobenzylguanidine has been used to diagnose and monitor the therapy of neuroblastoma (28).

Other tumors of the adrenal gland are quite rare in children. The most common of these is adrenocortical carcinoma. This tumor tends to be highly malignant and locally invasive, and the CT and ultrasound char-

Table 45.8. Cystic Abdominal Masses

Multicystic dysplastic kidney
Hydronephrosis (severe)
Enteric duplication cyst
Mesenteric cyst
Hydrops of the gallbladder
Choledochal cyst
Ovarian cyst
Urachal cyst
Pancreatic pseudocyst
Cerebrospinal fluid pseudocyst
Abscess/parasitic cyst
Lymphangioma
Teratoma/dermoid cyst
Tumor (necrotic)
Adrenal hemorrhage (resolving)

acteristics of the mass are similar to those of neuroblastoma. Benign adrenal masses such as adenomas and pheochromocytomas are very rare in children, as are congenital adrenal cysts.

Diffuse adrenal enlargement can occur with adrenocortical hyperplasia, which results in the adrenogenital syndrome; however, the adrenal glands may also appear normal in this condition. Wolman's disease is a rare lipidosis that results in enlarged, densely calcified adrenal glands. Plain films are usually diagnostic of this abnormality, although the enlarged calcified glands can also be demonstrated by ultrasound or CT. Wolman's disease is usually fatal at an early age.

Hepatobiliary Masses

A variety of cystic and solid masses may arise from the liver and biliary tract in children. Hydrops of the gallbladder and choledochal cysts both present as a cystic right upper quadrant mass (Table 45.8), and usually the conditions can be differentiated with ultrasound.

Acute Hydrops of the Gallbladder is a poorly understood condition in children that is thought probably to be secondary to transient, self-limiting obstruction of the cystic duct. This condition has been associated with the mucocutaneous lymph node syndrome, although in many cases the cause is unknown. Ultrasound shows a markedly enlarged, tender gallbladder with a thin wall. Occasionally, a similar appearance can be found with acute acalculous cholecystitis, although the gallbladder distension tends to be less pronounced, and gallbladder wall thickening is sometimes encountered. Transient distension of the gallbladder sometimes occurs in the neonate, particularly in premature infants. Prolonged total parental nutrition and sepsis have been implicated as possible etiologic factors.

Choledochal Cyst. Jaundice, pain, and a right upper quadrant mass comprise the classic triad of findings seen with a choledochal cyst, although young infants more commonly present with fluctuating jaundice, pain, and fever. The most common type of choledochal cyst consists of a localized, fusiform dilation of the common bile duct below the cystic duct. In many cases, choledochal cysts can be diagnosed by ultrasonography, appearing as a cystic mass in the porta hepatis, separate from the gallbladder and associated with dilated intrahepatic ducts (Fig. 45.68). ^{99m}Technetium-IDA scintigraphy can be used to demonstrate that the cyst communicates with the biliary tract, aiding in differentiation from other cystic abdominal masses (Table 45.8).

Hepatic Cysts are less common in infants and children than in adults; however, ultrasound and CT now allow diagnosis of these lesions more frequently than in the past. Solitary congenital cysts of the liver are usually encountered as an incidental finding at ultrasound or CT. Sonographically, they appear as sharply defined anechoic masses within the hepatic parenchyma. Such cysts rarely may be very large and pedunculated, and in such cases the hepatic origin of the cyst may be difficult to ascertain.

Multiple hepatic cysts most commonly occur in patients with the autosomal dominant (adult) form of polycystic kidney disease. The cysts are well defined and are of variable size. This form of hepatic cystic disease differs from the disease associated with the autosomal recessive (infantile) form of polycystic kidney disease, which is associated with increased periportal echogenicity due to hepatic fibrosis.

Acquired hepatic cysts may be solitary or multiple and are most commonly of infectious origin. Parasitic disease of the liver (i.e., echinococcal cysts, amebic abscess) most often presents as cystic lesions within the liver. These cysts most often contain some internal debris (Fig. 45.69), but occasionally the cysts may be difficult to differentiate from a simple congenital hepatic cyst. Pyogenic bacterial infections also occur and appear as cystic hepatic lesions. Such abscesses are more common in immunocompromised patients. Finally, resolving hematoma of the liver may also appear as a well-defined cystic lesion.

Hemangioendothelioma. Primary neoplasms of the liver are uncommon in infancy and childhood, and in the newborn and young infant, benign lesions predominate. The most common benign tumor encountered in infancy is the hemangioendothelioma. Hemangioendothelioma may be solitary or multiple and is associated with cutaneous hemangiomas in approximately 40% of cases. This tumor may be complicated by high-output cardiac failure, hemorrhage, hemolytic anemia, or thrombocytopenia due to sequestration of platelets within the tumor.

Ultrasound is the preferred initial screening technique in the evaluation of hepatic tumors; however,

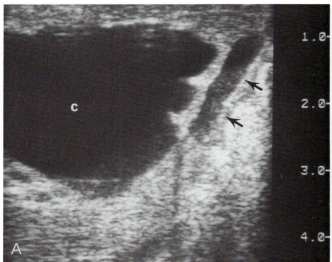

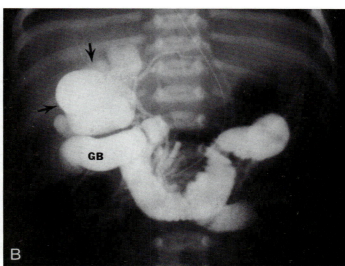

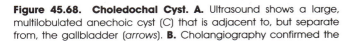

Figure 45.68. Choledochal Cyst. A. Ultrasound shows a large, multilobulated anechoic cyst (*C*) that is adjacent to, but separate from, the gallbladder (*arrows*). **B.** Cholangiography confirmed the presence of a large intrahepatic choledochal cyst (*arrows*) involving the right hepatic duct. *GB*, gallbladder.

further imaging is often required for the preoperative assessment of such tumors; CT, MR, and nuclear scintigraphy have all been used. In addition, arteriography continues to be of value in defining the vascular supply and drainage of the tumor.

The typical sonographic appearance of hemangioendothelioma consists of a complex mass containing large anechoic sinusoids and associated with large draining vessels (Fig. 45.70). Duplex and color flow Doppler ultrasound demonstrates the vascular nature of these tumors. The lesions produce a focal area of decreased radiotracer activity at scintigraphy, which concentrate the tracer used for blood pool imaging. On CT and MR, the lesion has an appearance similar to that seen with cavernous hemangiomas in adults. Cavernous hemangiomas are more common in older children and adolescents, and their imaging characteristics are the same as those seen in adult patients. *Mesenchymal Hamartoma* is an uncommon benign tumor that is most often seen in infants and young children. Hamartomas are usually solitary and, on sonography, appear predominantly cystic with multiple thin septae and sometimes intervening nodules of solid tissue. The CT appearance of hamartomas is variable, but often multiple areas of low attenuation are seen within the tumor mass. *Hepatic Adenomas* are rare in childhood but have been reported in association with Fanconi's anemia or glycogen storage disease type I. These tumors vary in echogenicity. *Focal Nodular Hyperplasia* most commonly presents as a mass-like hepatic lesion that also has a variable sonographic appearance and can be confused with hepatic adenoma. In some cases, scintigraphy using ^{99m}Tc-sulfur colloid demonstrates normal-to-increased tracer uptake within the lesion, dif-

ferentiating it from adenomas that do not concentrate the tracer.

Metastatic Disease. Beyond early infancy, malignant hepatic tumors are more common than benign tumors. Metastatic disease is more common than primary hepatic malignancy. Neuroblastoma is the most common childhood tumor to metastatize to the liver, followed by lymphoma, leukemia, and Wilms' tumor. Metastatic lesions are usually multiple, and their appearance on ultrasound, CT, and MR are generally nonspecific.

Hepatoblastoma and Hepatocellular Carcinoma. The most common primary malignant neoplasms of the liver in children are hepatoblastoma and hepatocellular carcinoma. Hepatoblastoma is a tumor of early childhood, presenting before 3 years of age. Hepatocellular carcinoma is more commonly seen in older children and adolescents. Sonographically, these tumors typically appear as single or multiple hyperechoic lesions, sometimes containing hypoechoic or anechoic areas due to hemorrhage or necrosis within the tumor mass. Invasion of the hepatic and/or or portal veins may be identified by ultrasound and is suggestive of the malignant nature of these tumors. On CT, the tumors appear as lesions of low attenuation with variable contrast enhancement (Fig. 45.71). Magnetic resonance imaging is comparable with CT for the initial diagnosis of these tumors; however, MR is more sensitive in the detection of postoperative tumor recurrence (29). Other less common primary malignant tumors in children include undifferentiated (embryonal) sarcoma and embryonal rhabdomyosarcoma of the biliary ducts. The latter tumor typically occurs in children between 2 and 5 years of age. When the tumor originates in a major bile

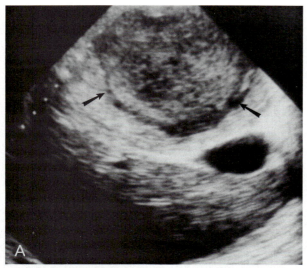

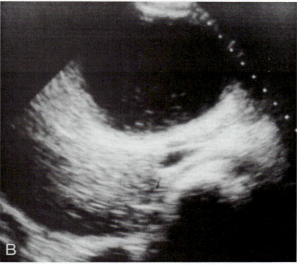

Figure 45.69. Amebic Abscess of the Liver. A. The initial ultrasound revealed a large complex mass (*arrows*) within the liver. Note that the mass is well defined with a sonolucent rim. **B.** With therapy, the abscess becomes predominantly anechoic with a few fine echoes in the dependent portion of the cyst.

duct, jaundice may be the presenting symptom. Those tumors that originate within the smaller intrahepatic ducts cannot be differentiated from other primary malignancies of the liver.

Splenomegaly

An enlarged spleen is a relatively common cause of a left upper quadrant mass in children. Splenic enlargement is most often secondary to some other systemic illness and common causes include hematologic diseases, infections, portal hypertension, and infiltrative diseases (e.g., mucopolysaccharidoses, reticuloendothelioses, leukemia, and lymphoma). In most cases, the imaging characteristics of the enlarged

spleen are nonspecific and insufficient for diagnosing the cause of splenomegaly.

In the newborn and young infant, splenomegaly most often occurs because of bacterial sepsis and infection. Hepatomegaly is generally also present. In older children, infections such as infectious mononucleosis, typhoid fever, and cat-scratch fever are more common. Splenic abscess formation is quite uncommon in children and is most often associated with an impaired immune system. Ultrasound is an excellent screening tool for splenic abscesses, which usually appear as multiple small, poorly defined and hypoechoic lesions.

Other cystic masses of the spleen are uncommon and include congenital epidermoid cysts, posttraumatic pseudocysts, and echinococcal cysts. Cystic lymphangiomatosis is a benign lymphatic malformation that may occasionally cause splenic enlargement. These lesions commonly have a characteristic, multiloculated cystic appearance sonographically. Other primary neoplasms of the spleen (e.g., hemangioma, hamartoma, angiosarcoma) are rare. Systemic malignancies such as lymphoma and leukemia commonly involve the spleen. One should be aware, however, that splenic involvement with tumors such as Hodgkin's disease does not necessarily result in splenic enlargement. Conversely, children with leukemia or lymphoma may have an enlarged spleen without true neoplastic involvement of the organ.

Splenic injury due to blunt abdominal trauma is common in the pediatric age group. Although CT is generally accepted to be the best initial imaging modality for splenic trauma, ultrasound can be used for follow-up. This is especially true now that a conservative, nonoperative approach to therapy of splenic trauma is becoming more common in children.

Splenic enlargement may also be encountered in the acute stages of splenic infarction. In children, infarction of the spleen most commonly occurs as a complication of sickle cell anemia, leukemia, or cardiac valvular disease. Acute splenic infarction results in decreased echogenicity sonographically and diminished contrast enhancement of the spleen on CT. A rare cause of splenic infarction in children is torsion of a wandering spleen. The abnormal position of the spleen is the primary clue to this diagnosis (Fig. 45.72).

Gastrointestinal and Pancreatic Masses

Enteric Duplication Cysts. A majority of the abdominal masses that arise from the GI tract or pancreas are cystic in nature. Enteric duplication cysts can involve any portion of the GI tract, but the most common location is the small bowel (specifically ileum). Duplication cysts are usually asymptomatic, although some cysts may contain ectopic gastric or pan-

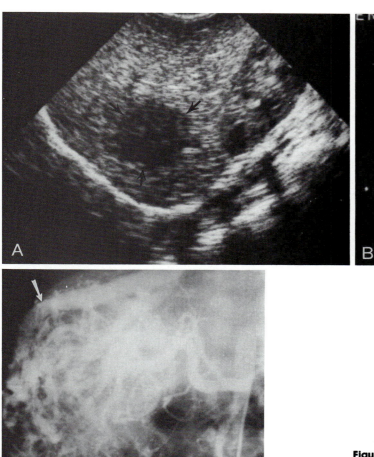

Figure 45.70.   Vascular Neoplasms of the Liver. A. Hemangioma. Ultrasound demonstrates a round, sonolucent mass (*arrows*) within the right lobe of the liver. This was a solitary hemangioma. **B.** Another patient with multiple sonolucent liver masses (*arrows*) representing hemangioendotheliomatosis. **C.** Hemangiomendothelioma. Arteriography demonstrates the marked vascularity (*arrows*) of this tumor. (Fig. 45.70**A** courtesy of C. Keith Hayden, Jr, M.D., Fort Worth, TX.)

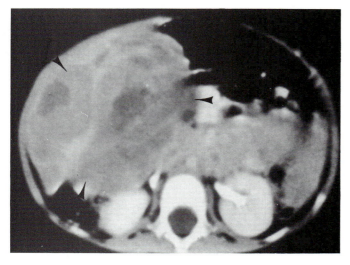

Figure 45.71.   Hepatoblastoma. A CT scan demonstrates a large inhomogeneous tumor within the right lobe of the liver (*arrows*).

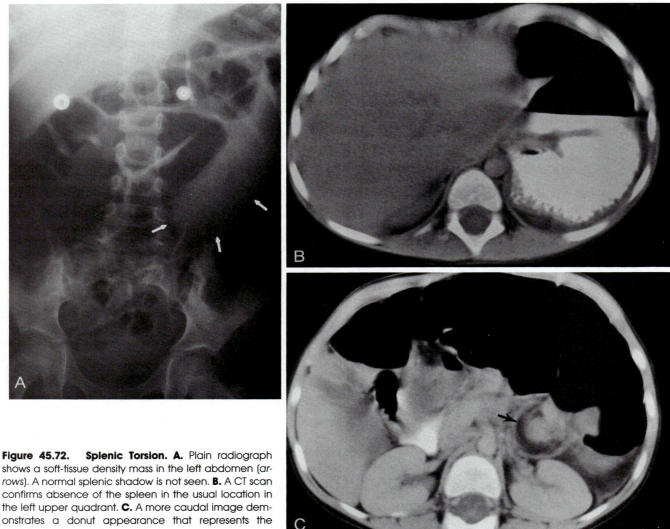

Figure 45.72.   Splenic Torsion. A. Plain radiograph shows a soft-tissue density mass in the left abdomen (*arrows*). A normal splenic shadow is not seen. **B.** A CT scan confirms absence of the spleen in the usual location in the left upper quadrant. **C.** A more caudal image demonstrates a donut appearance that represents the torsed splenic pedicle (*arrow*).

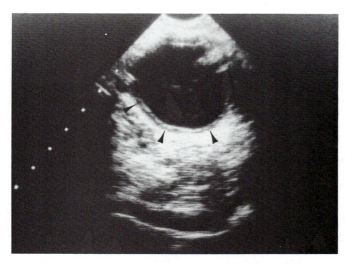

Figure 45.73. Enteric Duplication Cyst. Note the anechoic cyst with a well-defined wall that consists of an inner echogenic mucosal layer and a thin outer muscular layer (*arrows*).

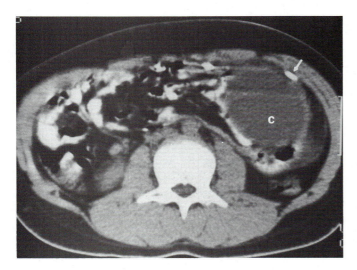

Figure 45.74. Cerebrospinal Fluid Pseudocyst. A CT scan demonstrates a loculated collection of fluid (C) in the left abdomen. Note the tip of the ventriculoperitoneal shunt lying adjacent to this fluid collection (*arrow*).

creatic tissue, which can lead to ulceration and hemorrhage. Occasionally, the cyst can act as a lead point for intussusception or volvulus.

Diagnosis of enteric duplication cysts is usually best accomplished by ultrasound. The cysts characteristically appear as simple anechoic round to oval masses with characteristic two-layered wall (30). The wall consists of an inner echogenic mucosal layer and a thin outer hypoechoic muscular layer (Fig. 45.73), and this appearance can be used to help differentiate duplication cysts from other types of cystic abdominal masses. Because most enteric duplication cysts do not communicate with the intestinal lumen, GI contrast studies are usually of little value. Cysts that con-

tain gastric mucosa are detectable by scintigraphy using ^{99m}Tc pertechnate.

Mesenteric and Omental Cysts. Congenital cysts of the mesentery and omentum are occasionally seen in the first decade of life and are now most often considered to be a form of lymphangioma. Typically, such cysts are thin-walled with multiple internal septations by ultrasound. The wall of the cyst consists of a single layer rather than the double layer seen with duplication cysts. Acquired mesenteric cysts are most often a complication of ventriculoperitoneal shunts used for the treatment of hydrocephalus. Generally, the cysts can be localized near the tip of the shunt tubing (Fig. 45.74).

Pancreatic Cysts. The most common cystic mass to arise from the pancreas is a pseudocyst secondary to pancreatitis. True congenital cysts of the pancreas are rare and occur chiefly in association with other multisystem diseases such as autosomal dominant polycystic kidney disease or Beckwith-Wiedenmann syndrome.

Solid Tumors of the GI tract are rather uncommon in infants and children. The most common malignant tumors of the small intestine include lymphosarcoma and Burkitt's lymphoma. Colonic neoplasms are rare; inflammatory polyps or polyps associated with one of the colonic polyposis syndromes are most common. Although carcinoma of the colon can occur in older children, tumors in infancy are more likely to be a leiomyoma, leiomyosarcoma, or lymphosarcoma. Tumors of the mesentery and omentum are primarily metastatic, usually neuroblastoma or lymphosarcoma.

Pancreatic Neoplasms are rare in children. The most common neoplasm is the benign islet cell adenoma (insulinoma), which is usually small and difficult to demonstrate. Other less common pancreatic neoplasms include adenocarcinoma, hamartoma, lymphangioma, and cystadenoma. Nesidioblastosis is an unusual condition in which the pancreas is diffusely infiltrated by primitive nesidioblasts, which cause hypoglycemia because of secretion of insulin. However, the imaging characteristics of this condition are not known.

Pseudomasses. Finally, a variety of pseudomasses in the abdomen may arise from the GI tract. These are primarily inflammatory in nature; the most common of these is the appendiceal abscess. In some children, once perforation occurs, the clinical findings improve and the symptoms may become remarkably mild. In such cases, unless the previous history of abdominal pain and fever is elicited, the abscess can be mistaken for an abdominal mass (Fig. 45.75). Sonographically, abscesses frequently appear as complex masses containing both cystic and solid components. Other intestinal pseudomasses include bowel

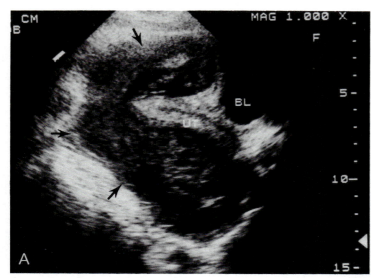

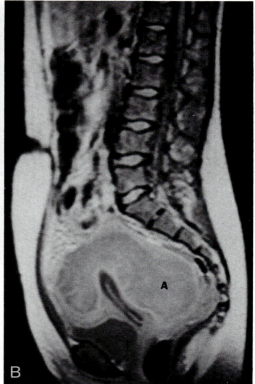

Figure 45.75. Appendiceal Abscess. A. Ultrasound revealed a large, elongated complex mass (*arrows*), that extended from the pouch of Douglas over the uterine fundus. *UT,* uterus; *BL,* bladder. **B.** Magnetic resonance imaging confirmed the presence of a large, high intensity abscess (*A*). This patient was only mildly symptomatic and was referred for evaluation of an "ovarian cyst."

thickening due to inflammatory bowel disease and intussusception. These pseudomasses have a characteristic sonographic and CT appearance, which has been described earlier in this chapter.

Masses of the Reproductive Organs

Ovarian Cysts. Abdominal and pelvic masses that arise from the reproductive system are very common in young females, and the majority of these masses arise from the ovaries. The most common ovarian mass in children and adolescents is a simple follicular or corpus luteum cyst (31, 32). Such cysts are common in neonates because of maternal hormonal stimulation and in adolescents. In many cases, such cysts remain asymptomatic and eventually spontaneously resolve without surgical intervention. Those cysts that are very large (greater than 5 cm) or that are complicated by hemorrhage or torsion may require aspiration or removal. Simple ovarian cysts sonographically appear as round or oval anechoic masses with a thin rim (Fig. 45.76**A**). In adolescents, hemorrhage into such cysts can cause pain. When this occurs, the cyst acquires a more complex sonographic appearance, which can be difficult to differentiate from other adnexal masses (Fig. 45.76, **B** and **C**).

A complex adnexal mass may be the result of a variety of conditions that generally must be differentiated on clinical grounds rather than imaging characteris-

tics. Infection and abscess formation due to pelvic inflammatory disease is not uncommon in adolescents, and ectopic pregnancy must always be considered in postmenarchal females. Ovarian neoplasms, overall, are uncommon in childhood. The most common ovarian tumor is the teratoma. Sonographically, teratomas can vary from an entirely cystic mass to a predominantly solid mass with internal cystic components. The characteristic appearance is a complex mass that contains both cystic, solid, and highly echogenic areas (due to calcifications or fat) (Fig. 45.77, **A** and **B**). A recognizable tooth within the mass is a pathognomonic plain film finding (Fig. 45.77**C**).

Although the majority of ovarian teratomas are benign, malignant teratomas do occur and are sometimes accompanied by ascites, intraperitoneal extension, and metastatic disease to the liver. Like ovarian cysts, ovarian tumors can lead to ovarian torsion. Teratomas that sonographically contain a larger component of solid tissue are more likely to be malignant. Less common ovarian neoplasms of childhood include dysgerminoma, cystadenomas and cystadenocarcinomas, and granulosa cell tumors.

Enlarged Uterus. An enlarged uterus is sometimes the cause of a palpable abdominal mass. Unsuspected pregnancy is not an uncommon cause of a pelvic mass in adolescents. Congenital vaginal obstruction leading to hydrometrocolpos usually presents either in the newborn period or at puberty. In most cases, ultrasound clearly identifies the en-

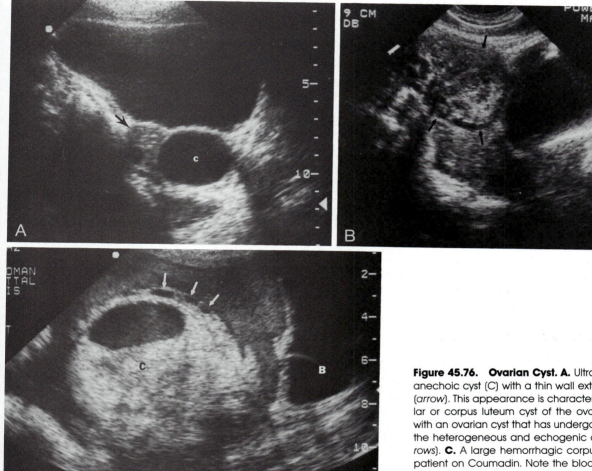

Figure 45.76.   Ovarian Cyst. A. Ultrasound shows a round, anechoic cyst (C) with a thin wall extending from the ovary (*arrow*). This appearance is characterisic of a simple follicular or corpus luteum cyst of the ovary. **B.** Another patient with an ovarian cyst that has undergone hemorrhage. Note the heterogeneous and echogenic clot within the cyst (*arrows*). **C.** A large hemorrhagic corpus luteum cyst (C) in a patient on Coumadin. Note the blood-fluid level within the cyst and several small follicles within the compressed and displaced ovary (*arrows*).

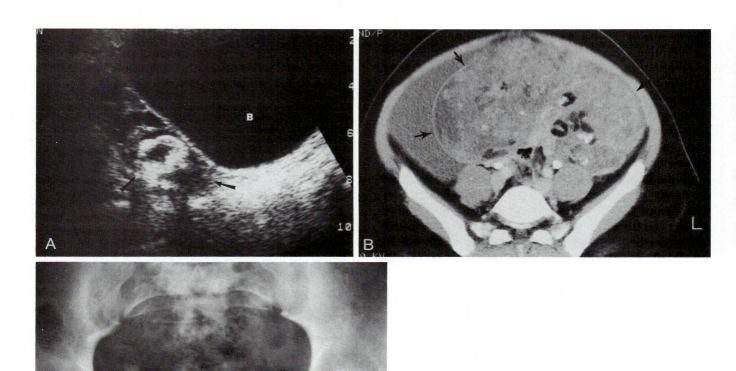

Figure 45.77.   Ovarian Teratoma. A. Ultrasound demonstrates a complex adnexal mass that contains both cystic and solid components as well as intensely echogenic areas of calcium and fat (*arrows*). *B,* bladder. **B.** A CT scan of a different patient with a very large ovarian teratoma. Note the heterogenous texture of this mass, with scattered calcifications and areas of fat density (*arrows*). **C.** The ovarian dermoid in this patient contains a formed calcification that closely resembles a tooth (*arrow*).

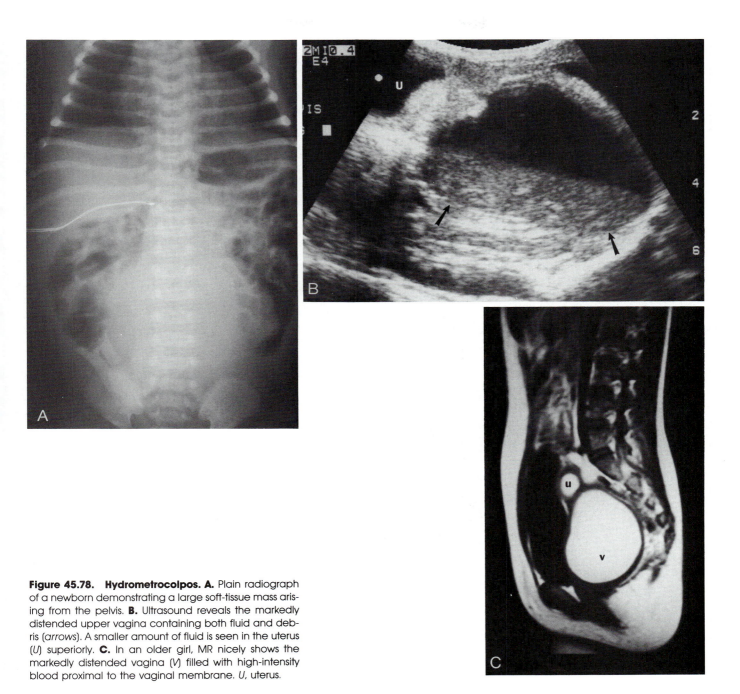

Figure 45.78. Hydrometrocolpos. A. Plain radiograph of a newborn demonstrating a large soft-tissue mass arising from the pelvis. **B.** Ultrasound reveals the markedly distended upper vagina containing both fluid and debris (*arrows*). A smaller amount of fluid is seen in the uterus (*U*) superiorly. **C.** In an older girl, MR nicely shows the markedly distended vagina (*V*) filled with high-intensity blood proximal to the vaginal membrane. *U*, uterus.

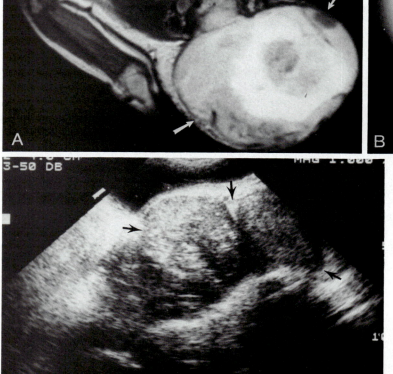

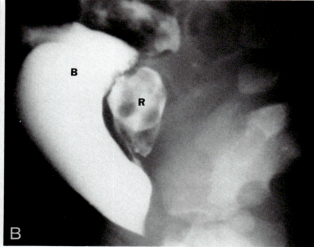

Figure 45.79.   Presacral Masses. A. Note the large complex [that extends from the presacral region (*arrows*). **B.** Another p[atient] with a soft-tissue mass in the presacral space that displace[s the] bladder (*B*) and rectum (*R*) anteriorly. **C.** Ultrasound sho[ws a] homogenously, moderately echogenic mass in the presacral sp[ace] (*arrows*) caused by neuroblastoma. (Fig. 45.79**A** courtesy of [ ] Boulden, M.D., Memphis, TN.)

larged uterus filled either with anechoic fluid in the newborn, or echogenic blood in adolescent patients (Fig. 45.78, **A** and **B**). The type of vaginal obstruction can also be suggested by ultrasound examination, particularly if a transperineal approach is used (33). Magnetic resonance imaging has also been shown to be useful for classifying the vaginal abnormality in older patients (Fig. 45.78**C**) (34). Uterine neoplasms are uncommon in children, but most are malignant. Rhabdomyosarcoma is the most common of these and generally arises from the anterior wall of the vagina. Rhabdomyosarcoma can also be present in the male pelvis, usually arising from the prostate gland or the trigone of the urinary bladder. Although these tumors can often be demonstrated sonographically, rhabdomyosarcoma frequently infiltrates the pelvic floor, and surrounding structures and CT or MR are usually preferable for determining the extent of the disease.

Presacral Masses

A wide variety of lesions can arise in the presacral space. In the newborn and young infant, the most

common presacral mass is a sacrococcygeal teratoma or dermoid. Like teratomas that occur elsewhere, sacrococcygeal teratomas frequently are calcified and sometimes contain formed calcifications such as teeth. The presence of calcium and fat within a presacral lesion virtually assures the diagnosis (Fig. 45.79**A**).

Neuroblastoma can also develop as a primary tumor of the presacral space (Fig. 45.79, **B** and **C**). Amorphous irregular calcifications are fairly common and characteristic of this tumor. Presacral neuroblastomas carry an improved prognosis over those that arise in the upper abdomen. Sacral chordomas are an uncommon neoplasm in this location. Plain radiographs demonstrate the destruction and expansion of the sacrum. Typical flocculant cartilaginous calcifications are often present. Most tumors of the presacral space are best demonstrated with MR or CT.

Anterior sacral meningoceles present as presacral masses that are usually associated with deformity of the sacral spine. This deformity usually consists of a crescent-shaped sacrum due to a concave lateral defect through which the meningocele extends. Anterior sacral meningocele is commonly seen with anorectal abnormalities and in patients with neurofibromatosis. Neuroenteric cysts are also occasionally seen in the presacral space and can also be associated with anterior sacral defects. Both of these conditions are nicely demonstrated by MR.

References

1. Swischuk LE, Hayden CK Jr, Stansberry SD. Sonographic pitfalls in imaging of the antropyloric region in infants. Radiographics 1989;9:437–447.
2. Shiels WE II, Maves CK, Hedlung GL, Kirks DR. Air enema for diagnosis and reduction of intussusception: clinical experience and pressure correlates. Radiology 1991;181:169–172.
3. Stein M, Alton DJ, Daneman A. Pneumatic reduction of intussusception: 5-year experience. Radiology 1992;183:681–684.
4. Alexander JE, Williamson SL, Seibert JJ, Golladay ES, Jimenez JF. The ultrasonographic diagnosis of typhlitis (neutropenic colitis). Pediatr Radiol 1988;18:200–204.
5. Kao SCS, Smith WL, Abu-Yousef MM, et al. Acute appendicitis in children: sonographic findings. AJR 1989;153:375–379.
6. Sivit CJ, Newman KD, Boenning DA, et al. Appendicitis: usefulness of US in diagnosis in a pediatric population. Radiology 1992;185:549–552.
7. Quillin SP, Siegel MJ. Appendicitis in children: color Doppler sonography. Radiology 1992;184:745–747.
8. Hayden CK Jr, Kuchelmeister J, Lipscomb TS. Sonography of acute appendicitis in childhood: perforation versus nonperforation. J Ultrasound Med 1992;11:209–216.
9. Haller JO. Sonography of the biliary tract in infants and children. AJR 1991;157:1051–1058.
10. Abramson SJ, Treves S, Teele RL. The infant with possible biliary atresia: evaluation by ultrasound and nuclear medicine. Pediatr Radiol 1982;12:1–5.
11. Majd M. ^{99m}Tc-IDA scintigraphy in the evaluation of neonatal jaundice. Radiographics 1983;3:88–99.
12. Couture A, Veyrac C, Baud C, Galifer RB, Armelin I. Evaluation of abdominal pain in Henoch-Schönlein syndrome by high frequency ultrasound. Pediatr Radiol 1992;22:12–17.
13. Hayden CK Jr, Swischuk LE, Fawcett HD, Rytting JE, McCord G. Urinary tract infections in childhood: a current imaging approach. Radiographics 1986;6:1023–1038.
14. Berdon WE. Contemporary imaging approach to pediatric urologic problems. Radiol Clin North Am 1991;29:605–618.
15. Shultz PK, Strife JL, Strife CF, McDaniel JD. Hyperechoic renal medullary pyramids in infants and children. Radiology 1991;181:163–167.
16. Hayden CK Jr, Swischuk LE. Renal cystic disease. Semin Ultrasound CT MR 1991;12:361–373.
17. White KS, Kirks DR, Bove KE. Imaging of nephroblastomatosis: an overview. Radiology 1992;182:1–5.
18. Gambino J, Caldwell B, Dietrich R, Walot I, Kangarloo H. Congenital disorders of sexual differentiation: MR findings. AJR 1992;158:363–367.
19. Burks DD, Markey BJ, Burkhard TK, Balsara ZN, Haluszka MM, Canning DA. Suspected testicular torsion and ischemia: evaluation with color Doppler sonography. Radiology 1990;175:815–821.
20. Atkinson GO Jr, Patrick LE, Ball TI Jr, Stephenson CA, Broecker BH, Woodard JR. The normal and abnormal scrotum in children: evaluation with color Doppler sonography. AJR 1992;158:613–617.
21. Kier R, McCarthy S, Rosenfield AT, Rosenfield NS, Rapoport S, Weiss RM. Nonpalpable testes in young boys: evaluation with MR imaging. Radiology 1988;169:429–433.
22. McHugh K, Stringer DA, Hebert D, Babiak CA. Simple renal cysts in children: diagnosis and follow-up with US. Radiology 1991;178:383–385.
23. Heij HA, Taets van Amerongen AHM, Ekkelkamp S, Vos A. Diagnosis and management of neonatal adrenal haemorrhage. Pediatr Radiol 1989;19:391–394.
24. Daneman A. Adrenal neoplasms in children. Semin Roentgenol 1988;23:205–215.
25. David R, Lamki N, Fan S, et al. Many faces of neuroblastoma. Radiographics 1989;9:859–882.
26. Forman HP, Leonidas JC, Berdon WE, Slovis TL, Wood BP, Samudrala R. Congenital neuroblastoma: evaluation with multimodality imaging. Radiology 1990;175:365–368.
27. Ruzal-Shapiro C, Berdon WE, Cohen MD, Abramson SJ. MR imaging of diffuse bone marrow replacement in pediatric patients with cancer. Radiology 1991;181:587–589.
28. Hibi S, Todo S, Imashuku S, Miyazaki T. ^{131}I-Meta-iodobenzylguanidine scintigraphy in patients with neuroblastoma. Pediatr Radiol 1987;17:308–313.
29. Boechat MI, Kangarloo H, Ortega J, et al. Primary liver tumors in children: comparison of CT and MR imaging. Radiology 1988;169:727–732.
30. Barr LL, Hayden CK Jr, Stansberry SD, Swischuk LE. Enteric duplication cysts in children: are their ultrasonographic wall characteristics diagnostic? Pediatr Radiol 1990;20:326–328.
31. Siegel MJ. Pediatric gynecologic sonography. Radiology 1991;179:593–600.
32. Surratt JT, Siegel MJ. Imaging of pediatric ovarian masses. Radiographics 1991;11:533–548.
33. Blask ARN, Sanders RC, Gearhart JP. Obstructed uterovaginal anomalies: demonstration with sonography: Part I. Neonates and infants. Radiology 1991;179:79–83.
34. Mintz MC, Grumbach K. Imaging of congenital uterine anomalies. Semin Ultrasound CT MR 1988;9:167–174.

Section X NUCLEAR RADIOLOGY

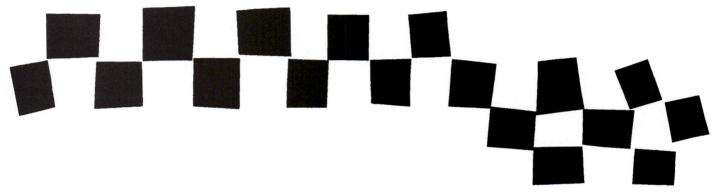

46

Introduction to Nuclear Medicine

Frederic A. Conte

CURRENT CLINICAL POSITION OF NUCLEAR MEDICINE

Regardless of where nuclear medicine is practiced, whether in the hospital-based radiology department, as a part of an imaging center, or found among the organ-specialist physicians (i.e., cardiologists), the understanding of nuclear medicine begins with the appreciation of its functional characteristics. X-ray, ultrasound, transmission computed tomography (CT), and even magnetic resonance imaging produce images with very high spatial resolution but which are predominantly anatomic in content. In other words, you can see the anatomy very well, but you cannot tell how well it is working. Pathology is inferred based upon the anatomic pattern. The strength of nuclear medicine imaging resides in its ability to portray the functional status of an organ or body part. As the first nuclear medicine images are viewed, there will be immediate disappointment with the lack of spatial resolution; but exploration of the image substance will make one quickly impressed with the high information content accessible to the trained eye. The contribution to patient care made by this functional information is matched by few other imaging modalities. Because of this, nuclear medicine procedures find themselves positioned in many diagnostic algorithms. This diagnostic capability will become evident as these pages are read.

FUTURE TRENDS

Nuclear medicine procedures utilize the concept of the tracer principle: a radioactive element, by itself or tied to another molecule, follows the biologic course of another species. The labeled species must act like the unlabeled species and not interfere with the process being studied. When imaging of the tracer is performed, the image reflects the biodistribution of the tracer, modified by physiologic, anatomic, and, if present, pathologic processes. As nuclear medicine procedures have waxed and waned in the face of changing diagnostic indications, the tracer principle has remained the driving force behind evolving nuclear imaging procedures. The tracer principle at the molecular level is being extended by new understanding of genetic and biochemical processes. As the biochemistry of these processes are exploited, additional tracers will be produced that are targeted to image such entities as specific biochemical receptors, DNA- and RNA-directed messengers, and genetic mapping. Current research with radioisotopes is vigorously pursuing many of these pathways: neuroreceptors such as D1 and D2 dopamine receptors; radiolabeled tumor antibodies directed toward colorectal, ovarian, breast, and prostate carcinomas, in addition to lymphoma and melanoma; and infectious disease evaluation using radiolabeled antibodies, such as antigranulocyte antibodies, and immune globins.

POSITRON EMISSION TOMOGRAPHY (PET)

Due to the scope of this text, discussion of PET imaging and its numerous radiopharmaceuticals will be limited. Despite superb, frontier-expanding radiopharmaceuticals, many uses are still investigational. The chances of a radiologist being involved in a multimillion dollar PET center (there were 65 PET centers as of 1992), although increasing, are still low. Suffice it to say, PET research and its positron agents create much of the basic science information base that serves as the precursor for development of more economical, nonpositron radionuclide agents (Tc-99m/iodine 123/In-111 labeled compounds). From the brain to the heart to various tumors, PET imaging has served as the reference standard to which radiopharmaceuticals based on gamma camera imaging have been tested. It will be this exact spin-off of PET agents to nonpositron analogs that will continue to nourish and assure a future of nuclear medicine as the next millennium is approached and entered.

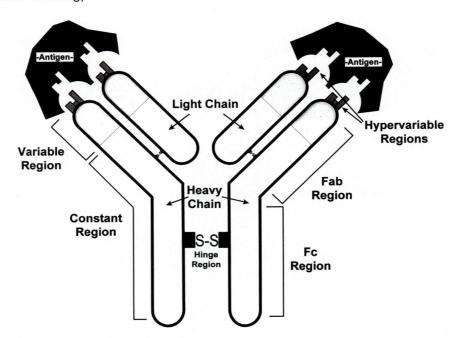

Figure 46.1. Monoclonal Antibody Structure. The basic antibody glycoprotein molecule consists of two identical heavy and light chains linked by a disulfide bridge. Each chain has a variable region responsible for antigenic binding, and a constant region involved in complement fixation and antibody-dependent cell toxicity. Each variable region, in turn, contains three hypervariable regions that form unique antigen-binding sites. The antibody can be fragmented into smaller units depending upon the cleavage plane. Enzymatic digestion produces either an F(ab')$_2$ fragment or two smaller Fab fragments and an Fc fragment. Fragment size dictates blood pool clearance rates, with the smaller ones clearly faster.

MONOCLONAL ANTIBODIES

As this book was going to press, the first imaging monoclonal antibody directed toward a tumor was approved by the FDA: OncoScint CR/OV (satumomab pendetide, Cytogen, Princeton, NJ). The result of 10 years of research, this immunoscintigraphic antibody has shown efficacy in determining the location and extent of extrahepatic malignant disease in patients with known colorectal or ovarian cancer.

Production of OncoScint CR/OV. Antibodies are glycoproteins (Fig. 46.1) called immunoglobulins produced by the plasma cells that originated as B lymphocytes sensitized to a foreign substance (antigen). The immunoglobulin response is termed "polyclonal" when numerous antibody species of varying affinity for the antigen-binding surfaces are produced. To achieve a monoclonal antibody population, a specific immunoglobulin-producing cell line is isolated. After fusing the sensitized B lymphocytes with immortal myeloma cells, large numbers of antibodies can be harvested by selectively culturing the hybridomas; this produces monoclonal antibodies directed toward the antigen of greatest interest. In the case of OncoScint CR/OV, the immunoglobulin G antibody-producing hybridoma is the result of rodent B lymphocytes sensitized to human cancer cells prior to incubation with the myeloma cell line. The antigen used is TAG-72 (*Tumor Associated Glycoprotein*), a high molecular weight glycoprotein expressed by the majority of colorectal and ovarian carcinomas. Indium-111 chloride is chelated to a carbohydrate molecule site-specifically attached to the constant region of the monoclonal antibody (Fig. 46.2). Some cross-reactivity is present between the OncoScint CR/OV antibody and other tumor cell lines such as nonsmall cell, breast, and gastrointestinal tract adenocarcinomas. Additionally, OncoScint CR/OV also reacts somewhat with mucin-secreting epithelial tissues such as salivary gland ducts, postovulatory endometria, and benign ovarian tumors.

The OncoScint CR/OV antibody is supplied as a kit vial to which In-111 chloride is added. Approximately 1 mg of antibody containing 5 mCi ^{111}In is intravenously injected. Imaging is usually initiated at 48–72 hours and may be extended to 120 hours as needed to evaluate for abnormal activity. Anterior and posterior planar images of the chest, abdomen, and pelvis are usually sufficient. When improved localization and contrast are needed, single-photon emission CT may be added, facilitating comparison of the antibody images with cross-sectional images from transmission CT.

The safety of OncoScint CR/OV has been demonstrated in over 500 injections. Adverse effects were observed in less than 4% of patients and consisted primarily of nonserious, readily reversible effects: fever, chills, hypotension, hypertension, rash, and pruritus.

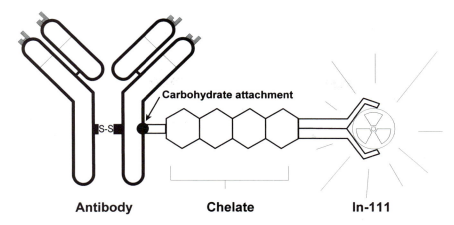

Figure 46.2. OncoScint CR/OV In-111 Structure. The immunoglob-ulin-G antibody directed against the TAG-72 antigen found on colorectal and ovarian tumors is linked via a carbohydrate attach-ment and chelate (pantetic acid) to the In-111 radionuclide. The linkage is very stable and does not interfere with the antigenic bind-ing by the hypervariable regions. The long half-life of In-111 (67.2 hours) permits serial imaging for up to 5–7 days.

Patients with hypersensitivity to products of murine origin and to In-chloride should not receive the anti-body. Its safety and efficacy in children has not been established. Pregnant or lactating women should be administered the labeled antibody only when the in-formation to be gained outweighs the potential risk from radiation and the antibody. Based on a 5 mCi injection, the estimated average absorbed radiation dose in adult patients is 12, 15, and 16 rads for the red marrow, liver, and spleen, respectively. Because of insufficient safety and efficacy data, as currently ap-proved by the FDA, OncoScint CR/OV is limited to sin-gle injection use only.

Using In-111 as the radionuclide attached to the antibody offers several advantages. The long half-life (67.2 hours) lends itself to serial imaging beyond 72 hours, during which time the background continues to clear. The relative availability of the radionuclide, which is cyclotron-produced, provides for a conve-nient kit preparation in many radiopharmaceutical labs. The "shake and bake" kit with In-111 and the site-specific attachment methodology results in a high-percentage chelation with the antibody.

Normal Distribution. Once injected, the OncoScint CR/OV monoclonal antibody circulates and attaches to TAG-72 molecules found on colorectal and ovarian adenocarcinomas. Because of the uptake of the antibody itself or of its breakdown products, other nondiseased sites of localized activity are also present. The normal pattern of biodistribution that emerges as the blood pool activity decreases includes the liver, where the whole immunoglobulin-G molecule is me-tabolized, spleen, bone marrow, kidneys (10% of activ-ity is excreted over 3 days), urinary bladder, testicles, breast nipples in females, and colon from excretion (Fig. 46.3).

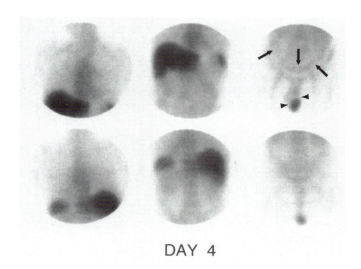

DAY 4

Figure 46.3. Normal Monoclonal Antibody Scan. The patient is a 57-year-old male who presented with diarrhea and was found to have multiple colonic polyps (tubular adenomas) on colonoscopy. Presurgical evaluation included a negative CT, a serum CEA of 6.2 ng/ml, and this normal monoclonal antibody scan. Anterior spot views were acquired at 96 hours after the injection of the tagged antibody. The normal biodistribution of the antibody is seen in the liver, spleen, bone marrow, cardiac blood pool, faintly in the bowel (arrows) and intensely in the testicles (arrowheads). (Case courtesy of Cytogen, Princeton, NJ, and Hani Abdel-Nabi, M.D., Buffalo VA Medical Center, Buffalo, NY.)

Other sites of nonspecific uptake have been re-ported: recent surgical wounds, corpus luteal cyst, salpingitis and colitis, bone fracture, gluteal folds, and normal colostomy stoma. With normal liver tak-ing up activity, a liver full of metastatic foci would, de-pending upon the activity of the metastases, present as either a liver full of holes or as one indistinguish-able from normal liver. Either way, the differential di-agnosis may be misleading.

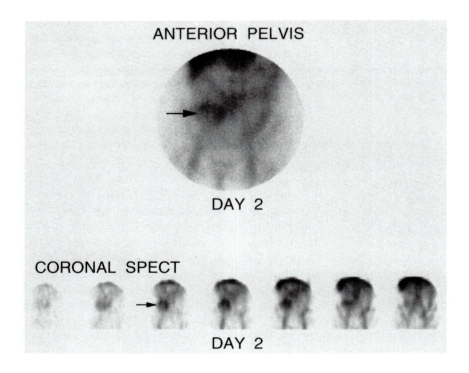

Figure 46.4. Abnormal Monoclonal Antibody Scan; Abdominal Uptake in Primary Colorectal Cancer. The patient is a 69-year-old woman who presented with heme-positive stools. A CT scan demonstrated a 5 × 6 cm cecal mass and a 1 × 3 cm left ischiorectal fossa mass. Colonoscopy was positive for well-differentiated adenocarcinoma of the cecum. The serum CEA level was 1.1 ng/ml. The antibody scan was performed at 48 hours. Anterior pelvic planar image and coronal single-proton emission CT (SPECT) images demonstrate abnormal increased activity in the right lower quadrant (*arrows*) corresponding to the cecal mass. Any possible confusion with bowel in a constipated individual can be resolved by repeat scanning after assuring a cathartic-induced bowel movement. Right hemicolectomy revealed an 11-cm tumor in the cecum that proved to be a mucinous adenocarcinoma with extension through the cecal wall and into the pericecal fat. (Case courtesy of Cytogen, Princeton, NJ, and Stanley Grossman, M.D., West Penn Hospital, Pittsburgh, PA.)

Table 46.1.   OncoScint CR/OV Multicenter Trial Results for Colorectal Cancer[a]

Number of patients evaluated	192
Sensitivity	69%
Specificity	76%
Positive predictive value	97%
Negative predictive value	19%
Occult disease (confirmed by surgery)	10%
Patient management	25%

[a]Adapted from Collier BD, ABdel-Nabi H, Doerr RJ, et al. Immunoscintigraphy performed with In-111-labeled CYT-103 in the management of colorectal cancer: comparison with CT. Radiology 1992;185:179–186.

Table 46.2.   Comparison of CT and OncoScint CR/OV for Colorectal Cancer[a]

Anatomic Site	Sensitivity (%)	
	OncoScint CR/OV	CT
Pelvis	74	57
Extrahepatic abdomen	66	34
Liver	41	84

[a]Adapted from Collier BD, Abdel-Nabi H, Doerr RJ, et al. Immunoscintigraphy performed with In-111-labeled CYT-103 in the management of colorectal cancer: comparison with CT. Radiology 1992;185:179–186.

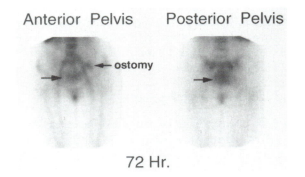

Anterior Pelvis   Posterior Pelvis

72 Hr.

Figure 46.5. Abnormal Monoclonal Antibody Scan; Pelvic Uptake in Recurrent Colorectal Cancer. The patient is a 36-year-old woman who had a primary rectal cancer resected 2 years previously and presented with rising CEA (5.3 ng/ml). A CT scan of the abdomen and pelvis was negative, as was a chest x-ray and colonscopy. The antibody scan was performed at 72 hours, with anterior and posterior views of the pelvis demonstrate an abnormal presacral collection of activity (*arrows*). A second focus, seen only on the anterior view, over the left ileum, corresponded to normal uptake by the patient's ostomy site (*arrow* labeled *ostomy*). An exploratory laparotomy revealed a pelvic mass pathologically shown to be recurrent invasive infiltrating adenocarcinoma. (Case courtesy of Cytogen, Princeton, NJ, and Drs. Amando Sardi and Lynn Witherspoon of the Ochsner Clinic, New Orleans, LA.)

Colorectal carcinoma is the third most common malignancy in the U.S. with 156,000 new cases and 58,300 deaths reported in 1992. In addition to a baseline carcinoembryonic antigen (CEA) level, initial preoperative staging is usually accomplished by chest radiography and contrast CT scans or magnetic resonance imaging, occasionally complemented by transrectal ultrasonography. Although the 5-year survival rate for localized disease is high (83–91%), that for regional and distant spread is much lower (50–60% and <7%, respectively). Of first recurrences, 50% occur in the extrahepatic abdomen and pelvis. Evaluation by colonoscopy and barium is limited to intraluminal disease and has a low yield. Serial postoperative serum CEA levels have been used with some success to monitor for recurrence, but one-third of patients with recurrence do not have elevated CEA levels. Even with an increasing CEA level, 30% of patients do not have disease by standard imaging, for which CT of the liver and abdomen is the current recommendation.

To evaluate the diagnostic efficacy of OncoScint CR/OV in a multicenter trail, 192 patients with primary or secondary colorectal carcinoma were imaged preoperatively with both CT and the monoclonal antibody. The sensitivity of OncoScint CR/OV for the detection of carcinoma, whether primary or recurrent, was 69% (Table 46.1), similar to the sensitivity of CT for detection (68%). Interestingly, combining the two imaging modalities raised the sensitivity to 88%. A negative predictive value of only 19% renders negative scans unreliable, but the high positive predictive value of 97% makes the positive monoclonal antibody scan potentially very helpful. When analyzed for anatomic site, the data (Table 46.2) showed OncoScint CR/OV superior in the extrahepatic abdomen and pelvis when compared to CT scans, which were better at evaluating the liver. When those patients with elevated CEA and a negative presurgical workup that included CT were separated, the accuracy of OncoScint CR/OV for detection of carcinoma was 74%. Two examples of typical positive monoclonal antibody scans for colorectal cancer are presented in Figures 46.4 and 46.5.

In summary, there are currently several clinical indications for the use of OncoScint CR/OV in the evaluation of primary and recurrent colorectal cancer. For primary disease, monoclonal antibody scanning may help in detecting synchronous lesions, determining the extent of regional disease, and finding occult metastases. It can be used judiciously in the evaluation of poor surgical candidates in whom metastasis would obviate exposing the patient to surgery. In the evaluation for tumor recurrence, the monoclonal scan can be useful in detecting occult disease, in verifying presumed resectable disease, and in clarifying equivocal CT/MR findings. Specifically, the antibody scan may differentiate recurrent disease from postradiation/postsurgical anatomic changes and determine the source of a rising serum CEA in patients with an otherwise negative workup.

Ovarian carcinoma is the fourth leading cause of death from female malignancy in the U.S., with 21,000 new cases and 13,000 deaths reported in

Table 46.3.   OncoScint CR/OV Multicenter Trial Results for Ovarian Cancer[a]

	Primary disease	Recurrent disease
Number of patients evaluated	103	
Sensitivity	95%	58%
Specificity	50%	60%
Positive predictive value	72%	83%
Negative predictive value	88%	28%
Occult disease (confirmed by surgery)	28%	35%
Adverse effects	<4%	

[a]Adapted from Krag DN. Clinical utility of immunoscintigraphy in managing ovarian cancer. J Nucl Med 1993;34:545–548.
From Surwit EA, Krag DN, Katterhagen JG, et al. Clinical assessment of In-111-CYT-103 immunoscintigraphy in ovarian cancer. Gynecol Oncol 1993;48:285–292.

Table 46.4.   Comparison of CT and OncoScint CR/OV for Ovarian Cancer[a]

	OncoScint CR/OV	CT
Sensitivity (%)	68	44
Primary	95	84
Recurrence	59	29
Specificity (%)	54	79
Primary	50	50
Recurrence	57	100
Carcinomatosis (%)	71	45

[a]Adapted from Krag DN. Clinical utility of immunoscintigraphy in managing ovarian cancer. J Nucl Med 1993;34:545–548.
From Surwit EA, Krag DN, Katterhagen JG, et al. Clinical assessment of In-111-CYT-103 immunoscintigraphy in ovarian cancer. Gynecol Oncol 1993;48:285–292.

1992. The 5-year overall survival rate is 39%. Staging of ovarian cancer is based on surgical findings at laparotomy since preoperative clinical staging by noninvasive imaging (CT, intravenous pyelogram, barium enema, chest x-ray, or ultrasound) is inadequate to detect small foci of tumor, particularly in the midabdomen, where more than 50% of metastatic lesions are located. Surgical staging by exploratory laparotomy does not detect extraabdominal tumors, is costly, and has a high complication rate. The most effective treatment for ovarian cancer is based upon complete surgical resection, although favorable response to chemotherapeutic agents has been demonstrated. Serum CA125 tumor antigen measurements are used to postoperatively monitor for recurrence. It is not used in the initial clinical staging because it does not predict disease extent or location and has a high false-negative rate.

In a multicenter trial, 103 patients were evaluated with CT and OncoScint CR/OV for either primary or recurrent ovarian cancer (Table 46.3). Surgery or biopsy was used to assess for the presence or absence of disease. The overall sensitivity for monoclonal antibody scanning was 68% versus 44% for CT (Table 46.4). Again, as with antibody imaging for colorectal cancer, a negative scan is not as reliable at predicting the absence of disease (28%) as is the positive scan at predicting the presence of disease (83%). Sensitivity for primary and recurrent disease was 95% and 59% for monoclonal antibody imaging versus 84% and 29% for CT. When the two modalities are compared for detection of carcinomatosis, the monoclonal scan's sensitivity was 71% versus 45% for CT (Table 46.4). Tumor was detected in 19 patients by antibody scanning where the CT was negative, while CT was able to detect two patients who had negative antibody scans. Of the patients with occult disease detected by antibody scanning, six had normal CA125 levels. Of the 17 patients with 19 false-positive sites, three were normal, five had benign ovarian tumors, one had nonadenocarcinoma tumor, and 10 had inflammatory tissues or adhesions.

In summary, there are several possible clinical indications for the use of OncoScint CR/OV in the evaluation of primary and recurrent ovarian cancer. Monoclonal antibody imaging may help to define the location and extent of extrahepatic disease, to detect occult disease (including miliary spread), and to limit the surgical approach and reduce morbidity. Antibody imaging appears to be superior to CT in the detection of carcinomatosis. Antibody imaging may prove useful in the early detection of recurrent ovarian cancer even in those patients with a normal CA125 serum level.

SUMMARY

Nuclear medicine procedures remain an integral part of the diagnostic armamentarium that the radiologist brings to bear on disease processes. The onus on the imaging specialist is to also become a valuable diagnostician. This is even more true given the ever-changing indications for the various imaging modalities that must meet cost-effective, acceptable risk-benefit ratios, as well as diagnostic and therapeutic efficacy. By maintaining a current knowledge base of indications for nuclear medicine procedures, the radiologist can be assured a position in providing the most appropriate service to the referring clinician and the most effective care for patients. The chapters that follow provide a firm didactic core of nuclear medicine on which the construction of this knowledge base can be built.

Special thanks to Denise Webber and Barbara Rogers of Cytogen Corporation for the use of the three cases used to demonstrate the clinical utility of OncoScint CR/OV.

Suggested Readings

1. American Cancer Society. Cancer Facts and Figures—1992. Atlanta: American Cancer Society, Inc. 1992:8.
2. Collier BD, Abdel-Nabi H, Doerr RJ, et al. Immunoscintigraphy performed with In-111-labeled CYT-103 in the

management of colorectal cancer: comparison with CT. Radiology 1992;185:179–186.

3. Collier DB, Foley DW. Current imaging strategies for colorectal cancer. J Nucl Med 1993;34:537–540.

4. Galandiuk S. Immunoscintigraphy in the surgical management of colorectal cancer. J Nucl Med 1993;34:541–544.

5. Goldenberg DM, Larson SM. Radioimmunodetection in cancer identification. J Nucl Med 1992;33:803–814.

6. Knight LC. Scintigraphic methods for detecting vascular thrombus. J Nucl Med 1993;34:554–561.

7. Krag DN. Clinical utility of immunoscintigraphy in managing ovarian cancer. J Nucl Med 1993;34:545–548.

8. Maynard CD. Medical imaging in the nineties: new directions for nuclear medicine. J Nucl Med 1993;34:157–164.

9. Serafini AN. From monoclonal antibodies to peptides and molecular recognition units: an overview. J Nucl Med 1993;34:533–536.

10. Surwit EA, Krag DN, Katterhagen JG, et al. Clinical assessment of 111-In-CYT-103 immunoscintigraphy in ovarian cancer. Gynecol Oncol 1993;48:285–292.

11. Texter JH, Neal CE. Current applications of immunoscintigraphy in prostate cancer. J Nucl Med 1993;34:549–553.

12. Wagner HN. The new molecular medicine. J Nucl Med 1993;34:165–166.

47

Essential Science of Nuclear Medicine

Frederic A. Conte
Jerrold T. Bushberg

DEFINITIONS

Difference Between γ-rays and X-rays

The electromagnetic spectrum of radiation can be divided into nonionizing and ionizing radiation. Nonionizing radiation includes commonly encountered forms of electromagnetic radiation such as visible light, microwave, and radiofrequencies (used in radio transmissions and in magnetic resonance imaging). The ionizing radiation includes x-rays and γ-rays used in diagnostic medical imaging. The primary difference between x-rays and γ-rays lies in their origin. X-rays are extranuclear in origin and can be produced from the interaction of bombarding photons or electrons with an atom; γ-rays are produced from within the atomic nucleus as an unstable nucleus transitions to a more stable state. The source of x-rays for diagnostic radiology is the x-ray tube, while the source of γ-rays for nuclear medicine is the radioactive or unstable nuclide (i.e., radionuclide) (Table 47.1). The production of images from these two sources is different and has a direct effect on the radiation dose delivered to a person. Diagnostic x-ray imaging is "transmission" imaging in which the x-ray photons from an external source traverse tissue where some photons are absorbed and some emerge to form the image. Each additional x-ray image requires an additional radiation exposure raising the dose to the patient. Nuclear medicine imaging with γ-rays is "emission" imaging in which the source resides within the patient and the photons are emitted and subsequently detected by the gamma camera imaging system. Emission imaging only requires additional acquisition time to obtain more images (views).

Ionizing radiation can also come in particulate form. The particle of medical interest is the β-particle, which is an electron but has its origin within an unstable nucleus as it transitions to reach a more stable state. As opposed to x-rays and γ-rays, β-particles interact quite easily with matter, traveling only a few centimeters in tissue while transferring their energy to the surrounding matter. Although not of imaging importance, it is this energy-transferring property that contributes to their ability to produce a high dose over a short range, thus providing for their therapeutic usefulness in such entities as Graves' disease and thyroid cancer.

Units

Various units to describe radiation and its effects have been established. Since the colloquial vernacular used in the scientific community is in transition between conventional units and the Système Internationale d'Unités (SI), a table of the old and new units with their conversion factors is provided in Table 47.2. Activity is used to describe the quantity of the

Table 47.1. Radionuclides[a]

Radionuclide (symbol)	Method of Production	Mode of Decay (%)	Principal Imaging Photons keV (abundance)	T$_P$1/2	Comments
Chromium-51 (Cr-51)	Neutron activation	EC (100)	320 (9)	27.8d	Used for in vivo red cell mass determinations, not utilized for imaging; samples counted in sodium iodide well counter
Cobalt-57 (Co-57)	Cyclotron produced	EC (100)	122 (86) 136 (11)	271d	Primarily used as a uniform flood field source for gamma camera quality control
Gallium-67 (Ga-67)	Cyclotron produced	EC (100)	93 (40) 184 (20) 300 (17) 393 (4)	78h	In practice, use the 93, 184, and 300 keV photons for imaging
Molybdenum-99 (Mo-99)	Nuclear fission (U-235)	β⁻ (100)	181 (16) 740 (12) 780 (4)	67h	Used as the source (parent) for Mo/Tc generators; not used directly as radiophamaceutical; 740 and 780 keV photons used to identify contamination of Tc-99m elution as "moly breakthrough"
Krypton-81m (Kr-81m)	Generator product	IT (100)	190 (67)	13s	The generator with its ultrashort lived parent (Rb-81, 4.6h) and high expense limit the use of this agent
Technetium-99m (Tc-99m)	Generator product	IT (100)	140 (90)	6.02h	This radionuclide, in kit form or as pertechnetate, accounts for more than 70% of all imaging studies
Indium-111 (In-111)	Cyclotron produced	EC (100)	171 (90) 245 (94)	2.8d (67.2h)	Principally utilized when optimal imaging occurs more than 24 hr after injection; both photons used in imaging
Iodine-123 (I-123)	Cyclotron produced	EC (100)	159 (83)	13.2h	Replaced I-131 for most diagnostic imaging applications to reduce radiation dose
Iodine-125 (I-125)	Neutron activation	EC (100)	35 (6) 27 (39) 28 (76) 31 (20)	60.2d	Used as I-125 albumin for in vivo blood/plasma volume determinations; not utilized for imaging, samples counted in well counter
Iodine-131 (I-131)	Nuclear fission (U-235)	β⁻ (100)	284 (6) 364 (81) 637 (7)	8.0d	Typical use now reserved for therapeutic applications; imaging is limited by high-energy photon (364 keV) and high patient dosimetry mostly from β⁻ particles
Thallium-201 (Tl-201)	Cyclotron produced	EC (100)	69-80 (94) 167 (10)	73.1h	The majority of clinically useful photons are low-energy x-rays (69-80 keV) form mercury 201 (Hg-201), the daughter of Tl-201
Xenon-133 (Xe-133)	Nuclear fission (U-235)	β⁻ (100)	81 (37)	5.3d	Xe-133 is a heavier than air gas; low abundance and energy of photon reduces image resolution
Fluorine-18 (F-18)	Cyclotron produced	β⁺ (97) EC (3)	511 (AR)	110 m	This radionuclide accounts for more than 80% of all clinical PET use; typically formulated as fluorodeoxyglucose (FDG)

[a]Legend: EC, electron capture; d, day; h, hours; β⁻, beta minus decay; IT, isomeric transition (i.e., γ-ray emission); s, sec; β⁺, beta plus decay; AR, annihilation radiation; m, minutes

Table 47.2. Conventional and SI Radiologic Units and Conversion Factors

Quantity	Conventional Units Name	Symbol	Multiply by the conventional units to obtain SI units	SI Units Name	Symbol	Example
Activity	Curie	Ci	3.7×10^{10}	Becquerel[a]	Bq	10 mCi = 370 mBq
Exposure	Roentgen	R	2.58×10^{-4}	Coulomb per kilogram	C/Kg	
Absorbed dose	Radiation absorbed dose	rad[b] (acronym)	10^{-2}	Gray[c]	Gy	100 rad = 1 Gy
Dose equivalent	Roentgen-equivalent man	rem (acronym)	10^{-2}	Sievert	Sv	100 rem = 1 Sv

[a]1 Bq = 1 disintegration/sec.
[b]1 rad = 0.01 joule/kg.
[c]1 Gy = 1 joule/kg.

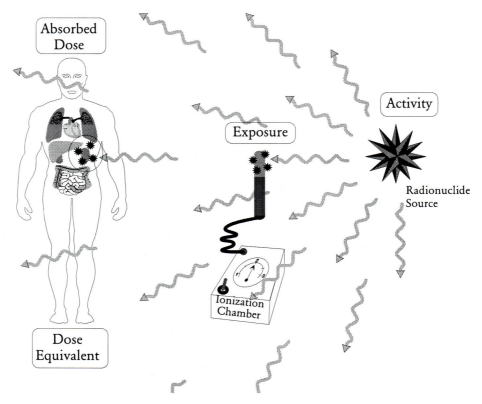

Figure 47.1. Graphical Representation of Radiation Units. The unit of measurement that is used to measure radioactivity is determined by where radioactivity is measured. *Activity* (curie/becquerel), whether occurring outside the body or inside, is measured at the source. *Exposure* (roentgen/coulomb per kilogram) is measured by an ionization chamber as the radioactivity transits air. *Absorbed Dose* (rad/gray) is a measure of radioactivity that has interacted with the tissue where it deposits its energy. *Dose Equivalent* (rem/Sievert) compares the effects on tissue by different types of radioactivity: α-particles, β-particles, and photons. The particles deposit more energy to the tissue than photons.

radionuclide being administered and represents the rate of nuclear transformations, denoted by curies (Ci) in conventional units and becquerels (Bq) in SI units. The roentgen is the unit utilized to express radiation exposure; this is a measure of the ability of x-rays and γ-rays to produce a given amount of ionization in a given volume of air. From a biologic point of view, the important consideration is how much of the radiation exposure results in energy deposited in an individual at a particular location, which is expressed as absorbed dose. Absorbed dose is the amount of energy deposited by ionizing radiation per unit mass in joules per kilogram; the conventional unit is the *radiation absorbed dose* (rad) and the SI unit is the gray (Gy). Since certain types of radiation are more biologically damaging than others, a radiation weighting factor (also called quality factor) is multiplied by the absorbed dose to yield the dose-equivalent, which is measured in rem (*roentgen equivalent man*) in conventional units and the Sievert (Sv) in SI units. The dose-equivalent unit allows comparison between the various ionizing radiation sources (photons, β-particles, α-particles). Because the quality factor is equal to 1 for photons and electrons, one roentgen approximately equals 1 rad in the diagnostic energy range for soft tissue, which approximately equals 1 rem (Fig. 47.1). That is, 1 R ~1 rad (0.01 Gy) ~1 rem (0.01 Sv).

Radiation Exposure

To the Worker. The total average exposure for an x-ray technician results in an annual dose equivalent of only 100–150 mrem, while for the nuclear medicine technician it is 200–300 mrem. The majority of whole-body radiation to a nuclear medicine worker comes from exposure to the dosed patient during imaging. Localized extremity exposure doses from radiopharmaceutical preparation and injection can be higher.

The primary risk from any increased radiation exposure is an increased risk for cancer. For each additional rem, the lifetime increased risk of cancer is approximately 5×10^{-4} (0.05%). With the cancer incidence risk in the general population at 33%, each additional rem will increase the risk by 0.05%. Therefore, an occupational whole-body dose of 1 rem (e.g., 100 mrem/year × 10 years = 1000 mrem) will increase the risk of developing cancer from 33% to

33.05%. With these numbers, several caveats to radiation exposure need to be remembered: any increased risk is spread over a lifetime; increased risks from exposure is additive; and the minimum latency of cancer is 5–8 years, with the mean for solid tissue tumors being closer to 20–25 years.

Since contamination in the workplace also increases radiation exposure to the worker, several guidelines can be followed to minimize contamination: follow universal precautions; wear protective clothing; use plastic-backed absorbent to restrict any spills; wash hands frequently; use covers over collimators that can be discarded if contaminated; monitor and wipe test frequently (see below); and avoid smoking, eating or drinking when handling radioactivity.

To the Patient. The average total annual radiation dose to the population in the United States is 370 mrem/year. Natural background radiation from atmospheric and terrestrial sources contributes 300 mrem/year (80%), while man-made sources, primarily from medical procedures, provide another 70 mrem/year (20%).

Since nuclear medicine procedures involve radionuclides and radiopharmaceuticals that are variably transient in the human body, dosimetric considerations include not only the initial activity administered but the biodistribution, the physical and biologic half-lives, as well as possible pathologic processes. On a relative scale, the dose to the whole body of most nuclear medicine diagnostic procedures is equivalent to one-third to four times the average annual dose-equivalent from natural background. That is, whole-body dose for nuclear medicine examinations range from 100 mrem for bone scan to 1.3 rem for Ga-67 procedure.

An additional dosimetry term that relates directly to the patient is the concept of "critical organ." The critical organ is the organ or tissue in a radiopharmaceutical procedure that receives the largest dose of radiation or that has the highest radiosensitivity. The dose to the critical organ depends on the radionuclide concentration within the organ, geometric factors, the effective retention in that organ, and the relative radiosensitivity of the organ. Interestingly, in many cases the dose to any organ (the target organ) comes as much from the organ itself as it does from the surrounding tissue (the source).

The pregnant patient faced with a diagnostic nuclear medicine procedure is a common problem. There are no absolute contraindications regardless of the diagnostic nuclear medicine examination being considered. Risk-versus-benefit evaluation determines the indication for the examination. If the radionuclide examination is indicated and cannot be postponed till after term, measures to minimize the dose can be employed such as halving the adult dose (and doubling the imaging time) and increasing hydration to enhance excretion.

A lactating female who is administered a radiopharmaceutical requires counseling to proscribe feeding her infant for a specified length of time. The guidelines for these lengths of time are based on the physical and biologic half-lives of the radionuclides (called effective half-lives), which, in turn, predict when the breast milk is safe to drink. The recommended times for succession of feeding are listed in Table 47.3. If the breast milk is measured, use the concentration values in the table to resume feeding; otherwise use the recommended times. For a quick, but very conservative, method to arrive at the time for cessation of breast feeding, a good rule of thumb is to use eight physical half-lives of the radionuclide, which will leave less than 1% of the radioactivity by the time breast feeding is resumed. Using this rule for ^{99m}Tc agents, 2 days would be recommended for cessation.

Radiation Safety in the Workplace

General Guidelines. The common goal of radiation safety principles is to minimize exposure to radiation, whether to the worker, patient, or public. Individuals exposed to radiation can limit their exposure by utilizing three very basic principles: time, distance, and shielding. Specifically, (a) limit the time, which, for the worker, can translate into being familiar enough with the procedure that it is performed efficiently thus minimizing exposure; (b) maximize the distance, observing the inverse square law where radiation exposure, like heat from a candle flame, drops off very rapidly as the intensity decreases with the square of the distance from the source; and (c) use shielding when possible. Shielding with thin lead aprons in diagnostic radiology is quite effective in stopping the low-energy photons. In nuclear medicine, because of the higher energy photons, shielding is confined to containers for the source activity, such as in preparation vials and syringes.

Regulations. The Nuclear Regulatory Commission (NRC) governs nuclear material and its products. By-products include reactor-produced radionuclides, such as molybdenum-99 (Mo-99) and iodine-131 (I-131). The NRC does not regulate accelerator-produced radioactive material; individual states govern their possession and use. The NRC licenses users (individuals or institutions) and governs many nuclear medicine proceedings, including the standards for protection against radiation (radiation protection program), waste disposal, surveys, instrumentation, and training requirements. Many states, after accepting the responsibility to regulate radioactive materials, become "agreement states" and license users and enforce regulations compatible with that of the NRC.

Table 47.3. Recommendations for Cessation of Breast Feeding after Administration of Radiopharmaceuticals to Mothers[a]

Radiopharmaceutical	Administered Activity	Imaging Procedure	Safe Breast Milk Concentration (μCi/ml)	Cessation of Breast Feeding till Breast Milk is Safe
Tc-99m sodium pertechnetate	10 mCi	Thyroid scan and Meckel's scan	8.2×10^{-2}	24 hr
Tc-99m kits (general rule)	5–25 mCi	All	8.2×10^{-2}	24 hr
Tc-99m DTPA	10 to 15 mCi	Renal scan	1.2×10^{-1}	16.8 hr
Tc-99m MAA	3 to 5 mCi	Lung perfusion scan	1.2×10^{-1}	9.6 hr
Tc-99m SC	5 mCi	Liver spleen scan	1.6×10^{-1}	14.4 hr
Tc-99m MDP	15 to 25 mCi	Bone scan	2.1×10^{-1}	16.8 hr
Ga-67 citrate	6-10 mCi	Infection and tumor scans	2.1×10^{-3}	4 weeks
Tl-201 chloride	3 mCi	Myocardial perfusion	2.4×10^{-3}	3 weeks
Sodium I-123	30 μCi	Thyroid uptake	1.2×10^{-4}	3 days
Sodium I-123	200 to 400 μCi	Thyroid scan	1.2×10^{-4}	5 days
Sodium I-131	5 μCi	Thyroid uptake	4.1×10^{-7}	68 days
Sodium I-131	10 mCi	Thyroid cancer metascan or Graves therapy	$4.1 + 10^{-7}$	(155 days) Discontinue[b]
Sodium I-131	29.9 mCi	Outpatient therapy for hyperfunctioning nodule	4.1×10^{-7}	(168 days) Discontinue[b]
Sodium I-131	100 mCi or more	Thyroid cancer treatment (ablation)	$4.1 + 10^{-7}$	(170 days) Discontinue[b]

[a]DTPA, diethylenetriaminepentaacetic acid; MAA, macroaggregated albumin; SC, sulphur colloid; MDP, methylene diphosphonate.
[b]Discontinuance is based not only on the excessive time recommended for cessation of breast feeding, but also on the high dose the breasts themselves would receive during the radiopharmaceutical breast transit.

The central goal of a radiation protection program is called ALARA, which promotes efforts to keep radiation exposures *as low as reasonably achievable*. As a requirement of the NRC, ALARA represents an administrative philosophy to encourage, enforce, teach, and observe all possible ways to minimize radiation doses and exposure. The ALARA program extends into personnel exposure (worker), misadministrations (patient), and environmental releases (general public) to achieve this dose minimization goal.

The NRC regulations that cover nuclear medicine are covered in the Code of Federal Regulations parts 19, 20, and 35. Part 19 covers the rights and responsibilities of workers to maintain a safe environment, and employers to educate their workers. Part 20 covers regulations of radiation protection for facilities to include dose limits for personnel and environment. Part 35 focuses on medical utilization of radiation sources, listing misadministration definitions and training requirements for authorized users. Board certification in diagnostic radiology or nuclear medicine suffices to qualify the individual as an authorized user in most states.

Safety Instruments

Two radiation detectors have a place in the radiation safety program of a department. The Geiger-Müller (GM) detector is a gas-filled survey meter that measures counts per minute. The GM meter is a very sensitive radiation detector that is useful for localizing very small quantities of activity, but will not accurately quantify it. Its primary use, therefore, is as a laboratory survey instrument in looking for contamination. The ion chamber, another gas-filled detector,

is used to accurately measure radiation exposure, especially at high levels. The ion chamber has several uses, including to quantify exposure levels, to assay doses prior to administration (dose calibrator, see later discussion), and to check packages for compliance with transportation regulations.

Radiopharmaceutical Possession and Handling

In general, compliance regulations require "cradle-to-grave" documentation of all radioactive substances. These requirements begin with an authorized individual ordering the radiopharmaceuticals, then setting standards for packaging and shipping, followed by procedures for the receipt of the package, and finally to demonstrating documentation of its use (patient or research) and disposal. Meticulous records of each step are imperative for adequate documentation of the "life" of a radioactive substance.

Radiation Monitoring

In a personnel monitoring program, all workers exposed to radiation wear either a thermoluminescent dosimeter or, more commonly, a film badge. For the film badge, the film is processed and the optical density is related to the radiation exposure. Depending upon the relative risk of exposure, reporting programs for personnel dosimeters can be established on a monthly (e.g., nuclear medicine technologists and angiographers) or a quarterly (e.g., mammography) basis.

The nuclear medicine workplace requires frequent monitoring for contamination. A typical monitoring program is as follows:

Daily   A GM survey meter is used to check over all work surfaces and trash. If any reading is 2 times background, then decontaminate (wash area) and resample until background reading, are less than twice background in unrestricted area (general public area). Dose rates in unrestricted areas must be less than 2 mrem/hr and less than 100 mrem/week; however, all potential exposures should be kept ALARA. Label all contaminated trash as radioactive and store for decay (10 physical half-lives).

Weekly Perform a radiation field survey using an ion chamber to survey controlled areas of the workplace.

Weekly Wipe test multiple sample areas of the workplace. Count in a multichannel analyzer attached to a multisample well counter using a wide energy window for 1 minute. Acceptable threshold is 200 disintegrations per minute per 100 cm^2 of surface area. If exceeded, then decontaminate and resample until within limits.

RADIOPHARMACEUTICALS
Functional Imaging

The major difference between images from radionuclides and those from x-ray sources is their greater functional information content. Most x-ray images carry a predominance of anatomic information; this is less true for Doppler ultrasonic images and magnetic resonance dynamic flow images. For nuclear medicine images, anatomic information is primarily inferred from the functional image. This functional image reflects not only the physiologic biodistribution (function) of the labeled tracer, but also the anatomic, pathologic, and artifact overlays present at the time of imaging. Recalling that the administered radiopharmaceuticals are delivered in tracer quantities to limit the absorbed dose, imaging is necessarily longer than for corresponding x-ray images.

Mechanism of Localization of Radiopharmaceuticals

A radiopharmaceutical is a compound to which a radionuclide is attached. The compound, sometimes in concert with the radionuclide, dictates the biodistribution of the radiopharmaceutical. Many radiopharmaceuticals act like analogs of natural biologic compounds, and thus localize via one of several methods. For example, ^{99m}Tc pertechnetate is analogous to the iodide molecule and distributes to the thyroid, salivary glands, stomach, and kidneys. Technetium-99m sulfur colloid acts like a colloid particle of approximately 1 micron and distributes throughout the reticuloendothelial system (liver, spleen, and bone mar-

row). Substituted iminodiacetic acid Tc-99m agents are analogous to bilirubin and are actively transported into hepatocytes and excreted into the biliary tree. See Table 47.4 for other examples.

Moly Generator

Nuclear medicine procedures are best served by a radionuclide that has a physical half-life long enough to allow for imaging in a reasonable amount of time, but not so long as to continue to radiate the patient much beyond that imaging. To provide for short-lived radionuclides, generators containing the parent material are constructed to provide an extended source of the daughter.

The most common radionuclide in nuclear medicine procedures, Tc-99m, comes from a generator, named for this parent-daughter relationship, the Mo-99 (molybdenum)-Tc-99m generator (also known as the Moly generator). Molybdenum-99 decays with a physical $T_{1/2}$ of 67 hours, while Tc-99m decays with a 6-hour $T_{1/2}$ (Fig. 47.2). The Mo-99 is adsorbed to an alumina column. As the Tc-99m evolves in place, it is easily removed from the column (eluted), as needed, by passing normal saline over the column, exchanging chloride for Tc-99m, in the form of sodium pertechnetate (Na Tc-99m O$_4$). Two types of Moly generators are commercially available (Fig. 47.3). The wet generator has a large reservoir of saline attached to one end of the column with which a vacuum bottle, attached to the other end, can extract the Tc-99m pertechnetate. The column is always "wet." The dry generator requires that a small saline vial be attached to one end, and a vacuum extraction vial to the other. The column is left "dry" after the elution.

After eluting (also known as milking) the Moly generator, the shorter-lived daughter, Tc-99m, begins immediately to reaccumulate on the column. This regrowth occurs at a predictable rate and dictates the yield at the subsequent elution (Fig. 47.4). The key times for regrowth and their yields include: 6 hours, 50% of activity; 23 hours, maximum activity. It can be readily appreciated from an inspection of the generator elution curve that eluting every 24 hours is both convenient and efficacious with respect to yield.

The quality control for the Moly generator consists of checking every elution for Mo-99 and aluminum breakthrough, that is, escape from the column. Although uncommon, the consequences of Moly breakthrough are important enough to mandate this quality control procedure for each elution. The assay for Moly breakthrough looks for the very high energy photons, 740 and 780 keV, emitted by Mo-99. The entire eluate is placed in a lead container, called a Moly Pig, that absorbs the majority of the 140 keV Tc-99m photons, but allows the higher energy Mo-99 photons to pass. This pig is then assayed in a dose calibrator

Table 47.4. Biodistribution: Mechanism of Localization of Radiopharmaceuticals[a]

Imaging Procedure	Radiopharmaceutical	Mechanism of Localization	Closest Biochemical Analog	Critical Organ (rad/mCi)
Lung perfusion scan	Tc-99m macroaggregated albumin (MAA)	Capillary blockade	Thrombo-embolus	Lungs (0.15–0.48)
Lung ventilation scan	Xe-133 gas	Compartment localization	Air	Trachea (0.64)
Bone scan	Tc-99m methylene diphosphonate (MDP)	Chemical adsorption onto bone crystal	Phosphate	Bladder (0.1–0.2)
Hepatobiliary scan	Tc-99m Iminodiacetic acid (IDA)	Active hepatocyte cellular transport	Bilirubin	Gallbladder (0.12–0.18)
Myocardial perfusion scan	Tl-201 Chloride	ATPase transport system	Potassium	Kidneys (0.4–0.9)
Labeled WBC scan	In-111 WBC Tc-99m HMPAO	Active migration of leukocyte to site of infection or inflammation after binding of radionuclide to intracellular component	Migratory leukocyte	Spleen (8.4–18.0) (0.79)
Renal scan	Tc-99m DTPA	Glomerular filtration	Inulin	Bladder (0.07–0.6)
	Tc-99m MAG3 (mertiatide)	Glomerular filtration and tubular secretion	p-Amino-hippurate (PAH)	
Thyroid	I-123	Active transport	Iodine	Thyroid (11.0–20.0)
Brain scan	Tc-99m HMPAO (hexametazime)	Lipophilic passive transport	Fatty Acid	Lacrymal gland (5.16)
Gated equilibrium blood pool scan	Tc-99m Labeled RBCs	Compartment Localization of RBC after Tc-99m binds to intracellular hemoglobin	RBC	Spleen (2.2)
Tumor imaging	Ga-67 Citrate	Unknown; iron receptor theory	Ferric ion	Colon (0.6–0.9)
	In-111 OncoScint monoclonal antibody (Satumomab Pendetide)	Antibody-antigen complex	Antibody	Spleen (3.2)
Meckel's scan	Tc-99m Pertechnetate	Active ion transport	Iodide	Thyroid (0.12–0.18)
Liver spleen scan	Tc-99m sulfur colloid	Reticuloendothelial phagocytosis	Colloid particle	Liver (0.2–0.4)

[a]WBC, white blood cells; HMPAO, hexamethylpropylamine oxine; DTPA, diethylenetriaminepentaacetic acid; MAG 3, mercaptoacetyltriglycine; RBC, red blood cells; ATPase, adenosine triphosphatase.

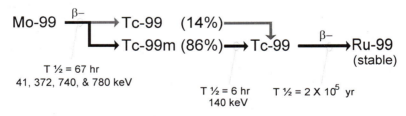

Figure 47.2. The Mo-99/Tc-99m Decay Scheme. The Mo-99 decays with both high-energy photons and β-particles (electrons). Fourteen percent of Mo-99 decays directly to Tc-99, while the other 86% produces metastable Tc-99m. Tc-99m gives up its 140 keV photon and reaches Tc-99.

with the Mo-99 button selected. The NRC limits are 0.15 Ci of Mo-99 per mCi of Tc-99m at the time of administration.

Aluminum breakthrough will cause Tc-99m kits to flocculate. These colloid particles will cause increased lung uptake on a sulfur colloid liver spleen scan and increased liver uptake on a bone scan. The quality control procedure to check for aluminum breakthrough is the colorimetric spot test where a drop of

eluate is placed on the colorimetric paper and compared with a standard. The maximum permissible amount of aluminum is 10 g/ml of eluate.

Radiochemical Purity

Many of the Tc-99m-based radiopharmaceuticals are produced by adding the generator elute, the "free" or unbound Tc-99m pertechnetate (TcO$_4$), to a "cold"

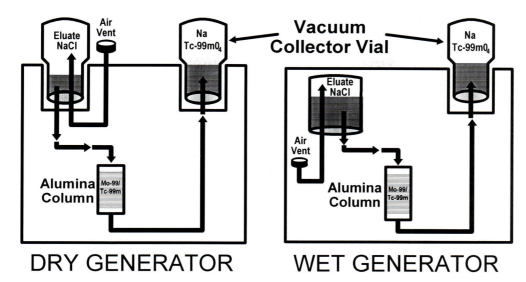

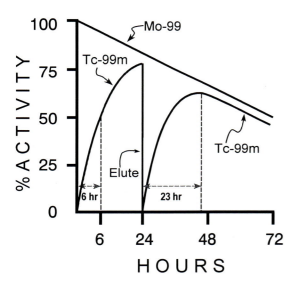

Figure 47.3.   Wet/Dry Generators. Both dry and wet generators use a vacuum collection vial; the difference is in the source of the NaCl eluate. The dry generator has a replaceable vial, while the wet generator has a fixed one. Both types of generators use the alumina column and are, therefore, susceptible to aluminum and Mo-99 (Moly) breakthrough. The end product is also the same: sodium pertechnetate (Na Tc-99mO₄).

Figure 47.4.   The Mo-99/Tc-99m Generator Elution Curves. The regrowth of the daughter (Tc-99m) on the column takes a predictable course after each elution. Inspection of the curves reveals that approximately 50% of the activity will be present 6 hours after an elution and that maximum activity is achieved at 23 hours after elution. This is convenient for a daily morning-scheduled elution and allows for an unplanned elutions by midday if needed.

kit containing the chelate (e.g., MDP, DTPA, DISIDA) and a reducing agent, usually stannous chloride. The reducing agent enables the Tc-99m with a valence of +7 to be reduced to +4 and react with the chelate. Some kits, such as sulfur colloid and MAG3, require heat to allow for the chelation to occur. Aside from the desired Tc-99m chelate, several radiochemical impurities can occur as a result of the introduction of either air or water into the kit vial. Air, which can in-

advertantly be introduced at the time of kit preparation, causes the oxidation of stannous chloride (Sn^{+2} to Sn^{+4}). This inhibits the reduction of Tc-99m, thus interfering with the complexation of the radiopharmaceutical. Water, which can be introduced prior to kit preparation, will hydrolyze stannous chloride to stannous hydroxide, a colloid. Another impurity, formed after kit preparation, is hydrolyzed reduced Tc-99m, also known as Tc-99m dioxide.

Radiochemical purity is defined as the percentage of the total radioactivity in a source that is present in the form of the desired chemical (i.e., the radiopharmaceutical). The Food and Drug Administration mandates testing of radiopharmaceuticals for radiochemical purity. Currently, radiochemical purity testing is required for HMPAO, teboroxime, sestamibi, and MAG3. The procedure to test for impurities involves separating the different species based on solubility using appropriate solvents. Various solvents and media are used in the separation method but the most common method is thin-layer chromatography, which consists of glass fiber strips impregnated with silica gel. After placing a drop of the radiopharmaceutical on the end (origin) of a thin-layer chromatography strip, the strip is placed, origin end down, in a shallow pool of solvent until the solvent front reaches the top. Since free Tc-99m is soluble in acetone and saline, it migrates with the solvent front, leaving behind the insoluble species for that particular solvent. In saline, both Tc-99m dioxide and Tc-99m tin colloid are insoluble and remain at the origin while the Tc-99m radiopharmaceutical migrates with any free Tc-99m to the top. In acetone, only the free Tc-99m migrates to the top, leaving behind all other species. By cutting the strips into an origin half and a solvent front half, each part of the total strip can be counted in a sodium iodide well counter. The total value of radiochemical impurities is calculated by subtracting from 100% the sum of the percentage of the various impurities present (free Tc-99m, Tc-99m tin colloid, and Tc-99m dioxide). No NRC limits are set for radiochemical purity, but the United States Pharmacopeia, which sets standards for pharmacies, has defined the lower limits of acceptability for purity at 95% for free Tc-99m, 92% for Tc-99m sulfur colloid, and 90% for all other Tc-99m radiopharmaceuticals.

Misadministrations

Misadministration of a radiopharmaceutical is a regulatory (NRC) definition. Misadministrations can be divided into those occurring during a diagnostic procedure and those occurring during a therapeutic procedure. Because of the inherent dosimetric potential, the radioiodines, I-123 and I-131, are identified specifically in the definition of misadministrations. The current NRC definition of misadministration is as follows:

1. For the radioiodines, I-123 and I-131, for dosages greater than 30 Ci, a diagnostic or therapeutic misadministration occurs when: (*a*) the dose is given to the wrong patient or the patient receives the wrong pharmaceutical, (*b*) the administered dose differs from the prescribed dose by more than 20% and that difference is greater than 30 Ci.
2. For all radiopharmaceuticals, other than the radioiodines, a diagnostic misadministration occurs when both: (*a*) the radiopharmaceutical is given to the wrong patient, or when the wrong radiopharmaceutical, wrong route of administration or wrong dose (other than is prescribed—no percentage specified) is given to a patient *and*, (*b*) the dose to the patient exceeds 5 rems or the dose to any organ exceeds 50 rems.
3. For all radiopharmaceuticals, other than the radioiodines, a therapeutic misadministration occurs when either: (*a*) the radiopharmaceutical is given to the wrong patient, or when the wrong radiopharmaceutical is given, or the wrong route of administration is used, or (*b*) the administered dose differs from that prescribed dose by more than 20%.

Federal law requires that misadministrations of radiopharmaceuticals be reported to the NRC no later than the next calendar day after the discovery of the misadministration. This must be followed by a written report within 15 days that details a number of items, including the cause of the misadministration and proposed corrective actions.

IMAGING AND DETECTORS OF RADIATION
Image Content

Almost all nuclear medicine procedures that produce images are accomplished with the gamma camera (also known as a scintillation camera). Since nuclear medicine images reflect the biodistribution of the radiopharmaceutical, interpretation of gamma camera images must be tempered with a knowledge of not only the patterns of normal and pathologic processes, but also with a knowledge of the influence of the individual patient's physiology, habitus, and positioning, as well as with the technical aspects of the examination. In nuclear medicine, technical aspects may take an overriding, and sometimes dangerously subtle, dominance in their contribution to the final image output. A mastery of the basic details of image acquisition combined with an awareness of the artifactual patterns will enable the interpreting physician to avoid erroneous conclusions caused by the myriad interplay of physiologic, anatomic, and technical factors.

Gamma Camera

The essential components in the construction of a gamma camera, as a photon is followed out of the patient, include the collimator, the sodium iodide crystal, the photomultiplier (PM) tubes, electronic positioning and correction circuitry, electronic pulse height analyzer (PHA), and output device (CRT, film, computer). Since photons emanate omnidirectionally from the patient, the lead collimator serves to select photons from a single projection, reducing the detection of scatter and other low-energy emissions. The γ-photons interact with the sodium iodide crystal, converting to a light flash that is proportional to its initial energy. To assess the amount of energy in the light flash, a bank of photomultiplier tubes juxtaposed to the crystal converts the light to a summed voltage (pulse) that, after massage by the electronic positioning and correction circuitry, is screened for photon energy by the pulse height analyzer for acceptance. The PHA is set by the console operator based on the administered radionuclide and its appropriate photon energy(ies). For those photons accepted by the PHA, a position indicator is output to the CRT, film, and/or computer matrix. This entire process, called an event, can take place in as little as 10^{-5} seconds.

Prior to PHA analysis, but after the positioning circuitry, the voltage event is subjected to various correction matrices. These are camera- and manufacturer-specific, but in essence are attempts to correct for slight variations in PM tube sensitivities and crystal properties that, together, can cause inaccuracies in PM voltage response and, subsequently, event positioning on the crystal. One or more correction matri-

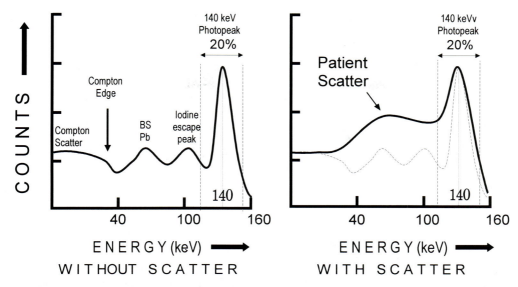

Figure 47.5. The Tc-99m Photospectrums. The left photospectrum displays the energies present from the radionuclide imaged by itself (without scatter), while the right photospectrum is from the radionuclide imaged from inside a patient (with scatter). The primary energies of the curve include: (*a*) *Compton Scatter* (0–50) keV; (*b*) *Compton Edge* at 50 keV—note that in the patient, scatter contributes to a broad increase in the 90–140 keV level; (*C*) Backscatter (*BS*)—primary gamma undergoes 180° scatter from behind the crystal, and upon reentering the crystal they are completely absorbed; (*d*) Lead x-ray Peak (*Pb*)—photoelectric absorption in lead shielding of camera housing causes 75–90 keV x-ray photons; (*e*) *Iodine escape peak* (112 keV)—iodine K-shell electons escape the sodium iodide crystal with an energy of 28 keV, therefore an incoming gamma of 140 keV would lose this much energy before it was registerd by the PM tubes (140–28 = 112 keV); (*f*) *Photopeak*—for imaging purposes, a 20% window over the 140 keV photopeak defines the limits of acceptance of detected energies. Note that some of the scatter photons from the patient are accepted, contributing to decreased image quality (loss of resolution).

ces can be present in a camera. Some of the more commonly found matrices include uniformity, energy, and linearity.

Photopeak

Although each radionuclide has one or more imaging photon energies (Table 47.1), interactions between the original photon and the patient and camera produce a wide range of energies that are all detected by the gamma camera. These various energies can be displayed by most gamma cameras using the multichannel analyzers, which plot frequency of event against photon energy. The desired photon energy is called the photopeak. The remainder of the detected energies are undesirable because they do not represent the true source of the radionuclide. This latter fact is due to scatter, and is the major source for decreased image quality. Comparing the photospectrum curves of the radionuclide by itself with that of the patient demonstrates dramatically the ability of the patient to contribute to scatter and, thereby, to image degradation (Fig. 47.5). Furthermore, the larger the patient and the greater the gamma camera distance to the patient, the greater is the scatter and image degradation.

As stated earlier, the PHA is used to select the desired photon energy by placing a "window" of acceptance of plus and minus 10% around the photopeak, thereby limiting the contribution of scatter to the image. Multiple windows can be simultaneously acquired in this manner as would be needed, for example, by gallium-67 (93, 184, and 300 keV) and indium-111 (172 and 247 keV).

Quality Control of the Gamma Camera

The quality control program of a nuclear medicine department must cover instrumentation (Table 47.5) as well as radiopharmaceutical preparation. The goal of quality control of a gamma camera is to assure both the uniform response of the detectors (PM tubes) and the correct location of the scintillation events occurring in the crystal.

The quickest and easiest check of a gamma camera is by the daily acquisition of an intrinsic (no collimator) flood image. A flood field image is obtained by exposing the entire crystal to either a uniform source of radioactivity, typically from either a point source, Tc-99m, or a commercially prepared sheet source, Co-57. Regardless of the source used, it must deliver count rates with less than 1% variation across the surface of the crystal. This is accomplished by positioning the point source at least 4 collimator crystal widths from the detector. The sheet source, which is placed on the detector face during the acquisition of the flood, is purchased with the manufacturer's guarantee that there is less than 1 % inherent variation. A visual in-

Table 47.5. Planar and SPECT Camera Recommended Quality Control Procedures

Procedure	Frequency	Camera System	Comment
Flood field	Daily	Planar	Intrinsically or extrinsically; intrinsic flood is acquired for 1 to 2 million counts with and without uniformity correction; percent difference should be less than 15% for most systems
Sensitivity	Weekly	Planar	Intrinsically or extrinsically; result is in counts per minute per curie
Spatial resolution	Weekly	Planar	Intrinsic or extrinsic; use bar phantom
Linearity	Weekly	Planar	Bar phanton or multiholed phantom
High count collimator flood	Weekly	SPECT	30 million counts for 64 × 64 matrix; 90 million counts for 128 × 128 matrix
Center of rotation (COR)	Weekly	SPECT	Corrected to less than 0.5 pixel for 64 × 64 matrix to less than 1.0 pixel for 128 × 128 matrix
Pixel calibration	Monthly	SPECT	Measurement of pixel size in both X and Y direction; used for attenuation correction
Jaszczak or Carlson phantom	Quarterly	SPECT	Commercially available phantoms that test total system performance

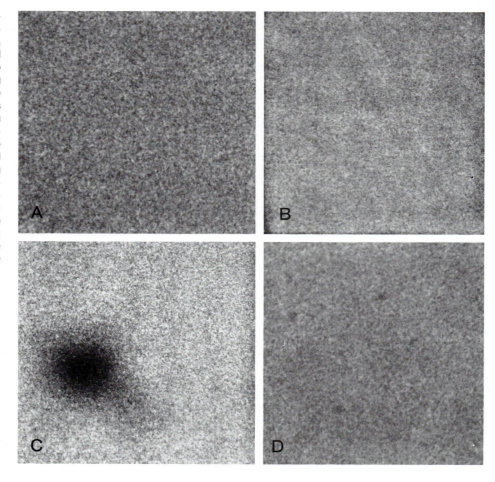

Figure 47.6. Intrinsic Floods. A. Normal uniform flood, with correction matrices applied. **B.** Same camera as in **A,** but with the correction matrices turned off. The correction matrices are able to compensate for sometimes striking nonuniformities in the flood field. These corrections are acceptable as long as they do not represent too great a data loss or prolong imaging times. **C.** Uncorrectable off-peak PM tube. The photopeak for this PM tube had drifted downward and the tube was accepting more counts than its neighbors **D.** Uncorrectable crystal hydration ("measles"). The dark spots are areas in the crystal where water has breached the manufacturer's water-tight seal to gain access to a hygroscopic sodium iodide crystal. The expensive crystal had to be replaced .

spection of the flood will give an adequate qualitative assessment of nonuniformities. Significant nonuniformities (5% or more) can be detected by the human eye. Results from quantitative analysis, performed by flood field-specific software, along with the flood image itself, can be logged into computer-based data bases for detection of subtle changes over time. If the pattern is abnormal, remedies include reloading correction matrices, replacing PM tubes, and addressing other electronic or mechanical problems (Fig. 47.6).

In a similar vein, a quantitative value of general camera performance can be obtained by comparing uniformity flood field images acquired with and without the uniformity correction. This difference value, termed "data loss," represents additional processing time imposed by the correction circuits to reach a set number of counts. Using a 1 million to 2 million count flood, the data loss can be calculated as the percentage difference between the time required to obtain an intrinsic flood with and without the uniformity cor-

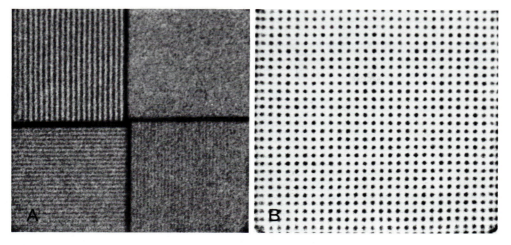

Figure 47.7. Spatial Resolution and Linearity of a Gamma Camera. Both of these floods were acquired without the collimator using a Co-57 sheet source over the phantom. **A.** Four-quadrant bar phantom. The distance between bars is equal within a quadrant, but progressively diminishes between quadrants. This bar flood demonstrates lack of visibility of the bars in the quadrant with the narrowest bars. Rotating the bars 90° will allow the entire crystal to be checked. Linearity can also be assessed with this phantom. **B.** Orthogonal-holed phantom. Pincushion (inward) and barrel (outward) distortion can easily be evaluated by visual inspection of this flood. Both are absent here.

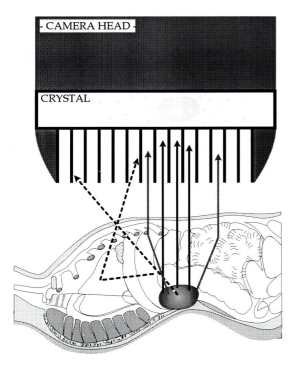

Figure 47.8. Function of a Collimator. The function of a collimator is to reduce scatter and correctly localize the source of the radionuclide in the patient. For example, a Tc-99m radiopharmaceutical localized primarily in the kidney will radiate 140 keV photons omnidirectionally. Those perpendicular to a parallel collimator will be detected at their corresponding anatomic location on the crystal. Because of the 20% window around the Tc-99m photopeak, some scatter photons (*solid gray lines*) will still be accepted and cause a slight degradation of image quality. But the majority of scatter, falling below the acceptance window (see photospectrums in Fig. 47.5), will be rejected because of either low energy or oblique incidence to the collimator (*dashed lines*).

rection turned on. Typically, differences under 15% are normal for most modern gamma camera systems. Greater differences significantly prolong imaging times and require either a reacquisition of the uniformity or other correction matrix or implicate a hardware electronic problem requiring a service call.

Two basic quality control procedures performed to assure correct positioning of events are spatial resolution and linearity (Fig. 47.7). These are generally performed weekly by acquiring a flood with a specially designed phantom sandwiched between a Co-57 sheet source and the camera, with or without the collimator. Alternatively, a Tc-99m point source at a 4-collimator distance can be substituted for the sheet source. Several commercial bar phantoms, such as PLES (parallel lines equal spaced) and four-quadrant, are available to assess spatial resolution using a series of equally spaced lead bars. Linearity can also be assessed by visual inspection of any of these straight bar phantoms, or can be individually assessed by other dedicated linearity phantoms such as an orthogonal holed phantom. Generally, inspection of these types of floods will reveal any linearity distortions such as pincushion or barreling.

Collimators

The collimator is composed of perforated lead or tungsten and is positioned on the face of the sodium iodide crystal detector. Its purpose is to reduce scatter and obliquely angled photons, allowing only those photons that pass through the collimator holes properly to be detected (Fig. 47.8). There are two basic collimator designs, pinhole and multihole (Fig. 47.9).

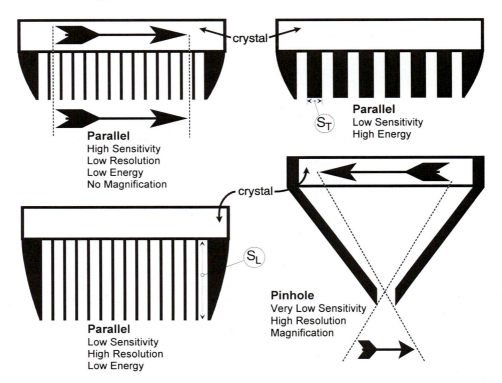

Figure 47.9. Collimator Types. Parallel multiholed collimators are the principle lead collimator used in nuclear medicine imaging. The septa (lead walls between the holes) confer the properties of resolution, energy, and sensitivity. The longer the septa, the higher the resolution. The wider the septa (S_T), the higher the energy that can be imaged without septal penetration of unwanted photons. The shorter the septa (S_l), the higher the sensitivity. The count rate is inversely proportional to the square of the septal length (S_l). Note the lack of magnification and distortion with parallel collimators, as opposed to the pinhole collimator.

The pinhole collimator is a single-holed collimator that allows only photons within the angle subtended by the pinhole to reach the detector. The geometry inverts the image and, depending upon its distance from the aperture, distorts it through magnification. Magnification translates into high-resolution images, but the small aperture lowers sensitivity and imposes long acquisition times to achieve adequate image photon statistics. The large cone of lead renders the pinhole collimator applicable across a large range of photon energies ranging from 140 keV (Tc-99m) to 364 keV (I-131). The pinhole collimator finds its major clinical use in imaging the thyroid and focal areas of the skeleton in a bone scan.

Multiholed collimators are classified as parallel, diverging, or converging. By far the most common of the multiholed collimators is the parallel collimator, which produces an image without distortion in a one-to-one correspondence with the source. The long axis of the holes of the collimator are perpendicular to the face of the crystal and parallel to each other, separated by lead septa of varying thickness. The physical design of the holes and septa dictates the sensitivity, energy range, and resolution of the parallel collimator. Thicker septa are used with higher energy photons to prevent septal penetration, but result in decreased sensitivity due to reduction of the crystal surface area exposed to holes. Deeper holes increase resolution by narrowing the field of view, but also decrease sensitivity by excluding more aberrant photons. Differences in septal and hole design create a functional classification, i.e., high-resolution collimator for bone scans, high-sensitivity/low-resolution collimator for flow imaging, and high-energy collimator for Ga-67/I-131 images. Most planar imaging (two-dimensional imaging as opposed to three-dimensional as in single-photon emission computed tomography (SPECT) is accomplished with parallel hole collimators, which includes bone, renal, hepatobiliary, and myocardial imaging.

The quality control for collimators is directed at assessing the integrity of the collimator. Imperfections from damaged septa in the collimator will introduce nonuniformities, causing image degradation. Aside from the visual inspection of the actual collimator, a high count extrinsic flood, performed periodically, may reveal more subtle defects.

Dose Calibrator

As a mandatory requirement by the NRC, all diagnostic and therapeutic doses must be assayed prior to administration. (See "Misadministrations for prescription limits.") The dose calibrator is an ionization

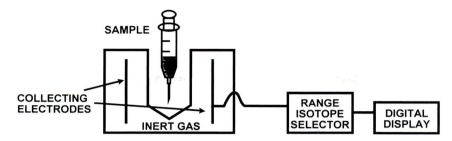

Figure 47.10. Dose Calibrator.

chamber, not a sodium iodide crystal. It is a cylinder that holds a defined volume of inert gas and a cylindrical collecting electrode (Fig. 47.10). A voltage applied across the electrodes will not pass current until the gas is ionized by radiation emitted from a radiopharmaceutical in the well. The measurement of the current is proportional to the activity of a given radionuclide. By calibrating to known radionuclides with known amounts of activity, the current can be equated to dose activity. A series of buttons imprinted with the radionuclide names resides on the face of the unit. A calibration factor is assigned to each button, unique for that particular radionuclide, to adjust the correct proportionality between current and activity. The dose calibrator will read activity with any button selected, but it is only accurate for the isotope for which it has been calibrated. As opposed to the well counter, which measures only in the curie range, the dose calibrator is capable of measuring quantities in the curie, millicurie, and microcurie ranges. The well counter, therefore, cannot act as a subsitute for a dose calibration.

Quality control for the dose calibrator consists of periodic checks on its performance. *Constancy,* performed daily, measures the activity of long-lived reference sources to look for deviations from expected values. Using long physical half-life isotopes such as Co-57 (120 keV) in the Tc-99m channel, and Cs-137 (662 keV) in the Mo-99 channel, the measured activity must agree with calculated activity ±5%. *Linearity,* performed quarterly, assesses the accuracy of measurements over a wide range of activity, usually from 10 µCi to the maximum administered dose, which in most laboratories is around 200 mCi. With a high activity Tc-99m source, a series of measurements is collected either over a 48-hour period of time, or by using commercially available simulated decay (leaded) cylinders. These measurements are compared with calculated (using decay factors) values and should agree within ±5%. *Accuracy,* performed annually, measures certified sources of different photon energies brought in from or referenced to National Institute of Standards and Technology (formerly the National Bureau of Standards). Sources include Co-57, Cs-137, and Ba-133. Their measurements must agree with

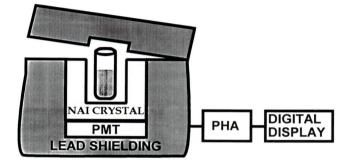

Figure 47.11. Sodium Iodide Well Counter.

known source measurements within ±5%. At installation and after repairs, *geometry* is evaluated to compensate for measurements made of sources in different volume dilutions or in different containers. Glass and plastic syringes can affect readings significantly. These calculated correction factors are applied to activity measurements by the operator, e.g., 2% added for volumes greater than 20 ml.

Sodium Iodide Well Counter

The sodium iodide well counter is used to quantify small amounts of activity in examinations such as an in vitro Schilling test or survey wipe tests. Constructed of a sodium iodide cylinder with a hole drilled in it, sitting on a single photomultiplier tube, and surrounded by lead on all sides, the design provides for good geometric and detection efficiency (Fig. 47.11). The quality control for the sodium iodide well counter consists of daily assessment of the high voltage and sensitivity. Additionally, resolution, chi-square, and linearity are checked quarterly.

Thyroid Uptake Probe

The thyroid uptake probe is used to quantitate the percentage of radioactive iodine taken up by the thyroid and to survey workers (called bioassay) for possible radioiodine contamination, most notably after radioiodine therapeutic administrations that may have resulted in some of the radioiodine entering the body (called internal contamination). Constructed of a single 2- or 3-inch thick sodium iodide crystal, 5 cm

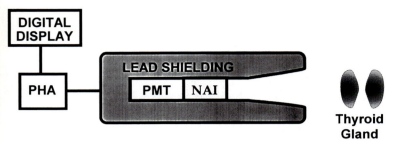

Figure 47.12.   Thyroid Uptake Probe.

in diameter, juxtaposed to a single photomultiplier, the field of view is defined by a cone-shaped, flat-field collimator (Fig. 47.12). No imaging is performed with this probe, only quantitative count measurements that are performed at a fixed crystal-to-patient distance. The quality control for the thyroid uptake probe is identical to that of the sodium iodide well counter.

SINGLE-PHOTON EMISSION CT (SPECT) IMAGING
Concept

In diagnostic radiology, computed tomography (CT) is achieved by the calculation (reconstruction) of a three-dimensional image from multiple x-ray transmissions through the body. To accomplish CT in nuclear medicine, the three-dimensional image representing the volume of distribution of the administered radiopharmaceuticals is reconstructed from detection of multiple emissions from the body. This form of CT is termed "single-photon emission computed tomography," or SPECT. Unlike x-ray CT, where one slice is acquired at a time, SPECT simultaneously acquires multislice raw data in the form of two-dimensional planar images.

There are two major advantages of SPECT over planar imaging: (*a*) image contrast is improved by minimizing the superimposition of activity present in a planar two-dimensional image, and (*b*) improved three-dimensional localization of radiopharmaceutical distribution results from the cross-sectional display of activity. Additionally, there is the theoretical advantage of being able to quantify the distribution of a radiopharmaceutical in the body. One disadvantage to SPECT needs to be noted. Because of the average increased detector-to-patient distance from the rotating camera head, spatial resolution is actually less in the tomographic images than in planar images.

Instrumentation of Rotational SPECT

Single-photon emission computed tomography can be accomplished by limited angle tomography, but rotational tomography is the dominant modality in the current clinical setting. In its elementary design, rotational tomography consists of a conventional gamma camera that is capable of orbiting the patient who lies on a table positioned on the axis of rotation. There is a commercial tendency to attach the camera to a gantry, as in most x-ray CT units, and to increase the number of camera heads from one to two or three. Rotating ring detectors can also be used in dedicated SPECT systems. All of these design modifications tend to optimize image quality.

Camera head orbits can be up to 360° and, depending upon the manufacturer, can be circular, elliptical, or body contouring. Noncircular orbits decrease the camera-to-patient distance and increase spatial resolution (Fig. 47.13). As the detector traverses its orbit, a series of planar images, referred to as projections or views, is acquired either continuously or at discrete angular intervals. These are the raw data used by the computer to reconstruct the tomographic images. Acquisition parameters are changed to tailor image acquisition to the patient and the clinical question to be addressed. Parameters under user control include the number of views, the time for each view, and the computer matrix size. Because of the low number of photons available for each projection during the single-camera SPECT acquisitions, a 64 × 64 matrix is usually optimal. The 128 × 128 matrices are usually reserved for very high photon flux scans, such as bone scans, or for multheaded SPECT systems.

The sum of the number of views, the time for each view, and the time for gantry movement is the total acquisition time. Most patients can tolerate acquisition times of 30–45 minutes. The greater the number of views, the better the image resolution and quality, provided each view has acquired enough counts to minimize statistical artifacts. Sixty views over 360° will produce an adequate SPECT image. Once the number of views has been chosen, the ability of the patient to lie still will dictate the time per view. For example, 60 stops over 360° at 30 seconds a stop with 5 seconds per gantry movement will require approximately 33 minutes to complete. Acquisition parameters must be selected to balance image quality with patient comfort. When choosing acquisition parameters, any patient motion will significantly degrade the reconstructed image.

The reconstruction from the raw planar data sets to the tomographic images is accomplished by high-speed computers. The most common method of reconstruction is the filtered backprojection. This method mathematically generates the three-dimensional volume from the planar data and then uses digital filters to alter noise and smooth and sharpen the images. The reconstruction method and choice of filters is generally vendor-specific but must be optimized for each particular camera/computer combination.

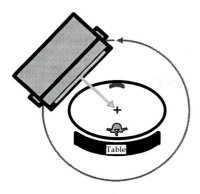
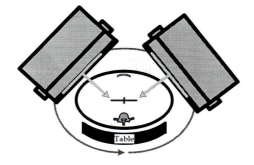

CIRCULAR ELLIPTICAL

Figure 47.13. The SPECT Orbits. Circular orbits are easy for the gantry to negotiate, but suffer from the increased detector-to-patient distance with loss of spatial resolution. By using noncircular orbits such as the elliptical one demonstrated here, the camera head-to-patient distance is minimized.

Immediately after the acquisition of the raw data, but before the reconstruction, a cine display of the raw data should be performed to detect any unsuspected patient motion that might prevent a valid SPECT reconstruction. The reconstructed image can be displayed in classical tomographic planes: transaxial, coronal, and sagittal. Cinematic display with the rotating three-dimensional images and volume-rendering are attempts that have been used to enhance localization of the activity.

Quality Control of SPECT Systems

The most important component of a SPECT system is the planar gamma camera. Any deficiencies in the planar capabilities of a SPECT system are amplified during the reconstruction process of the tomographic images. For example, an uncorrected flood-field nonuniformity defect or an off-peaked PM tube will produce subtle ring or blur artifacts in the three-dimensional images. In addition to the routine planar camera quality control, several SPECT-specific quality control procedures are necessary to minimize artifact formations (Table 47.5) Collimator imperfections will manifest as nonuniformities on the SPECT raw data. The effect of these collimator imperfections can be minimized by mathematically applying a statistically high count extrinsic (collimator) flood to each individual raw planar image prior to reconstruction. This extrinsic flood is computer acquired using a Co-57 sheet source, for 30 million counts when using a 64 × 64 matrix and for 90 million counts when using a 128 × 128 matrix.

The camera's mechanical center of rotation (COR) must be calibrated with the center of the computer's matrix as it is projected from the face of the crystal (Fig. 47.14). For various mechanical and electronic reasons, these are not perfectly aligned. An offset greater than half a pixel for a 64 × 64 matrix will re-

sult in loss of contrast and resolution, and distortion of the tomographic images. The COR calibration is performed by imaging a point or line source at multiple opposing intervals over 360°. The COR is then calculated by averaging the difference in the sets of offset of the source from the matrix center as seen by the opposing pairs of images. The COR value is stored by the computer for use during the ensuing reconstructions of the three-dimensional images. When this calibration factor is applied during reconstruction, the matrix centers are shifted to align with the mechanical rotational center. This COR calibration must be performed for each collimator, zoom factor, and matrix size used for SPECT acquisitions.

Attenuation correction refers to attempts to compensate for the loss of photons due to absorption as they traverse tissue. Photons arising from deeper tissues have greater attentuation. Attenuation correction compensates for these losses by adding counts back into the reconstructed slices. Attenuation correction for SPECT images is usually only performed for solid body parts such as the abdomen, pelvis, and head. It is not applied for the chest, where water and air density are not distributed evenly. Pixel size calibration prior to attenuation correction is a necessary quality control procedure to match the matrix size with the physical dimensions of the body part being imaged. Pixel calibration is easily performed by acquiring two point or two line sources separated by a known distance; the computer calculates and stores the pixels per millimeter of calibration factor for subsequent attenuation corrections.

As a general assessment of the total performance of a SPECT system, commercially available cylindrical phantoms can be imaged. Fluid-filled phantoms are designed so that after Tc-99m is added to the fluid, areas of cold and hot activity are present in varying dimensions. A subsequent SPECT acquisition, recon-

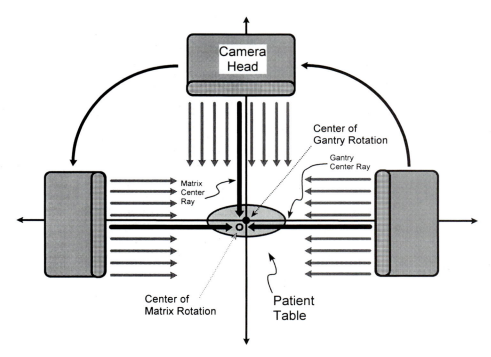

Figure 47.14. Center of Rotation. This illustration is diagrammatically exaggerated for teaching purposes. The COR represents the difference between mechanical center of rotation (*black dashed arrow/black dot*) and the center of the projected image matrix (*gray dashed arrow/black circle*). This difference must be adjusted to less than a half pixel for a 64 × 64 matrix to avoid SPECT reconstruction defects.

Table 47.6.   Comparison of SPECT and PET

	SPECT	PET
Principle of raw image formation	Collimation	Annihilation coincidence detection
Transverse slice reconstruction	Filter backprojection	Filter backprojection
Radionuclides	Tc-99m and other single photon emitting radionuclide	Positron emitters
Spatial resolution	12 mm (1 head) 7 mm (3 heads)	5 mm
Attenuation correction	Crude	Accurate (with a transmission source)
Scatter rejection	Good	Excellent
Cost	$400,000 (1 head) $700,000 (3 heads)	$2,000,000 (plus need for on-site cyclotron if nuclides other than F-18 and Rb-82 are to be used)

struction, and display of the phantom will test the SPECT system's contrast, resolution, field uniformity, and attenuation correction.

POSITRON EMISSION TOMOGRAPHY (PET)
Concept and Instrumentation

Whereas SPECT is designed for the detection and imaging of single-photon emitting radionuclides, PET deals with the detection and imaging of dual-photon positron-emitting (positive electron) radionuclides. These proton-rich radionuclides, such as carbon-11, nitrogen-13, oxygen-15, and fluorine-18, are short-lived, cyclotron-produced isotopes that decay by re-

leasing a positron from the nucleus. Once released, the positron travels only a few millimeters in tissue before combining with a negative electron and converting to annihilation radiation: two-ray photons of 511 keV each (energy equivalent of an electron's mass) emitted in 180° opposite directions. It is these annihilation photons that, when detected within a preset time window by a pair of opposed ring detectors, allow for accurate localization of the annihilation event by high-speed coincident circuitry along a line. From these lines, and using filters and computer reconstruction techniques, tomographic images of the distribution of the positron radionuclide can be calculated.

Advantages. Positrons have been labeled into compounds that have successfully produced PET images demonstrating physiologic and biochemical processes. This has been particularly true in the fields of cerebral and cardiac metabolism. These functional images enjoy higher resolution than SPECT affords, due in large measure to higher energy photons, efficient suppression of scattered radiation, and dedicated detector systems (Table 47.6).

Disadvantages. The high initial cost of a PET scanner, as well as the moderate investment in personnel necessary to operate the unit, have limited the proliferation of PET scanners. Additionally, some of the very short-lived positron radionuclides require an on-site cyclotron for their production.

Suggested Readings

Alazraki NP, Mishkin FS. Fundamentals of nuclear medicine. 2nd ed. New York: The Society of Nuclear Medicine, 1988:3–20.

English RJ, Brown SE. SPECT: single-photon emission computed tomography: a primer. 2nd ed. New York: The Society of Nuclear Medicine, 1990.

Graham LS. Quality Assurance for SPECT. In: Freeman LM, Wiessmann HS, eds. Nuclear medicine annual 1989. New York: Raven Press, 1989:81–108.

Kowalsky RJ, Perry JR. Radiopharmaceuticals in nuclear medicine practice. Norwalk, CT: Appleton & Lange, 1987.

Mettler FA, Guiberteau MJ. Essentials of nuclear medicine imaging. 3rd ed. Philadelphia: WB Saunders, 1991.

Romney BM, Nickloff EL, Esser PD, et al. Radionuclide administration to nursing mothers: mathematically derived guidelines. Radiology 1986;160:549–554.

Simmons GH, ed. The scintillation camera. New York: The Society of Nuclear Medicine, 1988.

Sorensen JA, Phelps ME. Physics in nuclear medicine. 2nd ed. Philadelphia: WB Saunders, 1987.

U.S. National Acadmy of Sciences. Report by the Committee on the Biological Effects of Ionizing Radiations ("BEIR-V"). Washington: National Accademy of Sciences/National Research Council, 1989.

48

Skeletal System Scintigraphy

Robert J. Telepak
Philip W. Wiest
Michael F. Hartshorne

Musculoskeletal imaging studies performed with gamma cameras and technetium-99m (Tc-99m) labeled diphosphonates are a staple of nuclear medicine. The bone scan is a map of osteoblastic activity that occurs in response to a variety of benign and malignant conditions. The bone scan is an excellent complement to other radiographic studies of the skeletal system. Blood flow is required to deliver the radiopharmaceutical to functioning osteoblasts. These assemble labeled diphosphonates into the hydration shell of hydroxyapatite crystals as they are formed and modified. Osteoclastic function is not measured by this technique.

TECHNICAL

Skeletal scintigraphy has a resolution of about 5 mm in the best conditions. Adult intravenous doses of 20 mCi (740 mBq) or more Tc-99m diphosphonates are adequate for static imaging 3—4 hours after injection. Vigorous osteoblastic activity in juvenile skeletons, healing fractures, pathologic conditions stimulating skeletal blood flow, and bone repair increase the bone labeling. The Tc-99m diphosphonates are excreted by glomerular filtration by the kidneys. In a normal subject, 50% is excreted by 2—4 hours, and up to 80% of the injected diphosphonate will be excreted by 24 hours. Normal renal function clears soft-tissue activity, which improves the quality of bone images. Decreased renal function for any reason degrades image quality. Waiting 3—4 hours before imaging is a compromise between remaining radioactivity and reduction of background around the skeleton. "Spot-view," "whole-body," and single-photon emission computed tomography (SPECT) imaging technology may be used. Technical factors influencing image quality are important but are beyond the scope of this discussion. The study should be modified as necessary to answer the clinical question for which the scan was ordered (Fig. 48.1).

TRAUMA

Trauma to the skeleton may be undetectable on standard radiographic examinations. The classic insufficiency (stress) fracture may be caused by overuse of the normal skeleton or normal use of weakened bone. Radiographically demonstrated trauma precedes scintigraphically detectable fracture healing by about 10 days. Decreased or normal osteoblastic activity is seen at the fracture site in this first phase of repair. The subsequent osteoblastic activity then shows as a "hot spot" weeks before the calcified callus appears on a radiograph (Fig. 48.2).

In an uncomplicated fracture, repaired bone returns to normal appearance as the callus at the fracture site remodels over a period of months. A complicated fracture in a weight-bearing bone healing with angulation may take many years to return to normal bone scan activity.

PROSTHETIC JOINTS

Prosthetic joint replacements, especially of the hip, may loosen and/or become infected. For about 6 months after surgery the bone around the prosthesis is expected to have increased osteoblastic activity. Thereafter, increased labeling correlates with infection, loosening, and heterotopic bone formation, depending upon the pattern of localization. Radiographs and occasionally radiolabeled white blood cell scans are required to evaluate abnormal findings (Fig. 48.3).

ARTHROPATHIES

Inflammation of a joint creates increased blood flow and increased radiopharmaceutical supplied to those portions of the bone bounded by the synovial capsule.

Increased bone labeling is seen in toxic synovitis, septic joints, inflammation associated with early degenerative conditions, and connective tissue arthropathies (Fig. 48.1). In early osteoarthropathy, high-resolution images detect increased subchondral bone labeling long before there are radiographic findings. Intense, abnormal labeling also is seen in neuropathic joints long before the abnormality is detected by radiographs.

OSTEOMYELITIS

In a large bone such as a tibia, acute hematogenous infection of bone that precedes radiographic ab-

normality can be sensitively and specifically diagnosed by three-phase bone scans. Early arterial flow seen seconds after injection (first phase), increased blood pool seen for a few minutes before bone labeling begins (second phase), and intense delayed labeling 3 or more hours after injection (third phase) is characteristic of early infection. This phenomena requires several days of symptoms before it develops. Radiographic changes may not be seen for 10–14 days. The scan is more difficult to read and not as specific when the target is small (like the bones of the foot) in comparison with the resolving power of the camera (Fig. 48.4). False-negative examinations

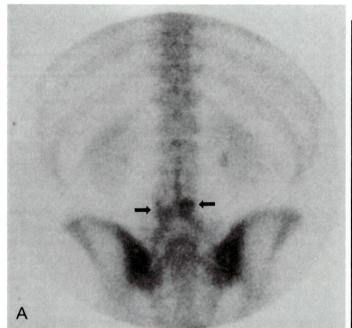

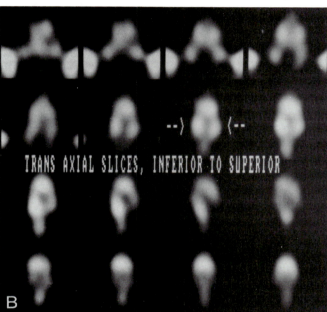

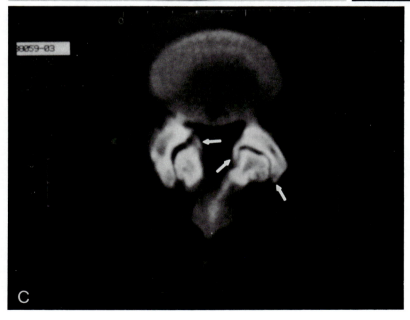

Figure 48.1. Single-photon Emission Computed Tomography-Enhanced Images of L4-5 Facet Degenerative Arthropathy. A. A planar, posterior image of the lumbar spine shows small areas of increased activity (arrows) in the lower lumbar spine in a patient with chronic low back pain. **B.** Transaxial images of the same lumbar spine start at the L5-S1 facet joint level and continue up to the L3-4 level. Note the conspicuity of the abnormality. Areas of increased bone labeling at the L4-5 facet joints are marked by arrows. **C.** The CT of the same level shows hypertrophic spurs (arrows) embracing the facet joints.

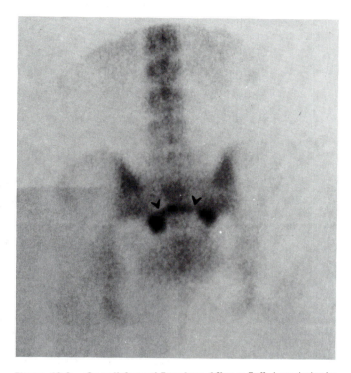

Figure 48.2.   *Occult Sacral Fracture After a Fall.* A posterior image of the pelvis shows a horizontal line of increased uptake (*arrowheads*) across the sacrum, which marks healing along a painful fracture that is invisible on radiographs.

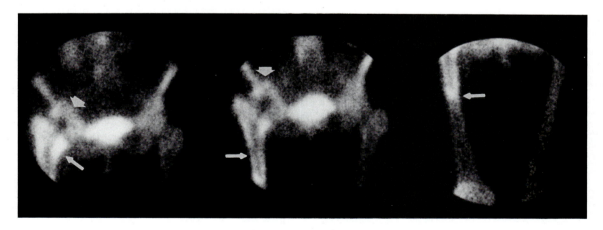

Figure 48.3.   Hip Prosthesis Loosening in a Patient with Hip Pain. Anterior images of the pelvis, hips, and femurs show intense labeling around the femoral (*arrows*) and acetabular (*arrowheads*) components of a 2-year-old total hip arthroplasty. Both had loosened without infection.

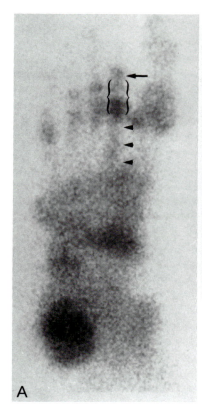

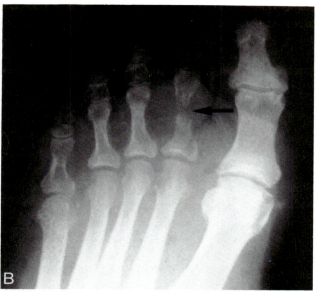

Figure 48.4. Osteomyelitis of the Second Toe and Metatarsal and Septic Second Metatarsal Phalangeal Joint. A. A plantar bone scan shows increased activity in the second proximal phalanx (*arrow*), metatarsal phalangeal joint (*brackets*), and second metatarsal (*arrowheads*) indicating reactive bone stimulated by the infection. Decreased activity distal to that point corresponds with necrotic tissue. **B.** A radiograph shows destructive changes in the second proximal phalanx (*arrow*), but appears normal in the second metatarsal phalangeal joint and metatarsal phalangeal shaft.

are reported in children when the duration of clinical illness is brief.

A cellulitis adjacent to bone is seen as soft-tissue areas of increased activity on the arterial and immediate blood pool phases with little or no increased activity in the bone on the third phase. In the peripheral skeleton where bones are small, it is frequently impossible to tell the difference between an infection adjacent to a bone with increased soft tissue and increased periosteal labeling from an infection within the bone. Bone scans may take months to nomalize after infections of bone are sterilized. A chronic infection of bone may be inseparable from normal healing demonstrated by bone scan.

VASCULAR PHENOMENA

There is a strong vascular influence on the labeling of bones. Increased blood flow stimulates increased osteoblastic *and* osteoclastic activity. The bone scan reflects the former effect. Common pathologic conditions such as tumor and trauma cause hyperemia and increased blood pooling with increased delivery of radiopharmaceuticals to the bone's osteoblasts. This is an appropriate response to injury. Reflex sympathetic dystrophy is an example of an inappropriate, increased vascular response to little or no injury (Fig. 48.5). A bone scan is a simple test of the vascular sta-

tus of a bone or bone graft. If osteoblasts are labeled, the blood supply must be intact. Acute avascular necrosis shows no labeling of the affected bone. Bone subjected to radiation therapy may lose blood supply and osteoblastic activity. Square-edged radiation portals produce typical areas of decreased labeling.

HETEROTOPIC BONE

Repair of soft-tissue injuries sometimes leads to the formation of heterotopic bone. Histologically, normal bone may form from differentiating fibroblasts after trauma. Muscle crush injuries healing with the formation of heterotopic bone (myositis ossificans) are readily labeled on bone scans weeks before the plain film shows signs of calcification. Soft tissues around joint prostheses, in paralyzed limbs, and in burn injuries are common sites of heterotopic bone formation.

METABOLIC CONDITIONS

Increased parathormone levels (or the presence of tumor-produced parathormone-like substances) simultaneously increase serum calcium and phosphate. Calcium/phosphate complexes precipitate in the thyroid gland, lungs, and stomach. This "metastatic calcification" is rarely seen on radiographs but is routinely visible on bone scans. Other generalized skeletal abnormalities such as tumoral calcinosis, hypertrophic

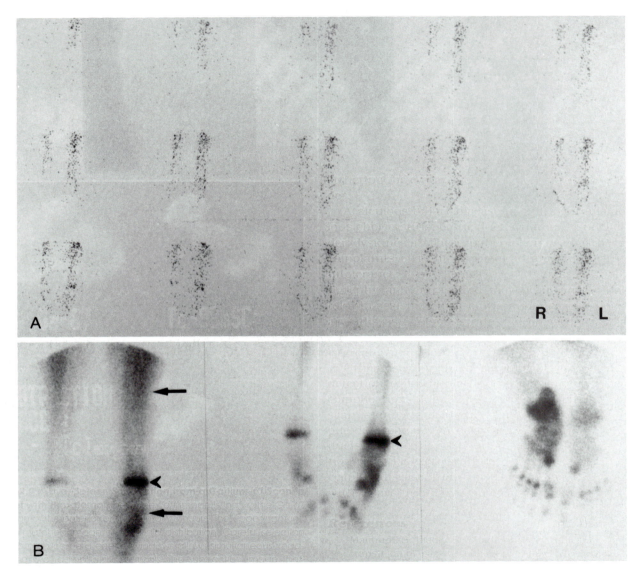

Figure 48.5.   Three-phase Bone Scan Showing Reflex Sympathetic Dystrophy in the Painful Left Ankle and Foot of a 13-year-old Child. A. The initial bolus, filmed at 1 second per frame in the anterior projection with heels together, arrives in the left foot (*L*) and ankle earlier than the right foot (*R*). **B.** The early blood pool image (*left*) shows greater blood pooling (*arrows*) in the same area. The 3-hour delayed images (*center* and *right*, anterior and plantar projections, respectively) show a generalized increase in bone labeling. Note the preferential labeling of the physeal plates, which is expected in a juvenile patient.

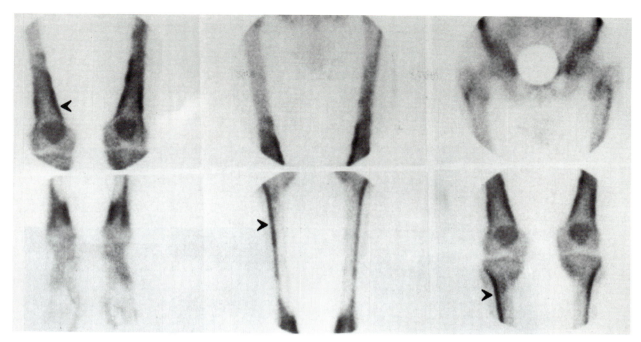

Figure 48.6. Hypertrophic Osteoarthropathy in a Patient with Carcinoma of the Lung and Bone Pain. A scan done to evaluate for metastases shows increased periosteal labeling (*arrowheads*), principally in the metaphyses of the lower extremity. The patient does not have metastases.

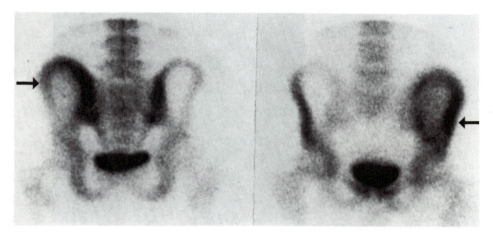

Figure 48.7. Paget's Disease of Bone. A posterior (left) and anterior (*right*) image of the pelvis of a 60-year-old man with carcinoma of the prostate. There is abnormal, increased uptake in the left hemipelvis (*arrows*), which is characteristic of pagetic bone. Radiographs (not shown) helped confirm that this is not metastatic cancer of the prostate.

osteoarthropathy, systemic mastocytosis, and many other diseases with calcification or ossification of tissues may be shown with bone scans (Fig. 48.6).

BONE DYSPLASIAS

Benign bone dysplasias frequently show the expected increase in labeling on bone scans. Paget's disease of bone, fibrous dysplasia, enchondromas, exostoses, and many other benign conditions of bone are detected by bone scan. Comparison with skeletal radiographs will clarify these multicentric diagnoses. An efficient way to screen the whole skeleton is the bone scan.

In the osteolytic phase of Paget's disease of bone, the radiographic changes are accompanied by marked increases in bone labeling. This repair continues with increased labeling during the radiographic stage of sclerotic, expansile pagetic bone (Fig. 48.7). The increased activity on bone scans may eventually disappear as repair is complete.

PRIMARY BONE TUMORS

There are two principle ways in which bone tumors are detected by bone scans. Osteosarcomas and chondrosarcomas may have abnormal osteoblastic or chondroblastic activity associated with the production of abnormal tumor calcification. This is a malignant process with the tumor itself being "hot." Metastases from calcifying or ossifying primary tumors to other

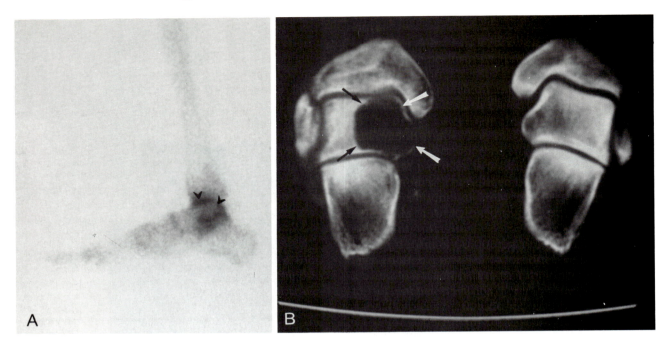

Figure 48.10. Aggressive Renal Cell Carcinoma Metastasis in the Talus. A. A medial projection bone scan of the ankle and foot shows a halo of increased activity (*arrowheads*) around the ankle joint. **B.** A CT scan of the ankles shows a scooped out lesion (*arrows*) of the right talus (image at left) where the metastasis has destroyed bone so fast that repair bone has no chance to form. The talus does not show a hot spot. The bone scan is abnormal because of hemarthrosis irritation of the synovium. Increased blood supplied to the inflamed synovium brings with it increased radiopharmaceutical, which labels all of the bones of the joint.

nonskeletal sites may also take up Tc-99m diphosphonates directly, making them readily detected by scintigraphy.

The Tc-99m diphosphonate may also be avidly concentrated by the normal osteoblasts reacting to the destructive presence of the primary tumor (Fig. 48.8). This common process makes the bone adjacent to tumors much more intense than the surrounding bone. Some malignancies may arise in the soft tissues adjacent to bone and invade through periosteum into the bone. In either case, the resulting reactive osteoblastic changes show the extent of invasion without showing the tumor itself.

An extremely destructive bone tumor may destroy bone more quickly than repair can be effected. Thus, a "cold" defect in a bone with a primary malignancy is an indication of an aggressive tumor. High-grade sarcomas may show this phenomenon.

METASTATIC MALIGNANCY

One of the principle uses of the bone scan is in the detection and monitoring of metastatic tumor involving the skeleton. The tumors monitored include prostate, lung, breast, thyroid, and renal carcinoma among many others. The majority of metastases afflict the axial skeleton in a pattern that reflects the distribution of the erythropoietic marrow. The likelihood of a metastasis peripheral to erythropoietic marrow is low. Most metastases are multiple at the time of discovery. Comparison bone scans at intervals of 3–6 months allow an accurate assessment of tumor spread (Fig. 48.9).

A knowledge of a given primary tumor's propensity to metastasize to the skeleton is helpful for scan interpretation. Confusion arises if an inexperienced observer cannot distinguish between common degenerative or posttraumatic changes and metastases. Merely counting the hot spots is of little value in the management of oncologic problems. Experience is necessary to judge metastatic disease in the skeleton.

As metastases progress and regress, increases in labeling reflect the status of repair bone, not the status of the metastases. Increased numbers and size of individual lesions usually indicates that the tumor load of the skeleton is expanding. Increased *intensity* of the individual lesions (in the absence of new lesions) frequently means that the tumor has become static and that the osteoblasts around it are engaged in vigorous repair. This "flare" response is usually a good indicator that a tumor has been checked by therapy.

Aggressive metastases may destroy bone so quickly that there is no repair (Fig. 48.10). Special attention should also be paid to those metastases in a critical, weight-bearing bone such as the femur. Early detection and treatment can prevent pathologic fractures that add to the suffering of a terminal illness.

Suggested Readings

Collier BD, Hellman RS, Krasnow AZ. Bone SPECT. Semin Nucl Med 1987;17:247–266.

Drane WE. Myositis ossificans and the three phase bone scan. AJR 1984;142:179–180.

Kozin F, Soin JS, Ryan LM, et al. Bone scintigraphy in the reflex sympathetic dystrophy syndrome. Radiology 1981;138:437–443.

Matin P. Bone scintigraphy in the diagnosis and management of traumatic injury. Semin Nucl Med 1983;8:108–122.

Maurer AH, Chen DCP, Carmago EE, et al. Utility of three-phase skeletal scintigraphy in suspected osteomyelitis: concise communication. J Nucl Med 1981;22:941–949.

Merkow RL, Jane JM. Current concepts of Paget's disease of bone. Orthop Clin North Am 1984;15:747–763.

McNeil BJ. Value of bone scanning in neoplastic disease. Semin Nucl Med 1984;14:277–286.

Orzel JA, Rudd TG. Heterotopic bone formation: clinical laboratory and imaging correlation. J Nucl Med 1985;26:125–132.

Rosenthal DI, Chandler HC, Azizi R, et al. Uptake of bone agents by diffuse pulmonary metastatic calcifications. AJR 1977;129:871–874.

Schauwecker DS. The scintigraphic diagnosis of osteomyelitis. AJR 1992;158:9–18.

Schuster HL, Sadowski D, Friedman JM. Radionuclide bone imaging as an aid in the diagnosis of fibrous dysplasia. J Oral Surg 1979;37:267–270.

Stevenson JS, Bright RW, Dunson GL, et al. Technetium-99m phosphate bone imaging: a method for assessing bone graft healing. Radiology 1974;110:391–396.

Subramanian G, McAfee JG, Blair RJ, et al. Technetium-99m-methylene diphosphonate—a superior agent for skeletal imaging: comparison with other technetium complexes. J Nucl Med 1975;18:744–755.

Sullivan DC, Rosenfield NS, Ogden J, Gottschalk A. Problems in the scintigraphic detection of osteomyelitis in children. Radiology 1980;135:731–736.

Tyler JL, Derbekyan V, Lisbona R. Early diagnosis of myositis ossificans with Technetium-99m diphosphonate imaging. Clin Nucl Med 1984;9:256–258.

Wellman H, Schauwecker D, Robb JA, et al. Skeletal scintiimaging and radiography in the diagnosis and management of Paget's disease. Clin Orthop 1977;127:55–62.

Weiss PE, Mall JC, Hoffer PB, et al. 99m Tc-methylene diphosphonate bone imaging in the evaluation of total hip prosthesis. Radiology 1979;133:727–729.

Williamson BR, McLaughlin RE, Wang GJ, et al. Radionuclide bone imaging as a means of differentiating loosening and infection in patients with a painful total hip prosthesis. Radiology 1979;133:723–725.

49

Pulmonary Scintigraphy and Thromboembolism

Rhonda A. Wyatt

ANATOMY AND PHYSIOLOGY

The primary function of the lung is gas exchange. Inspired air is transported via the bronchial tree to the alveoli where gas exchange occurs between the air and alveolar capillaries. Waste CO_2 dissolved in the blood diffuses into the alveoli and is exhaled. The inhaled O_2 diffuses across the alveolar cell membrane into the blood within the alveolar capillaries. The oxygenated blood travels from the pulmonary veins into the left heart and then into the systemic vasculature for distribution throughout the body.

The airways display a branching pattern, dividing from the trachea into the two mainstem bronchi, then into the lobar bronchi. The left mainstem bronchus divides into the left upper and lower lobe bronchi; the right mainstem bronchus divides into the right upper, middle, and lower lobe bronchi. Each of the lobes subdivides into segments (Fig. 49.1).

The right and left main pulmonary arteries branch in a pattern that follows that of the corresponding bronchus. The lungs also have a systemic arterial blood supply, the bronchial arteries. Two to four bronchial arteries arise from the aorta or intercostal trunk and follow the bronchial branching. They provide a blood supply for the bronchi, bronchioles, trachea, middle third of the esophagus, peribronchial connective tissue, peritracheal, hilar, and intrapulmonary lymph nodes, and the visceral pleura over the medial and diaphragmatic surfaces. The bronchial arteries anastamose with the pulmonary capillaries. They drain via bronchial veins into the azygous and hemiazygous veins and the pulmonary veins. The bronchial arteries provide 1–5% of the pulmonary blood flow.

It is important to learn the segmental anatomy of the lungs in order to interpret lung scans. The position of any ventilation or perfusion defects must be individually assessed to determine whether they correspond to the location of segments or subsegments of the lung. Pulmonary vascular diseases such as pulmonary embolism (PE) will have a segmental or subsegmental distribution pattern.

Although pulmonary ventilation occurs primarily through the branching bronchial system, there are other pathways by which distal alveoli can be aerated. The pores of Kohn connect adjacent alveoli while the canals of Lambert connect alveoli and respiratory, terminal, and preterminal bronchioles. These canals and pores permit collateral ventilation of alveoli whose airway has become blocked. This collateral air drift is dynamic and responds under neurohormonal control to factors such as pathologic events, gas tension, and drugs.

Ventilation and pulmonary blood flow are both affected by gravity. In the upright position, there is a gradient in blood flow from the apices to the lung bases with the apex receiving one-third of the blood volume the base gets. There is also a ventilation gradient when the patient is upright. The intrapleural pressure is less at the bases because of gravity. The more negative intrapleural pressure at the apices causes al-

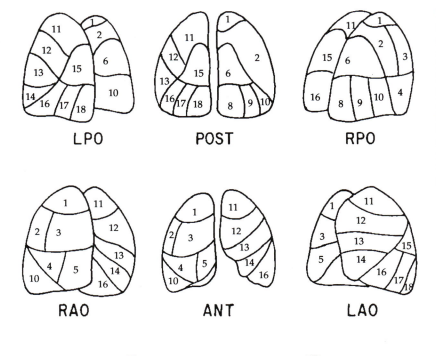

LPO   POST   RPO

RAO   ANT   LAO

R LAT   L LAT

Figure 49.1. Pulmonary Segment Anatomy. Bronchopulmonary segments of the right lung: *1*, apical; *2*, posterior; *3*, anterior; *4*, lateral; *5*, medial; *6*, superior; *7*, medial basal; *8*, posterior basal; *9*, lateral basal; *10*, anterior basal. Bronchopulmonary segments of the left lung: *11*, apical posterior; *12*, anterior; *13*, superior lingual; *14*, inferior lingual; *15*, superior; *16*, anterior medial basal; *17*, lateral basal; *18*, posterior basal. *LPO*, left posterior oblique; *POST*, posterior; *RPO*, right posterior oblique; *RAO*, right anterior oblique; *ANT*, anterior; *LAO*, left anterior oblique; *RLAT*, right lateral; *LLAT*, left lateral. (Adapted with minor modifications from Sostman HD, Gottschalk A. Diagnostic nuclear medicine. 2nd ed. Baltimore: Williams & Wilkins, 1988:513.)

veoli there to remain more open at expiration than basilar alveoli. Therefore, the basilar alveoli during a respiratory cycle undergoes a greater change in size, so greater gas exchange occurs in the base than the apex. Ventilation at the base is 1.5–2 times that in the apex. When a patient is in the supine position, the gradient shifts from superioinferior to anteroposterior. There is increased perfusion to the dependent posterior portions of the lungs (1).

Capillary perfusion and alveolar ventilation should match in order to maximize gas exchange. Any disease that produces localized hypoxia will cause autoregulatory mechanisms to divert blood flow away from that area. This prevents nonventilated areas from being perfused. Conversely, localized hypoperfusion rarely induces localized bronchoconstriction in humans. In humans, bronchospasm caused by local ischemia is transient. Primary vascular disorders such as pulmonary embolism, if unassociated with parenchymal consolidation or pulmonary infarction, usually have normal ventilation (1).

VENTILATION LUNG SCAN
Radiopharmaceuticals

Xenon-133. Several different agents have been used to perform ventilation lung (V) scans. Currently ^{133}Xe is the most widely used radioisotope for this purpose. It is a noble gas that is produced by fission of ^{235}U in a nuclear reactor. It has a half-life of 5.3 days and decays by beta minus emission. The emitted β-particle (374 keV) is responsible for most of the radiation dose delivered to the lungs by ^{133}Xe. The principle photon energy of ^{133}Xe is 81 keV . Ventilation scans are performed before perfusion lung scans. Compton scatter from the higher energy 99mTc macroaggregated albumin (MAA) would downscatter into the region of the 81 keV photopeak of the ^{133}Xe and thus interfere with the ventilation images. The soft tissues of the thorax readily attenuate the low-energy 81 keV photons of ^{133}Xe; therefore, ^{133}Xe images have poor resolution. The usual adult dose of ^{133}Xe for a ventilation scan is 10–20 mCi (370–540 mBq).

Xenon-127 is a cyclotron-produced isotope. It has a physical half-life of 36.4 days and decays by electron capture. The principle photon energies of ^{127}Xe are 203 keV (65%), 172 keV (22%), and 365 keV (18%). Because of the higher energy photons, ^{127}Xe ventilation scans can be performed after the perfusion scan; downscatter would not be a problem. Therefore, if the perfusion scan was normal, a ventilation scan would not be needed. If the perfusion scan was abnormal, the ^{127}Xe scan could be performed in the projection that best demonstrated defects on the perfusion scan. Because ^{127}Xe is cyclotron-produced, it is both expensive and not widely available. The usual adult ^{127}Xe

dose for a ventilation scan is 8–15 mCi (296–555 mBq).

The higher energy of ^{127}Xe necessitates the use of a medium-energy collimator. Therefore, using ^{127}Xe the collimator would have to be changed before the perfusion scan was performed. The higher energy photons and longer half-life of ^{127}Xe also require that more shielding be used and that the gas must be stored much longer for disposal.

Krypton-81m is the other noble gas that can be used for ventilation scans. It has a very short half-life of only 13 seconds. It is produced from a ^{81}Rb-^{81m}Kr generator. Krypton-81m decays by isomeric transition and has a 191 keV photon energy. The ^{81}Rb parent has a half-life of only 4.7 hours; therefore, the ^{81}Rb-^{81m}Kr generator has a short life span, approximately 1 day. Rubidium-81 is cyclotron-produced; therefore, the generator is relatively expensive and not widely available. As a result, using ^{81m}Kr is only practical at institutions that do a high volume of lung scans. The short half-life of ^{81m}Kr, however, eliminates the need for storage and disposal of radioactive gas. It can be vented into the room air as long as the room has good air circulation. The usual adult dose is 10–20 mCi (370–740 MBq).

Technetium-99m Aerosols. Ventilation scans can also be performed using aerosolized rather than gaseous agents. Radioisotope-labeled aerosols are produced by nebulizing radiopharmaceuticals into a fine mist that is then inhaled. Tecnetium-99m diethylene-triaminepentaacetic acid (DTPA) is the most commonly used radioaerosol. Indium-111 or ^{113m}In DTPA and colloids have also been used for this purpose. The main advantages of the ^{99m}Tc aerosols are that they are widely available, inexpensive, and have a 140 keV photopeak, which is ideal for imaging with a gamma camera. A shielded nebulizer produces a fine mist when air or oxygen is forced through a reservoir holding the radioisotope. The mist passes through a settling bag, which traps the larger particles. This mist is delivered to the patient via the nonrebreathing valve and is inhaled. This process, however, is inefficient; only 2–10% of the aerosolized radioisotope is deposited in the lungs. Of 30 mCi of ^{99m}Tc DTPA placed in the nebulizer, only 1–2 mCi actually make it to the lungs.

The site of deposition of the aerosolized particles within the lungs depends upon the size of the particle inhaled. The larger the particle, the more gravitational effect on the particle, and the more central the site of deposition. Particles larger than 2 microns localize in the trachea and pharynx. The current generation of aerosol nebulizers can produce microaerosols less than 0.5 microns in size. The microaerosol has particles small enough to reach the distal portions of the tracheobrochial tree. Using microaerosols, the aerosol localization reflects regional ventilation. Localized airway turbulence because of airway narrowing also plays a role in deposition of aerosol particles. The greater the turbulence the higher the likelihood of particles impacting the walls of an airway and depositing there. Therefore, patients with narrowed airways because of processes such as asthma, bronchitis, and chronic obstructive pulmonary disease (COPD) have more central deposition of the particles than normal. This can result in poor visualization of the peripheral lung fields in these patients. The clearance half-life of ^{99m}Tc aerosols from the lungs is 60–90 minutes. The half-life is shorter in tobacco smokers, only 20 minutes, because of increased alveolar permeability in smokers.

Dosimetry

The critical organ for ^{133}Xe is the trachea, which receives a dose of 0.64 rad/mCi. The lungs receive a dose of 0.01–0.04 rad/mCi while the whole-body absorbed dose is 0.001 rad/mCi. Xenon-127 has no particulate emission and its higher energy photons are absorbed less by soft tissues than ^{133}Xe. As a result, the dose to the lungs from ^{127}Xe is about one-third that of ^{133}Xe.

The critical organ for ^{81m}Kr ventilation scans is the lungs. Using ^{81m}Kr, the absorbed dose for the lungs is 0.05 rad per 20 mCi/min and for the whole body it is 0.001 rad per 20 mCi/min.

The lungs are also the critical organ for ventilation lung scanning using ^{99m}Tc aerosols. The lungs receive an absorbed dose of 0.1 rad/mCi, the bladder wall a dose of 0.18 rad/mCi, and the whole body a dose of 0.01 rad/mCi.

Technique

Ventilation scanning using radioactive gases requires special equipment to prevent leakage of the gas into the imaging room. Gas delivery systems are available that consist of a shielded spirometer, oxygen delivery system, and a xenon charcoal trap. The room in which ventilation scans are performed should be well ventilated and have negative pressure compared with its surroundings. Xenon is heavier than air and therefore tends to pool at floor level.

Xenon-133 Ventilation Scanning. Xenon is injected into the intake tubing or face mask and exhaled xenon vented to a xenon trap. Before a ^{133}Xe ventilation scan is performed, the patient is fitted with an air-tight face mask. While he or she takes a maximal inspiration, the ^{133}Xe is injected into the mask tubing. The patient then is asked to hold his or her breath as long as possible. A posterior 100,000 count image of the lungs is obtained. This is called the first-breath image. The ventilation system is switched so that the patient rebreathes the air ^{133}Xe

mixture. After the patient rebreathes the ^{133}Xe for 5 minutes, a posterior equilibrium image for 100,000 counts is performed. The distribution of ^{133}Xe activity on the equilibrium image represents the aerated lung volume. The ventilation system is readjusted so that the patient breathes in fresh air and exhales the ^{133}Xe mixture into a trap. Serial posterior 30-second washout images are obtained for 5 minutes. The ^{133}Xe should completely wash out of the lungs within 3–4 minutes. Since the lung bases are better ventilated than the apices, the ^{133}Xe washes out of the bases faster than the apices in a normal patient. If the patient is able to tolerate it, all images should be performed with the patient in an upright position.

Xenon-127 Ventilation Scanning is performed in the same manner as ^{133}Xe ventilation lung scans. A ^{127}Xe ventilation scan can be done after the perfusion scan because of the higher photon energy of ^{127}Xe. The ^{127}Xe ventilation scan would only be needed if the perfusion lung scan was not normal.

Krypton-81m Ventilation Scanning. The high-photon energy of ^{81m}Kr permits post-perfusion ventilation lung scans. Identical ^{81m}Kr images can be obtained after each perfusion scan image. Without moving the patient, after each perfusion image finished the patient inhales the ^{81m}Kr and the corresponding ventilation image is performed. This process is repeated until ventilation and perfusion images are obtained in all six positions. Using ^{81m}Kr, the ventilation images exactly match the positioning of the perfusion scan. However, because of its very short half-life, ^{81m}Kr activity in the lungs is proportional to regional ventilation. Krypton-81m images are equivalent to single-breath ^{133}Xe images. Krypton-81m decays before equilibrium occurs; therefore, washout and equilibrium images are not possible with ^{81m}Kr. Repeat images can also be performed if necessary because of the short half-life of ^{81m}Kr.

Technetium-99m Aerosol Ventilation Scanning. In this procedure, the patient inhales the nebulized aerosol while in the supine position to avoid an apex to base gradient from developing because of gravity. After inhaling the ^{99m}Tc aerosol for 3–5 minutes, the patient then sits upright and is imaged in the same positions as those performed during a perfusion lung scan. The ^{99m}Tc aerosol remains fixed in the lungs for several minutes after deposition; therefore, it is possible to obtain ventilation images in different positions using this agent. The exhaled aerosol is trapped in a filter that is stored until it has decayed sufficiently enough to dispose of it. The aerosol ventilation scan requires little cooperation from the patient; breath holding and taking deep breaths are not necessary as they are for ^{133}Xe scans. Aerosol ventilation lung scans can be performed more easily than other types of ventilation scans on patients on ventilators.

A ^{99m}Tc aerosol ventilation lung scan can be performed either before or after the perfusion lung scan. Technetium-99m aerosol has the same photon energy as the ^{99m}Tc MAA used for the perfusion scan because both contain ^{99m}Tc. If the perfusion scan is performed first, a small dose of ^{99m}Tc MAA, 0.5 mCi, and a large dose of ^{99m}Tc aerosol (30 mCi) are used. Approximately 3 mCi of the ^{99m}Tc aerosol will reach the lungs. If the ventilation scan is performed first, 5–10 mCi of ^{99m}Tc aerosol and 5 mCi of ^{99m}Tc MAA are administered. Perfusion defects that fill in on the ventilation scan are sought.

PERFUSION LUNG SCAN
Radiopharmaceuticals

Perfusion (Q) lung scanning is based on the principal of capillary blockade. Particles larger than the pulmonary capillaries (>8 microns) are injected intravenously and travel to the right heart where the venous blood mixes uniformly. The particles mixed in the blood pass from the right ventricle into the pulmonary circulation. Because they are larger than the capillaries, the particles lodge in the precapillary arterioles. The distribution of the particles within the lungs reflects the relative blood flow to the various pulmonary segments. Perfusion images, therefore, depict the regional perfusion of the lungs. Segments with decreased or absent blood flow will have diminished activity within them. Perfusion scans, therefore, simulate the process, embolization, which they are being used to diagnose.

Technetium-99m MAA is the radiopharmaceutical currently used to perform perfusion lung scans. Macroaggregated albumin is prepared by denaturing human serum albumin with heat. The MAA particles are very irregularly shaped molecules. The size of the MAA particles is determined by the exact conditions under which it is made. The size range and number of particles in most commercially available MAA kits is tightly controlled. Most of the particles are in the 20–40 micron size range; 90% of the particles are between 10 and 90 microns. Particles greater than 150 microns in size should not be injected since they will obstruct larger order arterioles. The size and number of particles in a kit can be checked by counting a sample volume from the kit in a hemocytometer under a light microscope. The ^{99m}Tc MAA is prepared by adding ^{99m}TcO$_4^-$ to the MAA kit. The volume and activity of the ^{99m}TcO$_4^-$ added to the kit determine the number of particles per mCi (mBq) in the ^{99m}Tc MAA solution. The biological half-life of ^{99m}Tc MAA particles in the lung is 2–9 hours. The MAA leaves the lungs by breaking down into smaller particles that pass through the alveolar capillaries into the systemic circulation where they are removed by the reticuloendothelial system. The physical half-life of ^{99m}Tc MAA is 6 hours.

Human Albumin Microspheres (HAM) have also been used to perform perfusion lung scans. The HAM particles are prepared by mixing human serum albumin with cottonseed oil and heating the mixture. The resulting particles are passed through fine sieves to get the desired size. The HAM particles are uniformly spherical in shape. The size range used for lung scanning was 10–45 microns. The biological half-life of ^{99m}Tc HAM particles is 7 hours and the physical half-life is 6 hours. There have been more problems with allergic reactions to HAM particles than MAA. The ^{99m}Tc HAM is rarely used in the United States for perfusion lung imaging.

A minimum of 60,000 particles must be injected to have enough particles to produce reliable statistics. Too few particles result in inhomogeneous distribution of particles, which could produce false-positive scans. Typically 200,000–500,000 particles are injected for a perfusion lung scan. There are approximately 280 million pulmonary arterioles/capillaries. Therefore, about 1 vessel in 1000 is occluded by the injected particles. In most patients there is a large margin of safety in perfusion lung scanning and it causes no significant alteration of pulmonary hemodynamics.

There are several categories of patients, however, who should receive a reduced number of particles during a perfusion scan. Occlusion of precapillary arterioles can worsen patients with severe pulmonary hypertension. Patients with known pulmonary hypertension should be given only 100,000 particles. Patients with known right-to-left shunts should also be administered fewer particles than normal. The shunt would allow the particles to bypass the lungs and become lodged in the systemic peripheral vascular beds. This would result in capillary blockade in critical organs such as the heart, kidneys, and brain. To minimize this, yet get an adequate study, these patients should also only be given 100,000 particles. Children should be injected with the 100,000 minimum number of particles because they have fewer pulmonary arterioles than adults. The kit can be made up as usual and a smaller dose given to the patient so that the total number of particles injected is reduced. Each perfusion image obtained would have to be recorded for a longer time interval to obtain statistics comparable with those with the higher normal dose. The kit could also be reconstituted with higher activity per unit volume ^{99m}TcO$_4^-$ than usual. This would result in more activity per particle. The normal 5-mCi dose could be administered, but fewer particles would be present. The kit manufacturer should provide instructions on the procedure to follow to alter the number of particles to be injected. Contraindications to perfusion lung scanning include severe pulmonary hypertension and known allergy to human serum albumin products.

Dosimetry

The normal adult dose administered is 3–5 mCi (111–185 mBq). The lung is the critical organ and receives and absorbed dose of 0.15–0.5 rad/mCi. The whole body and gonadal absorbed dose are 0.15 rad/mCi.

Technique

The syringe containing the ^{99m}Tc MAA should be gently agitated prior to injecting the patient to resuspend the particles. The patient should be injected in the supine position while taking slow, deep breaths to minimize visualization of the gravitational gradient on the pulmonary perfusion. Blood should not be drawn into the syringe to confirm the intravascular location of the needle tip. The aspirated blood may form clots, which would be labeled by the ^{99m}Tc MAA already present in the syringe. Injecting clumped ^{99m}Tc MAA particles and labeled clots both will result in multiple focal hot spots being scattered through the lung fields on the perfusion scan. This could result in poor visualization of the rest of the lung and perhaps cause missing of significant findings.

The patient should be imaged after the injection is completed on a large field of view, high-resolution gamma camera. If the patient's condition permits, he or she should be imaged in the upright position. The lungs are best expanded while upright, thereby improving the chance of visualizing small defects particularly at the lung base. A total of 500,000 count images should be obtained in the anterior, posterior, right lateral, left lateral, right posterior oblique, and left posterior oblique positions. Anterior oblique and decubitus views can be added if needed.

INDICATIONS FOR VENTILATION-PERFUSION LUNG SCANS

The indications for ventilation-perfusion lungs scans include suspicion of PE, follow-up of treated pulmonary embolism, evaluation of chronic lung disease activity and therapeutic response, preoperative estimation of postpneumonectomy lung function in lung carcinoma patients (split lung function), and evaluation of congenital pulmonary abnormalities.

NORMAL LUNG SCAN

Perfusion Scan. The lateral margins of both lungs on all views should be well-defined, smooth arcs with sharp costophrenic angles. Despite injecting the patient while supine, there will be a mild gradient in activity from the apex to the base because the lungs are thicker at their bases than at their apices. The tracer distribution should otherwise be homogeneous. If the patient's condition permits, he or she should be imaged in the upright position. The lungs are better expanded in the upright position; therefore, smaller defects particularly at the lung bases can be resolved in upright than supine position. The costophrenic angles should be sharp on all views (Fig. 49.2).

The heart may cause a curvilinear defect along the left medial lung border. The cardiac defect, however, should be smooth on all views. If it is triangular in shape, suspect that a perfusion defect abuts the normal cardiac defect. The hila can be prominent even in normal patients. Focal asymmetric hilar perfusion defects should be considered abnormal. Cardiomegaly, tortuosity of the aorta, and mediastinal or hilar enlargement will cause defects along the medial border of the lung. Defects because of mediastinal masses or structures would show corresponding defects on the ventilation scan, although usually less well defined. The apparent size and shape of the mediastinal mass or enlargement on the ventilation/perfusion (V/Q) scan should match the lesion present on chest x-ray.

Ventilation Scan. A normal ventilation scan has homogeneous radiopharmaceutical distribution throughout all lung fields on all three phases of the scan. A faint gradient from base to apex may also be seen in a ventilation lung scan since there is less lung parenchyma in the apex than the base. The first-breath ^{133}Xe image is often grainy in appearance because it has poor statistics; it reflects regional lung volume. The equilibrium images demonstrate aerated lung volume. In normal individuals, the first-breath and equilibrium images should look similar; the first-breath images will just have less activity. The equilibrium views are followed by the washout phase of the study. There should be rapid clearance of the ^{133}Xe from the lungs. The normal half-time for xenon washout is less than 1 minute. Xenon activity should have washed completely out of the lungs within 3 minutes. Retention of xenon in the lungs (trapping), whether focal or diffuse, is an indication of obstructive changes within the lungs (Fig. 49.3).

Xenon-127 scans appear similar to ^{133}Xe scans except that the borders on the images are sharper. The higher photon energy of ^{127}Xe is less attenuated by the soft tissues of the thorax than ^{133}Xe. Krypton-81m scans are essentially first-breath images because of the short half-life of ^{81m}Kr. The ^{81m}Kr images look similar to ^{133}Xe images except faint tracer activity may be visualized within the trachea on ^{81m}Kr scans.

Figure 49.2. Normal ^{99m}Tc MAA Perfusion Lung Scan. Images from left to right are, *top row*, posterior, left posterior oblique; *middle row*, *LT LAT* (left lateral), *LAO* (left anterior oblique), *ANT* (anterior); and *bottom row*, *RAO* (right anterior oblique), *RT LAT* (right lateral), *RPO* (right posterior oblique).

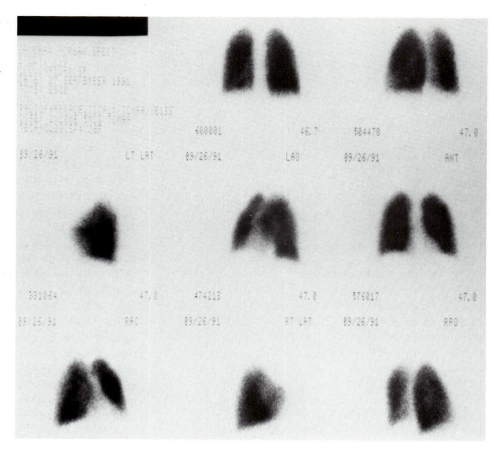

Figure 49.3. Normal ^{133}Xe Ventilation Lung Scan. *Insp*, inspiration; *Equil*, equilibrium; *RPO*, right posterior oblique; *LPO*, left posterior oblique.

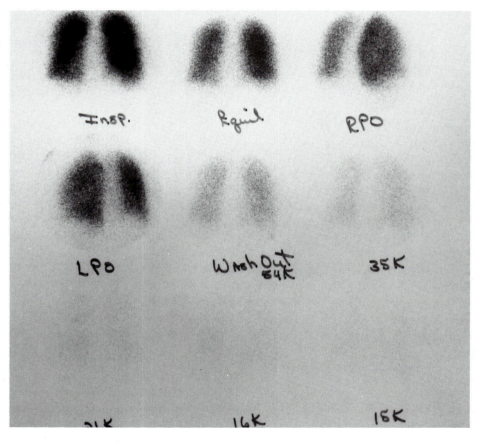

The ^{99m}Tc DTPA aerosol scan resembles the ^{99m}Tc MAA perfusion scans. Activity, however, is normally present on ^{99m}Tc aerosol within the trachea and mainstem bronchi. Central deposition of the ^{99m}Tc aerosol may occur in otherwise normal smokers. Swallowed ^{99m}Tc DTPA aerosol may be visualized within the esophagus and stomach.

ABNORMAL LUNG SCANS

Either ventilation or perfusion lung scans that have focal defects or inhomogeneity of tracer distribution are abnormal. Defects are areas of absent tracer localization on the scan. Focal perfusion defects should be compared with corresponding areas on the ventilation scan and vice versa. The relative size and shape of V/Q defects must then be correlated with the corresponding area on a recent chest x-ray. The correlative chest x-ray should not be more than 6–12 hours old. However chest x-ray findings even a few hours old may have changed significantly in a patient with deteriorating respiratory status. Infiltrates, effusions, pulmonary edema, or a pneumothorax may have developed, which could explain the deterioration and eliminate the need for a V/Q scan. The only time a chest x-ray is not essential for interpreting a V/Q scan is if the ventilation and perfusion scans are completely normal. A normal V/Q scan eliminates the possibility of a clinically significant pulmonary embolus.

Perfusion defects should be assessed to determine if they correspond to pulmonary anatomic segments. The shape, location, and size of the defect should fit that expected for a particular segment on all views. Perfusion defects that correspond to the segmental anatomy of the lung need to have their size assessed. A defect that represents less than 25% of a pulmonary segment is considered a small defect, 25–75% a moderate defect, and greater than 75% a large defect. The size of segmental defects and their number are used in the interpretation schemes for V/Q scans to assess the likelihood that the defects present represent pulmonary emboli. If the defect is nonsegmental in nature, then it should be compared with the chest x-ray to determine if a mass, effusion, mediastinal or hilar structure is responsible for the perfusion scan finding. The relative size and shape of a nonsegmental defect on the perfusion scan should be compared with its size and shape on chest x-ray and the ventilation scan.

Ventilation scans are also abnormal if areas of delayed xenon washin or washout are present. Defects present on the single-breath image may fill in later on the equilibrium images. This occurs when xenon bypasses obstructed pulmonary bronchioles through the pores of Kohn and canal of Lambert. Air drift through these alternate pathways permits the xenon to enter and leave the alveoli distal to the obstruction.

Movement by collateral air drift proceeds more slowly than through the bronchioles, resulting in delayed washin and washout. Normally, the xenon should wash completely out of the lungs within 3 minutes. Focal areas of abnormal retention therefore represents focal obstructive lung disease.

PULMONARY EMBOLISM

Incidence and Clinical Findings. Pulmonary embolism is one of the more common causes of death in the United States. Dahlen and Alpert (2) calculated that in 1975, 630,000 patients in America developed pulmonary emboli. They estimated that 30% of untreated patients died from the emboli, while only 10–16% of patients treated with anticoagulant therapy died. Although anticoagulants reduce the mortality from pulmonary emboli, they are not a benign form of therapy. Anticoagulants place patients at significant risk for bleeding and should not be prescribed if the diagnosis of thrombosis is uncertain.

Pulmonary emboli originate from thrombi in the deep venous system of the legs and pelvis. Predisposing factors for pulmonary emboli include prolonged immobilization, surgery—particularly within the pelvis or hips, history of prior PE, cardiac disease, estrogen therapy—particularly in smokers, and hypercoagualable states such as cancer and congenital defects in thrombolysis.

Pulmonary embolism is very difficult to diagnosis clinically. Dahlen and Alpert theorized that in 70% of patients who survived pulmonary emboli, the emboli had not been clinically suspected. The classic triad of dyspnea, hemoptysis, and pleuritic chest pain occurs in less than 20% of pulmonary emboli patients. The most common symptoms are dyspnea (79–84%), pleuritic chest pain (58–74%), cough (44–53%), hemoptysis (16–30%), and syncope (9–13%) (3). The Urokinase and Streptokinase Pulmonary Embolism Trials (USPE) and Prospective Investigation of Pulmonary Embolism Diagnosis (PIOPED) studies found a positive correlation between the size of the embolus and the likelihood of symptoms (4, 5). The relationship was stronger in the USPE than the PIOPED study. The symptoms associated with PE, however, are nonspecific. A wide range of diseases can cause symptoms such as chest pain or dyspnea. Pulmonary or cardiac infection or inflammation, cancer, and pneumothorax can all produce these findings.

Certain clinical signs are associated with PE. The USPE study found that 92% of patients with massive pulmonary emboli have tachypnea, 58% have rales, 44% have tachycardia, 43% have fever, and 32% have phlebitis; 53% have an increased pulmonic component of the second heart sound (4). However, the presence of these clinical signs and symptoms did not distinguish between patients with pulmonary emboli and those with other diseases. The symptoms had 85% sensitivity and 37% specificity in diagnosing pulmonary emboli (3).

A chest x-ray and electrocardiogram should be obtained in patients being evaluated for PE. Although these techniques cannot exclude the diagnosis of PE, they can help diagnose other processes that have similar clinical presentations, such as pneumothorax and myocardial infarction. The chest x-ray may be normal in a patient with a PE but, more commonly, peripheral infiltrates and/or pleural effusions are present. The classic finding for a PE is a wedge-shaped, pleural based infarct called a Hamptom hump. Wedge-shaped areas of oligemia (Westermark's sign) may be present distal to an embolus. If the patient develops acute cor pulmonale because of the pulmonary embolus, the electrocardiogram may show signs of right heart strain.

Nuclear Medicine Evaluation of PE.
Pulmonary angiography is considered the gold standard for the diagnosis of pulmonary embolism. However, it is an invasive, expensive procedure associated with slight risk for the patient. As a result angiography cannot be used as a screening test to rule out pulmonary embolism in patients with clinical findings compatible with that diagnosis. Anticoagulants are associated with their own risk; therefore, patients cannot be placed on this therapy indiscriminately. The V/Q scan has become the diagnostic method most commonly used to screen patients suspected of having pulmonary embolism. It has proven to be a sensitive indicator of clinically significant pulmonary emboli, is noninvasive, and is relatively easy to perform.

Classic V/Q findings for PE
are multiple, bilateral segmental pleural based perfusion defects in a patient with a normal ventilation scan (Fig. 49.4). However, most scans of patients with pulmonary emboli are not this clear-cut. Several different V/Q scan interpretation systems have developed that categorize scans in terms of probability of representing pulmonary emboli. Patterns of V/Q scan findings were assigned according to the likelihood that patients with that pattern would have emboli demonstrated on pulmonary angiography. Scans are read as normal, low, intermediate, or high probability for pulmonary embolism.

The V/Q Scan Interpretation.
The most widely used interpretive method is the Biello criteria. Biello et al. (6) in 1977, retrospectively compared V/Q scan findings with pulmonary angiography results. The perfusion scans were evaluated and any defects present assessed to find if they correlated with anatomic segments or subsegments of the lung. If the defects were subsegmental, they were sized. A defect was considered large if it corresponded to >75% of a lung segment, moderate if it represented 25–75% of a seg-

ment, and small if it was <25% of a segment. The ventilation scan was then assessed to determine if any ventilation defects were present and their location and size. The ventilation and perfusion scans were then compared to find if the defects matched in size and shape. The original Biello criteria did not take into account infiltrates on chest x-ray; however, recent modifications of this scheme factor chest x-ray abnormalities into the interpretation. Abnormalities on a recent chest x-ray should be assessed to determine if they are larger than, smaller than, or equal in size to any perfusion defects. The number and size of any perfusion defects as well as whether they match or are mismatched with abnormalities on the ventilation scan and the chest x-ray determines to which category a V/Q scan is assigned.

The different interpretation schemes such as Biello, modified Biello, and PIOPED are all based on applying this same process to viewing the V/Q scan. They differ in exactly which patterns of V/Q defects and chest x-ray findings is assigned a particular risk of representing PE. For example, under the modified Biello criteria a single moderate-sized, mismatched perfusion defect with a normal chest x-ray is intermediate in probability for PE, while under the PIOPED criteria it is low probability. The PIOPED authors used a modification of the Biello criteria that had more detailed categorization of the V/Q scan patterns. The PIOPED was a large, multicenter, prospective study of patients clinically suspected of having PE. All patients in this study had a V/Q scan, and those who had anything other than a normal V/Q scan underwent pulmonary angiography (5). Webber et al. (7) compared the Biello, McNeil, and PIOPED criteria in 96 patients who underwent V/Q scans and pulmonary angiography within 48 hours of each other. The PIOPED criteria had the most favorable likelihood ratio for predicting the presence of pulmonary emboli but the largest number of intermediate scans, while the Biello criteria had the most favorable likelihood ratio for predicting no emboli would be present on angiography. They concluded that "the Biello criteria represented the best compromise of the sets of criteria studied" (7). Table 49.1 has details of the modified Biello and PIOPED criteria.

A normal V/Q scan essentially rules out significant pulmonary emboli. Kipper et al. (8) did long-term follow-up of patients suspected of having pulmonary emboli who had normal V/Q scans (8). In their findings, 0/68 patients had clinical evidence of pulmonary emboli on follow-up. They concluded that patients with normal V/Q scans are unlikely to have clinically significant pulmonary emboli. Patients with matching V/Q defects caused by anatomic structures such as a tortuous aorta, cardiomegaly, and enlarged hila should

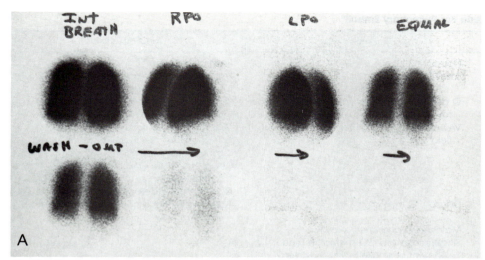

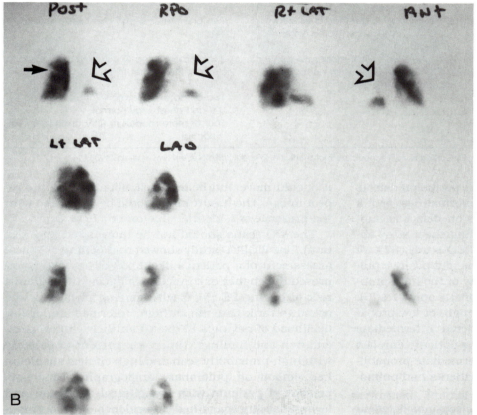

Figure 49.4. High Probability V/Q Scan. A. Normal ^{133}Xe ventilation scan. *Int Breath*, initial breath; *RPO*, right posterior oblique; *LPO*, left posterior oblique; *EQUAL*, equilibrium. **B.** ^{99m}Tc MAA perfusion scan demonstrates absence of perfusion to most segments of the right lung (*open arrows*). The left lung has multiple subsegmental defects (*small arrow*). *Post*, posterior; *RtLAT*, right lateral; *Ant*, anterior; *LtLat*, left lateral; *LAO*, left anterior oblique.

be considered as normal with regard to risk for PE if the scan is otherwise normal.

Under the modified Biello criteria, there are three patterns of V/Q scan that qualify as low-probability scans: multiple small subsegmental perfusion defects with normal ventilation scan and chest x-ray, matching ventilation and perfusion defects with no chest x-ray abnormalities in the corresponding region, and perfusion defects that are substantially smaller than corresponding ventilation or chest x-ray abnormalities (Fig. 49.5). Fourteen percent of patients with low-

probability scans, however, were found to have emboli if pulmonary angiography was performed in the PIOPED study. Several studies have been performed on patients with low-probability scans who were not anticoagulated; 0–0.6% of such patients demonstrated clinical evidence of PE on follow-up. Therefore, even if some patients with low-probability scans do have pulmonary emboli, most of these patients will do fine without anticoagulation.

The V/Q scans are categorized as high probability under the modified Biello classification if two or more

Figure 49.6. High-Probability V/Q Scan. A ^{133}Xe ventilation scan was normal. A ^{99m}Tc MAA perfusion scan demonstrates segmental defects on the right (*open arrows*) and moderate subsegmental defects on the left (*closed arrows*).

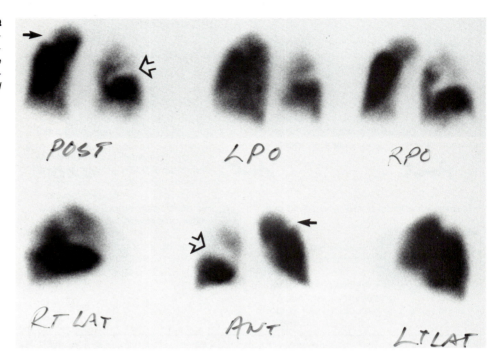

Figure 49.7. Intermediate-Probability V/Q Scan. A ^{133}Xe ventilation scan was normal. A ^{99m}Tc MAA perfusion scan demonstrates multiple bilateral small and moderate defects (*arrows*).

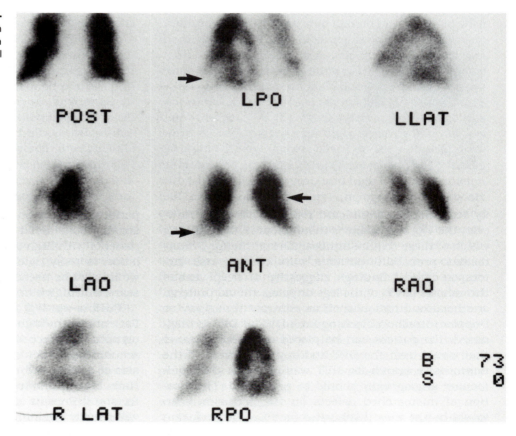

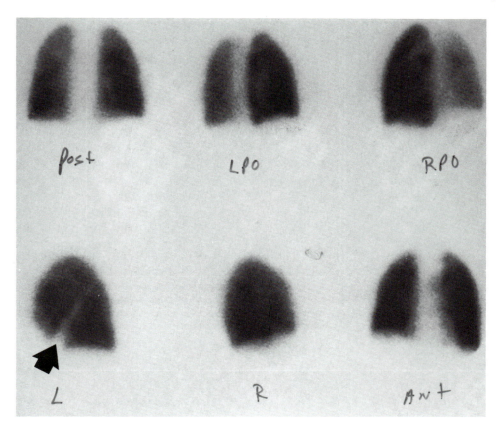

Figure 49.8. **Fissure Sign.** Low-probability ^{99m}Tc MAA perfusion scan demonstrates the fissure sign *(arrow)* on the left lateral view.

will improve and the less likely the scan will return to normal. Most young patients' scans will revert back to normal with a few weeks. Follow-up scans done within 2 weeks of the initiation of anticoagulation therapy may show new defects that do not represent recurrent emboli. Large central thrombi may fragment and produce small distal thrombi. Also emboli that were previously nonocclusive may become obstructive and show as new defects. The diagnosis of recurrent PE is more likely if multiple new large or moderate defects are present in areas that were previously normal.

False Positive V/Q Scans. Mismatched perfusion defects can represent chronic pulmonary emboli in patients with a remote history of PE. Follow-up V/Q scans after patients have been placed on anticoagulants can be useful as baselines in these patients. However, if no old scan is available, it is impossible to determine which emboli are old and which are new. Patients with a history of PE are at higher risk of having a PE than patients without such a history.

Mismatched perfusion defects can also be produced by extrinsic compression of the pulmonary vessels. Mass lesions in the mediastinum, hila, or pulmonary parenchyma may compress the pliable pulmonary vessels, particularly the veins. Adenopathy because of malignancies such as lung carcinoma and lymphoma or benign diseases like sarcoidosis or tuberculosis can impinge on the pulmonary vessels. Aneurysmal dilation of the thoracic aorta or congenital vascular ab-

normalities may rarely compress the pulmonary vascularity. The pulmonary vessels may also become entrapped and obstructed by mediastinal fibrosis.

The pulmonary vessels can be obstructed by nonthrombotic intraluminal processes. Malignancies such as renal cell carcinoma may grow intravascularly or may embolize to the pulmonary vessels. Sarcomas of the pulmonary arteries and lymphatic carcinomatosis have produced false-positive V/Q scans. Vasculitis, which results in obliterative lesions in the pulmonary vessel, such as Takayasu's arteritis and systemic lupus erythematosus can rarely cause false-positive scans. Radiation therapy can produce mismatched perfusion defects. These, however, are often geometric rather than segmental in shape.

False-negative V/Q Scans. Patients with true pulmonary emboli can have false-negative V/Q scans if the emboli are only partially occlusive. A pulmonary angiogram could show diagnostic intraluminal filling defects; however, if they do not completely obstruct the vessel they will not be demonstrated on the perfusion scan. Very small emboli may produce perfusion defects too small to be visualized on a perfusion scan.

ASTHMA

Asthma produces bronchospastic narrowing of the airways. This airway obstruction results in decreased ventilation in the affected areas. Focal segmental or subsegmental ventilation defects are present on the first-breath image during an acute asthma attack. These defects may wash in on the equilibrium images. If associated with mucus plug, the defects may persist. The bronchospasm induces localized hypoxia, which in turn produces localized vasoconstriction. Therefore, during an attack the perfusion scan will usually have defects that match the ventilation scan. The V/Q scan of an asthma patient successfully treated with bronchodilators will show improvement compared with scans performed during the attack. The transient nature of the V/Q defects caused by asthma helps distinguish them from the fixed defects because of COPD. Most V/Q defects caused by asthma will resolve with 24 hours of bronchodilator therapy.

LUNG CARCINOMA

Benign lung neoplasms, primary lung carcinomas, and metastatic disease to the lung all produce V/Q scan abnormalities. The location and size of the tumor determine the findings on the lung scan, not the tumor type. Therefore, solitary benign tumors cannot be distinguished from malignant ones on V/Q scans.

Extrinsic tumors that displace lung parenchyma such as mediastinal or chest wall tumors or focal parenchymal masses tend to produce matching V/Q defects. These V/Q defects do not correspond to segmental anatomy unless the mass has invaded or compressed a local branch of the bronchovascular tree. Tumors that do not cause vascular or bronchial obstruction or pleural effusions produce matched V/Q defects that correspond to the size and shape of the mass on chest x-ray.

Neoplasms that directly invade or compress pulmonary vessels have reduced or absent perfusion distal to the mass. This produces a wedge-shaped area of decreased or absent perfusion distal to the mass lesion itself. The compliant pulmonary vessels are more easily compressed than the cartilage-reinforced bronchi. Therefore, a common V/Q pattern seen with a lung tumor is a wedge-shaped area of reduced or absent perfusion distal to a nonsegmental perfusion defect with either normal ventilation or a ventilation defect matching only the mass itself. When a small perihilar lung carcinoma obstructs the pulmonary vessels but not the bronchi, a mismatched segmental or subsegmental perfusion defect occurs, which can be a false-positive sign for pulmonary embolism. Visualization of the mass lesion on the chest x-ray would be the clue to the true diagnosis.

If the carcinoma obstructs the adjacent bronchus or bronchiole as well as the pulmonary vessels, then the ventilation defect may again match the perfusion defect. An endobrochial lesion obstructing a bronchiole or bronchus would cause a mismatched wedge-shaped ventilation defect.

Perfusion lung scan is useful in preoperatively estimating lung carcinoma patients' postsurgical pulmonary function. It is used to estimate the fraction of the patient's pulmonary perfusion going to the lung that contains the carcinoma. The preoperative estimate of the postpneumonectomy FEV_1 as determined by a quantitative perfusion lung has been shown to correlate well with the postoperative FEV_1. A patient needs to have a postoperative FEV_1 of 800–1000 ml to have adequate lung function. A quantitative perfusion scan is performed in the same manner as a regular perfusion lung scan except that a single posterior image is obtained for a set time interval or fixed number of counts. Regions of interest are drawn around each lung and the counts over each are obtained. From this, the percentage of the total each lung contributes is calculated (Fig. 49.9). The preoperative FEV_1, multiplied by the percent perfusion going to the lung that will remain after pneumonectomy, is an estimate of the postoperative FEV_1.

CHRONIC OBSTRUCTIVE PULMONARY DISEASE

Chronic bronchitis and emphysema are common forms of COPD associated with smoking. Chronic bronchitis results in thickened mucosa, increased mucus production, and narrowed airways. Emphysema causes dilation and loss of alveoli. The alveoli lose their support and become narrowed and irregular. The narrowed airways result in increased airway resistance and reduced ventilation. On xenon ventilation scans, this produces delayed washin and washout. First-breath images may have defects that gradually fill in on the equilibrium phase. The xenon will wash out of the affected area more slowly than the rest of the lung and still be visible on images more than 3 minutes after the patient was switched to breathing air rather than xenon.

Patients with COPD frequently also have abnormal perfusion lung scans. Focal COPD changes can cause localized hypoxia within the lung, which in turn induces localized vasoconstriction. The inflammation and parenchymal destruction produced by chronic bronchitis or emphysema may narrow or damage alveolar or bronchiolar blood vessels and show as areas of reduced or absent activity on the perfusion scan. Therefore, regions of the lung that demonstrate obstructive changes on the ventilation scan will often have corresponding abnormalities on the perfusion scan. When the ventilatory changes are widespread, the perfusion scan may have a mottled appearance. The COPD patient may have normal perfusion scans if the ventilatory obstructive changes produce little hypoxia or vascular damage.

The COPD tends to affect the lung apices more than the bases. As a result, COPD V/Q scans show the ventilation and perfusion of the apices more involved

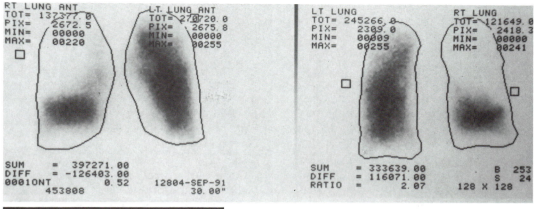

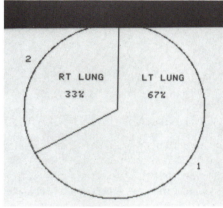

Figure 49.9. Quantitative Perfusion Lung Scan. The percentage of the pulmonary perfusion to each lung is calculated based on the relative counts over each lung on the posterior image.

than the bases. α_1-antitrypsin produces emphysematous changes, predominantly in the lower lobes. The obstructive changes on ventilation, therefore, occur mainly in the bases of the lungs rather than the apices as in COPD.

INFLAMMATORY/INFECTIOUS DISEASE OF THE LUNG

Areas of consolidation on chest x-ray because of pneumonia or pneumonitis will also be abnormal on a V/Q scan. The involved area will show as a defect on the ventilation scan. The consolidated airways will not ventilate and not have delayed washin. The resulting local hypoxia produces reflex vasoconstriction. Therefore, perfusion defects also occur in the consolidated region. The perfusion may be decreased or completely absent. Perfusion defects because of infiltrates are often smaller than the consolidated region on chest x-ray. If the perfusion defect appears larger than the chest x-ray abnormality, then pulmonary emboli may be present as well as the infiltrate.

THROMBUS DETECTION USING NUCLEAR MEDICINE

Thrombi from the deep venous system of the legs and pelvis are the source of pulmonary emboli. If the patient has signs or symptoms consistent with DVT, a

radionuclide venogram can be done to evaluate the deep veins of the legs and pelvis. This can be performed in conjunction with a perfusion lung scan. The ^{99m}Tc MAA normally used for the perfusion scan is divided between two syringes and injected into the veins on the dorsum of the feet instead of into the arm. The nuclear venogram is most sensitive for detecting thrombi above the knees.

In a normal study, the deep veins of the legs and pelvis will be visualized and should be symmetric (Fig. 49.10). The presence of deep venous thrombi is confirmed by obstruction of the veins with cutoff of activity and multiple collateral vessels (Fig. 49.11). Technetium-99m MAA can become impacted in a thrombus and show as a hot spot on the venogram. Hot spots, however, can also occur normally in the valves of the veins.

In the past, ^{125}I labeled fibrinogen and labeled platelets have been used to detect acute thrombi. However, neither technique proved very sensitive. Currently, studies are under way using antifibrin monoclonal antibodies (11). Preliminary results suggest that these antifibrin monoclonal antibodies are very sensitive and specific in detecting deep venous thrombi. However, heparin has been shown to reduce the intensity of uptake of the antifibrin monoclonal antibodies. Both ^{99m}Tc- and ^{111}In-labeled antifibrin monoclonal antibodies have been manufactured. Acute thrombi

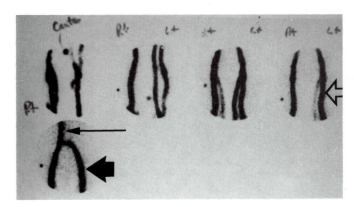

Figure 49.10.   Normal Nuclear Venogram. Technetium-99m MAA injected into dorsal foot veins bilaterally demonstrates the deep venous system of both legs. Images (*left to right*) begin at the knees and extend to the pelvis. The femoral veins (*open arrow*), iliac veins (*large closed arrow*), and inferior vena cava (*long arrow*) are well seen.

show as focal areas of asymmetric uptake within the deep venous system. If the preliminary results are confirmed in more extensive trials, antifibrin monoclonal antibodies may be a new, noninvasive method for detecting acute DVT. It may also be the only method capable of distinguishing between chronic and recurrent DVT.

SMOKE INHALATION

Many of the patients with serious burns also have inhalation injury of the lungs. Approximately 20–30% of patients admitted to a hospital for burns develop pulmonary complications; 70–75% of these patients die (1). Smoke consists of a mixture of toxic gases and particles. Inhalation of these toxins combined with thermal damage from the fire itself can produce severe pulmonary damage. A chest x-ray is insensitive in detecting early inhalation injury. There may be a lag period of 12–48 hours before the x-ray becomes abnormal (1).

Xenon in saline ventilation scans have proven useful in detecting inhalation lung injury (12). Xenon-133 under pressure will dissolve in saline. When injected intravenously, the xenon remains in solution until it reaches the lungs. In the alveolar capillaries, the xenon diffuses across the capillary membrane into the alveoli and is exhaled. Normally, the xenon washes out of the lungs in less than 2 minutes. Xenon, however, is retained in areas of inhalational injury. The xenon in saline study is 92% accurate in detecting lung injury.

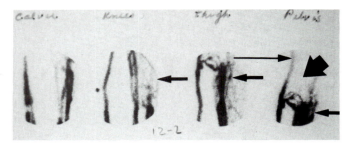

Figure 49.11.   Deep Venous Thrombosis. Nuclear venogram demonstrates cutoff of activity at the left knee with multiple collateral vessels (*small arrows*) visualized, indicating thrombosis of the left femoral and iliac veins. No radionuclide activity is present in the region of the left iliac vein (*large arrow*). Venous drainage from the left leg crosses the pelvis via collaterals to fill the inferior vena cava (*long arrow*).

References

1. Fraser RG, Paré JA, Paré PD, Fraser RS, Genereux GP. Diagnosis of diseases of the chest. 3rd ed. Philadelphia: WB Saunders, 1988:3–35,53–64,71–82,127–137.
2. Dahlen JE, Alpert JS. Natural history of pulmonary embolism. Prog Cardiovasc Dis 1975;17:259–270.
3. Palevsky HI. The problems of the clinical and laboratory diagnosis of pulmonary embolism. Semin Nucl Med 1991;21: 276–280.
4. Bell WR, Simon TL, DeMets DL. The clinical features of submassive and massive pulmonary emboli. Am J Med 1977;62:355–360.
5. The PIOPED Investigators. Value of the ventilation/perfusion scan in acute pulmonary embolism. Results of the Prospective Investigation of Pulmonary Embolism Diagnosis (PIOPED). JAMA 1990;263:2753–2759.
6. Biello DR, Mattar AG, McKnight RC, et al. Ventilation-perfusion studies in suspected pulmonary embolism. AJR 1979;133:1033–1037.
7. Webber MM, Gomes AS, Roe D, La Fontaine RL, Hawkins RA. Comparison of Biello, McNeil, and PIOPED criteria for the diagnosis of pulmonary embolism on lung scans. AJR 1990;154:975–981.
8. Kipper MS, Moser KM, Kortman KE, et al. Long term follow-up of patients with suspected pulmonary embolism and a normal lung scan. Chest 1982;82:411–415.
9. Sostman HD, Gottschalk A. The stripe sign: a new sign for diagnosis of nonembolic defects on pulmonary perfusion scintigraphy. Radiology 1982;142:737–741.
10. Juni JE, Alavi A. Lung scanning in the diagnosis of pulmonary embolism: the emperor redressed. Semin Nucl Med 1991;21:281–296.
11. Schaible TF, Alavi A. Antifibrin scintigraphy in the diagnostic evaluation of acute deep venous thrombosis. Semin Nucl Med 1991;21:313–324.
12. Lull RJ, Anderson JH, Telepak RJ, et al. Radionuclide imaging in the assessment of lung injury. Semin Nucl Med 1980;10:302–310.

50

Cardiovascular System Scintigraphy

Robert J. Telepak
Philip W. Wiest
Michael F. Hartshorne

Nuclear medicine applications in the cardiovascular system include maps of myocardial perfusion, gated ventricular functional studies of the blood pool in the ventricles, and detection and quantitation of intracardiac shunts.

MYOCARDIAL PERFUSION SCANS

Technique

Three gamma-emitting radiopharmaceuticals are readily available for mapping the flow of blood to the myocardium. The first, thallium-201 (Tl-201), an analog of K+ ion, is delivered to capillary beds by regional blood flow and actively pumped into viable cells by the Na+/K+ adenosine triphosphatase pump. Stress or dipyridamole challenge images should be acquired as soon after injection as possible. Washout of Tl-201 is measured by the effective half-life of Tl-201 in normal myocardium of about 4 hours. A complex "redistribution" of the isotope within the myocardium is governed by rates of washout from myocardial cells, renal excretion, and shifts of the isotope between muscle, visceral, and other compartments. Rest imaging is usually done 3–4 hours after injection.

Cyclotron production at a remote site (requiring shipping), a long physical half-life (73 hours), low energy, poorly penetrating photons (mostly 69–83 keV x-rays), and a relatively high absorbed dose (0.24 rad/mCi whole body) combine to make the usual dose of Tl-201 (2–5 mCi) a less than ideal agent for imaging. However, because of its active transport it is a more physiologic agent than the technetium-99m (Tc-99m)-labeled agents.

Technetium-99m is used to label the other two agents. The second radiopharmaceutical, Tc-99m sestamibi, is taken up by the perfused myocardium by passive diffusion and bound in the myocyte. There is no significant redistribution effect with this agent. Washout is negligible. Imaging is delayed for 45 minutes to 1 hour after stress (or dipyridamole challenge) to allow for biliary clearance (which reduces background activity around the heart). Because there is no redistribution, a repeat injection for resting images is commonly performed on a different day (Fig. 50.1.)

The third myocardial perfusion agent, Tc-99m teboroxime, is rapidly extracted from the blood by perfused myocardium but rapidly washed out as well. Because of this, imaging is done for a few minutes immediately after injection for both stress or rest images. Only a short interval (an hour) is needed between the two studies.

Both of the Tc-99m-labeled agents are prepared from Tc-99m pertechnetate and stocked pharmaceutical kits. They may be performed on an as-needed basis. Both are easy to image radiopharmaceuticals with good soft-tissue penetration (140 keV gamma energy) and a high photon flux from typical doses of 8–22 mCi.

Each of the perfusion agents may be imaged with planar techniques or with single-photon emission computed tomography (SPECT). Meticulous quality control of the stress and rest images is essential. The comparison of images requires identical repositioning so that the same areas of myocardium are compared. Poor positioning will lead to false-positive interpretations of ischemia and infarct.

The three principle coronary artery distributions of the left ventricle (LV)—left anterior descending artery, left circumflex artery, and posterior descending artery—normally provide equal intensity of myocardial labeling at any given level of cardiac work. Perfusion of the thin right ventricular wall is considerably less than that of the LV, but can be imaged with the same techniques.

Exercise, usually on a treadmill, or infusion of dipyridamole or adenosine are used in conjunction

Figure 50.1. Normal Exercise/Rest Planar Tc-99m Sestamibi Myocardial Scan. Anterior (*Ant*), left anterior oblique (*LAO*) 40°, LAO 70°, and left lateral (LLAT) planar views of a 380-pound patient, with the upper row representing stress and the lower row representing rest injections of the radiopharmaceutical. Note the superb image quality in spite of the patient's large size.

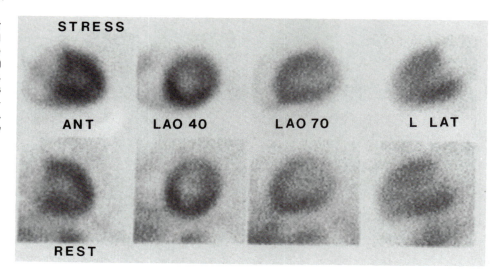

STRESS

ANT   LAO 40   LAO 70   L LAT

REST

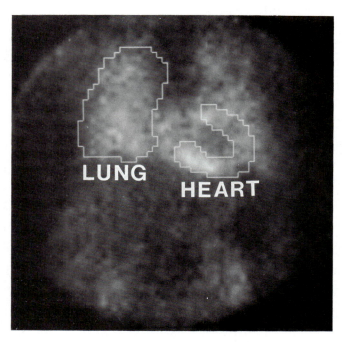

Figure 50.2. Abnormal Tl-201 Lung/Heart Ratio. This frame is an anterior projection acquired immediately after the start of a stress SPECT study. The lung:heart ratio of 0.77 is markedly elevated, indicating that the patient experienced heart failure during exercise.

with perfusion agents to increase delivery to the normal myocardium. Step-wise increases in physical exercise are monitored by sequential electrocardiogram (ECG), blood pressure, and pulse measurements and symptoms of angina. The radiopharmaceutical is injected under conditions of maximal exercise, which should be continued for 30–60 seconds beyond injection to obtain optimal mapping of stress perfusion.

Adequacy of the exercise challenge can be estimated simply from a calculation of the "double product" (DP) (systolic pressure × heart rate = DP). The DP correlates with an individual's myocardial work performed; duration of exercise and heart rate alone may not. There should be at least a doubling and preferably a tripling and an absolute rise to over 20,000 of the DP from rest to peak exercise.

For those patients who cannot perform physical exercise, coronary vasodilation can be pharmacologically forced. Intravenous dipyridamole or adenosine can vasodilate normal coronary arteries, but do not effectively increase flow through vessels that are stenosed.

In addition to clinical data (ECG, angina, etc.), the initial Tl-201 images of the chest and heart may help assess the heart's performance. High lung activity immediately after exercise usually indicates that left ventricular failure occurred during exercise. Dilation of the heart with exercise is another indicator of failure. Both phenomena have a severe prognosis for subsequent cardiac events (angina, infarction, arrythmia, and sudden deaths) (Fig. 50.2).

Interpretation

Reversible Ischemia. Images of the heart map relative regional perfusion. Areas of myocardium with poor blood supply, usually because of atherosclerosis, fail to increase labeling by the perfusion agent during exercise. The Tl-201 images delayed 3–4 to hours are compared with those from stress to detect redistribution that is indicative of reversible ischemia. A second injection of the Tc-99m perfusion agent produces images of resting perfusion. A reinjection of Tl-201 can also be used to record relative myocardial perfusion under resting conditions. The most important feature of the myocardial perfusion test is comparison of the stress and rest images to detect areas that are inadequately perfused at exercise yet viable. These areas are redundantly called reversibly ischemic.

Peri-infarct Ischemia. Ischemia detected by either exercise or pharmacologic dilation of normal ves-

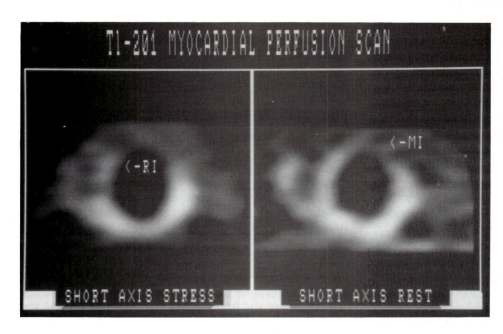

Figure 50.3. Abnormal Stress and 4-hour Rest Tl-201 SPECT Transaxial (Short Axis) Images. These images are through middle LV of the patient in Figure 50.2. Note that there is a dilated LV, a fixed defect in the anterolateral wall (diagonal branch of left anterior descending artery), and a reversible defect in the upper septal wall (septal perforators of left anterior descending artery).

sels usually corresponds with angiographic abnormalities in coronary arteries. Correction of the anatomic abnormality by either angioplasty, laser atherectomy, or coronary artery bypass surgery is expected to relieve the ischemia. A frequent location of ischemic tissue is immediately adjacent to an area of infarct. This is called periinfarct ischemia and may overlie or surround an infarct (Fig. 50.3).

Atypical Ischemia. Some arterial distributions have naturally recruited collaterals or bypass grafts that produce apparent discrepancies between angiographic and scintigraphic studies. Abnormal anatomy in a coronary artery may not produce hemodynamically significant changes in blood flow to the myocardium. Not all ischemia is produced by large vessel atherosclerosis. Capillary disease in diabetics, left bundle branch block, vasospasm, and vasculitis or myocardiopathy (dilated or hypertrophic) may produce ischemic myocardium even with normal arteries.

Hibernating Myocardium. Severe ischemia may be so slow to "reverse" on Tl-201 vessels that it will not be detected by rest images at 3–4 hours after exercise. Imaging at 24 hours or a Tl-201 second injection rest study may be required to detect extreme ischemia. The Tc-99m-labeled agents are routinely given as two separate injections, but there is evidence to suggest that rest injected Tl-201 studies may be best for detecting the severe ischemia that leads to a phenomenon known as "hibernating myocardium." Hibernating myocardium is important to diagnose as it simulates infarction by not contracting at rest. It remains viable, however, and will return to normal function after revascularization.

Ischemia may not be detected if there is inadequate exercise, inadequate pharmacologic challenge, or bal-

anced triple vessel disease. Fortunately, it is uncommon for all three coronary arteries to be hemodynamically compromised equally.

Myocardial Infarction produces layers of nonperfused scar tissue that are detected as areas of thin myocardium with decreased labeling at *both* exercise (or pharmacologic dilation of coronary arteries) *and* rest. The extent of an infarct, from subendocardial to transmural, is reflected by the size and degree of the perfusion defect. Technical artifacts from attenuation of the perfusion agent's radiation may be produced by SPECT tables, breast tissue, and subdiaphragmatic structures. These may appear as fixed defects superimposed on planar or SPECT images. This may lead to a false-positive reading of infarction. A false-positive interpretation of ischemia should not occur as long as the artifact does not change between stress and rest imaging.

A single myocardial perfusion scan cannot determine the age of an infarct. Acute infarcts usually appear larger than old infarcts when imaged with Tl-201. Temporarily damaged cells around infarcted cells, "stunned myocardium," will neither contract nor take up Tl-201 for a few days. As repair occurs, the apparent perfusion defect shrinks.

Acute infarcts may also be detected with Tc-99m pyrophosphate labeling. Ionized calcium released from myocytes forms dystrophic calcifications with phosphates and a "hot spot" is formed adjacent to infarcted tissue. Antimyosin antibodies labeled with Tc-99m or indium-111 (In-111) also localize on the fringes of acute infarctions. The need for imaging of acute infarction is clinically infrequent, usually when the patient has left bundle branch block. Contused myocardium is also detected with these techniques.

Figure 50.6. Normal Fourier Phase and Amplitude Images from the Same Patient in Figures 50.4 and 50.5. The lower (amplitude) image shows the relative displacement of blood in each chamber of the heart. The brightness of pixels depicts the relative degree of motion. The upper (phase) image shows the relative timing of contraction of each chamber. The histogram summarizes the number of pixels with a given phase angle. The cardiac cycle is represented on an arbitrary scale of −90° to 270°. Note that the *gray pixels* representing ventricular motion are tightly grouped around −30°, indicating synchronous contraction. Approximately 180° up the time scale, there is a cluster of *white* pixels corresponding to atrial motion.

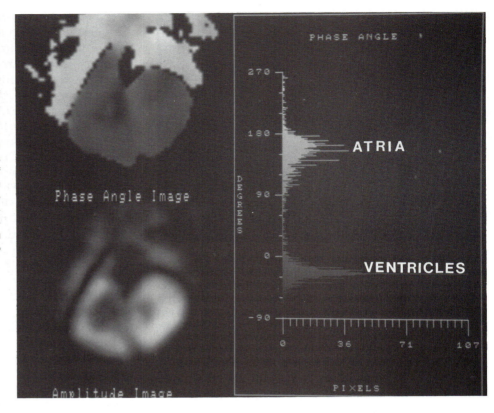

Table 50.1.   Exercise Radionuclide Ventriculogram—Relative Volumes and Cardiac Output[a]

Level	HR	BP	DP(K)	LVEF	LVEDV	LVESV	LVSV	CO
Rest	78	150	11.7	0.56	1.00	1.00	1.00	1.00
EX1	101	152	15.4	0.60	0.83	0.76	0.89	1.16
EX2	102	158	16.1	0.64	0.90	0.74	1.03	1.35
EX3	106	158	16.7	0.64	0.96	0.79	1.10	1.50
EX4	115	170	19.6	0.68	0.91	0.66	1.11	1.63
EX5	133	190	25.3	0.72	0.77	0.49	1.00	1.70
EX6	153	192	29.4	0.71	0.59	0.39	0.75	1.47
Post exercise	162	162	26.2	0.70	0.69	0.47	0.86	1.79

[a]This exercise radionuclide ventriculogram shows that the patient worked hard during six levels of bicycle exercise as the heart rate (HR) rose from 78 to 153, while systolic blood pressure (BP) rose from 150 to 192 with a resultant rise in double product (DP) from 11.7 to 29.4 K. The left ventricular ejection fraction (LVEF) rises appropriately from 0.56 to 0.71 at peak exercise. However, the ventricle fills poorly during exercise as relative end-systolic volume (LVESV) goes progressively down (normal) *but* relative end-diastolic volume (LVEDV) goes down (abnormal). The stroke volume (LVSV) changes little and the only improvement in cardiac output (CO) is the result of increased heart rate. Constrictive physiology limits endurance and exercise in this otherwise healthy individual. This is an example of the quantitative data inherent in nuclear medicine images.

than resting study. The patient must be cooperative and capable of exercising. The 2–3 minute periods for each exercise level usually supply a minimally acceptable amount of statistical counts in the images. Finally, a large amount of data must be processed and reviewed since each stage of the study is comparable with a usual resting study (Table 50.1).

Normal patients increase their LVEF and dV/DT significantly while decreasing their LV end-systolic volume. The relative cardiac output can be measured from one stage to another and rises with increasing work load. Abnormal exercise RVG response can be seen in several ways, such as an increase of LVEDV more than 10%, lack of increase or even a fall in LVEF with greater work loads, and development of wall motion abnormalities due to ischemia brought on by the exercise.

RIGHT VENTRICULAR STUDIES

First Pass Function Studies

Right ventricular function is more difficult to assess by the RVG study than is LV function. This is because labeled activity in the RV cannot be isolated as well from other chambers as can LV activity. For this

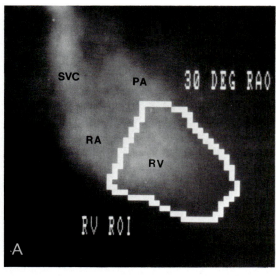
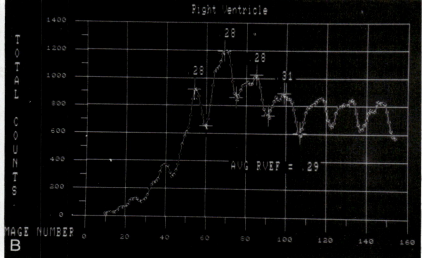

Figure 50.7. Right Ventricular First Pass Function Study. A. Fast dynamic right ventricular ejection fraction by first pass. The acquisition totaled 512 frames taken at 40-msec intervals in the right anterior oblique (*RAO*) projection as a radioactive bolus traversed the right atrium (*RA*) and ventricle (*RV*). An image of the *RV* is made by summing dozens of individual frames. A fixed region of interest (*ROI*) is drawn around the RV. *SVC,* superior vena cava; *PA,* pulmonary artery. **B.** A time activity curve from the ROI in **A** shows the relative volume of the ventricle rising and falling with diastole and systole. Peaks and valleys in the curve are flagged and beat by beat ejection fractions are averaged.

reason, RV function is best assessed by analyzing images from the first pass of a bolus through the right-sided chambers and lungs before overlapping left-sided chambers are seen. The patient is usually imaged in the right anterior oblique projection (Fig. 50.7). A bolus of up to 30 mCi of high specific-activity isotope must be very rapidly injected followed immediately by a nonradioactive flush dose. This activity will pass through the RV in three to eight heartbeats. Some systems allow acquisition as a gated study composed of these beats. Others allow retrospective reformatting of the first pass data into a cine loop display. These techniques yield a small amount of data compared with the many hundreds of beats in a resting RVG study. A region of interest is established around the RV and a time activity curve allows an RV ejection fraction to be measured for each beat. An average RV ejection fraction is calculated (Fig. 50.7).

If xenon-133 in saline is available for injection, a better RV evaluation is possible. During a slow infusion Xe-133 passes through the right side of the heart and into the lungs, where it immediately fills the alveoli and is exhaled. In this way, overlapping activity never enters the left side of the heart. A gated study over many seconds is possible. Data from many beats can be collected and processed in a manner identical to the standard RVG of the LV.

First Pass Flow Studies

The first pass study in an anterior projection can also be used to detect abnormalities of blood flow to one lung compared with the other. The effect of extrinsic compression on a pulmonary artery by a mediastinal or hilar mass can be easily detected, especially if Fourier phase analysis and display of the data is used. Abnormal blood flow to a lung segment such as is seen in pulmonary sequestration can be detected.

Left-to-right Intracardiac Shunts can be detected and quantified using a first pass imaging technique. Instead of using a region of interest over the RV for analysis, an area of lung is used. In a normal person, the bolus of activity passes into and out of the lung exponentially in a way that can be mathematically described by a gamma function. If a left-to-right shunt is present, some blood that has gone through the lungs to the left side of the heart reenters the right side of the heart and is pumped back into the lungs. This causes a prolongation of the washout of activity from the lung region of interest. A gamma-variate curve fitting method can be used to detect and quantify the amount of the left-to-right shunt. The method is sensitive to detect shunts with a ratio as low as 1.2: 1, far below the 2:1 shunt that can be detected by chest radiograph (Fig. 50.8).

Right-to-left Shunts can be detected by using a slow IV injection of macroaggregated albumin particles. In a normal person, less than 10% of the injected dose should pass through normal arteriovenous shunts in the lungs and be found in the systemic circulation. After injection, static images of the patient's whole body are performed. Regions of interest are taken over the lungs, head, neck, abdomen, and ex-

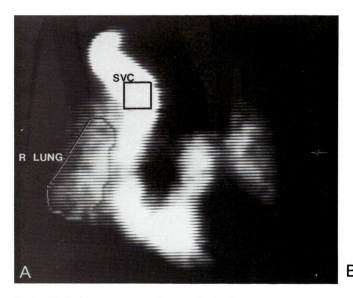

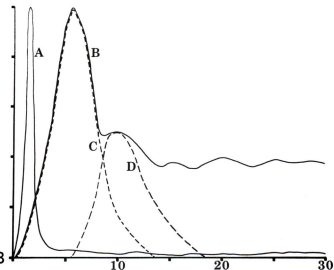

Figure 50.8.   Abnormal Left-to-right Shunt Study. Regions of interest are drawn around the superior vena cava (*SVC, square box*) and the right (*R*) lung on image data from a first pass flow study. Note lack of activity in the *LV* (*arrow*) in this summary of images from the dextrophase of the flow. **B.** Graph showing time activity curve of the activity within the two regions shown in **A.** *A* is the sharp bolus injection passing through the superior vena cava. *B* is the right lung time activity curve, which rises exponentially but does not follow the fitted gamma variate curve (*C*) on the way down. This indicates early recirculation due to a left to right shunt. The shunt is quantified by comparing the area under *C* with the area under the fitted recirculation gamma variate (*D*).

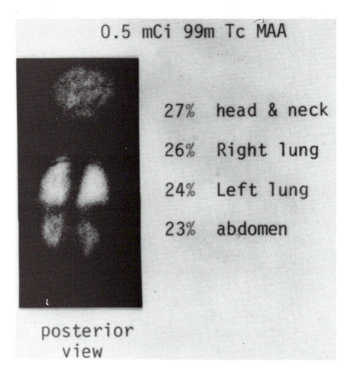

Figure 50.9.   Abnormal right-to-left shunt study. A significant portion of the injected Tc-99m macroaggregated albumin (*MAA*) particles are seen in capillary beds outside the lungs in the brain and kidneys. This indicates and measures the amount of shunted blood.

tremities. In this way, the amount of radioactivity outside the lungs in the systemic circulation can be quantified (Fig. 50.9). The study can be repeated at a later date to check progression.

Suggested Reading

Bacharach SL, Green MV, Borer JS. Instrumentation and data processing in cardiovascular nuclear medicine: evaluation of ventricular function. Semin Nucl 1979;9:257–274.

Berman DS, Kiat Hosen, Van Train, K, Garcia E, Friedman J, Maddahi J. Technetium 99m sestamibi in the assessment of chronic coronary artery disease. Semin Nucl Med 1991;21: 190–212.

Bonow RO, Dilszian V. T1-201 for assessment of myocardial viability. Semin Nucl Med 1991;21:230-241.

Green MV, Bacharach SL. Functional imaging of the heart: methods, limitations, and examples from gated blood pool scintigraphy. Progr Cardiovasc Dis 1986;28:319–348.

Jones RH. Use of radionuclide measurements of left ventricular function for prognosis in patients with coronary artery disease. Semin Nucl Med 1987;17:95–103.

Parker DA, Karvelis KC, Thrall JH, Froelich JW. Radionuclide ventriculography: methods. In: Gerson MC, ed. Cardiac nuclear medicine. New York: McGraw Hill, 1991:81–125.

Rozanski A, Berman DS. The efficacy of cardiovascular nuclear medicine exercise studies. Semin Nucl Med 1987;17:104–120.

Treves S, Parker JA. Detection and quantification of intracardiac shunts. In: Strauss HW, Pitt B, eds. Cardiovascular nuclear medicine. St Louis; CV Mosby, 1979:148–161.

51
Endocrine Imaging

Calvin L. Lutrin
William E. Brant

THYROID
Imaging Methods

Treatment of thyroid diseases requires the evaluation of thyroid function, thyroid anatomy, and tissue characterization of thyroid lesions (1, 2). Radionuclide imaging reflects the functional status of the thyroid as a whole as well as regional function within the gland. High-resolution ultrasound using 5.0–10 MHz linear array transducers provides excellent anatomic detail of the thyroid gland to assess size, parenchymal uniformity, and to screen for thyroid nodules. Ultrasound is an excellent modality to guide percutaneous aspiration biopsy to provide pathologic diagnosis of thyroid nodules. Computed tomography (CT) and magnetic resonance imaging (MR) supplement ultrasound by staging of invasive thyroid cancers, evaluating for postoperative recurrence of thyroid cancer, and determining the extent of goiter that extends into the thorax.

Radionuclide Studies assess the physiologic function of the gland and determine the activity of nodules. The commonest indication for performing a thyroid scan is to classify the functional status of a thyroid nodule as hyperfunctioning ("hot"), hypofunc-

tioning ("cold"), or indeterminate (sometimes called "warm"). Indeterminate nodules have the same significance as cold nodules. The defect caused by the lesion is obscured by activity in surrounding thyroid tissue. It is possible to detect nonpalpable abnormalities using a gamma camera with a pinhole collimator. Abnormalities smaller than 1 cm can be resolved. Iodine-123 is the agent of choice for most thyroid imaging (Table 51.1). The iodine is readily absobed from the gastrointestinal tract and trapped and organified in the thyroid. Technetium-99m pertechnetate can also be used for thyroid imaging. The disadvantage is a lesser target-to-background ratio and a requirement to perform an additional iodine study to exclude a technetium-avid carcinoma that demonstrates increased uptake. Iodine-131 is used to treat Graves' disease and for whole-body scans following thyroidectomy for thyroid carcinoma.

Radioiodine Uptake by the thyroid gland was used as a measure of thyroid function for many years. The advent of radioimmunoassay and the development of accurate methods of measuring serum levels of thyroid hormones and thyroid-stimulating hormone (TSH) provided a superior method of evaluating thyroid function. Now radioiodine uptake is done mainly for two reasons: (*a*) differentiating Graves' disease (uptake high, usually >40% at 24 hrs) from subacute or painless thyroiditis or factitious hyperthyroidism (uptake usually <2%), and (*b*) assisting in the calculation of the dose of radioactive iodine for treatment of Graves' disease. An oral dose of 100–400 μCi ^{123}I or 5–10 μCi ^{131}I is used for both uptake and imaging. A nonimaging uptake probe is used to obtain counts in neck phantom standard. At 24 hours, counts are obtained of the patient's neck and thigh as well as the background activity. In some laboratories measurements are also obtained at 4–6 hours.

$$\text{Uptake} = \frac{\text{Neck - thigh cpm}}{\text{Standard - background cpm}}$$

where cpm = counts per minute.

Normal = 10–30% at 24 hours (highly dependent on iodine intake).

Table 51.1. Radiopharmaceuticals Used for Thyroid Imaging

Isotope	Half-life	Principal Gamma Ray (keV)	Advantages	Disadvantages	Comments
I-123	13 hours	159	Physiologic Good organ-to-background ratio Same dose can be used for imaging and uptake	Expensive Image 4 hours after administration	
I-131	8 days	364	Cheap Widely available Long half-life	High radiation dose per mCi High-energy photon Unsuitable for gamma camera imaging	Whole-body scans used for evaluation of residual thyroid and metastatic disease in patients with thyroid cancer
Tc-99m	6 hours	140	Cheap Excellent imaging qualities	Requires separate dose of I-123 or I-131 for uptake measurements Must repeat imaging with I-123 if hot nodule found	

Anatomy and Physiology

The thyroid is located in the lower part of the neck. It consists of two lobes of approximately equal size (5 × 2 cm) positioned on either side of the trachea and connected across the midline by the thin thyroid isthmus (Fig. 51.1). A mild degree of asymmetry in size of the lobes is common. A pyramidal lobe extends upward from the isthmus in as many as 40% of individuals. Histologically, the thyroid gland is composed of follicular cells arranged in acini, with central collections of colloid. Larger pools of colloid ("colloid cysts") are commonly visualized with ultrasound (Fig. 51.2). Perifollicular cells ("C cells"), which produce calcitonin, comprise a small proportion of the cell population.

The lobes of the thyroid are between the carotid artery and jugular vein laterally and the trachea medially. They rest on the longus colli muscles posteriorly and are covered by the sternohyoid, sternothyroid, and prominent sternocleidomastoid muscles anteriorly. The esophagus may protrude from behind the trachea on the left side and must not be mistaken for a parathyroid or thyroid mass, or lymph node. With high-resolution imaging, the inferior thyroid artery and vein may be imaged between the thyroid and the longus colli.

Normal thyroid parenchyma is relatively homogeneous by all imaging modalities. Ultrasound demonstrates the parenchyma as homogeneous medium-to-high level echoes (Fig. 51.2). Computed tomography shows the thyroid to be of homogeneous high density because of its iodine content (Fig. 51.1). Because the thyroid is quite vascular, the gland enhances avidly with intravenous contrast administration. On T1-weighted MR images, the thyroid has lower intensity than fat and

higher intensity than muscle. With T2 weighting the signal intensity of the thyroid increases and the contrast differentiation from muscle is optimized.

The role of the thyroid gland is the production, storage, and release of thyroid hormones. Thyroid-stimulating hormone (TSH), produced by the pituitary gland, regulates the production and release of thyroid hormones. The secretion of TSH is, in turn, stimulated by hypothalamic thyrotropin-releasing hormone (TRH) and suppressed by circulating thyroxine (T_4) and triiodothyronine (T_3). Dietary iodide is absorbed in the stomach and upper small bowel. It is extracted from the blood stream by the follicular cells of the thyroid where it is used in the production of T_4 and T_3. Depending upon the dietary content, about 25% of ingested iodine is taken up by the thyroid and 75% is excreted in the urine. Recommended daily adult allowance for iodine is 100–150 μg. This is greatly exceeded in most developed countries such as the U.S. The daily intake of iodine in the United States may be as much as 500 μg. However, iodine deficiency is still endemic in certain parts of the world, particularly in the Andes, Himalayas, and inland areas of Europe and Africa.

Hypothyroidism

In endemic areas, hypothyroidism is usually caused by dietary iodine deficiency (with a goiter present) while in iodine-replete areas, the commonest noniatrogenic cause is chronic thyroiditis (Hashimoto's disease), in which a goiter is also usually present. Hyperthyroidism treated with radioactive iodine is another common cause (no goiter). Neonatal hypothyroidism is due to thyroid dysgenesis (agenesis,

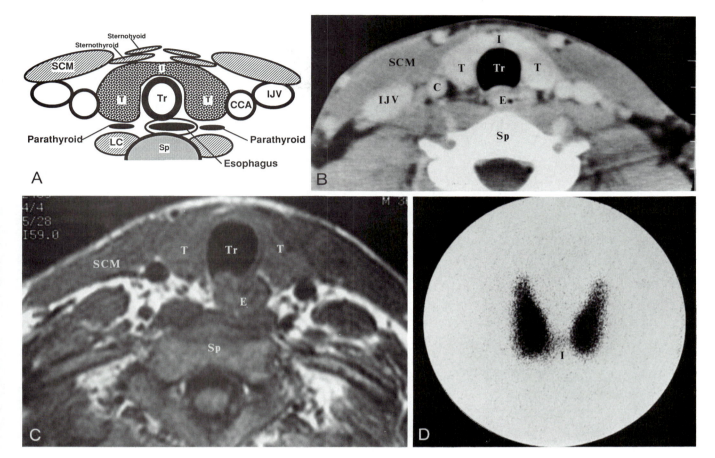

Figure 51.1. Normal Thyroid. Diagram (**A**), CT image (**B**), and T1-weighted MR (TR, 800; TE, 20) image (**C**) of the thyroid gland in cross-section. **D.** Normal ¹²³I scan. *T*, thyroid gland; *I*, isthmus of thyroid gland; *Tr*, trachea. *CCA* ; common carotid artery; *IJV*, internal jugular vein; *E*, esophagus; *SCM*, sternocleidomastoid muscle; *LC*, longus colli muscle; *Sp*, spine.

hypoplasia, or ectopia). The usual clinical features include weight gain, coldness, sluggishness, and dry skin. Laboratory findings include elevated serum TSH and low serum T_4.

Hyperthyroidism

The commonest cause of hyperthyroidism is Graves' disease (diffuse toxic goiter). Other causes include subacute or painless thyroiditis, toxic nodular goiter and factitious hyperthyroidism due to ingestion of thyroid hormone tablets. The usual clinical features include weight loss, increased appetite, tremor, irritability, heat intolerance, palpitations, muscle weakness, goiter, exophthalmus or stare. Laboratory findings include decreased serum TSH and elevated serum T_4.

Goiter

Goiter refers to the clinical finding of generalized thyroid enlargement. Goiter may be associated with increased, decreased, or normal thyroid hormonal function. On imaging studies, thyroid enlargement is best judged subjectively. Thickness of the isthmus greater than 1 cm is a reliable confirmatory sign of goiter. Goiters extending into the thorax can be accurately assessed by CT or MR. The causes of goiter include:

Multinodular goiter is a commonly used clinical term for adenomatous hyperplasia. Imaging studies show a diffusely abnormal enlarged nodular heterogeneous gland, or a pattern of multiple discrete nodules on a background of normal parenchyma.

Nontoxic goiter may be related to iodine deficiency, goitrogens in the diet, or deficiency of thyroid enzymes. The gland is usually soft and symmetric, but may appear multinodular with age.

Thyroiditis. All types of thyroiditis are characterized by rapid asymmetric glandular enlargement, with or without nodularity. Inflammatory changes may fixate the gland to adjacent structures and simulate malignancy.

Infection of the thyroid gland may be acute suppurative due to Gram-positive bacteria or subacute viral often involving only a portion of the gland. Suppurative infection is associated with hemorrhage, ne-

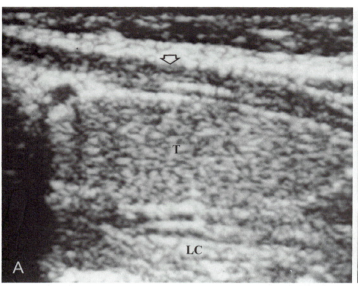

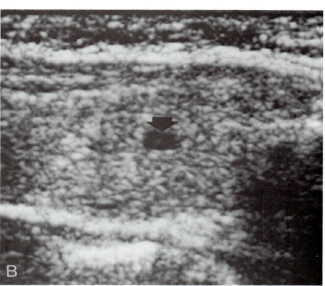

Figure 51.2. Normal Thyroid. A. Longitudinal ultrasound image demonstrates the normal midrange homogeneous echogenicity of the thyroid. The *arrow* identifies the sternothyroid muscle. *T*, thyroid;

LC, longus colli muscle. **B**. Longitudinal ultrasound shows a colloid cyst (*arrow*) in the right lobe of the thyroid. Colloid cysts are small (<5 mm), well defined, and of no clinical significance.

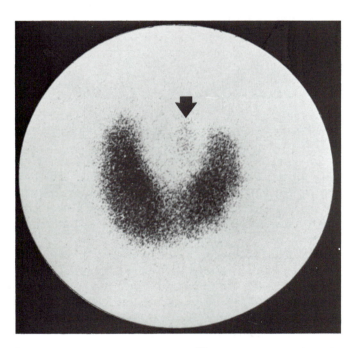

Figure 51.3. Graves' Disease. This ^{123}I scan demonstrates diffuse enlargement without nodules. A pyramidal lobe is visualized (*arrow*).

crosis, and abscess formation. Subacute viral infection usually causes focal edematous enlargement of the gland.

Graves' Disease is the most common cause of hyperthyroidism. It is an autoimmune disorder with thyroid-stimulating antibodies causing hyperplasia and hyperfunction of the thyroid gland. The gland is usually enlarged two- to three-fold, homogeneous, and without nodules (Fig. 51.3). Treatment options for

Graves' disease include subtotal thyroidectomy, antithyroid drugs (propylthiouracil, methimazole, and carbimazole), β-blockers such as propanolol for relief of hyperthyroid symptoms, and radioactive iodine.

The use of radioactive iodine in the treatment of hyperthyroidism has become the treatment of choice in the majority of patients. Iodine-131 in the form of sodium iodide has been in use for many years. It is given by mouth either as a capsule or as a liquid. After concentration in the thyroid, the high-energy β-particles and, to a lesser extent, gamma photons emitted from the ^{131}I nucleus deliver on the order of 5,000–10,000 rads to the adjacent thyroid cells. There is very little radiation to structures outside the thyroid gland. Most patients will become euthyroid after a single dose. Ten to 20% of patients require a second or third dose. Patients generally become euthyroid by 10–12 weeks after therapy and frequently become hypothyroid by 6–12 months. Estimation of the dose of ^{131}I is empiric. A commonly used formula is:

$$\text{Dose in mCi} = \frac{\text{100-150 } \mu\text{Ci/g} \times \text{wt of the gland in g}}{\text{fractional uptake} \times 1000}$$

resulting in a typical dose of approximately 5–15 mCi. The higher the dose, the quicker the response and the sooner the patient becomes hypothyroid. The smaller the dose, the longer it takes to become euthyroid and the later the development of hypothyroidism. However, it appears that hypothyroidism cannot be avoided, merely delayed by using small doses of ^{131}I.

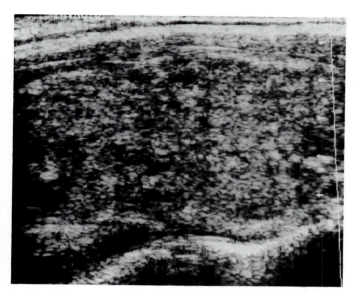

Figure 51.4. Hashimoto's Thyroiditis. Longitudinal ultrasound image of the right thyroid lobe demonstrates diffuse enlargement and a coarse granular pattern of parenchymal echogenicity.

Therefore, it has become a common policy to give larger doses of ^{131}I with the understanding that hypothyroidism, while not a goal of treatment, is inevitable and is easily treated. It is important to document that females of childbearing age are not pregnant prior to treatment as radioactive iodine crosses the placental barrier and will damage the fetal thyroid.

Complications, apart from permanent hypothyroidism, which is virtually universal, are uncommon. Transient worsening of thyrotoxicosis is fairly common. It occurs a few days to 2–3 weeks after treatment and is due to the release of preformed thyroid hormone from disrupted follicles. Occasionally patients develop symptoms of subacute thyroiditis, with pain and tenderness in the thyroid, often radiating to the ears or jaw. Temporary hypoparathyroidism and recurrent laryngeal nerve damage have been reported after radioactive iodine treatment; both are exceedingly rare. Though serious and life-threatening, thyroid storm is a very rare complication, more often seen after surgery in inadequately prepared patients. Carcinogenesis and genetic damage have not been observed.

Thyroiditis

All forms of thyroiditis may be mistaken for tumor because of rapid asymmetric enlargement and nodularity.

Subacute (Viral) Thyroiditis, also called de Quervain's or granulomatous thyroiditis, presents with thyroid pain and hyperthyroidism following an upper respiratory infection. Iodine uptake is usually decreased or absent in the acute stages. The disease runs a subacute course of a few weeks to a few months.

Hashimoto's Thyroiditis is the most common cause of goiter and primary hypothyroidism in adults in developed countries. It is an autoimmune disorder with circulating antithyroid antibody. Histology demonstrates diffuse lymphocytic infiltration of the gland. The thyroid is diffusely enlarged with abnormal texture and, frequently, discrete nodules (Fig. 51.4).

Riedel's Thyroiditis is a rare inflammatory fibrosing process that involves the thyroid and commonly extends into the neck. Radionuclide uptake is absent in involved areas.

Thyroid Nodules

The Problem. Thyroid nodules are extremely common, while thyroid cancer is relatively rare (3, 4). Nodules can be palpated in 4–7% of American adults who are asymptomatic for thyroid disease. Autopsy studies demonstrate thyroid nodules in 50% of patients with clinically normal thyroid glands. Ultrasound studies can detect thyroid nodules in 36–41% of middle-aged adults. Thyroid cancer, on the other hand, affects only 0.1% of the population. Thyroid cancer represents less than 1% of all cancer and is responsible for <0.5% of all cancer death. The ratio of thyroid nodules to thyroid cancer can be estimated at approximately 500:1. The challenge of clinical evaluation and imaging studies is to establish the likelihood of malignancy and to select out for surgery only those patients at high risk for thyroid malignancy.

Ultrasound is highly sensitive for the detection of thyroid nodules; however, its specificity for determining malignancy is low. Neither MR nor CT can improve that specificity. This is not surprising since the histologic differentiation of benign follicular adenoma from well-differentiated follicular carcinoma is based solely on identification of vascular invasion.

On the basis of radioiodine or technetium pertechnetate uptake during imaging, nodules may be classified as hypofunctioning (cold) (Fig. 51.5), relative to the rest of the gland, hyperfunctioning (hot) (Fig. 51.6), or indeterminate. In a patient with a nodular goiter the main concern is whether or not thyroid carcinoma is present. Single cold nodules have a 10–20% incidence of malignancy, while malignancy is exceedingly rare in hot nodules. A multinodular gland with one or more cold nodules may harbor cancer in up to 5% of patients. If technetium pertechnetate is used for imaging and a hot nodule is discovered, imaging should be repeated with I-123 as thyroid carcinoma may occasionally trap pertechnetate, resulting in a hot nodule. This nodule would be cold with I-123.

The differential diagnosis of thyroid nodules is as follows:

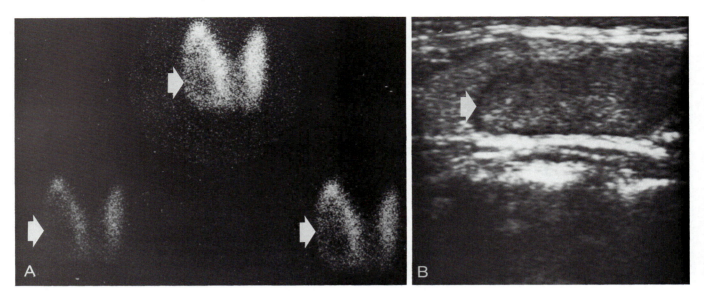

Figure 51.5. Cold Nodule—Follicular Adenoma. A. A ^{123}I scan photographed at three different intensities demonstrates a large hypofunctioning nodule (*arrows*) in the right thyroid lobe. **B.** Longitudinal ultrasound image of the right thyroid lobe reveals a well-defined solid nodule (*arrow*) with a hypoechoic rim.

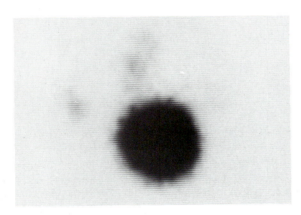

Figure 51.6. Hot Nodule. A hyperfunctioning adenoma demonstrates intense radionuclide activity with suppression of function of the remainder of the gland.

Follicular Adenoma is the most common benign neoplasm of the thyroid and represents about 20% of thyroid nodules. There are many subtypes based upon histologic criteria, including Hürthle cell adenoma, colloid adenoma, and others. Most are solitary, round or oval, and well encapsulated. Regressive changes are extremely common and greatly affect its imaging appearance. These include focal necrosis, hemorrhage, edema, infarction, fibrosis, and calcification (Fig. 51.7).

Adenomatous Hyperplasia is responsible for up to 50% of thyroid nodules. Adenomatous nodules, also called colloid nodules, are not true neoplasms but are the result of cycles of hyperplasia and involution of a thyroid lobule. They are frequently multiple, but one nodule may be dominant. Regressive changes are

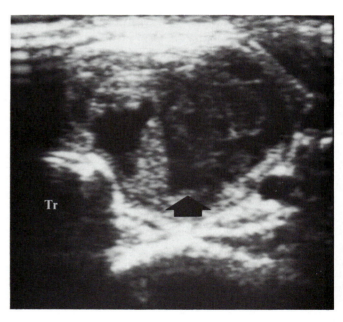

Figure 51.7. Degenerated Follicular Adenoma. Transverse ultrasound of the left lobe of the thyroid shows a well-defined mass (*arrow*) with large irregular areas of cystic degeneration. Regressive changes are common in follicular adenomas and adenomatous nodules. *Tr*, trachea.

common including necrosis, hemorrhage, cystic degeneration, and calcification.

Thyroid Cysts are extremely rare. Most cystic nodules found in the thyroid are actually cystic degeneration of an adenomatous nodule or a follicular adenoma.

Hemorrhagic Cysts also usually represent hemorrhage into an adenomatous nodule or a follicular

Table 51.2. Signs Suggesting Benignancy

Extensive cystic component
Multiple nodules
Hot on radionuclide scan
Peripheral calcification
Decrease in size following hormone therapy

Table 51.3. Signs Suggesting Malignancy

Imaging
  Solid nodule
  Cold on radionuclide scan
  Irregular contour
  Poor margination
  Size >4–5 cm
Clinical
  History of neck irradiation
  Age <20 years
  Male

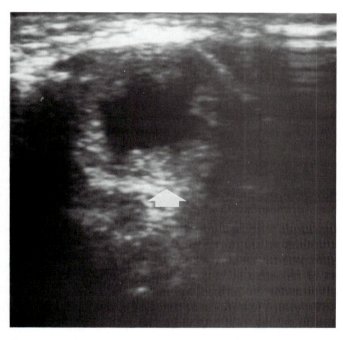

Figure 51.8. Papillary Carcinoma. Transverse ultrasound image demonstrates a well-defined nodule with a large cystic component (*arrow*). Histology revealed well-differentiated papillary carcinoma. Malignant nodules cannot be reliably distinguished from benign nodules by their appearance alone. Compare this figure with Figure 51.7.

adenoma. Hemorrhage into normal parenchyma also may produce a hemorrhagic cyst.

Thyroid Cancer. Malignant nodules cannot be reliably differentiated from benign nodules by any imaging method. Aspiration biopsy is required in every suspicious case. However, a number of criteria can be used to assess the relative risk of malignancy (Tables 51.2 and 51.3). Every assessment of thyroid nodules must consider all clinical and imaging features. A

nodule that is hot on radioiodine scan is extremely unlikely to be malignant. A nodule that is solitary and cold on scintigraphy has a 10–20% chance of being malignant. A history of neck irradiation, particularly in childhood, increases the risk of malignancy by five-fold to 10-fold. Nodules with extensive cystic component (>50% cystic), or well-defined peripheral calcification are unlikely to be malignant. Regression of nodule size following thyroid hormone therapy is a sign of a benign nodule. Large, predominantly solid nodules with irregular contour and poor margination are likely to be malignant. Punctate calcification is commonly present in both benign and malignant nodules and has no significance. A lucent peripheral halo usually represents compressed adjacent thyroid tissue and may be seen in both benign and malignant nodules. The histologic types of thyroid malignancy are as follows:

Papillary Carcinoma is the most common type, and is responsible for 75% of cases (Fig. 51.8). Patients are predominantly female (female:male = 4:1) with an average age of 45. The major route of spread is lymphatic to regional nodes, followed by hematogenous dissemination to lungs and bone.

Follicular Carcinoma represents 15% of cases, and is also more common in females. The primary route of spread is hematogenous to lung and bone. Prognosis is not as good as for papillary carcinoma.

Medullary Carcinoma arises from parafollicular cells (C cells) and is associated with multiple endocrine neoplasia (MEN II) in some cases. Calcitonin is a useful tumor marker. The prognosis is worse than for papillary or follicular carcinoma. The tumor spreads by both lymphatic and hematogenous routes. Although the tumor does not concentrate ^{131}I, metastases can be detected by thallium-201 (^{201}Tl), ^{99m}Tc(V) DMSA (dimercaptosuccinic acid, pentavalent form) and $^{123/131}$I-MIBG (metaiodobenzylguanidine). The last has also been used for treatment.

Anaplastic Carcinoma is an extremely lethal malignancy with no effective treatment and a 5-year survival rate of less than 4%. The tumor invades locally very aggressively and spreads early to distant sites.

When using ultrasound, nuclear medicine, CT, or MR for initial staging of thyroid malignancy or followup for recurrence, one must consider the common routes of spread of the specific type of malignancy to optimally plan the imaging study. The impressive contrast resolution of MR makes it excellent for determining involvement of muscles, larynx, esophagus, and other cervical structures by large in-

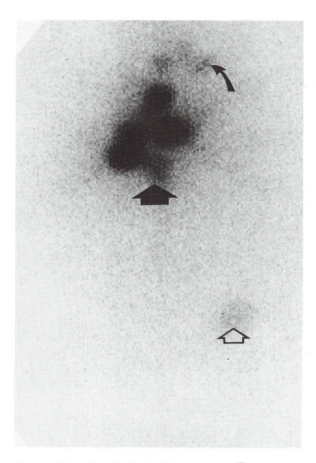

Figure 51.9. Lymph Node Metastases. A ^{131}I whole body scan postthyroidectomy shows intense radionuclide activity in papillary carcinoma lymph node metastases in the neck (*solid arrow*). Normal activity is present in the stomach (*open arrow*) and submandibular salivary glands (*curved arrow*).

vasive tumors. Recurrence of tumor may be demonstrated by MR. On T2-weighted images, tumor has high signal intensity, brighter than muscle, while fibrosis in the thyroid bed has low signal intensity, less than or equal to muscle (5). Lymph node involvement is determined primarily by size criteria. Normal lymph nodes in the neck are less than 10 mm in diameter. Som (6) provides an excellent review of the anatomy and description of cervical lymph nodes.

Whole-body radionuclide scans using ^{131}I are effective in demonstrating thyroid metastases and tumor recurrence following thyroidectomy for papillary carcinoma (Fig. 51.9). However, radionuclide whole-body scans are ineffective in medullary and anaplastic carcinoma because of the lack of iodine uptake by the tumor.

Radioiodine (^{131}I) scans of the whole body, neck, and chest are performed to determine the completeness of surgery and to evaluate the response to treatment. Uptake of ^{131}I in the thyroid bed frequently represents residual thyroid tissue. Salivary, stomach, bowel, and bladder activity represents physiologic traces of iodine distribution. Focal activity in the lungs, skeleton, or in the neck remote from the thyroid bed is pathologic. Nasal secretions may contain radioiodine. A contaminated pocket handkerchief should not be mistaken for a pelvic metastasis. Similarly, some breast uptake may occur. This should not be confused with lung metastasis.

Radioiodine Therapy. According to the Nuclear Regulatory Commission regulations, patients receiving 30 mCi or more of ^{131}I require hospitalization until the residual amount of ^{131}I falls below 30 mCi. Doses close to 30 mCi are frequently used on an outpatient basis to ablate residual thyroid postthyroidectomy. Some authors advocate larger doses on the grounds that 30 mCi is inadequate to ablate thyroid cancer. We believe the initial dose is not directed at the thyroid cancer but rather at normal residual thyroid tissue. Once that has been ablated, functioning thyroid cancer can be attacked. For the latter purpose, doses of 100–200 mCi are frequently used.

The patient should be hypothyroid with a serum TSH greater than 40 IU/ml prior to ablation. This is to ensure maximal stimulation of residual thyroid and/or thyroid cancer and thereby promote appropriate localization of the radioiodine. Iodine-rich foods such as shellfish, bread, and kelp should be avoided at least 1 week prior to therapy. A radiographic study with iodinated intravenous contrast will delay therapy by at least a month.

The frequency of side effects varies directly with the dose of radioiodine administered. Doses greater than 100 mCi may cause sialoadenitis. For this reason, patients should be encouraged to suck lemon drops or sour candy for 1–2 days posttherapy. Pulmonary fibrosis has been reported in patients who have had multiple doses of radioiodine therapy for extensive pulmonary disease. Leukemia has been reported in patients who have received in excess of 600 mCi total.

Metastasis. Metastatic disease to the thyroid gland is rare. The most common primary tumors to metastatsize to the thyroid are breast, lung, kidney, malignant melanoma, and lymphoma.

PARATHYROID

Parathyroid disorders are classified in terms of function, i.e., excessive parathyroid hormone (PTH) production or *hyperparathyroidism*, and insufficient PTH production or *hypoparathyroidism*. Imaging studies of the parathyroid glands are performed to localize parathyroid abnormalities in patients with hyperparathyroidism that has been confirmed clinically. There is no role for imaging in hypoparathyroidism. The causes of hyperparathyroidism are listed in Table 51.4.

Table 51.4. Causes of Hyperparathyroidism

Primary hyperparathyroidism
Solitary parathyroid adenoma, 85%
Parathyroid hyperplasia, 10%
Multiple parathyroid adenomas, 4%
Parathyroid carcinoma, 1%
Secondary Hyperparathyroidism
Diffuse or adenomatous parathyroid hyperplasia due to
calcium-losing renal disease
Tertiary Hyperparathyroidism
Autonomous parathyroid function resulting from long-standing
secondary hyperparathyroidism
Paraneoplastic Syndromes
Ectopic parathormone production
Bronchogenic carcinoma
Renal cell carcinoma

Imaging Methods

Because 80–85% of abnormal parathyroid glands are located near the thyroid, ultrasound is able to demonstrate the majority of these. Thyroid nodules may be sonographically similar to parathyroid adenomas, while degenerated parathyroid adenomas may mimic cystic thyroid masses. Ultrasound may be used for guiding needle biopsy. Cells of parathyroid origin can be readily differentiated from thyroid cells, while fluid aspirated from degenerated parathyroid nodules have high PTH levels. Magnetic resonance imaging or CT are generally required to demonstrate abnormal parathyroid tissue at ectopic sites: thymus (10–15%), posterior mediastinum (5%), retroesophageal (1%), within the carotid sheath (1%), and parapharyngeal (0.5%).

Technetium-thallium radionuclide subtraction imaging is also used to detect parathyroid adenomas with a sensitivity of about 75% and a specificity of 90% (2, 7). Thyroid tissue concentrates both technetium pertechnetate and thallium (Fig. 51.10). Parathyroid adenomas pick up ^{201}Tl but not ^{99m}Tc-pertechnetate. This is the basis for dual isotope imaging. First, the thallium images are acquired and then, without moving the patient, ^{99m}Tc-pertechnetate is administered and imaging at the technetium peak is performed. The technetium images are subsequently subtracted from the thallium images. A residual focus of activity indicates the presence of an adenoma. It is vital that the patient does not move at all, otherwise erroneous results will be obtained. False-positive results can be caused by thallium uptake in thyroid nodules, sarcoid lymph nodes, or metastases to the neck. Recently ^{99m}Tc-sestamibi has been used instead of thallium in some centers.

Anatomy

Most people (80%) have four parathyroid glands, two superior and two inferior. However, autopsy studies have demonstrated that 20% of individuals have three, five, or six parathyroid glands. The superior parathyroid glands arise from the fourth brachial pouch along with the thyroid gland and are seldom ectopic (8). The inferior parathyroid glands arise from the third brachial pouch along with the thymus and are more commonly ectopic, usually in the mediastinum. Normal glands measure $5 \times 3 \times 1$ mm in size. Because they are so small and flat, normal glands are not usually demonstrated by any imaging method. The normally located parathyroid glands are found posterior to the thyroid lobes superficial to the longus colli muscles (Fig. 51.1), and between the trachea and carotid sheath.

Parathyroid Adenoma

Parathyroid adenomas are characteristically oval in shape and 8–15 mm in greatest diameter. Their cellularity is homogeneous, giving a uniform internal appearance on all imaging modalities. On ultrasound, parathyroid adenomas are homogeneously hypoechoic (Fig. 51.11). Color Doppler ultrasound demonstrates hypervascularity. On MR T1-weighted images, adenomas show low intensity similar to muscle. On T2-weighted images, the adenomas showed high intensity similar to or greater than fat. Because adenomas may be isointense with fat, T2-weighted images alone provide an incomplete examination (5). Computed tomography is best performed with intravenous contrast to demonstrate the contrast-enhancing parathyroid nodules. Rarely, parathyroid adenomas may show cystic degeneration or calcification.

Multiple Gland Disease

Parathyroid hyperplasia cannot be differentiated from multiple parathyroid adenomas by imaging methods. Hyperplasia affects all of the parathyroid glands but is frequently asymmetric. The individual glands have the same imaging appearance as parathyroid adenomas.

Parathyroid Carcinoma

Carcinomas are usually larger than adenomas (at least 2 cm in size). The internal architecture is much more heterogeneous, with cystic degeneration more common. Invasion of adjacent muscle or vessels may be demonstrated. The differentiation of parathyroid carcinoma from a large adenoma can usually be made only histologically.

Ectopic Parathyroid

Ectopic parathyroids are most common in the anterosuperior mediastinum or low in the neck. Magnetic resonance imaging currently seems the modality

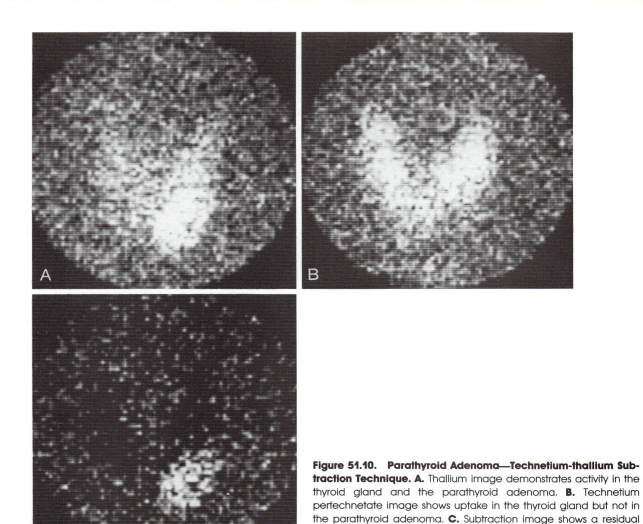

Figure 51.10. Parathyroid Adenoma—Technetium-thallium Subtraction Technique. A. Thallium image demonstrates activity in the thyroid gland and the parathyroid adenoma. **B.** Technetium pertechnetate image shows uptake in the thyroid gland but not in the parathyroid adenoma. **C.** Subtraction image shows a residual focus of activity, identifying a parathyroid adenoma at the lower pole of the left thyroid lobe.

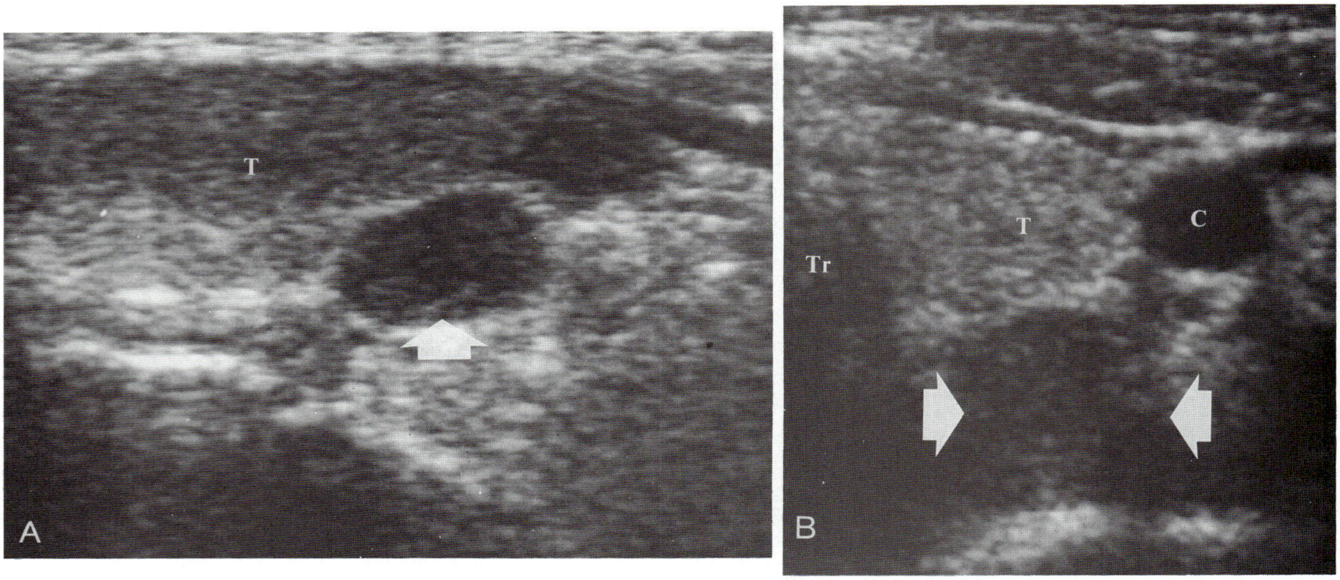

Figure 51.11. Parathyroid Adenoma. Longitudinal (**A**) and transverse (**B** ultrasound images demonstrate a parathyroid adenoma (*arrows*) at the lower pole of the left thyroid lobe. *T*, thyroid; *Tr*, trachea; *C*, common carotid artery.

of choice for identifying ectopic parathyroids. Reported sensitivities average 75%.

RADIONUCLIDE ADRENAL IMAGING

High-resolution *anatomic* imaging of the adrenal glands is performed by CT, MR, or ultrasound and is discussed in Chapter 29. Two groups of radiopharmaceuticals are available for *functional* imaging of hyperplastic or neoplastic adrenal disorders:

1. ^{131}I 6β-iodomethyl-19-norcholesterol (NP59); and,
2. ^{131}I-or ^{123}I MIBG.

The NP59, a cholesterol analog, is taken up by adrenal cortical tissue. Cholesterol is a common precursor of mineralocorticoids, glucocorticoids and androgens; MIBG is taken up by cells of adrenal medullary origin such as pheochromocytoma (Fig. 29.7). In addition, tumors of neural crest origin such as neuroblastoma and medullary thyroid cancer often concentrate MIBG. Note that NP59 and MIBG are available only for investigational use in the U.S., although they are available commercially in many other countries.

References

1. McDougall IR. Thyroid diseases in clinical practice. New York: Oxford University Press, 1992.
2. Sandler MP, Patton JA, Gross MD, et al. Endocrine imaging. Norwalk: Appleton & Lange, 1992.
3. Rojeski MT, Gharib H. Nodular thyroid disease: evaluation and management. N Engl J Med 1985;313:428–436.
4. James EM, Charboneau JW, Hay ID. The thyroid. In: Rumack CM, Wilson SR, Charboneau JW, eds. Diagnostic ultrasound. St. Louis: Mosby Year Book, 1991:507–523.
5. Higgins CB, Aufferman W. MR imaging of thyroid and parathyroid glands: a review of current status. AJR 1988;151:1095–1106.
6. Som PM. Lymph nodes of the neck. Radiology 1987;165:593–600.
7. Beierwaltes WH. Endocrine imaging: parathyroid, adrenal cortex and medulla, and other endocrine tumors. Part II. J Nucl Med 1991;32:1627–1639.
8. Reading CC. The parathyroid. In: Rumack CM, Wilson SR, Charboneau JW, eds. Diagnostic ultrasound. St. Louis: Mosby Year Book, 1991:524–539.

52

Gastrointestinal, Liver-Spleen, and Hepatobiliary Scintigraphy

Philip W. Wiest,
Robert J. Telepak,
Michael F. Hartshorne

GASTROINTESTINAL STUDIES
  Esophageal Imaging
  Gastroesophageal Reflux
  Gastric Imaging
  Gastrointestinal Bleeding Scintigraphy
  Meckel's Scan
LIVER AND SPLEEN STUDIES
  Liver Spleen Scan
  Heat-damaged Red Blood Cell Scan for Splenic Tissue
HEPATOBILIARY IMAGING

Nuclear medicine imaging studies can provide considerable information in the functional evaluation of the gastrointestinal system. Routine studies include hepatobiliary, gastrointestinal bleeding studies, and gastric emptying measurements. Other procedures that are less frequently ordered provide clinically valu-

able information. The order of presentation in this text is anatomic from proximal to distal.

GASTROINTESTINAL STUDIES

Esophageal Imaging

The esophageal transit study performed with swallowed technetium-99m (^{99m}Tc)-sulfur colloid is a seldom-ordered nuclear medicine examination. It has been reported to detect esophageal dysmotility in 50% of symptomatic patients with an otherwise normal evaluation for dysphagia (1).

The patient swallows a radioactive solid or fluid bolus while data are obtained via a computer. The esophagus is divided into three regions of interest (ROI)—upper, middle, and lower (Fig. 52.1**A**). Transit times are then calculated from time-activity curves representing the ROIs (Fig. 52.1**B**).

The normal esophagus demonstrates sequential activity from proximal to distal with no visualized esophageal activity remaining after 10 seconds. Re-

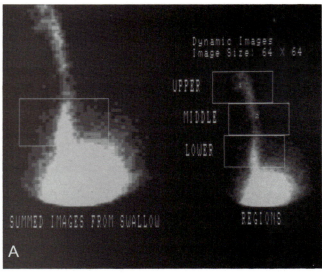
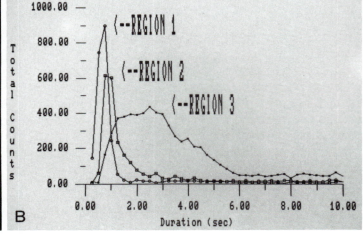

Figure 52.1. Normal Esophageal Transit Study. A. A composite image of the esophagus and stomach is used to generate ROIs around the upper, middle, and lower esophagus. **B.** Time-activity

curves for each region are displayed for 10 seconds after the swallow. Inspection of the curves allows calculation of the transit time.

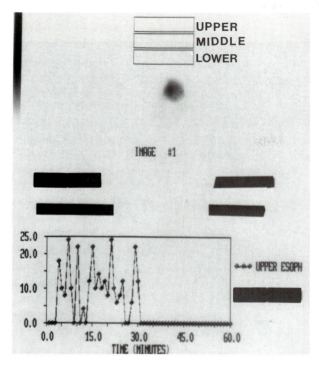

Figure 52.2. Abnormal GER Study. Three ROIs are established over the esophagus. A time-activity curve corresponding to the upper ROI for 60 minutes shows refluxed activity after 3 minutes, which continues for about 30 minutes.

gional analysis may differentiate between achalasia and scleroderma.

It is important to remember that esophageal scintigraphy is functional and does not provide detailed anatomic information. For this reason, barium studies or endoscopy is necessary to exclude the possibility of neoplasm or infection as the cause of impaired esophageal function.

Gastroesophageal Reflux

The evaluation of heartburn and atypical chest pain in the adult commonly raises the clinical question of gastroesophageal reflux (GER). In the pediatric population, failure to thrive and recurrent pneumonias often elicits the same question.

The most common diagnostic tool currently used in the diagnosis of GER is acid reflux monitoring. This examination unfortunately requires nasoesophageal intubation and 24 hour continuous recording. It is invasive and unwieldly, especially in the pediatric age group. Alternatives are few and fairly insensitive, with the exception of GER scintigraphy.

Gastroesophageal reflux scintigraphy is performed with acidified orange juice mixed with ^{99m}Tc-sulfur colloid (1). The acid decreases the lower esophageal sphincter pressure and also delays gastric emptying. Regions of interest are established via a computer to correspond to the stomach and segments (upper, mid-

dle, and lower) of the esophagus. In the pediatric population, ROIs over the lungs detect aspiration. Images may be recorded in adults with an abdominal binder that increases abdominal pressure sequentially in 10 mm Hg increments to a maximum of 100 mm Hg. Normal patients have no detectable GER activity. This examination is reported to have a 90% sensitivity in the detection of GER (Fig. 52.2).

Gastric Emptying

Gastric emptying is a complex physiologic process directed not only by neuroendocrine processes but also by a host of local factors. Food type and pH as well as food osmolality affect the rate of gastric emptying. Any process that interrupts this cycle can ultimately result in gastric stasis. Impaired gastric emptying can be caused by many disease states such as diabetes mellitus, electrolyte disturbances, postvagotomy syndromes, and some medications.

Excluding mechanical obstruction is important in diagnosing the cause of the patient's symptoms. Endoscopy or barium studies are superior in the detection of gastric ulcers, tumors, or bezoars. Gastric emptying scintigraphy has become the gold standard in the clinical evaluation of gastric motility (2). While it is a simple test to perform, interpretation is based upon complicated mathematical models. Solid food, liquids, or both are labeled with a radiotracer and consumed by the patient. Digital images of the stomach are acquired and a time-activity curve is generated (Fig. 52.3).

The normal half emptying time ($T_{1/2}$) of radioactive solids and liquids varies with the technique employed. In general, the normal $T_{1/2}$ is less than 90 minutes for solids and less than 60 minutes for liquids. Each laboratory should establish its own normal $T_{1/2}$ values.

Gastrointestinal Bleeding Scintigraphy

Patients who present with upper gastrointestinal bleeding are usually evaluated and often treated via endoscopy. The patient with lower gastrointestinal bleeding presents problems in diagnosis and therapy. Much confusion can be avoided if a systematic approach is utilized when evaluating lower gastrointestinal hemorrhage (Figs. 52.4–52.6).

At initial presentation, proctosigmoidoscopy should be performed to exclude hemorrhoidal bleeding. The next step is a gastrointestinal bleeding study with ^{99m}Tc-tagged red blood cells (3). Patients should be studied during the clinical period of maximal blood loss. Greatest success in localizing the source of hemorrhage occurs when patients require transfusion of at least two or more units of blood in the 24-hour period preceding gastrointestinal bleeding scintigraphy.

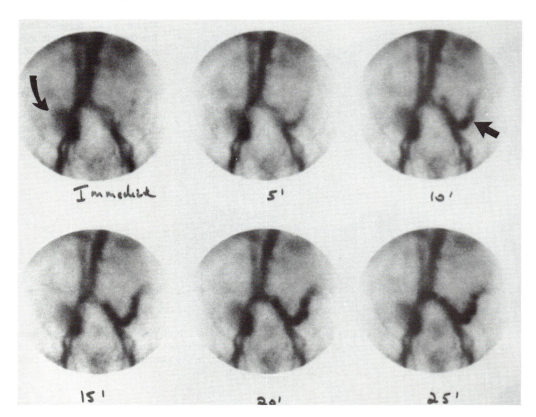

Figure 52.6. Distal Colon Bleeding in a Patient with Angiodysplasia. Images show a left lower quadrant hemorrhage (*arrow*). Note the blood pool in the transplanted kidney in the right iliac fossa (*curved arrow*).

uloendothelial system cells in the bone marrow are minimally seen. The liver/spleen scan has been recommended as an inexpensive and easy means to evaluate for focal or diffuse hepatic disease. Unfortunately, this scan lacks specificity. Radiotracer uptake may be abnormal in a multitude of diseases or simply a normal variant. Image resolution is poor even with modern gamma cameras. Lesions less than 1 cm are commonly missed. Single-photon emission computed tomography offers better resolution deep in the liver and spleen, but has predominantly been replaced in the evaluation of focal lesions by computed tomography and ultrasonography (Fig. 52.8).

Liver/spleen imaging remains useful for evaluation of liver and spleen size, configuration, and position. This may be beneficial in the evaluation of suspected hepatomegaly in patients with obstructive lung disease causing diaphragmatic flattening. Anatomic variants such as a Riedel's lobe of the liver are detectable. Liver spleen scans can be "subtracted" from other nuclear medicine studies to provide spatial information about the liver or spleen in relationship to a suspected abnormality. Indium-111 leukocyte scans (for infection) and gallium-67 scans (for inflammation or hepatoma) have physiologic uptake in the liver and spleen. Subtracting the liver/spleen scan from one of

these two scans confirms "hot" abnormalities adjacent to the liver or spleen (Fig. 52.9).

Alterations in perfusion and reticuloendothelial system function caused by cirrhosis and hepatitis are seen as a "shift" of activity to the spleen, bone marrow, and lungs. The liver/spleen scan provides information that helps monitor the disease process and efficacy of therapy (Fig. 52.10).

Heat-damaged Red Blood Cell Scan for Splenic Tissue

Technetium-99m-labeled red blood cells that have been damaged by heating are preferentially extracted from circulation by splenic tissue. Applications include diagnosis of polysplenia, splenosis, and confirmation of accessory splenic tissue.

HEPATOBILIARY IMAGING

Nuclear imaging of the gallbladder and biliary system is easily performed with ^{99m}Tc-labeled iminodiacetic acid compounds (5). Of the numerous iminodiacetic acid radiotracers that have been developed, ^{99m}Tc-diisopropyliminodiacetic acid (DISIDA) is one of the most commonly used. These radiopharmaceuticals are excreted unchanged into the biliary system,

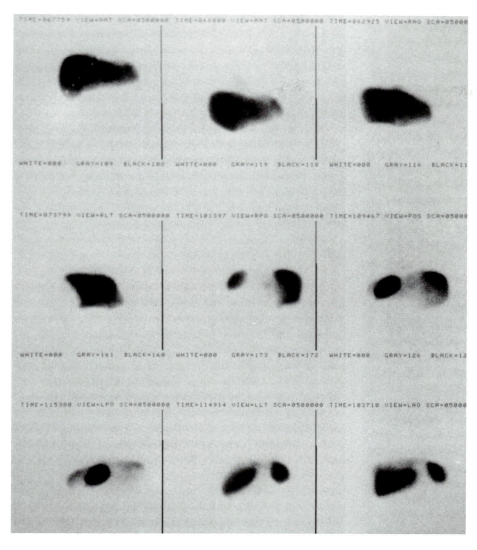

Figure 52.7. Normal Liver Spleen Scan. Sequential images begin with an anterior projection with a lead marker (row of cold dots) on the right costal margin. Subsequent images are anterior, right anterior oblique, right lateral, right posterior oblique, posterior, left posterior oblique, left lateral, and left anterior oblique from left to right, top to bottom. Note the homogeneous labeling of the liver and spleen and the relative size and position of these two organs in various projections.

even in the presence of elevated serum billirubin. Cholescintigraphy is the most requested use of hepatobiliary scans in the patient with suspected acute cholecystitis. A minimum of 2 hours fasting is recommended in preparation for this scan.

On hepatobiliary scans, it is normal to visualize prompt and homogeneous uptake of activity by the liver. This activity gradually decreases as the radiotracer is excreted into the biliary system and subsequently into the small bowel. Activity should be seen in the major extrahepatic ducts, gallbladder, and small bowel within 1 hour (Fig. 52.11).

Most patients with acute cholecystitis have a stone or stones obstructing the cystic duct. A small minority of patients, usually the chronically ill, have acalculous cholecystitis. The hallmark in the diagnosis of acute cholecystitis via cholescintigraphy is nonvisualization of the gallbladder at both 1- and 4-hour intervals after intravenous injection of the biliary agent. Chronic cholecystitis is diagnosed when the nonvisualized

gallbladder at 1 hour is seen at 4 hours. The nuclear medicine hepatobiliary examination has a 95% accuracy rate in the detection of acute cholecystitis (Fig. 52.12).

Increased blood flow on radionuclide angiograms of the gallbladder fossa aids in the diagnosis of acute cholecystitis. A "rim sign" on hepatobiliary scan images is seen as a band of increased activity around the gallbladder fossa, which represents poor excretion of radiotracer from inflamed hepatocytes. The rim sign is associated with gangrenous cholecystitis.

A pitfall in interpretation of acute cholecystitis may be caused by prolonged fasting with gallbladder distension. The radiopharmaceutical will not enter the already full gallbladder. This can be avoided by pretreating the patient with cholecystokinin. Cholecystokinin is a short-acting, natural hormone that causes prompt gallbladder contraction. After emptying, the gallbladder refills, allowing entry of the biliary agent.

Figure 52.8. Abnormal Liver/Spleen Scan, Anterior Projection. There are multiple round defects (*arrows*) in the liver that could represent tumor, cysts, abscesses, cavernous hemangiomas, or any of several other space-occupying lesions.

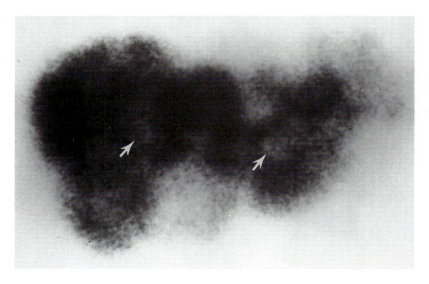

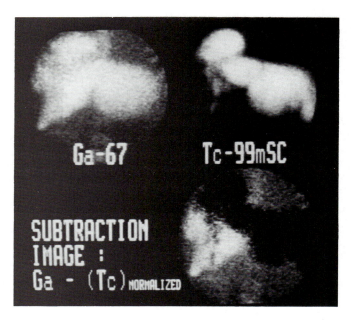

Figure 52.9. Liver/Spleen Subtraction from a Gallium-67 Scan in a Patient with Hepatoma. The *upper left* image is that of the Ga-67 distribution in the anterior projection at 48 hours. The *upper right image* is a matched image of a colloid distribution. Careful selection of the gamma camera energy windows allows simultaneous imaging of the two radiopharmaceuticals. The subtraction image (*bottom right*) shows the gallium-avid hepatoma, which does not label with the colloid.

Another common pitfall in this interpretation is the result of recent feeding with contraction of the gallbladder prior to the start of the hepatobiliary scan. In this case, the radiopharmaceutical may not enter the gallbladder. Morphine may be used to increase biliary pressure by contracting the sphincter of Oddi and shunting bile into the gallbladder.

A false-positive diagnosis of acute cholecystitis may also occur with previous cholecystectomy, tumor ob-

structing the cystic duct, and agenesis of the gallbladder.

Acalculous biliary disease includes chronic acalculous cholecystitis, cystic duct syndrome, and gallbladder dyskinesis. These patients present with similar complaints of right upper quadrant pain, fatty food intolerance, and epigastric distress. Cholescintigraphy and ultrasound may be normal. Cholecystokinin-assisted cholescintigraphy in acalculous biliary disease demonstrates decreased gallbladder contraction. The normal gallbladder ejection fraction is greater than 35%.

Other uses for the hepatobiliary scan include the detection of bile leaks in trauma and postoperative complications (Fig. 52.13). The excretion phase of the scan is important in evaluating hepatic and common bile duct patency. A delay in visualization of the bile ducts of more than 1 hour suggests obstruction. Caution must be exercised to differentiate severe hepatocellular disease from obstruction, as both present with delays in biliary visualization.

References

1. Malmud LS, Fisher RS. Radionuclide studies of esophageal transit and gastroesophageal reflux. Semin Nucl Med 1982;12:104–115.
2. Malmud LS, Fisher RS, Knight LC, Rock R. Scintigraphic evaluation of gastric emptying. Semin Nucl Med 1982;12:116–125.
3. Wiest PW, Hartshorne MF. Atlas of gastrointestinal bleeding (RBC) scintigraphy. In: Ziessman HA, Van Nostrand, eds. Selected atlases of gastrointestinal scintigraphy. New York: Springer-Verlag, 1992:35–74.
4. Royal HD, Drum DE. Liver-spleen scanning in benign disease. In: Mettler FA, ed. Radionuclide imaging of the GI tract. New York: Churchill Livingstone, 1986:83–134.
5. Ziessman HA. Atlas of cholescintigraphy: selective update. In: Ziessman HA, Van Nostrand D, eds. Selected atlases of gastrointestinal scintigraphy. New York: Springer-Verlag, 1992:1–34.

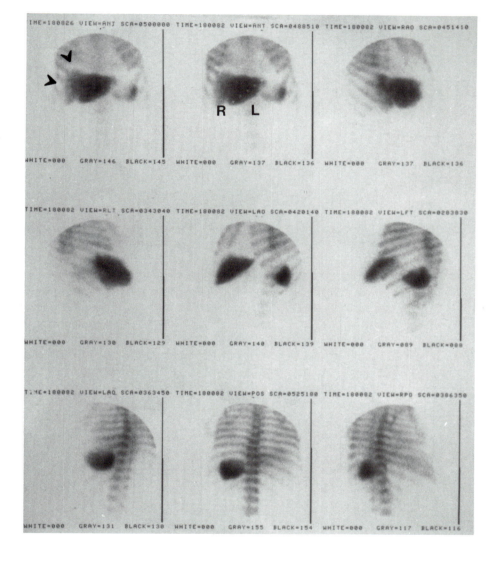

Figure 52.10. Abnormal Liver/Spleen Scan in a Patient with Cirrhosis. The liver is small and labels poorly. The left lobe of the liver (*L*) is better seen than the right lobe (*R*). Note the shift of the radiopharmaceutical to the bone marrow and spleen. Ascites separates the liver from the right ribs (*arrowheads*). Compare this figure with Figure 52.7.

Figure 52.11. Normal Hepatobiliary Scan. Images of the liver immediately after injection and at subsequent 5-minute intervals show rapid clearance of the blood pool followed promptly by central biliary duct and gallbladder (*arrow*) activity. Activity continues to fill the common bile duct (*arrowheads*) at 20 minutes and the small bowel (*curved arrow*) at 25 minutes.

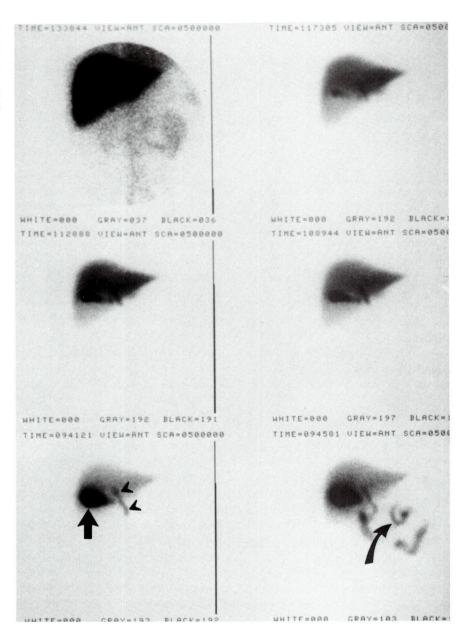

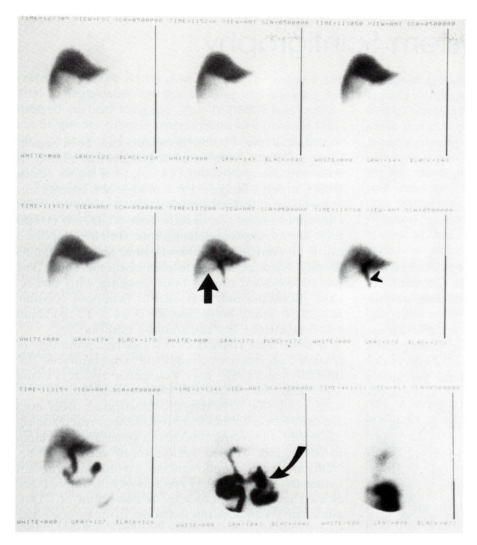

Figure 52.12. Acute Cholecystitis Diagnosed by Hepatobiliary Scan. **Figure 52.12. Acute Cholecystitis Diagnosed by Hepatobiliary Scan.** The first seven images were obtained during the 1st hour after injection of the biliary agent. The last two (anterior and right lateral in sequence) were performed 4 hours after injection. There is no entry of the radiopharmaceutical into the gallbladder (*arrow* on gallbladder fossa), though the bile progresses normally through the common bile duct (*arrowhead*) and small bowel (*curved arrow*).

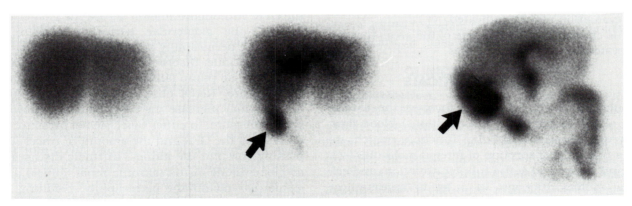

Figure 52.13. Biliary Leak after Cholecystectomy Detected by Hepatobiliary Scan. Images (*left to right*) obtained immediately, 30 minutes, and 1 hour after administration of the biliary agent show accumulation of bile in the area around the right lobe of the liver (*arrows*).

Recent advances in gamma camera technology and the increasing availability of SPECT allow for the ac-

centage of the dose administered. The choice of method depends on the clinical situation, the ability

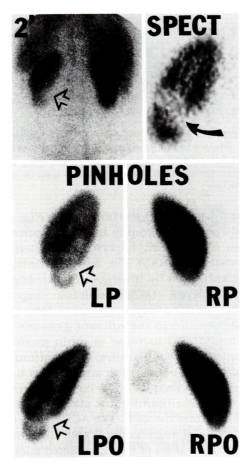

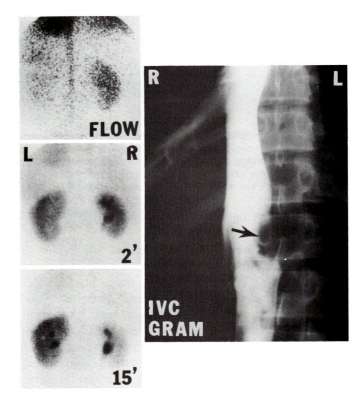

Figure 53.3.   Renal Mass. Tc-DTPA (2') posterior image (*upper left*) and Tc-DMSA pinhole images (*middle and lower*) demonstrate a renal contour abnormality (*open arrows*) of the lower pole of the left kidney. The SPECT image (*upper right*) demonstrates the true cortical defect (*curved arrow*) that corresponds to a renal tumor. *LP*, left posterior; *RP*, right posterior; *LPO*, left posterior oblique; *RPO*, right posterior oblique.

Figure 53.4.   Renal Vein Thrombosis. Posterior scintigrams (*left*) demonstrate normal flow, cortical uptake, and excretion for the right kidney. The left kidney is enlarged with severely diminished flow and a progressive rise in cortical tracer content through 15 minutes. The contrast inferior vena cavagram (*IVC GRAM*) (*right*) confirms thrombus in the left renal vein (*arrow*). Since 50% of patients with renal vein thrombosis develop pulmonary emboli, ventilation-perfusion scintigraphy should be considered.

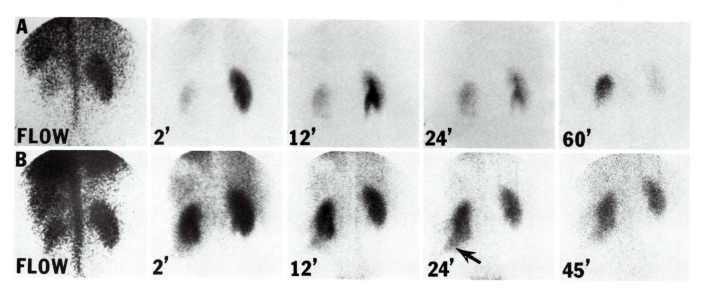

Figure 53.5.   Acute Tubular Necrosis. A. Posterior renal scintigrams 48 hours after left renal ischemia during a surgical procedure reveals diminished left renal flow and cortical function with slowly increasing cortical tracer retention through 60 minutes. GFR =74 ml/min (left = 19 ml/min, right = 55 ml/min). **B.** A study performed 1 month later reveals almost full resolution of the unilateral ATN. GFR = 94 ml/min (left = 42 ml/min, right = 52 ml/min). Extrarenal tracer activity (*arrow*) indicates a urine leak along a postoperative nephrostomy tract.

Figure 53.6. Renal Artery Stenosis—Scintigrams Posterior. A. Flow to the small right kidney is decreased (*image*) and delayed (*curve*). **B.** Right cortical Tc-DTPA activity (*top*) continues to rise during the first 12 minutes of the study. Orthoiodohippurate renography (*bottom*) (similar to Tc-MAG3) reveals the characteristic findings of delayed uptake and washout, characteristic of a severe RAS. **C.** Typical MAG3-captopril curves of a patient with compensated right RAS. Both curves are normal in the baseline study. This is because of efferent arteriolar constriction that is maintaining glomerular perfusion pressure and GFR (see text). After captopril, the right GFR has dropped and the cortical glomerular to pelvis transit time has become prolonged. This is evidenced by a prolonged time to peak, and a delayed washout on the stenotic side.

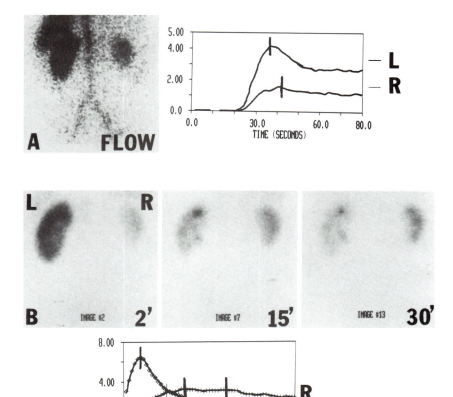

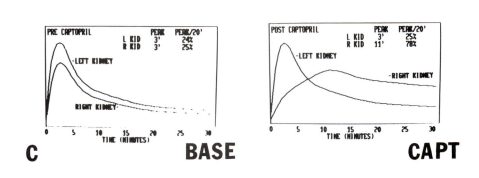

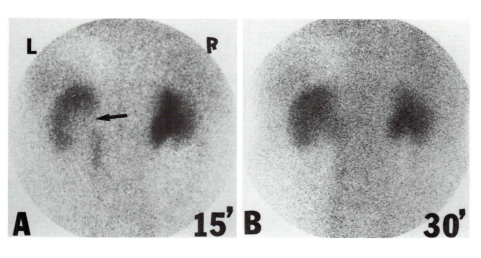

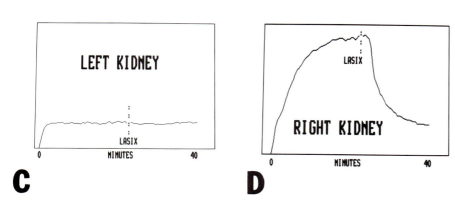

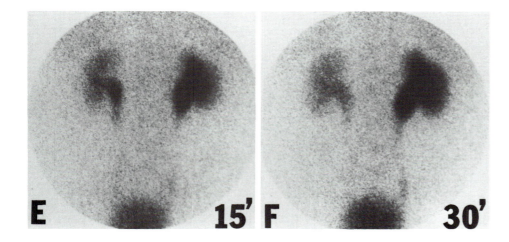

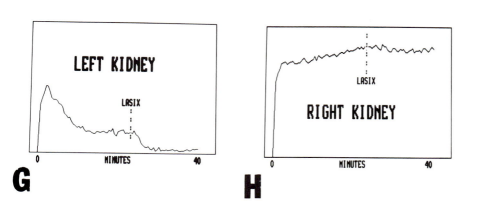

Figure 53.7. Furosemide Renography—Posterior Scintigrams. Furosemide (Lasix) administered at 15 minutes. A high-grade obstruction is seen on the left (**A, B, C**) with little tracer reaching the renal pelvis (*arrow*) and an absent furosemide response. On the right (**A, B, D**), a dilated but unobstructed renal pelvis empties rapidly following furosemide administration. A follow-up study many months later (**E to H**) demonstrates that, following surgery, the left kidney has returned to normal. However, the right kidney has developed a high-grade obstruction with poor furosemide response.

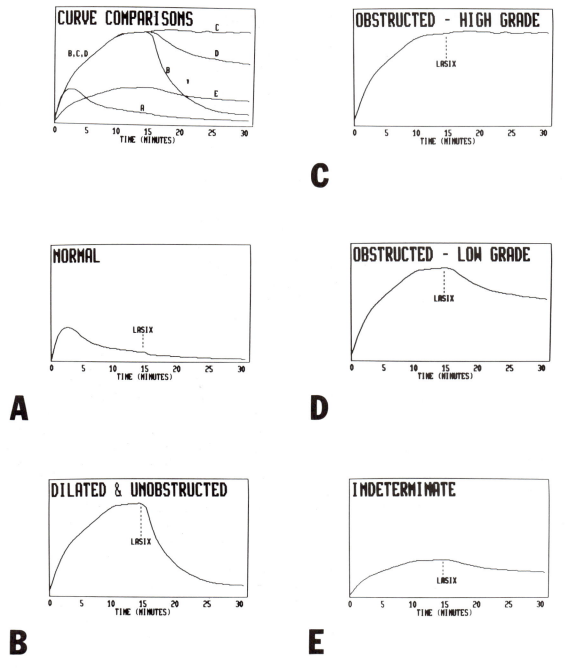

Figure 53.8.   Furosemide Curve Patterns. Normal (**A**), Dilated and unobstructed (**B**), high-grade obstruction (no Lasix response) (**C**). In a complete obstruction, no tracer would arrive at the renal pelvis. **D.** Low-grade obstruction. A partial response between that of curves **B** and **C** is seen. **E.** Indeterminate study. In a patient with a very large dilated collecting system or poor function in the kidney of interest, the furosemide dose may be insufficient to wash tracer from the collecting system. This curve represents a failed kidney that did not respond.

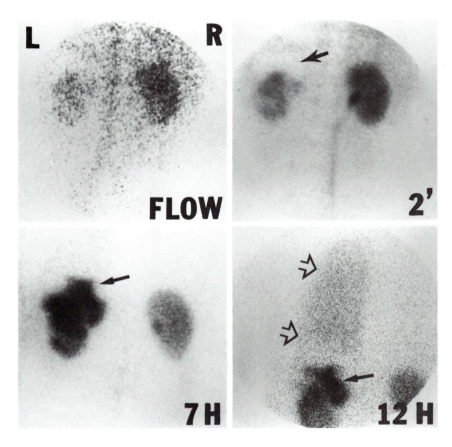

Figure 53.9. Renopleural Fistula—Posterior Scintigrams. The left kidney, contused in a motorcycle accident, demonstrates decreased perfusion (*FLOW*) and uptake (2'). A photon-deficient lesion (*arrows*) fills with tracer by 7 hours, indicating a traumatic urinoma. At 12 hours, tracer has moved from the urinoma through a renopleural fistula to the pleural space (*open arrows*).

the bladder must be emptied to avoid a false-positive study from ureteral reflux from a distended bladder.

When collecting system obstruction occurs, the postglomerular (Bowman's space) pressure rises and the GFR drops. Tubular damage occurs later than glomerular damage and takes significantly longer to reverse. The effects of acute obstruction on differential function are evaluated with Tc-DTPA (e.g., differential GFR), whereas chronic effects (e.g., scarring from pyelonephritis and serial differential function) are evaluated with Tc-DMSA static imaging. Renal imaging with Tc-MAG3 or Tc-DTPA reliably detects unilateral or bilateral urinary tract obstruction by demonstrating a dilated pelvocalyceal system and/or ureter with delayed drainage. When these findings are equivocal, such as in the case of a very large but unobstructed collecting system or decreased urine production, the routine study can be augmented with furosemide. In the absence of renal failure, the disappearance of tracer from the collecting system correlates with the severity of obstruction. In the adult a half-life of 15 minutes or less is normal, and a half-life greater than 20 minutes confirms obstruction.

Infection. In acute pyelonephritis, decreased parenchymal uptake of Tc-DMSA is seen either focally or diffusely within the normal renal contours. In chronic pyelonephritis, scarring occurs resulting in renal contour abnormalities with foci of diminished uptake. Renal or perinephric abscess and infected renal cysts may be imaged with ^{67}Ga or ^{111}In-WBC.

Renal Trauma (Fig. 53.9). Although largely supplanted by ultrasound and CT, radionuclide procedures do provide functional and anatomic information in the acute trauma patient. The use of Tc-DTPA and Tc-MAG3 permits assessment of aortic and renal flow and the functional integrity of the kidneys. Delayed images allow for the detection of urine leakage. The Tc-DMSA imaging demonstrates focal defects in contusion and renal infarction.

Ureteral Reflux (Fig. 53.10). Direct radionuclide cystography is the most sensitive imaging method for detecting ureteral reflux. The radiation dose is significantly lower than with other radiographic techniques. The agent TcO4, Tc-DTPA, Tc-MAG3, or Tc-sulfur colloid is instilled into the bladder and is followed by a continuous infusion of saline. With continuous computer acquisition during filling and voiding, even the most transient reflux can be seen. The bladder volume is reported when reflux occurs. The low radiation dose, compared with contrast cystography, is especially desirable in pediatric screening or when multiple studies are needed to evaluate progression of disease and response to therapy.

Renal Transplantation. Renal imaging of transplanted kidneys is performed to help distinguish

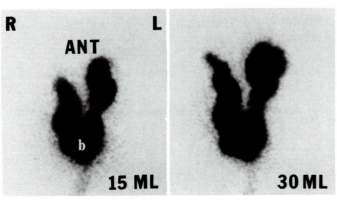

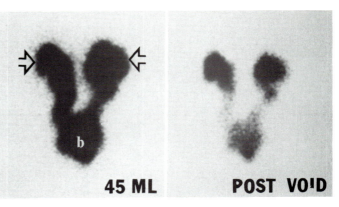

Figure 53.10.   Ureteral Reflux. Anterior scintigrams demonstrate reflux of tracer to the renal pelvis (*arrows*) immediately on the left and at 45 ml bladder volume on the right. *b*, bladder.

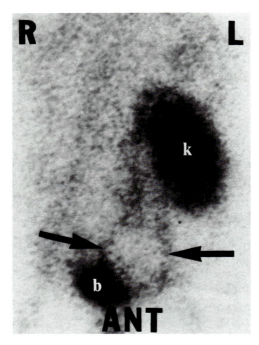

Figure 53.11.   Lymphocele in a Renal Transplantation Patient. A lymphocele is seen as a photopenic area (*arrows*) adjacent to the bladder (*b*) on this anterior scintogram. Because it is not obstructing the transplant ureter, it is probably not clinically significant. *k*, transplant kidney.

acute tubular necrosis from transplant rejection as well as to detect other posttransplant complications. In ATN, renal perfusion is relatively well preserved in comparison with the dramatic loss of renal function (GFR and cortical transit). Acute or chronic rejection results in a more balanced loss of perfusion and function because the damage is to small vessel perfusion with secondary and equivalent loss of function. Cyclosporine is a nephrotoxic drug used to combat rejection. The scintigraphic pattern of cyclosporine toxicity has been likened by some to that of ATN, and by others to that of rejection. As important as the pattern itself may be, even more significant are the time

course, the progression of sequential studies, and the correlation with clinical information. Acute tubular necrosis usually occurs during the 1st week, and acute rejection from the 1st to the 4th week following transplantation. Cyclosporine toxicity occurs later and only in patients taking cyclosporine. Chronic rejection is a late sequela, which eventually occurs to some degree in all transplants.

A myriad of additional postoperative complications are seen following transplantation. Some that are well investigated scintigraphically include renal artery and renal vein thrombosis, renal infarction, ureteral implant site obstruction or leakage, urinomas, and lymphoceles (Fig. 53.11).

Incidental Findings. Radiopharmaceuticals directed at other organ systems and accumulated by the kidneys may reveal unanticipated urinary tract abnormalities such as ureteral obstruction, urine leakage, abnormal renal position or shape, renal masses, and abnormal renal function. The kidneys are routinely demonstrated during skeletal imaging (Tc-MDP) and may also be seen during thyroid imaging (TcO4), blood pool imaging of the heart (Tc-RBC), and imaging for gastrointestinal bleeding (Tc-RBC). The kidneys are the main excretory route for 201-thallium and, during the first 24 hours after injection, for 67-gallium. Increased renal activity during lung perfusion imaging may be the result of a right-to-left intracardiac shunt.

TESTICULAR IMAGING

Testicular imaging is usually used to evaluate the acutely painful or swollen testicle (Fig. 53.12). Testicular torsion presents as a central hypovascular defect. As time passes, a hypervascular rim develops around the torsed testis and indicates loss of viability (delayed torsion). This rim may also be seen in abscess and hematoma. Epididymitis is hypervascular. Masses and

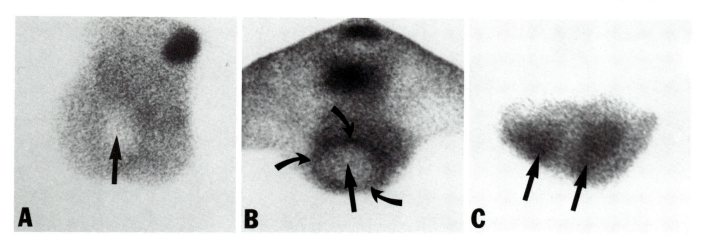

Figure 53.12. Imaging of the Painful Testis—Anterior Scintigrams. A. Testicular torsion is seen as a photon-deficient testis (*arrow*). **B.** The hyperemic rim (*curved arrows*) surrounding the photon-deficient testis occurs when the diagnosis of torsion is delayed ("missed") and correlates well with loss of testicular viability. **C.** Hyperemic inflammation occurs with epididymitis resulting in increased radionuclide accumulation in the epididymis, in this case bilaterally (*arrows*).

other testicular lesions are best evaluated with other modalities (Chapter 31).

Suggested Readings

Blue PW, Manier SM, Chantelois AE, et al. Differential diagnosis of prolonged cortical retention of radiotracer in technetium-99m DTPA renal scintigraphy (nuclear medicine atlas). Clin Nucl Med 1987;12:77–84.

Dondi M, Monetti N, Fanti S, et al. Use of Tc-99m-MAG3 for renal scintigraphy after angiotensin converting enzyme inhibition. J Nucl Med 1991;32:424–428.

Fogelman I, Maisey M. Renal. In: An atlas of clinical nuclear medicine. St. Louis: Mosby, 1988:217–373.

Freeman LM, Blaufox MD, eds. Genitourinary imaging update. In: Seminars in nuclear medicine (entire issue). Philadelphia: WB Saunders 1992:59–137.

Gottschalk A, Hoffer PB, Potchen EJ, eds. Diagnostic nuclear medicine. 2nd ed. Baltimore: Williams & Wilkins, 1988:927–992.

Mettler FA, Guiberteau MJ. Genitourinary system. In: Mettler FA, Guiberteau MJ, eds. Essentials of nuclear medicine imaging. 3rd ed. Philadelphia: WB Saunders, 1991:237–251.

McBiles M, Morita ET. Radionuclide imaging of the kidney, adrenals, and urinary tract. In: Davidson AJ, ed. Radiology of the kidney, 2nd ed. Philadelphia: WB Saunders, in press.

Sfakianakis GN. Nuclear medicine in congenital urinary tract anomalies. In: Freeman LM, ed. Nuclear medicine annual 1991. New York: Raven Press, 1991:129–192.

Sfakianakis GN, Vonorta K, Zilleruelo G, et al. Scintigraphy in acquired renal disorders. In: Freeman LM, ed. Nuclear medicine annual, 1992. New York: Raven Press, 1992:157–224.

54

Scintigraphic Diagnosis of Inflammatory Processes

John M. Bauman

The scintigraphic evaluation of inflammatory processes and tumors is extremely broad in scope and encompasses virtually all radiopharmaceuticals, imaging approaches, and inflammatory, benign and malignant diseases. Many of these topics have been discussed elsewhere and will not be further addressed. The focus of this discussion will be on the uses of gallium-67 and radiolabeled white blood cells (WBCs).

RADIOPHARMACEUTICALS

Gallium-67 (Ga-67) has been in use for over 20 years as a tumor and inflammation localizer after originally being introduced as a bone imaging agent. With principle photon energies of 93, 184, 296, and 388 keV and a poor photon yield per disintegration, Ga-67 is suboptimal as an imaging agent. Decay is by electron capture and the half-life is 78.1 hours. Typically, the three lower photopeaks are used for imaging and medium or high energy collimation is required.

Gallium-67 is administered as the citrate and is rapidly bound to transferrin and lactoferrin in vivo. Five to 8 mCi doses are recommended in infection workups; 10 mCi are recommended for tumor diagnosis. Higher doses are of particular help when single-photon emission computed tomography (SPECT) imaging is planned.

The biodistribution is variable depending on age, sex, prior transfusions, chemotherapy, lactation status, underlying disease process, and time of imaging. Imaging is typically performed at several times during the 6–72 hours after injection. Earlier times are used for evaluation of infectious processes; later times for the evaluation of malignancy. During the first 24–48 hours, approximately 15% of the administered dose is excreted in the urine. Subsequently another 10–20% is excreted by the colon (1). The normal Ga-67 study shows uptake in the liver, spleen, skeleton, lacrimal glands, salivary glands, genitalia, and, the kidneys and colon at the appropriate times (Fig. 54.1). Laxative administration helps to clear unwanted colonic activity.

The exact mechanisms of Ga-67 localization in inflammatory lesions and tumors are unclear, but three principle components have been cited: blood flow and local capillary status, incorporation and transfer by leukocytes, and bacterial ingestion. Mechanisms whereby certain tumors take up and concentrate Ga-67 are similarly unclear (1–4).

Indium-111-Labeled White Blood Cells (In-111-WBCs). Since the introduction of In-111-WBCs in 1976, a variety of labeling techniques have been reported. Typically, a WBC-rich, mixed cellular suspension from 60 ml of whole blood is incubated with In-111 oxine in a saline medium and injected. Autologous cells are usually used. However, in neutropenic patients and infants, ABO-compatible donor leukocytes may be used with appropriate type and crossmatch precautions. Since human immunodeficiency virus and hepatitis screening cannot be completed before injection of the donor cells, informed consent and careful donor selection are imperative. The procedure requires approximately 2.5 hours to perform.

Indium-111 is superior to Ga-67 in its imaging characteristics, with peaks of 173 keV (89%) and 247 keV (92%). It also decays by electron capture with a half-life of 67 hours. These energies require the use of a medium energy collimator but are easily imaged by the thinner crystals present in modern gamma cameras. The high target (abscess) to background ratios for In-111-labeled leukocytes provide excellent image contrast.

The spleen is the critical organ, receiving up to 20 rads per 0.5 mCi dose. There is no normal renal

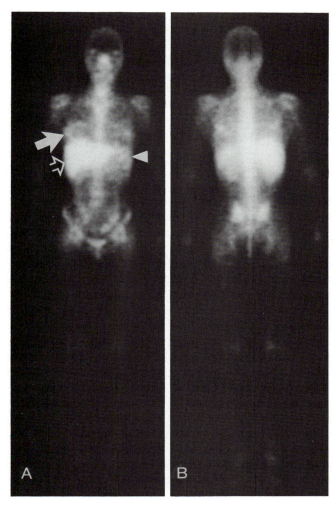

Figure 54.1. Normal Gallium Scan. A. Anterior view. **B.** Posterior view. The normal Ga-67 study has a variable appearance ranging from primarily soft-tissue localization to mostly skeletal uptake. Note the physiologic breast activity (*closed arrow*), which simulates the appearance of mildly abnormal pulmonary uptake in this middle-aged woman who was not lactating at the time of the study. The activity in the liver (*open arrow*) is much hotter than the activity in the spleen (*arrowhead*).

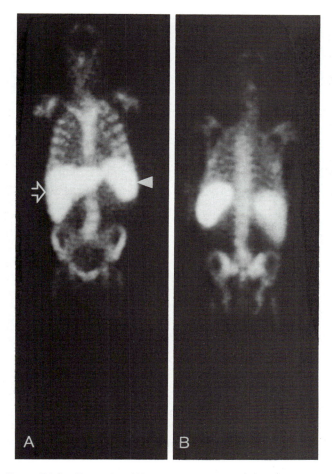

Figure 54.2. Normal In-111-WBC Scan in an Adult Male. A. Anterior view. **B.** Posterior view. Note the lumbar scoliosis. The activity in the spleen (*arrowhead*) is hotter than the activity in the liver (*open arrow*).

or intestinal excretion of In-111-labeled leukocytes, as is seen with Ga-67. Marrow activity is present because of normal cellular migration and marrow uptake of In-111. Moderate to marked lung activity is present on images obtained within 4 hours of injection. This activity represents margination of the cells in the lungs and is a physiologic response of the cells to contact with extracorporeal surfaces during labeling. Because of the low administered activity and the fact that a significant percentage of the cells are marginated early in the study, imaging is typically performed at 18—24 hours postinjection. A normal In-111 leukocyte scan at 18 hours post-injection is shown in Figure 54.2.

Technetium-99m-Labeled White Blood Cells.
Recently, leukocytes labeled with Tc-99m hexamethyl-

propylamine oxine (HMPAO) have been used to image inflammation (5–8). With the higher doses possible with Tc-99m and its shorter half-life of 6 hours, imaging is performed much earlier, at 1–6 hours postinjection. The biodistribution is similar to that of In-111-WBCs with four notable exceptions: renal, bladder, gallbladder, and intestinal activity are present because of excretion of the eluted Tc-99m complex. Hepatobiliary excretion with transit to gut is seen beginning about 3 hours after injection. Thus, gut and renal activity is less specific than with In-111-labeled cells. While clinical experience with Tc-99m-HMPAO-WBCs is not as extensive as with In-111-WBCs, most reports are encouraging. Indium-111 is cyclotron-produced and therefore not always available. The HMPAO, a lipophilic agent initially introduced as a brain blood flow imaging agent, is available in kit form for local compounding. The HMPAO offers the ability to provide abscess imaging at any time, although the labeling procedure requires as much time as indium-111 labeling.

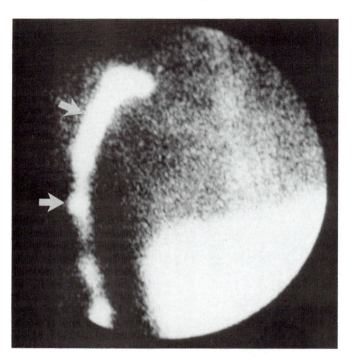

Figure 54.3. Septic Thrombophlebitis. Indium-111-WBC study demonstrates intense radionuclide activity in the right cephalic vein (*arrows*) in a patient with suspicion of intraabdominal sepsis. Septic thrombophlebitis was not suspected because the extremity was in a cast and the patient was taking narcotic analgesics.

INFLAMMATORY PROCESSES

Infection

Infection represents the most common class of inflammatory processes with which we are concerned. The orderly evaluation of a potentially infected patient requires a complete history, physical examination, and appropriate laboratory data before an imaging workup. Important questions to consider include the clinically likely sites and sources of infection, the duration of the infection, and the physiologic response the most likely organism(s) elicit in the host.

For the purposes of this discussion, acute pyogenic infection is that which has been present for 3 weeks or less and is associated with fever, leukocytosis, and immature leukocytes on the peripheral smear. Also included are acute exacerbations of a chronic illness with similar acute manifestations. Illnesses of greater duration or lacking leukocytosis and sustained fever should be considered chronic.

If the initial evaluation suggests a likely source or site of infection, the appropriate anatomic study should be performed, e.g., sonographic evaluation of the right upper quadrant. If localizing signs are absent and the chest radiograph and urinalysis provide no clue, scintigraphy is indicated. For acute processes, the radiopharmaceutical of choice is radio-

labeled autologous WBCs. The evaluation of chronic poorly localized infection is best performed using Ga-67 (9).

Acute Pyogenic Infections. Indium-111-labeled leukocytes have evolved to become the agent of choice in the evaluation of sepsis without localizing signs. Sensitivities and specificities of 85–95% have been reported, with some decline in specificity as the study has become more widely available (3, 10). Abnormal activity is graded relative to splenic activity. Foci of activity with an intensity similar to that of the spleen are regarded as abscess or phlegmonous tissue until proven otherwise. Abnormal activity of lesser intensity than the spleen should not be discounted in a severely ill patient. Chronicity of infection, treatment, host defenses, and other factors affect the amount of inflammation present, and therefore the chemotactic ability of a lesion. When abnormal activity is identified an anatomic study (computed tomography and ultrasound) may be of benefit in determining the need for percutaneous or surgical drainage.

In most patients, whole-body imaging should be performed since infectious foci will frequently be identified outside the area of clinical concern (Fig. 54.3). Upper abdominal infection may be difficult to diagnose because of normal hepatic and splenic activity. In such cases, concomitant imaging with Tc-99m sulfur colloid will help differentiate normal liver and spleen from adjacent or internal infection (Figs. 54.4 and 54.5). Similarly, other Tc-99m pharmaceuticals such as diethylene triaminepentaacetic acid (DTPA) and methylene diphosphonate (MDP) have been used successfully to localize infection to intra- or extrarenal sites and intra- or extraosseous sites, respectively. Such studies are optimally performed with the aid of computer subtraction techniques. Care should be taken, however, to use only the 247 keV peak of In-111 or to narrow the imaging window on the 173 keV peak when imaging after the injection of a Tc-99m agent. Otherwise the higher doses used with Tc-99m leads to acceptance of some Tc-99m counts into the lower window and may result in a false-positive diagnosis of infection.

Recently, Tc-99m-sulfur colloid has also been used to delineate the location of normal marrow or increased marrow activity in conjunction with In-111 leukocyte images in the evaluation of postoperative osteomyelitis (11, 12). This is an excellent technique since posttraumatic and postoperative bone recruits an increase in blood flow and, therefore, an increased delivery of labeled cells. The study may be misinterpreted as osteomyelitis unless the increased marrow activity is documented with the sulfur colloid study.

Lung activity on In-111-WBC images is nonspecific and may be seen in pneumonia, adult respiratory distress syndrome, congestive heart failure, endotox-

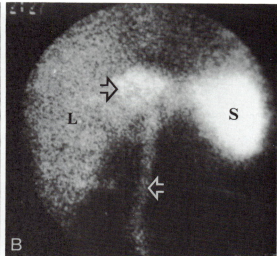

Figure 54.4. Abscess. A. Liver-spleen scan performed with Tc-99m sulfur colloid. **B.** Indium-111-WBC study performed to evaluate fever and leukocytosis following partial left hepatic lobectomy for cholangiocarcinoma. Note the operative bed abscess (*black arrow*) clearly defined by the combination of the two imaging modalities. Linear vertically oriented activity (*white arrow*) on the In-111-WBC study represents colonization of the surgical incision. *L*, liver; *S*, spleen.

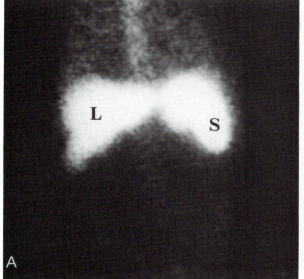

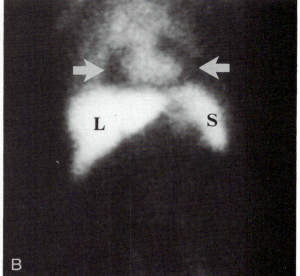

Figure 54.5. Unsuspected Pericardial Effusion. A. Indium-111-WBC study of the lower chest and upper abdomen performed to evaluate fever and leukocytosis. **B.** Technetium-99m-sulfur colloid image shortly after injection, with residual circulating colloid activity in the pulmonary and cardiac blood pool. The colloid study performed to exclude perisplenic abscess demonstrates a photopenic halo (*arrows*) completely surrounding the heart, indicative of pericardial effusion. *L*, liver; *S*, spleen.

emia, empyema, and other conditions. Abnormal lung activity should only be evaluated in light of clinical history and the chest radiograph, and then very carefully.

Liver and spleen activity mimics that of Tc-99m-sulfur colloid. Incidental findings such as cold defects due to metastases, radiation therapy, or benign lesions may be seen (Fig. 54.6). The patchy pattern of diffuse liver disease is also demonstrated (Fig. 54.7).

Intestinal activity is never normal on an In-111-WBC study but may represent swallowed leukocyte activity from respiratory tract infection, dental abscess, or other inflammatory oropharyngeal lesion.

Most urinary tract infections are diagnosed clinically, but occasionally a patient fails to respond promptly to therapy and clinical concern leads to a search for other causes (Fig. 54.8). Indium-111-WBCs are also useful in defining which (if any) cysts are in-

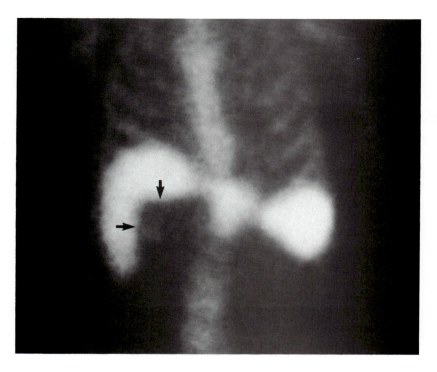

Figure 54.6. Radiation Therapy Portal. Anterior chest and upper abdomen from In-111-WBC study in patient being evaluated for fever and leukocytosis after surgery for carcinoma of the gallbladder. Note the rectangular "cut out" (*arrows*) from inferomedial aspect of the liver due to radiation therapy portal.

fected in patients with adult polycystic kidney disease and in confirming dialysis catheter infection.

The evaluation of osteomyelitis remains difficult and the literature is unclear as to the optimum imaging strategy (11–16). The three-phase bone scan remains preeminent in excluding osteomyelitis, although rare, false-negatives are seen in the first 24–72 hours of infection and in infants. Some authors recommend adding a fourth phase at 24 hours in an effort to enhance specificity, but this technique is not in widespread use. For the diagnosis of acute osteomyelitis, most would start with the three-phase bone scan, and if that were positive, follow with an In-111-WBC study or less commonly, Ga-67 (Fig. 54.9). In most cases, Ga-67 will not add sufficient specificity to the bone scan for diagnosis, but may be of benefit in assessing therapeutic response (Fig. 54.10).

Cold defects may be seen in the skeleton on In-111-WBC imaging because of osteonecrosis, absent blood flow, or marrow packing with malignant cells (Fig. 54.11). Less commonly, osteomyelitis may present as a cold defect due to compromise of the vascular supply with elevated intraosseous pressure (15).

Unlike Ga-67, normally healing wounds do not accumulate In-111-WBCs unless they are colonized (Fig. 54.4). Indium-111-WBCs are useful in evaluating vascular grafts for infection (Fig. 54.12). Caution is indicated in the first 6–8 weeks after graft placement because increased white cell activity is common with healing of tissues adjacent to the graft.

Acute Nonpyogenic Infection. Gallium-67 citrate remains the radiopharmaceutical of choice for the evaluation of all nonpyogenic inflammatory condi-

tions. While it can be used successfully in many of the acute pyogenic conditions just described, its suboptimal imaging characteristics and physiologic renal, intestinal, and wound accumulation have placed it in a second-string status for most acute infections.

The most notable exception is the evaluation of the febrile immunocompromised patient with a normal chest radiograph (2, 4, 17, 18). *Pneumocystis carinii* pneumonia (PCP) is highly prevalent in this population and frequently presents with fever, dyspnea, and normal chest radiographs. The Ga-67 scan in PCP demonstrates diffuse bilateral pulmonary activity that may antedate radiographic findings by 2 weeks. The Ga-67 study has a sensitivity approaching 100% for PCP in the acquired immunodeficiency syndrome (AIDS) population. Unfortunately, lung uptake of Ga-67 is extremely nonspecific and may be due to cytomegalovirus pneumonia, cryptococcosis, lymphoma, atypical mycobacterial infection, bacterial pneumonia, or nonspecific pneumonitis, among many others. Factors that enhance the specificity for PCP in any immunocompromised patient include a normal chest radiograph and markedly intense heterogeneous bilateral pulmonary activity (Fig. 54.13).

In the AIDS population, both *Mycobacterium tuberculosis* (Tb) and *M. avium-intracellulare* (MAI) are prevalent. The former is more frequent among intravenous drug abusers. Gallium-67 imaging reveals both pulmonary involvement and adenopathy. Again, however, the differential diagnosis is broad and includes lymphoma, cytomegalovirus, *Cryptococcus*, and bacterial lymphadenitis. It is important to

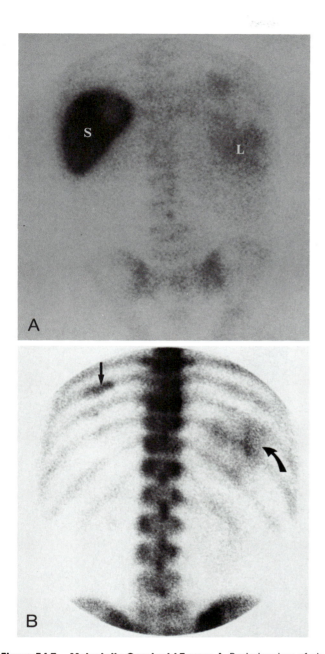

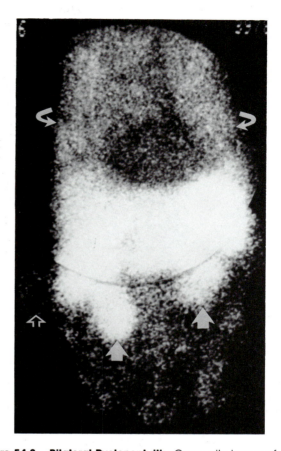

Figure 54.8. Bilateral Pyelonephritis. Composite image of anterior chest and abdomen demonstrates bilateral renal (*arrows*) and lung (*curved arrows*) activity due to pyelonephritis and adult respiratory distress syndrome secondary to sepsis. Activity adjacent to the patient's right side (*open arrow*) is located in an ostomy bag and was felt to be due to swallowed WBCs.

Figure 54.7. Metastatic Carcinoid Tumor. A. Posterior view of abdomen from In-111 study. The liver (*L*) is patchy, consistent with diffuse or multifocal disease. Photopenic defects are present in spleen (*S*) and bone marrow. **B.** Posterior bone scan image of the same area. Note the ill-defined soft-tissue activity (*curved arrow*) in the right upper quadrant corresponding to a photopenic defect in the liver, and focal areas of increased activity in the ribs (*straight arrow*) and spine. Metastatic carcinoid tumor involves the liver, spleen, and bone with calcification in the hepatic metastasis.

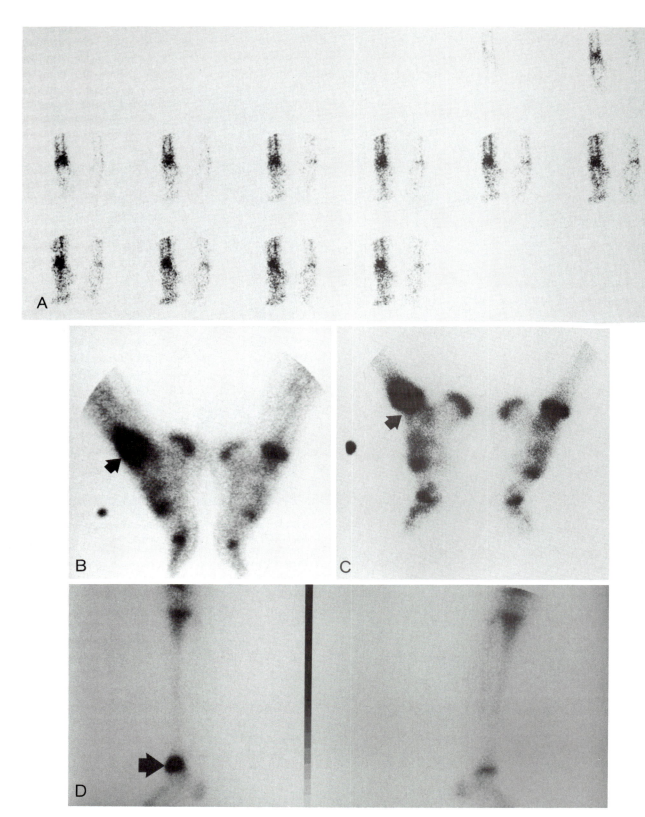

Figure 54.9. Acute Osteomyelitis in a 13-year-old Girl. Three-phase bone and Ga-67 scans. Radiographs were normal. **A.** Anterior view of arterial flow study of the feet and ankles with Tc-99m-MDP, 2 seconds per frame. Note the early and increased flow to the right foot and ankle. **B.** Blood pool image, marker indicates the right side. Note the markedly increased activity in the distal tibia (*arrows* in **B**, **C**, and **D**) extending to the physeal plate. **C.** Delayed static image in same view as **B**. **D.** Gallium-67 study of the same patient.

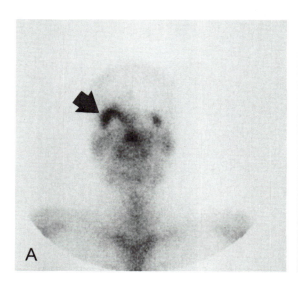
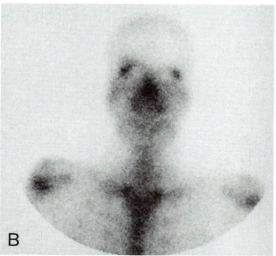

Figure 54.10. Osteomyelitis, Response to Therapy. A. Baseline Ga-67 scan in patient with proven right supraorbital rim osteomyelitis (*arrow*). **B.** Follow-up study demonstrating resolution after 6 weeks of therapy.

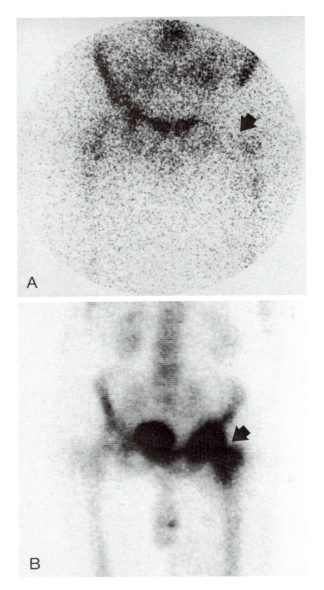

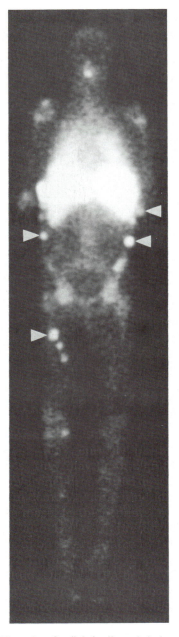

Figure 54.11.   Avascular Necrosis. A. Anterior image of the pelvis and hips from In-111-WBC study. Entire left proximal femur (*arrow*) is photopenic. **B.** Bone scan in the same patient demonstrates intense radionuclide activity in proximal left femur (*arrow*). Avascular necrosis of the left femoral head and neck complicated a chronic femoral neck fracture.

Figure 54.12.   Vascular Graft Infection. Anterior whole-body In-111-WBC image demonstrates multiple foci of infection (*arrowheads*) involving both axillofemoral vascular grafts and the right femoropopliteal graft. Bilateral lung activity is related to sepsis. Increased nasopharyngeal activity is seen with nasotracheal and nasogastric intubation as well as sinusitis.

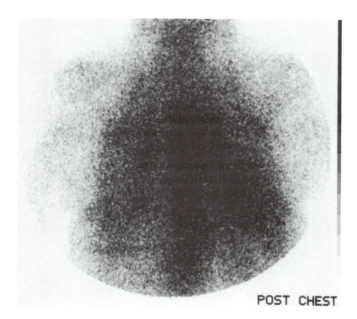

POST CHEST

Figure 54.13. *Pneumocystis carinii Pneumonia.* Gallium study of the chest demonstrates markedly increased heterogeneous pulmonary activity in a pattern that, in an AIDS patient with a normal chest radiograph, strongly suggests *P. carinii* pneumonia.

note that neither the lymphadenopathy of the AIDS-related complex nor Kaposi's sarcoma are Ga-67 avid.

Despite the foregoing discussion, careful consideration should be given to the use of a labeled WBC study prior to Ga-67 administration in immunocompromised patients since they are also susceptible to bacterial infections, and Ga-67 administration will preclude the use of labeled WBCs for at least 1 week (19).

Chronic Infection. Gallium-67 remains the radiopharmaceutical of choice for the investigation of low-grade chronic inflammatory processes. Such illnesses typically present as fever of unknown origin (FUO) in a relatively stable patient. Since a FUO by definition has been present for several weeks, labeled leukocyte scintigraphy would not be expected to be helpful. After history, physical examination, and routine laboratory data have been obtained, scintigraphy with Ga-67 is indicated. While the results are often nonspecific they may point toward additional diagnostic studies. The clinical differential diagnosis for FUO is extremely broad but includes chronic low-grade infections (e.g., fungus, tuberculosis, Epstein-Barr virus), malignancy (especially lymphoma and myeloproliferative disorders), vasculitides, collagen-vascular diseases, and endocrine disturbances.

Chronic osteomyelitis is a different cellular and clinical entity than acute osteomyelitis. As a result, the imaging approach is different, though still controversial. Most would begin with the three-phase bone scan, particularly in cases where the affected bone had been previously exposed to open trauma or surgi-

cal debridement. The bone study provides a better picture of the anatomy and physiology of the bone in the affected region. Subsequently, a Ga-67 study should be performed, with or without the aid of simultaneous Tc-99m bone imaging. Gallium-67 activity at the suspicious site is assessed in comparison with the bone scan activity. Excess Ga-67 activity suggests the presence of continued infection. The imaging diagnosis of chronic osteomyelitis has a relatively low sensitivity and specificity. White blood cell imaging would not be expected to be helpful unless there were acute indications of recrudescence of the infection to a more active state with recruitment of polymorphonuclear leukocytes to the lesion.

Noninfectious Inflammatory Processes

Inflammatory Bowel Disease. Both labeled WBCs and Ga-67 have been used to evaluate the extent and activity of inflammatory bowel disease (20). Since there is no physiologic intestinal or hepatobiliary excretion of In-111-WBCs, they are the radiopharmaceutical of choice. Excellent results have been obtained in the evaluation of the activity and extent of disease in both ulcerative colitis and Crohn's disease, although discriminating between them is not possible. Pseudomembranous colitis also provokes a profound inflammatory response (Fig. 54.14).

Imaging should be performed within 30–90 minutes of injection of the labeled cells. Serial imaging at 4 and 24 hours is recommended. The lesions of Crohn's disease and ulcerative colitis are intensely inflammatory and early cell migration to the most involved areas is the rule. Subsequently, the cells are transported to the lumen of the intestine and migrate with peristalsis. Thus, if early imaging is not performed it will be impossible to differentiate inflammatory foci from intraluminal activity. Delayed imaging is important because patients with inflammatory bowel disease are at high risk for abscess, and very active inflammatory bowel disease may mask the presence of concomitant abscess.

Interstitial Lung Disease. Gallium-67 imaging is an extremely sensitive indicator of inflammatory lung disease (2, 21). Gallium-67 uptake has been reported in sarcoidosis, interstitial pneumonitis in virtually all its forms and etiologies, drug reactions, collagen vascular disease, and pneumoconioses (Fig. 54.15). Unfortunately, a normal study does not absolutely exclude the possibility of low levels of inflammatory activity. Furthermore, the degree or pattern of activity is not diagnostic of specific illnesses. However, the degree of Ga-67 activity seems to reflect the severity of the underlying illness.

Gallium-67 imaging is most useful in sarcoidosis where it has been shown to correlate with pulmonary disease activity and response to therapy (Fig. 54.16).

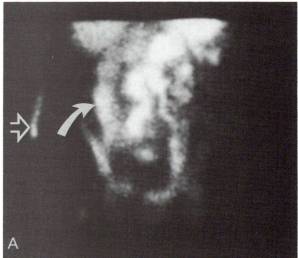
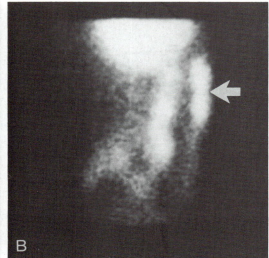

Figure 54.14.   Pseudomembranous Colitis. Anterior (**A**) and right lateral (**B**) views of the abdomen and pelvis from In-111-WBC study. An anterior surgical wound infection is present in the midline (*arrow*). Septic thrombophlebitis is present in the right upper extremity on the anterior view (*open arrow*). Diffuse colonic activity (*curved arrow*), best seen in the right colon, is due to pseudomembranous colitis in this patient on multiple broad-spectrum antibiotics.

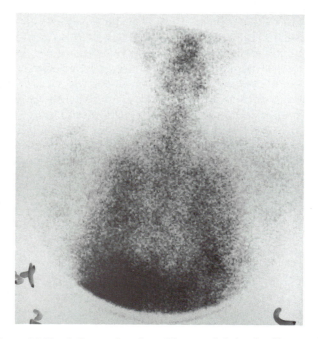

Figure 54.15.   Inflammatory Lung Disease. Anterior Ga-67 scan of the chest demonstrates bilateral increased activity in the lung due to bleomycin toxicity in a patient treated for lymphoma.

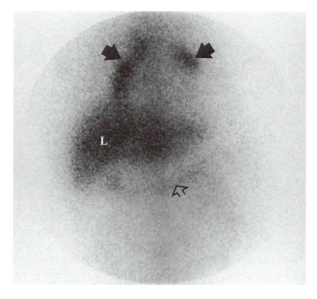

Figure 54.16.   Sarcoidosis. Anterior chest and abdomen from a Ga-67 study shows bilateral hilar adenopathy (*closed arrows*), a pattern characteristic for sarcoidosis. Nonvisualization of the spleen is a normal variant and faint bowel activity (*open arrow*) is physiologic. *L,* liver.

Furthermore, Ga-67 scintigraphy has been reported to be up to 97% sensitive for detection of active sarcoidosis when considering both pulmonary and extrapulmonary sites. It has not been proven whether Ga-67 imaging can provide prognostic information or therapeutic insight for other inflammatory lung diseases.

Since determining the relative pulmonary Ga-67 activity may be helpful in assessing the level of inflammatory activity present, an objective index of Ga-67 activity has been sought. Some authors have chosen to compare pulmonary activity with sternal activity, others have compared pulmonary activity with hepatic activity, and still others have used semiquantitative techniques involving computer acquisitions, SPECT, and whole-body imaging to report activity ratios (2). As a result, no uniform method for quantifying Ga-67 pulmonary activity is available. Therefore, when reporting Ga-67 activity, the specific scale and

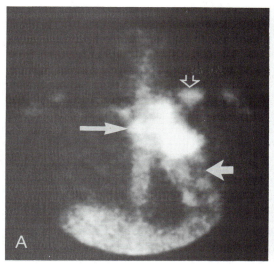
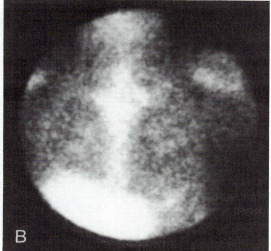
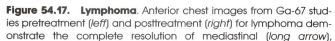

Figure 54.17.   Lymphoma. Anterior chest images from Ga-67 studies pretreatment (*left*) and posttreatment (*right*) for lymphoma demonstrate the complete resolution of mediastinal (*long arrow*), parenchymal (*short arrow*), and left supraclavicular nodal (*open arrow*) disease.

reference standard should be stated. For clinical work we use a scale of 0 to 3 in which pulmonary activity is subjectively graded against liver activity. In this schema, 0 represents no pulmonary activity, 1 represents activity greater than normal but less than liver activity, 2 represents activity equal in intensity to liver activity, and 3 signifies activity greater than that seen in the liver (22). Obviously, quantitative techniques using other organs as reference points assume a normal healthy reference organ.

Tumor Imaging with Ga-67

Gallium-67 has been widely investigated as a tumor imaging agent for over 30 years (1, 23, 24). Many early studies were performed on rectilinear scanners and early generation gamma cameras with relatively low doses in the range of 1–4 mCi. As a result, Ga-67 imaging has undergone a revival in recent years using higher doses of Ga-67 and SPECT instrumentation. The SPECT provides much higher contrast resolution than planar imaging and therefore detects abnormalities that would otherwise have been missed, even on modern high-resolution planar equipment. An increase in specificity with SPECT has also been reported. Whenever possible, SPECT imaging should be included in the evaluation of patients with malignancy. The principle malignancies where Ga-67 imaging has proved useful are Hodgkin's disease, non-Hodgkin's lymphoma and hepatocellular carcinoma. The usefulness of Ga-67 in other malignancies is controversial.

Lymphoma.   Planar Ga-67 imaging (Fig. 54.17) was 65–96% accurate in the staging of lymphoma in recent comparison studies using SPECT (1, 23, 24).

Relative Ga-67 uptake predicts the severity of the disease. The greater the magnitude of Ga-67 uptake in lymphoma, the more malignant the tumor. A baseline pretreatment study is mandatory since the Ga-67 study may be negative in low-grade non-Hodgkin's lymphoma, particularly lymphocyte predominant forms. Additionally, Ga-67 imaging is more specific than computed tomography in differentiating residual disease from posttreatment fibrosis in Ga-67 avid lymphoma. The exception is the pediatric population, where rebound thymic hyperplasia may result in significant Ga-67 uptake for several months.

Hepatoma.   With the advent of computed tomography and contrast-enhanced magnetic resonance imaging, the diagnostic problem of the cold defect on liver/spleen scintigraphy with Tc-99m-sulfur colloid would seem to be a thing of the past. Nonetheless there are no pathognomonic imaging characteristics for hepatocellular carcinoma (HCC) and differentiation from benign lesions such as adenoma and focal nodular hyperplasia remains problematic.

Gallium-67 scintigraphy in conjunction with radiocolloid and/or hepatobiliary imaging may provide physiologic clues to the correct diagnosis. Typically, HCC is Ga-67 avid but contains no Kupffer cells, and so does not accumulate radiocolloid. The differential diagnosis for the pattern of cold defect on radiocolloid study with corresponding "fill-in" on the Ga-67 study includes abscess and metastasis. As a result, hepatobiliary imaging is sometimes performed. Well-differentiated HCC may take up biliary agents albeit slower and to a lesser extent than surrounding normal liver, while poorly differentiated tumors will not. On delayed imaging, the HCC will be seen to retain the

Figure 54.18. Fibrolamellar Hepatocellular Carcinoma. Four anterior images of the liver. **A.** A Tc-99m sulfur colloid liver-spleen scan in a 22-year-old patient with a right upper quadrant mass demonstrates a large photopenic mass (*arrow*) in the inferolateral aspect of the right lobe. **B.** A Ga-67 study demonstrate "fill in" of the mass (*arrow*). **C.** Hepatobiliary scan, 5 minutes after injection, demonstrates limited patchy radionuclide activity in the mass (*arrow*) compared with the normal liver. **D.** Hepatobiliary scan, 70 minutes after injection. Normal liver has washed out; mass (*arrow*) still retains activity; incidental finding of intrahepatic gallbladder (*open arrow*).

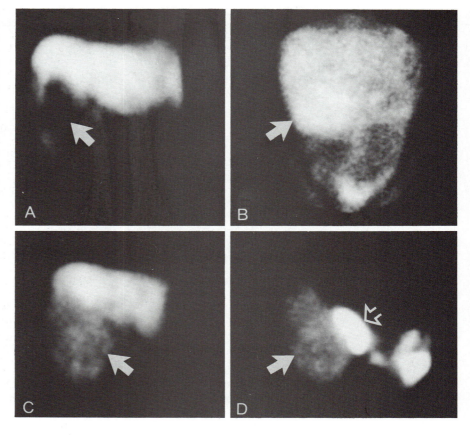

pharmaceutical because of the lack of connection to normal biliary radicles.

Hepatic adenomas rarely contain Kupffer cells, and so appear cold on radiocolloid studies. The hepatobiliary scan pattern for hepatic adenoma is the same as that for well-differentiated HCC, although some appear cold because of central scarring and hemorrhage.

Focal nodular hyperplasia may have normal, increased, or most commonly, decreased activity compared with normal liver on radiocolloid imaging.

It should be emphasized that in the context of hepatic lesions, Ga-67 avidity may be manifest as a normal-appearing liver despite the presence of a space-occupying lesion documented by another imaging modality. Given the relative prevalences in the United States of the other lesions in the differential diagnosis, a Ga-67 avid lesion should be viewed as HCC until proved otherwise by tissue diagnosis.

A separate clinical and pathologic entity is the fibrolamellar subtype of HCC that is seen in younger patients and may have a better prognosis (25). In contrast to typical HCC, which occurs most commonly superimposed on underlying cirrhosis or chronic active hepatitis, fibrolamellar HCC occurs in otherwise normal livers. It is important to suggest the diagnosis of fibrolamellar HCC early so that potentially curative resection can be undertaken without delay (Fig. 54.18).

Other Malignancies. Gallium-67 has been studied in a wide variety of malignant tumors with mixed results. Factors contributing to inconclusiveness include variable study design, low-dose Ga-67 imaging, older imaging equipment, inadequate documentation of disease, and patient selection criteria. Current controversies center around the usefulness of Ga-67 in melanoma and primary lung carcinoma (1, 23, 24). Undoubtedly, well-performed Ga-67 imaging will lead to better diagnosis in some patients with these diseases, but Ga-67 cannot stand alone as the single procedure of choice. The cost effectiveness of Ga-67 in a multimodality cancer evaluation has not been determined. A recent report indicates that Ga-67 may be useful in the evaluation of soft-tissue sarcomas (26).

FUTURE CONSIDERATIONS

Monoclonal antibody imaging of both inflammatory and malignant processes is an area of great clinical and research interest at present. Clinical trials with In-111 labeled immunoglobulin-G show promising results in the investigation of both acute and subacute infection (27). Clinical trials of both Tc-99m and In-111-labeled antibodies directed against breast, lung, and ovarian carcinoma as well as melanoma are under way (13). Recently, commercial approval was granted for the marketing of the B72.3 monoclonal antibody kit for imaging colorectal carcinoma with In-111.

SUMMARY

Scintigraphic imaging plays a pivotal role in the diagnosis of inflammatory and malignant conditions and will continue to do so in the foreseeable future. Optimal diagnosis requires careful consideration of the entire patient and the available imaging modalities. The scintigraphic techniques are best considered specific for inflammation rather than infection.

References

1. Halpern S, Hagan P. Gallium–67 citrate imaging in neoplastic and inflammatory disease. In: Freeman LM, Weissman HS, eds. Nuclear medicine annual 1980. New York: Raven Press, 1980:219–265.
2. Waxman AD. An update on the role of nuclear medicine in pulmonary disorders. In: Freeman LM, Weissman HS, eds. Nuclear medicine annual 1985. New York: Raven Press, 1985:199–231.
3. Froelich JW. Nuclear medicine in inflammatory diseases. In: Freeman LM, Weissman HS, eds. Nuclear medicine annual 1985. New York: Raven Press, 1985:23–71.
4. Bekerman C, Bitran J. Gallium-67 scanning in the clinical evaluation of human immunodeficiency virus infection: indications and limitations. Semin Nucl Med 1988;18:273–286.
5. Uno K, Yoshikawa K, Imazeki K, Minoshima S, Arimizu N. Technetium-99m HMPAO labeled leukocytes in inflammation imaging. Ann Nucl Med 1991;5:77–81.
6. Lantto EH, Lantto TJ, Vorne M. Fast diagnosis of abdominal infections and inflammations with technetium-99m-HMPAO-labeled leukocytes. J Nucl Med 1991;32:2029–2034.
7. Mountford PJ, Kettle AG, O'Doherty MJ, Coakley AJ. Comparison of technetium-99m-HMPAO leukocytes with indium-111-oxine leukocytes for localizing intraabdominal sepsis. J Nucl Med 1990;31:311–315.
8. Roddie ME, Peters AM, Danpure HJ, et al. Inflammation: imaging with Tc-99m HMPAO-labeled leukocytes. Radiology 1988;166:767–772.
9. Froelich JW, Swanson D. Imaging of inflammatory processes with labeled cells. Semin Nucl Med 1984;14:128–140.
10. Lamki LM, Kasi LP, Haynie TP. Localization of indium-111 leukocytes in noninfected neoplasms. J Nucl Med 1988;29:1921–1926.
11. Seabold JE, Nepola JV, Marsh JL, et al. Postoperative bone marrow alterations: potential pitfalls in the diagnosis of osteomyelitis with In-111-labeled leukocyte scintigraphy. Radiology 1991;180:741–747.
12. Schauwecker DS. The scintigraphic diagnosis of osteomyelitis. AJR 1992;158:9–18.
13. Kim EE, Haynie TP, Podoloff DA, Lowry PA, Harle TS. Radionuclide imaging in the evaluation of osteomyelitis and septic arthritis. Crit Rev Diagn Imag 1989;29:257–305.
14. Seabold JE, Nepola JV, Conrad GR, et al. Detection of osteomyelitis at fracture nonunion sites: comparison of two scintigraphic methods. AJR 1989;152:1021–1027.
15. Eisenberg B, Powe JE, Alavi A. Cold defects in In-111-labeled leukocyte imaging of osteomyelitis in the axial skeleton. Clin Nucl Med 1991;16:103–106.
16. Gupta NC, Prezio JA. Radionuclide imaging in osteomyelitis. Semin Nucl Med 1988;18:287–299.
17. Kramer EL, Sanger JJ. Nuclear medicine in the management of the AIDS patient. In: Freeman LM, ed. Nuclear medicine annual 1990. New York: Raven Press, 1990:37–57.
18. Vanarthos WJ, Ganz WI, Vanarthos JC, Serafini AN, Tehranzadeh J. Diagnostic uses of nuclear medicine in AIDS. Radiographics 1992;12:731–752.
19. Fineman DS, Palestro CJ, Kim CK, et al. Detection of abnormalities in febrile AIDS patients with In-111-labeled leukocyte and Ga-67 scintigraphy. Radiology 1989;170:677–680.
20. Froelich JW, Field SA. The role of indium-111 white blood cells in inflammatory bowel disease. Semin Nucl Med 1988;18:300–307.
21. Kramer EL, Divgi CR. Pulmonary applications of nuclear medicine. Clin Chest Med 1991;12:55–75.
22. Niden AH, Mishkin FS, Khurana MM. Gallium-67 citrate lung scans in interstitial lung disease. Chest 1976;69:266–268.
23. Yeh SD, Larson SM. Tumor imaging with monoclonal antibodies and gallium-67. Curr Opin Radiol 1989;1:508–517.
24. Bekerman C, Caride VJ, Hoffer PB, Boles CA. Noninvasive staging of lung cancer. Indications and limitations of gallium-67 citrate imaging. Radiol Clin North Am 1990;28:497–510.
25. Titelbaum DS, Burke DR, Meranze SG, Saul SH. Fibrolamellar hepatocellular carcinoma: pitfalls in nonoperative diagnosis. Radiology 1988;167:25–30.
26. Southee AE, Kaplan WD, Jochelson MS, et al. Gallium imaging in metastatic and recurrent soft-tissue sarcoma. J Nucl Med 1992;33:1594–1599.
27. Oyen WJ, Claessens RA, van der Meer JW, Rubin RH, Strauss HW, Corstens FH. Indium-111-labeled human nonspecific immunoglobulin G: a new radiopharmaceutical for imaging infectious and inflammatory foci. Clin Infect Dis 1992;14:1110–1118.

Central Nervous System Scintigraphy

James H. Timmons

TRADITIONAL BRAIN SCANS

The traditional nuclear medicine brain scan detects a breakdown in the blood-brain barrier. The normal blood-brain barrier protects the central nervous system by preventing entry of harmful substances. Materials are excluded on the basis of molecular size and chemical characteristics. Active transport mechanisms are present for certain key materials.

Radionuclides. Traditional brain scanning is typically performed with either 99m-technetium (^{99m}Tc) bound to diethylenetriaminepentaacetic acid (DTPA) (1) or glucoheptonate (GH) (2). Any agent that does not normally cross the blood-brain barrier can potentially be employed, although agents of cellular size (tagged red cells, for example) will be excluded even by a damaged blood-brain barrier. Pertechnetate may be used (3), but only if the patient is pretreated with 200–500 mg of potassium perchlorate. Perchlorate blocks the normal localization of pertechnetate in the choroid plexus, which might otherwise be mistaken for pathology (4).

Technique. A dose of 15–20 mCi of ^{99m}Tc-DTPA or GH is injected into an arm vein. Flow images are typically obtained at a rate of one image every 3 seconds for a total of 60 seconds, with the camera anterior to the head. Anterior, posterior, and lateral static images are subsequently obtained; vertex images are often useful. These are obtained by placing the camera at the vertex of the skull. A lead collar is employed to exclude radiation from radiopharmaceutical localized below the neck. Immediate static images are useful to evaluate blood pool abnormalities, while delayed static images after clearance of background activity are of greater value to detect breakdown of the blood-brain barrier.

Interpretation of static images depends primarily upon detecting or excluding radiopharmaceutical lo-

calization within the brain parenchyma. Some activity is invariably present from the radiopharmaceutical within the soft tissues of the scalp and within intracerebral blood vessels. Increased or asymmetric localization indicates breakdown of the blood-brain barrier. This finding is entirely nonspecific, being present in conditions as diverse as cerebral infarction, primary or metastatic tumor, and infectious processes. For this reason, clinical information is essential for interpretation. The presence of a lenticular photoenhanced (or occasionally photopenic) rim can be used to diagnose subdural hematoma.

The normal radionuclide angiogram is characterized by prompt symmetric perfusion. Asymmetric flow in the carotid arteries may indicate occlusive disease. The so-called flip-flop sign (decreased activity in the arterial phase, increased activity in the venous phase) may be seen in carotid occlusion. Vascular malformations, high-grade or vascular tumors, such as glioblastoma multiforme and meningioma, and inflammatory processes have increased flow. Low-grade or benign tumors, areas of porencephaly or edema, and occlusive processes have decreased flow. The complete absence of brain activity in the presence of prompt common carotid and scalp flow indicates brain death (5).

The traditional brain scan has largely been superseded by other techniques in current clinical practice. This change was not because of poor sensitivity of the technique. Indeed, brain scans performed with emission computed tomographic techniques (ECAT) or single-photon emission computed tomography (SPECT) compare favorably with computed tomography (CT) for detection of brain metastases (6, 7). The traditional brain scan was superseded because of the wealth of additional anatomic information available with CT and, subsequently, with magnetic resonance imaging (MR) (8), which improves specificity and provides valuable additional information. In the diagnosis of cerebral infarction, the ability of CT to detect hemorrhage is a significant competitive advantage over the traditional brain scan. The radionuclide angiogram, which often proved difficult to interpret, has largely been superseded by Doppler ultrasound techniques for occlusive disease and by CT or MR for other uses.

Despite its decline, familiarity with the traditional technique of brain scanning remains essential. A variety of radiopharmaceuticals used for other diagnostic purposes may cross a damaged blood-brain barrier, resulting in an incidental brain scan. It is important to understand the differential possibilities in this circumstance, especially in the patient undergoing bone scanning for metastatic disease. Brain scan may be the only method for confirming damage to the blood-brain barrier in patients who are morbidly obese, since these patients may exceed the weight limits for CT and MR scanners and may not fit within MR magnet bores. The potential for nonspecific localization must also be kept in mind when evaluating uptake of more advanced radiopharmaceutical agents, since this can be confused with specific (e.g., receptor-mediated) uptake.

Traditional radiopharmaceutical brain scans still have a limited diagnostic role in the evaluation of herpes encephalitis because of extremely high sensitivity for early inflammatory breakdown of the blood-brain barrier. This is especially true in centers where MR is not routinely available. The rapid proliferation and phenomenal technical advances in MR can be reasonably expected to eliminate even this use of the traditional scan. The traditional brain scan is of value in documenting brain death in potential organ transplant donors. In some regions, the absence of intracranial blood flow on a traditional brain scan is part of the legal definition of brain death (5). There is little doubt that more modern brain radiopharmaceuticals such as 99m-Tc hexamethylpropylamine oxine (HMPAO) are capable of providing the same information (9).

CEREBROSPINAL FLUID STUDIES

Cerebrospinal fluid (CSF) is formed in the choroid plexus as an ultrafiltrate of plasma. It flows from the ventricles through the foramina of the fourth ventricle and ascends over the convexities of the brain to be absorbed predominantly by the arachnoid villa. Processes that impede flow over the convexities or absorption of the fluid by the villi result in communicating hydrocephalus. Tracer techniques are ideal for imaging of this process, because they are injected in small amounts and do not alter the CSF flow. Processes that obstruct the outflow from a ventricle are more difficult to assess by these techniques because injection must be made directly into the ventricle. Patency and flow in therapeutic shunts and reservoirs can easily be evaluated by injecting tracer directly into the device.

Technique. The standard cisternogram is performed by intrathecal injection of a sterile, pyrogen-free radiopharmaceutical. The only approved agent currently marketed for this purpose is 111-indium DTPA (half-life = 2.8 days) (4). The injection of 0.5 mCi follows a spinal tap performed in the standard manner. Initial images may be obtained to ensure intrathecal injection. Subsequently, the radiopharmaceutical ascends to the basilar cisterns in approximately 4 hours and flows over the convexities within 24 hours in a normal individual. Images of the basilar cisterns are obtained at 4–6 hours. If images at 24 hours show ascent over the convexities with activity in the interhemispheric fissure and relative clearance of the basilar cisterns, imaging may be terminated. Otherwise, images should be obtained at 48 and 72 hours (10). Technetium-99m-based agents (half-life = 6 hours) are unacceptable because of the requirement for significantly delayed imaging (4).

Shunt and reservoir studies are performed by direct injection of the device with 0.5 mCi ^{111}In-DTPA in a small volume (11–13). Maintenance of sterile techniques during the injection is critical. It is also critical to understand the specific device being evaluated, as shunts often contain check valves and reservoir capacities are limited. A patient may also have several shunt tubes, some of which may be known to be occluded. In general, it is best to have direct input from the neurosurgeon involved in the case to ensure that the maximum amount of information is obtained (14).

Interpretation. Standard cisternography is performed primarily to evaluate for normal pressure hydrocephalus and for CSF leak. Normal pressure hydrocephalus is a form of communicating hydrocephalus classically associated with ataxia, dementia, and urinary incontinence (15, 16). Cisternography demonstrates early localization of activity within the lateral ventricles, persisting beyond 24 hours, and delayed clearance over the convexities (10). While these findings indicate an increased likelihood of a clinical response to shunting, they neither definitively establish the diagnosis nor reliably predict the outcome of shunting (17–19). The SPECT brain perfusion agents discussed subsequently may aid in determining response to CSF shunting (20). Other forms of communicating hydrocephalus (such as might result from radiation therapy or intrathecal chemotherapy) can also be evaluated with cisternography (21).

Cisternography has high sensitivity for CSF leak and remains the procedure of choice for this condition (22). The sensitivity results from the ability of tracer technique to detect very small amounts of activity. Imaging is performed between 1 and 3 hours after injection. Patient and camera position are chosen to maximize the likelihood of detection, with lateral views for CSF rhinorrhea and anterior views for CSF otorrhea. Cotton pledgets should be placed in the nostrils when evaluating CSF rhinorrhea. These are counted at 4–6 hours in a well counter. A serum sample from peripheral blood drawn concurrently is also counted. Pledget activity exceeding 1.5 times the serum concentration is evidence for CSF rhinorrhea (23).

Shunts are evaluated primarily for patency. If the proximal portion is occluded manually (or contains a check valve), flow through the distal limb can be evaluated. The tracer should flow freely into the peritoneum (for ventriculoperitoneal shunts) or atrium (for ventriculoatrial shunts). Delayed flow or persistent activity at the shunt tip suggests malfunction. Diffusion will typically allow determination of the level of obstruction even when flow is absent. Reservoir injection tests for proper placement, patency, and proper functioning of the reservoir. If the reservoir empties directly into the ventricle (such as an Omaya shunt placed for intrathecal chemotherapy), noncommunicating hydrocephalus may be excluded by normal progression of activity to the basilar cisterns and over the convexities. Ventriculospinal shunts may be evaluated only by direct injection of radiopharmaceutical into the ventricle.

FUNCTION BRAIN SCANS (SPECT)

Radiotracer techniques may be employed to evaluate blood flow in cerebral microvasculature. Agents suitable for this purpose include diffusable radiotracers such as 133-xenon, tracers which are actively taken up by neural tissues, and tracers which effectively function as "ideal microspheres." True microspheres that lodge in and thus obstruct capillaries are contraindicated as they would create a stroke. Therefore, these agents must cross the blood-brain barrier and be permanently retained by some chemical process such as ionic trapping, nonspecific protein binding, or chemical breakdown. Glucose consumption and blood flow are linked in normally functioning brain tissues and in most pathologic processes. Therefore, the relative localization of these agents in various cortical tissues gives a reasonable qualitative indication of relative function.

Radionuclides. Much of the early work in this area was performed with 133-xenon. This inhaled gas dissolves in blood to an extent adequate for imaging. The rapidity of perfusion and diffusion of this agent makes rapid imaging essential. Therefore, multiprobe-type cameras have predominantly been employed (24). This tracer is not well suited to rotating camera SPECT techniques. For this reason, and because of difficulties in handling and recovering a gaseous agent, this agent has largely been superseded by other radiopharmaceuticals (25). The radioxenon technique may also be difficult to apply reliably in small brain regions (26).

Iodinated amphetamines tagged with 123-iodine readily cross the blood-brain barrier, where they are taken up by presynaptic synaptosomes of neurons. Both uptake and blood-brain barrier diffusion are reversible. This agent, therefore, will slowly redistribute over time. Iodoamphetamine (iofetamine) is also immediately sequestered by and slowly released from the lung. This effectively yields slow intraarterial injection over a period of hours (27). Because of these phenomena, iodoamphetamine images represent integration of all brain activity from the time of injection until completion of imaging. Because 123-iodine is cyclotron-produced and has a relatively short half-life (13.2 hours), availability is sometimes a problem.

Technetium-99m-HMPAO is an agent of the "ideal microsphere" type. This agent crosses the blood-brain barrier and is trapped within the brain substance. The mechanisms proposed for trapping have included change in ionic state, binding to glutathione, and chemical decomposition (28). For purposes of scan interpretation, it is only necessary to understand that the agent essentially crosses the blood-brain barrier irreversibly. Unlike iodinated amphetamine, this agent provides a "snapshot" of brain activity for a short period after injection (approximately 10 minutes). The HMPAO is available as a kit that is combined with generator-produced pertechnetate prior to use. Availability is thus not problematic. Unfortunately, this agent is extremely unstable chemically in aqueous solution (29). It must be used immediately after preparation, which makes quality control procedures difficult. Other agents of this type are under development.

Technique. Iofetamine and HMPAO scans are typically performed with a rotating gamma camera. A 360° rotation with 60 steps and imaging times of 15–30 seconds per step are typical. Cameras specifically designed for brain work are available, including multiprobe and multihead scanners (30) (Fig. 55.1). However, a significant number of brain scanning referrals are required to justify purchase of this equipment. The agent is injected with the patient in a controlled stimulus state. This usually involves a supine, resting patient with closed eyes in a quiet room (or a room with white noise) and indirect lighting. The intravenous line should be established in advance and all instructions and questions should be dealt with prior to injection to avoid unintended stimulation of brain activity. While the integrative feature of iofetamine might be considered an advantage, it means that the patient must be injected in position on the imaging equipment and maintained in a controlled environment from injection through the end of scanning (Fig. 55.2, Color Plates). With HMPAO, the agent is stably bound approximately 10 minutes after injection, at which time the controlled stimulus state is no longer

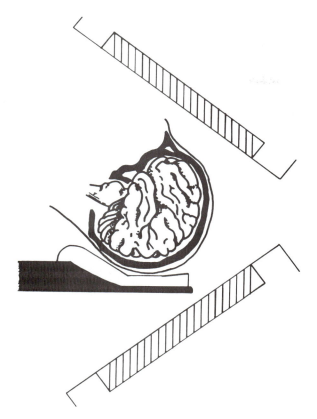

Figure 55.1. Dedicated Brain Scanning Camera. Line diagram demonstrates use of slant hole collimators to achieve improved resolution with a dual–head camera. The camera heads are tilted to compensate for the slant in the collimator. This reduces the average distance from the brain to the crystal face. It also flares the camera heads so that they clear the shoulders during rotation close to the head.

required. Only 4–6 mCi of iofetamine are injected, whereas 20 mCi of 99mTc-HMPAO are usually employed. Imaging with iofetamine thus requires less time and has improved counting statistics. A combination of reasons of convenience has made HMPAO the dominant imaging agent for functional brain SPECT.

Resolution depends on the distance from the collimator face to the subject. The shoulders of the patient prevent close orbit of a standard collimator about the head. Multiple solutions to this problem have been developed, including truncated collimators, slant hole collimators oriented obliquely to the axis of the head (Fig. 55.1), and focused collimators (30, 31). Reconstruction is similar to that performed for other SPECT images. Rigorous quality control is required for these as well as other SPECT studies (32).

Indications. The predominant uses for this technique are evaluation of dementia, identification of seizure foci, and evaluation of acute stroke. The identification of Alzheimer's disease is of special significance (33). Multiple other applications have been suggested but are beyond the scope of this chapter

(34). Unfortunately, even relatively successful applications have not resulted in significant increases in referral for brain SPECT in most hospitals. This may be due in part to a nihilistic attitude toward successful treatment of the disease processes detected, but may also be due in part to a prejudice in favor of techniques that reveal greater anatomic detail. This prejudice is unfortunate, because functional information is usually of greater value in the processes where SPECT functional brain imaging is applicable.

Interpretation. The extent of a stroke can be determined essentially immediately after its occurrence with functional brain scanning (Fig. 55.3, Color Plates) (35). This contrasts with several hours for MR and days for CT, respectively (8). Acute intervention is more feasible with immediate information on the extent of the infarction. Assessment of efficacy of therapy would also be more reliable. Until recently, however, therapy has been limited to anticoagulation and supportive care. Anticoagulation requires only exclusion of hemorrhage, which is best accomplished with CT. The development of effective therapies for early stroke could eventually catapult brain SPECT into the forefront of neuroimaging. Recent advances in molecular diffusion imaging may allow MR assessment of strokes acutely (36). The likelihood of extensive use of brain SPECT for stroke thus remains unclear.

The potential to predict risk of stroke is high with functional brain SPECT. By judicious use of acetazolamide (37) or inhaled carbon dioxide (38) to test vasodilatory reserve of cerebral vessels, it is possible to perform the equivalent of thallium coronary stress testing for cerebral vessels. Injection during vascular occlusion of a carotid artery can also test cross-circulation across the circle of Willis, demonstrating the precise areas of decreased perfusion during occlusion. This is the nuclear medicine version of the Matas test (39–41). The distribution of amobarbital injected for localization of speech and memory functions (the Wada test) may also be assessed accurately using functional agents as tracers (42). Vasospasm complicating subarachnoid hemorrhage (43) and cerebral angioplasty (44) may be assessed with SPECT. This should probably be considered the method of choice for vasospasm assessment, either alone or in combination with transcranial Doppler ultrasound.

Alzheimer's disease can be diagnosed with an accuracy of approximately 80% with functional brain scans (33). The typical pattern is decreased activity in parietal and posterior temporal regions bilaterally and symmetrically (Fig. 55.4, Color Plates). The findings may be asymmetrical. Logically, a positive diagnosis would be preferable to the tedious and low-yield procedures employed to exclude reversible causes of dementia. Unfortunately, referrals for this indication remain infrequent. This may be because of the absence of a

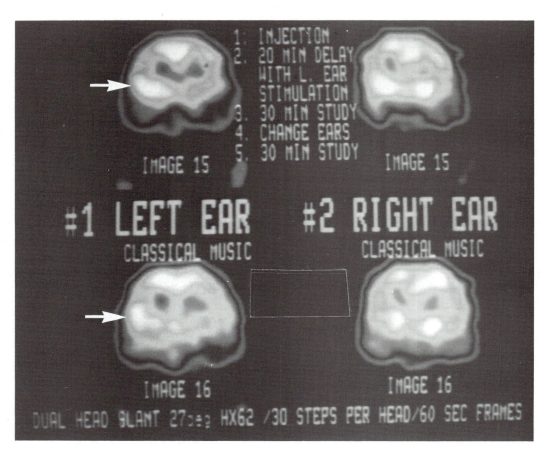

Figure 55.2 (Color Plates).   Brain Activation Study. Multiple coronal images from activation study using ^{123}I-iofetamine. The subject's right hemisphere is on the left side of the images. The images on the *left* were obtained while classical music was played into the left ear and white noise was played into the right ear during a 30-minute acquisition. Note the increased activity in the right temporal lobe (*arrows*). Fiber tracts crossing the midline activate the opposite side. Left temporal lobe activity remains low. The ear stimulation was then reversed (right, music; left, noise) and the scan was repeated without additional injection. The images on the *right* show the result. There is now increased activity in both temporal lobes. This experiment demonstrates the integrative nature of iofetamine brain scans. Activation at any point after injection may affect the final scan appearance. For this reason, care must be taken to avoid unintended stimulation of brain functions while using this agent. (All iofetamine images in this chapter were obtained during phase III trials of the agent. Modern equipment allows significant improvement in resolution.)

viable treatment for Alzheimer's disease at the current time. By demonstrating the absence of Alzheimer's changes, the test suggests patients who may have pseudodementia from depression and require a trial of antidepressant medication. The functional pattern in patients with multiple infarct dementia also tends to be distinct, with randomly scattered areas of decreased activity in brain parenchyma. Multiple infarct dementia may respond favorably to treatment of underlying causes (45).

The location of partial complex seizure foci can be predicted with some success by functional brain scans (46). Interictally, seizure foci tend to have a large aura or penumbra of decreased activity (Fig. 55.5, Color Plates). In simplistic terms, the brain tries to depress function in an erratically functioning area. Ictally, seizure foci have markedly increased blood flow and activity. Because of secondary activation and spread of the seizure foci, it is difficult to pinpoint the exact seizure focus without a dedicated ultrafast multiprobe or multihead camera. For this reason, one might reasonably predict that the technique will be applied mainly in larger referral centers that perform surgery for removal of seizure foci (47). Development of a water-soluble Tc-99m-based functional agent of the ideal microsphere type would significantly aid the use of SPECT imaging in this area. The Tc-99m-HMPAO is unstable in solution, requiring use immediately after reconstitution (29). Iofetamine has a short shelf life and suffers from problems of availability. Thus, truly ictal scans are difficult to reliably achieve. Currently, the technique will identify approximately 60–75% of partial complex seizure foci (48–50). This is significantly better than can be achieved with either MR or CT (47). The 18-fluorodeoxyglucose positron emission tomography (PET) remains the gold standard in this area, but SPECT, irrespective of agent, has proven equivalent in practice (48).

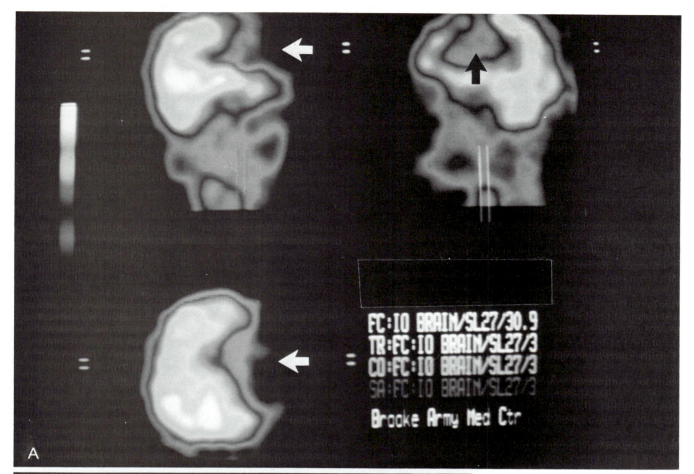

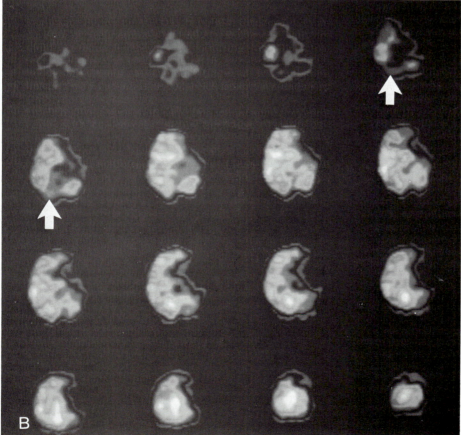

FC:IO BRAIN/SL27/30.9
TR:FC:IO BRAIN/SL27/3
CO:FC:IO BRAIN/SL27/3
SA:FC:IO BRAIN/SL27/3

Brooke Army Med Ctr

Figure 55.3 (Color Plates). Cerebral Infarction. A., Selected coronal (*left upper*), sagittal (*right upper*), and axial (*lower left*) images from a ^{123}I-iofetamine scan show a large region of absent perfusion (*arrows*) in the distribution of the left middle cerebral artery after cerebral infarction. **B.** Transaxial images reformatted into the plane of the orbitomeatal line (standard CT format) in the same patient. Note the decreased cerebellar activity on the side opposite the infarct (*arrow*), an example of crossed cerebellar diaschisis. This phenomenon results from decreased stimulation of the right cerebellum by the infarcted portion of the left cerebral hemisphere.

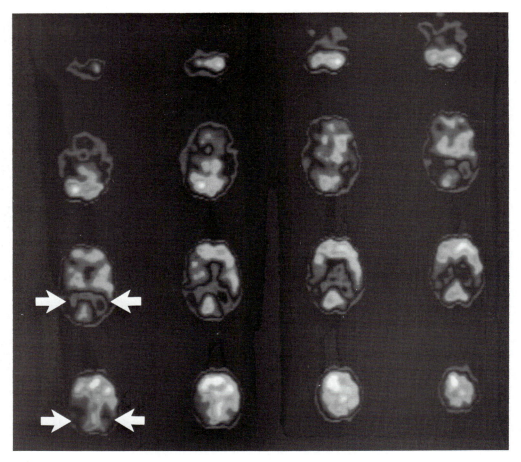

Figure 55.4 (Color Plates).   Alzheimer's Dementia. A ^{123}I-iofetamine scan in axial plane demonstrates bilateral decreased flow in the parietal and posterior temporal regions (*arrows*).

Positron emission tomography is still the leading imaging method for cerebral blood flow research. With separate agents for blood flow, cerebral blood volume, oxygen extraction fraction and metabolic rate (51), and glucose metabolism rate (52), PET allows a rather complete quantitative assessment of cerebral metabolism (53). Unfortunately, the technology is complicated and the cost is high. Routine clinical application of brain PET remains controversial. Where qualitative information is adequate, SPECT imaging has a distinct cost advantage. Meanwhile, MR methods for functional imaging are being developed. Both regional cerebral blood volume and regional cerebral blood flow changes can be identified with MR techniques. With the ability for simultaneous acquisition of anatomic information, MR eliminates the need for special techniques to obtain anatomic/functional correlation.

Positron emission tomography remains the procedure of choice for determining the localization of neurotransmitters and neuropharmaceuticals (54). Relatively straightforward organic synthesis of tagged transmitters and drugs that produce minimal changes in biodistribution and activity qualify PET methods superbly for this application. The SPECT labels for neurochemistry are possible (55), but the chemistry is more complicated. One must either use large transition metal tags requiring complicated syntheses or accept relatively labile tags of 123-iodine or 77-bromine and the availability problems associated with these radionuclides (56, 57). Both are significantly different from the low molecular weight substrates that they replace. This may have a significant effect on biodistribution and biochemistry, which must be proven to be similar to that of the original molecule before the results may be relied upon. Since MR contrast agents currently require paramagnetic or ferromagnetic transition metals, this limitation will also apply to MR of neurochemicals (58). However, MR spectroscopy in high-field magnets will have unique applications for in vivo chemistry (59–61).

The field of functional neuroimaging is progressing rapidly. The ultimate roles for MR, PET, and SPECT imaging are not yet clearly defined. The SPECT functional brain imaging will probably fill a clinical niche as a low-cost, qualitative (or semiquantitative) test of cerebral perfusion in evaluating and preventing stroke, dementia, and seizure disorders.

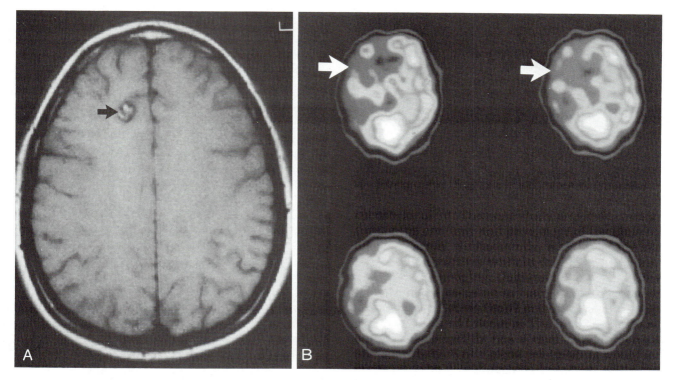

Figure 55.5 (Color Plates). Seizure Focus. A. Intermediate-weighted (proton density) MR image reveals prominent mixed signal right frontal lobe lesion (*arrow*), consistent with cavernous hemangioma. The patient suffers from a frontal lobe seizure disorder. **B.** Inter-ictal ^{123}I-iofetamine scan from the same patient shows an area of depressed flow/function (*arrows*) much larger than the underlying anatomic lesion.

References

1. Hauser W, Atkins HL, Nelson KG, et al. Technetium-99m-DTPA: a new radiopharmaceutical for brain and kidney scanning. Radiology 1970;94:679–684.

2. Waxman AD, Tanacescu D, Siemsen JK, et al. Technetium-99m-glucoheptonate as a brain scanning agent: critical comparison with pertechnetate. J Nucl Med 1976;17:345–348.

3. McAfee JG, Fueger CF, Stern HS, et al. 99mTc-pertechnetate for brain scanning. J Nucl Med 1964;5:811–827.

4. Chilton HM, Thrall JH. Radiopharmaceuticals for central nervous system imaging. Blood-brain barrier, function, receptor-binding, cerebral spinal fluid kinetics. In: Swanson DP, Chilton HM, Thrall JH, eds. Pharmaceuticals in medical imaging, New York: MacMillan Publishing, 1990;305–342.

5. Cowan RJ. Conventional radionuclide brain imaging in the era of transmission and emission tomography. Sem Nucl Med 1986;16:63–73.

6. Ell PJ, Deacon JM, Ducassou D, et al. Emission and transmission brain tomography. Br Med J 1980;280:438–440.

7. Hill TH, Lovett RD, McNeil BJ. Observations on the clinical value of emission tomography. J Nucl Med 1980;21:613–616.

8. Matthews VP, Barker PB, Bryan RN. Magnetic resonance evaluation of stroke. Mag Res Q 1992;8:245–263.

9. Galaske RG, Schober O, Heyer R. 99m-Tc-HMPAO and 123I-amphetamine cerebral scintigraphy: a new, noninvasive method in determination of brain death in children. Eur J Nucl Med 1988;14:446–452.

10. Harbert JC. Radionuclide cisternography. Semin Nucl Med 1971;1:90–106.

11. Harbert J, Haddad D, McCullough D. Quantitation of cerebrospinal fluid shunt flow. Radiology 1974;112:379–387.

12. Chervu S, Chervu LR, Vallabhajosyula B, et al. Quantitative evaluation of cerebrospinal fluid shunt flow. J Nucl Med 1984;25:91–95.

13. Hayden PW, Rudd TG, Shurtleff DB. Combined pressure-radionuclide evaluation of suspected cerebrospinal fluid shunt malfunction: a seven-year clinical experience. Pediatrics 1980;66:679–684.

14. Harbert JC. Radionuclide techniques in the evaluation of cerebrospinal fluid shunts. CRC Crit Rev Diagn Imag 1977;9:207–228.

15. Harbert JC, McCullough DC, Schellinger D. Computed cranial tomography and radionuclide cisternography in hydrocephalus. Semin Nucl Med 1977;7:197–200.

16. Kieffer SA, Wolff JM, Westreich G. The borderline scinticisternogram. Radiology 1973;106:133–140.

17. Stein SC, Langfitt TW. Normal-pressure hydrocephalus. Predicting the results of cerebrospinal fluid shunting. J Neurosurg 1974;41:463–470.

18. Hughes CP, Siegel BA, Coxe WS, et al. Adult idiopathic communicating hydrocephalus with and without shunting. J Neurology Neurosurg Psych 1978;41:961–971.

19. Messert B, Wannamaker BB. Reappraisal of the adult occult hydrocephalus syndrome. Neurology 1974;24:224–231.

20. Moretti J-L, Sergent A, Louarn F, et al. Cortical perfusion assessment with 123I-isopropyl amphetamine (123I-IAMP) in normal pressure hydrocephalus (NPH). Eur J Nucl Med 1988;14:73–79.

21. Grossman SA, Trump DL, Chen DCP, et al. Cerebrospinal fluid flow abnormalities in patients with neoplastic meningitis. An evaluation using 111Indium-DTPA ventriculography. Am J Med 1982;73:641–647.

22. Curnes JT, Vincent LM, Kowalsky RJ, et al. CSF rhinor-rhea: detection and localization with Tc-99m-DTPA. Radiology 1985;154:795–799.

23. McKusick KA, Malmud LS, Kordela A, et al. Radionuclide cisternography: normal values for nasal secretion of intrathecally injected 111In-DTPA. J Nucl Med 1973;14:933–934.

24. Lassen NA. Cerebral blood flow tomography with xenon-133. Semin Nucl Med 1985;15:347–356.

25. Ell PJ, Jarritt PH, Costa DC, et al. Functional imaging of the brain. Semin Nucl Med 1987;17:214–229.

26. Rezai K, Kirchner PT, Armstrong C, et al. Validation studies for brain blood flow assessment by radioxenon tomography. J Nucl Med 1988;29:348–355.

27. Creutzig H, Schober O, Gielow P, et al. Cerebral dynamics of N-Isopropyl (123I)p-iodoamphetamine. J Nucl Med 1986;27:178–183.

28. Suess E, Malessa S, Ungersbock K, et al. Technetium-99m-d,l-hexamethylpropyleneamine oxime (HMPAO) uptake and glutathione content in brain tumors. J Nucl Med 1991;32:1675–1681.

29. Hung JC, Corlija M, Volkert WA, Holmes RA. Kinetic analysis of technetium-99m d,l-HMPAO decomposition in aqueous media. J Nucl Med 1988;29:1568–1576.

30. Esser PD. Improvements in SPECT technology for cerebral imaging. Semin Nucl Med 1985;15:335–346.

31. Jaszczak RJ, Greer KL, Coleman RE. SPECT using a specially designed cone beam collimator. J Nucl Med 1988;29:1398–1405.

32. Greer K, Jaszczak R, Harris C, Coleman RE. Quality control in SPECT. J Nucl Med Technol 1985;13:76–85.

33. Holman BL, Johnson KA, Gerada B, et al. The scintigraphic appearance of Alzheimers's disease: a prospective study using technetium-99m-HMPAO SPECT. J Nucl Med 1992;33:181–185.

34. Alavi A, Hirsch LJ. Studies of central nervous system disorders with single photon emission computed tomography and positron emission tomography: evolution over the past 2 decades. Semin Nucl Med 1991;21:58–81.

35. Park CH, Madsen MT, McLellan T, Schwartzman RJ. Iofetamine HCL I-123 brain scanning in stroke: a comparison with transmission CT. Radiographics 1988;8:305–326.

36. LeBihan D. Molecular diffusion nuclear magnetic resonance imaging. Mag Res Q 1991;7:1–30.

37. Tikofsky RS, Hellman RS. Brain single photon emission computed tomography: newer activation and intervention studies. Semin Nucl Med 1991;21:40–57.

38. Keyeux A, Laterre C, Beckers C. Resting and hypercapneic rCBF in patients with unilateral occlusive disease of the internal carotid artery. J Nucl Med 1988;29:311–319.

39. Matsuda H, Higashi S, Asli IN, et al. Evaluation of cerebral collateral circulation by technetium-99m HMPAO brain SPECT during Matas test: report of three cases. J Nucl Med 1988;29:1724–1729.

40. Monsein LH, Jeffery PJ, van Heerden BB, et al. Assessing adequacy of collateral circulation during balloon test occlusion of the internal carotid artery with 99mTc HMPAO SPECT. AJNR 1991;12:1045–1051.

41. Peterman SB, Taylor A Jr, Hoffman JC Jr. Improved detection of cerebral hypoperfusion with internal carotid baloon occlusion and 99mTc-HMPAO cerebral perfusion SPECT imaging. AJNR 1991;12:1035–1041.

42. Jeffery PJ, Monsein LH, Szabo Z, et al. Mapping the distribution of amobarbital sodium in the intracarotid Wada test by use of Tc-99m HMPAO with SPECT. Radiology 1991;178:847–850.

43. Soucy JP, McNamara D, Mohr G, et al. Evaluation of vasospasm secondary to subarachnoid hemorrhage with technetium-99m-hexamethyl-propylene oxime (HMPAO) tomoscintigraphy. J Nucl Med 1990;31:972–977.

44. Lewis DH, Eskridge JM, Newell DW. Brain SPECT and the effect of cerebral angioplasty in delayed ischemia because of vasospasm. J Nucl Med 1992;33:1789–1796.

45. Meyer JS, Judd BW, Tawaklna T, et al. Improved cognition after control of risk factors for multi-infarct dementia. JAMA 1986;256:2203–2209.

46. Holman BL, Devous MD Sr. Functional brain SPECT: the emergence of a powerful clinical method. J Nucl Med 1992;33:1888–1904.

47. Rowland LP, Alavi A, Brook RH, et al. Surgery for epilepsy—National Institutes of Health concensus conference. JAMA 1990;264:729–737.

48. Devous MD Sr, Leroy RF, Homan RW. Single photon emission computed tomography in epilepsy. Semin Nucl Med 1990;20:325–341.

49. Rowe CC, Berkovic SF, Sia STB, et al. Localization of epileptic foci with postictal single photon emission computed tomography. Ann Neurol 1989;26:660–668.

50. Devous MD Sr, Leroy RF. Comparison of interictal and ictal regional cerebral blood flow findings with scalp and depth electrode seizure focus localization. J Cereb Blood Flow Metab 1989;9(suppl 1):S91.

51. Ter-Pogossian MM, Herscovitch P. Radioactive oxygen-15 in the study of cerebral blood flow, blood volume and oxygen metabolism. Semin Nucl Med 1985;15:377–394.

52. Alavi A, Dann R, Chawluk J, et al. Positron emission tomography imaging of regional cerebral glucose metabolism. Semin Nucl Med 1986;16:2–34.

53. Phelps ME, Mazziotta JC. Positron emission tomography: human brain function and biochemistry. Science 1985;228:799–809.

54. Wagner HN Jr. Quantitative imaging of neuroreceptors in the living human brain. Semin Nucl Med 1986;16:51–62.

55. Chabriat H, Levasseur M, Vidailhet M, et al. In-vivo SPECT imaging of D2 receptor with iodine-iodolisuride: results in supranuclear palsy. J Nucl Med 1992;33:1481–1485.

56. Kung HF. New technetium 99m labeled brain perfusion imaging agents. Semin Nucl Med 1990;20:150–158.

57. Kung HF, Ohmomo Y, Kung MP. Current and future radiopharmaceuticals for brain imaging with single photon emission computed tomography. Semin Nucl Med 1990;20:290–302.

58. Weissleder R, Bogdanov A, Papisov M. Drug targeting in magnetic resonance imaging. Mag Res Q 1992;8:55–63.

59. Petroff O, Prichard J, Alger J, et al. Cerebral intracellular pH by 31P nuclear magnetic resonance spectroscopy. Neurology 1985; 35:781–788.

60. Welch KMA, Helpern JA, Robertson WM, Ewing JR. 31P topical magnetic resonance measurement of high energy phosphates in normal and infarcted brain. Stroke 1985;16:151–154.

61. Duijn JH, Matson GB, Maudsley AA, et al. Human brain infarction: proton MR spectroscopy. Radiology 1992;183:711–718.

Index

Page numbers followed by *t* and *f* denote tables and figures, respectively.